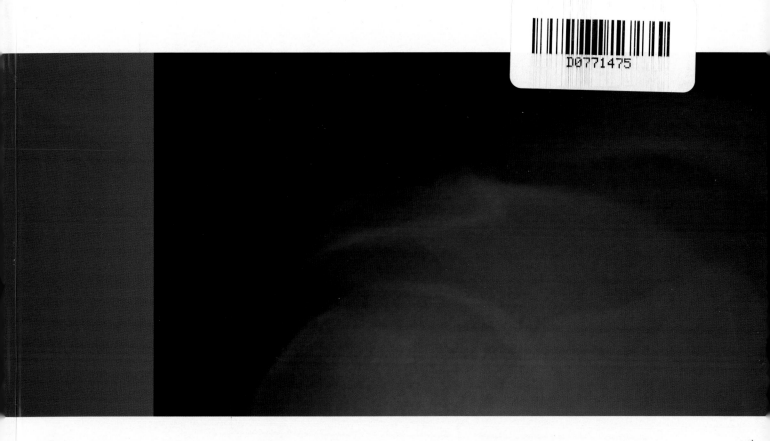

Essential Orthopaedics

Second Edition

Mark D. Miller, MD
S. Ward Casscells Professor of Orthopaedic Surgery
Department of Orthopaedics
University of Virginia
Charlottesville, Virginia

Jennifer A. Hart, MPAS, PA-C
Physician Assistant
Department of Orthopaedic Surgery
University of Virginia
Charlottesville, Virginia

John M. MacKnight, MD, FACSM
Professor of Internal Medicine
Medical Director and Primary Care Team Physician
Department of Athletics
University of Virginia
Charlottesville, Virginia

ELSEVIER

ESSENTIAL ORTHOPAEDICS, SECOND EDITION
ISBN: 978-0-323-56894-4

Notice

Practitioners and researchers must always rely on their own experience and knowledge in evaluating and using any information, methods, compounds or experiments described herein. Because of rapid advances in the medical sciences, in particular, independent verification of diagnoses and drug dosages should be made. To the fullest extent of the law, no responsibility is assumed by Elsevier, authors, editors or contributors for any injury and/or damage to persons or property as a matter of products liability, negligence or otherwise, or from any use or operation of any methods, products, instructions, or ideas contained in the material herein.

Previous editions copyrighted 2009.

Library of Congress Control Number: 2019934875

Content Strategist: Charlotta Kryhl
Senior Content Development Specialist: Rae Robertson
Publishing Services Manager: Catherine Jackson
Senior Project Manager: Kate Mannix
Design Direction: Brian Salisbury

Printed in China

Last digit is the print number: 9 8 7 6 5 4 3 2 1

1600 John F. Kennedy Blvd.
Ste 1600
Philadelphia, PA 19103-2899

 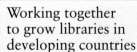

Working together
to grow libraries in
developing countries

www.elsevier.com • www.bookaid.org

To Ann Etchison, a smart lady and a great wife.
MDM

To my past teachers, from whom I learned what it takes to be a PA; to my current mentors, Drs. Diduch and Miller, from whom I gained my knowledge of orthopaedics; to all of the students I have encountered over the years from whom I learned that knowledge is ongoing; and to my husband, Joe, and my children, Jordyn, Julia, and Andrew, from whom I have learned everything else.
JAH

To my wife, Melissa, for her love, patience, and support. To my children, Abby, Hannah, Eliza, and JD, for their sacrifice and understanding. And to the memory of my parents for the inspiration to live a life of service.
JMM

Contributors

Sonya Ahmed, MD
Co-Director
Private Practice
Nilssen Orthopedics
Pensacola, Florida

James Alex, MD
Algone Sports and Regenerative Medicine
Wasilla, Alaska

R. Todd Allen, MD, PhD
Associate Professor of Orthopaedic
    Surgery
Director, UCSD Spine Surgery Fellowship
University of California San Diego
    Health System
San Diego, California

Annunziato Amendola, MD
Professor of Orthopaedic Surgery
Chief, Division of Sports Medicine
Duke University
Durham, North Carolina

Nicholas Anastasio, MD
Department of Physical Medicine &
    Rehabilitation
University of Virginia
Charlottesville, Virginia

Bradley M. Anderson
Research Assistant
Rothman Institute Spine Section
Philadelphia, Pennsylvania

D. Greg Anderson, MD
Professor of Orthopaedic Surgery
Thomas Jefferson University
Philadelphia, Pennsylvania

Kelley Anderson, DO, CAQSM
Assistant Professor of Orthopedics
University of Pittsburgh;
Primary Care Sports Medicine Physician
University of Pittsburgh Medical Center
Pittsburgh, Pennsylvania

Mark W. Anderson, MD
Professor of Radiology and Orthopaedic
    Surgery
Department of Radiology
University of Virginia
Charlottesville, Virginia

**Laurie Archbald-Pannone,
MD, MPH, AGSF, FACP**
Associate Professor of Internal Medicine
University of Virginia
Charlottesville, Virginia

Anthony J. Archual, MD
Resident Physician
Department of Plastic Surgery
University of Virginia
Charlottesville, Virginia

Michael Argyle, DO
Sports Medicine Physician
18th Medical Group
U.S. Air Force
Kadena Air Base, Japan

Joseph Armen, DO
Team Physician, Student Health Services
Sports Medicine Fellowship Program
    Director
Department of Family Medicine
East Carolina University
Greenville, North Carolina

Keith Bachmann, MD
Assistant Professor of Orthopaedic
    Surgery
University of Virginia
Charlottesville, Virginia

Geoffrey S. Baer, MD, PhD
Associate Professor of Orthopedics
    and Rehabilitation
University of Wisconsin
Madison, Wisconsin

Kaku Barkoh, MD
Spine Surgery Fellow
Department of Orthopaedic Surgery
University of Southern California
Los Angeles, California

Michael A. Beasley, MD
Instructor of Orthopedics
Harvard Medical School;
Division of Sports Medicine
Boston Children's Hospital
Boston, Massachusetts

Anthony J. Bell, MD
Assistant Professor of Orthopaedic
    Surgery and Rehabilitation
University of Florida College of Medicine
Jacksonville, Florida

David J. Berkoff, MD
Clinical Professor of Orthopedics and
    Emergency Medicine
University of North Carolina Chapel Hill
Chapel Hill, North Carolina

Anthony Beutler, MD
NCC Sports Medicine Fellowship
    Director
Injury Prevention Research Laboratory
CHAMP Consortium Professor
Department of Family Medicine
Uniformed Services University
Bethesda, Maryland

Matthew H. Blake, MD
Director of Sports Medicine
Department of Orthopedics and Sports
    Medicine
Avera McKennan Hospital & University
    Health Center
Sioux Falls, South Dakota

Jeffrey D. Boatright, MD, MS
Division of Hand and Upper Extremity
    Surgery
Department of Orthopaedic Surgery
University of Virginia
Charlottesville, Virginia

Benjamin Boswell, DO
ED Physician, Sports Medicine Fellow
Primary Care Sports Medicine Fellowship
Duke University
Durham, North Carolina

Seth Bowman, MD
Hand Fellow
Department of Plastic Surgery
University of Virginia
Charlottesville, Virginia

Robert Boykin, MD
Staff Physician
Blue Ridge Division
EmergeOrtho
Asheville, North Carolina

Rebecca Breslow, MD
Associate Physician, Primary Care
    Sports Medicine
Department of Orthopaedics
Brigham and Women's Hospital
Boston, Massachusetts

Thomas E. Brickner, MD
Team Physician
Department of Sports Medicine
University of North Carolina
Chapel Hill, North Carolina

Stephen Brockmeier, MD
Associate Professor of Orthopaedic
  Surgery
University of Virginia
Charlottesville, Virginia

**Per Gunnar Brolinson,
DO, FAOASM, FAAFP**
Vice Provost for Research
Professor of Family and Sports Medicine
Discipline Chair for Sports Medicine
Edward Via College of Osteopathic
  Medicine
Virginia Tech and Virginia College of
  Osteopathic Medicine
Blacksburg, Virginia

James A. Browne, MD
Associate Professor of Orthopaedic
  Surgery
Head, Division of Adult Reconstruction
University of Virginia School of
  Medicine
Charlottesville, Virginia

Chester Buckenmaier III, MD
Director, Defense & Veterans Center
  for Integrative Pain Management
Department of Military and Emergency
  Medicine
Uniformed Services University
Bethesda, Maryland

Jeffrey R. Bytomski, DO
Associate Professor of Community
  and Family Medicine
Duke University
Durham, North Carolina

Adam Carlson, MD
Assistant Professor of Rheumatology
University of Virginia School of
  Medicine
Charlottesville, Virginia

Wesley W. Carr, MD
Sports Medicin Physician
Uniformed Services University
Bethesda, Maryland

S. Evan Carstensen, MD
Staff Physician
Department of Orthopaedics
University of Virginia
Charlottesville, Virginia

Dennis Q. Chen, MD
Resident Physician
Department of Orthopaedic Surgery
University of Virginia
Charlottesville, Virginia

Mario Ciocca, MD
Director of Sports Medicine
Assistant Professor of Internal
  Medicine and Orthopaedics
University of North Carolina
Chapel Hill, North Carolina

Adam R. Cochran, MD
Hand Surgery Fellow
Department of Orthopedic Surgery
Virginia Commonwealth University
Richmond, Virginia

Alexander D. Conti, MD
Resident Physician
Department of Orthopaedic Surgery
West Virginia University
Morgantown, West Virginia

Minton Truitt Cooper, MD
Assistant Professor of Orthopaedic
  Surgery
University of Virginia School of Medicine
Charlottesville, Virginia

Gianmichel Corrado, MD
Sports Medicine Physician
Associate Program Director for Primary
  Care Sports Medicine Fellowship
Lecturer in Orthopedic Surgery
Harvard Medical School;
Head Team Physician
Northeastern University
Boston, Massachusetts

Quanjun (Trey) Cui, MD
G.J. Wang Professor of Orthopaedic
  Surgery
University of Virginia School of
  Medicine
Charlottesville, Virginia

Rashard Dacus, MD
Associate Professor of Orthopaedic
  Surgery
University of Virgnia
Charlottesville, Virginia

Jeffrey Dart, MD
Physician
Departments of Sports Medicine,
  Family Medicine
PeaceHealth
Vancouver, Washington

D. Nicole Deal, MD
Associate Professor of Orthopaedic
  Surgery
University of Virginia
Charlottesville, Virginia

Monika Debkowska, MD
Department of Orthopedic Surgery
Virginia Commonwealth University
Richmond, Virginia

Christopher DeFalco, MD
Community Physician Network
Orthopedic Specialty Care
Indianapolis, Indiana

Ian J. Dempsey, MD, MBA
Resident Physician
Department of Orthopaedic Surgery
University of Virginia
Charlottesville, Virginia

Christopher J. DeWald, MD
Assistant Professor of Orthopaedic
  Surgery
Director, Section of Spinal Deformity
Rush University Medical Center
Chicago, Illinois

**Kevin deWeber, MD, FAAFP,
FACSM**
Program Director, Sports Medicine
  Fellowship
Family Medicine of SW Washington
Vancouver, Washington;
Affiliate Associate Professor of Family
  Medicine
Oregon Health and Science University
Portland, Oregon;
Clinical Instructor of Family Medicine
University of Washington School of
  Medicine
Seattle, Washington

William Dexter, MD, FACSM
Division of Orthopedics and Sports
  Medicine
Maine Medical Partners
Portland, Maine;
Professor of Family Medicine
Tufts University School of Medicine
Boston, Massachusetts

Caleb Dickison, DO, CAQSM
Sports Medicine Physician
National Capital Consortium
Uniformed Services University of the
  Health Sciences
Bethesda, Maryland

Contributors

David Diduch, MD
Professor of Orthopaedic Surgery
Head Orthopaedic Team Physician
Division Head, Sports Medicine
University of Virginia
Charlottesville, Virginia

Robert J. Dimeff, MD
Professor of Orthopedic Surgery,
    Pediatrics, Family & Community
    Medicine
University of Texas Southwestern
    Medical Center
Dallas, Texas

Julie Dodds, MD
Clinical Associate Professor
Michigan State University
East Lansing, Michigan

Gregory F. Domson, MD, MA
Residency Director
Department of Orthopaedics
Virginia Commonwealth University
    Medical Center
Richmond, Virginia

Andrew S. Donnan III, MMSc
Physician Assistant, Distinguished Fellow
Spartanburg Regional Health Care
    System
Spartanburg, South Carolina

Jeanne Doperak, DO
Assistant Professor
Program Director, Primary Care Sports
    Medicine Fellowship
Associate Program Director, PM&R
    Sports Medicine Fellowship
Department of Orthopaedic Surgery
University of Pittsburgh
Pittsburgh, Pennsylvania

Jesse F. Doty, MD
Assistant Professor of Orthopaedic
    Surgery
University of Tennessee College of
    Medicine;
Director of Foot and Ankle Surgery
Erlanger Health System
Chattanooga, Tennessee

Thomas Ergen, MD
Resident Physician
Department of Orthopaedics
University of South Carolina
Columbia, South Carolina

David G. Fanelli, MD
Pennsylvania State University College
    of Medicine
Hershey Medical Center
Hershey, Pennsylvania

Gregory C. Fanelli, MD
Geisinger Sports Medicine and
    Orthopedic Surgery
Danville, Pennsylvania

Matthew G. Fanelli, MD
Geisinger Orthopedic Surgery
Danville, Pennsylvania

Patricia Feeney, DO, FAWM
Sports Medicine Fellow
Department of Family Medicine
Mountain Area Health Education Center
Asheville, North Carolina

**Christopher Felton, DO, CAQSM,
ATC**
Novant Health Primary Care Sports
    Medicine
Charlotte, North Caroline

Adam C. Fletcher, MD
Sports Medicine/Family Medicine
Winona Health
Winona, Minnesota

Jason A. Fogleman, MD
Foot and Ankle Fellow
Reno Orthopedic Clinic
University of California Davis
Reno, Nevada

Travis Frantz, MD
Resident Physician
Department of Orthopaedic Surgery
The Ohio State University Wexner
    Medical Center
Columbus, Ohio

Tyler W. Fraser, MD
Resident Physician
Department of Orthopedics
University of Tennessee
Chattanooga, Tennessee

Brett A. Freedman, MD
Associate Professor of Orthopedics
Mayo Clinic
Rochester, Minnesota

Ryan L. Freedman, MD, MS
Primary Care Sports Medicine
Department of Family Medicine
Clinical Associate
Department of Emergency Medicine
Duke University
Durham, North Carolina

Aaron M. Freilich, MD
Associate Professor of Orthopaedic
    Surgery
University of Virginia
Charlottesville, Virginia

Eric J. Gardner, MD
Mountain Vista Orthopedics
Greeley, Colorado

Trent Gause II, MD
Orthopaedic Surgeon
Department of Orthopaedic Surgery
University of Virginia
Charlottesville, Virginia

Nicholas E. Gerken, MD
Adult Reconstruction Fellow
Department of Adult Reconstruction/
    Orthopaedic Surgery
University of Virginia
Charlottesville, Virginia

Sanjitpal S. Gill, MD
Adjunct Assistant Professor
Department of Bioengineering
Clemson University
Clemson, South Carolina;
Orthopaedic Surgery
Medical Group of the Carolinas
Greer, South Carolina

Heather Gillespie, MD, MPH
Maine Medical Partners
Orthopedics and Sports Medicine
Portland, Maine;
Clinical Associate Professor
Tufts University School of Medicine
Boston, Massachusetts

Andrea Gist, MD
Resident Physician
Wake Forest Family Medicine
Winston-Salem, North Carolina

Victor Anciano Granadillo, MD
Department of Orthopaedics
University of Virginia Healthsystem
Charlottesville, Virginia

Anna Greenwood, MD
Resident Physician
Department of Orthopaedic Surgery
Virginia Commonwealth University
Richmond, Virginia

Kelly E. Grob, MD
Resident Physician
Department of Family Medicine
University of Virginia
Charlottesville, Virginia

F. Winston Gwathmey, Jr., MD
Associate Professor of Orthopaedic
    Surgery
University of Virginia
Charlottesville, Virginia

Michael Hadeed, MD
Resident Physician
Department of Orthopaedic Surgery
University of Virginia
Charlottesville, Virginia

Corey A. Hamilton, MD
Resident Physician
Department of Orthpaedics
University of South Carolina
Columbia, South Carolina

Kyle Hammond, MD
Assistant Professor
Departments of Orthopaedic Surgery,
    Sports Medicine
Emory University
Atlanta, Georgia

Jennifer A. Hart, MPAS, PA-C
Physician Assistant
Department of Orthopaedic Surgery
University of Virginia
Charlottesville, Virginia

Hamid Hassanzadeh, MD
Department of Orthopaedics
University of Virginia
Charlottesville, Virginia

Emanuel C. Haug, MD
Resident Physician
Department of Orthopaedic Surgery
University of Virginia
Charlottesville, Virginia

C. Thomas Haytmanek, Jr., MD
Attending Surgeon
Department of Orthopaedic Surgery
The Steadman Clinic
Vail, Colorado

Jonathan R. Helms, MD
Assistant Professor of Orthopaedic
    Surgery
University of Florida Health
    Jacksonville
Jacksonville, Florida

Shane Hennessy, DO
Primary Care Sports Medicine
University of Pittsburgh Medical Center
Pittsburgh, Pennsylvania

Donella Herman, MD, MEd
Primary Care Sports Medicine Physician
Sanford Orthopedics and Sports
    Medicine
Sanford Health
Sioux Falls, South Dakota

Joel Himes, DO
Fellow, Primary Care Sports Medicine
University of Pittsburgh Medical Center
Pittsburgh, Pennsylvania

Sarah Hoffman, DO, FAAP, CAQSM
Pediatric Sports Medicine Physician
Department of Orthopedics and Sports
    Medicine
Maine Medical Partners
South Portland, Maine;
Pediatric Hospitalist
Department of Pediatrics
Barbara Bush Children's Hospital
Portland, Maine;
Clinical Assistant Professor of Pediatrics
Tufts University School of Medicine
Boston, Massachusetts

Jarred Holt, DO
Sparrow Health System Sports Medicine
East Lansing, Michigan

Jason A. Horowitz, MD
Research Fellow
Department of Orthopaedic Surgery
University of Virginia
Charlottesville, Virginia

Thomas M. Howard, MD
Physician
Flexogenix
Cary, North Carolina

David Hryvniak, DO
Assistant Professor of Physical
    Medicine and Rehabilitation
Team Physician, University of Virginia
    Athletics
University of Virginia
Charlottesville, Virginia;
Team Physician, James Madison
    University Athletics
James Madison University
Harrisonburg, Virgin

Elizabeth W. Hubbard, MD
Department of Orthopaedic Surgery
Duke University Medical Center
Durham, North Carolina

Logan W. Huff, MD
Resident Physician
Department of Orthopaedics
University of South Carolina
Columbia, South Carolina

Brandon S. Huggins, MD
Orthopedic Surgery Resident
Department of Orthopedic Surgery
Greenville Health System
Greenville, South Carolina

Chad D. Hulsopple, DO
Assistant Professor of Family Medicine
Uniformed Services University of the
    Health Sciences
Bethesda, Maryland

Michael Hunter, MD
Department of Orthopaedic Surgery
Greenville Health System
Greenville, South Carolina

Mary C. Iaculli, DO
Martins Point Health Care
Portland, Maine

Jonathan E. Isaacs, MD
Herman M. & Vera H. Nachman
    Distinguished Research Professor
Chief, Division of Hand Surgery
Vice Chairman of Research and Education
Department of Orthopaedic Surgery
Virginia Commonwealth University
    Health System
Richmond, Virginia

Marissa Jamieson, MD
Resident Physician
Department of Orthopaedic Surgery
Ohio State Medical Center
Columbus, Ohio

Jeffrey G. Jenkins, MD
Associate Professor
Department of Physical Medicine and
    Rehabilitation
University of Virginia
Charlottesville, Virginia

Patrick Jenkins III, MD
Prompt Care
Division of Ambulatory Medicine
University Hospital
Augusta, Georgia

Darren L. Johnson, MD
Professor
Department of Orthopaedic Surgery
University of Kentucky
Lexington, Kentucky

Christopher E. Jonas, DO, FAAFP, CAQSM
Assistant Professor of Family Medicine
Uniformed Services University of the
    Health Sciences
Bethesda, Maryland

Carroll P. Jones, MD
Fellowship Director
Foot and Ankle Institute
OrthoCarolina
Charlotte, North Carolina

Contributors

Anish R. Kadakia, MD
Associate Professor of Orthopedic
Surgery
Fellowship Director, Foot and Ankle
Orthopedic Surgery
Northwestern University Feinberg
School of Medicine
Northwestern Memorial Hospital
Chicago, Illinois

Samantha L. Kallenback, BS
Steadman Philippon Research Institute
The Steadman Clinic
Vail, Colorado

Jerrod Keith, MD
Associate Professor
Divison of Plastic Surgery
University of Iowa Hospitals and Clinics
Iowa City, Iowa

Blane Kelly, MD
Surgeon
Department of Orthopaedics
Virgina Commonwealth/Medical
College of Virginia
Richmond, Virginia

Brian R. Kelly, MD
UT Southwestern Medical Center
Dallas, Texas

Jeremy Kent, MD
Assistant Professor of Family Medicine
University of Virginia
Charlottesville, Virginia

Michelle E. Kew, MD
Resident of Orthopaedic Surgery
University of Viriginia
Charlottesville, Virginia

A. Jay Khanna, MD, MBA
Professor and Vice Chair of
Orthopaedic Surgery
Department of Orthopaedic Surgery
Johns Hopkins University
Bethesda, Maryland

Patrick King, MD
Sports Medicine Fellow
Department of Family Medicine
Mountain Area Health Education Center
Asheville, North Carolina

Jason Kirkbride, MD, MS
Department of Physical Medicine and
Rehabilitation
University of Virginia
Charlottesville, Virginia

Amy Kite, MD
Department of Plastic and
Reconstructive Surgery
Virginia Commonwealth University
Richmond, Virginia

Alexander Knobloch, MD, CAQSM
Faculty Physician, Family Medicine
and Sports Medicine
David Grant Medical Center Family
Medicine Residency
Travis Air Force Base, California

Mininder S. Kocher, MD, MPH
Professor of Orthopaedic Surgery
Harvard Medical School;
Associate Director, Division of Sports
Medicine
Boston Children's Hospital
Boston, Massachusetts

Andrew Kubinski, DO, MS
Nonsurgical Orthopaedics and Sports
Medicine
Department of Private Diagnostic
Clinics, PLLC
Duke University
Durham, North Carolina

Justin Kunes, MD
Orthopedic Surgeon
Department of Orthopedic Surgery
Piedmont Medical Care Corporation
Covington, Georgia

Helen C. Lam, MD
Resident Physician
Department of Family Medicine
Kaiser Napa-Solano
Vallejo, California

Stephanie N. Lamb, MEd, ATC
VIPER Sports Medicine
559th Medical Group
JBSA-Lackland, Texas

Matthew D. LaPrade, BS
Steadman Philippon Research Institute
The Steadman Clinic
Vail, Colorado

Robert F. LaPrade, MD, PhD
Chief Medical Research Officer
Steadman Philippon Research Institute
The Steadman Clinic
Vail, Colorado

Leigh-Ann Lather, MD
Associate Professor of Orthopaedics
University of Virginia
Charlottesville, Virginia

Larry Lee, MD
Spine Surgery Fellow
Department of Orthopaedics, Spine
Center
University of Southern California
Los Angeles, California

Jeffrey Leggit, MD, CAQSM
Associate Professor of Family Medicine
Uniformed Services University of the
Health Sciences
Bethesda, Maryland

David Leslie, DO
Ochsner Sports Medicine Institute
Ochsner Health System
New Orleans, Louisiana

Xudong Li, MD, PhD
Associate Professor of Orthopaedic
Surgery
University of Virginia
Charlottesville, Virginia

Scott Linger, MD
Bloomington Bone & Joint Clinic
Bloomington, Indiana

**Catherine A. Logan, MD, MBA,
MSPT**
Orthopaedic Surgeon
Department of Orthopaedic Surgery
The Steadman Clinic
Vail, Colorado

Brian Lowell, MD
Department of Family Medicine
Southwest Peacehealth
Vancouver, Washington

Myro A. Lu, DO
Department of Family Medicine
Tripler Army Medical Center
Honolulu, Hawaii

Evan Lutz, MD, CAQSM
Sports Medicine Division Director
Department of Family Medicine
East Carolina University Sports Medicine
Greenville, North Carolina

Robert H. Lutz, MD
Team Physician
Davidson College Sports Medicine
Davidson, North Carolina

Matthew L. Lyons, MD
Orthopedic Surgeon
Department of Orthopedic Surgery
Kaiser Permanente Washington
Bellevue, Washington

John M. MacKnight, MD, FACSM
Professor of Internal Medicine
Medical Director and Primary Care
    Team Physician
Department of Athletics
University of Virginia
Charlottesville, Virginia

Steven J. Magister, MD
Resident Physician
Case Western Reserve University
Cleveland, Ohio

**Eric Magrum, DPT, OCS,
FAAOMPT**
Director, VOMPTI Orthopaedic
    Physical Therapy Residency
    Program
University of Virginia/Encompass
    Sports Medicine and Rehabilitation
Charlottesville, Viriginia

Harrison Mahon, MD
Resident Physician
University of Virginia
Charlottesville, Virginia

Aaron V. Mares, MD
Assistant Professor of Orthopaedic
    Surgery
Department of Orthopaedics
University of Pittsburgh Medical Center
Pittsburgh, Pennsylvania

Robert G. Marx, MD, MSc, FRCSC
Attending Orthopedic Surgeon
Hospital for Special Surgery;
Professor of Orthopedic Surgery
Weill Cornell Medical College
New York, New York

Scott McAleer, MD
University of Virginia School of Medicine
Charlottesville, Virginia

Melissa McLane, DO
Assistant Professor of Orthopaedic
    Surgery
University of Pittsburgh
Pittsburgh, Pennsylvania

**Michael McMurray, PT, DPT, OCS,
FAAOMPT**
Physical Therapist
University of Virginia/Encompass
    Sports Medicine and Rehabilitation
    Center
Charlottesville, Virginia

James Medure, MD
University of Pittsburgh
Pittsburgh, Pennsylvania

Todd Milbrandt, MD, MS
Associate Professor of Orthopedics
Consultant, Department of Orthopedic
    Surgery
Mayo Clinic
Rochester, Minnesota

Christopher Miles, MD
Associate Program Director of Primary
    Care Sports Medicine Fellowship
Assistant Professor of Family and
    Community Medicine
Wake Forest University School of
    Medicine
Winston-Salem, North Carolina

Mark D. Miller, MD
S. Ward Casscells Professor of
    Orthopaedic Surgery
Department of Orthopaedics
University of Virginia
Charlottesville, Virginia

Ryan D. Muchow, MD
Staff Pediatric Orthopaedic Surgeon
Department of Orthopaedic Surgery
Shriners Hospital for Children, Lexington;
Associate Professor of Orthopaedic
    Surgery
University of Kentucky
Lexington, Kentucky

John V. Murphy, DO
Primary Care Sports Medicine Fellow
Department of Orthopedics
University of Pittsburgh Medical Center
Pittsburgh, Pennsylvania

Tenley Murphy, MD
Associate Team Physician
Clemson University
Clemson, South Carolina

Lauren Nadkarni, MD
Primary Care Sports Medicine Fellow
Department of Family Medicine/Sports
    Medicine
Maine Medical Center
Portland, Maine

Michael T. Nolte, MD
Resident Physician
Department of Orthopaedic Surgery
Rush University Medical Center
Chicago, Illinois

Ali Nourbakhsh, MD
Spine Surgeon
Department of Orthopedics
WellStar Atlanta Medical Center
Atlanta, Georgia

Nathaniel S. Nye, MD
VIPER Sports Medicine Element Chief
559th Medical Group
JBSA-Lackland, Texas

Michael O'Brien, MD
Assistant Professor of Orthopedics
Boston Children's Hospital
Boston, Massachusetts;
Staff Physician
The Micheli Center for Sports Injury
    Prevention
Waltham, Massachusetts

Francis O'Connor, MD, PhD
Uniformed Services University
    Consortium for Health and Military
    Performance
Bethesda, Maryland

Matthew J. Pacana, MD
Resident Physician
Department of Orthopaedics
University of South Carolina
Columbia, South Carolina

Hugo Paquin, MD
Assistant Professor of Pediatrics
University of Montreal;
Attending Physician
Division of Pediatric Emergency
    Medicine
Centre Hospitalier Universitaire
    Sainte-Justine
Montreal, Quebec, Canada

Joseph S. Park, MD
Associate Professor
Foot and Ankle Division Head
Department of Orthopedic Surgery
University of Virginia Health System
Charlottesville, Virginia

Milap S. Patel, DO
Attending Physician
Northwestern Memorial Hospital
Chicago, Illinois

William Patterson, DO
Primary Care Sports Medicine Fellow
Department of Sports Medicine
Maine Medical Center
Portland, Maine

Sergio Patton, MD
University of Virginia
Charlottesville, Virginia

Venkat Perumal, MD
Assistant Professor of Orthopaedics
University of Virginia
Charlottesville, Virginia

Contributors

Christopher J. Pexton, DO
Family Medicine Physician
Peacehealth
Vancouver, Washington

Frank M. Phillips, MD
Professor and Spine Fellowship
Co-Director
Department of Orthopaedic Surgery
Rush University Medical Center
Chicago, Illinois

Jennifer Pierce, MD
Department of Radiology
University of Virginia
Charlottesville, Virginia

Tinnakorn Pluemvitayaporn, MD
Spine Unit
Department of Orthopaedic Surgery
Institute of Orthopaedics
Lerdsin Hospital
Bangkok, Thailand

Brian D. Powell, MD
Foot and Ankle Surgeon
Department of Orthopaedics
Ogden Clinic
Ogden, Utah

Bridget Quinn, MD
Department of Orthopedic Surgery
Boston Children's Hospital
Boston, Massachusetts

Kate Quinn, DO
Division of Sports Medicine
Maine Medical Partners Orthopedics
and Sports Medicine
South Portland, Maine

Rabia Qureshi, MD
Researcher
Department of Orthopedics
University of Virginia
Charlottesville, Virginia

Sara N. Raiser, MD
Resident Physician
Department of Physical Medicine &
Rehabilitation
University of Virginia
Charlottesville, Virginia

Justin J. Ray, MD
Resident Physician
Department of Orthopaedics
West Virginia University
Morgantown, West Virginia

Tracy R. Ray, MD
Director, Sports Medicine Primary Care
Department of Orthopedic Surgery
Associate Professor
Departments of Orthopaedic Surgery
and Community and Family
Medicine
Duke University
Durham, North Carolina

Scott Riley, MD
Department of Orthopaedic Surgery
Shriners Hospital for Children
Lexington, Kentucky

Mark Rogers, DO, CAQSM, FAAFP, FAOASM
Associate Professor of Family
Medicine
Discipline Sports Medicine
Edward Via College of Osteopathic
Medicine, Virginia Campus;
Team Physician
Department of Performance & Sports
Medicine
Virginia Tech
Blacksburg, Virginia

Mark J. Romness, MD
Associate Professor of Orthopaedic
Surgery
University of Virginia
Charlottesville, Virginia

Michael Rosen, DO
Adjunct Clinical Faculty
Osteopathic Surgical Specialties
Michigan State University
East Lansing, Michigan

Jeffrey Ruland, BA
Medical Student
University of Virginia School of Medicine
Charlottesville, Virginia

Robert D. Santrock, MD
Assistant Professor of Orthopaedics
West Virginia University
Morgantown, West Virginia

Thomas Schaller, MD
Program Director
Associate Professor
Department of Orthopedics
Greenville Health System
Greenville, South Carolina

David Schnur, MD
Private Practice
Plastic Surgery Clinic
Denver, Colorado

Andrew Schwartz, MD
Resident Physician
Department of Orthopaedics, Sports
Medicine, and Spine
Emory University
Atlanta, Georgia

Nicholas Sgrignoli, MD
Resident Physician
Family and Community Medicine
Wake Forest University
Winston-Salem, North Carolina

Stephen Shaheen, MD, CAQSM
Assistant Professor, Orthopedic
Surgery and Emergency Medicine
Primary Care Sports Medicine
Duke University Medical Center
Durham, North Carolina

Alan Shahtaji, DO, CAQ-SM
Associate Clinical Professor of Family
Medicine and Public Health
University of California San Diego
San Diego, California

Lisa A. Sienkiewicz, MD
Department of Orthopedics and
Rehabilitation
University of Wisconsin School of
Medicine and Public Health
Madison, Wisconsin

Anuj Singla, MD
Instructor
Department of Orthopaedic Surgery
University of Virginia
Charlottesville, Virginia

Bryan Sirmon, MD
Attending Surgeon
Georgia Hand, Shoulder & Elbow
Atlanta, Georgia

Jonathan P. Smerek, MS, MD
Associate Professor of Orthopaedics
Indiana University School of Medicine
Indianapolis, Indiana

W. Bret Smith, DO, MS
Director, Foot and Ankle Division
Department of Orthopedic Surgery
PH-USC Orthopedic Center;
Assistant Professor of Orthopedics
University of South Carolina
Columbia, South Carolina

Avinash Sridhar, MD
Family Medicine Resident
Department of Family Medicine
Mountain Area Health Education Center
Asheville, North Carolina

Michael S. Sridhar, MD
Assistant Professor of Orthopaedic
Surgery
Greenville Health System
Greenville, South Carolina

Uma Srikumaran, MD, MBA, MPH
Assistant Professor of Orthopaedic
Surgery
Johns Hopkins School of Medicine
Baltimore, Maryland

Siobhan M. Statuta, MD, CAQSM
Assistant Professor
Departments of Family Medicine and
Physical Medicine & Rehabilitation
Director, Primary Care Sports Medicine
Fellowship
Department of Family Medicine
University of Virginia
Charlottesville, Virginia

Andrea Stracciolini, MD
Department of Sports Medicine
Boston Children's Hospital
Boston, Massachusetts

Nicholas Strasser, DO
Clinical Faculty
Department of Family Medicine–Sports
Medicine
Edward Via College of Osteopathic
Medicine
Blacksburg, Viriginia

Jillian Sylvester, MD, CAQ
Saint Louis University Family Medicine
Residency
O'Fallon, Illinois

Vishwas R. Talwalkar, MD
Professor of Orthopaedic Surgery and
Pedatrics
University of Kentucky College of
Medicine;
Department of Orthopaedic Surgery
Shriners Hospital for Children
Lexington, Kentucky

Cole Taylor, MD, CAQSM, FAAFP
Clinic Chief, Sports Medicine
Fort Belvoir Community Hospital
Fort Belvoir, Virginia

John B. Thaller, MD
Director of Orthopaedics
Department of Orthopaedic Surgery
Maine General Medical Center
Augusta, Maine

Marc Tompkins, MD
Associate Professor of Orthopaedic
Surgery
University of Minnesota
Minneapolis, Minnesota;
TRIA Orthopaedic Center
Bloomington, Minnesota

Benjamin A. Tran
University of Virginia School of
Medicine
Charlottesville, Virginia

Obinna Ugwu-Oju, MD
Resident Physician
Department of Orthopaedic Surgery
Virginia Commonwealth University
Richmond, Virginia

Jon Umlauf, DPT
Department of Physical Therapy
Brooke Army Medical Center
Fort Sam Houston, Texas

Christopher E. Urband, MD
Orthopaedic Surgeon
Department of Orthopaedics
Torrey Pines Orthopaedics and Sports
Medicine
La Jolla, California

Ryan Urchek, MD
Fellow, Orthopaedic Sports Medicine
Emory University
Atlanta, Georgia

Kevin Valvano, DO
Primary Care Sports Medicine
Edward Via College of Osteopathic
Medicine, Virginia Campus;
Assistant Team Physician
Department of Performance and
Sports Medicine
Virginia Tech
Blacksburg, Virginia

Scott Van Aman, MD
Orthopedic Surgeon, Foot and Ankle
Orthopedic One
Columbus, Ohio

Corey Van Hoff, MD
Orthopaedic Trauma Surgeon
Orthopaedic One
Columbus, Ohio

Aaron Vaughan, MD
Sports Medicine Director
Department of Family Medicine
Mountain Area Health Education Center
Asheville, North Carolina

Janet L. Walker, MD
Professor of Orthopaedic Surgery
University of Kentucky College of
Medicine;
Attending Physician
Shriners Hospital for Children
Lexington, Kentucky

Nathan Wanderman, MD
Resident, Orthopedic Surgery Department
Mayo Clinic
Rochester, Minnesota

Jeffrey Wang, MD
Co-Director, University of Southern
California Spine Institute
Professor of Orthopaedic Surgery
Clinical Scholar
Department of Orthopaedics, Spine
Center
University of Southern California
Los Angeles, California

Robert P. Waugh, MD
Orthopaedic Surgeon
Coastal Orthopedic Associates
Beverly, Massachusetts

Justin L. Weppner, DO
Department of Physical Medicine and
Rehabilitation
University of Virginia
Charlottesville, Virginia

Brian C. Werner, MD
Assistant Professor of Orthopaedic
Surgery
University of Virginia
Charlottesville, Virginia

Andrea M. White, PA, MEd
Physician Assistant
Department of Orthopaedics
University of Virginia
Charlottesville, Virginia

Robert P. Wilder, MD, FACSM
Professor and Chair of Physical
Medicine and Rehabilitation
University of Virginia
Charlottesville, Virginia

George Lee Wilkinson III, BA
Scribe, Foot and Ankle
Department of Orthopedic Surgery
University of Virginia
Charlottesville, Virginia

Christina M. Wong, DO
Primary Care Sports Medicine Fellow
Department of Sports Medicine
Edward Via College of Osteopathic
Medicine
Blacksburg, Virginia

Contributors

Colton Wood, MD
Resident Physician
Family Medicine Residency Program
University of Virginia
Charlottesville, Virginia

Katherine Victoria Yao, MD
Assistant Professor of Clinical
    Rehabilitation Medicine
Weill Cornell Medical College
Cornell University;
Adjunct Assistant Professor of Clinical
    Rehabilitation and Regenerative
    Medicine
Columbia University College of
    Physicians and Surgeons;
Assistant Attending Physiatrist
Department of Rehabilitation Medicine
New York-Presbyterian Hospital
New York, New York

Seth R. Yarboro, MD
Assistant Professor of Orthopaedic
    Surgery
University of Virginia
Charlottesville, Virginia

S. Tim Yoon, MD, PhD
Associate Professor of Orthopedic
    Surgery
Emory University
Atlanta, Georgia

Dan A. Zlotolow, MD
Associate Professor of Orthopaedics
Thomas Jefferson University School of
    Medicine;
Attending Physician
Shriners Hospital for Children
Philadelphia, Pennsylvania

Contents

Contents

Contents

Contents

Contents

Video Contents

1

SECTION

General Principles

Chapter 1 How to Use This Book

Mark D. Miller, John M. MacKnight, Jennifer A. Hart

Welcome to what we hope will be the most comprehensive and useful textbook of orthopaedics you will ever own. Appreciating that the vast majority of orthopaedic care takes place not in the orthopaedic surgeon's office or operating room, but rather in a myriad of primary care settings, this work is designed to be a user-friendly reference to assist primary care physicians, physician's assistants, nurse practitioners, physical therapists, and athletic trainers. Having a reliable, thorough resource of clinical information is essential to ensure timely and appropriate management of all orthopaedic concerns. As such, we have produced *Essential Orthopaedics* to be your go-to resource in the clinic or the training room. The new edition also brings some exciting updates such as ICD-10-CM codes for the most common orthopaedic conditions, current concept updates, new composite figures, and even some new chapters to highlight the changes in the field. As you peruse the text, you will find that the initial sections are devoted to a number of general topics important to orthopaedic care. A review of orthopaedic anatomy and terminology is followed by information on the nuances of radiologic evaluation of orthopaedic conditions. Subsequent chapters are dedicated to such vital topics as pharmacology, impairment and disability, and principles of rehabilitation. Additional chapters are dedicated to special populations and conditions such as the obese, elderly, pediatric, and female and pregnant patients, and those with multiple comorbid conditions, arthritides, and trauma.

The remainder of the text is divided into major anatomic groups: shoulder, elbow, wrist/hand, spine, pelvis/hip, knee and lower leg, and ankle and foot, with a special section dedicated to pediatrics. Each section begins with an anatomic graphic that will direct you to likely diagnoses based on the location of the patient's symptoms or findings. The following pages include a review of regional anatomy, pertinent history that is characteristic for each anatomic area, a review of specific physical examination techniques, and practical management of imaging strategies.

Within each specific topic chapter you will find a consistent format designed to aid efficiency in finding the information that you need as quickly as possible. After alternative condition names and ICD-10-CM codes are provided, topic headings include Key Concepts, History, Physical Examination, Imaging, Additional Tests (if applicable), Differential Diagnosis, Treatment, Troubleshooting, Patient Instructions, Considerations in Special Populations, and Suggested Reading. We have placed great emphasis on including multiple drawings, photographs, and radiologic images to enhance the quality of each topic. In addition, we have added an accompanying DVD that covers in great detail the key orthopaedic physical examination techniques and procedures that any provider should know. We want you to feel comfortable that you have seen what you need to provide great care.

It is our sincere hope that you will find the latest edition of *Essential Orthopaedics* to be the finest orthopaedic reference for primary care providers of all types. Having a comprehensive reference designed for rapid access of information is crucial for busy practitioners. This text will help you find the right answer quickly and will help enhance your comfort with orthopaedic diagnosis, management, and appropriate referral. Musculoskeletal care accounts for a sizable percentage of medical encounters; let *Essential Orthopaedics* help enhance the care of every orthopaedic patient whom you see.

Chapter 2 Orthopaedic Terminology

Siobhan M. Statuta

Introduction

Orthopaedic complaints account for some of the most common presentations to physicians. A thorough working knowledge of basic anatomy, function, and movement is essential for prompt diagnosis and appropriate management of these conditions. The following terms are commonly used in orthopaedic practice. Mastery of these basic terms will allow the reader to better understand the material presented in the following chapters.

Anatomy

- *Allograft*: Tissue or specimen that comes from the same species but a different individual (e.g., cadaver grafts in reconstruction of the anterior cruciate ligament).
- *Anterior cruciate ligament*: The primary stabilizer that prevents anterior translation of the tibia on the femur, as well as for rotational movement. It is one of the most commonly injured knee ligaments. It heals poorly due to its limited blood supply and often requires surgical reconstruction.
- *Articular cartilage*: Hyaline cartilage that lines the end of long bones, forming the surface of a joint.
- *Autograft*: Tissue specimen that comes from the same individual but from a different anatomic site (e.g., bone–patellar tendon–bone or hamstring grafts in the reconstruction of the anterior cruciate ligament in the same individual).
- *Bipartite*: Meaning two parts, it refers to the anatomic variant in which the ossification centers of a sesamoid bone fail to properly fuse. Most commonly seen in the patella and sesamoids of the foot.
- *Diaphysis*: The shaft of a long bone composed of bone marrow and adipose tissue.
- *Discoid meniscus*: Anatomic variant in which the typical C-shaped fibrocartilage meniscus assumes a thickened, flat contour.
- *Epiphyseal plate (physis)*: The "growth plate." This hyaline cartilage structure is the site of elongation of long bones. Physes are inherently weak compared with the surrounding bone and thus are often sites of injury in developing children and adolescents.
- *Epiphysis*: The end of a long bone that ultimately forms the articular cartilage–lined edges of a long bone.
- *Labrum*: A fibrocartilage ring that surrounds the articular surface of a joint helping deepen and stabilize the joint (e.g., glenoid labrum of the shoulder and the acetabular labrum of the hip).
- *Lateral collateral ligament*: Primary knee stabilizer to varus stress.
- *Ligament*: Fibrous connective tissue attaching one bone to another. Provides structural support to the joint.
- *Medial collateral ligament*: The primary knee stabilizer to valgus stress.
- *Meniscus*: C-shaped fibrocartilage cushion in the knee; distributes load forces between the femur and tibia.
- *Metaphysis*: The portion of a long bone between the epiphysis and the diaphysis.
- *Posterior cruciate ligament*: The primary stabilizer that prevents posterior translation of the tibia to the femur and also contributes to rotary stability.
- *Tendon*: Fibrous connective tissue that attaches muscle to bone.
- *Triangular fibrocartilage complex*: A collection of ligaments and fibrocartilage located on the ulnar side of the wrist, which stabilizes the distal radius, ulna, and carpal bones.
- *Tuberosity*: A bony prominence that serves as the site of attachment for tendons and/or ligaments.

Injury

- *Apophysitis*: An overuse injury, caused by inflammation or repeated stress, at the attachment site of a tendon to bone. Commonly affected sites: tibial tubercle of the knee (Osgood-Schlatter disease), medial epicondyle in the elbow.
- *Bursitis*: Inflammation of the synovial sac (bursa) that protects the soft-tissue structures (muscles, tendons) from underlying bony prominences. Common areas of involvement include the shoulder (subacromial bursa), knee (prepatellar bursa), elbow (olecranon bursa), and hip (trochanteric bursa).
- *Dislocation*: Complete disassociation of the articular surfaces of a joint. Commonly affected sites: the patella, the glenohumeral joint.
- *Impingement*: The process by which soft tissues (i.e., tendons, bursae) are compressed by bony structures, often dynamic in nature. Frequently encountered in the shoulder and ankle.
- *Myositis ossificans*: Heterotopic bone formation at the site of previous trauma and hematoma formation. The most common site of involvement is the thigh following a contusion.
- *Osteoarthritis*: Degenerative condition that causes breakdown of articular cartilage and underlying bone. Results in joint pain, stiffness, and decreased range of motion.
- *Osteochondritis dissecans*: Injury (often traumatic) to a joint surface of bone that results in the detachment of subchondral bone from its overlying articular cartilage. Commonly affected sites include the knee, elbow, and ankle.
- *Salter-Harris*: Classification system used to categorize injuries to the growth plate (physis) in the skeletally immature:
  - Type I: Transverse fracture through the physis without other injury. Widening of the physis can be seen or radiographs may remain normal.

- Type II: Physeal fracture that extends into the metaphysis.
- Type III: Physeal fracture that extends into the epiphysis.
- Type IV: Fracture that involves the metaphysis, physis and epiphysis.
- Type V: Crush-type fracture that involves compression of the epiphyseal plate.
- *Spondylolisthesis*: The abnormal anterior or posterior translation of one vertebral body with respect to another.
- *Spondylolysis*: A fracture of the pars interarticularis of the vertebra usually due to repetitive stress. The lower lumbar vertebrae are most frequently affected.
- *Sprain*: An injury to the ligaments that support a joint. Mild injuries involve microscopic tearing; moderate injuries involve partial tearing of the ligament; severe insults involve complete disruption of the ligament.
- *Strain*: An injury to muscle or tendon around or attached to a joint. Grading scale is similar to sprains with mild injuries involving microscopic tearing, moderate injuries involving partial tearing of the muscle or tendon, and severe injuries resulting in complete disruption of muscle or tendon fibers.
- *Stress fracture*: Microscopic fractures in bone caused by isolated repetitive forces to a focal area. Bony breakdown occurs more rapidly than repair due to overuse or lack of recovery time.
- *Subluxation*: Partial dislocation of the articular surfaces of a joint.
- *Syndesmotic ankle ("high ankle") sprain*: Ankle sprain resulting in injury to the syndesmotic ligament that connects the tibia and fibula superior to the ankle joint proper. These injuries are generally more severe than routine ankle sprains.
- *Tendinitis*: Acute inflammation of a tendon. Symptoms are typically present for several weeks. Commonly affected sites include the shoulder, knee, elbow, and heel.
- *Tendinosis/tendinopathy*: Degenerative breakdown of the tendon and abnormal vascularization due to chronic, repetitive stress. Symptoms are often present for several weeks to months.
- *Tenosynovitis*: Inflammation of a tendon sheath. This can occur concomitantly with tendon involvement or independently.

Movement

- *Abduction*: Movement away from the body's midline.
- *Adduction*: Movement toward the body's midline.

- *Eversion*: Rotation of the foot or ankle outward away from midline.
- *Inversion*: Rotation of the foot or ankle inward toward midline.
- *Pronation*: Rotary movement described at the wrist, where the palm of the hand rotates from a superior facing position to one facing inferiorly. Similarly, at the ankle, the plantar aspect of the foot rotates outward or laterally.
- *Supination*: Rotary movement described at the wrist, where the palm of the hand rotates from an inferior facing position to one facing superiorly. Similarly, at the ankle, the plantar aspect of the foot rotates inward or medially.
- *Valgus*: Anatomic alignment of a joint where the distal portion is angulated away from the midline (i.e., knock knees).
- *Varus*: Anatomic alignment of a joint where the distal portion is angulated toward the midline (i.e., bowlegs).

Treatment

- *Arthrocentesis*: Aspiration of synovial fluid from a joint.
- *Arthroscopy*: A surgical technique that uses a small camera (arthroscope) in a joint space for the diagnosis and treatment of joint-related conditions.
- *Dry needling*: Technique in which needles are inserted into myofascial trigger points with the goal of improving muscle tension and pain.
- *Iontophoresis*: Process by which an electrical current is used to deliver a drug (often a corticosteroid) to the surrounding soft tissues or joint transdermally.
- *Physical therapy*: The branch of medicine that specializes in treatment, prevention, and functional optimization of disorders of the musculoskeletal system. It encompasses numerous treatment modalities including mobilization, strengthening, flexibility, massage, heat, and dry needling.
- *Rehabilitation*: The process of restoring one's health functionality.

Suggested Readings

Armstrong AD, Hubbard MC, eds. *Essentials of Musculoskeletal Care*. 5th ed. Rosemont, IL: American Academy of Orthopaedic Surgeons; 2016.

Miller MD, Thompson SR, eds. *DeLee & Drez's Orthopaedic Sports Medicine: Principles and Practice*. 4th ed. Philadelphia: Elsevier; 2015.

Thompson JC. *Netter's Concise Orthopaedic Anatomy*. 2nd ed (Updated Edition). Philadelphia: Elsevier; 2015.

Chapter 3 Imaging of the Musculoskeletal System

Mark W. Anderson

Key Concepts

- Imaging studies should be used as an adjunct to the history and physical examination.
- Obtain the least number of imaging studies needed to arrive at a diagnosis (or reasonable differential diagnosis).
- Each imaging modality has specific strengths and weaknesses that must be taken into account when considering which test to perform.

Imaging
Radiography

- *Technique:* A beam of x-rays is projected through the body to a detector that constructs a two-dimensional image based on the differential attenuation of the beam by various tissues.
- The primary modality for investigating the musculoskeletal system; it should be the first imaging study ordered for most indications.
- Four basic tissues are recognizable on a radiograph: metals, which are the densest structures on a film (this category includes bone because of its calcium content); air, which is the most lucent *(black)*; fat, which is *dark gray*; and soft tissue, which appears as *intermediate gray* (this category includes fluid that cannot be differentiated from muscle, etc.) (Fig. 3.1).
- At least two views are usually obtained, most often in the frontal and lateral projections (Fig. 3.2).

Strengths

- Relatively inexpensive
- Widely available

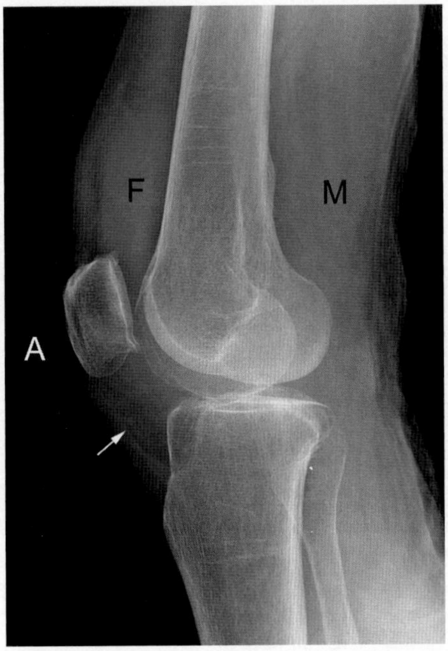

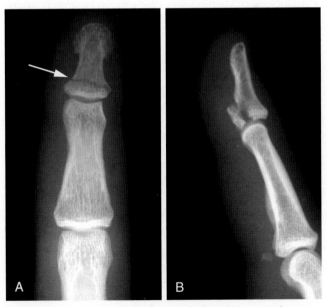

Fig 3.1 Radiography: Soft-tissue contrast. Lateral radiograph of the knee demonstrates dark, lucent air *(A)*; dark gray fat in Hoffa fat pad *(arrow)*; intermediate gray fluid in the suprapatellar bursa *(F)* related to a large joint effusion (note the similarity in density between the fluid and the hamstring muscles *[M]* posteriorly); and the relatively dense bones (related to their calcium content).

Fig 3.2 Radiography: Importance of obtaining more than one view. **(A)** Posteroanterior radiograph of the finger demonstrates a transverse fracture of the distal phalanx that does not appear to involve its articular surface *(arrow)*. **(B)** Corresponding lateral view reveals intra-articular extension and mild distraction along the fracture line.

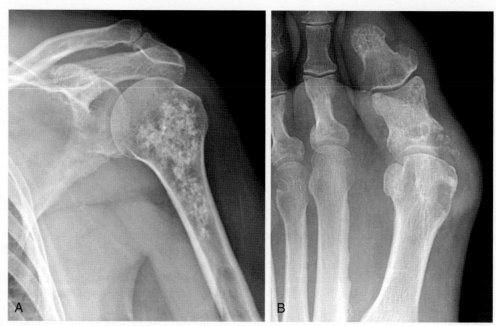

Fig 3.3 Radiography: Tumor and arthritis. **(A)** Frontal view of the shoulder reveals a coarse, sclerotic intramedullary lesion within the proximal humerus, compatible with a chondroid neoplasm, most likely an enchondroma. **(B)** Posteroanterior radiograph of the foot demonstrates classic findings of gout involving the first metatarsophalangeal joint including large marginal and para-articular erosions, calcific densities in the adjacent soft-tissue tophus, and relative sparing of the joint space.

- Evaluation of bone pathology (fracture, tumor, arthritis, osteomyelitis, metabolic bone disease) (Fig. 3.3)
- Assessment of orthopaedic hardware and fracture healing (Fig. 3.4)

Weaknesses

- Pathology of the medullary cavity (bone contusion, occult fracture, medullary tumor) (Fig. 3.5)
- Soft-tissue pathology
- Uses ionizing radiation

Computed Tomography

- *Technique:* An x-ray source is rotated around the patient, who is lying on a moving gantry, resulting in image "slices" in the transaxial plane.
- The data from these slices can then be viewed as axial images or used to create reformatted images in any plane (typically sagittal and coronal planes).
- Can be combined with intravenous (IV) contrast, which results in increased density (enhancement) in vessels and hypervascular tissues owing to its iodine content

Strengths

- Tomographic depiction of anatomy allowing for two- and three-dimensional reformatted images (Fig. 3.6)
- Depiction of complex fractures, especially those involving the spine and flat bones (pelvis and scapula) (Fig. 3.7)
- Evaluation of fracture healing
- Postoperative evaluation of the degree of fusion or hardware complications (Fig. 3.8)
- Can be combined with intrathecal or intra-articular contrast (computed tomography [CT] myelography and CT arthrography, respectively) (Fig. 3.9)

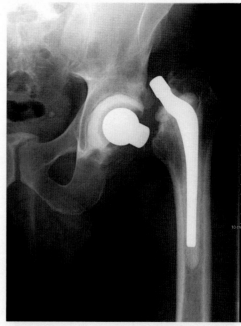

Fig 3.4 Radiography: Joint prosthesis. Frontal radiograph of the left hip shows prosthetic discontinuity of the femoral component at the junction of its head and neck with resulting superolateral migration of the proximal femur.

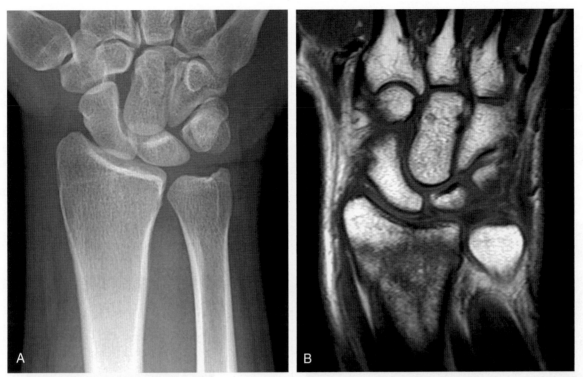

Fig 3.5 Radiography: occult fracture. **(A)** No discrete fracture is evident on this posteroanterior view of the wrist obtained after injury. **(B)** Coronal T1-weighted magnetic resonance image reveals numerous nondisplaced, low-signal-intensity fracture lines within the distal radius.

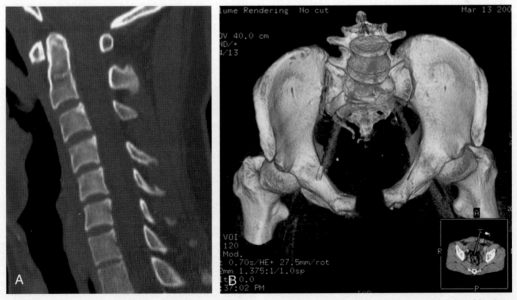

Fig 3.6 Computed tomography: Reformatted images. **(A)** Thin-slice computed tomography images obtained in the axial plane were combined to create this two-dimensional sagittal reconstructed image of the cervical spine. **(B)** A three-dimensional reformatted image of the pelvis depicts prominent diastasis of the symphysis pubis and less prominent widening of the right sacroiliac joint.

- Accurate demonstration of urate acid crystals using dual-energy CT allowing for a specific diagnosis of gout (Fig. 3.10)

Weaknesses

- Fracture detection in the setting of significant osteopenia (Fig. 3.11)
- Although CT produces much better soft-tissue contrast than radiographs, it is not as good as that obtained with magnetic resonance imaging (MRI).
- Uses ionizing radiation (unlike ultrasonography and MRI)

Radionuclide Scanning

- *Technique:* A bone-seeking radioactive material is injected intravenously (typically technetium-99m diphosphonate, a phosphorous analog that is taken up in areas of increased bone turnover such as tumor, infection, and fracture), and the patient is scanned 4 to 6 hours later, at which time whole-body images may be obtained.
- More localized, "spot" images may also be acquired in areas of specific clinical concern, and the use of single-photon emission tomography technology can produce tomographic images in the axial, sagittal, and coronal planes.
- Positron emission tomography scanning uses a metabolically active tracer, typically ^{18}F-fluorodeoxyglucose, a glucose analog that is taken up in tissues proportional to glucose use.

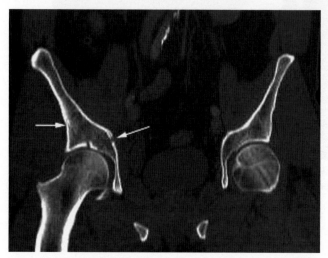

Fig 3.7 Computed tomography: Complex fractures. Coronal, two-dimensional reformatted image from a computed tomography scan of the pelvis demonstrates an essentially nondisplaced, comminuted right acetabular fracture *(arrows)*.

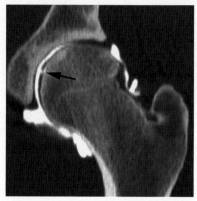

Fig 3.9 Computed tomography arthrogram. Coronal reformatted image from a computed tomography arthrogram of the left hip reveals a small cartilage flap along the medial femoral head *(arrow)*.

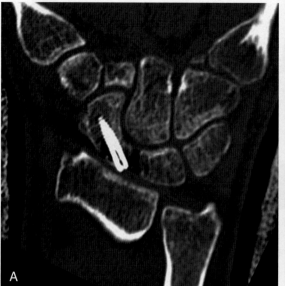

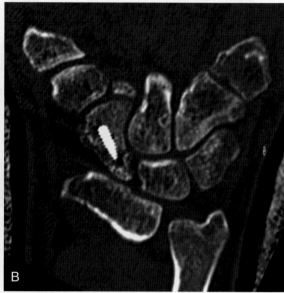

Fig 3.8 Computed tomography: Postoperative assessment. **(A)** and **(B)** Adjacent coronal reformatted images of the wrist reveal a nondisplaced scaphoid fracture transfixed with a surgical screw. Note the lack of metal-related artifact.

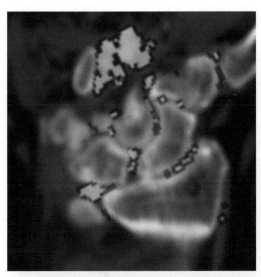

Fig 3.10 Dual energy computed tomography (CT): Gout. Color-coded coronal reformatted image from a dual energy CT examination demonstrates extensive monosodium urate deposition *(green foci)* throughout the wrist.

- Pathologic processes typically show increased metabolic activity and increased ^{18}F-fluorodeoxyglucose uptake.
- This modality also has theoretical value for the evaluation of a variety of neoplastic, infectious, and inflammatory conditions of the musculoskeletal system. Although promising results have been reported for some indications, the number of studies has been limited to date, and further investigation is needed.

Strengths

- Whole-body imaging allows rapid assessment of the entire skeleton; this is the study of choice to evaluate possible skeletal metastases.
- Provides physiologic information regarding the activity of a bone lesion (Fig. 3.12)
- High sensitivity

Weaknesses

- Relatively low specificity.
- Any process resulting in increased bone turnover (infection, tumor, fracture) may result in a focus of increased activity.
- False-negative examinations may occur in the initial 24 to 48 hours, especially in elderly patients.
- Insensitive for detecting multiple myeloma (plain radiographs are actually better for this purpose).
- Poor soft-tissue evaluation.
- Produces ionizing radiation.

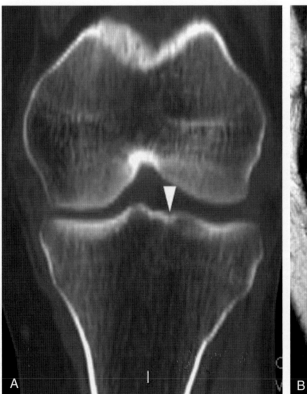
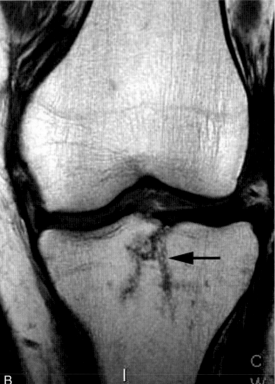

Fig 3.11 Computed tomography versus magnetic resonance imaging for a tibial plateau fracture. **(A)** Coronal reformatted computed tomography image of the knee reveals a very small cortical lucency *(arrowhead)* in the tibial plateau at the site of a nondisplaced fracture that is much better demonstrated using MRI as indicated by the *arrow* in **(B)**, a coronal T1-weighted image.

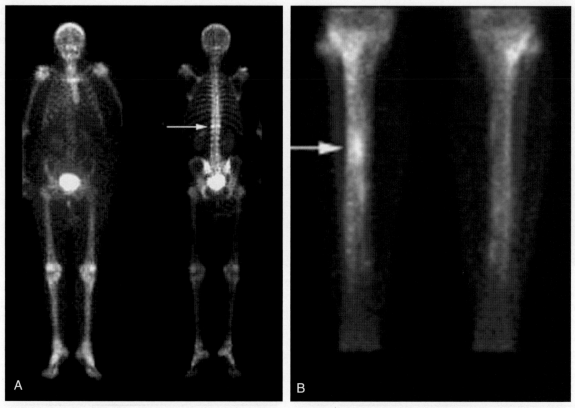

Fig 3.12 Bone scan. **(A)** Anterior and posterior whole-body bone scan images reveal focal uptake at the thoracolumbar junction *(arrow)* at the site of a pathologic fracture related to a vertebral metastasis. **(B)** Spot images of the lower legs from a bone scan in a different patient show abnormal uptake in the right mid-tibia at the site of a stress fracture *(arrow)*.

Ultrasonography

- *Technique:* Sound waves are passed into tissue via a handheld transducer, and the image is produced based on the pattern of returning waves.
- Tissues can be assessed in a dynamic, real-time fashion or on static images.
- Best if used for a specific clinical question (e.g., tendon laceration, evaluation of a soft-tissue mass, foreign body detection).
- Vascularity and flow dynamics can be assessed with Doppler ultrasound imaging.

Strengths

- Allows anatomic and dynamic functional evaluation of musculoskeletal tissues (e.g., tendon function, developmental dysplasia of the hip) (Fig. 3.13).
- Determining whether a soft-tissue mass is of a cystic or solid nature.
- Cystic masses appear as anechoic *(black)* structures with a sharp posterior wall and enhanced through transmission (owing to the lack of sound reflectors within the homogeneous fluid) (Fig. 3.14).
- Assessing the vascularity of a lesion.
- Real-time guidance for percutaneous interventional procedures.

- Foreign body detection (Fig. 3.15).
- No ionizing radiation.

Weaknesses

- Limited assessment of deeper tissues and bone
- Relatively time consuming and very operator dependent
- Limited field of view

Magnetic Resonance Imaging

- *Technique:* MRI is based on the fact that hydrogen protons within the body (most abundant in water and fat) will act like small bar magnets. The patient is placed in a strong magnetic field, and a small percentage of protons will align with the field.
- Energy, in the form of radio waves, is added to the tissue causing some of the protons to shift to a higher-energy state. When the radiofrequency source is turned off, the protons will relax back to their resting state and in the process release energy, again in the form of radio waves, which are detected and used to create the magnetic resonance image.
- The protons resonate differently in different tissues, based primarily on two tissue-specific factors called T1 and T2, and scanning parameters can be set to emphasize either factor, thereby producing T1-weighted and T2-weighted images, respectively.

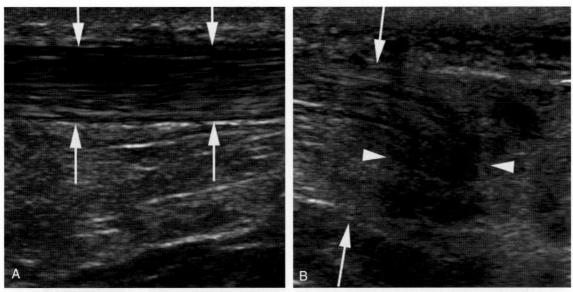

Fig 3.13 Ultrasonography: Tendons. (A) Longitudinal sonogram of a normal Achilles tendon *(arrows)*. (B) Longitudinal scan of the Achilles tendon in a different patient demonstrates diffuse thickening of the tendon *(arrows)* and an area of high-grade partial tearing *(arrowheads)*.

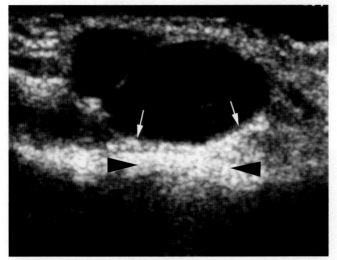

Fig 3.14 Ultrasonography: Ganglion cyst. Ultrasound scan of the finger reveals a small, bilobed ganglion cyst. Note the lack of internal echoes, sharp posterior wall *(arrows)*, and enhanced through transmission *(arrowheads)*, all of which are typical sonographic characteristics of a cyst.

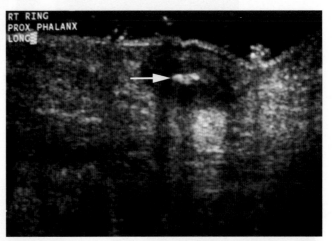

Fig 3.15 Ultrasonography: Foreign body. A small, echogenic foreign body *(arrow)* and surrounding hypoechoic *(dark)* reactive tissue is identified on this longitudinal sonogram of the finger.

- Each tissue displays a specific signal intensity on T1-weighted and T2-weighted images, allowing some degree of tissue characterization (Table 3.1 and Fig. 3.16).
- Using special techniques, the high signal from fat can be suppressed during scanning, thereby producing a fat-saturated image. This is especially useful for demonstrating marrow pathology on "fat-saturated" T2-weighted images, and areas of tissue enhancement after intravenous contrast administration on fat-saturated T1-weighted images (because gadolinium contrast results in increased T1 signal) (examples are shown in Figs. 3.17 and 3.18).

TABLE 3.1 **Tissue Characterization on Magnetic Resonance Images**

Tissue	T1	T2
Fluid	Dark	Bright
Fat	Bright	Intermediate
Tendon/ligament	Dark	Dark
Air	Black	Black

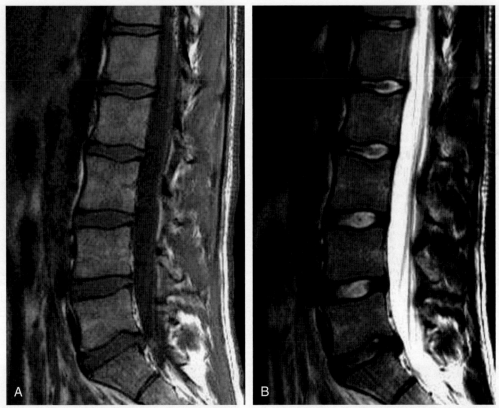

Fig 3.16 Magnetic resonance imaging: T1- and T2-weighted images. Sagittal T1-weighted **(A)** and T2-weighted **(B)** images of the lumbar spine illustrate the characteristic signal characteristics of fluid. Note the low signal intensity of the cerebrospinal fluid on the T1-weighted image and bright signal on the T2-weighted scan.

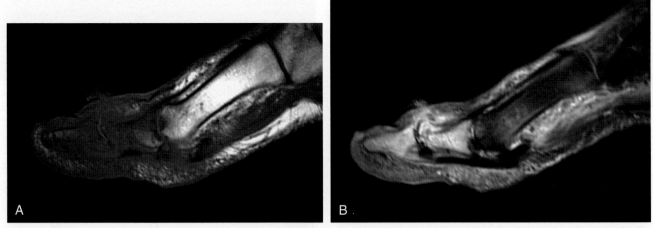

Fig 3.17 Magnetic resonance imaging: Osteomyelitis. Sagittal T1-weighted **(A)** and T2-weighted **(B)** images of the foot reveal abnormal, fluidlike signal throughout the marrow of the proximal and distal phalanges of the great toe compatible with osteomyelitis in this diabetic patient who had an adjacent cutaneous ulcer.

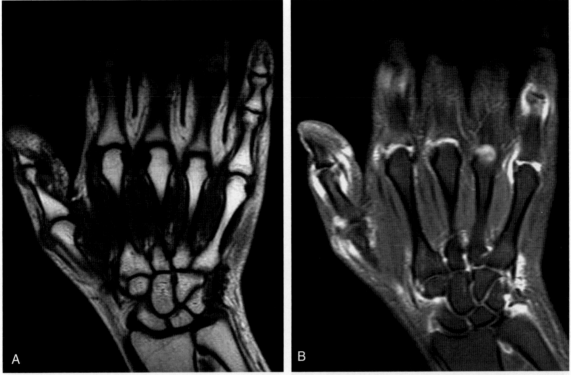

Fig 3.18 Magnetic resonance imaging: Use of intravenous contrast. **(A)** Coronal T1-weighted image before intravenous contrast administration shows no abnormality. **(B)** Coronal T1-weighted fat-saturated postcontrast image demonstrates prominent synovial enhancement throughout the joints of the hand and wrist, compatible with an inflammatory (rheumatoid) arthritis.

- Because of the strong magnetic field involved, contraindications to MRI include the presence of a cardiac pacemaker, a metallic foreign body in the orbit, certain vascular aneurysm clips and cochlear implants, and a metallic fragment (e.g., bullet) of unknown composition near a vital structure (e.g., spinal cord, heart), among other items. As a result, each patient should undergo a thorough screening process prior to scanning.

Strengths

- Images can be obtained in any plane and provide superb soft-tissue contrast, anatomic detail, and simultaneous demonstration of bones and soft tissues. As a result, it is the best single modality for evaluating most types of musculoskeletal pathology (Fig. 3.19, see also Figs. 3.17 to 3.18).
- The most sensitive modality for detecting marrow pathology (neoplastic marrow infiltration, bone contusion, occult fracture, tumor) (Figs. 3.20 and 3.21).

- The test of choice for evaluating neurologic deficits related to spinal trauma or neoplasm.
- Can be combined with gadolinium-based contrast agents injected either intravenously (to highlight tissues with increased vascularity) or directly into a joint (magnetic resonance arthrography) (Fig. 3.22, see also Fig. 3.18).
- No ionizing radiation.

Weaknesses

- Fractures of the posterior elements of the spine are difficult to detect with MRI.
- Assessment of fracture healing.
- Hardware (depending on type, may produce severe artifact, obscuring adjacent tissues) (Fig. 3.23).

Imaging Algorithms

- Please see Figs. 3.24 to 3.28.

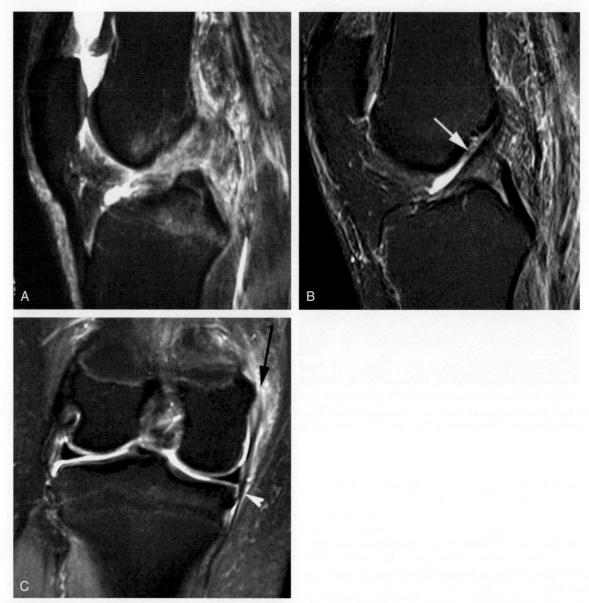

Fig 3.19 Magnetic resonance imaging: Ligament injuries. **(A)** Sagittal T2-weighted image with fat saturation demonstrates a complete rupture of the anterior cruciate ligament. Note the high signal edema and hemorrhage in the central intercondylar notch, as well as the absence of discernible ligament fibers. **(B)** A normal anterior cruciate ligament with taut, parallel fibers *(arrow)* is shown for comparison. **(C)** Coronal T2-weighted image with fat saturation shows a partial tear of the proximal medial collateral ligament *(arrow)*. Note the intact ligament fibers distally *(arrowhead)*.

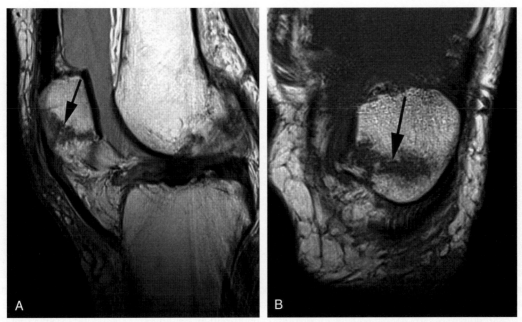

Fig 3.20 Magnetic resonance imaging: radiographically occult fracture. Sagittal (A) and coronal (B) T1-weighted images of the knee reveal a nondisplaced fracture in the lower pole of the patella (arrows). The fracture was not visible on radiographs. (This is the same patient as in Fig. 3.1.)

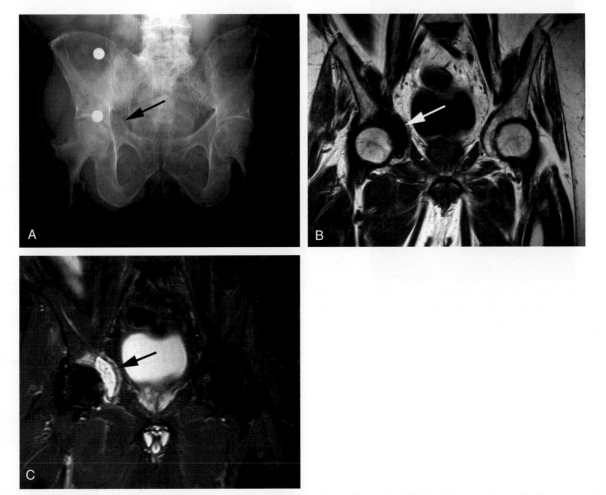

Fig 3.21 Magnetic resonance imaging: bone tumor. (A) Anteroposterior radiograph of the pelvis reveals subtle lucency in the right acetabulum (arrow) that could be potentially missed owing to the degree of diffuse osteopenia. Coronal T1-weighted (B) and fat-saturated T2-weighted (C) images demonstrate the lesion to much better advantage (arrows).

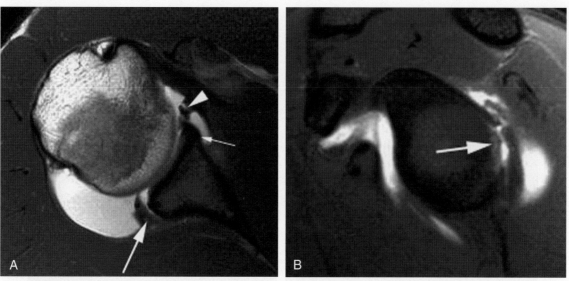

Fig 3.22 Magnetic resonance arthrography. **(A)** Axial T1-weighted image of the shoulder after an intra-articular injection of a dilute gadolinium solution reveals a posterior labral tear *(large arrow)*. Note also the normal labrum *(small arrow)* and middle glenohumeral ligament *(arrowhead)* anteriorly. **(B)** Oblique sagittal T1-weighted image with fat saturation confirms the posterior labral tear *(arrow)*.

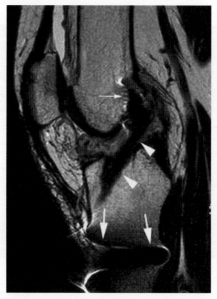

Fig 3.23 Magnetic resonance imaging: Metal artifact. Sagittal T2-weighted image of the knee after anterior cruciate ligament reconstruction demonstrates the normal anterior cruciate ligament graft *(arrowheads)*, as well as prominent low-signal artifacts related to associated metal hardware *(arrows)*. Note how these partially obscure and distort adjacent tissues.

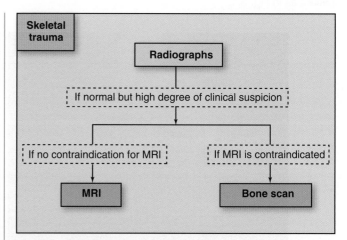

Fig 3.24 Skeletal trauma algorithm.

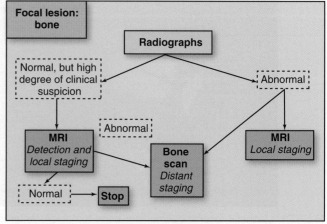

Fig 3.25 Focal lesion: Bone algorithm.

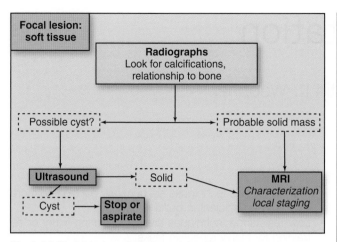

Fig 3.26 Focal lesion: Soft-tissue algorithm.

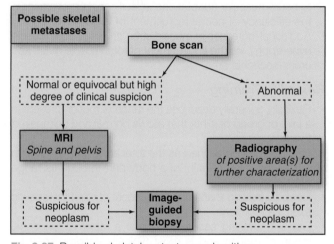

Fig 3.27 Possible skeletal metastases algorithm.

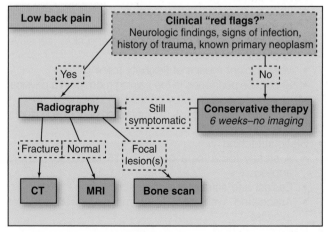

Fig 3.28 Low back pain algorithm.

Suggested Readings

Ahn JM, El-Khoury GY. Role of magnetic resonance imaging in musculoskeletal trauma. *Top Magn Reson Imaging.* 2007;18:155–168.

Collin D, Geijer M, Gothlin JH. Computed tomography compared to magnetic resonance imaging in occult or suspect hip fractures. A retrospective study in 44 patients. *Eur Radiol.* 2016;26:3932–3938.

Duet M, Pouchot J, Liote F, Faraggi M. Role for positron emission tomography in skeletal diseases. *Joint Bone Spine.* 2007;74:14–23.

Geijer M, El-Khoury GY. MDCT in the evaluation of skeletal trauma: principles, protocols, and clinical applications. *Emerg Radiol.* 2006;13:7–18.

Imhof H, Mang T. Advances in musculoskeletal radiology: multidetector computed tomography. *Orthop Clin North Am.* 2006;37:287–298.

Khoury V, Cardinal E, Bureau NJ. Musculoskeletal sonography: a dynamic tool for usual and unusual disorders. *AJR Am J Roentgenol.* 2007;188:W63–W73.

Kransdorf MJ, Bridges MD. Current developments and recent advances in musculoskeletal tumor imaging. *Semin Musculoskelet Radiol.* 2013;17:145–155.

Lalam RK, Cassar-Pullicino VN, Tins BJ. Magnetic resonance imaging of appendicular musculoskeletal infection. *Top Magn Reson Imaging.* 2007;18:177–191.

Love C, Din AS, Tomas MB, et al. Radionuclide bone imaging: an illustrative review. *Radiographics.* 2003;23:341–358.

Mhuircheartaigh NN, Kerr JM, Murray JG. MR imaging of traumatic spinal injuries. *Semin Musculoskelet Radiol.* 2006;10:293–307.

Nacey NC, Geeslin MG, Miller GW, Pierce JL. Magnetic resonance imaging of the knee: an overview and update of conventional and state of the art imaging. *J Magn Reson Imaging.* 2017;45:1257–1275.

Nicholau S, Yong-Hing CJ, Galea-Soler S, et al. Dual–energy CT as a potential new diagnostic tool in the management of gout in the acute setting. *AJR Am J Roentgenol.* 2010;194:1072–1078.

Papp DR, Khanna AJ, McCarthy EF, et al. Magnetic resonance imaging of soft-tissue tumors: determinate and indeterminate lesions. *J Bone Joint Surg Am.* 2007;89A(suppl 3):103–115.

Schoenfeld AJ, Bono CM, McGuire KJ, et al. Computed tomography alone versus computed tomography and magnetic resonance imaging in the identification of occult injuries to the cervical spine: a meta-analysis. *J Trauma.* 2010;68:109–114.

Tuite MJ, Small KM. Imaging evaluation of nonacute shoulder pain. *AJR Am J Roentgenol.* 2017;209:525–533.

Turecki MB, Taljanovic MS, Stubbs AY, et al. Imaging of musculoskeletal soft tissue infections. *Skeletal Radiol.* 2010;39:957–971.

Vande Berg B, Malghem J, Maldague B, Lecouvet F. Multi-detector CT imaging in the postoperative orthopedic patient with metal hardware. *Eur J Radiol.* 2006;60:470–479.

Chapter 4 Rehabilitation

Jeffrey G. Jenkins, Sara N. Raiser, Justin L. Weppner

Key Concepts

- Within a medical context, rehabilitation can be defined as a process by which the patient strives to achieve his or her full physical, social, and vocational potential.
- A formal medical rehabilitation program is most commonly used after an individual has experienced a loss of function due to an injury or disease process or as a side effect of necessary medical treatment (e.g., surgery).
- For rehabilitation to be successful, it is crucial that the patient, physician, and therapist(s) involved in the case share the same clearly defined functional goals; treatment will be directed toward the achievement of these goals.
- Although medical professionals provide direction and guidance during rehabilitation, the patient plays the most important active role in the program.
- The patient should give frequent feedback regarding effectiveness of interventions and any detrimental effects of treatment so that the rehabilitation plan and functional goals can be modified as needed throughout the rehabilitation process.
- Therapeutic exercise, physical modalities, and orthotic devices are the main components of a medical rehabilitation program for patients with musculoskeletal dysfunction.
- Physical therapists are trained to identify, assess, and work with the patient to alleviate acute or prolonged movement dysfunction. Most physical therapists use a combination of therapeutic exercise, physical modalities, manual manipulation, and massage to achieve the treatment goals.
- Occupational therapists are trained to identify, assess, and work with the patient to alleviate functional deficits in the areas of self-care, vocational, and avocational activities.

Therapeutic Exercise (Fig. 4.1)

- In most cases, therapeutic exercise should be taught and supervised, particularly during early stages, by a physical therapist.
- Occupational therapists are specifically trained to supervise exercises directly related to self-care, vocational, and avocational activities and are appropriate to refer to in these cases.
- Major categories of exercise include muscle strengthening (strength training), range of motion (flexibility), and neuromuscular facilitation.

Strength Training

- Both high-resistance/low-repetition and low-resistance/high-repetition techniques exist and can be effective.

- High-resistance techniques are generally considered more effective and efficient in building strength.
- Low-resistance techniques are useful during injury or as training for highly repetitive tasks.
- The most important factor in increasing strength in either case is to exercise the muscle to the point of fatigue.
- Observed effects of strength training occur primarily due to neuromuscular adaptations, specifically improvement in the efficiency of neural recruitment of large motor units.
- Additional increases in muscle strength result from muscle hypertrophy, via the enlargement of total muscle mass and cross-sectional area.

Flexibility Training

- Flexibility generally describes the range of motion present in a joint or group of joints that allows normal and unimpaired function.
- Flexibility can be defined as the total achievable excursion (within the limits of pain) of a body part through its range of motion.
- Flexibility training is an important aspect of most therapeutic exercise regimens.
- Flexibility training seeks to achieve a maximal functional range of motion and is most typically accomplished by stretching.
- Three categories of stretching exercises have been used.
- Passive stretching:
  - Uses a therapist or other partner who applies a stretch to a relaxed joint or limb
  - Requires excellent communication and slow, sensitive application of force
  - Very efficient means of flexibility training
  - Should be performed in the training room or in a physical or occupational therapy context
  - Potentially increases risk of injury when performed without due caution
- Static stretching
  - A steady force for a period of 15 to 60 seconds is applied.
  - Easiest and safest type of stretching
  - Associated with decreased muscle soreness after exercise
- Ballistic stretching
  - Uses the repetitive, rapid application of force in a bouncing or jerking maneuver
  - Momentum carries the body part through the range of motion until muscles are stretched to their limits.
  - Less efficient than other techniques because muscles contract during these conditions to protect from overstretching

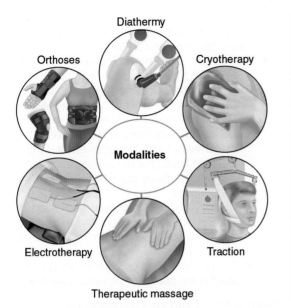

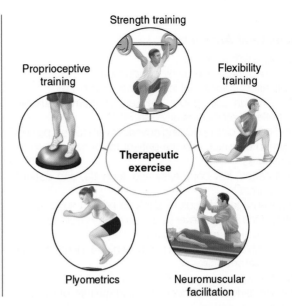

Fig 4.1 Therapeutic exercise and modalities.

- A rapid increase in force can cause injury.
- This type of stretching has been largely abandoned as a training technique.

Neuromuscular Facilitation
- Seeks to improve function through improved efficiency of the interplay between the nervous and musculoskeletal systems
- Neuromuscular facilitation techniques in flexibility training:
  - Isometric or concentric contraction of the musculotendinous unit followed by a passive or static stretch
  - Prestretch contraction of muscle facilitates relaxation and flexibility.
  - Examples include hold-relax and contract-relax techniques

Plyometrics
- Performance of brief explosive maneuvers consisting of an eccentric muscle contraction followed immediately by a concentric contraction
- This technique is primarily employed in the training of athletes.
- Should be approached with caution under the supervision of a trained therapist and begun at an elementary level
- Some studies demonstrate a decreased risk of serious injury during sports activity among athletes who receive plyometric training (e.g., reduction in the incidence of knee injuries in female athletes participating in a jump training program).

Proprioceptive Training
- Background:
  - Proprioceptive deficits have been shown to result from and predispose to injury.
  - Impairment of joint proprioception is believed to influence progressive joint deterioration associated with both rheumatoid arthritis and osteoarthritis.

- Proprioceptive exercises seek to improve joint position sense and thereby prevent injury.
- For example, a tilt or wobble board is commonly used after ankle ligamentous injury to reduce the incidence of recurrence.

Exercise Prescription
- A prescription for therapeutic exercise with a therapist should always include the following components:
  - Diagnosis
  - Frequency of treatment (i.e., number of sessions per week)
  - Specific exercises required
  - Precautions (includes restrictions on weight bearing and limb movement, as well as identification of significant tissue damage or other factors that may interfere with performance of specific exercises)
  - Contraindicated exercises or modalities (should include any specific motions, positions, or modalities that should be avoided to ensure appropriate tissue healing and patient safety without incurring further injury)
- Ideally, individual exercises are further defined by:
  - Mode: specific type of exercise (e.g., closed chain quadriceps strengthening)
  - Intensity: relative physiologic difficulty of the exercise (this is often best described in terms of the patient's rating of perceived exertion, ranging from very light to very hard)
  - Duration: length of an exercise session
  - Frequency: number of sessions per day/week
  - Progression: increase in activity expected over the course of training

Modalities: Heat, Cold, Pressure, Electrotherapy
- Physical agents: use of physical forces to produce beneficial therapeutic effects (see Fig. 4.1)

Heat
Superficial Heat Application

- Hot packs (hydrocollator)
  - Transfer of heat energy by conduction
  - Application: silicate gel in a canvas cover
  - When not in use, packs are kept in thermostatically controlled water baths at 70 to 80°C.
  - Used in terry cloth insulating covers or with towels placed between the pack and the patient for periods of 15 to 20 minutes
  - Advantages: low cost, easy use, long life, and patient acceptance
  - Disadvantages: difficult to apply to curved surfaces
  - Safety: One should never lie on top on the pack because it is more likely to cause burns.
  - Towels should be applied between the skin and the hydrocollator pack.
- Paraffin baths
  - Heat primarily by conduction: liquid mixture of paraffin wax and mineral oil
  - Helpful in the treatment of scars and hand contractures
  - Temperatures (52 to 54°C) are higher than hydrotherapy (40 to 45°C) but are tolerated well due to the low heat capacity of the paraffin/mineral oil mixture and lack of convection.
  - Treatments may include dipping, immersion, or, occasionally, brushing onto the area of treatment for periods of 20 to 30 minutes.
  - Safety: Burns are the main safety concern with paraffin treatment.
  - Visual inspection is important: The paraffin bath should have a thin film of white paraffin on its surface or an edging around the reservoir.

Diathermy (Deep Heating)

- Deep heating agents (diathermies) raise tissue to therapeutic temperatures at a depth of 3.5 to 7 cm.
  - Used for analgesic effects, decreasing muscle spasms, enhancing local blood flow, and increasing collagen extensibility
- Deep heating modality: therapeutic ultrasound (US)
  - US is defined as sound waves at a frequency greater than the threshold of human hearing (frequencies >20 kHz). Therapeutic US uses sound waves to heat tissues. A wide range of frequencies are potentially useful, but in the United States, most machines operate between 0.8 and 1 MHz.
  - US penetrates soft tissue well and bone poorly; the most intense heating occurs at the bone–soft tissue interface.
  - Treatments are relatively brief (5 to 10 minutes) and require constant operator attention.
  - Indications for therapeutic US:
    - Tendonitis, bursitis, muscle pain and overuse, contractures, inflammation, trauma, scars, and keloids
    - Fractures: low-intensity US (e.g., 30 mW/cm^2) accelerates bone healing and is approved by the U.S. Food and Drug Administration for the treatment of some fractures.

- Therapeutic US is typically avoided in the acute stages of an injury due to concerns that it may aggravate bleeding, tissue damage, and swelling.
- Therapeutic US contraindications:
  - Fluid-filled areas (i.e., eye and the pregnant uterus), growth plates, inflamed joints, acute hemorrhages, ischemic tissue, tumor, laminectomy site, infection, and implanted devices such as pacemakers and pumps
  - US is relatively contraindicated near metal plates or cemented artificial joints because the effects of localized heating or mechanical forces on prosthesis-cement interfaces are not well known.
- Phonophoresis
  - US may be used to deliver medication into tissues. The medication is mixed into a coupling medium, and US is used to drive (phonophorese) the material through the skin.
  - Corticosteroids and local anesthetics are most frequently used in the treatment of musculoskeletal conditions.

Therapeutic Cold or Cryotherapy

- Superficial only
- Used for analgesic effects, reduction of muscle spasm, decreasing inflammation, decreasing muscle spasticity/hyperactivity, vasoconstriction (reduction in local blood flow and associated edema)
- Ice massage used for treatment of localized, intense musculoskeletal pain (e.g., lateral epicondylitis)
- General indications:
  - Acute musculoskeletal trauma
  - Pain
  - Muscle spasm
  - Spasticity
  - Reduction of metabolic activity
- General contraindications and precautions:
  - Impaired circulation (i.e., ischemia, Raynaud phenomenon, peripheral vascular disease), hypersensitivity to cold, skin anesthesia, local infection
- Methods of application:
  - Ice packs and compression wraps are most common.
  - Sessions typically last 20 minutes.
  - Ice massage is a vigorous approach suitable for limited portions of the body. A piece of ice is rubbed over the painful area for 15 to 20 minutes.
  - Iced whirlpools cool large areas vigorously.
  - Vapocoolant and liquid nitrogen sprays produce large (as much as 20°C), rapid decreases in skin temperature and are used at times to produce superficial analgesia as well as in spray and stretch treatments.
- Trauma application:
  - Cooling applied soon after trauma may decrease edema, metabolic activity, blood flow, compartmental pressures, and tissue damage, and accelerate healing.
  - Rest, ice, compression, and elevation are the mainstays of treatment.
  - Cyclic ice application is often recommended (e.g., 20 minutes on, 10 minutes off) for 6 to 24 hours.
- Contrast baths
  - Two water-filled reservoirs, warm (43°C) and cool (16°C); alternate soaks; duration varies according to treatment protocol

- Used for desensitization and vasogenic reflex effects
- Mostly used on hands or feet; typical indications include rheumatoid arthritis and sympathetically mediated pain (reflex sympathetic dystrophy)

Traction

- Technique used to stretch soft tissues and to separate joint surfaces or bone fragments by the use of a pulling force.
- Based on available medical evidence, therapeutic use of spinal traction is generally limited to the cervical spine.
- The efficacy of lumbar traction is controversial.
- Traction has been shown to lengthen the intervertebral space up to 1 to 2 mm, but the lengthening is transient.
- Decreases muscle spasm, possibly by inducing fatigue in the paravertebral musculature
- May decrease neuroforaminal narrowing and associated radicular pain
- The patient should be positioned in 20 to 30 degrees of cervical flexion during traction to optimize the effect on the neural foramina.
- Therapeutic benefit is usually obtained with 25 pounds of traction (this includes the 10 pounds required to counterbalance the weight of the head).
- The duration of a treatment session is typically 20 minutes.
- The best results are obtained when a trained therapist administers manual traction in a controlled setting.
- Home cervical traction devices can be used (these typically use a pulley system over a door, and a bag filled with 20 pounds of sand or water).
- Home cervical traction devices should not be used without previous training and observation by a trained therapist or physician.
- Heat (hot packs) is helpful in decreasing muscle contraction and maximizing the benefit of treatment.
- Contraindications:
  - Cervical ligamentous instability resulting from conditions such as rheumatoid arthritis, achondroplastic dwarfism, Marfan syndrome, or previous trauma
  - Documented or suspected tumor in the vicinity of the spine
  - Infectious process in the spine
  - Spinal osteopenia
  - Pregnancy
- Cervical spinal traction should not be administered with the neck in extension, particularly in patients with a history of vertebrobasilar insufficiency.

Therapeutic Massage

- Causes therapeutic soft-tissue changes as a direct result of the manual forces exerted on the patient by a trained therapist
- Specific techniques can be helpful for musculoskeletal patients:
  - Deep friction massage
    - Used to prevent and break up adhesions after muscle injury
    - Friction is applied transversely across muscle fibers or tendons.
  - Soft-tissue mobilization
    - Forceful massage performed with the fascia and muscle in a lengthened position

- Effective as an adjunct to passive stretching in the treatment and prevention of contractures
- Myofascial release
  - Applies prolonged light pressure specifically oriented with regard to fascial planes
  - Typically combined with passive range of motion techniques to stretch focal areas of muscle or fascial tightness
- Contraindications:
- Should not be performed in patients with known malignancies, open wounds, thrombophlebitis, or infected tissues

Electrotherapy

- Transcutaneous electrical nerve stimulation (TENS)
  - Most common direct therapeutic application of electrical current
  - Used for its analgesic properties
  - The unit uses superficial skin electrodes to apply small electrical currents to the body.
  - Theorized to provide analgesia via the gate control theory of pain, in which stimulation of large myelinated afferent nerve fibers block the transmission of pain signals by small, unmyelinated fibers (C, A delta) at the spinal cord level
  - Signal amplitudes generally do not exceed 100 mA.
  - With initiation of treatment, TENS use is typically taught and monitored by a physical therapist. Once the patient is competent and confident in using the device (electrode placement, stimulator settings, duration of treatments), the unit can be used independently, outside the medical or therapy setting.
  - Common indications include posttraumatic/postsurgical pain, diabetic neuropathic pain, chronic musculoskeletal pain, peripheral nerve injury, sympathetically mediated pain/reflex sympathetic dystrophy, and phantom limb pain.
- Iontophoresis
  - Uses electrical fields to drive therapeutic agents through the skin into underlying soft tissue
  - Treatments in the musculoskeletal patient population typically use antiinflammatory agents and/or local anesthetics.
  - Conditions commonly treated include plantar fasciitis, tendinitis, and bursitis.
  - Most physical therapists are trained in this technique, although not all have access to the necessary equipment.
  - It is worth noting that, in most cases, injection enables a more efficient delivery of a greater concentration of the therapeutic agent in question.
- Electrical stimulation (E-stim)
  - At higher intensities than those used in TENS, E-stim can be used to maintain muscle bulk and strength.
  - Useful for immobilized limbs and for paretic muscles after nerve injury.
  - Evidence does not suggest that E-stim can strengthen otherwise healthy muscle.
  - Relative contraindications to E-stim include implanted or temporary stimulators (pacemakers, intrathecal pumps, spinal cord stimulators, etc.), congestive heart failure, pregnancy, skin sensitivity to electrodes, and actively

healing wounds near the stimulation site. Stimulation over the carotid sinus is also highly discouraged due to the propensity for vagal response.

Orthoses

- An orthosis is an external device that is worn to restrict or assist movement. Examples include braces and splints.
- Orthoses are typically prescribed and used for one or more of the following reasons:
- To rest or immobilize the body part: reduce inflammation, prevent further injury
- To prevent contracture: minimize loss of range of motion in a joint or limb
- To correct deformity: typically in conjunction with therapy or surgery
- To promote exercise: encourage strengthening of certain muscles and/or correct muscle imbalances
- To improve function
- Orthoses can be subdivided into static and dynamic devices.
  - Static orthoses keep underlying body parts from moving, thereby encouraging rest and healing via immobilization while preventing or minimizing deformity.
  - Dynamic orthoses have internal or external power sources that encourage restoration and/or control of joint movements.
- Orthoses are often named for the body parts that they incorporate (e.g., ankle-foot orthosis and wrist-hand orthosis).
- Prescriptions for orthotics should include the type (defined by incorporated limb segments/body parts) and a static/dynamic classification. If a dynamic orthosis is to be used, the prescription should specifically identify the motion(s) to be assisted or inhibited.
- Prefabricated, off-the-shelf orthotics can be effectively used in the treatment of most orthopedic injuries. Frequently encountered examples include knee and ankle braces prescribed for ligamentous injury or wrist splints for carpal tunnel syndrome.
- In special populations (e.g., hand trauma, nerve injury, partial limb loss, severe deformity), orthoses should be custom fitted by an orthotist or an appropriately trained occupational therapist.
- Orthotic use should generally be restricted to injured or dysfunctional limbs. Prophylactic bracing of joints is controversial.
- Indications for orthoses include:
  - Trauma (e.g., fracture, joint sprain)
  - Surgery (e.g., tendon repair, joint reconstruction)
  - Central or peripheral nervous system pathology (e.g., weakness, spasticity)
  - Painful disorders (e.g., rheumatoid arthritis, carpal tunnel syndrome)
- Orthoses and sports
  - There is no compelling evidence in the literature to support the use of prophylactic knee bracing in football players. In fact, both the American Academy of Pediatrics and the American Academy of Orthopaedic Surgeons have advised against the routine use of prophylactic knee bracing in football, in part due to data that actually showed an increase in anterior cruciate ligament injuries in brace wearers.

- There is some evidence that use of a semirigid ankle orthosis can decrease the risk of ligamentous injury in athletes, particularly those with a history of sprain.

When to Refer

- To a significant extent, the primary physician's own personal comfort level in managing a rehabilitation program determines the need for referral. However, some indications for referral include:
  - Patient's inability to progress functionally with the current therapy regimen
  - Suboptimally controlled acute or chronic pain
  - Painful or functionally disabling spasticity
  - Neuromuscular or musculoskeletal comorbidities (e.g., stroke, spinal cord injury, cerebral palsy, multiple sclerosis, rheumatoid arthritis, fibromyalgia, and chronic pain syndromes) that can compound functional deficits and/or complicate the process of progressing toward functional goals

Patient Instructions

- Your active participation in the rehabilitation process is the most important factor in determining the success of the program.
- Be involved in the development of functional goals for your rehabilitation program.
- Follow physician and physical therapist instructions as closely as possible.
- Give feedback to care providers as to the effectiveness of interventions as well as any side effects of treatment.
- Do not continue to do exercises or use modalities that worsen your symptoms or condition without checking with your physician.

Considerations in Special Populations

- Hand injuries
  - Whenever possible, a rehabilitation program for hand or wrist dysfunction should involve evaluation and treatment of the patient by a certified hand therapist.
  - Swelling will occur after any surgery or injury to the hand. Orthoses can potentially aggravate edema, and their use must be carefully monitored during this stage of rehabilitation to prevent loss of function.
- Sensory deficits
  - For obvious reasons, physical modalities and orthotic devices should be used with great caution in patients with sensory deficits (e.g., peripheral neuropathies, central nervous system disorders). Orthotic pressure over insensate areas must be minimized, and cryotherapy of these areas is contraindicated.
- Pregnancy
  - The safety of some physical modalities, including TENS and E-stim, has not been established in patients who are pregnant. Therapeutic US is absolutely contraindicated over the low back and abdomen of a pregnant woman.
- Diabetes
  - Many patients with diabetes will experience a decrease in blood glucose levels when beginning a new therapeutic

exercise regimen. Levels should be monitored closely and medications adjusted as necessary to avoid hypoglycemia.
- Elderly
  - Where possible, therapeutic exercise modalities prescribed for patients who are elderly should be chosen to minimize stress on the bones and joints.
- Pain
  - Pain is not a contraindication to therapeutic exercise, physical modalities, or the use of orthotic devices. However, significant worsening of pain or onset of new pain after initiation of treatment demands further investigation and/or referral.

Suggested Readings

Alfano AP. Physical modalities in sports medicine. In: O'Connor FG, Sallis RE, Wilder RP, St. Pierre P, eds. *Sports Medicine: Just the Facts*. New York: McGraw-Hill; 2005:405–411.

American Society of Hand Therapists (ASHT). *Splint Nomenclature Task Force: Splint Classification System*. Garner, NC: ASHT; 1991.

Hennessey WJ, Uustal H. Lower limb orthoses. In: Cifu DX, eds. *Braddom's Physical Medicine and Rehabilitation*. 5th ed. Philadelphia: Elsevier; 2016:249–274.

Kelly BM, Patel AT, Dodge CV. Upper limb orthotic devices. In: Cifu DX, eds. *Braddom's Physical Medicine and Rehabilitation*. 5th ed. Philadelphia: Elsevier; 2016:225–248.

Wilder RP, Jenkins JG, Panchang P, Statuta S. Therapeutic exercise. In: Cifu DX, eds. *Braddom's Physical Medicine and Rehabilitation*. 5th ed. Philadelphia: Elsevier; 2016:321–346.

Wolf CJ, Brault JS. Manipulation, traction, and massage. In: Cifu DX, eds. *Braddom's Physical Medicine and Rehabilitation*. 5th ed. Philadelphia: Elsevier; 2016:347–367.

Chapter 5 Special Populations: Geriatrics

Laurie Archbald-Pannone

ICD-10-CM CODES	
M15.0	Osteoarthritis (OA)
M67.90	Tendonoses
S46.019A	Rotator cuff strains
M77.0	Medial epicondylitis
M76.60	Achilles tendinitis
M23.309	Degenerative meniscus tears
T14.8XXA	Muscle strains
M84.40XA	Spontaneous fracture
M84.50XA	Non-traumatic fracture
M85.80	Osteopenia
M81.0	Osteoporosis

Key Concepts

- By 2030, approximately 20% of the U.S. population will be older than 65 years of age.
- Geriatric medicine is medicine focused on patients older than 65 years.
- Research has proven that regular exercise in the geriatric population provides many health benefits.
- Appropriate exercise is safe in the geriatric population and provides numerous health benefits.
- It is recommended that geriatric patients have 30 minutes of exercise at least 5 days each week.
- Although physiologic changes occur with aging, the capacity for the geriatric patient to exercise and improve strength, endurance, flexibility, and performance is maintained.
- Age-related changes in physiology affect metabolism of many medications, especially medications used to treat pain related to acute, chronic, or postoperative musculoskeletal conditions.
- With the increasing geriatric population, every health care provider must be familiar with the physiologic changes with aging, as well as common musculoskeletal conditions and the impact of comorbidities on these conditions.
- Physicians can support healthy lifestyles in the geriatric

  patient with an exercise prescription.

Physiologic Changes Associated With Aging

- Elderly adults have a decline in coordination, balance, and reaction time, as well as impaired vision, hearing, and short-term memory.

- Elderly adults have a decrease in bone mineral density, with losses as high as 3% per year in postmenopausal women and 0.5% per year in men older than 40 years.
- Elderly adults can develop sarcopenia, with an average 30% reduction in strength from age 50 to age 70 secondary to atrophy of type II muscle fibers, with associated decrease in tensile strength and increased stiffness of tendons and ligaments.
- Elderly adults also have weakening of articular cartilage and a decrease in elastic properties of intervertebral disks.
- Geriatric patients do not have increases of antidiuretic hormone (ADH) with activity to signal thirst and need for hydration.
- Body composition changes with age, leading to increased total body fat distribution that leads to increased retention of fat-soluble medication, such as those that cross the blood-brain barrier, as well as increased risk for dose stacking.
- With normal aging, there is a decrease in renal function (both number of functioning nephrons and incoming blood flow) in the geriatric population. Hepatic metabolism is not affected by normal aging. This change in renal function affects the types and doses of safe medications.
- Functional changes with aging can lead to impairment that can be assessed by determining a patient's ability to perform their activities of daily living (ADLs) (Box 5.1).
- As a person is less able to independently do their ADLs, their all-cause mortality risk increases with this functional decline.

Common Orthopaedic Conditions in the Geriatric Patient

- Older athletes experience fewer acute traumatic injuries than younger athletes during competition.
- The geriatric population has a high rate of falls—1 in 3 people over 65 years old is affected by falls. Falls result in moderate to severe injuries in approximately 25% of cases.
- The biggest risk factor for falls is a history of falls. A fall without injury is a critical opportunity to explore the cause of the fall so as to help prevent future falls that may result in injury.
- Osteoarthritis (OA) is the most common musculoskeletal condition in the geriatric population. OA can affect multiple joints and significantly impact a person's ADLs and general function.
- Secondary to the decrease in tensile strength and increase in stiffness of ligaments and tendons with aging, the geriatric

Activities of Daily Living

- Dressing
- Eating
- Ambulating
- Toileting
- Hygiene

patient is more likely to present with tendinoses such as rotator cuff strains, medial epicondylitis, and Achilles tendinitis.

- Geriatric patients are also more likely to have degenerative meniscus tears because of age-related collagen changes.
- Muscle strains are also common in the geriatric population secondary to a decrease in flexibility.
- Due to decrease in bone density, geriatric patients are at risk from spontaneous, nontraumatic, or minimally traumatic fractures.

Treating Chronic Osteoarthritis Pain in the Geriatric Patient

- Due to physiologic changes with normal aging, medication administration must be adjusted in the geriatric patient, as compared with a younger patient.
- In 2015 the American Geriatrics Society updated the Beers Criteria for medications to use with extreme caution in older adults.
- Due to age-related renal changes, nonsteroidal antiinflammatory drugs (NSAIDs) are not recommended for long-term use in the geriatric population. NSAIDs can be helpful for short-course treatment of acute pain or inflammation. Adverse effects commonly associated with NSAID use in the geriatric population include acute kidney injury, gastric bleeding, and peripheral edema.
- Acetaminophen can be used safely in the treatment of chronic arthritis pain in the geriatric patient. Regular dosing of scheduled acetaminophen can decrease pain level and act as a "narcotic-sparing medication" in chronic and postoperative pain control. Maximum dosing of acetaminophen in the geriatric patient is 3000 mg a day in divided doses of 1000 mg TID. All formulations of acetaminophen must be accounted for and be less than 3000 mg in any 1 day.
- Geriatric patients who are acutely ill are at risk for delirium from a variety of factors, including hospitalization, dehydration, medications, and postoperative state. Although pain medication, especially narcotic medication, can be associated with delirium, untreated pain is also associated with delirium.
- Short-course narcotic pain medication at appropriate dosing can be used in the geriatric population with close monitoring for side effects. Narcotic-induced constipation is a common side effect in this population and can be treated with a promotility stimulant laxative such as senna.
- A key principle in dosing medication in elderly population is "start low, go slow." Start a medication at a low therapeutic dose and slowly titrate up while reevaluating for effect and adverse effects in the geriatric patient.

- Often geriatric patients are on multiple medications, and polypharmacy (>3 medications) is frequent in this population. The addition of any new medication, as well as the dose, frequency, and duration of the medication, must account for the geriatric patient's comorbidities and other medications.
- A geriatrician can assist in the management of medications and comorbidities associated with elderly patients. Studies have shown that the rate of delirium is decreased in postoperative units that comanage elderly patients with geriatric physicians and an interdisciplinary team.

Benefits of Exercise in the Geriatric Patient

- Exercise can impact the rate and extent of functional decline.
- It is recommended that geriatric patients have approximately 30 minutes of exercise at least 5 days each week.
- Exercise programs that include balance, flexibility, and strength exercises have been shown to significantly reduce the number of falls in the geriatric population.
- Light to moderate exercise training has been shown to decrease systolic blood pressure.
- Endurance training is associated with improved insulin sensitivity, and regular exercise has been shown to decrease depressive symptoms.
- Weight-bearing exercise has been shown to attenuate bone density loss in several studies.
- A regular exercise program has been shown to improve OA pain and improve function in this population.

Promoting Safe Exercise for the Geriatric Patient

- To promote safe exercise, a preparticipation screening evaluation can assess for cardiovascular risk factors prior to initiating or escalating an exercise program.
- Established cardiovascular screening guidelines for masters' level athletes should be followed with particular attention to key clinical risks such as family history of sudden death, exertional syncope, exertional dyspnea, chest pain, or hypertension. The cardiovascular exam should focus on identification and characterization of heart murmurs, peripheral pulse quality, and stigmata of Marfan's syndrome.
- Geriatric patients can work under direct monitoring of a physical therapist or personal trainer to first establish an exercise regimen before transitioning to working independently.
- After medical clearance for exercise, prescribe an exercise regimen that is consistent with that individual's cognitive and functional abilities.
- Proper hydration and nutrition must be maintained for optimal function. Hydration is especially important due to a decrease in thirst perception that is part of normal aging.

Exercise Prescriptions for the Geriatric Patient

- After cardiac clearance, an exercise prescription is an excellent way to promote a healthy lifestyle in an elderly patient.

BOX 5.2 **Exercise Prescription**

An exercise prescription should specify the following:

- Exercise frequency
- Intensity of exercise
- Type(s) of exercise
- Duration of exercise session
- Progression of exercise program

  Exercise prescription goals

- At least 5 times each week
- At least 30 min sessions
- Increase daily exercise time by 10 min every week until at a maximum of 60 min per day
- Moderate activity can be defined at a participant's ability to carry on a conversation while engaged in exercise (approximately 50% maximum heart rate)

- An exercise prescription should include the recommended frequency, intensity, type, duration, and progression of exercise (Box 5.2).
- Exercise prescriptions should also take acute and chronic medical conditions into account, such as avoiding high-impact activities in patients with severe OA.
- Exercise prescriptions should account for a patient's level of function, cognition, and goals of care. Improvement in ADLs can lead to decrease risk of frailty.

Geriatric Patient Instructions

- A regular exercise program with balance, flexibility, and strength components provides numerous health benefits.

- A screening evaluation should be done before initiating an exercise program to ensure a safe plan and determine a need for monitored exercises or any limitations.

Suggested Readings

Anderson LA, Deokar A, Edwards VJ, et al. Demographic and health status differences among people aged 45 or older with and without functional difficulties related to increased confusion or memory loss, 2011 Behavioral Risk Factor Surveillance System. *Prev Chronic Dis.* 2015;12:140429.

Barbour KE, Stevens JA, Helmick CG, et al. Falls and fall injuries among adults with arthritis—United States, 2012. *MMWR Morb Mortal Wkly Rep.* 2014;63(17):379–383.

Concannon LG, Grierson MJ, Harrast MA. Exercise in the older adult: from the sedentary elderly to the masters athlete. *PMR.* 2012;4(11):833–839.

Faul M, Stevens JA, Sasser SM, et al. Older adult falls seen by emergency medical service providers: a prevention opportunity. *Am J Prev Med.* 2016;50(6):719–726.

Fick DM, Semla TP, Beizer J, et al. American Geriatrics Society 2015 updated Beers criteria for potentially inappropriate medication use in older adults. *J Am Geriatr Soc.* 2015;63(11):2227–2246.

Maron B, Araujo C, Thompson P, et al. Recommendations for preparticipation screening and the assessment of cardiovascular disease in master athletes. *Circulation.* 2001;103:327–334.

Roddy E, Zhang W, Doherty M, et al. Evidence-based recommendations for the role of exercise in the management of osteoarthritis in the hip or knee—the MOVE consensus. *Rheumatology.* 2005;44:67–73.

Snowden M, Steinman L, Carlson WL, et al. Effect of physical activity, social support and skills training on late-life emotional health: a systematic literature review and implications for public health research. *Front Public Health.* 2015;2:213.

Chapter 6 Special Populations: Disabled

David Hryvniak, Jason Kirkbride

ICD-10-CM CODES
Z73.6   *Limitation of activities due to disability*
Z74.09 *Other reduced mobility*
F79   *Unspecified intellectual disabilities*

Key Concepts

- A disability, as defined by the World Health Organization (WHO), is a condition (either mental or physical) that limits the ability of a person to perform an activity in the range considered normal for a human being.
- An impairment, as defined by the WHO, is "any loss or abnormality of psychological, physiological or anatomical structure or function" and is used by the International Paralympic Committee to create their competition classification system.
- Nearly 60 million Americans have some type of disability according to 2010 U.S. Census Bureau data—an increase of 2.2 million since 2005.
- Musculoskeletal diseases are some of the major causes of disability in the United States and the world.
- The benefits of a regular exercise program can be obtained by those with disabilities, but 54% of people with disabilities engage in no leisure-time physical activity compared with just 32% of their peers without disabilities and are 4 times more likely to suffer from cardiovascular disease among adults ages 18 to 44 years.
- Physicians who have disabled patients must encourage physical activity while being mindful of both the limitations of the disability and common injury patterns either unique to the disability or the result of the activity type.
- Physicians must also be aware of societal and environmental factors that hinder the activities of disabled persons and provide tools to eliminate obstacles as necessary.

Background

- A disabled sports program was started for wheelchair athletes in the 1950s, borne from a need to rehabilitate war veterans
- The first Paralympic Games were held in Rome in 1960. The Paralympics were games established for athletes with either a physical disability or visual impairment.
- The Special Olympics began in 1960 and has since grown to involve more than 5.7 million athletes in 172 different countries. The games are for those athletes with mental retardation regardless of physical ability.

- The International Paralympic Committee was established in 1989 to act as the representative body of adaptive sports.
- The Rehabilitation Act of 1973 aided in bringing physical activity programs to most disabled people regardless of participation in competitive sports.
- Currently, there are a myriad of programs promoting physical activity for the disabled, including the Special Olympics, the United States Association of Blind Athletes, the National Wheelchair Athlete Association, the National Association of Sports for Cerebral Palsy, and Adaptive Sports USA.
- In addition, the Centers for Disease Control and Prevention sponsor several programs, such as Healthy People, aimed at improving physical fitness and promoting healthy lifestyles for disabled persons.

Musculoskeletal Disabilities

- Several different types of disabilities exist (Box 6.1).
- Musculoskeletal disabilities are among the most common types and affect social functioning and mental health, further worsening a patient's quality of life.
- The burden to the health care system from musculoskeletal disabilities worldwide is significant and is growing.
- The Bone and Joint Decade was established worldwide to help prevent musculoskeletal disability and improve the quality of life for those with musculoskeletal disease.

Common Injuries in the Disabled

- According to data from the Special Olympics, the injuries sustained in disabled athletes are similar to those sustained in their nondisabled peers, with musculoskeletal injuries accounting for the majority of medical tent visits during competition.
- When a physician performs a preparticipation physical examination on a disabled athlete, it is important to identify abnormalities that predispose to injury.
- The relationship of Down syndrome to atlantoaxial instability requires that all Down syndrome athletes obtain lateral cervical spine x-rays in flexion, extension, and neutral: the atlantodens interval must be less than 5 mm. If the radiographs are abnormal, then participation in contact sports is precluded.
- All traumatic paraplegic or quadriplegic athletes should undergo a stress test before participation in high-demand sports (i.e., basketball, track).
- The athlete should be examined for any skin abnormalities including pressure sores. If pressure sores are present, the athlete cannot compete.

BOX 6.1 Types of Disabilities[a]

Visual impairment
Hearing impairment
Mental retardation
Autism
Spinal cord injuries
Cerebral palsy
Muscular dystrophy
Multiple sclerosis
Chronic pain
Osteoarthritis
Traumatic brain injury
Limb loss
Depression
Dementia
Stroke
Addiction
Diabetes mellitus
Obesity

[a]This is a partial list. The definition of disability encompasses any condition that prohibits an individual from performing an activity in the range considered normal for a human being.

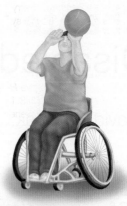

Benefits of athletic activity

↑ Quality of life

↑ Mental health

↑ Social function

↓ Incidence of diabetes

↓ Incidence of heart disease

Resources for patients:
- National Organization on Disability www.nod.org
- National Center on Physical Activity and Disability www.ncpad.org
- International Paralympic Committee www.ipc.org
- Adaptive Sports USA www.adaptivesportsusa.org

Fig 6.1 The benefits of sports participation for the disabled population and patient resources.

- Other medical conditions should be carefully documented. These include seizure disorders, congenital and acquired cardiovascular disease, visual problems, and allergies.

Treatment

- Following a preparticipation physical, physical activity should be encouraged for all individuals with disabilities because it has been demonstrated to improve overall health.
- Education should be provided to prevent injuries specific to the disabled athlete.
  - Prevention of skin breakdown should be attempted through the use of protective clothing, avoidance of moist clothing, and frequent skin checks.
  - Prevention of overuse injuries is increasingly important in wheelchair-bound athletes because they are increasingly dependent on upper extremities for mobility and activities of daily living (ADLs).
  - Spinal cord–injured athletes are more susceptible to heat illness due to impaired thermoregulation and should additionally be educated about risks of autonomic dysreflexia and boosting.
- A disabled patient's attitude toward physical activity has been shown to be the strongest predictor of future physical activity.
- A strong support system has been shown to limit an individual's disability.
- A multidisciplinary approach involving physical therapists, physicians, social workers, occupational therapists, and others provides the disabled athlete the most benefit.

Patient Instructions

- A disability should not preclude an individual from obtaining the benefits of living a healthy lifestyle.

- There are online resources and community programs that can help to provide access to services offered to help people with a disability summarized in Fig. 6.1.

Suggested Readings

Batts KB, Glorioso JE, Williams MS. The medical demands of the special athlete. *Clin J Sport Med*. 1998;8:22–25.

Billinger S, Arena R, Bernhardt J, et al. Physical activity and exercise recommendations for stroke survivors: a statement for healthcare Professionals from the American Heart Association/American Stroke Association. *Stroke*. 2014;45:2532–2553.

Birrer R. The Special Olympics athlete: evaluation and clearance for participation. *Clin Pediatr (Phila)*. 2004;43:777–782.

Brooks P. The burden of musculoskeletal disease—a global perspective. *Clin Rheumatol*. 2006;25:778–781.

Carmona R. *Disability and Health 2005: Promoting the Health and Well-Being of People with Disabilities*. Rockville, MD: Department of Health and Human Services, Centers for Disease Control and Prevention; 2005.

Global Alliance for Musculoskeletal Health of the Bone and Joint Decade (website). Available at www.bjdonline.org. Accessed April 5, 2018.

Klenck C, Gebke K. Practical management: common medical problems in disabled athletes. *Clin J Sport Med*. 2007;17(1):55–60.

Kosma M, Ellis R, Cardinal B, et al. The mediating role of intention and stage of change in physical activity among adults with physical disabilities: an integrative framework. *J Sport Exerc Psychol*. 2007;29:21–38.

Hawkeswood JP, O'Connor R, Anton H, Finlayson H. The preparticipation evaluation for athletes with disability. *Int J Sports Phys Ther*. 2014;9(1):103–115.

Lerman J, Sullivan E, Barnes D, Haynes R. The Pediatric Outcomes Data Collection Instrument (PODCI) and functional assessment of patients with unilateral upper extremity deficiencies. *J Pediatr Orthop*. 2005;25:405–407.

Pelliccia A, Quattrini FM, Squeo MR, et al. Cardiovascular diseases in Paralympic athletes. *Br J Sports Med*. 2016;50(17):1075–1080.

Platt L. Medical and orthopaedic conditions in Special Olympics athletes. *J Athl Train*. 2001;36:74–80.

Price MJ, Campbell IG. Effects of spinal cord lesion level upon thermoregulation during exercise in the heat. *Med Sci Sports Exerc*. 2003;35:1100–1107.

Pueschel SM, Scola FH, Perry CD, Pezzullo JC. Atlanto-axial instability in children with Down syndrome. *Pediatr Radiol*. 1981;10:129–132.

Storheim K, Zwart J. Musculoskeletal disorders and the Global Burden of Disease study. *Ann Rheum Dis*. 2014;73:949–950.

U.S. Department of Health and Human Services. *The Surgeon General's Call to Action to Improve Health and Wellness of Persons with Disabilities*. Rockville, MD: U.S. Department of Health and Human Services, Office of the Surgeon General; 2005.

Vallaint PM, Bezzubyk I, Daley ME. Psychological impact of sport on disabled athletes. *Psychol Rep*. 1985;56:923.

Warms C, Belza B, Whitney J. Correlates of physical activity in adults with mobility limitations. *Fam Community Health*. 2007;30(2 suppl):S5–S16.

World Health Organization. *The Burden of Musculoskeletal Conditions at the Start of the New Millennium*. Technical Report Series 919. Geneva: World Health Organization; 2003.

World Health Organization. *International Classification of Functioning, Disability and Health: ICF*. Geneva: World Health Organization; 2001.

Chapter 7 Special Populations: Pediatrics

Mark Rogers, Kevin Valvano

ICD-10-CM CODES
X50.3 *Overexertion from repetitive movements*
R62.50 *Development arrested or delayed (child)*
N91.2 *Amenorrhea*
Z71.3 *Dietary counseling and surveillance*
E58 *Dietary calcium deficiency*
Z71.83 *Exercise counseling*

Key Concepts

- More than 60 million American young people of all ages participate in organized sports today.
- Youth sports are now more competitive than previously. Many children play at competitive levels at younger ages, often specializing in a single sport at a younger age. These athletes may even follow a year-round cycle of practice, private training, and events for that sport.
- Sports-related injuries have been increasing among young people, becoming the leading cause of all injuries in adolescents, as well as the leading reason for adolescents to visit health care providers. Many of these injuries present because of overtraining and overuse.
- Skeletal growth, physiologic development, and the psychological changes of puberty can influence which sports activities adolescent athletes choose and how well they perform.
- There is growing interest in training and conditioning programs for young athletes. Well-designed and supervised training programs have shown significant value and are safe for all youth athletes, including prepubertal children.
- Primary care providers should encourage age- and developmentally appropriate physical activities for their young patients and should provide anticipatory guidance to parents, with the goal of choosing activities that are fun, safe, and rewarding.
- Providers should be able to assess young people's "sports readiness," via their cognitive, social, and motor development, to determine if they can meet the demands of the specific sport and level of competition that they desire.

Trends in American Youth Sports

- Over the past several decades, the numbers of children and adolescents involved in formal youth sports have nearly tripled (Table 7.1). The increase in female participants has been greater than that of male participants, although males still outnumber females in absolute numbers.

- The increase in female participation is associated with Title IX, a 1972 federal law that mandated equal athletic facilities and programs for females and males.
- This has led to a greater acceptance of girls and women in competitive sports and the ascension of female sports figures as role models.
- The athletic focus has shifted away from the recreational component of sports to that of increased competition resulting in participation earlier in life, single-sport specialization, and an increase in frequency and intensity of training at younger ages.
  - Traditionally, coaches and (less so) parents are the driving forces behind single-sport specialization.
  - Specialization can limit development of various physical and mental athletic skill sets.
- The most frequently cited reasons for younger children's participation in organized sports are to have fun, learn new skills, test abilities, and experience excitement.
  - Receiving individual awards, winning games, and pleasing others are ranked lower.

Sports Injuries

- Sports injuries are the most common type of injury in adolescents, and sports-related injury is the leading reason for adolescent visits to primary care providers.
- The highest incidence of sports-related pediatric injuries occurs in the 5- to 14-year-old age range.
  - These children are less coordinated, have slower reaction times, and are less proficient than older children and adults in assessing and avoiding the risks of sports.
  - Most sports-related overuse injuries in young athletes are related to musculoskeletal and physiologic immaturity due to underdeveloped muscles, ligaments, and bones.
    - In other words, immature epiphyses are weaker than the surrounding soft tissue (muscles and ligaments), allowing significant stress to cause a traumatic epiphyseal fracture.
- Injury risk is greatest during times of poor physical condition, usually at the beginning of sports seasons. Other factors increasing the risk of injury include rapid increases in activity over short periods of time, athletes playing above their skill/age level, improper rest, and poor adaptation to the increased demands of their sport.
- Most, if not all, of these risk factors can be observed in the increased specialization, intensity, and year-round athletic activity of the pediatric athletic population.
- Recent analyses revealed (1) elite athletes specialized in their respective sports at a later age than the nonelite

TABLE 7.1 Numbers of High School–Age American Boys and Girls Involved in Organized Sports

Group	1971	1996	2006	2016
Boys	3,670,000	3,700,000	4,321,000	4,560,000
Girls	294,000	2,500,000	3,022,000	3,400,000
Total	3,960,000	6,200,000	7,342,000	7,960,000

population and (2) professional baseball players surveyed did not feel sport specialization was required prior to high school to master their skills (as indicated in an early sport specialization article [Wilhelm et al., 2017]).

Growth and Maturation

- Preparedness for particular sports, capabilities for training, and skills development are all directly related to age-specific maturation in children's neuromuscular, cardiovascular, and cognitive systems.
- By age 6 years, most children have acquired sufficient physical skills to participate in some organized sports.
- Gaining experience in a variety of sports is important for the young athlete to enable them to acquire a mix of skill sets and to keep physical activity interesting and fun.

Developmental Levels and Readiness for Sports at Various Prepubertal Ages

- Selection of appropriate athletic activities for children should be guided by knowledge of the developmental skills and limitations of specific age groups.

Ages 3 to 5 Years

- Focus on learning basic skills such as running, swimming, tumbling, throwing, and catching.
- It is recommended that direct competition should be avoided; fun play should be emphasized.

Ages 6 to 9 Years

- Focus on developing fundamental sports skills with limited emphasis on direct competition.
- To learn additional fundamental skills and work toward a transition to direct competition, sports like swimming, running, and gymnastics can be tried.
  - Note: Children have a short attention span, limited memory development, and do not easily make rapid decisions; they need simple, flexible rules and short instruction times.

Ages 10 to 12 Years (Prepubertal Years)

- With the mastery of basic skills, children can now compete in activities and are able to learn more complex motor skill patterns.
  - Children begin to develop their sense of confidence, esteem, and self-awareness. At these ages, body image and popularity are distinguished, and successful mastery of new skills become closely linked to child's self-esteem.
- They have the cognitive, social, and emotional maturity to handle modest competitive pressure and complex

skill sports such as football, basketball, soccer, and field hockey.
  - Can accept increasing emphasis on game tactics and strategy

Many changes occurring during puberty can affect children's athletic performance. The exact timing of these changes can be affected by genetics, endocrine function, nutritional status, and amounts and types of exercise.

Athletic and Sports Issues of Puberty
Co-Ed Youth Teams

- Muscle strength, speed, and skills are usually nearly equal in boys and girls until age 10 to 11 years, and sports activities can still be coeducational due to these similarities.
- Girls generally begin their pubertal changes at approximately 10 years of age, approximately 2 years before boys.
- By age 12 to 13 years, pubertal differences start to affect the skill and strength involved in sports, and depending on the sport, these differences may affect whether girls and boys should continue to play and compete together.

Physiologic Changes of Puberty

- Capacities for both aerobic and anaerobic exercise are beginning to increase, which allow longer and more intense periods of exercise to be tolerated.
  - Aerobic capacity: Greater maximum oxygen uptake (VO_{2max})
    - Due to increases in pulmonary ventilation and cardiac output and to more efficient extraction and use of oxygen by muscle
  - Anaerobic capacity: allows for short, intense bursts of activity
- Note: The downside of these physiologic changes is that although pubertal children are less limited by body fatigue and can thus exercise longer, they are also more capable of overexercising, which can lead to overuse injuries.

Musculoskeletal Changes of Puberty

- Changing body contours during early puberty can lead to physical awkwardness, which may be associated with increased chances of injury, especially in early adolescence when new skills have not caught up with new capacities and new growth.
- Flexibility and joint hypermobility are increased, which increases the risk of glenohumeral and patellar subluxation and dislocation.

Bone Density and Calcium Needs

- During early puberty, bone mineral density begins to increase in both boys and girls.
- The calcium needs of all adolescents are great during puberty, due to the deposition of calcium into rapidly growing bone.
  - Adolescents accrue 40% of their eventual adult bone mass during puberty.
- Recommended calcium intake for adolescents is 1300 mg/day (amenorrheic females may need up to 1500 mg/day).

Linear Growth

- Linear growth begins first in the long bones of the extremities and can contribute to a temporary clumsiness that can have an impact on the athletic performance of younger

TABLE 7.2 Average Timing of Pubertal Changes in Linear Growth (Height)

Specific Pubertal Change	Girls	Boys
Increasing height velocity begins	9 years	11 years
Peak height velocity and timing	9 cm/year, at Tanner stage 2–3	10 cm/year, at Tanner stage 3–4
Duration of growth spurt	24–36 months	24–36 months
Average age at complete skeletal maturity	14 years	16 years

adolescents (Table 7.2). The child who previously exhibited strong skills may suddenly appear to be less coordinated. Puberty-related increases in height velocity usually begin in girls at approximately 9 years of age and in boys at approximately 11 years of age.

- The preadolescent and adolescent growth spurt, which can last for 24 to 36 months, accounts for approximately 20% of final adult height.

Epiphyseal Growth Plates and Other Vulnerable Anatomic Sites

- In early puberty, areas of rapid cell production include (1) articular surfaces, (2) physes (growth plates), and (3) apophyses. The relative weakness of these areas compared to adjacent ligaments, tendons, and bone make these sites more susceptible to injury, including fracture.
- Articular Surfaces
  - Examples include osteochondritis dissecans and patellofemoral syndrome.
- Physes and Apophyses
  - Physes are responsible for the linear growth of bones, while apophyses are responsible for growth at tendinous insertion sites.
    - Physeal fractures represent 15-30% of all childhood fractures.
  - Apophysites include Sever disease (calcaneus), Osgood-Schlatter and Sinding-Larsen-Johansson diseases (Chapter 221), and Iselins disease (fifth metatarsal).
  - Physeal and epiphyseal injuries include little league shoulder (Chapter 218), little league elbow (Chapter 219), and spondylolysis and spondylolisthesis (Chapter 223).
    - These are self-limited and usually resolve with a temporary reduction in activity.
- Additional injuries can result from overuse, lack of skills, lack of appropriate protective equipment, improperly learned (or taught) techniques, and/or excessive performance expectations.

Injury Prevention

- Regular conditioning, stretching regimens, and light strength training can be particularly beneficial in prevention of injuries (especially lower extremity injuries).

- There has been a recent increase of training facilities focusing on proper lifting and sports-related techniques, rather than growth and power, at younger ages.
- Young athletes, regardless of gender, should avoid power lifting until the growth plates are closed, due to an associated with avulsion fractures at the growth plates.

Weight Increases During Puberty

- Puberty-related weight increases account for approximately 50% of adult total body weight.

Weight Changes in Girls

- Lean body mass decreases during puberty to 75% of the total body weight, due to increases in body fat.
- Maximum weight velocity occurs approximately 6 months before their linear growth (height) spurt.
- Hip enlargement decreases waist-to-hip ratio.

Body Image

- Body image concerns in young female athletes may arise because of higher levels of fat in this population.
- Sports where low body fat is valued include dancing, gymnastics, cheerleading, figure skating.
  - Loss of self-esteem and eating disorders are a particular risk in this age group.

Weight Changes in Boys

- Lead body mass increases to approximately 90% of total body weight due to higher androgen levels.
- On average, boys end up with 1.5 times the lean body mass and one-half the body fat of girls.
- Muscle mass accounts for 54% of boys' body weight, making the average male athletes stronger and faster than the average female athletes.

Training and Conditioning

- The purpose of all athletic training programs for young athletes should include improvement of skills, speed, flexibility, strength, conditioning, maintenance of good nutrition, and attention to hydration.
  - Benefits of training and conditioning include greater muscle strength, power, and coordination and a lower risk of athletic injuries (especially knee injuries).
    - Training is a noncompetitive (or less competitive) means of improving conditioning, strength, and coordination.
    - Training can improve athletic performance, increase bone density, promote weight loss, and enhance children's self-esteem.
    - Training can promote a healthy lifestyle that can last into adulthood.

Training Guidelines

- Successful training programs should include qualified adult supervision, no/low weight to focus on technique, and enjoyment.
  - Age: No minimum age for participation in a youth resistance training program
    - Need emotional maturity to accept and follow directions (~7 to 8 years old)

- Instruction: Training should include sufficient instruction and supervision in proper techniques and equipment use.
  - Adult supervisors should stress positive attitude, character building, teamwork, and safety.
- Results: Improvement of baseline strength and muscle tone by 40-50% over a 6-week period.
  - Prepubertal athletes: training increases strength and neuromuscular adaption but will not result in muscle hypertrophy.
  - Pubescent athletes: training will result in larger muscle mass, due to increasing testosterone, especially with increasing weights and resistances.
- Conditioning: should start at least 6 weeks before beginning a sports season.
  - Two to three times per week on nonconsecutive days (to allow a day of rest between sessions)
  - Warm-ups and cool-downs, including stretching, should be part of each session.
  - One to 3 sets of 6 to 15 repetitions with light weights on a variety of exercises, starting with a small number of exercises
  - Gradual increase in weights, number of repetitions, and number of exercises
  - Core exercise should be supplemented by some form of cardiovascular activity for 30 to 40 minutes three to four times weekly.

Suggested Readings

Anderson SJ, Harris SS. *Care of the young athlete*. Elk Grove Village, IL: American Academy of Pediatrics; 2010.

Benjamin HJ, Glow KM. Strength training for children and adolescents: what can physicians recommend? *Physician Sports Med*. 2003;31:19–25.

Coon ER, Young PC, Quinonez RA, et al. Update on pediatric overuse. *Pediatrics*. 2017;139(2).

Feeley BT, Agel J, Laprade RF. When is it too early for single sport specialization? *Am J Sports Med*. 2015;44(1):234–241.

Greydanus DE, Patel DR, Pratt HD. *Essential Adolescent Medicine*. New York: McGraw Hill Professional; 2011.

Kraemer WJ. *Strength Training for Young Athletes*. Champaign, IL: Human Kinetics; 2005.

Marques A, Santos R, Ekelund U, Sardinha LB. Association between physical activity, sedentary time, and healthy fitness in youth. *Med Sci Sports Exerc*. 2015;47(3):575–580.

Metzl JD. *Sports Medicine in the Pediatric Office*. Elk Grove Village, IL: American Academy of Pediatrics; 2017.

Metzl JD, Shookhoff C. *The Young Athlete: A Sports Doctor's Complete Guide for Parents*. New York: Time Warner; 2002.

Patel DR, Soares N, Wells K. Neurodevelopmental readiness of children for participation in sports. *Transl Pediatr*. 2017;6(3):167–173.

Rosenbloom C. Youth athletes: nourishing young bodies and minds. *Nutr Today*. 2016;51(5):221–227.

Stracciolini A, Casciano R, Friedman HL, et al. A closer look at overuse injuries in the pediatric athlete. *Clin J Sport Med*. 2015;25(1):30–35.

Strasburger VC, Brown RT, Braverman PK. *Adolescent Medicine: A Handbook for Primary Care*. Philadelphia: Wolters Kluwer; 2015.

Wilhelm A, Choi C, Deitch J. Early sport specialization: effectiveness and risk of injury in professional baseball players. *Orthop J Sports Med*. 2017;5(9):232596711772892.

Chapter 8 Special Populations: Obesity

Siobhan M. Statuta, Colton Wood

ICD-10-CM CODE
E66.9   Obesity, unspecified

Key Concepts

- According to 2016 World Health Organization data, worldwide obesity has nearly tripled since 1975 with nearly 650 million obese adults worldwide.
- Most recent estimates, according to the 2015–16 National Health and Nutrition Examination Survey (NHANES), reveal that 39.8% of the US adult population is obese (a body mass index [BMI] >30; Fig. 8.1).
- The US government's agenda for building a healthier nation—Healthy People 2020—has set a national goal to decrease obesity prevalence to <30.5% in adults and <14.5% in youth by the year 2020.
- Obesity has been implicated in many musculoskeletal conditions, including knee osteoarthritis and meniscal tears, hip fractures, medial epicondylitis, rotator cuff tendinitis, carpal tunnel syndrome, and postural instability. Obesity leads to a greater need for surgical intervention and yet also predisposes to higher rates of postsurgical complications.
- Obesity is a risk factor for the development of chronic medical diseases including diabetes, hypertension, cardiovascular disease, stroke, chronic pain, numerous cancers, sleep apnea, infertility, birth defects/miscarriages, asthma, and other respiratory illnesses.
- Weight loss, combined with physical exercise and cognitive-behavioral therapy, can help treat both the musculoskeletal conditions and chronic medical diseases caused by obesity.

Demographics

- The BMI is a calculation used in the classification of obesity and compares weight to height parameters (weight [kg]/height [m^2]). A BMI of 25 to 30 is classified "overweight," whereas a BMI >30 is "obese" (Fig. 8.2).
- In 2016, 39.8% of US adults met criteria for obesity: a nearly 10% increase from survey data for the period 1999–2000 (see Fig. 8.1).
- The prevalence of obesity is higher in certain adult populations: middle-aged adults (40 to 59 years) compared with younger adults (20 to 30 years) and non-Hispanic blacks.
- The percentage of obese youth in the US has also risen over the years to an estimated 18.5% in 2016: a 4.6% jump from the 2000 data. This elevated prevalence is in stark contrast to the data from the late 1960s, when rates of overweight and obese children combined were under 5%.

Obesity and Musculoskeletal Conditions

- The risk of knee osteoarthritis increases with an increasing BMI. A longitudinal study demonstrated that a BMI >24.7 in patients ages 20 to 29 years predicted three times the risk of knee osteoarthritis later in life than a BMI <22.8 in that same group.
- While a high BMI has been associated with knee osteoarthritis, it has not been associated with hip or ankle osteoarthritis, suggesting that mechanical factors cause the knee to experience greater forces during weight-bearing activities. It is estimated that every 1 lb of body weight places 4 to 6 lbs of additional pressure across each knee joint.
- Retrospective reviews of anterior cruciate ligament reconstructions have shown that higher BMIs significantly predict the extent of intra-articular injury seen during arthroscopic procedures.
- According to the Canadian Joint Replacement Registry: the need for total knee arthroplasty was 8.5 times greater in patients with BMI >30, 18.5 times greater in patients with BMI >35, and 32.7 times greater in patients with BMI >40.
- In addition to accelerated wear and tear of joints, all-cause musculoskeletal injuries are also 15% higher in overweight individuals and 48% higher in obese individuals.
- A high BMI can affect other areas of the body. A case control study found that rates of rotator cuff tendinitis requiring surgery were twice as likely in obese patients compared with those of normal weight. The risk of surgery rose with an increasing BMI, ranging from a 120% increased risk in moderately obese patients to a 300% increased risk in those with a BMI >35.
- Obesity has been found to be an independent risk factor for medial epicondylitis in women in a Finnish population study involving 5000 patients.
- Carpal tunnel syndrome is twice as likely in obese people compared with those of average weight. This is hypothesized to be due to excess adipose tissue compressing the median nerve and altered mechanics secondary to girth.
- Difficulty with balance has been correlated with increasing weight.

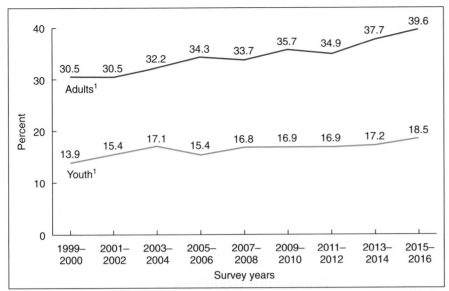

Fig 8.1 US obesity trends in adult and childhood populations. (Modified from Hales CM, Carroll MS, Fryar CD, Ogden CL. Prevalence of obesity among adults and youth: United States, 2015–2016. *NCHS Data Brief*. 2017;288:1–8.)

[1]Signficant increasing linear trend from 1999–2000 through 2015–2016.
NOTES: All estimates for adults are age adjusted by the direct method to the 2000 US census population using the age groups 20–39, 40–59, and 60 and over.
Access data table for this figure at: https://www.cdc.gov/nchs/data/databriefs/db288_table.pdf#5.
SOURCE: NCHS, National Health and Nutrition Examination Survey, 1999–2016.

BMI	19	20	21	22	23	24	25	26	27	28	29	30	31	32	33	34	35
Height							Weight (pounds)										
4'10" (58")	91	96	100	105	110	115	119	124	129	134	138	143	148	153	158	162	167
4'11" (59")	94	99	104	109	114	119	124	128	133	138	143	148	153	158	163	168	173
5' (60")	97	102	107	112	118	123	128	133	138	143	148	153	158	163	168	174	179
5'1" (61")	100	106	111	116	122	127	132	137	143	148	153	158	164	169	174	180	185
5'2" (62")	104	109	115	120	126	131	136	142	147	153	158	164	169	175	180	186	191
5'3" (63")	107	113	118	124	130	135	141	146	152	158	163	169	175	180	186	191	197
5'4" (64")	110	116	122	128	134	140	145	151	157	163	169	174	180	186	192	197	204
5'5" (65")	114	120	126	132	138	144	150	156	162	168	174	180	186	192	198	204	210
5'6" (66")	118	124	130	136	142	148	155	161	167	173	179	186	192	198	204	210	216
5'7" (67")	121	127	134	140	146	153	159	166	172	178	185	191	198	204	211	217	223
5'8" (68")	125	131	138	144	151	158	164	171	177	184	190	197	203	210	216	223	230
5'9" (69")	128	135	142	149	155	162	169	176	182	189	196	203	209	216	223	230	236
5'10" (70")	132	139	146	153	160	167	174	181	188	195	202	209	216	222	229	236	243
5'11" (71")	136	143	150	157	165	172	179	186	193	200	208	215	222	229	236	243	250
6' (72")	140	147	154	162	169	177	184	191	199	206	213	221	228	235	242	250	258
6'1" (73")	144	151	159	166	174	182	189	197	204	212	219	227	235	242	250	257	265
6'2" (74")	148	155	163	171	179	186	194	202	210	218	225	233	241	249	256	264	272
6'3" (75")	152	160	168	176	184	192	200	208	216	224	232	240	248	256	264	272	279

Fig 8.2 Body mass index (BMI) table. (Data from National Heart, Lung and Blood Institute. *Clinical Guidelines on the Identification, Evaluation, and Treatment of Overweight and Obesity in Adults: The Evidence Report*. Bethesda, MD: NIH Publications; 1998.)

Treatment

- Treatments supported by the most rigorous evidence include dieting (net calorie deficit 500 to 1000 kcal/day for >6 months) and physical exercise (>30 minutes of moderate-intensity exercise most days of the week).
- A goal to lose 1 to 2 lbs/week or 10% of body weight in 6 months is both safe and attainable.
- No clear difference in sustained weight loss has been demonstrated between any dietary approach (i.e., low fat vs. low carb vs. Mediterranean diet).
- If further therapy is needed beyond diet and exercise, pharmacotherapy and/or psychotherapy with cognitive-behavioral therapy are good first steps.
- Effective weight-reducing agents include orlistat, phentermine, lorcaserin, and naltrexone with bupropion. Importantly, ephedra and ephedrine should not be prescribed due to risk of death and disability; both are currently banned in the United States.
- Bariatric surgery is an option for patients with BMI >40 who have failed first-line diet/exercise/pharmacologic options; it is also an option for patients with BMI >35 who also have severe comorbidities.
- Prevention of obesity will help decrease the prevalence of many of the aforementioned musculoskeletal conditions.
- For those individuals who are overweight or obese with knee osteoarthritis, several randomized, controlled trials have demonstrated a decrease in osteoarthritis symptoms with weight loss. The Framingham study demonstrated that a weight loss of just 11 pounds was associated with a 50% reduction in arthritis symptoms.
- It has been demonstrated that weight loss by diet alone decreases symptoms of knee osteoarthritis.
- Physical therapy incorporating quadriceps and hip muscle strengthening has been associated with a decrease in knee osteoarthritis symptoms.

Patient Instructions

- A 6-month trial of exercise (with physical therapy playing an integral role), diet, and behavioral therapy (psychotherapy

for cognitive-behavioral therapy) is a good first-step strategy with a goal of losing 1 to 2 lbs/week, or 10% of body weight in the first 6 months.
- A nutritionist or registered dietician is an invaluable resource for education and assisting with meal planning according to one's palate and medical concerns.
- Close follow-up with a primary care provider for intensive behavioral counseling and motivational interviewing has shown strong correlations with weight loss efficacy.
- Consistency in dietary modifications, physical activity, and doctor visits are correlated with greater patient outcomes/successes.
- Obesity is a risk factor for several diseases from diabetes and hypertension to knee osteoarthritis and rotator cuff tendinitis.
- A weight loss of as little as 5 kg can drastically help with musculoskeletal and medical conditions caused by obesity.

Suggested Readings

American Academy of Orthopaedic Surgeons: *Obesity linked to increased risk for orthopaedic conditions and surgical complications*. AAOS Online Newsroom, 2014. Available at http://newsroom.aaos.org/media-resources/Press-releases/obesity-link-to-increased-risk-for-orthopaedic-conditions-and-surgical-complications.htm. Accessed April 5, 2018.

Hales CM, Carroll MD, Fryar CD, Ogden CL. Prevalence of obesity among adults and youth: United States, 2015–2016. *NCHS Data Brief*. 2017;288:1–8.

Mihalko WM, Bergin PF, Kelly FB, Canale ST. Obesity, orthopaedics, and outcomes. *J Am Acad Orthop Surg*. 2014;22(11):683–690.

Sabharwal S, Root MZ. Impact of obesity on orthopaedics. *J Bone Joint Surg Am*. 2012;94(11):1045–1052.

Summerbell CD, Cameron C, Glasziou PP. Advice on low-fat diets for obesity. *Cochrane Database Syst Rev*. 2008;(3):CD003640.

World Health Organization: *WHO obesity and overweight data fact sheet*. WHO Media Center, 2017. Available at http://www.who.int/mediacentre/factsheets/fs311/en/. Accessed April 5, 2018.

Chapter 9 Special Populations: Comorbidities

Adam C. Fletcher

ICD-10-CM CODES
E10.4 *Diabetes mellitus type 1*
E11.8 *Diabetes mellitus type 2*
I10 *Essential hypertension*
I26.10 *Atherosclerotic coronary artery disease*
E66.0 *Obesity due to excess calories*

Key Concepts

- Comorbid conditions are increasingly common in today's patient population.
- A multitude of comorbid conditions can affect both a patient's ability to participate in physical activity and recovery from injury.
- While physical activity can reduce an individual's risk of developing or worsening their comorbid conditions, exercise should be recommended in a safe manner.
- Health care providers must be able to safely develop an exercise program and encourage its execution in patients with a variety of diseases.
- Treatment of patients with increasing numbers of comorbidities becomes more complex. All of the following recommendations should be evaluated on a case-by-case basis with the complete patient situation in mind.
- A variety of physical activities have been categorized based on intensity regarding static and dynamic components as seen in Fig. 9.1, which can be helpful when making exercise recommendations.

Diabetes Mellitus

- Exercise safety and recommendations differ depending on the underlying cause of diabetes mellitus (DM), traditionally classified as type 1 and type 2.
- Individuals with DM have an increased risk of specific orthopaedic concerns, including adhesive capsulitis of the shoulder, carpal tunnel syndrome, and Charcot foot.

Type 1 Diabetes Mellitus (5-10% of Patients With Diabetes Mellitus)

- Type 1 DM is due to autoimmune destruction of insulin-secreting β-cells, resulting in a lack of insulin production.
- Disease onset typically occurs in childhood, although it can develop at any age.
- Physical activity should be recommended for all individuals with type 1 DM.

- Various insulin and carbohydrate intake adjustments may be required to maintain a euglycemic state during physical activity due to variability in exercise intensity and duration.
- Blood glucose should be checked before exercise, with a goal level between 90 and 250 mg/dL.
- If blood glucose level is less than 90 mg/dL, 15 to 30 g of carbohydrates should be ingested prior to exercise, with subsequent rechecks throughout activity.
- If blood glucose level is greater than 250 mg/dL, the individual should test for ketones. If positive, exercise should be avoided. If negative, low- to moderate-intensity exercise can be started. If glucose level is greater than 350 mg/dL, consider insulin correction.
- Carbohydrate-based foods should be readily available during exercise as needed.
- Continuous glucose monitoring (CGM) is becoming more popular as technology advances. At this time, these devices should be used only as an adjunct to more traditional finger stick methods due to concerns regarding accuracy and calibration.

Type 2 Diabetes Mellitus (90-95% of Patients With Diabetes Mellitus)

- Type 2 DM is related to a reduction in circulating insulin along with insulin resistance.
- Onset has traditionally occurred in adulthood, although type 2 DM is becoming increasingly prevalent in the pediatric population.
- Prediabetes or impaired fasting glucose occurs when glucose levels are elevated beyond normal but do not reach the threshold for DM diagnosis.
- Exercise has been shown to prevent or delay onset of type 2 DM in individuals with prediabetes.
- In individuals in the late stages of DM, exercise has been shown to decrease insulin resistance and allow better blood glucose control.
- Low- or moderate-intensity programs are considered generally safe for well-controlled patients with DM who remain asymptomatic.
- While physical activity is encouraged in all patients with type 2 DM, special consideration should be given when additional comorbidities exist:
  - Microalbuminuria/diabetic nephropathy—high-intensity activity should be avoided 24 hours before urine collection to avoid falsely elevated results.
  - Peripheral neuropathy—daily foot checks and routine foot care are required, including keeping feet dry and protected to avoid foot ulcers. Maximizing

	A. Low (<40% Max O₂)	B. Moderate (40-70% Max O₂)	C. High (>70% Max O₂)
III. High (>50% MVC)	Bobsledding/Luge*†, Field events (throwing), Gymnastics*†, Martial arts*, Sailing, Sport climbing, Water skiing*†, Weight lifting*†, Windsurfing*†	Body building*†, Downhill skiing*†, Skateboarding*†, Snowboarding*†, Wrestling*	Boxing*, Canoeing/Kayaking, Cycling*†, Decathlon, Rowing, Speed-skating*†, Triathlon*†
II. Moderate (20-50% MVC)	Archery, Auto racing*†, Diving*†, Equestrian*†, Motorcycling*†	American football*, Field events (jumping), Figure skating*, Rodeoing*†, Rugby*, Running (sprint), Surfing*†, Synchronized swimming†	Basketball*, Ice hockey*, Cross-country skiing (skating technique), Lacrosse*, Running (middle distance), Swimming, Team handball
I. Low (<20% MVC)	Billiards, Bowling, Cricket, Curling, Golf, Riflery	Baseball/Softball*, Fencing, Table tennis, Volleyball	Badminton, Cross-country skiing (classic technique), Field hockey*, Orienteering, Race walking, Racquetball/Squash, Running (long distance), Soccer*, Tennis

Increasing Dynamic Component ⟶

Increasing Static Component ↑

Fig 9.1 Classification of sports. (Modified from Mitchell JH, Haskell W, Snell P, Van Camp SP. Task Force 8: classification of sports. *J Am Coll Cardiol*. 2005;45:1364–1367. In Levine BD, Baggish AL, Kovacs RJ, et al. Eligibility and disqualification recommendations for competitive athletes with cardiovascular abnormalities: Task Force 1: Classification of Sports: Dynamic, Static, and Impact. A Scientific Statement from the American Heart Association and American College of Cardiology. *J Am Coll Cardiol*. 2015;66[21]:2350–2355.)

non–weight-bearing activity may reduce potential trauma to the feet.

- Autonomic neuropathy—utilize caution with exercise in hot environments and rapid postural changes. Use ratings of perceived exertion (RPE) in the setting of blunted heart rate response to monitor exercise intensity.
- Diabetic retinopathy—regular follow-up with ophthalmology is required.
  - Mild nonproliferative disease—all activities are considered safe.
  - Moderate/severe nonproliferative disease—avoid activities that significantly elevate blood pressure (high static activities such as powerlifting).
  - Unstable proliferative disease—avoid jumping and jarring activities, due to increased risk of vitreous hemorrhage and retinal detachment.
- Vascular disease
  - Recent myocardial infarction or stroke—exercise should be initiated in a cardiac rehabilitation program with initial low intensity and progression under supervision.
  - Exertional angina—heart rate should be maintained at least 10 beats per minute below symptom development. Exercise stress test can be helpful in determining individual threshold.
- All medications to treat type 2 DM are considered generally safe with exercise.

- Medication dose adjustments may be required with insulin and insulin secretagogues if previous exercise-induced hypoglycemia has occurred.

Hypertension

- Hypertension is the most common cardiovascular condition in competitive athletes.
- Accurate blood pressure sampling is critical for correct diagnosis. See Box 9.1 for complete details.
- A 24-hour ambulatory blood pressure monitor may be helpful in equivocal cases.
- The definitions of blood pressure classifications are now defined by the 2017 Guideline for High Blood Pressure in Adults as defined in Table 9.1. Recently evidence is lowering the definitions of hypertension.
- A thorough screening for secondary causes of hypertension and evidence of end organ damage should be performed, which should include the following:
  - History should inquire about substance use that can provoke hypertension, including nonsteroidal antiinflammatory medications (NSAIDs), stimulant medications including those for attention deficit disorder, and street drugs including amphetamines and anabolic steroids.
  - Focused physical examination to look for a Cushingoid body habitus and abdominal bruits.

BOX 9.1 Guidelines for Clinic (or Office) Blood Pressure Measurement

Posture

- BP obtained in the seated position is recommended. The subject should sit quietly for 5 min, with the back supported in a chair, with feet on the floor and the arm supported at the level of the heart, before BP is recorded.

Circumstances

- No caffeine should be ingested during the hour preceding the reading, and no smoking during the 30 min preceding the reading
- A quiet, warm setting should be available for BP measurements.

Equipment

- Cuff size
  - The bladder should encircle and cover at least 80% of the length of the arm; if it does not, use a larger cuff. If bladder is too short, misleadingly high readings may result.

Manometer

- Use a validated electronic (digital) device, a recently calibrated aneroid or mercury column sphygmomanometer.

Technique

- Number of readings
  - On each occasion, take at least two readings, separated by as much time as is practical. If

readings vary by >10 mm Hg, take additional readings until two consecutive readings are within 10 mm Hg.
- If the arm pressure is elevated, take the measurement in one leg to rule out aortic coarctation (particularly in patients <30 years of age).
- Initially, take pressures in both arms; if the blood pressures differ, use the arm with the higher pressure.
- If the initial values are elevated, obtain two other sets of readings at least 1 week apart.

Performance

- Inflate the bladder quickly to a pressure 20 mm Hg above the systolic BP, as recognized by the disappearance of the radial pulse; deflate the bladder at 2 mm Hg/s.
- Record the Korotkoff phase I (appearance) and phase V (disappearance) sounds. If the Korotkoff sounds are weak, have the patient raise the arm, then open and close the hand 5–10 times, and then reinflate the bladder quickly.

BP, Blood pressure.

From Black HR, Sica D, Ferdinand K, White WB. Eligibility and disqualification recommendations for competitive athletes with cardiovascular abnormalities: Task Force 6: hypertension. A scientific statement from the American Heart Association and the American College of Cardiology. *J Am Coll Cardiol.* 2015;66(21):2393–2397.

TABLE 9.1 2017 Guideline for High Blood Pressure in Adults

Definition	Systolic BP	Diastolic BP
Normal	<120 mm Hg	<80 mm Hg
Elevated	120–129 mm Hg	<80 mm Hg
Stage 1 hypertension	130–139 mm Hg	80–89 mm Hg
Stage 2 hypertension	>140 mm Hg	>90 mm Hg

BP, Blood pressure.

- Laboratory studies should screen for additional comorbid diseases including dyslipidemia, diabetes mellitus, and chronic renal disease.
- Twelve-lead electrocardiogram to evaluate for left ventricular hypertrophy.
- Consider echocardiogram in individuals with Stage 2 hypertension or other findings of end organ damage.
- Cardiac stress testing is not universally required in the absence of exertional symptoms.
- Exercise has been shown to reduce both systolic and diastolic blood pressure; therefore exercise should be a recommended part of the treatment plan.

- Individuals with Stage 1 hypertension and no evidence of end organ damage should be allowed to participate fully in all physical activity.
- Individuals with Stage 2 hypertension may participate only if blood pressure is controlled and there is no evidence of end organ damage. These individuals should avoid high static sports, including weight lifting, wrestling, and boxing if poorly controlled.
- Individuals with any evidence of end organ failure should be evaluated by a health care provider, and exercise recommendations should be made on an individual basis.
- The use of antihypertensive agents may limit an athlete's exercise performance. This is especially true with β-blockers and diuretics, which should be avoided in competitive athletes.

Atherosclerotic Coronary Artery Disease

- Atherosclerotic coronary artery disease (ASCAD) is the leading cause of sudden cardiac death in adult athletes.
- Physical activity has been shown to positively affect additional risk factors, including obesity, diabetes, and hypertension; however, individuals should see their physician for a preparticipation evaluation.

- Evaluation should include a maximal exercise stress test and echocardiogram, which serve to identify exercise tolerance, any signs of inducible ischemia or electrical instability, and their left ventricular ejection fraction (LVEF). Stress testing should be performed while taking home medications, including beta-adrenergic blocking medications.
- Individuals with a LVEF of greater than 50% who remain asymptomatic and have no findings of ischemia or electrical instability on stress testing can participate in all athletic activities.
- Individuals who do not meet the above criteria should be restricted to low dynamic and low/moderate static competitive sports (e.g., golf, billiards, bowling, archery, walking).
- Individuals with worsening symptoms of ischemia should be restricted from physical activity until further evaluation by a health care provider is performed, including repeat cardiac stress testing and consideration of advanced procedures to identify significant stenosis of coronary arteries.
- Aggressive lipid-lowering treatment should be initiated with high-intensity statin therapy in all individuals with ASCAD.
- After a myocardial infarction, a patient should be enrolled in a cardiac exercise and rehabilitation program, which has been shown to reduce overall mortality by as much as 25%.

Obesity

- Obesity is more comprehensively outlined in Chapter 8.
- Obesity is defined as a body mass index greater than 30. Overweight is characterized by a body mass index between 25 and 30.
- The prevalence of obesity has continued to rise.
- Obesity is associated with significant morbidity and mortality, including increased cardiovascular mortality, diabetes, hypertension, dyslipidemia, and stroke. It also increases one's risk of gallbladder disease, sleep apnea, and a number of cancers including breast, colon, and prostate cancer.
- All individuals with obesity should be encouraged to adopt an exercise program, and limitations should be guided by additional comorbidities.
- In addition to exercise, dietary calorie restriction is oftentimes required to reduce body mass index.
- A 5-10% weight loss reduction can help reduce the risk of developing comorbid conditions such as hypertension, knee osteoarthritis, and diabetes mellitus.

Patient Instructions

- A routine exercise program has been shown to help treat common medical conditions such as hypertension, diabetes, coronary artery disease, and obesity.

- In all situations, new aerobic activity should be initiated at low intensity and volume with a gradual increase as tolerated unless contraindicated by a comorbidity.
- To promote a healthy lifestyle, individuals should participate in at least 150 minutes of aerobic activity each week, ideally with no more than two days off between exercise sessions.
- Physical activity should also include resistance, flexibility, and neuromotor exercises.

Suggested Readings

Bauman AE. Updating the evidence that physical activity is good for health: an epidemiological review 2000–2003. *J Sci Med Sport*. 2003;7:6–19.

Colberg SR, Sigal RJ, Yardley JE, et al. Physical activity/exercise and diabetes: a position statement of the American Diabetes Association. *Diabetes Care*. 2016;39(11):2065–2079.

Flegal K, Graubard B, Williamson D, Gail M. Cause-specific excess deaths associated with underweight, overweight, and obesity. *JAMA*. 2007;298:2028–2037.

Garber CE, Blissmer B, Deschenes MR, et al. American College of Sports Medicine position stand. Quantity and quality of exercise for developing and maintaining cardiorespiratory, musculoskeletal, and neuromotor fitness in apparently healthy adults: guidance for prescribing exercise. *Med Sci Sports Exerc*. 2011;43(7):1334–1359.

James PA, Oparil S, Carter BL, et al. 2014 Evidence-based guideline for the management of high blood pressure in adults: report from the Panel Members Appointed to the Eighth Joint National Committee (JNC 8). *JAMA*. 2014;311(5):507–520.

MacKnight J. Exercise considerations in hypertension, obesity, and dyslipidemia. *Clin Sports Med*. 2003;22:101–121.

Maron BJ, Mitchell JH eds. 26th Bethesda Conference: recommendations for determining eligibility for competition in athletes with cardiovascular abnormalities. *J Am Coll Cardiol*. 1994;24:845–899.

Maron BJ, Zipes DP, Kovacs RJ, et al. Eligibility and disqualification recommendations for competitive athletes with cardiovascular abnormalities: preamble, principles, and general considerations: a scientific statement from the American Heart Association and American College of Cardiology. *Circulation*. 2015;132(22):e256–e261.

Pescatello LS, Franklin BA, Fagard R, et al. American College of Sports Medicine position stand. Exercise and hypertension. *Med Sci Sports Exerc*. 2004;36(3):533–553.

Thompson PD, Buchner D, Pina IL, et al. Exercise and physical activity in the prevention and treatment of atherosclerotic cardiovascular disease. *Circulation*. 2003;107:3109–3116.

Whelton PK, Carey RM, Aronow WS, et al. 2017 ACC/AHA/AAPA/ABC/ACPM/AGS/APhA/ASH/ASPC/NMA/PCNA Guideline for the prevention, detection, evaluation, and management of high blood pressure in adults: a report of the American College of Cardiology/American Heart Association Task Force on Clinical Practice Guidelines. *J Am Coll Cardiol*. 2018;71:e127–e248.

Chapter 10 Special Populations: Female Athletes

Siobhan M. Statuta, Kelly E. Grob

ICD-10-CM CODES

FEMALE ATHLETE TRIAD

N91.2 *Amenorrhea, unspecified*
F50.9 *Eating disorder, unspecified*
M85.9 *Disorder of bone density and structure, unspecified*

EXERCISE AND PREGNANCY
Z34 *Normal Pregnancy*

Female Athlete Triad

Key Concepts

- The female athlete triad is a syndrome of three tightly interwoven conditions: low energy availability (with or without disordered eating or an eating disorder), menstrual dysfunction, and low bone density.
- For each condition, the athlete may fall somewhere on the continuum between the normal healthy end and the pathologic end of the spectrum.
- It is unclear how widespread the triad is. Prevalence is variable by sport—those with highest energy expenditure, sports with an aesthetics component, or those in which a lean physique is preferable have the highest prevalence.
- Early detection and intervention are key to preventing progression to serious sequelae.
- The International Olympic Committee introduced a similar syndrome titled *Relative Energy Deficiency in Sport (RED-S)*. This syndrome applies to female and male athletes alike, athletes with disabilities, and those across ethnicities. Instead of it being a triad, this is a more widely encompassing concept, with low energy affecting a broad array of physiological systems.
- Although some standard approaches exist to apply science to return-to-play decision making, these methods have inherent weaknesses and continue to be refined as more evidence emerges. Taking an individualized approach to each athlete case scenario is imperative to appropriately consider the unique circumstances that influence safe return to sport.

Screening

- Current guidelines recommend screening as part of the preparticipation physical evaluation, although the panel of question varies by organization.

- Any risk factor identified during screening should immediately prompt further evaluation.
- Late-stage findings such as amenorrhea, stress fracture, or signs of an eating disorder may be what triggers further medical evaluation, as much of the early pathology occurs silently.

History

- Dietary/energy inquiries: eating habits, caloric intake, dietary restrictions, disordered eating patterns, recent weight changes (intentional?), changes in training schedule, athlete knowledge regarding "energy balance."
- Menstrual history to help determine age of menarche, pattern of regularity, lapses, severity, birth control use, and purpose of initiation (i.e., regulation of menses vs. contraception).
- Any history of significant bone pain or injury, even if not officially diagnosed.
- Other: unexplained fatigue, cold intolerance, lightheadedness, drop in athletic performance, mental status, stressors in life, medications/supplements, sleep patterns.

Physical Examination

- Primarily a clinical diagnosis made from the athlete's history; the physical examination is often normal.
- There may be findings suggestive of an eating disorder, including bradycardia, hypotension (particularly orthostatic hypotension), dental enamel erosion, parotid gland hypertrophy, Russell sign (callus on finger from self-induced vomiting), cold/discolored hands and feet, and lanugo hair or skin dryness. Assess appropriateness of the Tanner stage.
- Often, the presenting athletic concern is a stress fracture; thus the exam will be consistent with findings of bony stress injury.

Imaging

- If concerned about a stress fracture, appropriate images should be obtained.
- The presence of certain factors in the history must be evaluated when considering the need to further assess bone mineral density (BMD). These include number of stress fractures suffered, the location and risk stratification of these fractures, age of menarche, menstrual history and regularity, and/or the presence of an officially diagnosed eating disorder. The test of choice for evaluating BMD is with a dual-energy x-ray absorptiometry (DEXA) scan.

Additional Tests

- Consider obtaining a panel of electrolytes, serum proteins, liver enzymes, complete blood count with differential, ferritin, erythrocyte sedimentation rate, thyroid function tests, vitamin levels, and a urinalysis to investigate an athlete with disordered eating or clinical eating disorder.
- Workup to exclude other causes of amenorrhea may include pregnancy test, follicle-stimulating hormone and luteinizing hormone, prolactin, and thyroid function studies.
- Consider free serum testosterone and dehydroepiandrosterone sulfate (DHEA-S) if evidence of androgen excess is seen on physical examination.
- To further evaluate estrogen levels in the body, a serum estradiol or progesterone challenge test may be helpful. Athletes with functional hypothalamic amenorrhea are likely to be hypoestrogenic and may fail to have expected normal withdrawl bleeding with the challenge test.
- Additional testing for primary amenorrhea should be based on personal and family history, as well as exam findings.

Differential Diagnosis

- Other causes of amenorrhea include, but are not limited to, pregnancy, thyroid disease, pituitary or adrenal tumor/disease, polycystic ovarian syndrome, premature ovarian failure, and Turner syndrome (primary amenorrhea).
- Hyperparathyroidism and excess glucocorticosteroid use may result in decreased bone mineral density and recurrent stress fractures.
- Consider other causes of low energy availability including eating patterns, dietary choices, or malabsorption syndromes such as celiac disease, autoimmune disease, or malignancy.

Treatment

- To reverse this condition, energy availability *must* increase; thus modifications in diet and exercise need to occur. A written contract may be necessary in at-risk athletes to ensure minimal criteria are being met to continue training and competition.
- Adequate nutrition, optimal energy availability, and healthy body weight should be the primary focus of treatment to restore regular menses and improve bone mineral density (Fig. 10.1).
- A multidisciplinary treatment team is imperative and should include a health care provider, a registered dietitian/nutritionist, and, for athletes with clinical eating disorders, a mental health professional specializing in these disorders (see Fig. 10.1).
- Contemplate vitamin supplementation if warranted due to limited dietary intake.

Troubleshooting

- Prevention of the female athlete triad through education should be the goal of those caring for at-risk athletic populations. Athletes, coaches, and parents must be informed about the triad and the wide array of negative impacts it imparts. Taking an "eat to perform" approach lends itself well to athletes, often providing a motivating stance toward nutrition.
- Provide age-appropriate counseling on energy/caloric needs and nutritional requirements, including calcium and vitamin D.
- In pediatric and adolescent athletes, special attention must be given to education regarding maximizing bone mineral accrual while still possible.
- Female athletes should be educated about the detrimental effects of resultant secondary amenorrhea.
- Screening is essential for early detection and intervention. The preparticipation examination is often the ideal time to screen women. Questions regarding menstrual, diet, and exercise history should be included. Any endorsed amenorrhea or oligomenorrhea needs to be further investigated. A history of disordered eating, pathologic weight control practices, or stress fracture should also prompt further workup.

Patient Instructions

- Returning to a state of optimal energy balance is very likely to improve endurance and athletic performance.
- Absence of menstruation should not be considered a desirable convenience, but rather an indication that the body does not have enough energy available to continue normal physiologic function. Spontaneous return of menses is an indicator of improving energy availability.
- Restoring optimal energy balance through good nutrition and monitoring of activity is essential to long-term bone health.

Exercise and Pregnancy

Key Concepts

- Exercise, with some modifications, has very few risks and is beneficial to most pregnant women.
- It is best for an obstetrical provider to evaluate a pregnant patient prior to initiation or continuation of exercise.
- Exercise during pregnancy promotes physical fitness, aides weight management during pregnancy, can decrease the risk of gestational diabetes, and can promote general mental health. In the later trimesters, it can reduce back pain, shorten labor, and reduce the risk of caesarean section.
- Both absolute and relative contraindications to aerobic exercise during pregnancy exist. Similarly, there are specific warning signs to terminate exercise during pregnancy.
- Some normal physiologic changes to the musculoskeletal system during pregnancy may lead to discomfort; modifications should be made.
- Close obstetrical monitoring of athletes is essential particularly in the pregnant competitive athlete.

History

- Before providing an exercise prescription during pregnancy, factors such as patient's age, general physical condition, and prepregnancy exercise regimen must be considered.

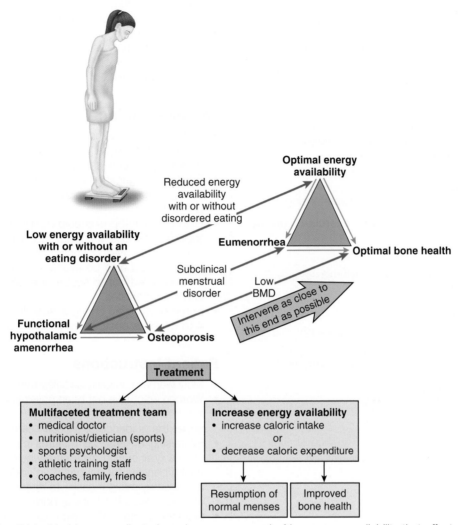

Fig 10.1 The female athlete triad is a complicated syndrome composed of low energy availability that affects menstrual regularity and bone health. Each individual component is located on its own continuum. Treatment is guided by a comprehensive treatment team, with the main focus on increasing energy availability.

Any history of orthopaedic injuries or musculoskeletal issues as well as risk factors for cardiovascular disease should be assessed. Inquire about current medications, medical history (including the presence of pulmonary disease, diabetes), and obstetric history.

- Patients should be educated regarding the warning signs, when to stop exercise, and when to seek medical attention (Box 10.1).

Physical Examination

- Pregnancy requires routine obstetrical visits and observation of healthy progression. Normal physiological responses result in changes in heart rate, cardiac output, and blood volume—all of which will shift vitals and exercise tolerance.
- Any findings that might exclude a patient from exercise should be noted. (Absolute and relative contraindications to exercise during pregnancy are found in Box 10.2.)

BOX 10.1 Warning Signs to Terminate Exercise While Pregnant

Vaginal bleeding
Dyspnea before exertion
Dizziness
Headache
Chest pain
Muscle weakness
Lower leg pain or swelling
Preterm labor
Decreased fetal movement
Amniotic fluid leakage

Adapted from the American College of Obstetricians and Gynecologists Committee Opinion No. 650.

BOX 10.2 **Contraindications to Aerobic Exercise in Pregnancy: Absolute and Relative**

Absolute contraindications to exercise during pregnancy:

- Hemodynamically significant heart disease
- Restrictive lung disease
- Incompetent cervix/cerclage
- Multiple gestation pregnancy at risk of premature labor
- Persistent second- or third-trimester bleeding
- Placenta previa after 26 weeks' gestation
- Premature labor during current pregnancy
- Ruptured membranes
- Preeclampsia-/pregnancy-induced hypertension

Relative contraindications to exercise during pregnancy:

- Severe anemia
- Unevaluated maternal cardiac arrhythmia
- Chronic bronchitis
- Poorly controlled type 1 diabetes
- Extreme morbid obesity
- Extreme underweight (body mass index <12)
- History of extremely sedentary lifestyle
- Intrauterine growth restriction in current pregnancy
- Poorly controlled hypertension
- Orthopaedic limitations
- Poorly controlled seizure disorder
- Poorly controlled hyperthyroidism
- Heavy smoking

Adapted from the American College of Obstetricians and Gynecologists Committee Opinion No. 650.

Imaging

- No other imaging, besides routine ultrasound during pregnancy, needs to be performed.

Additional Tests

- No further workup is needed for exercise during pregnancy.
- Further evaluation is warranted for any concerning symptoms, including vaginal bleeding, contractions, loss of fluid, dyspnea, lightheadedness, headaches, chest pain, and swelling.

Treatment

- Encourage exercise during pregnancy for all women without known contraindications.
- Competitive athletes may require closer monitoring during strenuous training with particular attention to adequate hydration/caloric intake.
- Physiologic changes of pregnancy, including weight gain, altered center of gravity, and musculoskeletal laxity, may require modification of activity for continued comfort during exercise.
- Any history or risk factor for preterm labor may well require reduction of activity for competitive athletes during the second/third trimester, as physical activity can increase the likelihood of contractions.
- Avoid the use of nonsteroidal antiinflammatory medications in pregnant women. Alternative modalities such as cryotherapy, bracing, acetaminophen, and physical therapy are deemed helpful and safe.

Troubleshooting

- Although exercise is generally considered safe during pregnancy, the goal should be to maintain rather than drastically increase the pregnant woman's level of fitness.
- Education regarding increased fluid and nutritional needs during pregnancy exercise as well as heat management is critical.
- High-contact sports should be avoided during pregnancy (including ice hockey, boxing, soccer, basketball). Sports that involve fall risk (skiing, surfing, gymnastics, and horseback riding) should also be avoided. Pregnant women should be counseled not to scuba dive, sky dive, or participate in hot yoga/pilates.
- Some physiologic changes seen in pregnancy persist for 4 to 6 weeks postpartum (longer if breastfeeding).

Patient Instructions

- Most women can exercise safely throughout their pregnancy.
- Women who have not been physically active may initiate a low-intensity exercise program gradually during pregnancy under the guidance of a health care provider.
- Exercising at least 30 minutes most days of the week (with a goal of 150 minutes a week) can provide multiple health benefits for a woman. In addition, regular physical activity may make it easier to restore prepregnancy levels of fitness once the baby is born.
- Contact sports, sports with risk of falling, sports in high-temperature or high-altitude environments, and those where you lie on your back after the first trimester should be avoided.

Suggested Readings

Female Athlete Triad

De Souza MJ, Nattiv A, Joy E, et al. 2014 Female Athlete Triad Coalition consensus statement on treatment and return to play of the female athlete triad. *Br J Sports Med.* 2014;48(4):289.

Mountjoy M, Sundgot-Borgen J, Burke L, et al. The IOC consensus statement: beyond the Female Athlete Triad—Relative Energy Deficiency in Sport (RED-S). *Br J Sports Med.* 2014;48(7):491–497.

Williams NI, Statuta SM, Austin A. Female Athlete Triad: future directions for energy availability and eating disorder research and practice. *Clin Sports Med.* 2017;36(4):671–686.

Exercise and Pregnancy

American College of Obstetricians and Gynecologists. Physical activity and exercise during pregnancy and the postpartum period. American College of Obstetricians and Gynecologists Committee Opinion No. 650. *Obstet Gynecol.* 2015;Reaffirmed 2017.

Borg-Stein J, Dugan SA. Musculoskeletal disorders of pregnancy, delivery and postpartum. *Phys Med Rehabil Clin N Am.* 2007;18:459–476.

Gregg VH, Ferguson IIJE. Exercise in pregnancy. *Clin Sports Med.* 2017;36(4):741–752.

Paisley TS, Joy EA, Price RJ. Exercise during pregnancy: a practical approach. *Curr Sports Med Rep.* 2003;2:325–330.

Chapter 11 Special Populations: Athletes

Jeremy Kent, Scott McAleer

Key Concepts

- A substantial portion of the population competes in athletic events at the grade school, high school, collegiate, master, recreational, and professional levels.
- A preparticipation physical examination should be performed annually in any individual competing in sporting events to ensure safe play.
- A team physician at the event needs to be able to stabilize and triage injuries as necessary.
- Treating athletes requires knowledge of return-to-play guidelines.

Demographics

- The National High School Sports-Related Injury Surveillance System offers the most comprehensive epidemiologic data for the 2005–06 to 2015–16 school years.
- An estimated 7.8 million adolescents participated in high school sports in 2014–15.
- High school athletes suffered approximately 1.4 million injuries during the 2015–16 school year, at an injury rate of 2.32 per 1000 athlete exposures (AE).
- More than 460,000 student athletes compete at the collegiate level in 25 different sports.
- The National Collegiate Athletic Association (NCAA) uses a Web-based Injury Surveillance System (ISS) to collect data on injuries, injury rates, and AEs (Fig. 11.1).

Preparticipation Examination

- Annual preparticipation physical evaluations (PPE) have not been proven to prevent sports-related morbidity/mortality; however, they may help detect conditions that predispose athletes to illness and injury.
- PPEs should include a personal history of injury/illness and a family history of cardiac pathology or sudden cardiac death.
- The physical exam should at minimum assess blood pressure, vision, cardiovascular, and musculoskeletal systems.
- At this time, routine ECG and echocardiogram screening of asymptomatic, low-risk athletes is not recommended.
- Certain athlete populations at greater risk for sudden cardiac death (i.e., football, men's basketball) may be considered for ECG screening.
- The 36th Bethesda Conference offers additional information regarding eligibility and disqualification criteria for competitive athletes with cardiovascular abnormalities.
- The PreParticipation Physical Evaluation Monograph, 4th edition, should be reviewed for disease-specific participation guidelines.
- The provider should consider preseason baseline concussion testing using computer-based neurocognitive batteries if resources are available.

Sport-Specific Injuries

- No-time-loss (NTL) injuries are defined as those resulting in participation restriction <24 hours.
- Severe injuries are defined as participation restriction >28 days or early termination of season.
- Football
  - Data collected from the NCAA Injury Surveillance Program (NCAA-ISP) from the 2004 to 2009 academic years revealed that:
    - Over half (55.9%) of all injuries were reported during regular practices, although the highest injury rates occurred during competitions and scrimmages.
    - The most common injuries were sprains and strains (50.6%) of the lower extremity.
    - Most sprains involved the lateral ligament complex of the ankle and medial collateral ligament (MCL)/anterior collateral ligament (ACL) of the knee.
    - Common injury mechanisms included contact with another player while tackling or being tackled, and noncontact/overuse.
    - See Suggested Reading for the 2017 interassociation consensus recommendations on Year-Round Football Practice Contact for College Student-Athletes.
    - Concussions account for about 6% of injuries in collegiate athletics and 7% in the National Football League.
- Soccer
  - Data collected from the NCAA-ISP from the 2009 to 2015 academic years.
  - Majority of men's and women's soccer injuries occurred to the lower extremity and included ankle sprains, knee sprains, upper leg strains, and hip/groin strains.
  - Overall injury rates during competition and practice did not differ between men and women.
  - Rate of concussion caused by ball contact was 2.43 times higher in women than men, thought as due to weaker neck musculature and level of contact.
  - Approximately 50% of all soccer injuries were NTL.
  - Women suffered a higher percentage of severe injuries compared to men (9.2% vs. 5.1%)

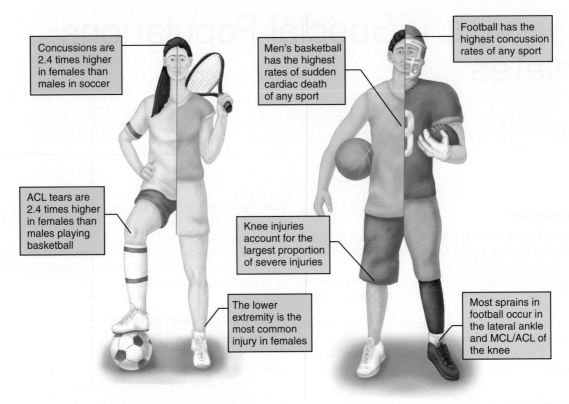

Fig 11.1 Injury rates from the The National Collegiate Athletic Association Injury Surveillance Program. *ACL,* Anterior collateral ligament; *MCL,* medial collateral ligament.

- Basketball
  - Data collected from the NCAA-ISP from the 2009 to 2015 academic years.
  - The majority of injuries in men's and women's basketball were to the lower extremity, with ankle sprains (17.9% and 16.6% of all injuries, respectively) being the most common.
  - Knee injuries accounted for the largest proportion of severe injuries, and the rate of knee internal derangement was approximately 35% higher in women than men.
  - The number of ACL tears was almost 2.5 times higher in women than men.
  - NTL injuries accounted for 57.7% and 52.3% of men's and women's basketball injuries, respectively.
- Tennis
  - Data collected from the NCAA-ISP from the 2009 to 2015 academic years.
  - The overall injury rate for men's and women's tennis was just under 5/1000 AEs.
  - Competition injury rates were higher than practice injury rates for both men's and women's tennis.
  - The majority of injuries in men's and women's tennis were to the lower extremities (47.0% and 52.4%, respectively), followed by the trunk (16.6% and 17.6%, respectively) and shoulder/clavicle (14.4% and 11.9%, respectively).
  - The most common specific injury for men's and women's tennis was sprain of the lateral ankle ligament complex.
  - The proportion of severe injuries reported in men's tennis was disconcerting, with about one of every nine injuries categorized as severe.

Treatment

- Treatments are as outlined in the corresponding chapters in the text.
- Include goals for return to play in treatment plan.
- Emphasize coordination between physicians, physical therapists, athletic trainers, and other components of the medical team.

Performance

- Athletes at all competitive levels will push the limits of personal performance.
- Sports psychology and sports nutrition are resources for athletes looking to improve.
- Athletes may also turn to performance-enhancing drugs. Counseling athletes on the safety and legality of these substances is necessary.

Suggested Readings

Bernhardt DT, Roberts WO. American academy of pediatrics. In: *PPE: Preparticipation Physical Evaluation.* 4th ed. Elk Grove Village, IL: American Academy of Pediatrics; 2010.

Drezner JA, O'Connor FG, Harmon KG, et al. AMSSM position statement on cardiovascular preparticipation screening in athletes: current evidence, knowledge gaps, recommendations and future directions. *Br J Sports Med.* 2016;[Epub ahead of print].

Kerr ZY, Simon JE, Grooms DR, et al. Epidemiology of football injuries in the national collegiate athletic association, 2004-2005 to 2008-2009. *Orthop J Sports Med.* 2016;4(9):2325967116664500.

Lynall RC, Kerr ZY, Djoko A, et al. Epidemiology of national collegiate athletic association men's and women's tennis injuries, 2009/2010-2014/2015. *Br J Sports Med.* 2016;50(19):1211–1216.

Maron BJ, Zipes DP, Ackerman MJ. 36Th bethesda conference: eligibility recommendations for competitive athletes with cardiovascular abnormalities. *J Am Coll Cardiol.* 2005;45(8):1312–1375.

Mirabelli MH, Devine MJ, Singh J, Mendoza M. The preparticipation sports evaluation. *Am Fam Physician.* 2015;92(5):371–376.

National Collegiate Athletic Association (NCAA): Online Resource for the NCAA. Available at http://www.ncaa.org.

National Collegiate Athletic Association Sports Science Institute (NCAA SSI): Year-Round Football Practice Contact Recommendations. Available at http://www.ncaa.org/sport-science-institute/year-round-football -practice-contact-recommendations. Accessed April 24, 2018.

National High School Sports-Related Injury Surveillance Study: 2016-2017 School Year. Available at http://www.ucdenver.edu/academics/colleges/ PublicHealth/research/ResearchProjects/piper/projects/RIO/Pages/ Study-Reports.aspx. Accessed February 13, 2018.

Roos KG, Wasserman EB, Dalton SL, et al. Epidemiology of 3825 injuries sustained in six seasons of national collegiate athletic association men's and women's soccer (2009/2010-2014/2015). *Br J Sports Med.* 2017;51(13):1029–1034.

Zuckerman SL, Wegner AM, Roos KG, et al. Injuries sustained in national collegiate athletic association men's and women's basketball, 2009/2010-2014/2015. *Br J Sports Med.* 2018;52(4):261–268.

Chapter 12 Trauma: Principles of Fracture Management

David J. Berkoff, Christopher Felton

ICD-10-CM CODES
S12 *Fractures to the neck*
S22 *Fractures to the rib, sternum, and thoracic spine*
S32 *Fracture of lumbar spine and pelvis*
S42 *Fracture upper arm or shoulder*
S52 *Fracture of forearm*
S62 *Fracture of wrist, hand, finger*
S72 *Fracture of femur*
S82 *Fracture of lower leg, including ankle*
S92 *Fracture of foot, toe (except ankle)*

Key Concepts

- A fracture represents a disruption of bone continuity, either complete or partial.
- Fractures are most commonly the result of trauma.
- They can be due to an abnormal force applied to a normal bone or a normal force applied to an abnormal bone.
- In patients without trauma, these injuries can be related to overuse, osteoporosis, or diseases related to abnormal bone formation.
- Fractures can result in gross or microscopic destruction of the bone matrix.
- Fractures that compromise neurovascular structures or have the potential to become open injuries must be emergently treated with immediate reduction of the fracture and/or dislocation.
- An open fracture is defined as one with a disruption of the skin overlying a fractured bone allowing contact with the external environment.
- A closed fracture has intact overlying skin.
- Lacerations or abrasions require evaluation for possible underlying open fracture and/or joint involvement, particularly those over bony prominences.
- Accurate fracture description is important for both proper diagnosis and treatment (Table 12.1).

History

- Fractures most commonly occur from an acute traumatic injury.
- The mechanism of injury (e.g., direct blow, rotation, fall) should be used to guide accurate evaluation of the injury.
- Trauma may be minor particularly if underlying bone abnormality is present.
- Patients frequently complain of pain and loss of function typically at the site of fracture.

- Severity, type, and quality of pain vary widely among patients and should not be used to determine if fracture is present.
- Pain without obvious fracture should prompt consideration of stress fractures in the setting of repetitive trauma or in those with abnormal bone formation or osteoporosis.

Physical Examination

- Carefully inspect injury to determine skin integrity for open or closed status of fractures.
- Palpate injured area for crepitus, swelling, and deformity.
- Evaluate for and document any bony deformity identified on examination
- Assess neurovascular integrity and document thoroughly both before and after any manipulation of the fractured bone.
- Fractures that result from high-energy trauma require careful evaluation for compartment syndrome, especially in the setting of crush injuries.
- Always examine the joint above and below to identify potential occult injuries.

Imaging

- Plain radiographs (multiple orthogonal planes) frequently identify acute and chronic fractures.
- Stress fractures, nondisplaced fractures, and other subtle fractures may not be visible on plain radiographs initially, and may require further evaluation either acutely or during timely follow-up evaluations to fully assess for bony injury.
- Computed tomography (CT) can be used to further describe fractures and better identify fracture fragments, displacement, and angulation. CT is also often helpful before surgical management.
- Magnetic resonance imaging (MRI) is also used to further identify occult fractures, stress fractures, and insufficiency fractures, and to better evaluate the soft-tissue structures that surround the fractured bone.
- Ultrasound can also be used to identify both acute fracture (cortical breaks can be visualized) and abnormalities seen in stress fractures (cortical thickening, periosteal reaction and increased vascularization).
- Proper fracture description requires a consistent and logical approach and includes skin integrity, anatomic location, fracture line orientation, angulation, and displacement (see Table 12.1).
- Always obtain repeat radiographs after splinting/reducing to evaluate changes in fracture orientation.

TABLE 12.1 Fracture Description

Fracture Descriptor	Type	Pathologic Description
Anatomic location	Epiphyseal	End of bone
	Metaphyseal	Flared portion of bone between diaphysis and epiphysis
	Diaphyseal	Shaft of long bone
	Physeal (growth plate)	Salter-Harris classifications I–V describe fractures involving the growth plate
Orientation of fracture line	Transverse (Fig. 12.1)	Fracture perpendicular to long axis of bone
	Oblique (Fig. 12.2)	Angular fracture down long axis of bone
	Spiral (Fig. 12.3)	A complex fracture line that encircles shaft of bone (twisting fracture)
	Longitudinal	Along long axis of bone
	Segmental (Fig. 12.4)	Free-floating fracture segment bordered by fracture lines
	Torus (Fig. 12.5)	Buckling of the cortex without breaking bone on other side (pediatric)
	Greenstick (Fig. 12.6)	Fracture with disruption through one cortex while the other side remains intact (pediatric)
	Pathologic	Fracture of bone with underlying disease
Fragments	Simple	2 fragments
	Comminuted (Fig. 12.7)	>2 fragments
	Avulsion (Fig. 12.8)	Fragment of bone torn away from the main mass of bone
	Compression (Fig. 12.9)	Collapse of a bone, most often a vertebra
Position/displacement (described distal segment relative to proximal)	Nondisplaced	Fracture fragments are aligned
	Displaced (Fig. 12.10)	Fracture fragments are separated
	Nonangulated	Anatomic alignment preserved
	Angulated (Fig. 12.11)	Fragments without usual anatomic alignment
	Shortened (bayonette)	Described as the number of centimeters of overlap
	Rotated	Description of distal fragment relative to proximal

Differential Diagnosis

- See Table 12.2.

Treatment (Fig. 12.12)

- Initial treatment should focus on accurate diagnosis to ensure proper immediate and long-term planning for fracture care.
- Pain control is essential for patient comfort and to aid in patient cooperation for splinting and/or reductions.
- Closed reduction employing traction and realignment is used for many displaced fractures.
- Splinting and/or casting are used to maintain anatomic alignment in both simple fractures and those requiring reduction/relocation.
- Repeat imaging is required after reduction or splinting to assess and document postreduction changes in bony alignment.
- Referral or consultation for further management or urgent/ emergent treatment should be considered if (1) open reduction and internal fixation are required, (2) closed reduction is not possible, (3) there are open fractures, (4) neurovascular compromise is present, or (5) the severity and complexity of fracture require more definitive treatment than can initially be provided.

Troubleshooting

- Recognizing compartment syndrome due to acute injury or casting injury too tightly is imperative.
- Malunion, nonunion, stiffness, and neurovascular injury should all be comprehensively evaluated and discussed with the patient before treatment and discharge.
- The potential for long-term complications, including the development of arthritis and loss of motion in a fractured joint, should be discussed with the patient.

Patient Instructions

- Rest, ice, elevation, splinting, and nonsteroidal antiinflammatory drugs.
- Nonsteroidal antiinflammatory drugs may inhibit bony healing in long bones; therefore, they should be used sparingly

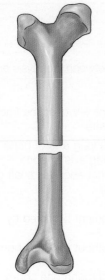

Fig 12.1 Transverse fracture.

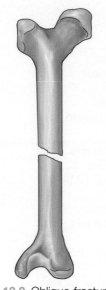

Fig 12.2 Oblique fracture.

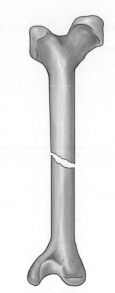

Fig 12.3 Spiral fracture.

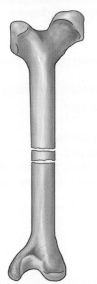

Fig 12.4 Segmental fracture.

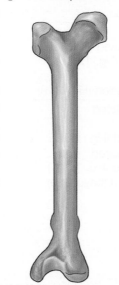

Fig 12.5 Torus fracture.

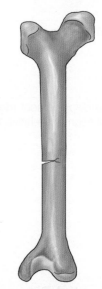

Fig 12.6 Greenstick fracture.

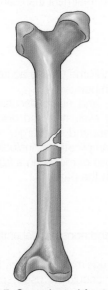

Fig 12.7 Comminuted fracture.

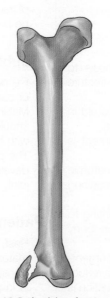

Fig 12.8 Avulsion fracture.

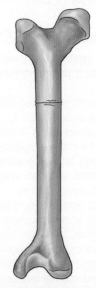

Fig 12.9 Compression fracture.

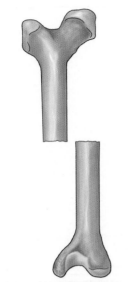

Fig 12.10 Displaced fracture.

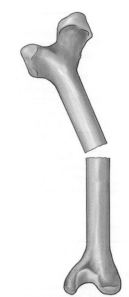

Fig 12.11 Angulated fracture.

TABLE 12.2 Differential Diagnosis

Diagnosis	History	Symptoms/Signs	Radiographic Evaluation
Fracture	Trauma with or without deformity	Pain, swelling, deformity, loss of function	Radiographs for uncomplicated, computed tomography or magnetic resonance imaging for complicated/operative fractures
Contusion	Direct blow to body part	Pain, swelling, ecchymosis, decreased function	Negative for fracture
Sprain	Excessive force applied to a joint causing ligamentous injury	Point tenderness, swelling, ecchymosis, minimal range of motion	May be negative or show avulsion fracture at site of ligamentous insertion, joint space widening
Strain	Overexertion or overstretching of muscle leading to damage of muscle/tendon complex	Pain, swelling, ecchymosis, decreased range of motion, palpable defect if complete disruption	Negative for fracture
Dislocation	Dependent on specific type of dislocation	Pain, gross deformity, decreased range of motion; possible neurovascular deficits	Shows disarticulation of involved bones with possible accompanying fracture

and with a clear understanding of their role in fracture management.

- Weight-bearing status and use limitations must be clearly outlined to the patient.
- Ensure prompt and appropriate follow-up care for patients with fractures that threatened neurovascular structures, required closed or open reduction, may be unstable, are at high risk of nonunion, or have been splinted or casted.
- Make patients aware of signs of possible compartment syndrome such as increasing pain, pain on passive range of motion, pain out of proportion to injury, paresthesia, pallor, and weakness. If any of these signs are present, the patient should seek immediate orthopaedic evaluation.

Considerations in Special Populations

- Normal radiographs alone do not rule out stress fractures in sports medicine patients who are subject to repetitive impact injuries.
- In the elderly or others with osteoporosis, there may not be a defined traumatic event that precedes a fracture.
- In the pediatric population, tenderness overlying a growth plate can be a nondisplaced Salter-Harris type I fracture, which requires appropriate treatment to ensure optimal outcomes.

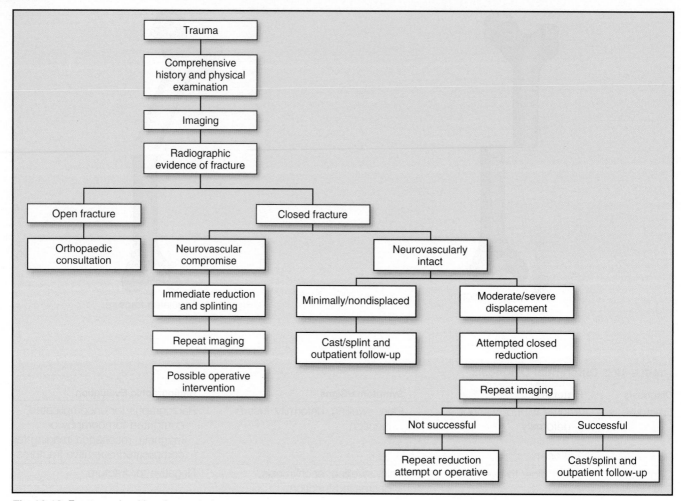

Fig 12.12 Fracture algorithm for acute trauma.

Suggested Readings

Buckwalter JA. Fracture principles. In: Griffen LY, eds. *Essentials of Musculoskeletal Care*. 3rd ed. Rosemont, IL: American Academy of Orthopaedic Surgeons; 2005:62.

Egol KA, Koval KJ, Zuckerman JD, eds. *Handbook of Fractures*. 5th ed. Philadelphia: Lippincott Williams & Wilkins; 2015.

Eiff MP, Calmbach WL, Hatch RL. *Fracture Management for Primary Care*. 3rd ed. Philadelphia: Elsevier; 2011.

Geiderman JM. General principles of orthopedic injuries. In: Marx JA, Hockberger RS, Walls RM, eds. *Rosen's Emergency Medicine: Concepts and Clinical Practice*. 8th ed. Philadelphia: Elsevier; 2013.

Green NE, Swiontkowski MF, eds. *Skeletal Trauma in Children*. 4th ed. Philadelphia: Saunders; 2009.

Menkes J. Initial evaluation and management of orthopedic injuries. In: Tintanalli JE, Kelen GD, Stapczynski S, eds. *Emergency Medicine: a Comprehensive Study Guide*. 8th ed. New York: McGraw-Hill; 2016.

Miller MD, Thompson SR, eds. *DeLee and Drez's Orthopaedic Sports Medicine: Principles and Practice*. 34th ed. Philadelphia: Elsevier; 2014.

Perron AD, German CA, et al. Approach to musculoskeletal injuries. In: Harwood-Nuss AL, Wolfson AB, Linder CH, eds. *Clinical Practice of Emergency Medicine*. 6th ed. Philadelphia: Lippincott Williams & Wilkins; 2015:237.

Chapter 13 Trauma: Compartment Syndrome

Stephen Shaheen, Jeffrey R. Bytomski

ICD-10-CM CODES
M79.Ax   *Compartment syndrome, nontraumatic*
T79.Ax   *Compartment syndrome, traumatic*
(Both require an expansion of the placeholder "x" for transformation into a billable code)

Key Concepts

- Skeletal muscles are contained within distinct osseofascial compartments throughout the body.
  - Compartment syndrome is caused by an increase in pressure within these relatively noncompliant compartments.
- Compartment syndrome can be acute or chronic.
  - Acute compartment syndrome (ACS) is an emergency and can lead to permanent functional loss if not treated.
  - Chronic exertional compartment syndrome usually presents with exercise-induced symptoms that resolve with rest.
- Elevated compartment pressures in ACS can result from internal or external factors.
  - Internal: Fluid accumulation within the compartment, secondary to hemorrhage or edema, diminishes the space available for the muscles and nerves.
  - External: Compression or traction of the limb can lead to change in the size/volume of the compartments.
- Epidemiology
  - 3.1 per 100,000 in Western populations
  - Male-to-female predominance of 10:1, which is believed to be reflective of the increased male presence in acute trauma
  - Higher incidence in younger (<35 years old) men, which may reflect the increased muscle mass within the compartments in this population
  - Equal incidence of both high- and low-energy injuries
  - Fractures are the most common cause of ACS (69% of cases)
    - Occurs in both open and closed fractures
    - Most common fractures
      - Tibial diaphyseal fractures
        - 1-11% incidence of ACS (approximately 40% of all compartment syndromes)
      - Forearm (radius/ulna) diaphyseal fractures
        - 3% incidence of ACS
      - Distal radius fractures
        - 0.25% incidence of ACS

- Etiology
  - Fractures
  - Soft-tissue trauma/crush injury
  - Vascular injury
  - Bleeding diatheses or anticoagulation leading to hemorrhage/hematoma
  - Burns (soft-tissue contracture)
  - Constrictive circumferential dressings/casts
  - Skeletal traction for fracture reduction
  - Fluid extravasation (e.g., intravenous fluids, contrast dye)
  - Intramedullary reaming during fracture fixation (forces blood and marrow into surrounding compartments)
  - Surgical positioning (through direct pressure or certain positioning; i.e., Lloyd-Davies for colorectal surgery)
  - Prolonged recumbent position leading to limb compression (e.g., drug overdose)
  - Reperfusion after prolonged ischemia
  - Abscess/infection
- Pathophysiology
  - Increased intracompartmental pressure results in a progressive pathologic pathway:
    - Alteration in arteriovenous pressure gradient
    - Diminished capillary perfusion
    - Cellular anoxia
    - Muscle and nerve ischemia
    - Tissue necrosis
    - Functional impairment of the limb
  - Elevated intracompartmental pressure leads to a reduction in venous outflow, which in turn increases interstitial pressure, contributing to edema formation—a continuously worsening cycle.
  - Tissue ischemia can also lead to an increase in vascular permeability and exacerbate the intracompartmental pressure elevations.
    - The innermost muscle fibers are the first to become ischemic, with progression to peripheral muscle involvement in a centrifugal fashion.
  - The magnitude and duration of elevated intracompartmental pressure that determines the extent of muscle and nerve ischemia and necrosis.
- Locations
  - Upper extremity
    - Shoulder girdle
    - Arm (two compartments: anterior and posterior)
    - Forearm (three compartments: dorsal, volar, and mobile wad)
    - Hand (10 compartments)

- Lower extremity
  - Buttock
  - Thigh (three compartments: anterior, posterior, and adductor)
  - Leg (four compartments: anterior, lateral, superficial, and deep posterior)
    - most common location
  - Foot (nine compartments)
- Spinal musculature

History

- ACS is a clinical diagnosis that is supported by compartment measurements; making the diagnosis and deciding when to treat can be a challenge.
- A high clinical suspicion must be maintained so that the diagnosis is not missed.
- It is important to understand the mechanism of injury; ACS most often occurs after a traumatic event.
- Inquire about other risk factors such as age, anticoagulants, bleeding diatheses (i.e., hemophilia), or other medical comorbidities (i.e., neuropathy, hypotension, or shock).

Physical Examination

- Swelling, discoloration, or blistering of the skin (Fig. 13.1)
- Limb compartment palpation/manual compression to estimate tension
- Active and passive motion of involved limb
- Muscle strength
- Sensory function
- Vascular status:
  - Close monitoring with serial examinations is critical because the development of compartment syndrome can occur over hours to days.
  - The diagnosis is made by considering the entire clinical picture, because no examination finding is pathognomonic.
  - Individually the classic P signs (*p*ain, *p*ulselessness, *p*aresis/*p*aralysis, *p*aresthesias, *p*ressure, and *p*allor) can be absent or equivocal. However, together, the constellation of signs and symptoms including severe or intensifying pain, firm compartments, and sensory changes are strong indicators of an ACS.

Early Signs

- Pain:
  - Pain with passive movement—one of the most sensitive signs (Fig. 13.2)
  - May not be elicited in the involved extremity if the patient has altered mental status, a concomitant nerve injury, other distracting injuries, or received anesthesia
  - Severe or progressive pain, especially with an increasing narcotic requirement
- Pressure:
  - Increased tension of muscle compartments may be the only sign
  - Difficult to quantitate clinically—assessment subjective and unreliable
    - Deep posterior compartment cannot be palpated
- Paresthesias (Fig. 13.3):
  - Herald ischemia of the nerves within the involved compartments
    - Occurs early because nerves are sensitive to anoxia
  - Can progress to hypoesthesia and, later, irreversible motor and sensory loss
  - Can also be present with nerve injuries and are not specific for ACS

Late Signs

- Paresis/paralysis (Fig. 13.4)
  - Difficult to distinguish between direct muscle/nerve injury or inhibition secondary to pain
  - Found in established, late-stage compartment syndrome—full recovery is doubtful
- Pallor/pulselessness
  - Palpable pulse can be misleading and does not rule out compartment syndrome.
  - Peripheral pulses and capillary refill are always found unless a vascular injury is present.

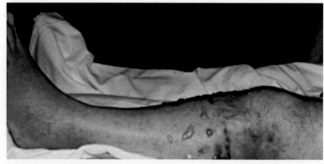

Fig 13.1 Appearance of acute compartment syndrome. (From Amendola A, Twaddle BC. Compartment syndromes. In: Browner BD, Jupiter JB, Levine AM, Trafton PG, eds. *Skeletal Trauma: Basic Science, Management, and Reconstruction*. 3rd ed. Philadelphia: Saunders; 2003:271.)

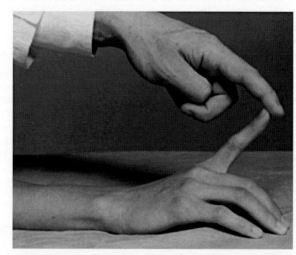

Fig 13.2 Passive stretch test. (From Amendola A, Twaddle BC. Compartment syndromes. In: Browner BD, Jupiter JB, Levine AM, Trafton PG, eds. *Skeletal Trauma: Basic Science, Management, and Reconstruction*. 3rd ed. Philadelphia: Saunders; 2003:271.)

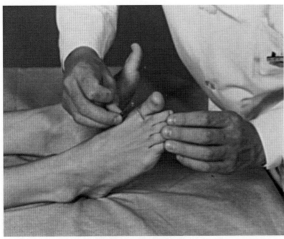

Fig 13.3 Sensory assessment of first dorsal webspace. (From Amendola A, Twaddle BC. Compartment syndromes. In: Browner BD, Jupiter JB, Levine AM, Trafton PG, eds. *Skeletal Trauma: Basic Science, Management, and Reconstruction*. 3rd ed. Philadelphia: Saunders; 2003:272.)

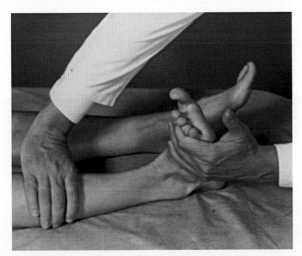

Fig 13.4 Muscle strength testing. (From Amendola A, Twaddle BC. Compartment syndromes. In: Browner BD, Jupiter JB, Levine AM, Trafton PG, eds. *Skeletal Trauma: Basic Science, Management, and Reconstruction*. 3rd ed. Philadelphia: Saunders; 2003: 272.)

- Ischemia in compartment syndrome is secondary to decreased capillary perfusion, not interruption of arterial inflow.
- Consider an angiogram if pulses cannot be found.

Imaging

- Radiographs
  - To diagnose fractures
- Angiogram
  - If pulses are absent and vascular injury is suspected
- Near-infrared spectroscopy, magnetic resonance imaging, scintigraphy, laser flow Doppler scan
  - No proven diagnostic utility in the setting of ACS

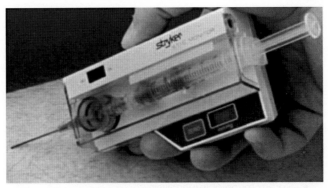

Fig 13.5 Stryker solid-state transducer intracompartment catheter. (From Amendola A, Twaddle BC. Compartment syndromes. In: Browner BD, Jupiter JB, Levine AM, Trafton PG, eds. *Skeletal Trauma: Basic Science, Management, and Reconstruction*. 3rd ed. Philadelphia: Saunders; 2003:281.)

Additional Tests

- Compartment pressure monitoring
  - Only objective measurement
  - Most commonly a solid-state transducer intracompartment (STIC) catheter in acute situations (Fig. 13.5)
  - Resting compartment pressures: 0 to 8 mm Hg
  - Record the compartment pressure at the level of the fracture where the pressures are the highest
    - pressure varies significantly if as little as 5 cm from the fracture
  - Measure all four compartments in leg injuries
    - anterior compartment is most commonly affected
    - anterior and deep posterior compartments typically have the highest pressures
- Absolute pressure
  - Controversy existed regarding the actual pressure at which compartment syndrome developed; pressures of 30, 40, and 50 mm Hg had been proposed as the indicators for fasciotomy.
    - These pressures were selected because they exceeded the normal capillary blood pressure of 20 to 30 mm Hg.
  - Variations in tolerance to elevated intracompartmental pressure have been observed among individuals, believed to be secondary to differences in systemic blood pressures.
- Pressure differential
  - Pressure at which ischemia occurs has not been delineated; studies now indicate that the difference between compartment pressure and diastolic blood pressure (ΔP) determines muscle perfusion.
    - ΔP = (diastolic blood pressure) − (intracompartmental pressure)
      - Difference of less than 30 mm Hg has been supported as the point at which tissue perfusion pressure is compromised
  - Postischemic muscle is more vulnerable to elevation in pressures—hypoxic changes are observed at a ΔP of less than 40 mm Hg.

- Laboratory studies
  - Complete blood count with differential
    - Can detect extensive blood loss/extravasation or be used as an indicator of infection
  - Chemistry panel with blood urea nitrogen/creatinine
    - Evaluate for electrolyte abnormalities and assess renal function
  - C-reactive protein/erythrocyte sedimentation rate
    - If infection suspected
  - International normalized ratio/prothrombin time and partial thromboplastin time
    - To evaluate for anticoagulant use, coagulopathy
  - Serum myoglobin/urinalysis
    - Evaluate for rhabdomyolysis

Differential Diagnosis

- Vascular or neurogenic claudication: pain relieved with rest or pain related to position
- Venous insufficiency: leg discoloration, varicose veins, heart disease
- Deep vein thrombosis: consider duplex scan to rule out
- Lymphedema/congestive heart failure: frequently pitting is present with palpation
- Hematoma: focal swelling, history of trauma
- Neuropathy: consider if history of diabetes, other neuropathic conditions
- Tenosynovitis: pain with passive stretch and tenderness along path of tendons, focal swelling of digit
- Deep infection/abscess/pyomyositis/cellulitis/necrotizing fasciitis: history of penetrating trauma, open wound, monitor for sepsis, elevated infection markers
- Complex regional pain syndrome: chronic, mild swelling, hypersensitivity
- Stress fracture: history of repetitive athletic activity or distance running

Treatment

- Remove compressive dressings or cast, if present.
- Maintain limb at level of heart or below—elevation may impede optimal limb perfusion.
- Avoid systemic hypotension.
- Apply supplemental oxygen to assist in preventing tissue hypoxia.
- Surgical fasciotomy
  - Lower leg (Figs. 13.6 and 13.7)
    - Must decompress all four compartments.
    - One or two incision techniques are available.
      - Incisions 16 cm in length have been shown to be required for adequate decompression.
    - Avoid injury:
      - Anterior and lateral fascial incisions: superficial peroneal nerve
      - Deep posterior compartment: tibial nerve, posterior tibial vessels
  - Thigh
    - Often can be adequately decompressed through a single lateral incision.
      - Second medial incision may be necessary to release the adductor compartment.

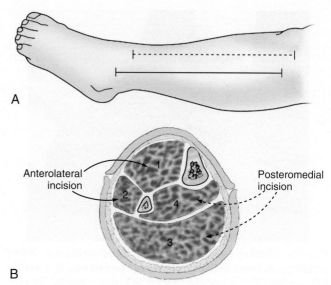

Fig 13.6 **(A)** Illustration of two-incision fasciotomy technique for the lower leg. Incisions should be at least 16 cm in length. **(B)** Axial diagram of the lower leg demonstrating how all four compartments can be decompressed through the two-incision technique. (Adapted from Amendola A, Twaddle BC. Compartment syndromes. In: Browner BD, Jupiter JB, Levine AM, Trafton PG, eds. *Skeletal Trauma: Basic Science, Management, and Reconstruction*. 3rd ed. Philadelphia: Saunders; 2003:286.)

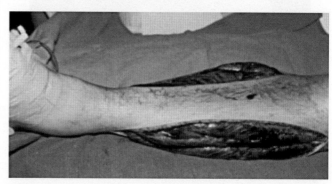

Fig 13.7 Lower extremity fasciotomy incisions. (From Amendola A, Twaddle BC. Compartment syndromes. In: Browner BD, Jupiter JB, Levine AM, Trafton PG, eds. *Skeletal Trauma: Basic Science, Management, and Reconstruction*. 3rd ed. Philadelphia: Saunders; 2003:287.)

- Arm
  - Anterior and posterior incisions
  - Rarely, the deltoid muscle must be released separately.
- Forearm (Figs. 13.8 and 13.9)
  - Volar incision from the wrist to the elbow first; then reassess dorsal compartment pressure
    - Often the volar incision is enough to decompress both
  - If the pressures remain elevated, a separate, second dorsal incision can be made.
- Hands and feet
  - Two dorsal incisions, over the second and fourth metacarpals or metatarsals

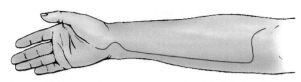

Fig 13.8 Anterior fasciotomy incision of the forearm. (Adapted from Amendola A, Twaddle BC. Compartment syndromes. In: Browner BD, Jupiter JB, Levine AM, Trafton PG, eds. *Skeletal Trauma: Basic Science, Management, and Reconstruction*. 3rd ed. Philadelphia: Saunders; 2003:283.)

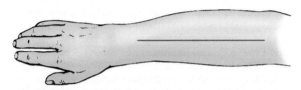

Fig 13.9 Dorsal fasciotomy incision of the forearm. (Adapted from Amendola A, Twaddle BC. Compartment syndromes. In: Browner BD, Jupiter JB, Levine AM, Trafton PG, eds. *Skeletal Trauma: Basic Science, Management, and Reconstruction*. 3rd ed. Philadelphia: Saunders; 2003:284.)

- Foot may require a separate medial incision to adequately decompress the plantar and hindfoot compartments.
- Management of fasciotomy wounds
  - Primary skin closure is avoided to ensure adequate compartment decompression.
  - Vacuum-assisted closure dressings are now frequently used to cover wounds and may assist in reducing tissue edema.
  - Operating room reassessment of tissue viability in 24 to 48 hours
    - Necrotic tissue must be debrided to reduce the risk of infection.
    - Delayed skin closure may be performed at this time if swelling has adequately resolved.
      - Split-thickness skin grafts may be required to cover wounds.
- Treatment algorithm (Fig. 13.10)

When to Refer
- No role for conservative management
- Definitive management is surgery.
  - An orthopaedic surgeon should be promptly consulted if the diagnosis of ACS is suspected.

Prognosis
- Compartment syndrome is a surgical emergency.
- Surgical decompression should be performed as soon as the diagnosis is made.
  - Ideal time for fasciotomy is within 6 hours of onset.
  - Can be difficult to determine the onset or duration
- Muscles can withstand 4 to 6 hours of anoxic insult.

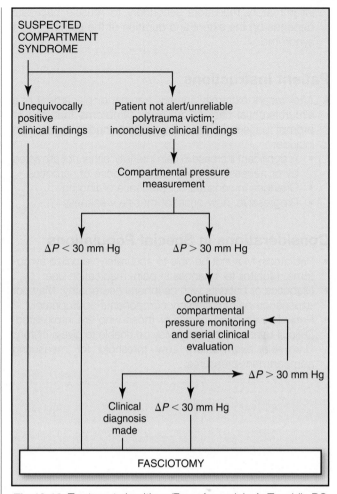

Fig 13.10 Treatment algorithm. (From Amendola A, Twaddle BC. Compartment syndromes. In: Browner BD, Jupiter JB, Levine AM, Trafton PG, eds. *Skeletal Trauma: Basic Science, Management, and Reconstruction*. 3rd ed. Philadelphia: Saunders; 2003:274.)

- After 6 hours, complete functional recovery cannot be guaranteed; beyond 8 to 12 hours, damage is irreversible.
- Once paralysis and sensory deficits are present (6 to 8 hours), delayed fasciotomies are not recommended—the necrotic tissue becomes a medium for infection.

Complications
- Muscle necrosis
- Muscle and tendon scarring
- Volkmann's ischemic contractures
- Delayed fracture healing
- Infection
- Permanent weakness or sensory loss, especially around the incision sites
- Amputation for insensate or nonfunctional limb or severe infection
- Crush syndrome/reperfusion injury: acute renal failure and organ damage from release of myoglobin and other

inflammatory mediators secondary to muscle necrosis; depends on the extent and duration of the compartment syndrome

Patient Instructions

- After recent extremity surgery, trauma, or placement of a circumferential cast or dressing, symptoms that should prompt patients to seek immediate medical evaluation include:
  - A significant increase in pain intensity, either not alleviated by or necessitating an increasing dose of narcotics
  - Changes in sensation or presence of tingling
  - Progressive, new onset of muscle weakness

Considerations in Special Populations

- Pediatrics: May not be able to accurately verbalize symptoms. Monitor for changes in pain, medication use.
- Diabetics or patients with peripheral neuropathy: May not experience pain or sensory components appropriately.
- Patients with head injuries or those who are intoxicated: Difficult to assess clinically. May be unable to give a history. Unreliable examination. Low threshold for measuring compartment pressures.

Suggested Readings

Amendola A, Twaddle BC. Compartment syndromes. In: Browner BD, Jupiter JB, Levine AM, Trafton PG, eds. *Skeletal Trauma: Basic Science, Management, and Reconstruction*. 3rd ed. Philadelphia: Saunders; 2003:268–292.

Elliot K, Johnstone A. Diagnosing acute compartment syndrome. *J Bone Joint Surg Br*. 2003;85B:625–632.

Garner MR, Taylor SA, Gausden E, Lyden JP. Compartment syndrome: diagnosis, management, and unique concerns in the twenty-first century. *HSS J*. 2014;10(2):143–152.

Jobe MT. Compartment syndromes and Volkmann contracture. In: Azar FM, Beaty JH, Canale ST, eds. *Campbell's Operative Orthopaedics*. 13th ed. Philadelphia: Elsevier; 2017:3722–3733.

Konstantakos EK, Dalstrom DJ, Nelles ME, et al. Diagnosis and management of extremity compartment syndromes: an orthopaedic perspective. *Am Surg*. 2007;73(12):1199–1209.

McQueen M. Compartment syndrome. In: Bucholz RW, Heckman JD, Court-Browne C, eds. *Rockwood and Green's Fractures in Adults*. 6th ed. Philadelphia: Lippincott Williams & Wilkins; 2005:425–443.

Olson S, Glasgow R. Acute compartment syndrome in lower extremity musculoskeletal trauma. *J Am Acad Orthop Surg*. 2005;13:436–444.

von Keudell AG, Weaver MJ, Appleton PT, et al. Diagnosis and treatment of acute extremity compartment syndrome. *Lancet*. 2015;386(10000):1299–1310.

Whitesides TE, Heckman MM. Acute compartment syndrome: update on diagnosis and treatment. *J Am Acad Orthop Surg*. 1996;4(4):209–218.

Chapter 14 Trauma: Heterotopic Ossification and Myositis Ossificans

Mario Ciocca

ICD-10-CM CODES
M61.50   *Myositis ossificans*
M89.8X9   *Heterotopic ossification*

Key Concepts

- Refers to abnormal deposition of lamellar bone in soft tissue structures; often associated with trauma but may result from a number of other etiologies
- First described nearly 1000 years ago in the healing of fractures.
- Formation closely resembles the physiology of fracture healing.
- Tissues with a heightened or prolonged inflammatory response to injury are prone to heterotopic ossification.
- The true mechanism for the development of heterotopic ossification is uncertain, although prerequisites needed for development include
  - A signaling protein (bone morphogenic protein) secreted from cells of injured tissue or inflammatory cells
  - A supply of mesenchymal cells that can differentiate into osteoblasts or chondroblasts
    - An appropriate environment conducive to osteogenesis
- Posttraumatic heterotopic ossification occurs most frequently in the hip. Elbow injuries are the second leading cause.
- More common in males

History

- Recent trauma or surgery followed by pain and an increase in joint stiffness
- Usually develops 3 to 12 weeks after injury

Physical Examination

- Joint erythema, warmth, edema, and limited range of motion

Imaging

- Radiographic abnormalities can be seen within 18 to 21 days but may take 4 to 5 weeks to develop and should be present by 8 weeks.
- Nuclear medicine bone scan is the most sensitive imaging modality for early heterotopic ossification and can be used to indicate whether the lesion is active or has matured. It is usually positive by 2 to 4 weeks and can be used to predict the optimal timing for surgical resection.
- Ultrasound can detect heterotopic ossification sooner than radiographs, computed tomography, or magnetic resonance imaging, and enables early identification and treatment.
- Magnetic resonance imaging is not typically used but can identify a nonspecific soft-tissue mass within the first few weeks. Magnetic resonance imaging may be useful in the preoperative setting to help describe relationships to other structures.
- Computed tomography can delineate zonal pattern of calcification and can be diagnostic before radiographs.
- Computed tomography with three-dimensional reconstruction may be used for preoperative planning.

Additional Tests

- Sedimentation rate may be elevated in the early stages.
- Alkaline phosphatase elevates after 3 weeks, reaches 3.5 times normal at 4 weeks, peaks at 11 to 12 weeks, and normalizes when the bone matures.
- Calcium decreases briefly and then normalizes when serum alkaline phosphatase increases.
- Prostaglandin E_2 excretion in a 24-hour urine collection may be increased.
- Creatinine kinase may be elevated.

Differential Diagnosis

- Clinically the early inflammatory stage may be confused with cellulitis, deep venous thrombosis, thrombophlebitis, or osteomyelitis.
- An early lesion may be misdiagnosed as a soft-tissue osteosarcoma, whereas a late lesion may be mistaken for parosteal osteosarcoma.
- Differential diagnosis may also include abscess, soft tissue recurrence of giant cell tumor of bone, extraskeletal osteosarcoma, and melorheostosis.

Treatment
Early (Prevention After Injury)

- Gentle range of motion within a pain-free zone
- Nonsteroidal antiinflammatory drugs have been effective after total hip arthroplasty. The mechanism of action includes inhibition of differentiation of mesenchymal cells into osteogenic cells and suppression of the prostaglandin-mediated inflammatory response.
  - Indomethacin often used for 2 to 6 weeks
  - Selective cyclooxygenase (COX)-2 inhibitors may be equally effective

- Radiation
  - Has been effective prophylactically for perioperative care of total hip arthroplasty
  - May inhibit the differentiation of pluripotent mesenchymal cells into osteoblasts
  - Complications include soft tissue contracture, delayed wound healing, and theoretically malignancy
  - Equally effective as nonsteroidal antiinflammatory drugs

Later (If Heterotopic Ossification Develops)

- Physical Therapy
- Bisphosphonates
  - Have been effective in neurogenic heterotopic ossification
  - May be effective in other forms of heterotopic ossification including burns and spinal cord injury
  - Mechanisms include
    - Inhibition of precipitation of calcium phosphate
    - Delaying aggregation of hydroxyapatite crystals
    - Blocking conversion of calcium phosphate into hydroxyapatite
  - May develop rebound and bone growth after discontinuation due to resumption of osteoid mineralization while osteoclast function remains suppressed
  - May need long-term treatment (at least 6 months)
- Radiation has been used in heterotopic ossification related to spinal cord injury and in conjunction with removal of heterotopic ossification
- Extracorporeal shock wave therapy has been used successfully
- Surgery
  - Indications
    - Peripheral nerve compromise due to compression
    - Persistent pain
    - Impaired range of motion not amenable to conservative measures
  - Need to combine with nonsteroidal antiinflammatory drugs and/or radiation
  - Resection can generally be performed after 6 to 9 months and usually after bone matures.
  - Earlier resection with secondary prophylaxis with single-dose radiation or nonsteroidal antiinflammatory medications may be safe.

- Early surgical intervention may provide more effective rehabilitation and dramatic improvements in patient function.

When to Refer

- Refer to surgeon for indications listed.

Troubleshooting

- Delayed treatment of an initial injury may increase the risk of developing heterotopic ossification.
- Removal of ectopic bone before maturation may lead to an increased risk of recurrence.

Patient Instructions

- Educate on the importance of early rest, ice, compression, and elevation and stretching.
- Educate on earlier treatment leading to quicker recovery and less risk of heterotopic ossification.
- Inform physician if pain, swelling, or loss of motion persists or recurs, or a mass can be felt.

Specific Clinical Entities
Myositis Ossificans

- Usually occurs after muscle contusion but can be secondary to strain or repetitive use (Fig. 14.1)
- Incidence 9-20% and related to severity of contusion
- Most common in adolescent or young adult males
- Most common sites are larger muscle groups including quadriceps, thigh adductors, and brachialis
- After trauma, a mass may appear 1 to 2 days later, reach 4 to 10 cm after 1 to 2 months, and then mature and harden. It may become smaller but rarely disappears.
- Should be suspected if pain and swelling do not resolve 4 to 5 days after a muscle contusion
- Physical exam includes tenderness, swelling, decreased range of motion, and warmth. A firm mass may be palpated later.
- Treat contusion with rest, ice, compression, and elevation, and place muscle in the stretch position.

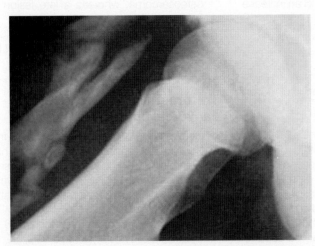

- Occurs in large muscle groups after contusion/strain
- Rx contusion: rest, ice, compression, elevation, and place muscle in stretch position
- Aspirate hematoma
- NSAIDs for prophylaxis
- Suspect myositis ossificans:
  - Swelling and tenderness persist
  - Decreased ROM
  - Mass palpated

Fig 14.1 Myositis ossificans. *NSAID,* Nonsteroidal antiinflammatory drug; *ROM,* range of motion.

- If hematoma present, may need to aspirate.
- Nonsteroidal antiinflammatory drugs have been used to treat muscle contusions (2 to 6 weeks) as preventive treatment for myositis ossificans.
- Ultrasound or heat should be avoided in the acute phase of a muscle contusion.
- Refer for surgery if the patient is symptomatic with muscle atrophy and/or decreased joint motion.

Heterotopic Ossification of Hip

- Most common site
- High incidence after open reduction of acetabular fractures or total hip arthroplasty
- Prophylactic radiation or nonsteroidal antiinflammatory drugs can reduce incidence.
- Risk factors include male sex, previous history of heterotopic ossification of either hip, ankylosing spondylitis, obesity, older age, and osteoarthritis.
- Generally asymptomatic but can cause stiffness, pain, and impaired function
- Can also occur after hip arthroscopy, although incidence is lower

Heterotopic Ossification After Elbow Trauma

- Can occur after distal humerus fracture, Monteggia fracture, olecranon fracture, radial head fracture, dislocation, and fracture-dislocation
- Risk of developing is 16-20% with a fracture/dislocation (Fig. 14.2)
- Risk increased with multiple reduction attempts
- Risk increases with fracture severity
- Most common extrinsic cause of elbow contracture

- Symptoms include pain, stiffness, sensory loss, weakness, and possibly a palpable mass.
- Usually present 6 weeks after injury
- Those at risk of developing heterotopic ossification may receive preventive nonsteroidal antiinflammatory drugs or radiation after injury.
- If functionally limiting, can treat surgically combined with prophylactic nonsteroidal antiinflammatory drugs or radiation
- Also seen from chronic use involving ulnar collateral ligament
  - Chronic stress leading to edema and inflammation followed by scarring, calcification, and ossification
  - Smoothly marginated and usually measures 4 to 5 mm × 1 to 2 mm
  - May have associated partial or complete tear of the ligament
  - May develop heterotopic ossification on medial epicondyle side after reconstruction of ulnar collateral ligament

Pellegrini-Stieda Syndrome

- Refers to ossification in the medial collateral ligament of the knee; may also involve the adductor magnus tendon (Fig. 14.3)
- Usually occurs adjacent to medial femoral epicondyle
- First described in the early 1900s
- Usually develops 3 to 4 weeks after injury
- Medial side swelling, pain, stiffness, and possibly a palpable mass.
- May be due to direct or indirect injury

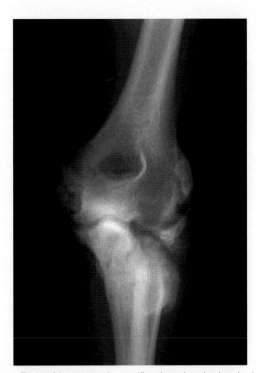

Fig 14.2 Risk of heterotopic ossification developing is 16-20% with a fracture/dislocation.

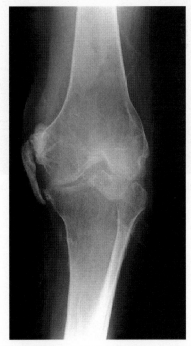

Fig 14.3 Pellegrini-Stieda syndrome refers to ossification in the medial collateral ligament of the knee and may also involve the adductor magnus tendon. (From Altschuler B. *Pellegrini-Stieda Syndrome*, vol. 354. Copyright 2006 Massachusetts Medical Society. All rights reserved.)

- May be a type of myositis ossificans, but theories of origin include
  - Hematoma formation that later calcifies
  - Direct metaplasia of the ligament
  - An avulsion fragment with subperiosteal proliferation of bone
  - Traumatic tear of the adductor magnus tendon with periosteal new bone formation
- Ossification may occur in as many as 3% of knee injuries.
- Calcification may increase in size or may eventually recede.
- Surgical removal is indicated for a painful mass or a large mass that limits motion.

Heterotopic Ossification of Tibiofibular Syndesmosis

- Calcification of the syndesmosis can develop as a complication of fracture or ligamentous injury (Fig. 14.4).

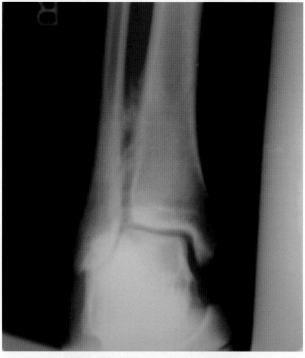

Fig 14.4 Calcification of the syndesmosis can develop as a complication of injuries to the ankle.

- Increased incidence in males, use of syndesmotic screw, tibiotalar dislocation, and Weber Type-C fractures
- Can occur in syndesmotic sprains whether treated conservatively or surgically
- Can be seen 3 to 12 months after injury
- Persistent pain and a palpable mass develop
- May lose range of motion in plantar and dorsal flexion
- If symptomatic, can undergo operative excision, although there is a risk of recurrence

Blast Injury

- Recent increase due to increased survival rate from rapid medical care in combat areas
- Incidence over 60% in combat-related amputation
- War-traumatized tissue contains elevated levels of osteogenic progenitor cells and upregulation of multiple osteogenic genes
- Causes difficulty in rehabilitation and long-term prosthetic use

Suggested Readings

Bedi A, Zbedu RM, Bueno VF, et al. The incidence of heterotopic ossification after hip arthroscopy. *Am J Sports Med*. 2012;40(4):854–863.

Dey D, Wheatley BM, Cholok D, et al. The traumatic bone: trauma-induced heterotopic ossification. *Transl Res*. 2017;186:95–111.

Edwards DS, Clasper JC. Heterotopic ossification: a systematic review. *J R Army Med Corps*. 2015;161:315–321.

Keschner MT, Paksima N. The stiff elbow. *Bull NYU Hosp Jt Dis*. 2007;65:24–28.

Marvan J, Dzupa V, Krbec M, et al. Distal tibiofibular synostosis after surgically resolved ankle fractures: an epidemiological, clinical and morphological evaluation of a patient sample. *Injury*. 2016;47:2570–2574.

Mulligan SA, Schwartz ML, Broussard MF, Andrews JR. Heterotopic calcification and tears of the ulnar collateral ligament: radiographic and MR imaging findings. *AJR Am J Roentgenol*. 2000;175:1099–1102.

Nauth A, Giles E, Potter BK, et al. Heterotopic ossification in orthopaedic trauma. *J Orthop Trauma*. 2012;26(12):684–688.

Niitsu M, Ikeda K, Iijima T, et al. MR imaging of Pellegrini-Stieda disease. *Radiat Med*. 1999;17:405–409.

Sferopoulos NK, Kotakidou R, Petropoulos AS. Myositis ossificans in children: a review. *Eur J Orthop Surg Traumatol*. 2017;27:491–502.

Shukla DR, Pillai G, McAnany S, et al. Heterotopic ossification formation after fracture-dislocations of the elbow. *J Shoulder Elbow Surg*. 2015;24:333–338.

Walczac BE, Johnson CN, Howe BM, et al. Myositis ossificans. *J Am Acad Orthop Surg*. 2015;23:612–622.

Wang JC, Shapiro MS. Pellegrini-Stieda syndrome. *Am J Orthop*. 1995;24:493–497.

Chapter 15 Arthritides

Adam Carlson

ICD-10-CM CODES
M19   Osteoarthritis
M10   Gout
M11   Calcium Pyrophosphate Deposition Disease
M05   Rheumatoid Arthritis
L40.5 Psoriatic Arthritis
M02   Reactive/Postinfective Arthritis
M32   Systemic Lupus Erythematosus

Key Concepts (Fig. 15.1)

- A healthy articular joint such as the hip or knee is composed of two bony surfaces lined with hyaline cartilage that are surrounded by a joint capsule. The capsule is lined with a thin synovial membrane that is no more than a few cell layers thick.
- Articular joints move freely and painlessly with a low coefficient of friction due to the smooth surfaces of articular cartilage and the lubricating properties of synovial fluid.
- Joint pain due to arthritis arises from damage to articular surfaces and tension on the joint capsule from effusions. Joint damage can occur from several different processes including mechanical stresses over time, trauma, crystal deposition, primary joint inflammation, and primary joint infection.
- The hallmarks of inflammatory joint pain include stiffness and pain that are most pronounced in the morning. These symptoms improve with activity and return after periods of rest. Prolonged stiffness is a key historical feature of inflammatory joint pain. Morning stiffness typically lasts more than 1 hour in individuals with inflammatory joint disease.
- In contrast to inflammatory joint pain, mechanical joint pain is typically worse with activity and improves with rest. Morning stiffness may be present, though it tends to improve within 30 minutes of activity.
- Additional features are important to consider as they may help narrow the differential diagnosis. Important features of arthritis include the duration of symptoms, the number of joint involved, the size of joints involved, symmetry of joint involvement, pattern of onset (episodic, additive, migratory, etc.), and axial involvement (SI joints and spine; Boxes 15.1 to 15.3).
- Acute (<2 weeks) joint pain and swelling requires a rapid workup and must include synovial fluid analysis including gram stain and cultures to evaluate for a bacterial infection suggestive of septic arthritis. Septic arthritis may lead to rapid joint damage and can be life threatening if left untreated.

Osteoarthritis

- Osteoarthritis (OA) arises due to degeneration of joint surfaces from mechanical stress over time or from prior trauma. Articular cartilage loss exposes underlying bone, ultimately resulting in the downstream activation of pain/sensory nerve endings in the subchondral bone.

History

- The hips, knees, and the first metatarsophalangeal joint (MTP) of the foot are the most common lower extremity joints affected. The first carpometacarpal joint (CMC), distal interphalangeal joints (DIPs), and proximal interphalangeal joints (PIPs) of the hands are the most commonly affected joints in the upper extremity. In the absence of trauma or other conditions, osteoarthritis is uncommon in the wrist, shoulder, and ankle.
- Pain related to osteoarthritis is worse with use of the involved joint and improves with rest.
- Stiffness typically resolves within 30 minutes of activity.

Physical Examination

- Vital signs
  - Usually normal
- Gait
  - Often antalgic with lower extremity joint involvement
- Joints
  - Joint effusions may be present
  - Bony swelling may be observed due to osteophyte formation.
  - Joints affected by osteoarthritis are rarely warm to touch. Joint temperature should be assessed by comparing the temperature of the joint to a neighboring large muscle group. Normal joints are cooler than the area over normal muscle bellies.
  - Joint range of motion may be limited, with pain at the endpoints of motion. On hip examination, internal rotation will often elicit pain when hip OA is present
  - Joint lines may be tender to palpation
  - Joint crepitations may be present.
  - Ligament stability is usually unaffected in early disease but may occur in late disease.

Imaging

- Radiographic hallmarks of osteoarthritis include joint space narrowing (which may be asymmetric in weight bearing joints), osteophytes, joint line sclerosis, and subchondral cysts (Fig. 15.2).

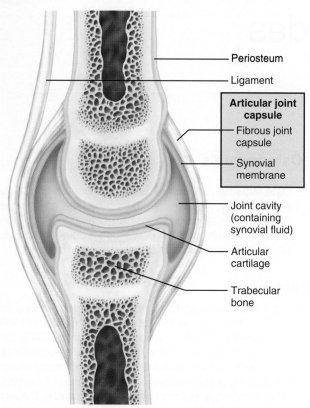

Fig 15.1 Anatomy of a synovial joint. (Redrawn from Mescher AL. *Junqueira's Basic Histology Text & Atlas*. 13th ed. New York: McGraw-Hill; 2013.)

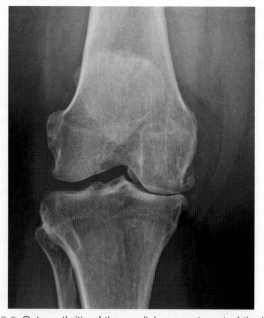

Fig 15.2 Osteoarthritis of the medial compartment of the knee. Classic radiographic features seen here include asymmetric joint space narrowing, osteophyte formation, and joint line sclerosis.

BOX 15.1   Causes of Acute Arthritis

Acute Monoarthritis

Septic arthritis
    Gonococcal
    Nongonococcal
Acute crystalline arthritis
    Gout
    Pseudogout (acute CPPD)
Trauma

Acute Oligoarthritis

Septic arthritis
    Gonococcal—often migratory
    Nongonococcal—up to 25% of cases involve >1 joint

Lyme Arthritis

Postinfectious arthritis
    Rheumatic fever
    Reactive arthritis
Acute sarcoid—Lofgren syndrome

Acute Polyarthritis

Viral infections
    Parvovirus B19
    Acute hepatitis B
    Hepatitis C
    HIV
Acute sarcoid—Lofgren syndrome
Atypical manifestations of systemic autoimmune disease
    Rheumatoid arthritis
    Psoriatic arthritis
    Systemic lupus

BOX 15.2   Causes of Chronic Noninflammatory Arthritis

Osteoarthritis
Internal and periarticular derangements
    Meniscal
    Ligament
    Tendon
    Labrum
Osteochondrosis dissecans
Osteonecrosis
Neuropathic arthritis (Charcot joint)

- Magnetic resonance imaging is more sensitive than plain films at detecting osteoarthritis and may show chondral defects and subchondral bone edema.
- Bone scans have no utility in the workup of osteoarthritis

Additional Tests

- Synovial fluid analysis will demonstrate either normal or noninflammatory joint fluid with <2000 white blood cells (WBCs; Table 15.1).

TABLE 15.1 Synovial Fluid Characteristics

Type of Fluid	WBC Count (cells/mm^3)	Clarity and Viscosity	Example
Normal	<500	Clear and viscous	Normal
Noninflammatory	500–2000	Translucent and viscous	Osteoarthritis
Inflammatory	2000–50,000	Opaque and watery	Rheumatoid arthritis Spondyloarthritis Crystalline disease
"Septic"	>50,000	Opaque and viscous	Bacterial infection Crystalline disease

BOX 15.3 Causes of Chronic Inflammatory Arthritis

Chronic Monoarthritis

Infection
    Gonococcal
    Nongonococcal
    Lyme arthritis
    Fungal arthritis
    Mycobacterial arthritis
    Syphilis
Tophaceous gout

Chronic Oligoarthritis

Tophaceous gout
Spondyloarthropathy
    Psoriatic arthritis
    Reactive arthritis
    Ankylosing spondylitis
    IBD related arthropathy
Rheumatoid arthritis
Systemic lupus erythematosus
Infection
    Lyme

Chronic Polyarthritis

Rheumatoid arthritis
Systemic lupus and related conditions
Spondyloarthropathy
Drug induced
    Lupus (hydralazine and others)
    Periostitis (voriconazole)
Tophaceous gout
Adult-onset Still's
Systemic vasculitis
Paraneoplastic

Differential Diagnosis

- Joint sprain
- Periarticular injury (e.g., tendonitis or bursitis)
- Ligament injury
- Meniscal/labral injury
- Osteochondritis dissecans
- Osteonecrosis/avascular necrosis (AVN)

Treatment

- Nonpharmacologic Therapy
  - Weight loss and activity modification can reduce stress across lower extremity joints.
  - Physical therapy strengthens the musculature that supports the affected joint.
  - Braces may assist in off-loading affected joints (e.g., unloader brace for knee OA).
- Pharmacologic Therapy
  - Acetaminophen is the safest first-line agent.
  - Nonsteroidal antiinflammatory drugs (NSAIDs) are often effective and can be combined with acetaminophen. Topical diclofenac is approved for hand and knee osteoarthritis and can be used in individuals with renal insufficiency or significant gastritis in whom NSAIDs are contraindicated.
  - Oral corticosteroids should be avoided in osteoarthritis.
  - Intra-articular injections often rapidly reduce pain but have been shown to lead to accelerated thinning of cartilage.
  - Intra-articular viscosupplementation with hyaluronic acid derivatives has been shown to reduce symptoms in mild to moderate arthritis and does not appear to contribute to progression of cartilage loss.
- Surgery—advanced disease only
  - Joint replacements are reasonably well tolerated and effective in the shoulder, hip, and knee.
  - CMC arthritis in the hand often improves with resection of the trapezoid.

Acute Crystalline Arthropathies (Gout and Pseudogout)

- Gout and pseudogout arise in response to precipitation of crystals in and around joints. There are acute and chronic forms of each condition. The acute manifestations of these two conditions are similar and only differentiated by identification of the causative crystal on microscopic analysis of the synovial fluid.

History

- Acute flares of crystalline arthritis typically over the course of hours to days.

- Patients report warm, swollen, and exquisitely painful joints that are sensitive even to light touch.
- Involvement of the first metatarsophalangeal joint (called "podagra") is highly characteristic of gout.

Physical Examination

- Vital signs
  - May have increased heart rate due to pain and may have low-grade fevers
- Skin
  - Affected joint is often warm to the touch and exquisitely tender
  - Patients with chronic gout may have tophi (fingers, toes, olecranon bursae, and heels)
- Gait
  - Antalgic with lower extremity joint involvement
- Joints
  - Warm and very tender to touch; may mimic an infected joint.
  - The range of motion is extremely limited due to pain and joint swelling.

Imaging

- Radiographs may be notable only for evidence of effusion in early disease.
- Chronic gout results in characteristic erosions. Erosions in chronic gout are often nonmarginal. They have an ovoid shape often with overhanging edges and sclerotic margins (so-called rat bite lesions; Fig. 15.3).
- Pseudogout is an acute manifestation of calcium pyrophosphate deposition disease (CPPD). This condition can lead to chondrocalcinosis, which is typically seen in the fibrocartilage structures of the knee and wrist (Fig. 15.4).

Additional Tests

- There is no role for a uric acid level in diagnosing acute gout. It is helpful in managing chronic gout.
- Synovial fluid analysis with polarizing microscopy is essential to establish a diagnosis.
  - Gout crystals are needle shaped with bright negative birefringence (yellow when plane of polarization is parallel to axis of crystal).
  - CPPD crystals are rhomboid shaped with faint positive birefringence (blue when plane of polarization is parallel to axis of crystal).

Differential Diagnosis

- Septic arthritis
- Cellulitis/septic bursitis
- Acute trauma
- Atypical manifestation of rheumatoid arthritis (RA) and similar conditions

Treatment

- Acute treatment for both gout and pseudogout are the same. Medical comorbidities may guide choice of agent.

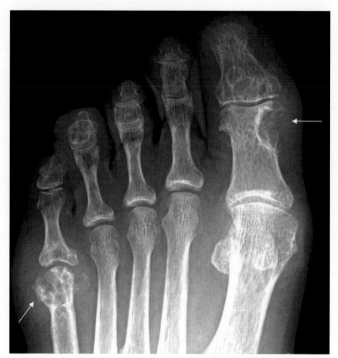

Fig 15.3 Chronic tophaceous gout. Gouty erosions are often nonmarginal with sclerotic margins and overhanging edges, as seen in the proximal phalanx of the great toe *(horizontal arrow)*. There is a tophus over the fifth metatarsophalangeal joint, where there is erosive disease at the joint and focal areas of calcification in the soft tissue *(diagonal arrow)*.

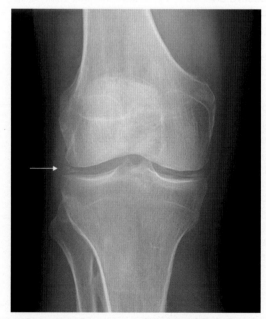

Fig 15.4 Chondrocalcinosis is a radiographic feature of calcium pyrophosphate deposition disease. It is commonly seen in the fibrocartilaginous menisci of the knee, appearing as thin radiopaque bands *(white arrow)*.

- Oral NSAIDs
- Oral corticosteroids (prednisone 20 to 60 mg daily for acute flares)
- Use caution with intraarticular steroids as septic arthritis can precipitate flares of crystalline disease.
- Colchicine (two 0.6 mg pills at first sign of flare and then one 0.6 mg pill 1 hour later followed by one 0.6 mg daily thereafter)
- Chronic gout is addressed with dietary changes and pharmacologic therapy that lowers the serum uric acid.

Rheumatoid Arthritis

- RA is a systemic autoimmune condition whose primary manifestation is an inflammatory arthritis. It affects approximately 1% of the US population and is more common in women than men (3:1).

History

- Gradual onset of inflammatory joint symptoms over the course of weeks to months. Pain and stiffness tend to be worse in the morning and improve with activity only to return with rest.
- Symmetrical joint involvement with a predilection for the wrists, metocarpophalangeal joints (MCPs), and MTPs. It spares the DIPs in contrast to OA, psoriatic arthritis, and gout.
- General fatigue and malaise may be present though fever is uncommon.

Physical Examination

- Vital signs
  - Usually normal
- Gait
  - May be antalgic if lower extremity joints are affected
- Skin
  - Skin nodules may present in RA
- Joints
  - Involved joints are warm and swollen
  - Progressive disease results in characteristic joint deformities such as ulnar deviation at the MCPs, and boutonniere and swan neck deformities in the fingers.

Imaging

- Bilateral hand and foot films are recommended at baseline. Hand views should include PA and Norgaard ("ball-catcher") views.
- Early radiographic changes include soft-tissue swelling and periarticular osteopenia.
- With more advanced disease there may be uniform joint space narrowing (Fig. 15.5), marginal erosions, and deformities (Fig. 15.6).
- RA involves the spine only at C1-C2, where it can lead to atlantoaxial instability. There is a risk of cord compression, especially with forceful neck extension, as occurs with intubation.

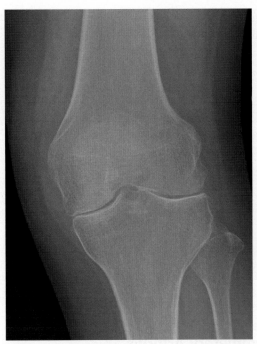

Fig 15.5 Rheumatoid arthritis. In contrast to osteoarthritis, inflammatory arthritis in the knee leads to uniform joint space narrowing throughout all compartments. Inflammatory arthritis is often associated with periarticular osteopenia.

Additional Tests

- Auto-antibodies help define the disease and provide prognostic information.
  - A rheumatoid factor (RF) is approximately 70% sensitive and 70% specific for RA.
  - An anticyclic citrullinated peptide (CCP) is 70% sensitive but >90% specific for RA.
- Acute phase reactants: sedimentations rate (ESR) and C-reactive protein (CRP)

Differential Diagnosis

- Systemic lupus
- Psoriatic arthritis
- Reactive arthritis
- Acute parvovirus
- Chronic gout
- Chronic CPPD

Treatment

- At diagnosis, all RA patients should be referred to a rheumatologist and receive a trial of methotrexate, which is a disease-modifying antirheumatic drug (DMARD). An alternative DMARD to methotrexate is leflunomide.
- RA will often respond to modest doses of prednisone in the range of 5 to 10 mg daily.
- NSAIDs can help with pain but do not control the disease.

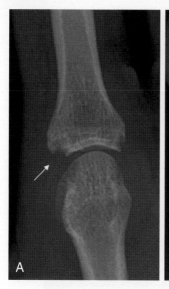
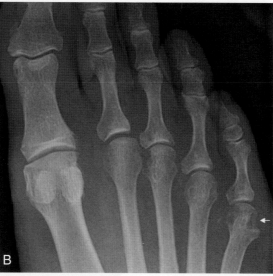

Fig 15.6 Rheumatoid arthritis. The early erosions of rheumatoid arthritis *(arrows)* occur at the joint margins and have predilection for **(A)** the second and third MCPs in the hands, and **(B)** fourth and fifth metatarsophalangeal joints in the feet.

Other Conditions Associated With Inflammatory Arthritis
Lyme Arthritis

- Lyme disease is caused by the spirochete *Borrelia burgdorferi,* which is transmitted by a tick vector. Lyme is endemic to specific geographic regions of the United States, including New England, the Mid-Atlantic, and parts of the Midwest (notably Wisconsin).
- Lyme disease occurs in separate phases. Acute Lyme is characterized by the target-shaped rash of erythema migrans that occurs at the site of inoculation. The organism may spread, causing disseminated disease that can affect multiple organ systems including the heart, joints, and nervous system.
- An important manifestation of disseminated Lyme infection is an inflammatory arthritis. The weight-bearing joints, typically the knees, are involved. Lyme arthritis is often migratory, with pain moving between affected joints. Inflammation in the joint is caused by the presence of the spirochete in the joint.
- An initial diagnosis is often made with Lyme serologies in the right clinical context. Synovial fluid can be sent for a polymerase chain reaction analysis, which detects bacterial nucleic acid.
- Lyme arthritis should be suspected only in individuals who have lived or traveled in areas where the spirochete is endemic.
- First-line therapy for Lyme arthritis includes 28 days of doxycycline in adults and 28 days of Amoxicillin in children and pregnant women
- Reinfection can occur after treatment.

Systemic Lupus Erythematosus

- Systemic lupus erythematosus (SLE) is a multisystem autoimmune disease that commonly affects the skin, serosal surfaces of the heart and lung, joints, kidneys, and blood cell lines.
- It is more common in women, with a 9:1 female predominance affecting women of childbearing age.

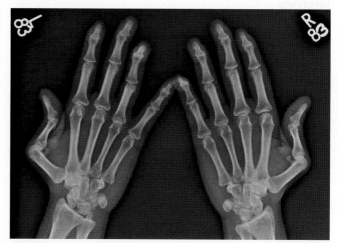

Fig 15.7 Jaccoud arthropathy. Systemic lupus is associated with a nonerosive inflammatory arthritis of the hands that leads to reducible ulnar deviation and swan neck deformities.

- Joint involvement can mimic RA, though erosions are not typically seen. With hand involvement, it is more likely to see the characteristic Jaccoud arthropathy characterized by reducible ulnar deviation and swan neck deformities (Fig. 15.7).
- Blood tests are critical in establishing a diagnosis of lupus. An antinuclear antibody (ANA) is a highly sensitive (>95%) but relatively nonspecific test for lupus.
- First-line therapy includes hydroxychloroquine and systemic steroids. Additional therapy is indicated if there is internal organ involvement.

Psoriatic Arthritis

- Psoriatic arthritis (PsA) belongs to a larger group of conditions known as the inflammatory spondyloarthropathies. These include ankylosing spondylitis, inflammatory bowel disease (IBD)–associated arthritis, and reactive arthritis. These conditions can affect the spine and sacroiliac joints, though peripheral arthritis is more common in PsA.

- PsA and the other spondyloarthropathies affect not only joints but also tendons and ligaments, leading to tenosynovitis and enthesitis. The entheses are special anatomical sites where tendons and ligaments insert onto bone.
- PsA develops most often in individuals with preexisting psoriasis. In a small minority of cases, the inflammatory arthritis predates the cutaneous manifestations.
- Men and women are equally affected.
- Joint involvement in the peripheral joints mirrors RA, with the notable exception that PsA often involves the DIPs in the hands and feet.
- Severe PsA can lead to dramatic deformities of the hands and feet. The classic radiographic deformity of PsA is the pencil-in-cup deformity.
- Therapy also mirrors that of RA OTE: Systemic steroids should be avoided in PsA if possible, as they are associated with severe rebound of skin and joint disease when tapered.

Reactive Arthritis

- In contrast to PsA, reactive arthritis (ReA) usually affects the larger joints, including knees and ankles.
- Reactive arthritis follows infections of various types, the most common of which include urethritis from chlamydia and enterocolitis due to campylobacter
- There is a variant of poststreptococcal reactive arthritis that must be differentiated from acute rheumatic fever.
- Reactive arthritis can be associated with conjunctivitis and a characteristic set of skin findings, including a psoriaform rash on the palms and soles known as keratoderma blennorrhagia.
- Reactive arthritis usually has a self-limited disease course and can be managed with NSAIDs alone. Persistent disease may require steroids and DMARDs. Sulfasalazine is the first-line agent if a DMARD is necessary.

Imaging

- Avascular necrosis of the knees, hips, and shoulders can be seen in lupus independent of steroid exposure.

- The spondyloarthropathies often have spine and sacroiliac involvement. A Ferguson view is recommended when assessing for sacroiliitis.

Troubleshooting

- Always perform arthrocentesis on an acutely warm and swollen joint in order to rule out septic arthritis. Synovial fluid analysis should include a cell count and differential, crystal analysis, and gram stain and culture

Considerations in Special Populations

- Monitor elderly patients closely for side effects of NSAIDs including gastrointestinal bleeding and renal function. Joint pain and disability have a negative effect on balance; canes and walkers—when used appropriately—lessen the chance of falling but require training.
- Any joint effusion in a child requires urgent attention.

Suggested Readings

Hochberg MC, Altman RD, April KT, et al. American College of Rheumatology 2012 recommendations for the use of nonpharmacologic and pharmacologic therapies in osteoarthritis of the hand, hip, and knee. *Arthritis Care Res (Hoboken)*. 2012;64(4):465–474.

Khanna D, Khanna PP, Fitzgerald JD, et al. American College of Rheumatology guidelines for management of gout. Part 2: therapy and antiinflammatory prophylaxis of acute gouty arthritis. *Arthritis Care Res (Hoboken)*. 2012;64(10):1447–1461.

Margaretten ME, Kohlwes J, Moore D, Bent S. Does this patient have septic arthritis? *JAMA*. 2007;297(13):1478–1488.

Singh JA, Saag KG, Bridges SL Jr, et al. 2015 American College of Rheumatology guideline for the treatment of rheumatoid arthritis. *Arthritis Care Res (Hoboken)*. 2016;68(1):1–25.

Chapter 16 Infections (Septic Joint, Septic Arthritis, and Osteomyelitis)

Joseph Armen, Evan Lutz

Osteomyelitis

Key Concepts

- Acute osteomyelitis is an acute infection of bone without the development of necrotic bone (sequestra). The duration is variable, but the condition usually evolves over several days to weeks.
- Chronic osteomyelitis is a long-term infection of bone with the presence of dead bone (the sequestrum). Common features include reactive bony encasement of the sequestrum (involucrum), local bone loss, and the possibility of sinus tract development if there is extension of the infection through cortical bone.
- The pathogenesis can include hematogenous spread of bacteria, contiguous spread from a soft-tissue infection, and local inoculation after surgery or trauma.
- Hematogenous spread has a biphasic distribution, occurring in children due to their unique bone anatomy and in patients older than the age of 50 who have increased risk factors for bacteremia.
- The long bones are most often involved in children. In adults, the vertebrae and sternoclavicular and sacroiliac bones are most commonly involved.
- This is a difficult disease to diagnose; testing must be tailored to the clinical scenario and may require bone biopsy for definitive diagnosis.
- When present, positive blood cultures with typical radiographic changes obviate the need for a bone biopsy.

History

- Signs and symptoms can vary with duration of disease.
  - Acute osteomyelitis
    - Typically has an insidious onset over several days to a week with bone pain, tenderness, warmth, and swelling
    - Fevers can be present, and pain occurs with and without movement. Complaints can be vague and nonspecific, with few constitutional symptoms.
  - Chronic osteomyelitis
    - May be subtle with few symptoms. There may be a history of chronically developing skin changes or ulcerations, bone pain, or concomitant medical issues including diabetes and peripheral vascular disease.
    - Easily recognized if there is a draining sinus along with recurrent pain, erythema, and swelling in someone with a known history of osteomyelitis

Physical Examination

- Acute osteomyelitis
  - Children
    - If hematogenous in origin, likely to have fever and local signs of inflammation
    - A limp or refusal to walk may be observed if the spine, pelvis, or lower extremity is involved. Pseudoparalysis may occur when the upper extremity is involved.
  - Adults
    - Usually present with vague, nonspecific pain and few constitutional symptoms
    - Limitation of joint motion, swelling, erythema, fever, and a symptomatic effusion
- Chronic osteomyelitis
  - External physical findings may be minimal; however, soft-tissue inflammation and tenderness may develop.
  - Persistent drainage through a sinus tract or fistula, low-grade fever, chronic pain, local bone loss, and mild systemic symptoms may be present.

Imaging

- Plain radiographs
  - Acute osteomyelitis
    - Two to three weeks are required for bone changes to be evident.
    - The triad of soft-tissue swelling, bone destruction, and periosteal reaction is specific.
  - Chronic osteomyelitis
    - Bone sclerosis, periosteal bone formation, and sequestra are the primary findings.
- Ultrasonography
  - Findings may include a fluid collection adjacent to the bone and periosteal elevation by more than 2 mm with thickening.
  - Larger studies are needed to evaluate the sensitivity and specificity of this modality.

TABLE 16.1 Common Organisms in Osteomyelitis Based on Age and Chronic Conditions

Osteomyelitis Type	Age	Likely Microorganism
Acute and chronic osteomyelitis	Newborn to 4 months	Group A and B streptococcus, *Staphylococcus aureus*, *Enterobacter*
	4 months to 4 years	*S. aureus*, *Haemophilus influenzae*, *Escherichia coli*, group A streptococcus
	4 years to adults	Group A streptococcus, *Staphylococcus epidermidis*, *Pseudomonas*, *Serratia marcescens*
Special populations	Immunocompromised	*Bartonella henselae*, *Aspergillus*, *Mycobacterium avium-intracellulare*, *Candida albicans*, anaerobes, *Mycobacterium tuberculosis*
	Sickle cell disease	*Salmonella*, *Streptococcus pneumoniae*

Data from Carek PJ, Dickerson LM, Sack JL. Diagnosis and management of osteomyelitis. *Am Fam Physician*. 2001;63:2413–2420.

- Computed tomography
  - Detects cortical destruction, periosteal reaction, intraosseous gas, soft-tissue extension
- Magnetic resonance imaging
  - Provides anatomic detail when planning surgical débridement and identifying abscesses
  - High sensitivity and negative predictive value; shows bone marrow edema within 3 to 5 days of infection
  - Especially advantageous when evaluating vertebral or foot osteomyelitis
- Three-phase bone scan
  - Historically considered the test of choice when evaluating acute osteomyelitis if plain radiographs are normal. The scan generally turns positive in 2 to 3 days.
  - More useful when metal hardware limits the quality of MRI images
  - Osteomyelitis results in increased uptake in all three phases, making it useful when differentiating from cellulitis but limited in differentiating from gouty arthritis and conditions with high bony turnover.

Additional Tests

- Laboratory studies
  - Complete blood count—leukocytosis common in acute, but not chronic, osteomyelitis
  - Erythrocyte sedimentation rate/C-reactive protein—may be markedly increased
  - Monitoring can be useful to detect relapses.
- Cultures
  - Blood (positive in 50% of cases-of-acute osteomyelitis)
- Bone biopsy
  - The gold standard is an open bone biopsy with histopathologic examination and cultures.

Differential Diagnosis

- Cellulitis
- Gout
- Acute leukemia
- Bone malignancy
- Septic arthritis
- Rheumatic fever
- Bone infarct (i.e., sickle cell disease)

Treatment

- At diagnosis
  - Debridement of necrotic bone and empiric antibiotics to cover suspected organisms based on patient age, severity of disease, and comorbid conditions (Table 16.1)
  - Neurosurgical decompression for those with vertebral osteomyelitis and epidural abscess
- Later
  - Definitive antimicrobials chosen based on culture and sensitivity results when available
  - Parenteral antibiotics are traditionally continued for 4 to 6 weeks.
  - In chronic osteomyelitis, oral quinolones for 6 to 8 weeks can be considered.

When to Refer

- Atypical infectious agents
- Difficulty in differentiating osteomyelitis from other diagnoses

Prognosis

- A good result can be expected with successful early treatment in an immunocompetent host.
- Progression to a chronic state is more common when the lower extremities are involved and in diabetics.

Troubleshooting

- The diagnosis of acute osteomyelitis cannot be excluded if the plain films are negative.
- False-positive magnetic resonance imaging results can occur with either a bone infarct or healed osteomyelitis.
- The sensitivity of a needle biopsy is especially low in the postoperative or posttrauma patient.
- Osteomyelitis in hip, pelvis, and vertebral locations tend to manifest few signs and symptoms.

Patient Instructions

- Follow your physician's instructions regarding treatment including antibiotic duration.

- As symptoms improve, physical therapy may be recommended to help the affected joint or limb regain function and flexibility.
- Notify your physician if symptoms persist or recur or new symptoms develop.
- Alert your physician if the drugs used for treatment produce side effects.

Considerations in Special Populations

- Sickle cell disease
  - Difficulty in differentiating bony crisis pain from osteomyelitis
  - *Salmonella* is the most common infectious organism involved.
- Diabetes
  - Underlying osteomyelitis is often missed in diabetic foot ulcers.
  - Magnetic resonance imaging is the imaging modality of choice for diabetic foot ulcers.

Septic Arthritis

Key Concepts

- Also referred to as infectious arthritis
- Many pathogens can be involved, including bacteria, viruses, spirochetes, mycobacteria, and fungi.
- Bacterial pathogens are most significant because of their rapidly destructive nature.
- Two major classes of bacterial arthritis are gonococcal and nongonococcal.
  - Gonococcal
    - *Neisseria gonorrhoeae*: most frequent among younger, sexually active individuals
  - Nongonococcal
    - *Staphylococcus aureus*: overall, the most common cause among adults and children older than 2 years of age
    - Aerobic gram-negative rods: seen in the very young, the very old, intravenous drug users, and the immunosuppressed population
    - Polymicrobial and anaerobes: usually a consequence of trauma or an abdominal infection
- There are three types of prosthetic joint infections: early, delayed, and late.
  - Early—less than 3 months; typically involves *S. aureus*
  - Delayed—3 to 24 months; coagulase-negative *S. aureus* and gram-negative rods
  - Late—>24 months; due to seeding from hematogenous spread
- Joints can be infected by three mechanisms:
  - Direct inoculation
  - Contiguous spread from infected periarticular tissue
  - Hematogenously
- Previously damaged joints are most susceptible, particularly arthritic joints with synovitis.
- Articular cartilage damage occurs due to the particular organism or host response.

History

- Fever, extra-articular manifestations and/or underlying joint disease may be present.
- Acute onset of joint pain is typical.
- Monoarticular involvement is common.
- Risk factors include history of intravenous drug use, sexually transmitted infections, prosthetic joint surgery, arthroscopy, chronic disease, and immunosuppression.

Physical Examination

- Findings can vary, but may include
  - General—fever, tachycardia
  - Inspection—erythema, rash involving overlying skin
  - Palpation—warmth, joint effusion
  - Range of motion—pain and/or restriction of active and passive motion

Imaging

- Plain radiographs
  - Evidence of demineralization may be present within days of onset.
  - Bony erosions and narrowing of the joint space followed by osteomyelitis may be seen within 2 weeks.
- Ultrasonography
  - Can be helpful in identifying joint effusions and guide needle aspirations
- Computed tomography/magnetic resonance imaging
  - Better when evaluating the sacroiliac and sternoclavicular joints along with the spine
  - Best when ruling out osteomyelitis, periarticular abscess, or other soft-tissue extensions
- Radionuclide scans
  - Helpful in identifying infections in deep-seated joints (i.e., the hip and sacroiliac joints)
  - Nonspecifically localizes other regions affected by inflammatory processes

Additional Tests

- Arthrocentesis with synovial fluid analysis (Table 16.2)
- Laboratory tests
  - Complete blood count with differential
  - Erythrocyte sedimentation rate/C-reactive protein
- Cultures
  - Blood and synovial fluid along with urethral, pharyngeal, and/or rectal if clinically indicated
  - Echocardiogram if positive blood cultures for staphylococcus to rule out endocarditis

Differential Diagnoses

- Still's disease
- Rheumatic fever
- Lyme disease
- Transient synovitis
- Gout
- Pseudogout

TABLE 16.2 Synovial Fluid Analysis

Synovial Fluid	Color	Clarity	WBC (mL)	PMN (%)	Crystals	Culture
Normal	Clear	Transparent	<200	<25	Negative	Negative
Noninflammatory	Straw to yellow	Transparent	2000	<25	Negative	Negative
Inflammatory	Yellow	Translucent	2000–50,000	>70	May be positive	Negative
Septic[a]	Variable	Opaque	>50,000	>90	May be positive	85-95% positive[b]
Hemorrhagic	Red	Bloody	200–2000	50–75	Negative	Negative

[a]Glucose and lactate dehydrogenase levels have low sensitivity/specificity to confirm or exclude the diagnosis of septic joint.

[b]85-95% positive cultures for nongonococcal arthritis and 25% for gonococcal arthritis.

PMN, Polymorphonuclear neutrophil; *WBC*, white blood cell count.

TABLE 16.3 Likely Infecting Organism and Empirical Antibiotic Treatment of Septic Arthritis

Age	Likely Organism	Initial Antibiotic Regimen
Neonate	*Staphylococcus aureus,* group B streptococcus	Oxacillin + gentamicin
Child <5 years	*S. aureus*, group A streptococcus, *Streptococcus pneumoniae*, *Haemophilus influenzae*	Second-generation cephalosporin
5 years to adolescence	*S. aureus*	Oxacillin
Adolescence to adulthood	*Neisseria gonorrhoeae*	Ceftriaxone
Older adults	*S. aureus*	Oxacillin or cefazolin + aminoglycoside

Data from Griffin LY, ed. *Essentials of Musculoskeletal Care*. 3rd ed. Rosemont, IL: American Academy of Orthopaedic Surgeons; 2005:115.

- Osteoarthritis
- Rheumatoid arthritis
- Psoriatic arthritis
- Osteomyelitis
- Pseudoseptic reaction (after an intra-articular injection)

Treatment

- At diagnosis
  - Parenteral antibiotics
    - Initial choice is based on clinical judgment of causative organism (Table 16.3) and is modified if necessary based on culture and sensitivity results.
  - Frequent local aspirations
    - When synovial fluid rapidly reaccumulates and causes symptoms
  - Surgical drainage
    - To be considered if the hip is involved and/or medical therapy fails over a 2- to 4-day period
  - Rest, immobilization, elevation, local hot compresses, and early passive and active range-of-motion exercises as pain tolerates
- Later
  - Physical therapy may be needed to address functional limitations or impairments
  - Frequent outpatient follow-up visits to help recognize adverse outcomes or recurrence
  - Consider prosthetic replacement

When to Refer

- Failed arthrocentesis
- Joint that is difficult to aspirate (i.e., the hip and sacroiliac joints)
- Atypical infectious agents

Prognosis

- 5-10% death rate, usually from respiratory complications of sepsis
- 50% of adults have residual decreased range of motion and chronic pain, especially if treatment is delayed.
- Predictors of poor outcome include age older than 60, involvement of the hip or shoulders, underlying rheumatoid arthritis, positive cultures after a week of appropriate therapy, and a delay of more than 1 week before initiating treatment.

Troubleshooting

- Fever is common, but may be absent in as many as 20% or more of patients, especially if they are immunosuppressed or are taking corticosteroids or antipyretics.
- A superimposed cellulitis is a relative contraindication to arthrocentesis.
- An undiagnosed chronic monoarthritis requires arthroscopy and a synovial biopsy.

- Patients taking warfarin can undergo arthrocentesis if their International Normalized Ratio is less than 4.

Patient Instructions

- Educate yourself about the disease and risk factors and seek medical attention if needed for early diagnosis and treatment.
- Sometimes treatment requires hospitalization, and patient participation in developing a treatment plan can be beneficial.
- Once the infection is under control, exercises can strengthen joints and muscles and improve the range of motion.

Considerations in Special Populations

- Pediatric
  - Negative clinical predictors include fever; non–weight bearing on the affected joint; white blood cell (WBC) count greater than 12,000; and an erythrocyte sedimentation rate greater than 40.
  - Joint destruction or physeal damage is possible.
- Geriatric
  - Be aware of drug interactions between prescribed antibiotics and long-term medications.
  - Renal dosing of antibiotics when appropriate.
  - Instruct patients with prosthetic joints to recognize early signs of joint infection.

Suggested Readings

Osteomyelitis

Aloui N, Nessib N, Jalel C. Acute osteomyelitis in children: early MRI diagnosis. *J Radiol*. 2004;85:403–408.

Burnett MW, Bass JW, Cook BA. Etiology of osteomyelitis complicating sickle cell disease. *Pediatrics*. 1998;101:296–297.

Carek PJ, Dickerson LM, Sack JL. Diagnosis and management of osteomyelitis. *Am Fam Physician*. 2001;63:2413–2420.

Gold RH, Hawkins RA, Katz RD. Bacterial osteomyelitis: findings on plain radiography, CT, MR, and scintigraphy. *AJR Am J Roentgenol*. 1991;157:365–370.

Karchevsky M, Schweitzer ME, Morrison WB, Parellada JA. MRI findings of septic arthritis and associated osteomyelitis in adults. *AJR Am J Roentgenol*. 2004;182:119–122.

Lew DP, Waldvogel FA. Osteomyelitis. *N Engl J Med*. 1997;336:999–1007.

Norden C, Gillespie WJ, Nade S. *Infections in Bones and Joints*. Boston: Blackwell Scientific; 1994.

Septic Arthritis

Donatto KC. Orthopedic management of septic arthritis. *Rheum Dis Clin North Am*. 1998;24:275–286.

Frank G, Mahoney HM, Eppes SC. Musculoskeletal infections in children. *Pediatr Clin North Am*. 2005;52:1083–1106, ix.

Griffin LY, ed. *Essentials of Musculoskeletal Care*. 3rd ed. Rosemont, IL: American Academy of Orthopaedic Surgeons; 2005:115.

Mararetten ME, Kohlwes J, Moore D, Bent S. Does this patient have septic arthritis? *JAMA*. 2007;297:1478–1488.

Shmerling RH, Delbanco TL, Tosteson AN, Trentham DE. Synovial fluid tests. What should be ordered? *JAMA*. 1990;264:1009–1014.

Simon RR, Koenigsknecht SJ. Septic arthritis of the hip joint. In: *Emergency Orthopedics: The Extremities*. 4th ed. New York: McGraw-Hill; 2001:404–406.

Chapter 17 Neurovascular Disorders: Arterial Conditions in Athletes

Mario Ciocca

ICD-10-CM CODES

SUBCLAVIAN ARTERY/AXILLARY ARTERY OCCLUSION

G45.8   *Other transient cerebral ischemic attacks and related syndromes*

I74.2   *Embolism and thrombosis of arteries of the upper extremities*

QUADRILATERAL SPACE SYNDROME

S44.30xa *Injury of axillary nerve, unspecified arm, initial encounter*

HYPOTHENAR HAMMER SYNDROME

I73.89   *Other specified peripheral vascular diseases*

ILIAC ARTERY OCCLUSION

I74.5   *Embolism and thrombosis of iliac artery*

ADDUCTOR CANAL SYNDROME

S76.209a *Unspecified injury of adductor muscle, fascia and tendon of unspecified thigh, initial encounter*

POPLITEAL ARTERY ENTRAPMENT SYNDROME

I77.89   *Other specified disorders of arteries and arterioles*

Subclavian Artery/Axillary Artery Occlusion

Key Concepts

- The axillary artery arises from the subclavian artery at the outer border of the first rib and courses deep to the pectoralis minor muscle.
- The subclavian artery is susceptible to compression from a cervical rib, anomalous first rib, or overdeveloped scalene muscles.
- Axillary artery occlusion develops secondary to pressure from the overlying pectoralis minor muscle in the overhead position.
- The axillary artery may also be compressed by the humerus when the shoulder is in the cocked position (Fig. 17.1).
- An axillary artery aneurysm (usually at the origin of the posterior humeral circumflex artery) or distal embolization may develop.

History

- Symptoms may include claudication, fatigue, and night pain
- Sudden onset of numbness, coolness, and cold intolerance in the hand may be secondary to distal embolization.

Physical Examination

- Tenderness over pectoralis minor muscle area
- May have diminished distal pulses that are usually position dependent
- Provocative tests for thoracic outlet syndrome may be positive.
- Weakness or sensory deficits are rare.

Imaging

- Radiographs may demonstrate a cervical rib, a long transverse process, or other bone abnormalities that may cause thoracic outlet syndrome.
- Duplex ultrasonography can evaluate flow and presence of aneurysm.
- Computerized tomography arteriography and magnetic resonance arteriography can confirm diagnosis and evaluate surrounding musculoskeletal anatomy.
- A definitive diagnosis can be made with an arteriogram in the symptom-provoking position.

Treatment

- In the absence of complete thrombosis, aneurysm, or embolism, treatment can be conservative with strengthening and stretching of scalene and pectoralis minor muscles and strengthening of the posterior scapular stabilizers.
- Initial treatment for occlusion and aneurysm includes anticoagulation.
- Surgical treatment may include segmental vascular excision, bypass with a venous graft, and thoracic outlet decompression.

Quadrilateral Space Syndrome

Key Concepts

- Quadrilateral space bordered by the teres minor muscle superiorly, teres major muscle inferiorly, proximal humerus laterally, and long head of the triceps muscle medially (Fig. 17.2).

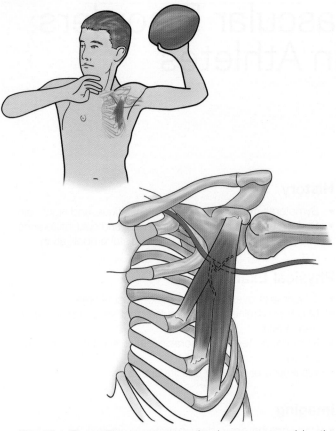

Fig 17.1 The axillary artery may also be compressed by the humerus when the shoulder is in the cocked position.

- The posterior humeral circumflex artery arises from the distal third of the axillary artery and enters the quadrilateral space with the axillary nerve.
- This space is compressed when the shoulder is in the abducted and externally rotated position.
- Possible etiologies include:
  - Repetitive activity causing abnormal fibrous bands and/or muscular hypertrophy
  - Traction on the posterior humeral circumflex artery by the pectoralis major muscle
  - Tethering of the posterior humeral circumflex artery to the proximal humerus, placing it at risk of traction injury
  - Space-occupying lesions such as glenoid labral cysts
  - Glenohumeral instability

History

- Typically occurs in a 20- to 40-year-old overhead-throwing athlete.
- Symptoms often related to compression of the axillary nerve
- May complain of poorly localized shoulder discomfort, deltoid weakness, arm fatigue in the overhead position, paresthesia to the lateral arm, and night pain
- Throwing often affected
- Coolness, pallor, or cyanosis may occur with ischemia secondary to mechanical injury to the posterior circumflex humeral artery.

Physical Examination

- Localized tenderness over the quadrilateral space
- Re-creation of the pain when the shoulder is placed in forward flexion, abduction, and external rotation for 1 to 2 minutes

- Quadrilateral space borders
  - Teres minor
  - Teres major
  - Proximal humerus
  - Long head of triceps
- Compression of posterior humeral circumflex artery
- History: poorly localized pain, arm fatigue, paresthesia
- PE: tenderness in space, reproduce symptoms with provocative maneuvers
- Rx: stretch, NSAIDs, corticosteroid injection, surgical decompression

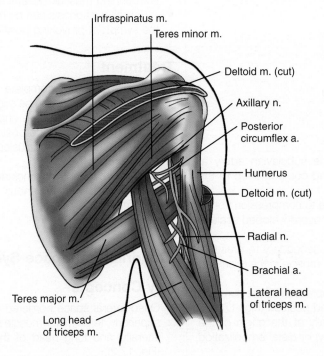

Infraspinatus m.

Teres minor m.

Deltoid m. (cut)

Axillary n.

Posterior circumflex a.

Humerus

Deltoid m. (cut)

Radial n.

Brachial a.

Lateral head of triceps m.

Teres major m.

Long head of triceps m.

Fig 17.2 Quadrilateral space syndrome. *a*, Artery; *m*, muscle; *n*, nerve; *NSAIDs*, nonsteroidal antiinflammatory drugs.

Imaging

- Radiographs to rule out other pathology
- Magnetic resonance imaging can reveal teres minor muscle atrophy and fat infiltration and rule out other etiologies.
- Subclavian arteriography may show posterior humeral circumflex artery occlusion when the arm is abducted and externally rotated.
- Magnetic resonance angiography is not useful because it is positive in as many as 80% of asymptomatic shoulders that are placed in abduction and external rotation.

Differential Diagnosis

- Cervical spine disorders
- Rotator cuff pathology
- Thoracic outlet syndrome
- Suprascapular neuropathy

Treatment

- Initial treatment
  - Activity modification
  - Stretching into horizontal adduction and internal rotation
  - Rotator cuff muscle strengthening
  - Active-release soft-tissue massage technique to the quadrilateral space
  - Nonsteroidal antiinflammatory drugs
  - Corticosteroid injection
- Later (if not improved after 3 to 6 months)
  - Surgical decompression with release of fibrous bands via a posterior approach
  - Thrombolysis and surgical intervention indicated sooner if acute thrombus

Hypothenar Hammer Syndrome

Key Concepts

- Overuse injury involving ulnar artery or palmar arch
- Area where ulnar artery crosses hypothenar muscles is susceptible to blunt trauma
- Artery is superficial and immobile and can be compressed against hook of hamate
- Seen in athletes from many different sports
- 90% involve dominant hand
- Long finger most prone to ischemia

History

- May complain of pain, cold sensitivity, numbness, cramping with activity, or acute paleness

Physical Examination

- Thrill or bruit may be present
- Positive Allen test

Imaging

- Ultrasonography can reveal occlusion or decrease blood flow
- Contrast angiography gold standard

Differential Diagnosis

- Raynaud disease
- Autoimmune disease
- Buerger disease
- Arterial embolus

Treatment

- Treatment includes:
  - Equipment modification
  - Vasodilator medication
  - Thrombolytic medication
  - Catheter directed thrombolytic therapy
  - Intravascular vasodilators
- Surgery indicated for symptomatic ischemia, vascular damage to multiple digital arteries, or aneurysm formation

Iliac Artery Occlusion

Key Concepts

- Flow limitations may be due to lumen narrowing from endofibrotic thickening of the intima or from kinking of the vessel.
- Arterial endofibrosis is due to intimal hyperplasia in the absence of inflammatory or atherosclerotic lesions.
- Factors inducing endofibrosis or kinking include mechanical stress from extreme hip flexion, excessive length of artery, fixation of artery to surrounding tissues, and compression from psoas hypertrophy.
- Most often seen in highly trained cyclists but can also occur in speed skaters, runners, and triathletes
- The flow limitations will progress in 80% of patients.
- Endofibrotic lesions most often affect the external iliac artery, but may affect the common iliac artery and the femoral artery.

History

- Symptoms usually develop in the mid-20s.
- Claudication in buttock/thigh that quickly disappears at rest
- Paresthesia of leg and plantar aspect of foot
- Cramping at maximal effort, which may affect multiple muscles
- Loss of power
- Usually affects the left side but may be bilateral

Physical Examination

- Examination is often normal.
- Auscultation over the anterior hip at rest

- A bruit with hip extended has good specificity for flow limitation.
- A bruit with the hip flexed is more sensitive for flow limitation.
- Auscultation after exercise is not useful, because femoral bruits are heard in normal subjects.
- Ankle brachial index recorded within 5 minutes of stopping exercise is usually reduced. Can assess difference from contralateral side if symptoms are unilateral.

Imaging

- Duplex ultrasonography with hip flexion, hip extension, psoas contraction, and after exercise can detect kinking and intravascular lesions.
- Magnetic resonance angiography combined with hip flexion best delineates kinking in the common iliac artery. Magnetic resonance angiography can also assess excessive vessel length when the hip is extended and evaluate for intravascular lesions.
- Angiography is less useful for evaluating intravascular lesions because they are often located eccentrically.

Treatment

- Conservative
  - Decrease amount and intensity of exercise
  - For cyclists, change the cycling position to decrease hip flexion and do not actively pull pedal upward.
- Surgical release of the iliac artery
  - Used for vessels that kink during hip flexion
  - The artery is released from the vascular sheath and the underlying surface, and the vessel is left intact.
  - Psoas branches and fibrous tissue ligated
  - Low complication rate with quick return
  - Will need further treatment if vessel diameter less than 70% compared with unaffected side or kinking due to excessive vascular length
- Vascular reconstruction
  - Shortening of vessel: done for kinking due to excessive vessel length
  - Endarterectomy or replacement by venous graft
- Percutaneous transluminal angioplasty
  - May provide short-term relief
  - Does not address vessel length and may result in dissection
- Stenting
  - May provide short-term relief
  - Complications include stent migration or fracture and arterial damage.
  - May induce intimal hyperplasia

Adductor Canal Syndrome

Key Concepts

- Chronic exertional compression of the superficial femoral artery

- Canal bordered by the vastus medialis anterolaterally, adductor longus and magnus posteriorly, and sartorius medially
- Compression can be caused by fibrous bands, anomalous musculotendinous band, or hypertrophied adductor magnus or vastus medialis
- Can lead to vessel injury, thrombus, and limb ischemia
- Seen in runners and skiers

History

- Symptoms may include exercise-induced claudication, paresthesia, or pallor.

Physical Exam

- If thrombus develops, may have loss of pulse.
- Exercise ankle-brachial index (ABI) may be abnormal.

Imaging

- Doppler ultrasonography, computed tomography angiography, magnetic resonance angiography, and contrast arteriography may be used to establish diagnosis.

Treatment

- If acute thrombus, then catheter thromboembolectomy or catheter-directed thrombolysis.
- Surgery includes resection/release of the external compression and patch angioplasty or bypass of the affected artery.

Popliteal Artery Entrapment Syndrome

Key Concepts

- Most common arterial cause of leg pain in athletes
- The popliteal artery may be entrapped due to an anatomic variation that may include compression from an accessory medial head of the gastrocnemius muscle and an aberrant course of the popliteal artery.
- Entrapment may also be functional with no anatomic variation other than a hypertrophied gastrocnemius muscle.
- The condition may be bilateral in 25-38%
- Male predilection and age usually less than 30
- Has been seen in young, healthy athletes including runners, soccer, football, basketball, tennis, and rugby players, and weight lifters
- Needs to be treated early to prevent complications such as stenosis, thrombosis, aneurysm, and distal emboli

History

- Claudication pain in the calf or anterior leg that increases with the intensity of exercise and quickly resolves when exercise stops
- Other symptoms may include calf cramps, swelling sensation, coldness, or paresthesia (tibial nerve distribution).
- Lack of risk factors for peripheral vascular disease

Physical Examination

- Examination at rest is usually normal.
- May have popliteal bruit accentuated with active ankle plantar flexion or passive dorsiflexion and may increase after exercise
- Dorsalis pedis and posterior tibial artery pulses are normal in the neutral position but may diminish or disappear during passive dorsiflexion or active ankle plantar flexion.

Imaging

- Duplex ultrasonography of the popliteal artery with provocative maneuvers including passive dorsiflexion and active plantarflexion may reveal compression of the artery and a reduction of the velocity waves of arterial flow.
- Computed tomography angiography or magnetic resonance angiography can confirm a positive ultrasound.
- Magnetic resonance angiography can be used to differentiate functional from anatomic entrapment.
- Angiography is gold standard and performed with provocative maneuvers

Differential Diagnosis

- Lumbar disc disease
- Buerger disease
- Exertional compartment syndrome
- Tendinitis
- Cystic disease of the popliteal artery (mucoid cysts in the vessel adventitia, usually in men in their mid-40s)
- Popliteal artery injury due to trauma

Treatment

- Anatomic—Treatment is surgical and includes resection of causative muscle and venous bypass graft.
- Functional—Initial treatment is conservative with rest and stretching followed by surgery if indicated.

Suggested Readings

Aval SM, Durand P Jr, Shankwiler JA. Neurovascular injuries in the athlete's shoulder: part II. *J Am Acad Orthop Surg*. 2007;15:281–289.

Brown SN, Doolittle DA, Bohanon CJ, et al. Quadrilateral space syndrome: the Mayo Clinic experience with a new classification system and case series. *Mayo Clin Proc*. 2015;90(3):382–394.

Corneloup I, Labanere C, Chevalier L, et al. Presentation, diagnosis, and management of popliteal artery entrapment syndrome: 11 years of experience with 61 legs. *Scand J Med Sci Sports*. 2017;1–7.

De Mooij T, Duncan AA, Kakar S. Vascular injuries in the upper extremity in athletes. *Hand Clin*. 2015;31:39–52.

Peach G, Schep G, Palfreeman R, et al. Endofibrosis and kinking of the iliac arteries in athletes: a systematic review. *Eur J Vasc Endovasc Surg*. 2012;43:208–217.

Perlowski AA, Jaff MR. Vascular disorders in athletes. *Vasc Med*. 2010;15(6):469–479.

Pham TT, Kapur R, Harwood MI. Exertional leg pain: teasing out arterial entrapments. *Curr Sports Med Rep*. 2007;6:371–375.

Rajasekaran S, Kvinlaug K, Finnoff JT. Exertional leg pain in the athlete. *PM R*. 2012;4:985–1000.

Reeser JC. Diagnosis and management of vascular injuries in the shoulder girdle of the overhead athlete. *Curr Sports Med Rep*. 2007;6:322–327.

Chapter 18 Neurovascular Disorders: Nerve Entrapment

Thomas E. Brickner

ICD-10-CM CODES
G58.9 *Nerve entrapment*
G62.9 *Neuropathy*

Key Concepts

- Peripheral nerve injuries due to mechanical constriction or deformation
- Pathophysiology is most often ischemic due to capillary hypoperfusion resulting from the constrictive force.
- May be due to tight anatomic passageways, space-occupying masses, external compressive forces, trauma, and inflammation
- May produce sensory and/or motor symptoms with atrophy
- Pattern of involvement is typically focal and mononeuritic
- Seddon classification of nerve injuries (mild to severe)
  - Neurapraxia: demyelination of axon sheath
  - Axonotmesis: axonal disruption with intact epineurium
  - Neurotmesis: complete disruption

Conditions

- Median nerve
  - Sites of compression: bicipital aponeurosis in antecubital fossa, between two heads of pronator teres (pronator syndrome), origin of flexor digitorum superficialis (FDS), carpal tunnel in wrist
  - Pronator syndrome
    - Proximal, ventral forearm pain and paresthesias of radial 3.5 digits
    - Tinel's sign at proximal forearm, pain with resisted pronation and/or FDS of third finger
  - Anterior interosseous syndrome
    - No sensory symptoms, purely motor
    - May have proximal, volar forearm pain
    - Abnormal pinch (OK) sign d/t weakened flexor pollicis longus (FPL) and flexor digitorum profundus (FDP) of second and third fingers
  - Carpal tunnel syndrome
    - Paresthesias in radial 3.5 digits
    - Positive Tinel and Phalen signs at wrist
    - Weakness in thumb abduction, grip, or pinch
- Radial nerve
  - Sites of compression: radial tunnel between heads of supinator, arcade of Frohse
  - Radial tunnel syndrome/posterior interosseous nerve syndrome (PIN)

- Aching pain in supinator and extensor tendon group 3 to 5 cm distal to lateral epicondyle
- Weakness upon metacarpophalangeal extension and of extensor carpi ulnaris (PIN)
- Ulnar nerve
  - Sites of compression: cubital tunnel at the posteromedial elbow, arcade of Struthers, Guyon's canal in wrist
  - Cubital tunnel syndrome
    - Aching pain at medial elbow
    - Paresthesias of ulnar 1.5 digits
    - Weakness of dorsal interosseous and abductor digiti minimi muscles
- Lateral antebrachial cutaneous nerve
  - Site of compression: lateral free margin of bicipital aponeurosis
  - Terminal sensory branch of musculocutaneous nerve
  - Supplies sensation over radial half of forearm
- Femoral nerve
  - Sites of compression: inguinal ligament, lumbar plexus due to mass
  - Sensory over anteromedial thigh and leg
  - Weakness of quadriceps muscle and knee jerk reflex
- Saphenous nerve
  - Site of compression: exit point of subsartorial fascia in medial distal thigh
  - Branch of femoral nerve
  - Purely sensory: knee and lower leg medially
- Lateral femoral cutaneous nerve (meralgia paresthetica)
  - Site of compression: near attachment of inguinal ligament to anterior superior iliac spine
  - Paresthesias over anterolateral thigh
- Peroneal nerve
  - Sites of compression: fibular head, anterior tarsal tunnel at ankle
  - Divides into deep peroneal nerve (DPN) and superficial peroneal nerve (SPN) branches near fibular neck
    - Deep: paresthesias of first web space, weakness to ankle/toe dorsiflexion
    - Superficial: paresthesias of lateral distal leg and dorsum of foot, weakness to eversion
- Posterior tibial nerve
  - Sites of compression: popliteal fossa due to mass, posterior tarsal tunnel behind medial malleolus (tarsal tunnel syndrome)
  - Proximal lesion: calf pain, plantar flexion weakness
  - Distal lesion: heel and plantar foot paresthesias
- Interdigital neuroma (Morton neuroma)
  - Site of compression: metatarsal heads
  - Pain radiating into toes

- Sural nerve
  - Site of compression: distal lateral leg
  - Sensory over lateral foot and heel

Imaging

- Magnetic resonance imaging
  - Identify space-occupying masses
  - Evaluate anatomy for hypertrophy, bony constrictions/spurring, anomalous structures
  - Evaluate signal change of muscles suggesting denervation atrophy
  - Visualize pathologic characteristics of nerves
    - Focal enlargement
    - Hyperintense signal on T2 images
    - Altered fascicular pattern
- Ultrasonography
  - Allows dynamic study for assessment of nerve compression
  - Does not show pathologic changes within nerves
  - Focal enlargement proximally and flattened at entrapment site

Diagnostics

- Electromyography (includes needle electrode examination and nerve conduction studies)
  - Detect peripheral nervous system lesions, site of pathology, severity, chronicity, and pathophysiology
  - Abnormalities may take weeks to fully develop after injury and may be completely unrevealing in mild cases.
- Nerve conduction studies
  - Measures conduction velocities, latencies, amplitude, and areas of nerve function
  - Demonstrates changes indicative of demyelination and/or axonal loss

- Needle electrode examination
  - Evaluates muscle spontaneous and intentional activity
  - Fibrillation potentials are evidence of denervation.
  - Alterations of motor unit action potentials are seen with neurogenic lesions.

Differential Diagnosis

- Tendinitis, epicondylitis, and arthritis
  - Provocative testing helpful in differentiating
- Endocrine/metabolic (diabetes mellitus, hypothyroidism), vasculitis, toxic, nutritional, infectious (acquired immunodeficiency syndrome), medications
  - Typically multifocal and symmetrical

Treatment

- External devices such as splints and padding
- Antiinflammatory drugs and injections
- Stretching and postural adjustments
- Activity modifications
- Hydrodissection with ultrasound guidance
- Surgical intervention
  - Releases, transpositions, decompressions

Suggested Readings

Cass S. Upper extremity nerve entrapment syndromes in sports: an update. *Curr Sports Med Rep*. 2014;13(1):16–21.

Gasparotti R, Padua L, Briani C, Lauria G. New technologies for the assessment of neuropathies. *Nat Rev Neurol*. 2017;13:203–216.

Meadows JR, Finnoff JT. Lower extremity nerve entrapments in athletes. *Curr Sports Med Rep*. 2014;13(5):299–306.

Peck E, Strakowski J. Ultrasound evaluation of focal neuropathies in athletes: a clinically-focused review. *Br J Sports Med*. 2015;49:166–175.

Chapter 19 Osteoporosis and Osteopenia

John M. MacKnight

ICD-10-CM CODES
M81.0   *Osteoporosis*
M85.80 *Osteopenia*

Key Concepts

- Osteopenia and osteoporosis are common skeletal disorders characterized by decreased bone mass, disruption of bony microarchitecture with loss of trabeculae, diminished bone strength, and an increased risk of fracture.
- Both conditions arise from inadequate bone development/deposition, excessive bone breakdown, or a combination of both.
- Relative estrogen deficiency in pre-menopause or frank estrogen deficiency in postmenopause are important causative factors, as estrogen plays a central role in skeletal homeostasis and bone mineral density (BMD).
- In the vast majority of cases, osteoporosis arises as a natural consequence of aging, though a number of other causative factors may impact overall bone health (Box 19.1).
- Based on World Health Organization (WHO) criteria (see the following), 20-30% of postmenopausal women in the United States have osteoporosis, with more than 1.3 million fractures per year attributable to the disease.
- Using the same criteria, it is estimated that 1 to 2 million men have osteoporosis and 8 to 13 million men have osteopenia.

History

- Osteoporosis is considered a "silent disease" until an insufficiency fracture occurs.
- The National Osteoporosis Foundation has established guidelines to aid practitioners in identifying patients for whom BMD testing is appropriate (Box 19.2).
- Assessment of clinical risk factors (Box 19.3) is an important starting point in evaluating a patient with low BMD; the most readily recognized risk factors are increasing age and female gender.
- Trabecular bone in vertebral bodies, the neck of the femur, and the distal radius are most frequently affected by osteoporosis.
- Vertebral body fractures are the most common manifestation of osteoporosis, typically presenting with acute onset of severe thoracic or lumbar back pain often with minimal trauma.

Physical Examination

- Osteoporosis has few diagnostic signs, but there are a number of findings that can alert the practitioner to the possibility of disease and/or increased fracture risk.
- Poor visual acuity and depth perception, decreased proprioception, decreased proximal muscle strength, and an impaired "get up and go" test are all risk factors for fall and fracture in older patients.
- Kyphotic deformity of the spine is a late sequela of vertebral fractures.

Imaging

- BMD testing remains the cornerstone of osteoporosis diagnosis and assessment of response to treatment.
- Central dual-energy x-ray absorptiometry (DEXA) is the standard for BMD testing.
  - T-score—established by WHO to compare the standard deviation (SD) difference between patient BMD and a young adult reference group:
    - T-score 0 to –1.0—normal
    - T-score –1.1 to –2.4—osteopenia
    - T-score –2.5 or below—osteoporosis
    - Every 1 SD decrease in BMD is associated with a two- to threefold increase in fracture risk
  - Z-score—compares patient BMD to a group of age-matched peers
    - Typically utilized in young and premenopausal patients
    - A Z-score < –2.0 is considered "below the expected BMD for age" and should prompt a search for secondary causes of bone loss.
- Fracture Risk Assessment Tool (FRAX) uses femoral neck BMD data from DEXA scans to calculate the 10-year probability of hip fracture and major osteoporotic fracture for untreated patients between the ages of 40 and 90 years. FRAX cannot be used in the premenopausal population.
- High-resolution peripheral quantitative CT (HR-pQCT) uses three-dimensional data to provide a true volumetric assessment of bone density that differentiates healthy bone microarchitecture from suboptimal bone.
- Peripheral technologies such as peripheral quantitative computed tomography, peripheral dual-energy x-ray absorptiometry, and quantitative ultrasonography are increasingly being used for screening purposes. However, WHO criteria should not be applied to these measurements.

Additional Tests

- All patients diagnosed with osteoporosis should undergo basic laboratory testing for secondary causes of osteoporosis

BOX 19.1 Secondary Causes of Osteoporosis

Endocrine

Adrenal insufficiency
Cushing syndrome
Eating disorders
Endometriosis
Hyperparathyroidism
Hyperprolactinemia
Hyperthyroidism
Hypogonadism
Diabetes Mellitus

Gastrointestinal/Nutrition

Inflammatory bowel disease
Vitamin D and/or calcium deficiency
Anorexia nervosa
Celiac disease
Malabsorption syndromes
Pancreatic insufficiency

Marrow Disorders

Hemochromatosis
Leukemia
Lymphoma
Mastocytosis
Multiple myeloma
Pernicious anemia

Miscellaneous Causes

Ankylosing spondylitis
Idiopathic hypercalciuria
Idiopathic scoliosis
Multiple sclerosis
Rheumatoid arthritis

BOX 19.2 Who Should Be Tested

National Osteoporosis Foundation

- All women aged 65 and older regardless of risk factors
- Younger postmenopausal women with one or more risk factor(s) (other than being white, postmenopausal, and female)
- Postmenopausal women who are considering therapy if bone mineral density testing would facilitate the decision
- Postmenopausal women who present with fractures (to confirm the diagnosis and determine disease severity)

including complete blood counts, serum calcium, phosphorus, magnesium, alkaline phosphatase, creatinine, parathyroid hormone, 25-hydroxy vitamin D levels, thyroid-stimulating hormone, and testosterone in men.
- Other tests such as serum and urine electrophoresis to screen for multiple myeloma and screening tests for hypercortisolism and malabsorptive syndromes should be obtained in appropriate clinical settings.
- Measurement of 24-hour urinary calcium may be helpful in identifying calcium malabsorption or idiopathic hypercalciuria, both of which may contribute to low BMD.
- Routine use of N-telopeptide or other bone turnover markers is generally unnecessary in treated osteoporotic women.

BOX 19.3 Risk Factors for Osteoporotic Fractures

Major Risk Factors in White Women

- Personal history of fracture as an adult
- History of fragility fracture in a first-degree relative
- Low body weight (<127 pounds)
- Current smoking
- Use of oral corticosteroid therapy for >3 months

Additional Risk Factors

- Premature menopause (<45 years)
- Primary or secondary amenorrhea
- Primary and secondary hypogonadism in men
- Impaired vision
- Prolonged immobilization
- Dementia
- Excessive alcohol consumption (>2 drinks/day)
- Low calcium intake
- Recent falls
- Poor health/frailty

Differential Diagnosis

- Osteomalacia or impaired bone mineralization may present with low BMD and fractures.
- Patients with osteoporosis may have superimposed osteomalacia due to vitamin D deficiency and/or calcium malabsorption.

Treatment

- The management of osteoporosis is multifactorial and includes a combination of lifestyle modifications, nutritional counseling, and pharmacologic interventions.
- Lifestyle modifications:
  - All patients should pursue a combination of weight-bearing exercises and strength training.
  - Patients with severe mobility impairment should be referred for physical therapy.
  - All patients should be advised on fall prevention measures including proper lighting in all rooms, removal of area rugs and floor clutter, use of walking devices as deemed appropriate, avoidance of uneven walking surfaces.
  - Smoking cessation and moderate alcohol consumption
- Nutritional counseling
  - Patients should consume 800 to 1000 IU of vitamin D daily with a goal vitamin D serum value of 30 ng/mL or higher.
  - Patients should also get 1000 to 1200 mg of elemental calcium daily through supplements and/or dietary sources.
- Pharmacologic therapy
  - The National Osteoporosis Foundation (NOF) recommends the following guidelines:
    - Pharmacologic treatment for postmenopausal women with a history of fragility fracture or with osteoporosis based upon BMD measurement (T-score ≤ −2.5)
    - Pharmacologic treatment of high-risk postmenopausal women with T-scores between −1.0 and −2.5 who have a high-risk FRAX score indicating a 10-year probability of hip fracture of ≥3% or of combined major osteoporotic fracture of ≥20%.

- Pharmacologic treatment options include bisphosphonates, recombinant human parathyroid hormone (teriparatide), and hormone therapy.
- In general, bisphosphonates and teriparatide have been shown to be most efficacious in increasing BMD and decreasing future fracture risk.
- For postmenopausal women with osteoporosis, oral bisphosphonates should be considered first-line therapy for most based on efficacy, cost, and long-term proven safety.
  - Of the available bisphosphonates, oral alendronate and risedronate and intravenous zoledronic acid and ibandronate are most commonly used.
  - Daily oral bisphosphonates have been associated with an increased incidence of gastrointestinal side effects including heartburn and dysphagia. This increased incidence has not been observed with the weekly or monthly formulations.
  - Intravenous formulations are associated with flu-like symptoms for the first 24 to 48 hours after medication administration. No long-term side effects have been described.
  - There have been isolated case reports of osteonecrosis of the jaw in patients treated with oral bisphosphonates for osteoporosis, but the incidence is very low (0.7 cases per 100,000 person-years of exposure).
- Teriparatide is the only anabolic agent currently approved for the treatment of osteoporosis. Composed of the amino terminal portion of the human parathyroid hormone molecule, it binds to the parathyroid hormone 1 receptor and results in the recruitment of quiescent bone-forming osteoblasts.
- Estrogen replacement improves BMD, decreases fracture risk, and improves menopausal symptoms in postmenopausal women. After publication of the Women's Health Initiative and the Million Women Study, use decreased due to concerns about potential risks of breast cancer, cardiac disease, and stroke. Because of these concerns and the availability of alternative osteoporosis therapies for use in the postmenopausal population, estrogen replacement is no longer considered a first-line agent for postmenopausal osteoporosis.

Prognosis

- Bisphosphonates and teriparatide have been shown to decrease fracture risk at the spine by 40-70% and at the hip by 30-50%.
- Untreated patients with a history of an insufficiency fracture have a nearly 50% chance of having a second fracture within 2 to 3 years of the initial event.

Troubleshooting

- Close follow-up is required to assess compliance and response to treatment.
- A DEXA scan 1 year after treatment initiation is recommended to document the response to therapy.
- Once an adequate response is observed, including an increase in BMD and a fracture-free state, monitoring with DEXA may be done every 2 years.

- Patients with a poor response to therapy should be rescreened for secondary causes of osteoporosis.

Patient Instructions

- Osteoporosis is a chronic condition that requires long-term follow-up and treatment.
- Adherence to treatment modalities including lifestyle, nutritional, and pharmacologic interventions is crucial for success.

Considerations in Special Populations

- The geriatric population is most commonly affected due to the normal decrease in BMD with aging.
- Other particular populations at risk include:
  - Patients with rheumatologic disorders, particularly those treated with glucocorticoids
  - Patients with a history of malabsorptive syndromes including celiac sprue, inflammatory bowel disease, and gastric bypass
  - Women with a history of breast cancer or men with a history of prostate cancer treated with anti-hormonal therapy
  - Survivors of childhood cancer
  - Female athletes with a history of amenorrhea
  - Immobilized patients

Acknowledgment

The author would like to recognize Theresa Guise and Ailleen Heras-Herzig for their contributions to the original manuscript of this chapter.

Suggested Readings

Binkley N, Bilezikian JP, Kendler DL, et al. Summary of the international society for clinical densitometry 2005 position development conference. *J Bone Miner Res*. 2007;22:643–645.

Black DM, Rosen CJ. Clinical practice: postmenopausal osteoporosis. *N Engl J Med*. 2016;374:254–262.

Cosman F, de Beur SJ, LeBoff MS, et al. Clinician's guide to prevention and treatment of osteoporosis. *Osteoporos Int*. 2014;25:2359–2381.

Crandall CJ, Newberry SJ, Diamant A, et al. Comparative effectiveness of pharmacologic treatments to prevent fractures: an updated systematic review. *Ann Intern Med*. 2014;161:711–723.

Kohrt WM, Bloomfield SA, Little KD, et al. American college of sports medicine position stand: physical activity and bone health. *Med Sci Sports Exerc*. 2004;36:1985–1996.

Looker AC, Borrud LG, Dawson-Hughes B, et al. Osteoporosis or low bone mass at the femur neck or lumbar spine in older adults: United States, 2005-2008. *NCHS Data Brief*. 2012;93:1–8.

National Institutes of Health (NIH). NIH consensus development panel on osteoporosis prevention, diagnosis and therapy. *JAMA*. 2001;285:785–795.

Pentyala S, Mysore P, Pentyala S, et al. Osteoporosis in female athletes. *Int J Clin Ther Diagn*. 2013;1(1):5–11.

World Health Organization. *Assessment of fracture risk and its application to screening for postmenopausal osteoporosis: report of a WHO study group*. Available at http://apps.who.int/iris/handle/10665/39142. Accessed March 28, 2018.

Chapter 20 Tumors

Gregory F. Domson, Anna Greenwood

A tumor can be thought of as any mass in the soft tissues or bone that otherwise should not be there. Upon initial identification, a systemic approach to the evaluation of these lesions aids in providing a timely diagnosis and proper referral.

Evaluation and Staging
History and Physical Examination

The history and physical examination are the first steps in evaluating any bone lesion or soft-tissue mass. Age is integral to the development of a differential diagnosis. Whereas a bone lesion in an older patient is most likely to be a metastatic lesion, younger patients are more likely to present with primary bone tumors (Table 20.1).

Hallmark Signs and Symptoms
- Insidious onset of pain, especially at night and at rest
- Systemic symptoms including fatigue, night sweats, fevers, and unintentional weight loss
- Enlarging mass or limb asymmetry

Physical Examination
- Note any masses and their features (firm vs. soft, fixed vs. mobile, deep vs. superficial).
- Examine the entire extremity and perform a thorough neurovascular examination. Subtle changes may be present secondary to the mass effect of the lesion. Note any thrill or bruit.
- Examine regional lymph nodes, which are the third most common sites of musculoskeletal tumor metastases after the lungs and bones.

Imaging
Conventional Radiographs
- Initial step in evaluation of all lesions, bone or soft tissue.
  - Obtain orthogonal views (anterior-posterior and lateral) of the entire bone and adjacent joints involved.
- Note what the lesion is doing to the bone and how the bone appears to be reacting.
  - A large expansile lesion with cortical disruption, no clear margins, and corresponding soft-tissue mass is more likely to be malignant.
  - A small, well-circumscribed lesion with intact cortices and no soft-tissue mass is more likely to be benign.
- Note the location of the lesion within the bone (epiphysis vs. metaphysis vs. diaphysis, cortical vs. intramedullary), as different lesions have a propensity to form in certain regions of the bone.

Bone Scan
- Used to detect multifocal and/or distant sites of bone disease.
- Multiple myeloma, lymphoma, and metastatic renal cell or thyroid carcinomas may appear cold on bone scan.

Computed Tomography
- Chest computed tomography (CT) to evaluate for lung metastases (the predominant site of metastatic disease) and regional adenopathy.
- Chest and abdomen/pelvis CT to evaluate for primary site in case of metastatic lesions.
- Primary method of evaluating certain bone lesions, for example, osteoid osteoma.

Magnetic Resonance Imaging With Contrast
- Primary method of evaluating characteristics of both bone and soft-tissue lesions
- Demonstrates anatomic relationship of mass and surrounding structures

Positron Emission Tomography
- Useful for detecting metastatic or recurrent disease (particularly sarcoma) and tumor response to chemotherapy

Tumors of the Bone
The American Cancer Society reports that there were approximately 2400 cases of primary bone cancer in 2007. The incidence of all bone tumors and tumor-like conditions is unknown, as many benign lesions are either not ever identified or not reported. A lesion may go undetected until found incidentally on radiographs performed for a remote complaint or after trauma. Any painful lesion or lesion resulting in a pathologic fracture requires further investigation. In addition, large lesions, lesions in critical weight-bearing areas (e.g., subtrochanteric femur), and lesions with associated periosteal reaction or soft-tissue mass require evaluation. The radiographic appearance of benign, benign aggressive, and malignant lesions may demonstrate significant overlap.

Common Benign Bone Lesions
Osteoid Osteoma
- Benign lesion characterized by significant pain, which may lead to secondary physical examination findings such as scoliosis (painful), limb length inequality, and synovitis/joint effusions, depending on location.
- Typical age range is 10 to 30 years, and the most common locations are the long bones of the lower extremity and the posterior elements of the spine.

- A hallmark feature is night pain, often causing awakening, and marked symptomatic improvement with nonsteroidal antiinflammatory drugs/aspirin.
- Radiographically, a small lucent lesion (<1 cm) surrounded by a reactive area of dense cortical bone that can be further delineated with CT (Fig. 20.1).
- Osteoid osteomas will gradually burn out, so the pain can be managed with long-term nonsteroidal antiinflammatory medications. Many patients, however, prefer intervention, and the nidus can be removed surgically or destroyed with radiofrequency ablation.

Osteoblastoma

- Benign bone-forming tumor presenting in the second or third decade with progressive pain that is not worse at night and does not improve with nonsteroidal antiinflammatory drugs (NSAIDs).
- Occur most commonly in long bones and posterior elements of the spine.
- Radiographically, these lesions are >2 cm, geographic and radiolucent, with a thin rim of sclerotic, reactive

TABLE 20.1 Common Ages of Presentation

Age (Years)	Tumor
<5	Metastatic (especially metastatic nephroblastoma and nephroblastoma)
5–30	Ewing sarcoma
5–20	Osteosarcoma
10–25	Chondroblastoma
10–20	Osteochondroma
5–15	Simple bone cyst
10–20	Aneurysmal bone cyst
2–16	Nonossifying fibroma
20–40	Giant cell tumor
>40	Myeloma
>40	Metastatic carcinoma (breast, prostate, thyroid, kidney, lung)
>50	Chondrosarcoma
>50	Chordoma

bone. Variable ossified matrix. Can appear aggressive with periosteal reaction and soft-tissue mass.
- Magnetic resonance imaging (MRI) demonstrates relationship of tumor to surrounding structures.
- Treatment includes extended intralesional curettage with adjuvant treatment (e.g., phenol, liquid nitrogen, argon beam) and grafting of the defect. En bloc excision may be necessary in aggressive or recurrent lesions. Recurrence rates vary from 10% to 20%.

Osteochondroma

- Benign cartilage-forming tumor, also known as an osteo-cartilaginous exostosis, identified incidentally or due to discomfort from soft-tissue impingement in young adults. Most often solitary but may be multiple when part of the multiple hereditary exostosis syndrome, an autosomal dominant condition.
- Radiographically, the lesions are broad based (sessile) or stalk-like (pedunculated) with corticomedullary continuity (Fig. 20.2).
- The pathologic cap of the lesion is composed of cartilage that is subject to the same growth regulation as the physes, so osteochondromas grow until skeletal maturity.
- Low risk of degeneration to a secondary chondrosarcoma. Any growth after cessation of skeletal maturity or increasing size of the cartilage cap is a cause for concern and may indicate malignant transformation.
- Surgical excision for symptomatic or suspicious lesion.

Enchondroma

- Benign cartilaginous tumor found, often incidentally, within the medullary canal of virtually any bone in the third or fourth decade. The most common location is the hand, where they can present with pathologic fracture (Fig. 20.3).
- Radiographs reveal a circumscribed lesion with good margination. Speckled calcifications, minimal endosteal thinning, and (very) mild bone expansion may be found.
- These lesions can be part of a genetic syndrome, characterized by multiple enchondromas—Ollier disease or Maffuci syndrome.
- Low risk of malignant transformation to low-grade chondrosarcoma. Risk increased significantly in setting of enchondromatosis (Ollier disease, Maffuci syndrome).
- Treatment typically consists of serial radiographs with curettage and bone grafting reserved for clinically aggressive or symptomatic lesions.

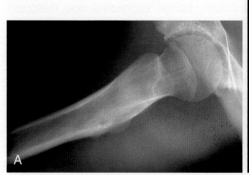

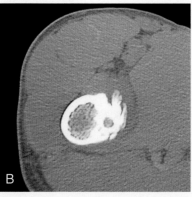

Fig 20.1 (A) Radiograph of the right proximal femur demonstrates a well-circumscribed lytic lesion on the posterior cortex of the femur. **(B)** Axial slice of a computed tomography scan of the proximal femur further delineates the reactive bone around a radiolucent nidus that is less than 1.5 cm.

A B

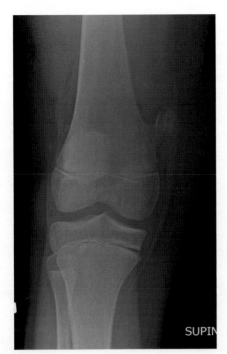

Fig 20.2 Radiograph of the knee of a skeletally immature patient with a pedunculated osteochondroma off of the medial distal femur. Note the continuity between the medullary cavity of the femur and the osteochondroma.

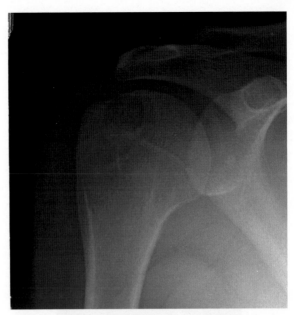

Fig 20.4 Located in the proximal humerus epiphysis and extending into the metaphysis is a well circumscribed lytic lesion with slight cortical expansion visible laterally, consistent with a chondroblastoma.

Chondroblastoma

- Benign, locally aggressive bone tumor typically found in the epiphysis of long bones, most often around the knee, proximal humerus, or proximal femur
- Present in the second or third decades of life with joint pain and swelling.
- Radiographs reveal a destructive epiphyseal lesion with a thin sclerotic rim, often with stippled or punctate calcification (Fig. 20.4).
- Treatment consists of an extended curettage and grafting. Recurrences rates of up to 30%.
- Can rarely metastasize to the lung, where treatment is wedge resection.

Giant Cell Tumor

- Aggressive benign lesion arising in the metaphyseal-epiphyseal region of long bones of patients 20 to 40 years old whose primary complaint is of pain. Most common around the knee.
- Radiographically a lytic, metaphyseal/epiphyseal lesion that typically extends to the subchondral surface of the bone (Fig. 20.5) without a clear sclerotic rim and, in some cases, associated with a soft-tissue mass.
- Treatment is generally intralesional curettage plus adjuvant treatment (chemical/thermal ablation) followed by defect reconstruction with cement and/or bone graft.
- Can rarely metastasize to the lung, so chest radiograph is a routine part of the initial evaluation and follow-up.

Malignant Lesions of the Bone
Metastatic Carcinoma

- Most common cause of a lytic bone lesion in a patient over 40 years old and 25 times more common than sarcomas.
- The five carcinomas that metastasize to bone most commonly are breast, prostate, kidney, lung, and thyroid.

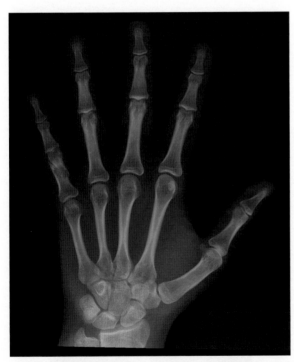

Fig 20.3 A radiograph of the left hand demonstrates a pathologic fracture through an enchondroma of the proximal phalanx of the small finger. The enchondroma is a well-defined lucent lesion with characteristic "popcorn" stippling internally and cortical thinning radially predisposing to a pathologic fracture.

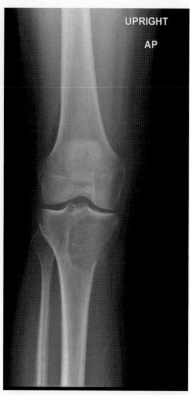

Fig 20.5 Radiograph of the right knee illustrates the characteristic appearance of a giant cell tumor of the proximal tibia—an eccentric lytic lesion within the epiphysis/metaphysis, which borders subchondral bone and expands the medial tibial cortex.

- Can occur in any bone, but most common locations are the thoracic and lumbar spine.
- Radiographically metastatic lesions may be blastic, lytic, or mixed (Fig. 20.6).
- Treatment includes multidisciplinary approach with chemotherapy and radiation therapy, along with surgical stabilization in cases of pathologic or impending pathologic fractures or resection in cases of isolated metastases.
- Prognosis is often poor, especially for metastatic lung cancer.

Multiple Myeloma

- Second most common cause of lytic bone lesions in adults.
- Radiographically well-defined, punched-out lytic lesions (Fig. 20.7) occurring in any bone.
- Present with systemic symptoms of anemia (due to replacement of bone marrow with tumor) and hypercalcemia (from bone lysis) or with pathologic/impending pathologic fractures. Found to have a monoclonal protein spike on urine and serum protein electrophoresis.
- Treatment is multidisciplinary, including medical oncology, radiation oncology, and orthopaedics.

Osteosarcoma

- Most common primary sarcoma of bone presenting predominately in the skeletally immature, with a second peak in the elderly in association with preexisting conditions such as Paget disease.
- The knee is the most commonly involved site (distal femur > proximal tibia), followed by the proximal humerus.

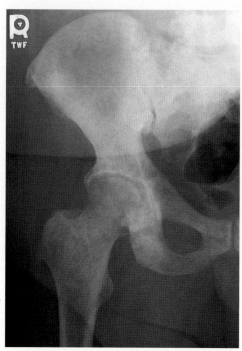

Fig 20.6 The mottled appearance of the right proximal femur and acetabulum on this pelvis radiograph is due to metastatic breast cancer, which often causes mixed lesions with both blastic and lytic characteristics.

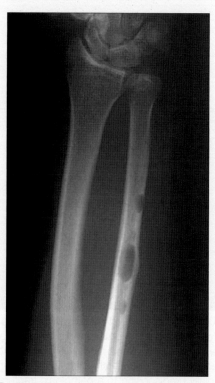

Fig 20.7 Radiograph of the forearm of demonstrates multiple well-defined "punched-out" lytic lesions within the ulna due to multiple myeloma.

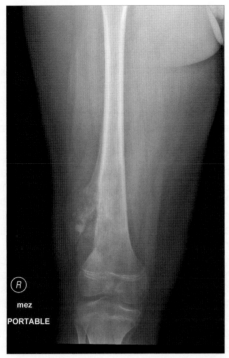

Fig 20.8 A radiograph of the right distal femur of a skeletally immature patient with an osteosarcoma of the distal femur metaphyseal/diaphyseal region. A large mixed blastic and lytic lesion is present with an extensive soft-tissue mass. A Codman triangle, characteristic of osteosarcomas, is visible on the lateral surface of the femur.

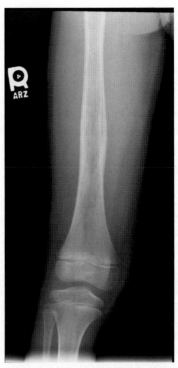

Fig 20.9 An Ewing sarcoma classically occurs in the femoral diaphysis, causing a periosteal reaction described as "onion skin" or "sunburst" pattern, as well as giving the femur a moth-eaten appearance, as illustrated in this radiograph of the femur of a skeletally immature individual.

- Three subtypes: classic (central), parosteal (parallel to the bone, low grade), and periosteal (arising from the periosteum).
- Radiographically, classic osteosarcoma (OSA) lesions (Fig. 20.8) consist of a mixed lytic and blastic picture leading to a "sunburst" appearance with bone spicules forming a radial pattern, as well as triangular elevation of the periosteum at the edge of the lesion (Codman triangle). Lesions are best visualized on MRI. The entire bone should be imaged with MRI to rule out the presence of a skip lesion in the marrow.
- Treatment consists of neoadjuvant chemotherapy followed by wide (margin free of tumor) resection and further chemotherapy. The 5-year survival rate is generally 70%-80%.
- Local recurrence is approximately 10%, and metastases occur primarily to the lungs.

Chondrosarcoma

- Malignant primary bone tumor of chondroid origin. May arise from a preexisting benign cartilage lesion such as an enchondroma or osteochondroma.
- Occur primarily in patients over 50 years of age, with the pelvis, ribs, femur, and proximal humerus being the most common locations.
- Radiographically, chondrosarcomas are destructive lesions that cause cortical thinning and generally contain rings and arcs or "popcorn" calcifications classic for cartilaginous tissue. Further evaluated with MRI.

- Most commonly metastasize to lung.
- Treatment is wide resection with tumor-free margins, as chondrosarcomas are relatively insensitive to radiation and chemotherapy. Overall prognosis depends on the grade.

Ewing Sarcoma

- Second most common primary sarcoma in children. Approximately 80% of cases present in patients younger than 20 years of age.
- High-grade tumor composed of small round blue cells with characteristic t(11,22) gene translocation resulting in EWS:FLI1 fusion, oncogene.
- Clinical presentation may mimic that of osteomyelitis, with fever, pain, swelling, anemia, leukocytosis, and elevated sedimentation rate. Common locations include the femur, pelvis, and scapula.
- Radiographically, diffuse, permeative lesions with classic "onion skin" appearance (multiple thin layers of periosteal reaction; Fig. 20.9). A soft-tissue mass, often very large, is generally present and best seen on MRI.
- Treatment includes surgical resection, plus radiation and possibly chemotherapy, depending on tumor location and resectability. Overall prognosis is about 70% survival rate at 5 years.

Soft-Tissue Tumors

Soft-tissue masses in the extremities are most commonly benign; however, malignant tumors do occur in both children and adults, and delay in diagnosis can affect morbidity and mortality. Evaluation of these lesions includes a careful history and physical examination, appropriate imaging (typically plain radiographs and an MRI), and histologic evaluation as appropriate. Biopsy should be performed under the guidance of the treating surgeon. The classic MRI findings of a soft-tissue sarcoma are intermediate intensity on T1 and bright and heterogenous on T2-weighted images. Included below is a brief overview of the most common soft-tissue tumors.

Benign Soft-Tissue Lesions
Lipoma

- Common, benign soft-tissue masses composed of mature white adipocytes, which is slow growing, typically asymptomatic, and <5 cm.
- Multiple subtypes, including angiolipoma, spindle cell lipoma, and pleomorphic lipoma, exist. The must common presentation is a subcutaneous lesion noted by an adult.
- Radiographically may be visible as a radiolucent mass in the soft tissue, very rarely with subtle calcifications. MRI is often diagnostic, as the mass is isointense to fat on all sequences and does not enhance with gadolinium. Intramuscular lipomas may exhibit internal stranding, raising concern for low-grade liposarcomas.
- Treatment includes observation or marginal excision.

Hemangioma

- Benign vascular malformations presenting in all age groups (most common <30 years old), affecting any portion of the vascular system (arterial or venous) and located superficial (capillary) or deep (cavernous)
- Symptoms include aching pain that varies with activity and palpable mass of variable size depending on posture or activity level.
- Radiographically, mass may contain small mineral densities (phleboliths). MRI reveals a lesion with indistinct margins, often infiltrative into the surrounding musculature, with bright signal areas on T1-weighted sequences (fatty areas) and a more diffuse, "bag of worms," bright appearance on T2-weighted sequences (dilated venous channels).
- Treatment is generally observation (infantile hemangiomas involute by age 7), with intervention reserved for symptomatic lesions, including sclerotherapy, embolization, or surgical resection.

Peripheral Nerve Sheath Tumor

- Benign lesions in peripheral nerves of adults, the most common of which are schwannoma (neurilemmoma) and neurofibroma.
  - A schwannoma typically presents as a painless mass (possibly with a Tinel sign) on the flexor surfaces of the extremities. Composed of Schwann cells. Extremely rarely undergo malignant transformation.
  - Neurofibromas can occur sporadically, usually presenting in third to fifth decade, or in the setting of neurofibromatosis type 1 in patients <20 years old. Sporadic neurofibromas are generally solitary asymptomatic masses with low propensity to become malignant. Plexiform neurofibromas are pathognomonic for NF1 and have a 10% risk of malignant transformation.

- MRI can often differentiate between schwannomas and neurofibromas. Schwannomas are eccentric to the nerve fibers while neurofibromas are found central to the nerve fibers. Both are seen in continuity with a nerve.
- Treatment involves excision of the tumor when symptomatic. In the case of a schwannoma, the nerve can generally be spared. A neurofibroma, however, generally involves multiple fascicles, and excision may sacrifice the nerve, resulting in a neural deficit. Recurrence after excision is rare.

Extraabdominal Desmoid Tumor

- Benign, locally aggressive tumor that presents as an enlarging mass that is firm and fixed and may be symptomatic due to mass effect on adjacent neurovascular structures. Common locations include the shoulder girdle, chest wall, and thigh. May be solitary or multiple in the same extremity.
- Radiographically, long-standing lesions juxtaposed to bone may result in bone remodeling or even invasion of the cortex. MRI is mainstay in diagnosis and reveals a lesion that varies between well circumscribed and infiltrative in nature.
- Nonoperative management of symptomatic inoperable lesions includes low-dose chemotherapy or tamoxifen. Wide resection and radiotherapy is indicated for symptomatic or recurrent lesions. Local recurrence is common.

Malignant Soft-Tissue Lesions
Fibrosarcoma

- Malignant fibrogenic tumor presenting as enlarging painless mass in patients 30 to 80 years of age. Most common soft-tissue sarcoma in adults.
- Radiographs are nonspecific and reveal a soft-tissue density. MRI is also nonspecific but generally reveals a heterogeneous soft-tissue mass that invades the surrounding tissues, displacing neurovascular structures by mass effect.
- Treatment is wide resection of the lesion with perioperative radiation.

Liposarcoma

- Second most common soft-tissue sarcoma, which presents as painless deep mass in patients 50 to 80 years of age, most commonly in the lower extremity.
- There are multiple subtypes that range from low-grade to very high-grade, aggressive lesions. The most common subtype is the well-differentiated (low-grade) lesion (i.e., atypical lipomatous tumor), followed by the myxoid (intermediate-grade) subtype.
- Radiographs reveal a soft-tissue mass possibly with mineralization/calcification within the lesion. MRI appearance of low-grade lesions is similar to lipomas, while high-grade tumors appear similar to other high-grade soft-tissue sarcomas (isointense to muscle on T1, bright and heterogeneous on T2; Fig. 20.10), although there may be evidence of a fatty signal in part of the mass.
- Myxoid liposarcoma may metastasize to the retroperitoneum, so the workup should include CT of the abdomen and pelvis as well as chest.
- Treatment is marginal resection in low-grade lesions and wide local excision and radiation in higher-grade lesions.

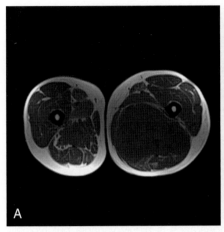
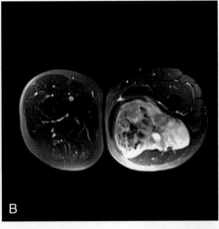

Fig 20.10 High-grade soft-tissue sarcomas, regardless of the cell type, generally exhibit similar characteristics on magnetic resonance imaging—isointense to muscle on T1-weighted imaging (A) and hyperintense and homogeneous on T2-weighted images (B).

Prognosis ranges from a 5-year survival rate of nearly 100% in low-grade lesions to less than 50% in high-grade lesions.

Rhabdomyosarcoma

- Malignant tumor originating from primitive mesenchymal cells, which is the most common sarcoma in children. Presents as a rapidly enlarging painless mass in the head/neck, retroperitoneum, or genitourinary tract, most commonly.
- Four histologically distinct types: embryonal, alveolar, botryoid, and pleomorphic.
- MRI appearance is similar to other sarcomas.
- Can metastasize to lymph nodes and to bone marrow. Bone marrow biopsy is therefore part of the initial evaluation after diagnosis is made.
- Treatment for pediatric rhabdomyosarcoma includes chemotherapy and wide resection. Rhabdomyosarcoma in adults, most commonly pleomorphic subtype, is not sensitive to chemotherapy and is treated with wide resection and radiation. Prognosis for embryonal and alveolar subtypes is 60%-80% 5-year survival, but for botryoid and pleomorphic it is only about 25%.

Synovial Sarcoma

- Most common sarcoma in young adults (15–40 years old), which presents as a slow-growing painless mass most often in the lower extremities.
- Radiographs may reveal calcifications within the mass. MRI demonstrates a heterogenous mass, which is often well circumscribed and may be cystic in appearance.
- Treatment includes wide resection with adjuvant radiation. Prognosis is generally poor, with a 5-year survival rate of approximately 50% and a 10-year survival rate of approximately 25%.

Tumor-Like Lesions
Simple Bone Cyst/Unicameral Bone Cyst

- Nonneoplastic intramedullary lesion filled with serous or serosanguineous fluid identified incidentally or due to pathologic fracture primarily in children. Occurs in the metaphysis adjacent to the physis, most commonly in the proximal humerus.
- Radiographs show a central, lytic, and well-demarcated lesion of the metaphysis with symmetric cortical thinning.

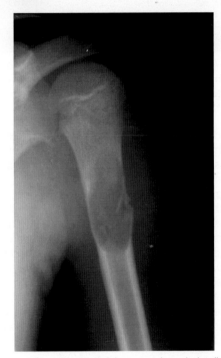

Fig 20.11 A radiograph of a left humerus in a skeletally immature patient demonstrates the classic features of a unicameral bone cyst, including the "fallen leaf" sign indicating pathologic fracture through the thinned cortex of the cyst.

"Fallen leaf" sign indicates fracture (Fig. 20.11). MRI confirms a cystic lesion.
- Treatment can be observation or immobilization after fracture, injection of steroids or marrow substitutes, or curettage and bone grafting. Lesions can recur; however, at skeletal maturity, UBCs will often decrease in size and heal in with bone.

Aneurysmal Bone Cyst

- Nonneoplastic cystic lesion of bone composed of blood-filled spaces separated by soft-tissue septae, which appear in all age groups but are most common in the first two decades. Present with pain and swelling. Neurologic deficits may be present with spinal lesions.

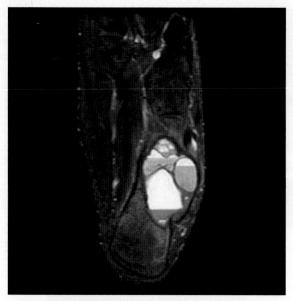

Fig 20.12 A magnetic resonance imaging of the calcaneus shows a well-defined multiloculated lesion with fluid-fluid levels characteristic of an aneurysmal bone cyst.

- Arise commonly in the metaphysis of the long bones (tibia, femur, humerus) and in the posterior elements of the spine.
- Can arise de novo or secondarily to other lesions (giant cell tumor, osteoblastoma, chondroblastoma, fibrous dysplasia).
- Radiographs reveal a lytic, usually eccentric, expansile lesion that is typically well marginated. Expansion into the soft tissue is common, but a thin bony rim around the lesion is generally present. Hot on bone scan, and MRI shows the classic, multilobulated lesion with fluid/fluid levels (Fig. 20.12).
- Treatment is extended intralesional curettage (with or without adjuvant treatment) and bone grafting, after fracture healing in the setting of pathologic fracture. Prognosis is very good, with recurrence of approximately 5-10% in appropriately treated lesions.

Fibrous Dysplasia

- Benign fibro-osseous lesion occurring in one (monostotic, 80%) or multiple (polyostotic, 20%) bones due to failure in normal bone mineralization. Monostotic lesions are usually incidental findings in the proximal femur, rib, maxilla, or tibia most commonly. Pathologic fractures can occur.
- Polyostotic form is associated with endocrine abnormalities such as McCune-Albright syndrome.
- Radiographically, nonaggressive, geographic lesion with ground-glass appearance, often with mild expansion of the bone and thinning of the cortex. Long-standing lesions of the proximal femur may result in deformity (shepherd's crook). A bone scan is generally warm. MRI and CT are

rarely warranted but will demonstrate a central lesion with minimal surrounding edema.
- Treatment is observation or surgical stabilization in symptomatic lesions or lesions at risk of fracture. 1% risk of malignant transformation.

Eosinophilic Granuloma

- Part of the spectrum of lesions that constitute Langerhans cell histiocytosis, a neoplastic proliferation of Langerhans cells. Solitary lesion that presents most commonly with pain and swelling.
- Occurs primarily in those younger than 30 years of age but can present at any age. Most common sites are the skull, femur, and pelvis. Vertebral body lesions may present with collapse (vertebra plana) and neurologic symptoms.
- Radiographic appearance is highly variable but typically shows lytic, geographic, well-marginated lesions, often with periosteal new bone formation. MRI is nonspecific but may show adjacent soft-tissue mass.
- Treatment depends on location and symptoms, as it is a self-limiting process, and includes steroid injections, low-dose irradiation, and curettage and bone grafting.

Paget Disease

- Condition of abnormal bone remodeling marked by increased osteoclastic bone resorption. Presents in individuals more than 50 years old with bone pain and in some cases associated deformity or pathologic fracture or large joint osteoarthritis. Can affect almost any bone, but the pelvis, spine, skull, femur, and tibia are the most common locations and can be monostotic or polyostotic.
- Radiographs demonstrate coarsened trabeculae with thickened cortices, enlargement of the bone, and both lytic and blastic changes in the bone. Very hot on bone scan, and MRI generally shows a moderately increased T2-weighted signal, with a low to moderately low T1-weighted appearance.
- Treatment is generally observation for asymptomatic lesions and bisphosphonates for symptomatic Paget disease. Bony changes may require surgery for progressive skeletal deformity or pathologic fracture or joint arthroplasty for advanced arthritis.
- Less than 1% malignant transformation (OSA, fibrosarcoma, or chondrosarcoma); however, 5-year survival of <10% in these cases.

Suggested Readings

Bullough PG. *Orthopaedic Pathology*. 5th ed. St. Louis: Elsevier; 2010.

Fischgrun JS, ed. *Orthopaedic Knowledge Update 9*. Rosemont, IL: American Academy of Orthopaedic Surgeons; 2007.

Goldblum JR, Folpe AL, Weiss SW, eds. *Enzinger and Weiss's Soft Tissue Tumors*. 6th ed. Philadelphia: Elsevier; 2014.

Schwartz HS, ed. *Orthopaedic Knowledge Update: Musculoskeletal Tumors 2*. Rosemont, IL: American Academy of Orthopaedic Surgeons; 2007.

Chapter 21 Pain Management: Acute Pain

Wesley W. Carr, Chester Buckenmaier III, Francis O'Connor

ICD-10-CM CODES
Codes vary by location of the pain
G89.1 *Acute pain, not elsewhere classified*
G89.11 *Acute pain due to trauma*
G89.18 *Other acute postprocedural pain*

General Information

- Acute pain is the physiologic response and experience to noxious stimuli that can become pathologic, is normally sudden in onset, time limited, and motivates behaviors to avoid actual or potential tissue injuries (Acute Pain Medicine Shared Interest Group).

Etiology and Pathogenesis

- Pain is multifactorial and dependent on both physiologic and psychologic components.
- Traditional attempts to delineate acute and chronic pain, while clinically helpful, may neglect potential pathophysiologic links between the two.
- Commonly used systems include:
  - Time course, where an upper limit of 3 to 6 months is ascribed to acute pain
  - Qualitative descriptors, where perioperative, traumatic, obstetric, etc., usually refer to acute pain processes and cancer, noncancer, neuropathic, etc., typically apply to chronic pain
- Categorizing pain as physiologic or pathologic may be more appropriate
  - Physiologic (adaptive pain)
    - Most common type of acute pain (e.g., surgery, trauma)
    - Relies on peripheral nociceptor activation by noxious stimuli (e.g., extreme temperatures, pressure, inflammatory cytokines and chemokines)
    - Afferent pathways transmit peripheral impulses to the central nervous system
    - Efferent pathways modulate the response to noxious stimuli to locate and interpret the intensity of pain, avoid or minimize additional tissue damage, and support behavioral modifications to promote recovery and function.
  - Pathologic (maladaptive pain)
    - Less common cause of acute pain; usually associated with chronic pain (e.g., migraines, stroke, spinal cord injury)
    - Described as neuropathic pain or dysfunction of the somatosensory system

- The pain experience is significantly impacted by anxiety, depression, pain catastrophizing, fear avoidance, previous experience with pain, culture, and beliefs.

History and Physical

- A thorough history is essential, given the subjective and individualized nature of pain.
- The simple mnemonic, OLD CARTS, covers most components of a pain history (Onset, Location/radiation, Duration, Character, Aggravating factors, Relieving factors, Temporal association, Severity).
- It is additionally helpful to ascertain associated symptoms (e.g., nausea and vomiting), effect on activities and sleep, relevant medical history, previous and current treatments, and factors influencing the patient's response to treatment (e.g., beliefs, knowledge, and expectations of pain and its management).
- Physical examination becomes more important when history is limited by critical illness, age, communication barriers, or cognitive impairment.
- Provocative maneuvers such as Spurling test, Tinel sign, Phalen test, straight leg raise, and slump test may reveal less apparent neurogenic involvement.
- Findings suggestive of pain include increased respiratory rate, heart rate, blood pressure, palmar sweating, intracranial pressure, and agitation.

Diagnosis

- Measurement of pain is a greater diagnostic dilemma than determining the presence or absence of pain.
- Routine assessment of pain has been shown to improve pain management.
- Avoid reliance on unidimensional pain scales (e.g., pain intensity), as they may be interpreted differently by patients and providers, neglect psychosocial components of pain, or overlook the assessment of pain with and without movement.
- Multidimensional assessments of pain, such as the Defense and Veterans Pain Rating Scale (DVPRS), are preferred when possible.
- Poorly controlled pain despite adequate attempts at analgesia should always prompt reconsideration of the underlying diagnosis.

Treatment

- Always consider the impact a treatment option may have on daily function, occupation, and athletic performance.

- Multimodal analgesia delivered in a multidisciplinary approach is ideal.
  - Multimodal analgesia refers to the administration of ≥2 medications or interventions with unique mechanisms of action that work in additive or synergistic fashion to reduce adverse effects or dose of any one medication or technique.
- Integrative medicine
  - Acupuncture, massage, biofeedback, and physical therapy—among other techniques—are effective primary and adjunct therapies with an extremely favorable side-effect profile compared to pharmacologic pain management approaches.
- Acetaminophen
  - Avoid concomitant administration of acetaminophen-containing medications.
  - Hepatotoxicity is exceedingly rare when daily dose is less than 4000 mg.
- Nonsteroidal antiinflammatory drugs (NSAIDs)
  - Use at lowest dose and duration to avoid cardiovascular adverse effects.
  - Use with caution in patients at risk for or with known renal impairment.
  - Nonselective NSAIDs increase the risk of minor and major bleeding after surgery.
  - Administration of ibuprofen reduces the protective effects of low-dose aspirin.
  - The effect on bone healing is unclear.
- Opioids
  - Calculate total daily morphine milligram equivalent given variable potency.
- Adverse effects of opioids are dose-related, so minimizing dosage is the goal.
- Tramadol and tapentadol are weak opioid agonists that are effective for neuropathic pain, and both have lower rates of adverse effects and abuse.
- Corticosteroids
  - Systemic dexamethasone may reduce postoperative pain and opioid requirement, but risk in surgical patients has not been studied.
  - Regional corticosteroids (e.g., shoulder, epidural, knee, etc.) are effective for short-term pain relief, but adverse effects may outweigh benefits.
- Local anesthetics
  - Systemic administration of lidocaine has good evidence as a preventive analgesic.
  - The use of local anesthetics in regional anesthesia techniques (both single injection and continuous) can provide profound perioperative pain control.
- N-methyl-D-aspartate (NMDA) receptor antagonists
  - Systemic administration of ketamine has good evidence as a preventive analgesic.
  - Perioperative use of ketamine lowers the incidence of chronic postoperative pain.
- Anticonvulsants
  - Gabapentin and pregabalin are effective for neuropathic pain and reduce postoperative pain and opioid requirements.
- Antidepressants
  - Tricyclic antidepressants (TCAs) and serotonin-norepinephrine-reuptake inhibitors (SNRIs) are effective for neuropathic pain and fibromyalgia.

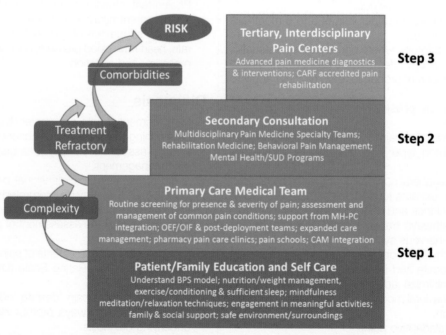

Fig 21.1 Stepped Care Model for Pain Management. *BPS,* Biopsychosocial; *CAM,* complementary and alternative medicine: *CARF,* Commission on Accreditation or Rehabilitation Facilities; *MH-PC,* Primary Care-Mental Health; *OEF,* Operation Enduring Freedom; *OIF,* Operation Iraqi Freedom; *PACT,* Patient Aligned Care Team; *SUD,* substance use disorders. (Reprinted from U.S. Department of Veterans Affairs/Department of Defense. *VA/DoD Clinical Practice Guideline for Opioid Therapy for Chronic Pain.* <www.healthquality.va.gov/guidelines/pain/cot/>; 2017 Accessed February 2018.)

- Bisphosphonates and salmon calcitonin
  - Salmon calcitonin has been shown to reduce acute phantom limb pain.
  - Pamidronate is effective for osteoporotic vertebral compression fracture pain.
- Alpha-2 agonists
  - Systemic administration of clonidine and dexmedetomidine has good evidence as a preventive analgesic, but bradycardia and hypotension may preclude their use.
- Inhalational agents
  - Nitrous oxide and methoxyflurane have evidence as rapid acting analgesics.

Complications and Prognosis

- Transitional care from the inpatient to outpatient setting is an area prone to error.
- The VA/DoD stepped care model is useful in developing individualized pain treatment plans (Fig. 21.1).
- Opioid use disorder after postoperative opioid prescription use is as high as 10%.
- 35-80% of people with opioid use disorder report their first exposure to opioids occurring after treatment of diagnosed pain, including postoperative pain.

- Pain is a continuum, and almost all chronic pain begins as acute pain that fails to resolve.

Suggested Readings

Buckenmaier C. *Military Advanced Regional Anesthesia and Analgesia Handbook*. Government Printing Office; 2009.

Buckenmaier CC 3rd, Galloway KT, Polomano RC, et al. Preliminary validation of the defense and veterans pain rating scale (DVPRS) in a military population. *Pain Med*. 2013;14(1):110–123.

Chou R, Gordon DB, de Leon-Casasola OA, et al. Management of postoperative pain: a clinical practice guideline from the American pain society, the American society of regional anesthesia and pain medicine, and the American society of anesthesiologists' committee on regional anesthesia, Executive committee, and administrative council. *J Pain*. 2016;17(2):131–157.

Polomano RC, Galloway KT, Kent ML, et al. Psychometric testing of the defense and veterans pain rating scale (DVPRS): a new pain scale for military population. *Pain Med*. 2016;17(8):1505–1519.

Schug SA, Palmer GM, Scott DA, et al. Acute pain management: scientific evidence, fourth edition, 2015. *Med J Aust*. 2016;204(8):315–317.

Tighe P, Buckenmaier CC 3rd, Boezaart AP, et al. Acute pain medicine in the United States: a status report. *Pain Med*. 2015;16(9):1806–1826.

Chapter 22 Pain Management: Chronic Pain

Jillian Sylvester, Chester Buckenmaier III, Francis O'Connor

ICD-10-CM CODES
(Codes will vary by location of pain.)
G84.4 *Chronic pain syndrome*
G89.2 *Chronic pain, not elsewhere classified*

Epidemiology

- Approximately 15-22% of Americans suffer from chronic pain.
- Chronic pain costs society approximately $600 billion annually: $261 to $300 billion in health care costs and $297 to $336 billion in related compensation costs, lost wages, and reduced productivity.
- More than 400 million workdays are lost each year secondary to chronic pain.
- Evaluations for spine and musculoskeletal disorders account for approximately 70 million physician office visits and 130 million outpatient, hospital, and emergency department (ED) visits annually.

Definitions

- Pain is an unpleasant sensory and emotional experience arising from actual or potential damage to tissue. It can be influenced by genetics, epigenetic biological processes, psychological responses, and societal and cultural norms.
- Chronic pain is ongoing or recurrent pain, lasting more than 3 months or beyond the usual course of acute injury, that adversely affects the individual's well-being.
- In chronic pain, the structural and chemical function of the nervous system is altered through sensitization, which makes it physiologically distinct from acute pain (see Chapter 21), although acute pain can lead to chronic pain through a process termed *chronification*.
- Chronic pain may be nociceptive, neuropathic, or mixed. It serves no evolutionary function but contributes to the development and persistence of disability.
  - Nociceptive pain: derived from detection of potentially damaging noxious stimuli by nociceptors
    - Often described as Somatic, Referred, Radicular, or Postoperative
    - Persistent pain of unclear etiology may be due to underlying malignancy
  - Neuropathic pain: generated without adequate stimulation of sensory nerves
    - Caused by nerve injury, and can affect both peripheral and central nervous systems
    - Can occur in conjunction with nociceptive pain

History

- It is important to establish good clinical rapport with the patient, first achieved during the initial encounter.
- Collect a comprehensive history. Special focus should be given to:
  - Clinical course of pain (onset and inciting source of pain, how the pain has evolved since its onset, etc.)
  - Pain functional and emotional impairment along with pain intensity should be assessed (see Defense and Veterans Pain Rating Scale [DVPRS], Chapter 21). Measuring only pain intensity to quantify pain and guide therapy is no longer acceptable.
  - Pain character to help distinguish between types of pain (burning or electric shocks consistent with neuropathic pain versus cramping, classically describing nociceptive visceral pain)
  - Aggravating and alleviating pain factors (e.g., associations of pain with activities, weather, stressors, or mood)
  - Associated symptoms (such as weakness, numbness, loss of function, bladder, or bowel incontinence)
  - Previous pain treatments and their effect on the patient's function
- Assess for impact of pain on social, physical, occupational, and sexual function, and overall quality of life. Use of validated scores such as National Institutes of Health (NIH) Patient-Reported Outcomes Measurement Information System (PROMIS) self-report measures can help quantify this impact.
- Obtain past medical history:
  - Psychiatric
    - There is a bidirectional relationship between chronic pain and depression.
    - Studies have shown individuals with chronic pain are at an increased risk of depression, and those with depression are at an increased risk for chronic pain.
    - Many medications used for management of psychiatric conditions can affect chronic pain symptoms and treatment options.
  - Substance Abuse
    - Addiction in the setting of chronic pain can complicate the evaluation and treatment of the presenting complaint.
    - The prevalence of substance abuse in those with chronic pain is 2-25%.
    - It is important to screen for a personal or family history of substance abuse.
    - The risk of drug use or abuse should be quantified using a validated screening tool (e.g., Opioid Risk Tool [ORT]).

- Medical Illness
  - Medical comorbidities requiring use of certain chronic medications may limit treatment options (drug-drug interactions, medication side effects, etc.).
- Outside influences such as ongoing litigation and disability claims can complicate the clinical picture. It may be necessary to explore competing self-interest issues hindering therapeutic goals.

Physical Examination

- Physical examination will vary based on patient's report of pain symptoms.
- Vital signs (typically not elevated with chronic pain as they are in acute pain)
- Evaluation of all chronic musculoskeletal pain should include a systematic assessment of:
  - Gait, posture, muscular symmetry or atrophy, observed rashes
  - Range of motion and strength testing
  - Neurologic evaluation of light touch, pinprick, and deep-tendon reflexes
    - Allodynia is the experience of pain from non-painful stimuli (e.g., light touch). Allodynia should raise suspicion for underlying neurologic cause of pain.
  - Provocative maneuvers (e.g., Spurling test evaluating for nerve root disorder; straight-leg-raise evaluation for lumbosacral nerve root lesion; Patrick sign evaluating for sacroiliac joint pain or intra-articular hip pathology; Tinel sign evaluating for peripheral nerve irritation via direct percussion)
- Psychological evaluation, including signs of nonorganic pain

Imaging

- Imaging is rarely warranted and depends on the chronic pain complaint.

Additional Tests

- Additional tests are typically only warranted to evaluate for neurologic or vascular etiologies of pain.

Treatment

- Multidisciplinary care is the mainstay of treatment for optimal outcomes, including pharmacologic treatments, interventions (e.g., integrative medicine and injections in select patients), rehabilitation, and psychological treatments. The stepped care model for pain (Chapter 21) should be utilized to guide therapy. Surgery for pain is reserved for patients where other options are ineffective or inappropriate.
- Providers should discuss and establish goals of care early within the treatment course and educate patients that complete pain resolution may not be feasible. A focus on improved function with concomitant pain reduction is a more reasonable approach for patients with chronic pain.
- Active patient self-care is very important for successful treatment and outcomes. Self-directed treatments can include weight loss, smoking cessation, home physical therapy, and regular exercise programs.
- Nonpharmacologic and non-opioid pharmacologic therapy are the preferred treatments for chronic pain management.

Opioid Crisis

- There has been a significant increase in the use of prescription opioids to treat chronic, noncancer pain.
  - Approximately 1 in 5 patients with noncancer pain diagnoses are prescribed opioids in office-based settings.
  - Primary care providers prescribe about half of dispensed opioid pain relievers.
  - Sales of prescribed opioids in the United States has nearly quadrupled since 1999, with no overall change in the amount of pain reported by Americans.
  - Despite the surge in prescribing, there is no evidence to support the use of long-term opioids for the management of chronic pain.
- In 2015, more than 2 million Americans abused prescription opioids; more than 15,000 died from related overdoses. In 2016, more than 61.8 million people were prescribed opioids.

Nonpharmacologic Treatment

- Behavioral/Cognitive: psychotherapy, cognitive behavioral therapy, mindfulness, sleep education
  - Cognitive treatments have been shown to be more effective than pharmacologic intervention.
- Physical: graded exercise, physical therapy, massage, acupuncture, chiropractic manipulations, TENS units, heat/cold modalities
- Education: promoting self-treatment and self-efficacy to achieve improved pain outcomes
- Injections: may be both therapeutic and diagnostic, helping to isolate the pain drivers in musculoskeletal pain. Examples of injections include:
  - Epidural steroid injections for lumbar or cervical radicular pain
  - Facet injections (intra-articular or medial branch blocks) for axial pain
  - Joint injections (including sacroiliac, hip, shoulder joint injections)
  - Trigger point injections for myofascial pain
- Advanced specialty pain procedures (e.g., intrathecal pumps or spinal cord stimulation and/or surgery can be warranted in some instances for refractory pain, depending on pathology)

Pharmacologic, Non-Opioid Treatment

- Characterization of pain can help direct non-opioid pharmacologic therapy.
  - Nociceptive Pain
    - Nonsteroidal antiinflammatory drugs (NSAIDs; e.g., ibuprofen, naproxen, diclofenac, ketorolac) or acetaminophen
    - Antispasmodics (e.g., cyclobenzaprine, tizanidine, baclofen)
  - Neuropathic Pain or Co-occurring Pain Syndromes (e.g., fibromyalgia)
    - Serotonin norepinephrine reuptake inhibitors (SNRIs [e.g., venlafaxine, duloxetine])

- Serotonin selective reuptake inhibitor (SSRIs [e.g., fluoxetine, paroxetine])
- Gabapentinoids (e.g., gabapentin, pregabalin)
- Tricyclic antidepressants (TCAs [e.g., amitriptyline, imipramine])
- Co-occurring Psychiatric Conditions
  - SNRIs and SSRIs can be effective treatments for neuropathic pain and/or mood enhancement.
  - Prazosin can be an effective treatment for both pain and posttraumatic stress disorder.
  - Exercise caution with prescribing TCAs or opioids in individuals at risk of suicide.

Pharmacologic, Opioid Treatment

- Opioids should never be the first-line treatment for chronic pain, and should be administered in conjunction with non-opioid adjuvant therapies. There is no evidence that long-term opioid therapy benefits chronic pain, although significant evidence is available concerning the morbidity associated with this approach.
- Patient selection for chronic opioid therapy is critical to reduce risk of dependence and adverse effects.
  - Patients with cancer-related pain or other conditions resulting in significant pain, where previous non-opioid multimodal therapies have been tried, are reasonable candidates for chronic opioid therapy.
  - Patients with mechanical back pain, centralized pain syndromes (e.g., fibromyalgia), and chronic headache should not be prescribed chronic opioids.
- Before initiating chronic opioid therapy:
  - Screen for addiction risk using verified methods, such as the ORT.
  - Complete a baseline urine drug toxicity screen.
  - Check for active or previous opioid and benzodiazepine usage through states' electronic Prescription Drug Monitoring systems.
  - Consider use of a written Sole Provider Agreement to limit sources of opioid prescriptions.
  - Counsel patients on the risks and benefits of opioid use for chronic pain management.
  - Establish treatment goals and continue opioid therapy only if achieving clinically meaningful improvements in physical and emotional function that outweigh risks to patient safety.
- When initiating opioid therapy in an opioid-naïve person, clinicians should ensure other pain management options have been exhausted (Pain Stepped Care Model). Start with the lowest effective dosage.
  - Dosages should be titrated up slowly to an effective dose. Once reaching an effective dose, providers should critically consider further dose escalations due to risk of paradoxical hyperalgesia and tolerance.
  - If tolerance is suspected, changing opioid medications can be an effective way of restoring analgesia.
- Opioids should never be prescribed with benzodiazepines due to risk of significant adverse effects.

When to Refer

- Clinicians should strongly consider specialty care consultation prior to initiating treatment of chronic pain in pregnant women, children, individuals with substance use disorders, or severe psychiatric comorbidities.

Considerations in Special Populations

- Polypharmacy is a risk in all patients, more so in the elderly, those with comorbid psychiatric conditions requiring medical therapy, and those with prior/current substance abuse. Take care to ensure prescribed treatments do not react with existing therapies.
- Careful titration of medications is important in the elderly to account for age-related changes in kidney function and a higher predisposition to cognitive changes.
  - Many of the medicines used to treat chronic pain are on the BEERS List for limited use in elderly populations.
- Many of the above drug therapies are contraindicated in pregnancy, as are certain types of acupuncture and chiropractic manipulation. Ensure therapy is safe in pregnancy before starting.

Suggested Readings

Bajwa ZH, Wootton RJ, Warfield CA, eds. *Principles and Practice of Pain Medicine*. 3rd ed. New York: McGraw-Hill Education; 2017:56–68.

Centers for Disease Control and Prevention: *Annual surveillance report of drug-related risks and outcomes—United States, 2017*. Surveillance Special Report 1. Centers for Disease Control and Prevention, U.S. Department of Health and Human Services. August 2017. Available at https://www.cdc.gov/drugoverdose/pdf/pubs/2017-cdc-drug-surveillance-report.pdf. Accessed April 5, 2018.

Dowell D, Haegerich TM, Chou R. CDC guideline for prescribing opioids for chronic pain—United States, 2016. *JAMA*. 2016;315(15):1624–1645.

Jamison RN, Serraillier J, Michna E. Assessment and treatment of abuse risk in opioid prescribing for chronic pain. *Pain Res Treat*. 2011;2011:941808.

NIH National Institute on Drug Abuse: *Sample Patient Agreement Forms (website)*. Available at https://www.drugabuse.gov/sites/default/files/files/SamplePatientAgreementForms.pdf. Accessed April 5, 2018.

Qaseem A, Wilt TJ, McLean RM, et al. Noninvasive treatments for acute, subacute, and chronic low back pain: a clinical practice guideline from the American college of physicians. *Ann Intern Med*. 2017;166(7):514–530.

Tauben D. Nonopioid medications for pain. *Phys Med Rehabil Clin N Am*. 2015;26(2):219–248.

U.S. Department of Health and Human Services: *Patient-Reported Outcomes Measurement Information System (PROMIS) Self-Reporting Tools (website)*. Available at http://www.nihpromis.org/default. Accessed April 5, 2018.

Von Korff M, Saunders K, Thomas Ray G, et al. De facto long-term opioid therapy for noncancer pain. *Clin J Pain*. 2008;24(6):521–527.

Webster LR: *Opioid Risk Tool (website)*. 2005. Available at https://www.drugabuse.gov/sites/default/files/files/OpioidRiskTool.pdf. Accessed April 5, 2018.

Chapter 23 Pain Management: Complex Regional Pain Syndrome

Nathaniel S. Nye, Stephanie N. Lamb

ICD-10-CM CODES

G90. 511	*CRPS type I upper limb, right*
G90.512	*CRPS type I upper limb, left*
G90.521	*CRPS type I lower limb, right*
G90.5322	*CRPS type I lower limb, left*
G56.41	*Causalgia (CRPS type II) upper limb, right*
G56.42	*Causalgia (CRPS type II) upper limb, left*
G57.71	*Causalgia (CRPS type II) lower limb, right*
G57.72	*Causalgia (CRPS type II) lower limb, left*

Key Concepts

- Complex regional pain syndrome (CRPS) is a regional neuropathic pain that does not follow the usual distribution of a dermatome or nerve territory.
- Associated with abnormal sensory, autonomic, motor, and/ or trophic changes
- Most commonly develops after distal limb trauma or surgery
- CRPS diagnosed clinically using the Budapest criteria, which was approved by International Association for the Study of Pain (IASP) in 2012

History

- Usually occurs 4 to 6 weeks after inciting event
- Risk factors: female, postmenopausal, recent distal radius fracture, ankle dislocation and/or intra-articular fracture, immobilization, high levels of reported pain after trauma
- Pain is commonly felt deep within the limb and is described as burning, searing, or shooting; worsens with movement, contact, temperature variation, and stress.
- Four symptom categories: sensory, vasomotor, sudomotor/ edema, motor/trophic (Table 23.1)

Physical Examination

- Inspect area carefully and compare findings with contralateral limb (see Table 23.1).
- Observe gait and posture for any compensatory movements and guarding.
- Inspect extremity for edema, changes in hair/nail growth, and skin color/appearance.
- Assessment of skin temperature, tone, and texture.
- Evaluate range of motion, strength, and reflexes.
- Neurologic: pinprick, light touch, temperature, deep somatic pressure.

Imaging

- No specific test or imaging can diagnose or exclude CRPS.
- Primary goal of diagnostic/medical tests is to exclude other diagnoses.
- MRI and triple phase bone scan may show findings suggestive of CRPS.

Differential Diagnosis

- Peripheral neuropathy (e.g., diabetic neuropathy, carpal tunnel syndrome)
- Thoracic outlet syndrome (especially vascular subtype)
- Peripheral vascular disease
- Deep vein thrombosis (e.g., Paget Schroetter syndrome)
- Autoimmune arthritis
- Raynaud disease
- Fibromyalgia
- Bacterial infection (skin, muscle, joint, or bone)
- Erythromelalgia

Treatment

- Requires multidisciplinary approach, individualized to the patient
- Goal of all therapies is to improve function and relieve pain (Fig. 23.1).
- Prevention: Vitamin C supplementation after distal limb fracture or surgery may be effective in reducing risk of developing CRPS.

Pharmacologic Treatment

- First-line, low-risk medications: topical analgesics, NSAIDs, corticosteroids
- Second-line medications: anticonvulsants (e.g., gabapentin), antidepressants, α-adrenergic antagonists (e.g., clonidine), bisphosphonates, calcitonin, opioids (use with caution)
- Additional medication options involve greater risk and require the involvement of pain specialist.
  - Ketamine has been shown to be effective in reducing pain; however, evidence is limited and optimal dosage and duration of treatments are still unknown.
  - Regional sympathetic blockade (e.g., stellate ganglion) has shown promise in small trials.

Interventional Techniques

- Neuromodulation: includes noninvasive options (e.g., transcutaneous electrical nerve stimulation, or TENS) and

TABLE 23.1 Budapest Clinical Diagnostic Criteria for Complex Regional Pain Syndrome

Criteria	Clinical Categories of Signs and Symptoms
1 Continuing pain, which is disproportionate to any inciting event	Sensory—hyperalgesia, hypoesthesia, allodynia
2 Must report at least one symptom in three of the four clinical categories	Vasomotor—skin color or temperature changes/asymmetry
3 Must display at least one sign at the time of assessment in two or more of the four clinical categories	Sudomotor/edema—edema and/or sweating changes and/or sweating asymmetry
4 There is no other diagnosis that better explains the signs and symptoms	Motor/trophic—decreased range of motion and/or motor dysfunction (weakness, tremor, dystonia) and/or trophic changes (hair, nail, skin)

invasive procedures (e.g., implanted spinal cord stimulation, dorsal root ganglion stimulation, and deep brain stimulation)
- Surgical sympathectomy; amputation

Physical Therapy/Occupational Therapy
- Normalize movement patterns and manage pain-related fear of moving the extremity.
- Graded motor imagery and mirror box therapy are effective in reducing pain and disability.

Psychological Interventions
- Build coping mechanisms, confidence, and commitment to the rehabilitation process.
- Assess for concomitant axis I disorders that could complicate the rehabilitation process.

When to Refer
- Immediate referral to specialists for multidisciplinary management is crucial once CRPS is suspected, as it is believed earlier treatment may prevent some cases from becoming chronic.

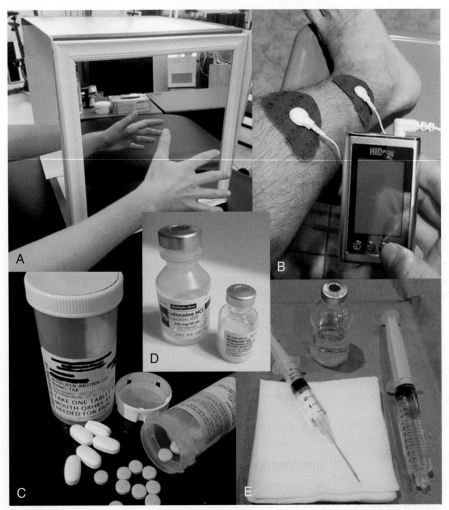

Fig 23.1 Examples of treatments for complex regional pain syndrome. (A) Mirror box therapy. (B) Transcutaneous electrical nerve stimulation (TENS). (C) Oral medications. (D) Injectable lidocaine and triamcinolone. (E) Ketamine infusion.

Prognosis

- Highly variable; most cases resolve within a few months to a year.
- Approximately 10-20% of cases become chronic and refractory to any therapy.
- Delayed diagnosis and inadequate management are associated with prolonged recovery.

Troubleshooting

- A diagnosis of CRPS should not be given in cases of pain isolated to proximal joints (hip/shoulder) or in cases where symptoms are isolated to the head/torso.

Patient Instructions

- Patients should be encouraged to be an active participant in therapy.
- Take time to ensure the patient understands the diagnosis and reasoning behind therapies.

Considerations in Special Populations

- CRPS can affect children/adolescents, but presentation may differ slightly from adult patterns.
- Diagnosis based on the same clinical criteria as adults (Budapest criteria)
- Psychological issues more prominent in children (e.g., depression/anxiety, eating disorders)
- Skin temperature in affected limb is generally cooler in children than adults at presentation.

- Education, physical therapy, and psychotherapy are considered first line of treatment.
- The majority of children have a favorable outcome.

Suggested Readings

Birklein F, O'Neill D, Schlereth T. Complex regional pain syndrome: an optimistic perspective. *Neurology.* 2015;84:89–96.

Birklein F, Schlereth T. Complex regional pain syndrome—significant progress in understanding. *Pain.* 2015;156:S94–S103.

Borsook D. Ketamine and chronic pain—going the distance. *Pain.* 2009;145(3):271.

Bruehl S. Complex regional pain syndrome. *BMJ.* 2015;350:1–13.

Bussa M, Mascaro A, Cuffaro L, Rinaldi S. Adult complex regional pain syndrome type I: a narrative review. *PM R.* 2017;9(7):707–719.

Carr AC, McCall C. The role of vitamin C in the treatment of pain: new insights. *J Transl Med.* 2017;15:77.

Goh EL, Chidambaram S, Ma D. Complex regional pain syndrome: a recent update. *Burns Trauma.* 2017;5(1):2.

O'Connell NE, Wand BM, McAuley J, et al. Interventions for treating pain and disability in adults with complex regional pain syndrome. *Cochrane Database Syst Rev.* 2013;(4):CD009416.

Picarelli H, Sterman-Neto H, De-Oliveira ML, Teixeira MJ. Neuromodulation in treating complex regional pain syndrome: a critical review of the evidence. *J Neurol Neurosci.* 2017;8:1.

Smart KM, Wand BM, O'Connell NE. Physiotherapy for pain and disability in adults with complex regional pain syndrome (CRPS) types I and II. *Cochrane Database Syst Rev.* 2016;(2):CD010853.

Wertli MM, Brunner F, Steurer J, Held U. Usefulness of bone scintigraphy for the diagnosis of complex regional pain syndrome 1: a systematic review and bayesian meta-analysis. *PLoS ONE.* 2017;12(3):e0173688.

Chapter 24 Pain Management: Novel and Alternative Therapies for Chronic Pain

Jeffrey Leggit, Caleb Dickison

ICD-10-CM CODES
G89.4 *Chronic pain syndrome*
G89.2 *Chronic pain, not elsewhere classified*

Key Concepts

- Chronic pain is defined as pain present longer than 3 months. A direct correlation between tissue pathology and the degree and duration of pain does not always exist.
- Rather than thinking in terms of a "cure," the goal is to maximize function while avoiding morbidity from medications or procedures. A holistic, multimodal approach is advocated.
- This chapter will focus on an integrative approach that combines conventional with nonmainstream and novel practices.
- Many integrative treatments lack rigorous evidence; however, if the patient is following prescribed therapies, the integrative treatment is not harmful, and the patient is perceiving a benefit, they should be allowed to continue.
- Patients must understand that health insurance may not cover some of these treatments, although a flexible spending account can offset some costs if available.
- The patient as well as his or her support system should be involved in the care plan, and the patient should be empowered to set goals to achieve self-actualization.
- Patients should have regularly scheduled follow-up appointments to discuss the effectiveness of treatments as well as discussions of further management options if treatments are not having the desired effect.
- Restoration of normal sleep patterns is paramount in the treatment plan.

History

- Location and type of pain will depend on medical condition and will vary significantly.
- Performing a thorough history and physical exam is essential to making the correct diagnosis and treatment plan. It is also important to consider contributing factors such as socioeconomic class, previous treatments, comorbidities including psychological/mental illness, as well as social and occupational status.

Physical Examination

- Physical exam will depend on location and etiology of pain.
- The exam should be thorough and include a full neurological exam to verify the correct location and diagnosis of pain.

Imaging

- Often when considering nonmainstream treatments, advanced imaging has already been performed. Additional imaging should only be done if it will change management or assist in clarifying diagnosis.

Additional Tests

- Will vary widely based on type of pain, and could be used to verify diagnosis or rule out other conditions.
- Electrodiagnostic studies may be helpful for certain types of nerve conditions.
- Vascular studies can be done if there is a concern for vascular diseases.
- If history and physical exam are concerning for systematic disease, laboratory studies should be performed.
- A sleep study may be needed to diagnose an organic sleep disorder.

Treatments

- Acupuncture
  - There are multiple theories of its mechanism of action, but none to date have been proven. In its most simplistic terms, it interrupts the pain signal to the central nervous system (CNS).
  - In general it is very safe, although there are case reports of perforated organs, chiefly pneumothorax.
  - There are a multitude of acupuncture techniques related to the combination of points chosen, length of treatment, manipulation/stimulation of the needle, and frequency of treatment.
  - Although there are protocols, each patient responds differently and the acupuncturist should be flexible in their interventions.
  - Patients can continue all other therapies while receiving acupuncture, but the goal would be to minimize or eliminate medications and/or procedures.

- Referrals for acupuncture treatment should include the diagnosis, previous treatments attempted, as well as ongoing treatments.
- The physician's and patient's goals should be communicated to the consultant.
- The proper expectation must be set, which is that acupuncture is an adjunct to the treatment plan.
- There is controversy whether dry needling can be considered a form of acupuncture and, as such, whether practitioners require the same rigor of training as acupuncturists. The same needle is used in both, but in dry needling the needle is passed multiple times into a symptomatic area, not necessarily an acupuncture point, and no external stimulation is provided. The procedure can be painful, often producing an ecchymosis. Benefit is felt to arise from stimulating beneficial local effects in the tissues.
- Injections
  - Targeted injections can be a useful adjunct when accessible pain generators have been clearly localized.
  - Multiple studies have shown placement failure rate as high as 70% for palpation guided only injections depending on location. Therefore it is recommended that ultrasound guided injections be performed when injecting the specific agents described below. Refer to Box 24.1 for locations and indications of injections.
    - **Dextrose prolotherapy**: Mechanism of action is not completely understood, with several theories being proposed. It appears to cause an inflammatory response or destroys neo-neurovascular structures leading to pain improvement. 12.5-25%

BOX 24.1 **Injection Indications**

Prolotherapy

Low back pain
Tendinopathies
    Lateral epicondylosis
    Achilles tendinopathy
    Hip adductor tendinopathy
    Plantar fasciitis
Osteoarthritis

Botulinum Toxin

Cervical dystonia
Migraine
Hemifacial spasm
Low back pain
Myofascial pain
Piriformis
Exertional compartment syndrome

Platelet-Rich Plasma (PRP)

Tendinopathies
    Lateral epicondylosis
    Patellar tendinosis
    Achilles tendinopathy
Muscle strain/contusion
Osteoarthritis
Ligaments—additional studies needed

---

concentrations are injected either peri- or intratendonous or intra-articularly. Ligamentous injections are advocated by some as well.
- **Botulinum toxin (BTX):** A newer adjunct treatment that has shown promise for certain conditions. BTX is theorized to effect peripheral sensitization and possibly have an effect on central sensitization through pain transmission and modulation. BTX does not cross the blood-brain barrier and has no direct effect on CNS. Caution is advised when injected around the muscle tendon junction and judicious doses are recommended. Intra-articular injection for osteoarthritis has shown much promise, and the dose is adjusted for the size of joint ranging from 50 to 200 units.
- **Platelet-rich plasma (PRP)** has been a recent topic of much research and discussion. There are multiple variables to consider in regard to PRP use that impact on efficacy, including platelet concentration, leukocyte-rich versus leukocyte-poor, and viability of the platelets. To date it is unclear which preparation has the most efficacy. PRP can be effective in chronic tendinopathy treatment and possibly osteoarthritis, but has still not been proven to be effective for other conditions.
- Prolotherapy and PRP patients typically will have some discomfort for several days after an injection due to a proinflammatory response. Most common complications of injections are related to placement, which again highlights the need to be performed under ultrasound guidance. Otherwise, few complications have been reported from PRP or prolotherapy. BTX has been associated with polyradiculoneuritis and skin reactions.
- Manual Therapy
  - Osteopathic manual therapy (OMT) is based on multiple concepts of how the body functions and ways to treat dysfunctions of the body. The body is considered a unit and has the ability to self-heal. Structure and function are interrelated and affect one another.
  - OMT can be performed on multiple areas of the body for treatment of pain.
  - OMT involves evaluating the patient for structural dysfunctions that are contributing to pain and adjusting those dysfunctions to restore normal function.
  - For consistency and safety, it is recommended that only doctors of osteopathy who routinely perform OMT do these types of treatments.
  - Chiropractic and manual treatments by physical therapists are distinctly different than OMT, although each of these treatments can have a role for chronic pain.
  - Massage therapy is another useful adjunct and continues to be studied as an effective treatment for chronic pain.
- Dietary/Supplements
  - Curcumin, the active ingredient in turmeric, has been found equivalent to nonsteroidal antiinflammatory drugs (NSAIDs) for pain relief in knee osteoarthritis and rheumatoid arthritis in several trials. Doses range from 500 to 1500 mg/day and combining with black seed oil improves absorption.
  - Alpha lipoic acid in dosages 600 to 1200 mg/day have been found beneficial for chronic peripheral neuropathic pain and is generally regarded as safe.

- Vitamin D supplementation to achieve a level of ≥30 ng/mL has shown some efficacy in improving musculoskeletal pain with little toxicity.
- Mind/Body
  - Cognitive behavioral therapy is recommended for chronic pain management and has strong evidence supporting use. It can be administered by a trained therapist or via online resources (http://www.alustforlife.com/mental-health/therapies/cbt/top-5-online-cbt-course). Both approaches have ample studies showing their efficacy.
  - Prayer and therapeutic use of a patient's spiritual belief system are also highly encouraged.
  - Yoga and tai chi are recommended for the treatment of chronic neck/back pain, headache, rheumatoid arthritis, and general musculoskeletal pain
  - Biofeedback training from a qualified therapist can be helpful in managing stress
  - Reiki is a Japanese therapy technique for stress reduction and relaxation.
  - Other mind/body options with varying evidence:
    - Art therapy, dance therapy, therapeutic breathing, meditation, hypnosis, mindfulness, guided imagery journaling, virtual reality games, exercise of the nonpainful limb, mirror therapy
- Electronic Devices
  - Noninvasive neuromodulation can be used for chronic intractable pain. This device combines a traditional TENS unit with pulsed radiofrequency.
  - Alpha-stim along with a traditional TENS unit are efficacious for chronic pain.
  - Low-level laser therapy has been shown to be effective for multiple different types of chronic pain, but it is lacking long-term data as well as standard of care for treatment.
- Medical Cannabis
  - Medical cannabis may be an effective treatment in appropriate patients and is being used more frequently for the treatment of chronic pain.
  - Currently evidence is still lacking, and the risks versus benefits need to be further studied.
  - The physician should consult their privileging organization and state licensing board for current regulations.

When to Refer

- Consider surgical consultation if any surgical indication is identified.
- If any concern for psychological/mental component to chronic pain, a psychiatric consult should be placed.

Prognosis

- Will vary significantly based on diagnosis and cause of chronic pain. Often the goal of novel treatments is management of pain versus complete cure.

- If treatments are providing relief of pain, they can be continued as long as patient would like.

Troubleshooting

- There are limited side effects of all the listed treatments, but these should be discussed with the patient. The patient should be monitored closely for side effects at the time of initial treatment.
- If the patient does not have improvement of symptoms with one treatment, it is reasonable to do a trial of another treatment.
- If the patient is not having improvement of symptoms, recommend stopping treatment and considering other options.
- Ensure sleep architecture is normalized.

Patient Instructions

- In-depth risks and benefits need to be discussed with the patient, as well as an explanation of the procedure with the patient.
- The concept of managing the pain to be functional must be understood as opposed to being pain free.

Considerations in Special Populations

- These novel treatments are considered safe in most populations, but should be discussed with individual patients to verify no contraindications.
- Certain treatments, specifically that require movement, may be difficult for patients with decreased range of motion. These treatments will need adjustments to allow patients to participate.

Suggested Readings

Benzon H, Rathmell J, Wu CL, eds. *Practical Management of Pain*. 5th ed. Philadelphia: Elsevier; 2014.

Harmon K, Drezner J, et al. Platelet-rich plasma therapy and autologous blood. In: O'Connor F, Casa DJ, Davis BA, eds. *ACSM's Sports Medicine: A Comprehensive Review*. Philadelphia: Lippincott Williams & Wilkins; 2013:512–519.

Hill KP, Palastro MD, Johnson B, Ditre JW. Cannabis and pain: a clinical review. *Cannabis Canabinoid Res*. 2017;2(1):96–104.

Licciardone JC, Gatchel RJ, Aryal S. Recovery from chronic low back pain after osteopathic manipulative treatment: a randomized controlled trial. *J Am Osteopath Assoc*. 2016;113(6):144–155.

Nahin RL, Boineau R, Khalsa PS, et al. Evidence-based evaluation of complementary health approaches for pain management in the United States. *Mayo Clin Proc*. 2016;91(9):1292–1306.

Rabago D, Slattengren A, Zqierska A. Prolotherapy in primary care practice. *Prim Care*. 2010;37(1):65–80.

Rakel D, ed. *Integrative Medicine*. 4th ed. Philadelphia: Elsevier; 2018.

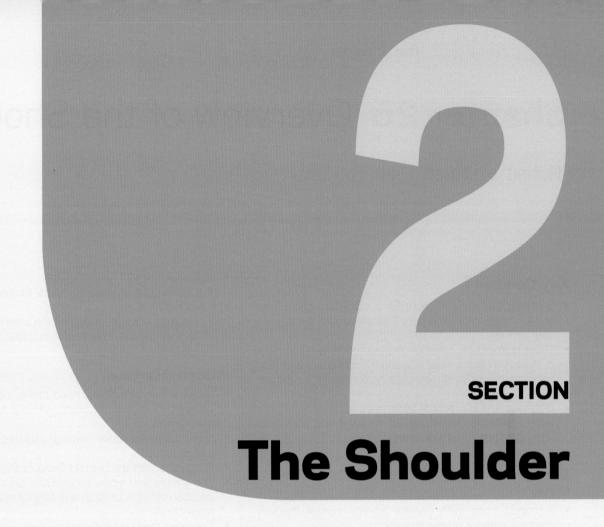

SECTION 2

The Shoulder

Chapter 25 Overview of the Shoulder

Robert J. Dimeff, Brian R. Kelly

Key Concepts

- Shoulder problems account for a significant percentage of musculoskeletal disorders that present to the primary care provider.
- The anatomy of the shoulder complex with its extreme range of motion, inherent instability, and multiple pain generators can lead to significant diagnostic challenges for the primary care provider.
- Diagnosis and appropriate treatment can easily be attained with knowledge of the relevant anatomy and correlation history and physical examination.

Bones

Clavicle

- S-shaped bone with convex anterior border medially, concave anterior border laterally.
- Only bone to connect the upper extremity to the axial skeleton.
- Functions as a strut to maintain distance between shoulders by opposing gravity and muscle action.
- Stabilizes the glenohumeral (GH) joint and upper extremity anteriorly and protects the medial brachial plexus.
- Eighty percent of fractures occur at the medial and lateral junction secondary to inherent weakness in this area.

Scapula

- Flat, triangular bone composed of the body, spine, acromion, glenoid fossa, scapular neck, and coracoid process.
- Provides numerous sites for muscular attachment.
- Approximates with posterolateral aspect of thorax between the second and seventh ribs.
- Body
  - Posterolateral aspect of thorax between the second and seventh ribs.
  - Functions mainly to serve as site for muscle attachment.
- Spine
  - Posterior crest that divides the scapula body and ends laterally at the flattened acromion.
  - Separates scapula into supraspinous and infraspinous fossae.
- Acromion Process
  - Lateral extension of scapular spine that articulates with distal end of the clavicle.
- Glenoid Fossa
  - Inverted, comma-shaped, to articulate with humerus
  - Slightly concave fossa covered with hyaline cartilage
  - Has a larger radius of curvature than the humerus
- Scapular Neck
  - Constriction of scapula medial to glenoid fossa
- Coracoid Process
  - Hooked, bony projection off the anterior surface, medial to the scapular neck, which projects anteriorly and laterally

Proximal Humerus

- Nearly spherical humeral head that is inclined 130 to 150 degrees in relation to shaft, with 20 to 30 degrees of retroversion
- One-third has articular cartilage directed medial, superior, and posterior.
- Articulates with the glenoid fossa of the scapula
- The greater and lesser tuberosities are sites for muscular insertion of the supraspinatus and subscapularis muscles, respectively.
- The intertubercular (bicipital) groove between tuberosities houses the long head of the bicep tendon.

Joints and Ligaments

Sternoclavicular Joint

- Only articulation between upper limb and axial skeleton.
- Joint has ball and socket qualities, although least stable of all major joints.
- Allows clavicle 35 degrees of elevation, 35 degrees of forward/backward motion, and 50 degrees of rotation.
- The costoclavicular, interclavicular, and sternoclavicular ligaments and the intra-articular fibrocartilage disc provide stability.

Acromioclavicular Joint

- Only articulation between clavicle and scapula.
- Transmits forces from extremity to axial skeleton and supports upper extremity, allowing for 40 degrees of rotation during arm elevation.
- Superior and inferior acromioclavicular ligaments control anterior and posterior stability, providing principal restraints to axial and posterior translation.
- Coracoclavicular ligaments include the lateral trapezoid and medial conoid ligaments, limiting anterior and posterior scapular rotation, respectively.

Glenohumeral Joint

- Greatest mobility of all joints, although stability sacrificed to maintain range of motion
- Stability conferred by interaction of bony, ligamentous, and muscle constraints

- 0.3 mm of superior/inferior translation, 5 mm of anterior/posterior translation

Glenoid

- Bony base from lateral scapula
- Thicker peripheral articular cartilage allows for "concavity compression" (suction) effect to enhance stability.

Labrum

- Ring of dense fibrous triangular shaped tissue that deepens glenoid by 2.5 mm, with thickening of periphery to increase joint congruity and stability
- Attachment site of GH ligaments and long head of biceps tendon

Glenohumeral Capsule

- Twice the surface area of the humeral head, lined with synovium
- Limited joint fluid volume, resulting in negative intra-articular pressure, which assists with joint stability
- Acts as "check rein" for GH articulation when placed under tension near extremes of range of motion

Glenohumeral Ligaments

- Composed of the superior, medial, and inferior GH ligament
- Collagenous thickening of shoulder capsule, providing static stability to the GH joint
- Assists in controlling anterior/posterior and superior/inferior translation of the humerus
- Primary stabilizer at extremes of shoulder motion

Coracohumeral Ligament

- Static suspensory function for the humeral head and glenoid with arm at side
- Provides restraint to inferior translation and reinforces rotator cuff interval

Coracoacromial Ligament

- Contributes to the roof of the GH joint

Transverse Humeral Ligament

- Connects greater and lesser tuberosities
- Maintains long head of bicep tendon in the intertubercular groove

Scapulothoracic Articulation

- Provides for movement of scapula on chest wall, although not a true joint

Muscles
Rotator Cuff Muscles

- Includes the supraspinatus, infraspinatus, teres minor, and subscapularis
- Serve as primary active stabilizers of the GH joint
- Active contraction of these muscles compresses humeral head within the glenoid.
- See Table 25.1 for a summary of relevant shoulder musculature.

TABLE 25.1 Summary of Relevant Shoulder Musculature

Muscle	Action on Shoulder
Supraspinatus	Initiates shoulder abduction, depresses humeral head with deltoid contraction, compresses humeral head within glenoid
Infraspinatus	Primary external rotator of shoulder. Upper fibers abduct, lower fibers adduct
Teres minor	External rotation and adduction
Subscapularis	Internal rotation, assists with abduction, adduction. Flexion and extension depending on arm position
Biceps brachii	Flexion of shoulder and elbow, primary supinator of forearm
Coracobrachialis	Flexion and adduction
Pectoralis major	Flexion, adduction, and internal rotation
Pectoralis minor	Draws scapula forward and downward
Subclavius	Draws shoulder down and forward
Deltoid	Primary mover of shoulder, abducts, anterior fibers flex and internally rotate shoulder, posterior fibers extend and externally rotate shoulder
Triceps brachii	Extends elbow. Long head extends and adducts shoulder
Teres major	Adducts, extends, and internally rotates
Serratus anterior	Rotates scapula, stabilizes and draws scapula forward
Rhomboids	Draw scapula medial, depress shoulder
Levator scapulae	Elevate and rotate scapula
Latissimus dorsi	Extends, adducts, and internally rotates
Trapezius	Raises, lowers, rotates, and adducts scapula

Neurovascular Structures and Bursae
Brachial Plexus

- Originates as roots from the anterior and primary divisions of cervical nerves 5 through 8 and thoracic nerve 1
- Divides further into upper, middle, and lower trunks
- Trunks then form the anterior and posterior divisions, which lead to the medial, lateral, and posterior cords
- The cords give rise to the terminal branches of the musculocutaneous, median, ulnar, radial, and axillary nerves.

Axillary Artery

- The subclavian artery becomes the axillary artery at the first rib.
- Multiple major branches from the axillary artery supply the shoulder region.
- Axillary artery becomes the brachial artery at the lower border of the teres major tendon.

Bursae

- Function as lubrication sacs to decrease friction between musculoskeletal structures.
- Include the subacromial, subdeltoid, subscapular, biceps, and scapulothoracic bursae.

Shoulder Biomechanics

- Result of four joints moving synchronously and simultaneously.
- Humerus moves twice as fast and far as scapula.
- Shoulder range of motion:
  - Abduction 180 degrees; adduction 45 degrees
  - Flexion 160 degrees; extension 45 degrees
  - Internal rotation 90 degrees; external rotation 100 degrees
- Scapula
  - Elevation and depression, protraction and retraction
- Sternoclavicular joint
  - Rotation 35 degrees with anterior and posterior arm movement
  - Elevation 35 degrees with arm abduction between 30 degrees and 90 degrees
  - Rotation 45 degrees along long axis after 70 to 80 degrees of arm elevation
- Acromioclavicular joint:
  - 20 degrees of rotation during the first 20 degrees and last 40 degrees of arm elevation
- Scapulothoracic articulation:
  - Arm elevation involves the sum of GH and scapulothoracic motions.
  - No scapular motion during the first 60 degrees of flexion or 30 degrees of abduction; then synchronous with 2 degrees of scapulothoracic motion for each 3 degrees of GH motion.
- GH joint:
  - Responsible for most of shoulder motion
  - Two-thirds of abduction and forward flexion, nearly all of adduction and extension, all of rotation
  - Pattern of motion is a combination of gliding and rolling.
  - Stability is conferred by the interaction of bony, ligamentous, and muscular constraint systems that control the movement of the instant center of motion of the GH joint.
  - Static stabilizers include bone (glenoid and humerus), labrum, GH ligaments, GH joint capsule, concavity-compression effect, and finite joint volume.
  - Dynamic stabilizers include passive muscle bulk acting as a physical barrier, and muscular contraction providing compressive force and stiffening of the joint capsule while redirecting the joint reactive force to the center of the glenoid.

TABLE 25.2 Biomechanics of Shoulder Muscles

Action	Responsible Muscles
Flexion	Primary: Anterior deltoid, coracobrachialis Secondary: Clavicular head of pectoralis major, biceps
Extension	Primary: Latissimus dorsi, teres major, posterior deltoid Secondary: Teres minor, long head of triceps
Abduction	Primary: Middle portion of deltoid, supraspinatus Secondary: Anterior and posterior portions of deltoid, serratus anterior
Adduction	Primary: Pectoralis major, latissimus dorsi Secondary: Teres major, anterior portion of deltoid
External rotation	Primary: Infraspinatus, teres minor Secondary: Posterior portion of deltoid
Internal rotation	Primary: Subscapularis, pectoralis major, latissimus dorsi, teres major Secondary: Anterior portion of deltoid
Scapular elevation	Primary: Subscapularis, pectoralis major, latissimus dorsi, teres major Secondary: Rhomboid major, rhomboid minor
Scapular depression	Serratus anterior and lower trapezius
Scapular retraction	Rhomboid major and rhomboid minor
Scapular protraction	Serratus anterior

- See Table 25.2 for a summary of biomechanics of shoulder muscles.

History

- Severity of pain, instability, weakness, deformity, loss of motion, or disability
- Symptom onset: acute or chronic
- Activities that aggravate or relieve symptoms
- Quality of pain and presence of night, exertional, or radiating pain
- Paresthesias, or "dead arm"
- Looseness, slipping sensation, shoulder popping out of joint
- Muscle atrophy or fatigue
- Clicking, catching, grinding, grating
- Edema, cyanosis, coolness
- Trauma or overuse factors
- Neck, upper extremity, or other associated musculoskeletal complaints

TABLE 25.3 Description of Physical Examination Components

Test	Physical Maneuvers	Likely Diagnosis if Positive Test
Neer impingement sign	Arm forcibly flexed to overhead position	Subacromial impingement of humerus against coracoacromial arch
Cross arm test	Forward elevation to 90 degrees with active adduction	Acromioclavicular joint arthritis
Hawkin impingement sign	Forward flexion of the shoulder to 90 degrees with internal rotation	Impingement of supraspinatus tendon
Sulcus sign	Inferior traction of the arm by pulling on elbow or wrist	Widened sulcus consistent with inferior instability
Apley scratch test	Patient touches inferior and superior aspects of opposite scapula	Loss of range of motion secondary to rotator cuff disorder
Apprehension test	Arm is abducted to 90 degrees and externally rotated, anterior force applied to humerus	Anterior GH instability
Relocation test	Posterior force applied with arm in position of apprehension test	Improvement of pain consistent with anterior instability
Yergason test	Elbow flexed to 90 degrees with resisted forearm supination	Bicep tendonitis or bicep instability
Speed maneuver	Elbow flexed 20–30 degrees with humerus flexed to 60 degrees	Bicep tendonitis if pain with resisted forward flexion of arm
Spurling test	Spine extended with head rotated to affected shoulder while axially loaded	Cervical nerve root disorder
Drop sign	Arm abducted 90 degrees, externally rotated until resistance met, patient holds	Rotator cuff tear likely if unable to hold external rotation
Lift-off test	Patient places hand on lower back, attempts to lift off	Pain or inability represents subscapular muscle disorder
O'Brien's test	Arm forward flexed to 90 degrees, arm adducted 10–15 degrees, downward force, patient resists	Possible anterior superior labral tear if more pain with thumb down than palm up
Jerk test	Arm abducted to 90 degrees and internally rotated, axial load placed on humerus and arm then adducted	Sudden jerk likely represents humeral head sliding off glenoid
Bear hug test	Arm internally rotated to position of palm atop opposite shoulder, patient resists examiner pulling hand with an external rotation force	Subscapularis tear if weak

GH, glenohumeral.

- Other relevant historical information includes age, occupation, avocation, handedness, sports demands, loss of throwing velocity or accuracy, general medical health and medications, presence of connective tissue diseases, workers' compensation issues, or pending litigation.

Physical Examination (Video 25.1)

- Inspection: atrophy, swelling, discoloration
- Range of motion: symmetric, compensatory changes
- Palpation: focal tenderness, deformities
- Strength: assess throughout the upper extremity, upper back, and neck
- Assessment for impingement and stability
- Neurovascular examination: sensation and reflexes
- Evaluation of the ipsilateral elbow and neck
- See Table 25.3 for a description of specific physical examination components.

Suggested Readings

Bahk M, Keyurapan E, Tasaki A, et al. Laxity testing of the shoulder. *Am J Sports Med*. 2007;35(1):131–144.

Baker CL, Merkley M. Clinical evaluation of the athlete's shoulder. *J Athl Train*. 2000;35(3):256–260.

Ebell MH. Diagnosing rotator cuff tears. *Am Fam Physician*. 2005;71(8):1587–1589.

McFarland EG, Selhi H, Keyurapan H. Clinical evaluation of impingement: what to do and what works. *J Bone Joint Surg Am*. 2006;88:432–441.

Myers TH, Zemanovic JR, Andrews JR. The resisted supination external rotation test. *Am J Sports Med*. 2005;33(9):1315–1320.

Quillen DM, Wuchner M, Hatch R. Acute shoulder injuries. *Am Fam Physician*. 2004;70(10):1947–1954.

Woodward TW, Best TM. The painful shoulder, part i. Clinical evaluation. *Am Fam Physician*. 2000;61(10):3079–3089.

Chapter 26 Anterior Shoulder Instability

Lauren Nadkarni, Heather Gillespie, William Dexter

ICD-10-CM CODES
M25.31X *Instability of shoulder joint*
M25.3 *Other instability of joint*
S43.01X *Anterior subluxation and dislocation of humerus/shoulder*
S43.00X *Unspecified subluxation and dislocation of shoulder joint*
S43.30X *Dislocation of shoulder girdle*
M24.41X *Recurrent shoulder dislocation*

Key Concepts

- Shoulder instability is defined as excessive translation of the humerus over the glenoid surface to the point that it is symptomatic.
- Both static (glenoid fossa, labrum, joint capsule, ligaments) and dynamic (rotator cuff, long head of the biceps muscle, deltoid muscle) stabilizers are needed to improve the stability of the glenohumeral joint, which is naturally shallow.
- The least stable position of the shoulder is abduction with external rotation, causing anterior subluxation or dislocation.
- Anterior dislocation causes traumatic instability, often with a Bankart lesion (avulsion of the anterior capsule–labral complex below the midline of the glenoid and may include a bony avulsion). Dislocation may also be associated with a Hill-Sachs lesion (injury to the posterolateral aspect of the humeral head).
- Bony lesions >20% of the articular surface may contribute to recurrent dislocations and instability.
- Comorbidities include capsular tearing or stretching, rotator cuff tears (primarily in older patients with primary dislocations), and axillary nerve injuries.
- Chronic, repetitive microinjury, as in the overhead throwing athlete, can result in acquired anterior instability from stretching of the joint capsule or recurrent micro-subluxation of the glenohumeral joint.
- Rates of anterior instability after a primary dislocation vary from 17% to 100%.
- Rates of instability are higher in men and patients younger than 20 years old. Instability decreases with age but may increase again in the elderly as a result of increasing rotator cuff problems.
- Instability can lead to recurrent dislocations.

History

- The diagnosis of anterior instability is primarily clinical and may not be frankly traumatic, but there may be history of joint laxity or prior dislocation or subluxation.
- The patient may complain of shoulder discomfort with contact and overhead activities, often without any restriction of range of motion.
- A history of Marfan syndrome or other hyperlaxity condition in the athlete or immediate family is important to document. However, this does not necessarily increase the risk of recurrent instability after surgical repair.

Physical Examination

- The physical examination should include inspection for any swelling or malformations, palpation for tenderness and regions of anesthesia in the axillary nerve distribution, active and passive range of motion, strength, and neurovascular testing, as well as specific tests to assess for instability.
- A decrease in mobility following an anterior dislocation is primarily from pain versus an anatomic restriction. The strength of the shoulder girdle and arm should be tested and any weaknesses noted.
- The apprehension test (see Video 28.1 in Chapter 28) is done with the patient supine or sitting with shoulder abducted and externally rotated to 90 degrees. Apprehension indicates a positive test, as pain can also be elicited with primary impingement.
- Jobe's apprehension-relocation test (see Video 28.1 in Chapter 28) is done after a positive apprehension test. Posterior force is applied to the anterior humeral head, which alleviates the pain and/or apprehension.
- A load-and-shift test and a crank test have also been shown to predict labral tears, which are common in anterior instability.

Imaging

- An initial radiograph is important to diagnose a bony Bankart or Hill-Sachs lesion.
- Obtain anteroposterior radiographs of the shoulder in neutral rotation (assess the lower rim of the glenoid) and internal rotation (assess impaction of the humeral head, or Hill-Sachs lesion), an axillary view in external rotation at 90 degrees, and a profile glenoid view to detect glenoid lesions (Fig. 26.1).
- An apical oblique view (Garth view) is helpful for visualizing both glenoid bone loss and Hill-Sachs lesions with limited manipulation of the shoulder.
- Bankart lesions are nearly ubiquitous in patients with recurrent anterior instability.
- Hill-Sachs lesions are more associated with recurrent dislocations versus subluxation.

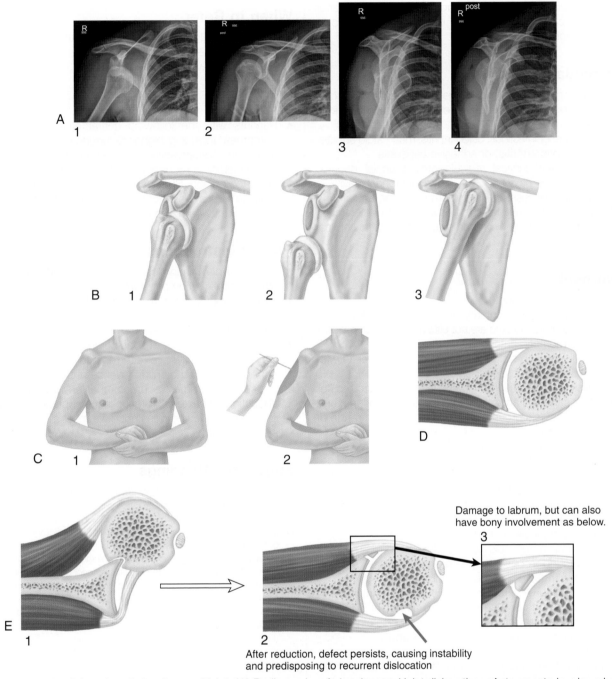

Fig 26.1 Anterior dislocation of glenohumeral joint. **(A)** Radiographs of glenohumeral joint dislocations. Anteroposterior views before *(1)* and after *(2)* reduction. Y views before *(3)* and after *(4)* reduction. **(B)** Schematic of dislocations. *(1)* Subcoracoid dislocation (most common); *(2)* Subglenoid dislocation; *(3)* Subclavicular dislocation (uncommon). **(C)** Important physical exam findings include *(1)* humeral head prominence, shoulder flattened, forearm internally rotated, and elbow flexed, and *(2)* evaluating for sensation in axillary nerve (superior) and musculocutaneous nerves (forearm). **(D)** Normal shoulder anatomy (humeral head on right). **(E)** Mechanism of bony injuries with anterior dislocation. *(1)* Initial injury with dislocation; *(2)* Hill Sachs lesion *(red arrow)*; *(3)* Bankart lesion *(black arrow)*.

- Computed tomography (CT) is an excellent tool for the diagnosis of bony lesions, but it may not be necessary if radiographs are negative. CT may help confirm the presence of a very small humeral fracture or inferior glenoid lesions.
- Magnetic resonance imaging is useful in detecting labral lesions and in assessing a nonbony Bankart lesion.

- Magnetic resonance arthrography is superior to magnetic resonance imaging in diagnosing labral tears.
- Arthrography or arthroscopy can visualize labral or glenohumeral ligament injuries.
- Arthroscopy is done only after all other imaging is negative but the clinical history is still highly suspicious. Direct

visualization of anatomic damage indicative of anterior instability can be obtained, and it may be possible to fix the damage concurrently.

Differential Diagnosis

- Trauma or mechanical: impingement, rotator cuff pathology, labral tears, bicipital tendinitis, or acromioclavicular joint injuries
- Inflammatory or infectious: osteoarthritis, rheumatoid arthritis, bursitis, septic arthritis, or adhesive capsulitis
- Referred pain: cervical radiculopathy, brachial neuritis, biliary disease, blood or gas in the peritoneal cavity, a subphrenic abscess, splenic trauma, cancer, apical lung diseases, angina pectoris, or an acute myocardial infarction
- Other: thoracic outlet syndrome (especially with cervical rib)

Treatment

- Conservative treatment:
  - Recommended for primary dislocations in patients older than 20 years old who are not elite athletes or in patients with atraumatic anterior instability
  - Immobilize with sling for a range of 1 to 6 weeks with early mobilization exercises
  - Physical rehabilitation, including isometric exercises (for grip, scapular stabilization, and the biceps, triceps, and deltoid muscle groups) and then isotonic and range of motion exercises
  - Return to play regimen
- Surgical treatment:
  - Options include arthroscopic stabilization, open stabilization, or coracoid transfer (Latarjet) procedures.
  - Arthroscopic repair is as effective as an open approach, though large glenoid or Hill-Sachs defects may have a better prognosis with an open approach.
  - Following arthroscopic repair, better functional outcomes were found in patients greater than 24 years old and those with fewer preoperative dislocations (<8).
  - Consider surgical repair for athletes who participate in contact sports or who have more than 20-25% bone loss at the intra-articular surface, regardless of whether they have had previous shoulder instability.
- Outcomes:
  - No significant difference in global patient satisfaction between conservative and operative approaches, but there is limited evidence available.

When to Refer

- Consider surgical intervention for elite athletes or recurrent instability, as recurrence of dislocation is less frequent with surgery than without it.

Prognosis

- Patients with the following characteristics have worse outcomes, including higher recurrence rates for dislocations with conservative management: younger patients, family history of recurrent instability, bony Bankart lesion, Hill-Sachs lesion, SLAP (superior labrum, anteroposterior) tear, humeral avulsion of the glenohumeral ligaments, and anterior labroligamentous periosteal sleeve avulsions.

Patient Instructions

- Return-to-play timing can range from weeks to months after a rehabilitation program.
- Ideal criteria for return to play include little or no pain and nearly normal range of motion, strength, functional ability, and sport-specific skills.
- 37-90% of athletes with shoulder instability who return to play in-season will have recurrence of instability
- Although there is no solid evidence of their efficacy, there are several commercial braces that are available to limit abduction and external rotation in the apprehensive patient or in the patient who does not quite meet all the previously stated criteria.

Suggested Readings

Donohue MA, Owens BD, Dickens JF. Return to play following anterior shoulder dislocation and stabilization surgery. *Clin Sports Med.* 2016; 35(4):545–561.

Gasparini G, De Benedetto M, Cundari A, et al. Predictors of functional outcomes and recurrent shoulder instability after arthroscopic anterior stabilization. *Knee Surg Sports Traumatol Arthrosc.* 2016;24(2):406–413.

Thompson SR, Al-Saati MF, Litchfield RB. Anterior shoulder instability. In: Miller M, Thompson SR, eds. *Delee and Drez's Orthopaedic Sports Medicine: Principles and Practice.* 4th ed. Philadelphia: Elsevier; 2015.

Watson S, Allen B, Grant JA. A clinical review of return-to-play considerations after anterior shoulder dislocation. *Sports Health.* 2016;8(4): 336–341.

Chapter 27 Posterior Shoulder Instability

Mark Rogers, Nicholas Strasser

ICD-10-CM CODES

M25.311	*Posterior shoulder instability, right shoulder*
M25.312	*Posterior shoulder instability, left shoulder*
S43.024A	*Posterior dislocation humeral head, initial encounter, right shoulder*
S43.025A	*Posterior dislocation humeral head, initial encounter, left shoulder*
S43.025D	*Posterior dislocation humeral head, subsequent encounter (right and left shoulders)*
S43.025S	*Posterior dislocation humeral head, sequela (right and left shoulders)*
S43.021A	*Posterior subluxation humeral head, initial encounter, right shoulder*
S43.022A	*Posterior subluxation humeral head, initial encounter, left shoulder*
S43.021D	*Posterior subluxation humeral head, subsequent encounter, right shoulder*
S43.022D	*Posterior subluxation humeral head, subsequent encounter, left shoulder*
S43.021S	*Posterior subluxation humeral head, sequela, right shoulder*
S43.022S	*Posterior subluxation humeral head, sequela, left shoulder*

Key Concepts

- Posterior shoulder instability describes a variety of conditions ranging from acute traumatic dislocation to chronic subluxation (Fig. 27.1).
  - Dislocation: humeral head is forced out of glenoid cavity.
  - Subluxation: posterior movement of humeral head without complete escape from the glenoid rim; usually reduces spontaneously
- Nonacute posterior instability is divided into three groups:
  - Recurrent dislocation
  - Recurrent subluxation
  - Pain with forward flexion, adduction, internal rotation, which is a position of instability
- Approximately 50% of recurrent posterior instability has had an inciting injury, and up to 5% of patients with shoulder instability include a posterior element.
- Posterior instability is often a result of subluxation more than dislocation.

- Acute traumatic posterior instability usually occurs with a posterior force while the arm is in a position of instability.
  - Can be seen with electrocution, high-energy trauma, and seizure activity
- Less than 5% of shoulder dislocations are posterior.
- Chronic dislocations are those diagnosed more than 6 weeks from initial trauma.
- Undiagnosed posterior dislocation can lead to chronic loss of range of motion.
- Associated humeral head fractures may prevent self-reduction of acute posterior dislocations.
- Posterior instability can be associated with posterior labral injury, posteroinferior capsular ligament damage, and/or poor rotator cuff function.
- Glenoid hypoplasia or lack of normal concavity may increase the risk of multiple types of shoulder instability.

History

- Obtain mechanism of injury (traumatic versus atraumatic), focus on arm position or activities that reproduce symptoms, and delineate between voluntary and involuntary instability.
- Symptoms can range from mild discomfort with sport-specific activity to severe diffuse pain with limited range of motion and inability to perform activities of daily living.

Physical Examination

- Without an inciting trauma, strength and range of motion may be normal.
- Forward flexion, adduction, and internal rotation may reproduce pain or instability in patients with posterior instability.
- Testing for instability may include the posterior apprehension test, jerk test, Kim test, sulcus sign, and posterior load and shift test (Fig. 27.2).
- Atraumatic posterior instability may present with a positive dimple sign—a small skin indentation 1 cm medial and inferior to the posterior angle of the acromion.
  - 65% of female and 50% of male athletes may present with atraumatic, nonpainful posterior instability on exam.
- Patients presenting with recurrent instability should also be tested for general ligament laxity, evidenced by elbow hyperextension greater than 10 degrees, genu recurvatum greater than 19 degrees, and ability to touch both thumbs to the ipsilateral forearm.

- Traumatic presentations may lack obvious physical deformity.
  - The affected arm is often guarded in adduction and internal rotation against the abdomen.
  - There are usually active and/or passive limitations with forward flexion, external rotation, and forearm supination.

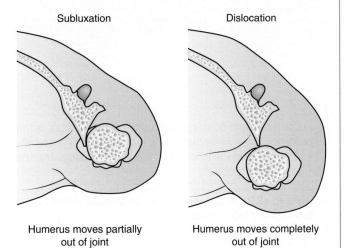

Subluxation

Dislocation

Humerus moves partially out of joint

Humerus moves completely out of joint

Fig 27.1 Posterior instability.

- A displaced humeral head often causes swelling and prominence of the coracoid.
- Long head of the biceps, rotator cuff, and periarticular musculature can be painful.
- Grading of posterior instability is based on the amount of translation of humeral head in relation to the glenoid.
  - Grade 0: no translation
  - Grade 1+: humeral head movement to but not over the glenoid
  - Grade 2+: humeral head translation over the glenoid rim with spontaneous reduction
  - Grade 3+: complete dislocation even after removal of translating force

Imaging

- Posterior dislocations are best confirmed with x-rays, specifically axillary, scapular Y, or transscapular views.
- The West Point and Stryker notch views serve as specific options to assess for bony abnormalities of the glenoid (e.g., Bankart lesions) and the humeral head (e.g., Hill-Sachs deformities), respectively.
  - Axial views can be challenging to obtain with acute dislocations; however, apical oblique, Velpeau, or

Upper Extremity Posterior Shoulder Instability

- **Mechanism of Injury**
  - Repetitive posterior loading (football linemen, overhead athletes, swimmers)
  - High energy trauma
  - Electrocution
  - Seizure

- **Physical Exam**
  - Pain with position of instability (forward flexion, adduction, internal rotation)
  - Positive posterior load and shift test, jerk test, posterior apprehension test

- **Treatment**
  - Reduction of any dislocation
  - Early rehabilitation
  - Surgical consult for suspected muscle or nerve injury, fracture, labral tear, or resistant pain

- **Late Sequela**
  - Chronic pain
  - Limited range of motion

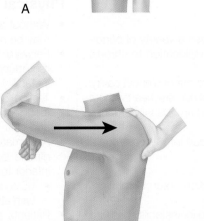

Posterior dislocation

Acromion

Glenoid

Humerus

A

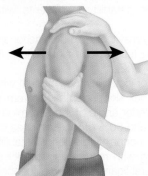

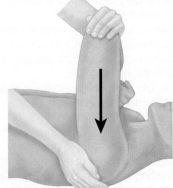

B   Posterior load and shift test

Jerk test

Posterior apprehension test

Fig 27.2 (A) Right shoulder anatomy showing posterior dislocation. (B) Examples of posterior shoulder instability testing.

modified axial radiographs may be obtained with the patient in a sling.
- If the patient is unable to tolerate modified axillary views, CT scan is indicated.
- Traumatic dislocations and concern for possible reverse Bankart lesions on x-ray imaging would justify MRI with arthrography for additional detailed soft-tissue assessment.
  - Reverse Bankart lesion: tear of the posteroinferior aspect of the capsulolabral complex
- CT or MRI can assess glenoid morphology; however, CT with intra-articular contrast may provide the greatest detail, and may be useful for surgical planning.

Differential Diagnosis
- Shoulder impingement
- Rotator cuff injury
- Labral injury
- Glenohumeral arthritis
- Suprascapular and long thoracic nerve entrapment or palsies
- Scapular instability
- Frozen shoulder

Treatment
- At time of trauma, avoid any painful motions or activities.
- Acute dislocations may require guided reduction under anesthesia.
- Atraumatic instability and first-time dislocations are best treated with rehabilitation.
  - Emphasize rotator cuff, posterior deltoid, and scapular stabilizer strengthening.
- May attempt nonoperative treatment for posterior dislocations diagnosed within 6 weeks of injury and with a humeral head defect less than 20%.

When to Refer
- Failure to reduce acute dislocation
- Suspected nerve or muscle injury
- No improvement with rehabilitation and nonoperative care over 6 months (less with instabilities of traumatic origin associated with lesions in the capsulolabral or bone complex)
- Recurrent pain or dislocations

Prognosis
- Up to 80% of posterior instability can be treated nonsurgically.
- Younger age, delayed time from onset to diagnosis, and inciting traumatic event with possible associated reverse Bankart lesion increase the risk for recurrent instability and failed nonoperative therapy.

Troubleshooting
- Traumatic dislocations may lead to brachial plexus lesions, fracture of the humeral surgical neck or tuberosities, or injury to the glenoid rim.
- Voluntary recurrent posterior instability is classically associated with psychogenic disorders and secondary gain.

Patient Instructions
- Dedication to physical therapy and a home rehabilitation plan improves the chances of full return to activity and long-term function.
- Avoid all voluntary dislocations.
- Do not progress physical activity of the affected shoulder until cleared by a medical professional.

Special Population
- High-risk athletes for posterior instability include football linemen, overhead athletes, swimmers, and weight lifters.
- Athletes should achieve full strength, full active and passive range of motion, and pain-free sport specific activity before being cleared for full participation.
- With traumatic injuries in patients over 40 years old, consider concurrent rotator cuff tears.
- Nonsurgical rehabilitation is standard of care for geriatrics, patients with limited disability, or patients with low functional expectations.

Suggested Readings

Alepuz E, et al. Treatment of the posterior unstable shoulder. *Open Orthop J*. 2017;11:826–847.

Díaz Heredia J, Ruiz Iban MA, Ruiz Diaz R, et al. The posterior unstable shoulder: natural history, clinical evaluation and imaging. *Open Orthop J*. 2017;11:972–978.

Millett PJ, Clavert P, Hatch GF 3rd, Warner JJ. Recurrent posterior shoulder instability. *J Am Acad Orthop Surg*. 2006;14:464–476.

Robinson C, Aderinto J. Posterior shoulder dislocations and fracture-dislocations. *J Bone Joint Surg Am*. 2005;87A:639–651.

Steinmann S. Posterior shoulder instability. *Arthroscopy*. 2003;19(1 suppl): 102–105.

Chapter 28 Multidirectional Shoulder Instability

Helen C. Lam, Christopher E. Jonas

ICD-10-CM CODES
M25.311 *Other shoulder instability, right*
M25.312 *Other shoulder instability, left*
M25.319 *Other shoulder instability, unspecified*
M24.819 *Other joint derangement, not elsewhere classified, shoulder region*

Key Concepts

- Classically defined as symptomatic involuntary instability of the glenohumeral joint in two or more directions (anterior and/or posterior, and inferior) with minimal or no causative trauma (Fig. 28.1).
- There is no pathognomonic finding indicative of multidirectional instability, and no objective standardized criteria have been established.
- The term *laxity* refers to increased potential of a joint to sublux or dislocate, whereas the term *instability* refers to laxity that is also symptomatic.
- May be classified as congenital, or secondary to a single traumatic event, or recurrent microtrauma.
- Congenital cases typically present at an earlier age and are commonly bilateral.
- Microtraumatic, overuse injuries are common in the athletic population.
- Increased shoulder laxity may be an independent risk factor for instability.
- The primary pathologic issue appears to be generalized laxity of the shoulder capsule (Fig. 28.2), characterized by redundant capsular tissue resulting in increased glenohumeral volume.
- Other contributing factors include deficient shoulder proprioception, muscle control; biomechanical abnormalities; and irregular bony, labral, or ligamentous anatomy.
- It is rare for multidirectional instability to be present in the absence of hyperlaxity; this may be found in an individual with multiple traumatic events leading to instability in multiple directions.

History

- The onset of symptoms may or may not be related to an injury or recurrent traumatic events.
- Symptoms reported are often vague, including activity-related pain, fatigue, and sense of apprehension. A presenting symptom of actual instability is less common.
- Correlation of symptoms with arm position is important to ensure accurate diagnosis. Inferior instability leads to symptoms when carrying objects. Anterior instability symptoms occur with the arm overhead in an abducted and externally rotated position. Posterior instability occurs with the arm in an adducted position and when reaching.
- Patients who can voluntarily dislocate can demonstrate instability on their own, in either one or multiple directions; this usually develops before skeletal maturity and is less commonly associated with trauma.
- Atraumatic instability may be associated with connective tissue disorders such as Marfan syndrome, osteogenesis imperfecta, benign hypermobility syndrome, or Ehlers-Danlos syndrome.
- Symptoms are common in the midportion of shoulder range of motion and may affect activities of daily living. Patients may frequently change their lifestyle by avoiding certain aggravating positions or developing compensatory routines to avoid inciting symptoms.
- Associated with repetitive overhead sports, including swimming, gymnastics, and baseball pitching.
- Athletes may present with indistinct symptoms leading to decreased performance, lack of confidence in shoulder function, or painful execution of shoulder activity.

Physical Examination

- The examination should begin with the contralateral shoulder for comparative laxity and enhanced patient understanding; observe for any asymmetry, abnormal motion, scapular winging, or atrophy.
- The presence of multidirectional instability should be evaluated after traumatic dislocation of any nature, when pain has subsided.
- Tests for recurrent instability include apprehension and relocation testing (which may be normal or painful; Fig. 28.3A, Video 28.1), the sulcus sign, the load-and-shift test, the Gagey hyperabduction test (indicative of inferior laxity if passive abduction is >105 degrees or if there is marked >20 degrees difference in hyperabduction of the contralateral shoulder), and the jerk test (a positive test is indicated by sharp pain in the shoulder).
- Shoulder laxity testing should include the anterior and posterior drawers.
- Assessment for generalized ligamentous laxity should be performed.
- The four Beighton criteria for generalized ligamentous laxity include:
  - Hyperflexibility of the thumb to touch ipsilateral forearm (see Fig. 28.3B)

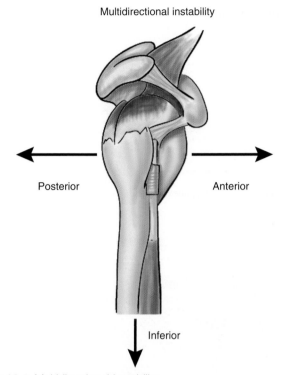

Fig 28.1 Multidirectional instability.

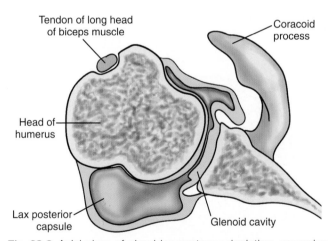

Fig 28.2 Axial view of shoulder anatomy depicting excessive laxity of posterior capsule.

- Hyperextensibility of the metacarpophalangeal joint of the little finger beyond 90 degrees
- Hyperextension of the elbows and knees beyond 10 degrees
- The ability to forward bend and place the hands on the floor without bending the knees
- The presence of laxity alone on physical examination is insufficient to diagnose multidirectional instability, as subluxation of the humeral head on the glenoid rim should be symptomatic (on examination and during activity) for further treatment to be considered.

Imaging

- Standard radiographs for multidirectional instability may include scapular anteroposterior with external rotation of the humeral head, true anteroposterior with internal rotation, West Point, and Stryker notch views of both shoulders.
- West Point view (obtained with patient prone with affected arm hanging off the table while shoulder is abducted to 90 degrees with elbow bent and x-ray beam is directed 25 degrees caudal and medial) and Stryker notch views (obtained with patient supine with forward flexion of the arm to 100 degrees with the x-ray beam centered over the coracoid with 10 degrees of tilt toward the head) are more sensitive to assess for bony abnormalities of the glenoid (e.g., Bankart lesion) and the humeral head (e.g., Hill-Sachs lesion), respectively.
- Normal radiographs do not exclude a diagnosis of multidirectional instability.
- Computed tomography may be used for detailed evaluation of bony anatomy, which may be appropriate after traumatic events or if bone abnormality identified on plain films requires further evaluation.
- Magnetic resonance imaging with arthrography is the most sensitive and specific imaging modality for assessment of a labral injury, capsular tears, and increased joint volume.
- Musculoskeletal ultrasound can be used to dynamically evaluate for increased capsular volume, rotator cuff or other tissue tears, impingement, and other differential causes of shoulder pain.

Differential Diagnosis

- Rotator cuff injury
- Impingement
- Labral tear
- Suprascapular and long thoracic nerve entrapment/palsies
- Cervical radiculopathy
- Scapular winging
- Glenohumeral or acromioclavicular arthritis

Treatment

- At diagnosis
  - Relative rest and activity modification to aid pain control
  - Temporary use of acetaminophen or nonsteroidal antiinflammatory drugs for pain control.
  - These should be used at the lowest effective dose for the shortest effective duration.
  - Gentle, pain-free range of motion therapy is encouraged.
- Later
  - Rehabilitation that emphasizes strengthening and improved tone and coordination of the deltoid, rotator cuff, pectoralis major, and periscapular musculature should theoretically compensate for lack of stability and help in active control of the shoulder.
  - Incorporate assessment and correction of abnormal scapular motion, as scapular dyskinesis is often found in patients with traumatic or microtraumatic glenohumeral instability.

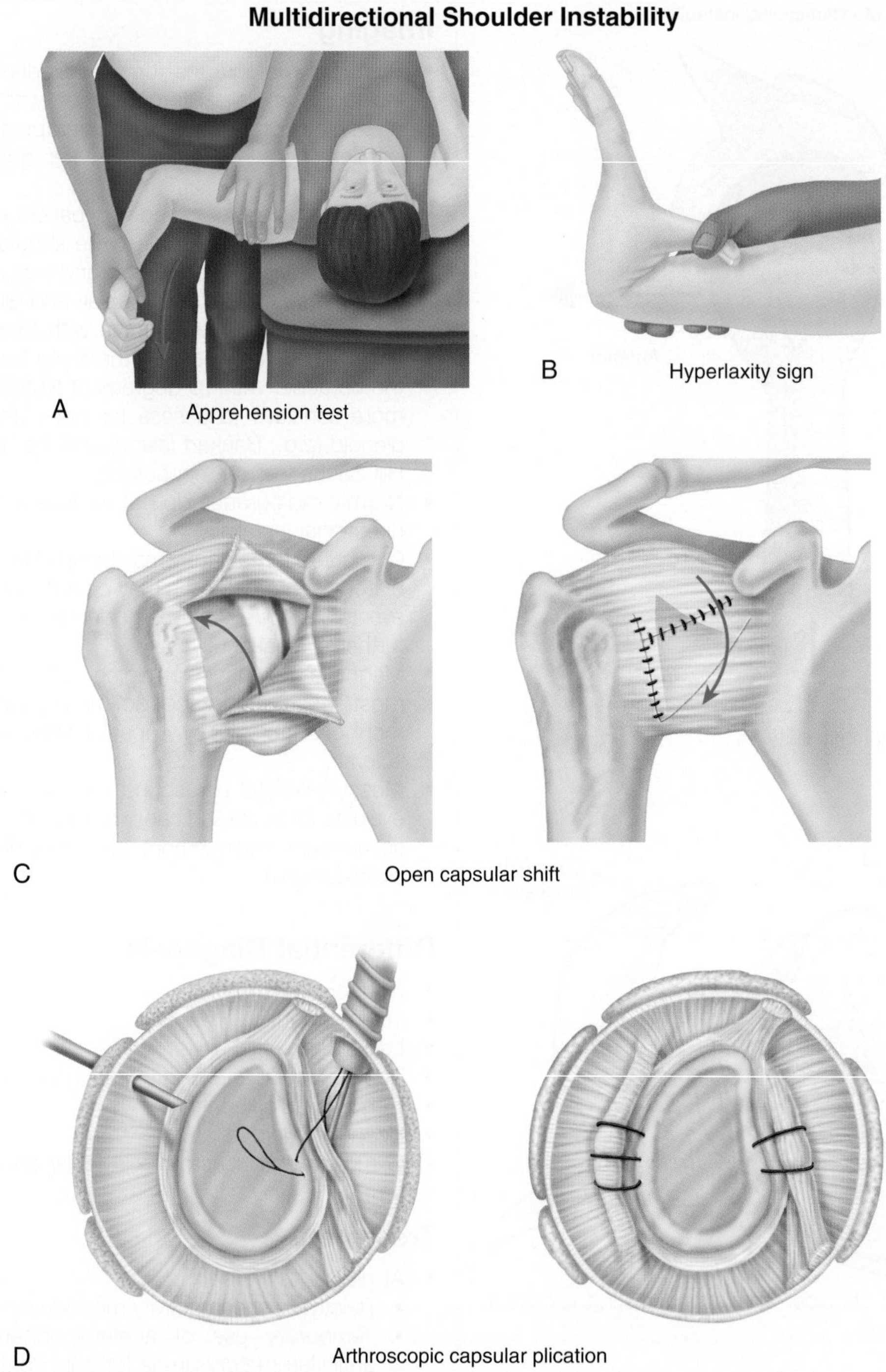

Multidirectional Shoulder Instability

Fig 28.3 Multidirectional shoulder instability. **(A)** Apprehension test. **(B)** Hyperlaxity as demonstrated by hyperflexibility of the thumb to touch ipsilateral forearm. **(C)** Open capsular shift surgery: An incision is made along the front of the joint, and the subscapularis is detached. The shoulder capsule is then identified and split; the inferior shoulder capsule is brought up, and then the superior portion is pulled down to decrease the volume of the shoulder joint. **(D)** Arthroscopic capsular plication: Small incisions are made and sutures placed through the shoulder capsule are sewn upon themselves to tighten the capsular tissue.

- Reconditioning, particularly in athletes, should include core training and evaluation/treatment of other hyperlax joints (if present) to prevent injury.

When to Refer

- Failure to improve with 6 to 12 months of therapy with recurrent pain or dislocations
- Axillary or other nerve injuries
- Suspected or confirmed vascular compromise
- Bony injury present on radiographs
- Surgery is commonly deferred in patients who have not reached full skeletal maturity.

Prognosis

- Approximately 20% of patients require surgical intervention.
- Surgical correction holds better promise for athletes with single shoulder involvement, whereas bilateral repairs are less successful.
- Patients of high school and college age may fare worse than an older patient population, although it is unknown whether this is due to higher physical demands or a natural history of improvement of instability with age.
- Voluntary dislocators are typically poor surgical candidates.
- When surgery is indicated, shoulder stabilization surgery can be performed. Arthroscopic plication or open capsular shift are the most common surgical procedures (see Fig. 28.3C and D).
  - Arthroscopic surgery has advantages of limited scarring, less incidence of subscapularis tendon damage, and trend toward higher rates of return to sport.
  - Isolated thermal capsulorrhaphy has largely fallen out of favor.

Troubleshooting

- Preceding trauma should be properly evaluated for the presence of fractures.
- Rarely, secondary bursitis or tendonitis may cause difficulty in rehabilitation efforts.
  - Treat with acetaminophen or oral nonsteroidal anti-inflammatory drugs or consider subacromial corticosteroid injections.

Patient Instructions

- Full return to activity and long-term function is more likely with dedication to physical therapy and home rehabilitation programs.
- Avoid any voluntary dislocation.
- Do not attempt physical exertion of the affected arm until properly cleared.

Considerations in Special Populations

- Return-to-play guidelines for athletes have been more thoroughly studied in anterior dislocation; recommendations include achieving at least 90% of normal strength and motion as well as performing sport-specific activity without pain.
- Athletes who use overhead throwing motions, particularly pitchers, with instability require extra attention to rehabilitation of lower extremity and core musculature as an element of their return to activity.

Suggested Readings

Longo UG, Rizzello G, Loppini M, et al. Multidirectional instability of the shoulder: a systematic review. *Arthroscopy*. 2015;31(12):2431–2443.

Merolla G, Cerciello C, Chillemi C, et al. Multidirectional instability of the shoulder, clinical presentation, and treatment strategies. *Eur J Orthop Surg Traumatol*. 2015;25:975–985.

Ren H, Bicknell RT. From the unstable painful shoulder to multidirectional instability in the young athlete. *Clin Sports Med*. 2013;32:815–823.

Saccomanno MF, Fodale M, Capasso L, et al. Generalized joint laxity and multidirectional instability of the shoulder. *Joints*. 2013;1(4):171–179.

Walz D, Berge AJ, Steinbach L. Imaging of shoulder instability. *Semin Musculoskelet Radiol*. 2015;19:254–268.

Warby SA, Pizzari T, Ford JJ, et al. The effect of exercise-based management for multidirectional instability of the glenohumeral joint: a systematic review. *J Shoulder Elbow Surg*. 2014;23:128–142.

Witney-Lagen C, Hassan A, Doodson C, et al. Arthroscopic plication for multidirectional instability: 50 patients with minimum of 2 years of follow up. *J Shoulder Elbow Surg*. 2017;26:e29–e36.

Chapter 29 The Overhead-Throwing Athlete

William Patterson, Sarah Hoffman, William Dexter

Key Concepts

- The overhead throw involves complex motions through the shoulder, elbow, and wrist.
- Proper mechanics involve distribution of energy through the kinetic chain from the lower extremity push-off, to pelvic and torso rotation, and into elbow extension and shoulder rotation.
- Lower extremity propulsion and body rotation produce 50% of the velocity of a throw.
- Inadequate leg and core strength necessitates increased upper extremity forces to achieve high velocities. This places the thrower at increased risk of injury.
- Extreme forces placed on the shoulder and elbow during repetitive throws often cause microtrauma to the surrounding soft tissues, leading to overuse injuries.
- There are many different techniques of throwing mechanics, yet the "classic throw" (baseball throw) is the most common.
- Injuries can occur in traditional throwing sports (e.g., baseball) as well as repetitive overhead motion sports (e.g., swimming and tennis).
- Different sports and types of projectiles require different types of throws (e.g., a football pass differs from a baseball pitch).
- Decreased range of motion, lower joint forces, and lower velocity of football pass when compared to baseball pitch.
- Different sports can yield different injuries (e.g., football injuries are typically from trauma whereas baseball injuries are typically due to overuse).
- Isolating what phase of the throw the pain or dysfunction is in can be helpful in diagnosis.

Phases of the Classic Throw

- The throw is generally divided into six phases:
  - Wind-up
  - Early arm cocking (stride)
  - Late arm cocking
  - Arm acceleration
  - Arm deceleration
  - Follow-through
- Wind-up phase
  - Purpose is to begin to build potential energy.
  - Uses very little energy
  - Requires motion through the hip and torso to generate full potential energy
  - The wind-up phase begins with the throw initiation and ends as the stride leg moves toward the target (Fig. 29.1A and B).
  - Few injuries occur during this phase.

- Early arm cocking phase (stride)
  - Purpose is to initiate the vector of force at the target and begin transition of potential energy to kinetic energy.
  - The early arm cocking phase (or stride phase) begins with hand separation and ends when the foot contacts the ground (see Fig. 29.1C).
  - The hind foot pushes off, and the pelvis and torso rotate to move the thrower toward the target.
  - Shoulder movements include glenohumeral abduction, external rotation, and scapular upward rotation.
  - Almost no injuries occur during this phase, but lack of flexibility and proper positioning can lead to overloading of the shoulder in later phases.
- Late arm cocking phase
  - Purpose is to produce maximal external rotation of the shoulder to allow for full transfer of force to the object being thrown.
  - Begins as the stride foot contacts the ground and ends as shoulder internal rotation begins (Fig. 29.2A)
  - Maximal external rotation occurs at the shoulder.
  - This can lead to impingement between the superior rotator cuff and the labrum.
  - The inferior glenohumeral ligament and the long head of the biceps muscle prevent anterior translation of the humeral head.
  - The rotator cuff muscles contract to center the humeral head on the glenoid.
  - Strong valgus forces applied to medial elbow
  - Wrist and hand in hyperextension position
- Acceleration phase
  - Purpose is to transfer all the energy from the trunk to the object being thrown in a vector toward the target.
  - Begins with shoulder internal rotation and ends with ball release (see Fig. 29.2B)
  - Most forceful phase
  - Transition of trunk from hyperextension to forward flexion
  - Wrist goes from hyperextension to neutral
  - Large rotational torque placed on the soft tissues of the shoulder
  - Elbow extension begins, causing increased elbow forces. Maximal valgus stress is in this phase.
  - Humerus should be aligned in the plane of the scapula.
  - Ulnar collateral ligament is under maximal valgus stress, preventing elbow instability.
- Deceleration phase
  - Purpose is to dissipate excess energy from acceleration phase that was not transferred to the thrown object.

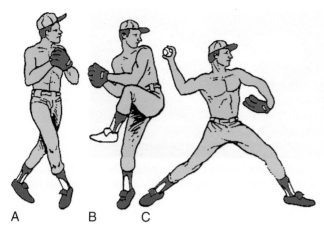

Fig 29.1 The sequence of motion of the early phases of throwing from throw initiation (A), to the windup (B), and then into the early cocking phase (C). (Modified from Park S, Loebenberg ML, Rokito AS, Zuckerman J, The shoulder in baseball pitching: biomechanics and related injuries—part 1. *Bull Hosp Joint Dis.* 2002–2003;61:68–79.)

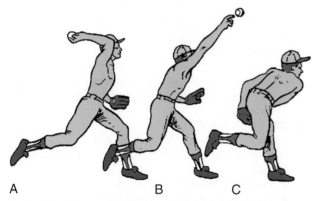

Fig 29.2 The sequence of motion of the late phases of throwing from the late cocking phase (A), to the acceleration phase (B), and ending with the deceleration phase and follow-through (C). (Modified from Park S, Loebenberg ML, Rokito AS, Zuckerman J. The shoulder in baseball pitching: biomechanics and related injuries—part 1. *Bull Hosp Joint Dis.* 2002–2003;61:68–79.)

- Begins at ball release and ends when shoulder reaches maximal internal rotation and terminal elbow extension (see Fig. 29.2C).
- Rotator cuff muscles contract to oppose internal rotation and glenohumeral distraction.
- Large traction force applied to the long head of the biceps to decelerate extending elbow.
- A longer deceleration phase reduces risk of injury, as this spreads the dissipation of energy out over a longer path.
- Follow-through phase
  - Purpose is to finish dissipation of energy from deceleration phase and return to a "ready" position for another action.

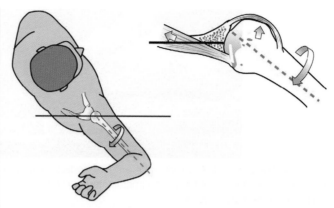

Fig 29.3 Internal impingement of the undersurface of the rotator cuff against the posterior aspect of the labrum in maximum external rotation and abduction. (From Braun S, Kokmeyer D, Millett P. Shoulder injuries in the throwing athlete. *J Bone Joint Surg Am.* 2009;91:966–978.)

- Begins at maximal shoulder internal rotation and ends when thrower returns to a balanced stance (see Fig. 29.2C)
- Arm adducted across the body
- Movements of trunk flexion and lead knee extension help dissipate deceleration force into large muscle groups.
- No primary injuries occur during this phase; however, the thrower may experience elbow pain if posterior impingement is limiting full elbow extension.

Pathology
Shoulder Injuries

- Extreme external rotation can cause anterior laxity of the glenohumeral joint capsule, leading to instability and impingement (Fig. 29.3).
- Internal impingement syndrome: anterior instability during external rotation causes the rotator cuff tendons and the labrum to be pinched between the greater tuberosity of the humeral head and the posterior superior glenoid.
- Internal impingement may lead to a variety of problems: rotator cuff tendon fraying, chondromalacia of the humeral head, superior labrum anteroposterior lesions/tears (SLAP).
- Subacromial impingement may occur as the humerus is internally rotated (see Chapter 33).
- Younger pitchers typically have internal impingement, whereas older pitchers tend to have subacromial impingement.
- Anterior laxity can increase strain on the biceps tendon, causing bicipital tendonitis (see Chapter 31).
- Laxity can develop in the posterior shoulder capsule as microtears occur during resisted glenohumeral distraction.
- Posterior laxity produces instability and painful glenohumeral subluxation (see Chapter 28).
- Rotator cuff injuries
  - Eccentric rotator cuff forces may eventually lead to tears (see Chapter 34).
  - Repeated impingement may lead to tears (as discussed previously).
  - Articular sided tears at the junction of the infraspinatus and supraspinatus are commonly found.

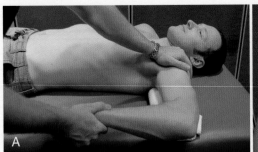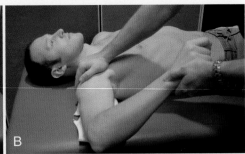

Fig 29.4 The physical examination of a right-handed throwing patient with glenohumeral internal rotation deficit. **(A)** The left side depicts normal left shoulder glenohumeral internal rotation. **(B)** The right side shows an approximately 30-degree internal rotation limitation of the right shoulder.

- Labral tears
  - SLAP lesions (see Chapter 30).
  - During deceleration phase, traction occurs at insertion of long head of biceps.
  - Often occur concomitantly with rotator cuff tears
- Glenohumeral internal rotation deficit (GIRD)
  - Glenohumeral internal rotation deficits caused by posterior capsular tightness can also contribute to internal impingement.
  - Glenohumeral internal rotation deficits should be suspected if internal rotation range of motion is decreased in the throwing arm compared with the nonthrowing arm (Fig. 29.4).
  - A difference of >25 degrees from the nonthrowing arm is associated with increased risk of injury.
  - Can lead to internal impingement and eventually articular sided rotator cuff tears and SLAP tears
  - Athletes generally respond well to physical therapy regimens focused on stretching of the posterior capsule.
- Scapulothoracic impingement can occur if proper scapular kinetics are not addressed.
  - Typically noted during the cocking phase
- Little league shoulder (proximal humeral epiphysiolysis; see Chapter 218)
- Sick scapula and scapular dyskinesis

Elbow Injuries

- Extreme elbow forces cause medial tension and posterior/lateral compression injuries.
- Medial injuries:
  - UCL injury (see Chapter 58)
  - UCL reconstruction (a.k.a. Tommy John surgery) is a common treatment in the overhead throwing athlete for UCL injury.
  - Flexor/pronator mass strain (see Chapter 56)
  - Ulnar neuropathy (see Chapter 61)
  - Medial epicondyle apophysitis; "Little league elbow" (see Chapter 219)
  - Repetitive stress during late cocking and acceleration phases of throwing
  - Excessive elbow extension may also produce avulsion injuries of the lateral epicondyle apophysis.
- Posterior and lateral injuries:
  - Triceps tendinopathy, olecranon apophysitis or triceps tendon avulsion (see Chapter 225)

- Osteochondral defect of elbow (see Chapter 53):
  - Compression of radio-capitellar joint can increase risk of osteochondral injury.
  - Occurs in adolescent throwers and typically produces lateral elbow pain
- Valgus extension overload (VEO) syndrome:
  - During acceleration phase, posteromedial elbow pain can result from extension of elbow under valgus load, compressing posteromedial aspect of the olecranon against the olecranon fossa.
  - Can be associated with osteophyte formation and loose bodies
  - Consider diagnosis in the setting of range of motion deficits (loss of terminal extension) and UCL laxity (pain between 30 degrees of flexion and terminal extension)
- Olecranon stress fracture:
  - Same causes as VEO (previously)
- Panner disease (osteochondrosis of the elbow; see Chapter 220):
  - Pediatric throwers (~ age 7 to 12)
  - Focal lesion in subchondral bone of capitellum and overlying articular cartilage

Other Pathology

- Axillary-subclavian vein thrombosis (Paget-Schroetter syndrome)
  - Often can present as swelling of the affected arm
  - Associated with repetitive overhead activity leading to trauma of the endothelium of the subclavian vein
  - Can be related to anatomic variants associated with thoracic outlet syndrome
  - Thrombophilic conditions increase risk

Treatment

- At diagnosis
  - In most cases, activity modification/limit throwing
  - Formal physical therapy
  - Disease-specific exercises (see related chapters)
  - Preservation of full shoulder and elbow range of motion
  - Appropriate lower extremity strength including hip external rotators and abductors as well as adequate core strength are important
  - Biomechanical and kinetic chain evaluation imperative

- Later
  - May need adjustment in throwing motion
  - Formal throwing assessment to identify poor mechanics is recommended
  - Maintenance strengthening program to prevent muscular fatigue
  - Glenohumeral internal rotation deficits treatment focused on restoring internal rotation
  - Affected arm abducted 90 degrees and externally rotated 90 degrees, and elbow flexed 90 degrees; contralateral arm applies internal rotation force to throwing arm to stretch out contracted posterior glenohumeral ligament ("sleeper stretch")

Troubleshooting

- Weak core and lower extremity strength increases shoulder and elbow stress, leading to frequent injury.
- Evaluating the complete kinetic chain for abnormalities can provide insight into the cause of the injury.
- Following pitch count restriction will help prevent many overuse injuries.
- Resting between throwing episodes is essential to avoid repetitive soft-tissue microtrauma.

Patient Instructions

- Follow defined pitch count restrictions, which are provided according to age.
- Learning proper throwing mechanics will help avoid increased shoulder and elbow strain, which can lead to injury.
- Notify a physician early if a problem occurs to limit serious injury.

Suggested Readings

Ahmad C, El Attrache N. Valgus extension overload syndrome and stress injury of the olecranon. *Clin Sports Med*. 2004;23:665–676.

Braun S, Kokmeyer D, Millett P. Shoulder injuries in the throwing athlete. *J Bone Joint Surg Am*. 2009;91:966–978.

Cain E, Dugas R, Wolf R, Andrews J. Elbow injuries in throwing athletes: a current concepts review. *Am J Sports Med*. 2003;31:621–635.

Fleisig GS, Andrews JR, Cutter GR, et al. Risk of serious injury for young baseball pitchers: a 10-year prospective study. *Am J Sports Med*. 2011;39:253–257.

Jobe C, Coen M, Screnar P. Evaluation of impingement syndrome in the overhead-throwing athlete. *J Athletic Train*. 2000;35:293–299.

Kuremsky M, Cain EL Jr, Dugas JR, Andrews JR. Elbow throwing injuries. In: Miller MD, Thompson SR, eds. *DeLee & Drez's Orthopaedic Sports Medicine: Principles and Practice*. 4th ed. Philadelphia: Elsevier; 2015: 784–795.

Meyers J, Laudner KG, Pasquale MR, et al. Glenohumeral range of motion deficits and posterior shoulder tightness in throwers with pathologic internal impingement. *Am J Sports Med*. 2006;34:385–391.

Park P, Loebenberg ML, Rokito AS, Zuckerman J. The shoulder in baseball pitching: biomechanics and related injuries—part 1. *Bull Hosp Joint Dis*. 2002–2003;61:68–79.

Park P, Loebenberg ML, Rokito AS, Zuckerman J. The shoulder in baseball pitching: biomechanics and related injuries—part 2. *Bull Hosp Joint Dis*. 2002–2003;61:80–88.

Major League Baseball: *Pitch count guidelines*. Available at http://m.mlb .com/pitchsmart/pitching-guidelines/. Accessed April 5, 2018.

Raasch WG. Baseball. In: Madden CC, Putukian M, McCarty EC, Young CC, eds. *Netter's Sports Medicine*. 2nd ed. Philadelphia: Elsevier; 2018:580–585.

Zheng N, Eaton K. Shoulder rotational properties of throwing athletes. *Int J Sports Med*. 2012;33:463.

Zheng N, Fleisig G, Barrenine S, Andrews J. Biomechanics of pitching. In: Hung GK, Pallis JM, eds. *Biomechanical Engineering Principles in Sports*. New York: Springer; 2004:209–256.

Chapter 30 Superior Labral Injuries

Brian Lowell, Kevin deWeber

ICD-10-CM CODE
S43.43 *Superior labrum anterior to posterior (SLAP) lesion*

Key Concepts

- The anatomy of glenohumeral (GH) joint is complex, and stability is provided from a combination of the capsule, tendons, muscles, bones, and the labrum.
  - The labrum acts by increasing the surface area for humeral head contact and provides attachment sites for the glenohumeral ligament and the tendon of the long head of the biceps.
  - Composed of fibrocartilage and dense fibrous collagenous tissue.
  - The superior aspect is more mobile than the inferior portion that is tightly attached to the glenoid rim.
  - Multiple anatomic variations exist, including congenitally absent portions of the labrum, different anchor sites for the glenohumeral ligament, different biceps tendon origins, and superior labral recesses.
- There are currently 10 described SLAP lesions, of which the 4 originally described by Snyder are the most common (Fig. 30.1).
- SLAP lesion development consists of an internal rotation deficit, tightening of the posterior capsule, posterior superior glenohumeral shift, maximization of external rotation forces at the biceps anchor and superior labral attachment, and "peel back" of the labrum. Alterations in scapular movements (dyskinesis) exacerbate this mechanism.
- The true incidence of SLAP injury is relatively low, occurring in approximately 3% to 6% of all arthroscopic shoulder cases.

History

- SLAP lesions occur with acute injuries or chronic degradation.
  - Acute injuries can occur via compression due to a fall on an outstretched arm or onto an adducted shoulder, traction from a swift pull, or via humeral head shearing, such as during vehicle accidents from seat belt restraint.
  - Chronic injuries occur with repetitive overhead motions that result in microtrauma accumulation; throwers and swimmers are at high risk for such injuries.
- Symptoms can include pain with overhead motions, loss of strength with certain arm movements, and a sensation of catching, clicking, or popping deep within the shoulder; patient experience is highly variable.

- A high index of suspicion is required when evaluating for a SLAP lesion. Other shoulder injuries coexist in about 85% of cases (glenohumeral instability, rotator cuff and bicipital tendon pathology), which can confound the diagnosis.

Physical Examination

- Examination maneuvers are generally inaccurate; there is no gold standard clinical test.
- Combinations of clinical tests provide higher accuracy. Combining 2 tests from a group with relatively high sensitivity (compression rotation test, anterior apprehension test, or O'Brien test) with 1 test from a group with relatively high specificity (Yergason test, biceps load test II, or Speed test) results in sensitivity and specificity of nearly 75% and 90%, respectively.
- Relatively High Sensitivity Tests:
  - Compression rotation test: with patient supine, the patients arm is abducted to 90 degrees and the elbow is flexed to 90 degrees, while the examiner applies axial force to humerus. With axial pressure, the arm is internally and externally rotated. Positive if pain or clicking is noted.
  - Anterior apprehension test: with patient supine, examiner passively externally rotates the humerus to end range with the shoulder in 90 degrees of abduction. Positive if pain or sensation of instability are noted.
  - O'Brien test (Video 30.1): with patient standing the arm is flexed to 90 degrees with elbow in full extension. With an adducted arm to 10 degrees and an internally rotated humerus, the examiner applies downward force to arm as patient resists. Patient then fully supinates arm and repeats resistance. Positive if pain is elicited with internal rotation and reduced with external rotation (supination).
- Relatively High Specificity Tests:
  - Yergason test: with patient standing with elbow at 90 degrees of flexion, patient supinates forearm against examiner's resistance, while examiner palpates long head of biceps tendon. Positive if pain at biceps tendon.
  - Biceps Load Test II (Video 30.2): with patient supine, examiner grasps patient's wrist and elbow. The arm is abducted to 120 degrees and fully externally rotated, with elbow held in 90 degrees of flexion and forearm supinated. Examiner then resists elbow flexion by patient. Positive if pain is noted.
  - Speed Test: with patient seated, elbow extended and forearm in full supination, the clinician resists active forward flexion from 0 to 60 degrees. Positive if pain is increased in the shoulder and the patient localizes the pain to the bicipital groove.

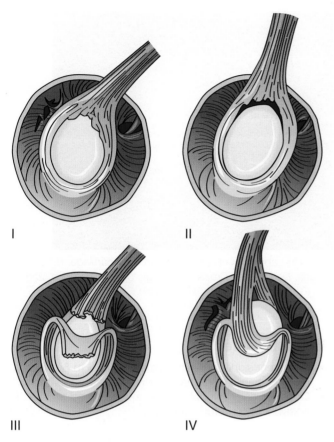

Fig 30.1 Snyder classification for SLAP lesions. Type I is degenerative fraying of labrum, type II is a detached labral/biceps complex, type III is a bucket-handle tear, and type IV is a bucket-handle tear with extension into the biceps. (Modified from Snyder SJ, Karzel RP, Del Pizzo W, et al. SLAP lesions of the shoulder. *Arthroscopy.* 1990;6:274–279, Fig. 21K-8.)

I

II

III

IV

Imaging

- Plain radiographs are useful in identifying bony pathology such as fracture, glenohumeral arthritis, AC joint arthritis, and tendinous calcific deposits.
- Ultrasound is useful in evaluating for coexistent injuries (biceps tendon, rotator cuff tendons, joint capsule, and acromioclavicular joint) but is insensitive for labral pathology. Joint effusion, bicipital sheath effusion, and paralabral cysts are secondary findings that suggest intra-articular pathology, which may include SLAP lesion.
- Magnetic resonance imaging (MRI) and magnetic resonance arthrography (MRA) are the mainstays in imaging for SLAP lesions.
  - Arthrography with intra-articular contrast medium improves imaging by outlining the intra-articular and synovial surfaces through slight distension of the capsule (Fig. 30.2).
  - Direct (intra-articular) MRA is superior to plain MRI and vascular contrast-enhanced MRI for detecting SLAP lesions with respect to both sensitivity and specificity.
  - 3-Tesla MRI improves diagnostic accuracy compared to 1.5-Tesla imaging.
- The gold standard for diagnosis of a SLAP lesion is direct visualization via arthroscopy. Evaluation of the biceps labral complex should be done with a probe as it may appear normal with just visualization (Fig. 30.3).

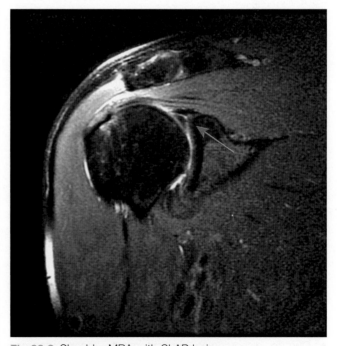

Fig 30.2 Shoulder MRA with SLAP lesion.

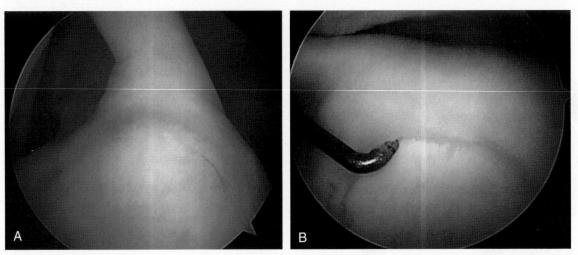

Fig 30.3 Arthroscopy picture of two common types of glenoid labrum. **(A)** Labrum continuous with articular cartilage. **(B)** Labrum has a meniscus-like structure. (From DeLee JC, Drez D Jr, Miller MD, eds. *De Lee and Drez's Orthpaedic Sports Medicine*, 2nd ed. Philadelphia: Saunders, 2003, p. 1047, Fig 21K-2.)

- Computed tomography arthrography (CTA) is rarely used in detection of SLAP lesions as specificity is low.

Differential Diagnosis

- Glenohumeral arthritis
- Rotator cuff impingement, tendinopathy or tear
- Biceps tendinopathy or partial tear
- Acromioclavicular joint arthritis
- Paralabral ganglion cyst
- Internal impingement syndrome (posterior pain)

Treatment

- Ideal treatment of these injuries remains unclear.
- In general, conservative treatment is indicated prior to surgical intervention.
  - Relative rest from aggravating activities.
  - Physical therapy with a focus on endurance and strengthening of the rotator cuff and scapular stabilizers, posterior capsule stretching, and anterior capsular strengthening to assist with limitations on internal rotation (Fig. 30.4).
  - Consideration of antiinflammatory medications or intra-articular corticosteroid injection for pain control.
  - A history of trauma or participation in overhead activities is strongly associated with failure of nonoperative treatment.
- Operative: evaluation with diagnostic arthroscopy and treatment is indicated if conservative therapy does not appropriately manage symptoms.
- While there is no uniform approach to SLAP lesion surgical repair, several options are available (arthroscopic debridement, SLAP repair/fixation, tenotomy of the long head of the biceps tendon, and tenodesis of the long head of the biceps tendon).
- Due to discouraging surgical results (poor outcomes with respect to return to previous level of play, and surgical complications) with SLAP repair, biceps tenodesis is becoming more prevalent.

When to Refer

- Persistent significant symptoms despite 3 to 6 months of quality rehabilitation and other conservative treatments.
- Consider early referral in elite and overhead athletes for possible faster return to sports.

Prognosis

- Contact athletes typically returned to sport quicker than overhead athletes and had a greater percentage of athletes return to their prior level of play. The evidence is rather unfavorable for overhead athletes returning to prior level of play status post SLAP repair (40-70%).
- Return to play and returning to previous level of play were limited in pitchers compared with other positional players.
- Individuals with isolated SLAP lesions (very rare) returned to activity much quicker (2.6 months) than individuals with concomitant shoulder pathology (6 months).
- Age appears to affect outcomes, as younger athletes have better outcomes overall.

Troubleshooting

- Failure of conservative therapy should prompt one to consider advanced imaging (MRI vs MRA) if it has not yet been obtained.
- MRI and MRA are not perfect imaging modalities. Normal anatomic shoulder variants occur and may confound imaging results. The gold standard for diagnosing SLAP lesions is via arthroscopy. One must have a high index of suspicion when considering SLAP lesion.
- If no labral pathology is identified, broaden the differential to include cervical or brachial plexus pathology

Patient Instructions

- Therapy is largely patient directed. Best outcomes come with great compliance to exercise regimen.

Posterior capsule stretching and mobility

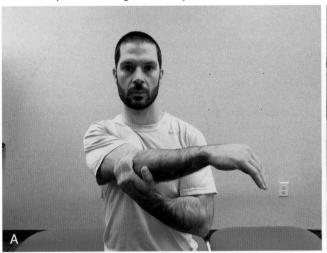

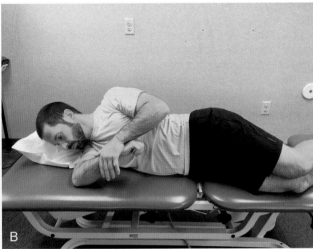

Periscapular strengthening and rotator cuff function

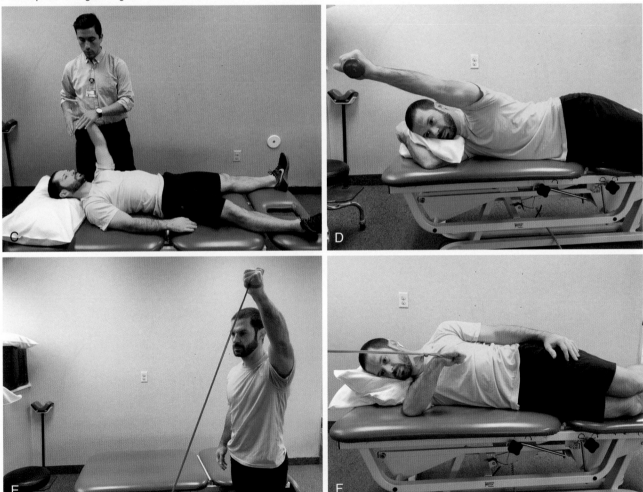

Fig 30.4 Conservative physical therapy maneuvers. From *top* to *bottom*, *left* to *right*: **(A)** horizontal adduction, **(B)** sleeper stretch, **(C)** balanced position-rhythmic stabilization, **(D)** side laying flexion (lower trapezius), **(E)** standing (D2) flexion and resisted internal rotation in sleeper position **(F)**. (Photos courtesy of Chris Garcia, PT, DPT, OCS, CSCS.)

- With the exception of overhead athletes, literature recommends significant conservative approach due to complications associated with surgical repair.
- Surgical repair of the superior labrum comes with complications. One should discuss and consider all surgical options available and outcomes associated with each option prior to making a surgical decision.

Suggested Readings

Abrams G, Safran M. Diagnosis and management of superior labrum anterior posterior lesions in overhead athletes. *Br J Sports Med*. 2010;44:311–318.

Manske R, Prohaska D. Superior labrum anterior to posterior (SLAP) rehabilitation in the overhead athlete. *Phys Ther Sport*. 2010;11:110–121.

Oh JH, Kim JY, Kim WA, et al. The evaluation of various physical examinations for the diagnosis of type II superior labrum anterior to posterior lesion. *Am J Sports Med*. 2008;36:353–359.

Popp D, Schoffl V. Superior labral anterior posterior lesions of the shoulder: current diagnostic and therapeutic standards. *World J Orthop*. 2015;6(9):660–671.

Rangavajjula A, Hyatt A, Raneses E, et al. Return to play after treatment of shoulder labral tears in professional hockey players. *Phys Sportsmed*. 2016;44(2):119–125.

Symanski JS, Subhas N, Babb J, et al. Diagnosis of superior labrum anterior-to-posterior tears by using MR imaging and MR arthrography: a systemic review and meta-analysis. *Radiology*. 2017;285:101–113.

Chapter 31 Biceps Tendon Injury

Christopher Miles, Andrea Gist, Nicholas Sgrignoli

ICD-10-CM CODES
M75.20 *Bicipital tendonitis, unspecified laterality*
M66.829 *Spontaneous rupture of other tendons, unspecified upper arm*

Key Concepts

Biceps anatomy
- The biceps brachii is composed of two muscles. The long head of the biceps tendon (LHBT) originates on the supraglenoid tubercle and attaches to the superior labrum.

Proximal Biceps Injury

- Injury is common in overhead athletes.
- Bicipital tendinitis
  - An overuse syndrome caused by repetitive overload of the biceps tendon from elbow flexion and supination; often occurs with impingement syndrome.
- Rupture
  - Ninety-six percent of biceps ruptures involve the proximal LHBT, 3% the distal head, and 1% the short head.
  - Most common in older individuals (ages 40 to 60 years), affecting more men than women.
  - Biceps tendinitis may predispose to rupture.
  - Most ruptures result in a characteristic "Popeye" muscle appearance.
- Biceps tendon subluxation/dislocation across the bicipital groove can be caused by a tear in the subscapularis tendon

History

Patients will often complain of anterior shoulder pain that increases with overhead activities, elbow flexion, and/or supination. Later in the course of the disease, pain may be more notable at night or while resting. Pain often radiates distally and can be compounded by concomitant impingement syndrome or rotator cuff tendinitis. In the setting of proximal biceps tendon rupture, most patients recall a single acute injury with an audible "pop" noted by the patient.

Physical Examination

- **Inspection:** Evaluate for "Popeye" appearance of biceps muscle caused by retraction of the LHBT distally (Fig. 31.1). Ecchymosis may be noted if injury is relatively acute.
- **Palpation:** Bony palpation of the sternoclavicular joint, intrinsic shoulder bones, and cervical spine is recommended. Soft-tissue palpation should include palpation of the long and short heads of the biceps muscle, the rotator cuff muscles, and the anterior and posterior capsules.
  - With bicipital tendinitis, point tenderness with palpation of long head tendon at the bicipital groove is common. Point tenderness should move in conjunction with the bicipital groove as the examiner rotates the affected arm. Comparing the contralateral shoulder is helpful.
- **Range of motion:** Both passive and active range of motion of the shoulder and elbow should be evaluated. In the acute setting, motion may be limited secondary to pain.
- **Neurovascular examination:** Sensation and distal pulses of the upper extremity should be evaluated.

Special Tests

- **Speed test:** With the affected shoulder in 90 degrees of forward flexion, the forearm is extended and supinated. The examiner then applies a downward pressure on the palm. A positive test is pain over the bicipital groove (sensitivity [Sn] 54%, specificity [Sp] 81%).
- **Yergason test:** The elbow is flexed at 90 degrees with the forearm in pronation with active resistance against supination. A positive test is pain over the bicipital groove or subluxation of the LHBT at the bicipital groove (Sn 41%, Sp 79%).
- **Ludington test:** Patient places both hands behind head with interlocking fingers, flexing biceps muscles. A positive test is pain at the bicipital groove or a notable subluxing tendon. This may elicit the "Popeye" sign (see Fig. 31.1).
- **Upper cut:** Shoulder in neutral position with forearm at 90 degrees and supinated. The patient creates an upper-cut motion while the examiner resists while allowing for movement. A positive test is pain or popping over the anterior shoulder during the resisted movement (Sn 73%, Sp 78%). One study found that combining the uppercut test with tenderness at the bicipital groove demonstrated the most value to diagnostic accuracy.
- Consider testing for concomitant rotator cuff tears and labral tears.

Imaging

- **Radiographs:** Anteroposterior and axillary views are typically negative but should be obtained to evaluate for acromioclavicular (AC) joint or glenohumeral bony pathology. A fisk view (tangential projection of bicipital groove) can be used to evaluate bicipital groove pathology.
- **Musculoskeletal ultrasonography** for the diagnosis of biceps pathology is a low-cost tool. It is highly accurate in diagnosing complete tears, subluxations, and dislocations (Sn 96%, Sp 100%). It is more difficult to diagnose partial tears with ultrasonography.

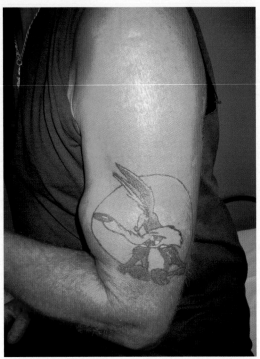

Fig 31.1 "Popeye" muscle seen in proximal biceps tendon rupture. (From Johnson DL, Mairs SD, eds. *Clinical Sports Medicine.* St. Louis: Mosby; 2006:237.)

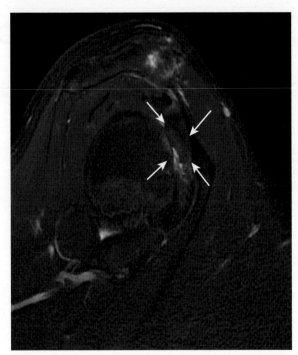

Fig 31.2 Magnetic resonance imaging T2 FS sagittal oblique image showing enlarged biceps tendon (tendinosis) with increased signal intensity and surrounding fluid. *Arrows* reflect enlarged tendon and surrounding edema.

- **Magnetic resonance imaging (MRI)** can be used to diagnose tendinitis (Fig. 31.2) and should be considered in young athletes and patients with persistent pain to evaluate for intra-articular pathology (associated superior labral anteroposterior lesion) or rotator cuff tear. MRI has been found to be only 27% sensitive in diagnosing partial LHBT tears.
- **Magnetic resonance arthrogram** can increase sensitivity of diagnosing biceps pathology; however, it is more invasive and requires experienced personnel to administer and interpret the study.

Differential Diagnosis

Rotator cuff tear or impingement, subacromial bursitis, labral tear, glenohumeral arthritis or instability, adhesive capsulitis, cervical radiculopathy, and coracoid impingement syndrome.

Treatment

Biceps tendinitis
- Relative rest, nonsteroidal antiinflammatory drugs (NSAIDs), and physical therapy.
- Local corticosteroid injection may be attempted in persistent cases and may be assisted by ultrasound guidance (Fig. 31.3). Injections require risk–benefit discussion given the increased risk of tendon rupture.
- Patients with biceps tendinitis should also be evaluated and treated for overlapping pathology in surrounding structures such as rotator cuff, AC joint, etc., to maximize recovery.

Proximal biceps tendon rupture
- At time of presentation the patient should be instructed on relative rest, including no lifting >10 lbs. Immobilization, NSAIDs, and ice may be helpful until inflammation abates.

Subacute management of biceps tendon rupture
- Choice of conservative versus surgical treatment must take into account patient age, occupation, and level of physical activity. Biceps tendon rupture usually responds well to physical therapy. Patients can usually expect normal range of motion, grip strength, and pronation; however, they may experience up to 20% reduction in supination strength.
- Surgical tenodesis is controversial and is usually reserved for young, active patients or those patients whose occupation requires maximal supination and flexion strength. Techniques for tenodesis range from a completely open technique to arthroscopy. Fixation by suture anchors, screws, or bone tunnels is common (see Fig. 31.3).
- Tenotomy may also be an option for older patients with minimal physical demands, patients that are not concerned with the resulting cosmetic deformity, or patients without time for lengthy rehabilitation.

When to Refer

- The overall recommendation is to take a patient-centered approach. One may consider surgery for young people with high standards for activity, elite athletes, young manual laborers, or people unwilling to experience any cosmetic defect. Early intervention is recommended in this group.

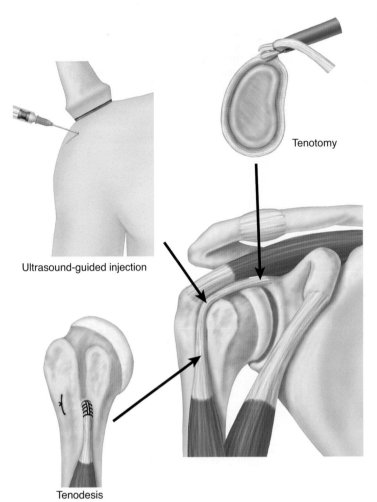

Tenotomy

Ultrasound-guided injection

Tenodesis

Fig 31.3 Invasive intervention options for proximal tendon injury, including ultrasound-guided injection, tenotomy, and tenodesis.

Prognosis

- In biceps tendinitis, the prognosis is generally good, depending on patient adherence to treatment.
- Research has found no difference between patients managed operatively and nonoperatively.
- Patients experience similar satisfaction with tenodesis or tenotomy.

Troubleshooting

- Patients should be counseled comprehensively on non-operative and surgical options and expected outcomes of both to make an informed decision.
- Patients choosing nonoperative management will need close follow-up to ensure progression toward recovery and to address potential concerns about living with this injury.
- Counsel patients that corticosteroid injections are an option for inflammation relief, but it should not be relied upon chronically given risk of tendon rupture.

Patient Instructions

- Adherence to physical therapy to restore strength, flexibility, and range of motion is crucial.

Considerations in Special Populations

- Biceps tendon injury should be considered in any overhead- or underhand-throwing athletes presenting with anterior shoulder pain.
- Tenodesis of bicep tendon rupture should be considered in active patients less than 40 years old or an older patient whose occupation, such as carpentry or other physically demanding job, requires full supination strength.
- In athletes with time constraints or the geriatric population, tenotomy is a reasonable treatment option after the patient has been counseled and accepts the possible deformity if the long head retracts into the arm. This has been successfully conducted in NFL players with this condition.

Suggested Readings

Armstrong A, Teefey SA, Wu T, et al. The efficacy of ultrasound in the diagnosis of long head of the biceps tendon pathology. *J Shoulder Elbow Surg*. 2006;15:7–11.

Burkhead WZ Jr, Habermeyer P, Walch G, Lin K. The biceps tendon. In: Rockwood CA Jr, Matsen FA III, eds. *The Shoulder*. 4th ed. Philadelphia: WB Saunders; 2009:1309–1360.

Carr RM, Shishani Y, Gobezie R. How accurate are we in detecting biceps tendinopathy? *Clin Sports Med*. 2016;35(1):47–55.

Chalmers PN, Verma NN. Proximal biceps in overhead athletes. *Clin Sports Med*. 2016;35(1):163–179.

Hanypsiak BT, Delong JM, Guerra J. Proximal biceps tendon pathology. In: Miller MD, Thompson SR: *DeLee and Drez's Orthopaedic Sports Medicine*. Philadelphia: Elsevier; 2015:569–584.

Rosas S, Krill MK, Amoo-Achampong K, et al. A practical, evidence-based, comprehensive (PEC) physical examination for diagnosing pathology of the long head of the biceps. *J Shoulder Elbow Surg*. 2017;26(8):1484–1492.

Schickendantz M, King D. Nonoperative management (including ultrasound guided injections) of proximal biceps disorders. *Clin Sports Med*. 2016;35(1):57–73.

Wilk KE, Hooks TR. The painful long head of the biceps brachii: nonoperative treatment approaches. *Clin Sports Med*. 2016;35(1):75–92.

Chapter 32 Pectoralis Major Muscle Rupture

John V. Murphy, James Medure, Aaron V. Mares

ICD-10-CM CODES

S43.491A	*Other sprain of right shoulder joint, initial encounter*
S43.492A	*Other sprain of left shoulder joint, initial encounter*
S43.499A	*Other sprain of unspecified shoulder joint, initial encounter*
S46.819A	*Strain of other muscles, fascia and tendons at shoulder and upper arm level, unspecified arm, initial encounter*
S29.011A	*Strain of muscle and tendon of front wall of thorax, initial encounter*
S29.011D	*Strain of muscle and tendon of front wall of thorax subsequent encounter*
S29.011S	*Strain of muscle and tendon of front wall of thorax sequela*

Key Concepts

- Composed of two heads: clavicular (segmented) and sternal (uniform), with sternal being more proximal and posterior (Fig. 32.1).
- Innervated by the medial and lateral pectoral nerves (C5-T1).
- 365 cases of pectoralis muscle rupture have been reported in the medical literature between 1822 and 2010, with 76% reported after 1990.
- Pectoralis rupture is almost exclusively in men in third and fourth decade of life.
- Main function is adduction, forward elevation of shoulder (clavicular head), and internal rotation (sternal head).
- Management of tear is typically surgical in the young active population; however, for partial tears, nonsurgical management options may be utilized.
- Acute tear <6 weeks and chronic tear is >6 weeks duration.
- Rupture tends to occur at low speeds with the arm abducted and externally rotated, which puts significant stretch on the inferior fibers.
- Locations of tears (most to least common): humeral insertion, musculotendinous junction, muscle belly, bony avulsion, and sternal origin (Fig. 32.2).

History

- Often occurs in male weight lifters performing bench-press exercises.
- May have an audible "pop" or "snap" with immediate sharp or tearing pain.

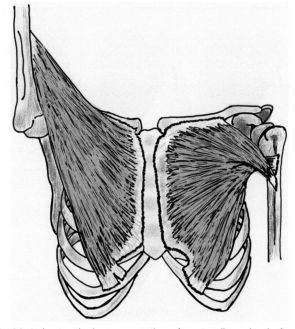

Fig 32.1 Anatomical representation of pectoralis major. Left arm in anatomical position and left arm in full forward flexion. (Original artwork by Jim Medure.)

- Sharp tearing pain with resisted internal rotation and adduction.
- Most often occurs during the eccentric phase of contraction as more tension is generated than during the concentric phase.
- Often present with acute pain, swelling and weakness of shoulder adduction, and internal rotation from a rapid eccentric load.

Physical Exam

- Pain, swelling, and ecchymosis of anterior chest wall, axilla, and arm.
- May have asymmetry of medial prominence of the muscle belly, which may represent hematoma formation or retracted muscle belly, which is more obvious with a chronic tear (Fig. 32.3).
- This also may obscure the axillary fold or cause a webbed appearance of the thinned out anterior axilla (see Fig. 32.3).
- May have palpable defect in muscle belly, which may be enhanced by contraction of the muscle in 90-90 shoulder

133

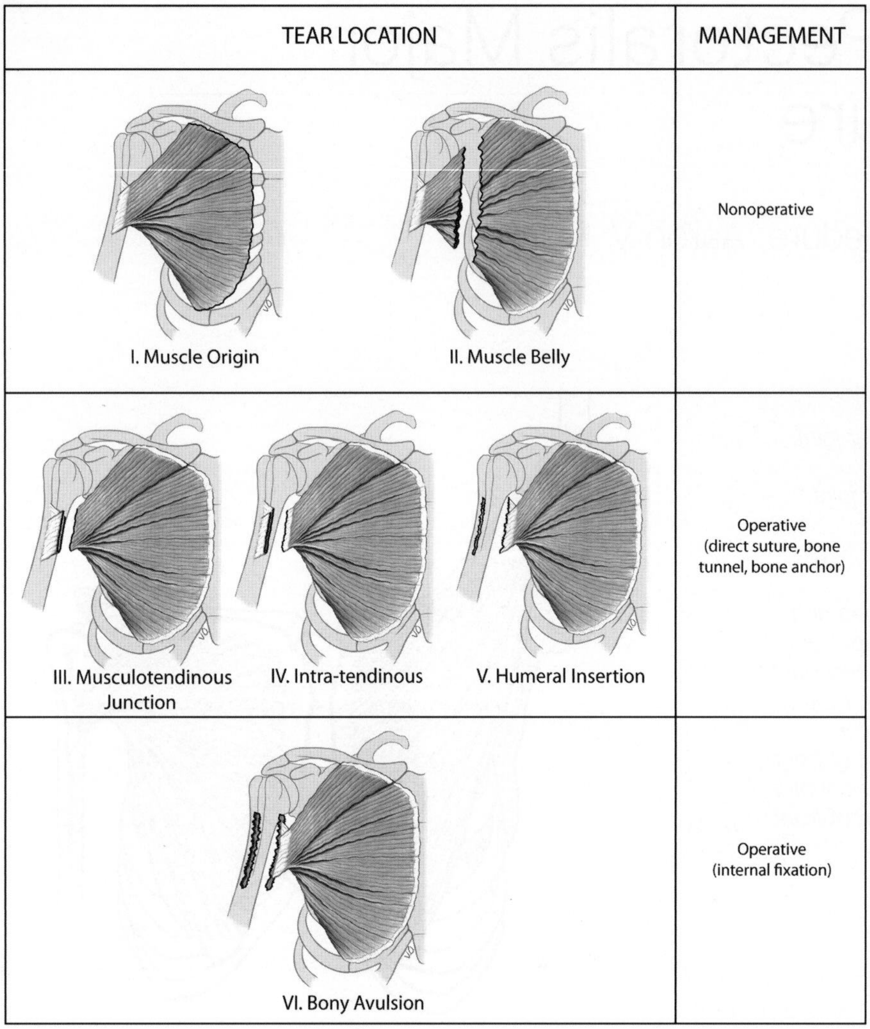

TEAR LOCATION		MANAGEMENT
I. Muscle Origin	II. Muscle Belly	Nonoperative
III. Musculotendinous Junction	IV. Intra-tendinous V. Humeral Insertion	Operative (direct suture, bone tunnel, bone anchor)
VI. Bony Avulsion		Operative (internal fixation)

Fig 32.2 Locations of ruptures with appropriate management. (From Elmaraghy AW, Devereaux MW. A systematic review and comprehensive classification of pectoralis major tears. *J Shoulder Elbow Surg*. 2012; 21[3]:412–422. Courtesy Valerie Oxorn.)

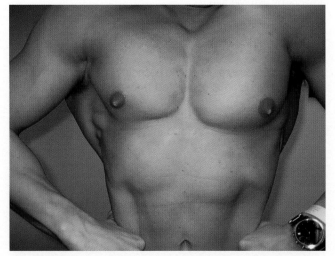

Fig 32.3 Patient with acute pectoralis major muscle rupture illustrating the asymmetry of the axilla and anterior chest as well as the webbed axillary fold. (Courtesy Brett D. Owens, MD, West Point, NY. In Haley CA, Zacchilli MA. Pectoralis major injuries: evaluation and treatment. *Clin Sports Med*. 2014;33(4)739–756, Fig. 3.)

abduction and elbow flexion in either shoulder internal or external rotation positions.
- Results in weakness with adduction and internal rotation.
- Important to differentiate from other chest and shoulder injuries (Table 32.1).

Imaging

- Radiographs often negative unless avulsion has occurred. Recommend: true anteroposterior (AP), scapular Y, and axillary lateral views.
- Ultrasound can identify quickly the location and severity of tear, as well as hematoma formation.
- Both ultrasound (Figs. 32.4 and 32.5) and MRI (Figs. 32.6 and 32.7) can identify and classify tear:
  - Timing: acute (<6 weeks) versus chronic (>6 weeks)
  - Location (muscle, musculotendinous junction, tendon or insertion)
  - Extent: thickness (partial or full) and width (complete or incomplete)
- MRI may better show severity and location. Acute tears enhanced with T2-weighted images and chronic tears with T1-weighted images.

TABLE 32.1 Differential Diagnoses

Condition	Differentiating Feature
Pectoralis muscle strain	No ecchymosis or palpable defect
Biceps tendon injury	Weakness +/– pain with elbow flexion
Rotator cuff injury/impingement	Shoulder limited ROM/weakness, pain with overhead motion
Shoulder dislocation	No palpable defect, shoulder in internal rotation and adduction with sulcus sign
Chest wall contusion	No defect with resisted shoulder adduction
Rib fracture	Pain on inspiration
Medial pectoral nerve entrapment	Pain without palpable defect, insidious onset

ROM, Range of motion.

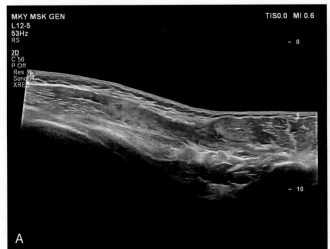
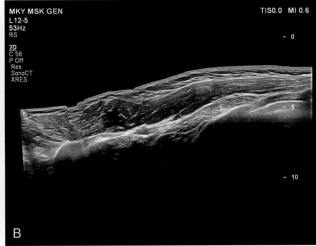

Fig 32.4 Ultrasound extended field of view of pectoralis rupture **(A)** and normal pectoralis **(B)**. (Courtesy Dr. Kenji Yamazaki.)

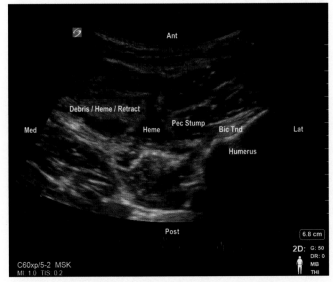

Fig 32.5 Ultrasound long-axis labeled view of pectoralis rupture and hematoma. (Courtesy Dr. Kenji Yamazaki.)

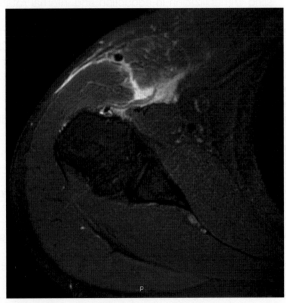

Fig 32.6 Axial magnetic resonance imaging view of pectorals tear. (Courtesy Dr. Kenji Yamazaki.)

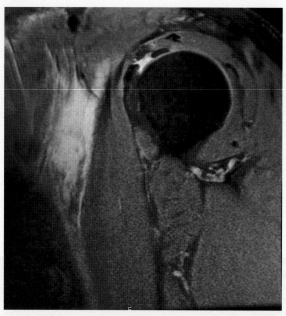

Fig 32.7 Sagittal view magnetic resonance imaging of pectorals tear. (Courtesy Dr. Kenji Yamazaki.)

Treatment (Fig. 32.8)

- Nonoperative:
  - Utilized for contusions, partial tendinous tears, muscle belly tears, and complete tendinous tears for sedentary individuals.
  - Results in functional recovery but often a visible cosmetic defect.
  - Includes rest, ice, analgesia, control of hematoma, and sling immobilization in adduction and internal rotation (for comfort).
  - Consider ultrasound-guided orthobiologic (platelet-rich plasma [PRP]/autologous conditioned plasma [ACP]/ stem cells) injection to intramuscular or partial tear to assist in healing if choosing conservative treatment.
  - First 2 weeks: passive range of motion (ROM).
  - 2 to 6 weeks: gradual increase in active ROM.
  - 6 to 8 weeks: begin light resistance exercise with gradual progression.
  - 3 to 4 months: may return to resistance training.
  - 5 to 6 months: return to contact sport if regained full ROM and strength.
  - If failing to progress over the first 3 to 4 months, consider surgical evaluation.
- Operative:
  - Provides the best outcome for strength, cosmesis/ satisfaction, and return to play.
  - Complete tears at the tendon insertion, intratendinous, or myotendinous junction should all be repaired.
  - Rehabilitation postrepair.
  - After repair, sling immobilization for 6 weeks.

- Weeks 1 to 6 should be pendulum exercises but avoid abduction and external rotation.
- Weeks 6 to 12, progress through all planes of motion starting with gentle passive techniques.
- Should develop full active range of motion (AROM) around 3 months and begin light resistance.
- By 6 months should be back to unrestricted activity.

Prognosis

- Operative treatment is generally recommended to ensure full restoration of strength and to return to previous activity level.
- Delayed reconstruction not recommended due to muscle retraction and involution of tendon, which may not allow for surgical reconstruction.
- ROM is often regained with surgical or nonsurgical treatment.

When to Refer

- Referral to orthopaedic specialist recommended quickly to assess the severity of the injury.
- Surgical referral necessary when any tendinous insertion or musculotendinous tear is suspected, or if cosmesis is a concern.

Troubleshooting

- Risks and benefits of surgical intervention must be discussed with the patient.
- Although rare, complications include weakness (due to damage to pectoral nerve), cosmetic deformity, hematoma, infection, abscess formation, and myositis ossificans.
- Adequate rehabilitation necessary to regain strength and ROM, as well as to prevent rotator cuff or shoulder complications.

Patient Instructions

- Stop exercising and immobilize the arm if possible to prevent further injury.
- Apply ice to area to decrease pain and swelling.
- Seek primary care provider or orthopaedic specialist evaluation.
- Adhere to the rehabilitation protocol/plan to optimize regain of function.

Considerations in Special Populations

- Weightlifting/powerlifting
- Power sports: American football and rugby players
- Male gender
- Young military personnel
- Use of anabolic steroids can weaken tendon fibers while disproportionately enlarging muscle tissue.
- Further risk factors for injury include: inappropriate activity, abnormal biomechanics, muscle weakness/imbalance, muscle tightness, poor posture affecting humeral head position with forceful eccentric activity.

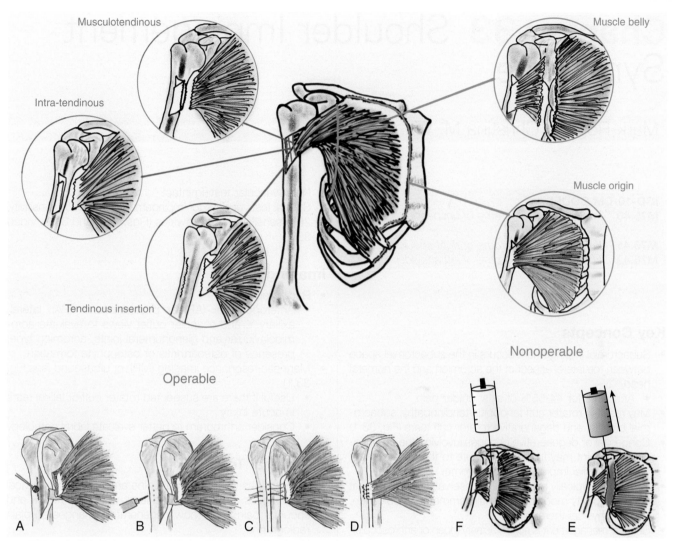

Fig 32.8 Locations of ruptures with appropriate treatment options. **(A to D)** represents appropriate surgical repair of pectoralis rupture. **(E and F)** represents hematoma drainage +/– orthobiologic (platelet-rich plasma [PRP]/autologous conditioned plasma [ACP]/stem cells) injection into tear site to assist with healing. (Original artwork by Jim Medure.)

Suggested Readings

Aarimaa VA, Rantanen J, Heikkila J, et al. Rupture of the pectoralis major muscle. *Am J Sports Med*. 2004;32:1256–1262.

Boggess B, Mooreman C. Partial pectoralis tear treated with orthobiologics: a case report. *Curr Sports Med Rep*. 2017;16(2):74–76.

Chiavaras MM, Jacobson JA, Smith J, Dahm DL. Pectoralis major tears: anatomy, classification, and diagnosis with ultrasound and MR imaging. *Skeletal Radiol*. 2014;44(2):157–164.

Elmaraghy AW, Devereaux MW. A systematic review and comprehensive classification of pectoralis major tears. *J Shoulder Elbow Surg*. 2012;21(3):412–422.

Hanna CM, Glenny AB, Stanley SN, Caughey MA. Pectoralis major tears: comparison of surgical and conservative treatment. *Br J Sports Med*. 2001;35:202–206.

McEntire J, Hess WE, Coleman S. Rupture of the pectoralis major muscle. *J Bone Joint Surg Am*. 1972;54A:1040–1047.

Ohashi K, El-Khoury MD, Albright J, Tearse D. MRI of complete rupture of the pectoralis major muscle. *Skeletal Radiol*. 1996;25(7): 625–628.

Petilon MD, Carr DR, Sekiya JK, Unger DV. Pectoralis major muscle injuries: evaluation and management. *J Am Acad Orthop Surg*. 2005;13: 59–68.

Provencher MT, Handfield K, Boniquit NT, et al. Injuries to the pectoralis major muscle diagnosis and management. *Am J Sports Med*. 2010;38(8):1693–1705.

Rehman A, Robinson P. Sonographic evaluation of injuries to the pectoralis muscles. *AJR Am J Roentgenol*. 2005;184:1205–1211.

Schepsis AA, Grafe MW, Jones H, Lemos M. Rupture of the pectoralis muscle: outcome after repair of acute and chronic injuries. *Am J Sports Med*. 2000;28:9–15.

Sherman SL, et al. Biomechanical analysis of the pectoralis major tendon and comparison of techniques for tendo-osseous repair. *Am J Sports Med*. 2012;40(8):1887–1894.

Zvijac J, Schurhoff M, Hechtman KS, Uribe J. Pectoralis major tears: correlation of magnetic resonance imaging and treatment strategies. *Am J Sports Med*. 2006;34:289–294.

Chapter 33 Shoulder Impingement Syndrome

Mark Rogers, Christina M. Wong

ICD-10-CM CODES
M75.40 *Impingement syndrome of unspecified shoulder*
M75.41 *Impingement syndrome of right shoulder*
M75.42 *Impingement syndrome of left shoulder*

Key Concepts

- Subacromial impingement occurs in the subacromial space between the lateral aspect of the acromion and the humeral head
  - Accounts for 44-65% of all shoulder pain
- May result in rotator cuff tendonitis/tendinopathy, subacromial bursitis, and degenerative rotator cuff tears (Fig. 33.1)
- Congenital or degenerative changes involving the acromioclavicular joint may further contribute to the development of subacromial impingement syndrome.
- Symptoms typically resolve with conservative management such as activity modification, antiinflammatory medication, and/or physical therapy.
- Surgical management is acromioplasty (open or arthroscopic)/subacromial decompression

History

- Insidious onset of throbbing or aching pain of the anterolateral shoulder
- Typically no history of an acute injury
- Participation in repetitive overhead activities
- Painful range of motion, worse with forward flexion and abduction above the level of the shoulder (90 degrees)
- No radicular symptoms or sensory deficits

Physical Examination

- Inspection: Usually no visible shoulder abnormalities or asymmetry compared with opposite side, unless scapular winging or dyskinesia present (see Chapter 41)
- Palpation: May have tenderness on palpation lateral to the acromion or upon compression of subacromial space
- Range of motion: Overall preserved, but pain reported on forward flexion and in mid-range of abduction (70 to 130 degrees, the "painful arc of abduction")
- Strength testing: Usually equal to opposite side unless apparent strength loss due to pain from another cause, such as rotator cuff tendinitis

- Neurovascular testing intact
- Special tests positive for impingement: Neer (92% sensitivity, 26% sensitivity) and Hawkins (Figs. 33.2 and 33.3; Video 33.1)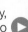

Imaging

- Radiographs
  - Anteroposterior (AP) or posteroanterior (PA), lateral, axillary Y, and scapular outlet views to evaluate acromioclavicular and glenohumeral joints, acromion type, presence of osteoarthritis or osteophyte formation
- Magnetic resonance imaging (MRI) or ultrasound (see Fig. 33.1)
  - Useful if there are suspected rotator cuff or labral tears in acute injury
  - Consider arthrogram to better evaluate labral pathology

Additional Tests

- Radiographs of the cervical spine are indicated if cervical pathology is suspected in patients with vague neck and shoulder pain; may show degenerative changes on plain radiographs
- Diagnostic injection of 1% lidocaine in the subacromial space improves pain with Hawkins and Neer tests

Differential Diagnosis

- See Table 33.1.

Treatment
Conservative Management

- Nonsteroidal antiinflammatory drugs (oral or topical)
- Ice on affected area 20 to 30 minutes every 2 hours or after activity
- Activity modification (i.e., limit overhead activity, modify repetitive activity)
- Physical therapy for stretching/range of motion and rotator cuff strengthening to improve scapular position and motion
- For mild symptoms, it may be preferential, pending patient compliance, to give the patient a home exercise program
- Follow-up in 4 to 6 weeks

Corticosteroid Injection

- Depending on progress with above conservative measures, a corticosteroid injection into the subacromial space and bursal area may be offered (see Fig. 33.1)

Shoulder Impingement

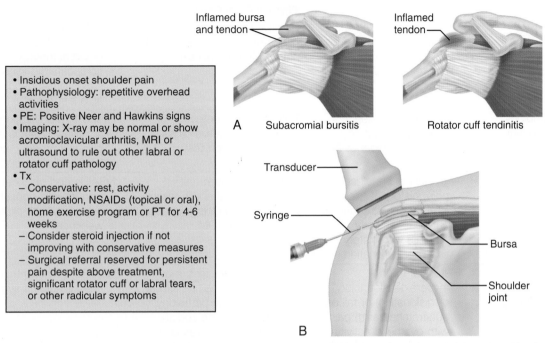

- Insidious onset shoulder pain
- Pathophysiology: repetitive overhead activities
- PE: Positive Neer and Hawkins signs
- Imaging: X-ray may be normal or show acromioclavicular arthritis, MRI or ultrasound to rule out other labral or rotator cuff pathology
- Tx
  - Conservative: rest, activity modification, NSAIDs (topical or oral), home exercise program or PT for 4-6 weeks
  - Consider steroid injection if not improving with conservative measures
  - Surgical referral reserved for persistent pain despite above treatment, significant rotator cuff or labral tears, or other radicular symptoms

A   Subacromial bursitis

Inflamed bursa and tendon

Inflamed tendon

Rotator cuff tendinitis

Transducer

Syringe

Bursa

Shoulder joint

B

Fig 33.1 (A) *Left,* Subacromial bursitis; *Right,* Rotator cuff tendinitis. (B) Evaluation of the subacromial space with ultrasound and ultrasound guided steroid injection. *MRI,* Magnetic resonance imaging; *NSAIDs,* nonsteroidal antiinflammatory drugs.

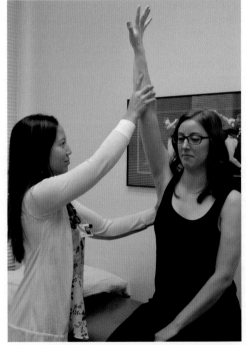

Fig 33.2 Neer sign. Pain with passive forward elevation of affected arm to 180 degrees with the arm externally rotated.

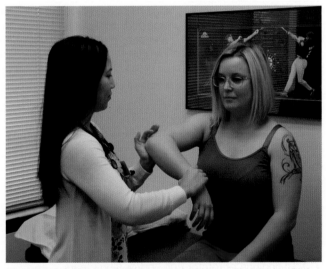

Fig 33.3 Hawkins sign. Pain is reproduced with passive flexion of the affected arm at 90 degrees and flexion of the elbow at 90 degrees. The arm is then internally rotated.

TABLE 33.1 Differential Diagnosis

Condition	History	Physical Exam Findings	Treatment
Impingement syndrome	Gradual onset; pain with overhead movement; pain mostly on anterolateral shoulder; night pain	Positive impingement signs (Hawkins and Neer); ROM and strength usually normal	First line: modification of activities, NSAIDs and physical therapy; subacromial corticosteroid injection, and subacromial decompression as a last resort
AC joint pathology (arthritis, sprain)	Fall on affected side (sprain); pain on anterior shoulder at AC joint	Pain on direct palpation of AC joint; positive cross-arm adduction test;	First line: modification of activities, NSAIDs and physical therapy; consider AC joint corticosteroid injection
Rotator cuff tear	Anterolateral shoulder pain; history of trauma in acute tears; consider cuff tear in elderly patients with history of shoulder dislocation,	Positive drop arm test; decreased strength testing on involved muscle group; decreased ROM	NSAIDs and physical therapy; orthopaedic consult, especially with profound weakness
Labral tear (superior labrum anterior-posterior [SLAP])	History of trauma (hyperextension injury or dislocation) or fall on outstretched arm; pain with overhead activity (i.e., throwing athletes); mechanical symptoms	Positive O'Brien test; may have exam findings similar to rotator cuff pathology; there is not one specific test for labrum, rather a combination of + tests.	NSAIDs, physical therapy; may need surgery if symptomatic
Frozen shoulder (adhesive capsulitis)	Stiffness, limited AROM and PROM; pain at rest or with minimal movement	Limited ROM, both active and passive	Physical therapy for mobilization/ROM; may need surgery if physical therapy fails
Cervical disc disease/radiculopathy	Vague neck pain (upper trapezius muscle) and shoulder pain; pain radiating down arm	Pain with neck ROM testing; may have weakness of affected shoulder/arm; + arm abduction test, positive Spurling maneuver	NSAIDs, oral steroids, physical therapy; may need surgery for severe symptoms/nerve compression or if physical therapy fails

AC, Acromioclavicular; *AROM*, active range of motion; *NSAIDs*, nonsteroidal antiinflammatory drugs; *PROM*, passive range of motion; *ROM*, range of motion.

- Repeat physical exam maneuvers after injection for a better assessment
- Continue physical therapy for 4 to 6 weeks before reevaluating

When to Refer

- Persistence or worsening of pain despite 4 to 6 months of conservative therapy
- MRI findings of rotator cuff and/or labral tears
- Coexisting cervical disc disease/radiculopathy

Prognosis

- Good with conservative therapy, in the absence of other shoulder/neck pathology

Troubleshooting

- Internal impingement is a condition found in overhead or throwing athletes in whom the posterior superior capsule of the shoulder is impinged when the arm is in the abducted and externally rotated position as in the cocking phase of throwing. This results from overall excessive laxity of the capsule as a function of repetitive throwing or overhead activities.
- Perform a cervical spine examination to rule out cervical pathology.

Patient Instructions

- Avoid overhead activities in the acute phase and modify activity to adapt to work or sport
- Take antiinflammatory medications as needed for pain and inflammation
- Consider using ice or a corticosteroid injection to help modify pain with physical therapy
- With the potentially chronic or recurring symptoms of impingement syndrome, it is important to continue exercises at home even after reduction or resolution of symptoms

Considerations in Special Populations

- In the athletes who use overhead throwing motions, glenohumeral and scapular stabilization, in addition to rotator cuff strengthening exercises, is key to the management of internal impingement symptoms
- Osteopathic manipulative therapy, including muscle energy and facilitated position release techniques, may be an alternative treatment to help improve range of motion and pain
- In the elderly patient, if there is no improvement after several weeks of conservative therapy, evaluation with MRI for rotator cuff tears may be considered

Suggested Readings

Almekinders L. Impingement syndrome. *Clin Sports Med*. 2001;20:491–504.

Armstrong A. Evaluation and management of adult shoulder pain: a focus on rotator cuff disorders, acromioclavicular joint arthritis, and glenohumeral arthritis. *Med Clin North Am*. 2014;98(4):755–775.

Burbank KM, Stevenson JH, Czarnecki GR, Dorfman J. Chronic shoulder pain: part II. Treatment. *Am Fam Physician*. 2008;77(4):493–497.

Cain EL Jr, Meis RC. Internal impingement. In: Johnson DL, Mair SD, eds. *Clinical Sports Medicine*. Philadelphia: Mosby; 2006:227–234.

Campbell RS, Dunn A. External impingement of the shoulder. *Semin Musculoskelet Radiol*. 2008;12(2):107, 127–135.

Codsi M. The painful shoulder: when to inject and when to refer. *Cleve Clin J Med*. 2007;74:473–488.

Cowderoy GA, Lisle DA, O'Connell PT. Overuse and impingement syndromes of the shoulder in the athlete. *Magn Reson Imaging Clin N Am*. 2009;17(4):577–593.

King JJ, Wright TW. Physical examination of the shoulder. *J Hand Surg Am*. 2014;39(10):2103–2112.

Koester M, George M, Kuhn GM. Shoulder impingement syndrome. *Am J Med*. 2005;118:452–455.

Morrison DS, Frogameni AD, Woodworth P. Non-operative treatment of subacromial impingement syndrome. *J Bone Joint Surg Am*. 1997;79A:732–737.

Natsis K, Tsikaras P, Totlis T, et al. Correction between the four types of acromion and the existence of enthesophytes: a study on 423 dried scapulas and review of the literature. *Clin Anat*. 2007;20:267–272.

Chapter 34 Rotator Cuff Tear

Jeremy Kent, Sergio Patton

ICD-10-CM CODES
M75.1   *Rotator cuff tear or rupture, not specified as traumatic*
M75.11 *Incomplete rotator cuff tear or rupture not specified as traumatic*
M75.12 *Complete rotator cuff tear or rupture not specified as traumatic*

Key Concepts

- Rotator cuff tears may result from acute trauma but more commonly develop insidiously due to chronic overuse or degeneration.
- Tears can be classified based on location, size, magnitude of tendon retraction, muscle atrophy, and fatty infiltration.
- Rotator cuff tears occur in less than 7% of patients younger than 40 years but are present in 45-50% of the population older than 70.
- Acute shoulder dislocation in patients older than 40 results in a rotator cuff tear in approximately 25% of cases.
- Conservative management is preferred for partial tears, as no definitive benefit has been proven with early surgical intervention.
- Etiologic factors
  - Trauma
  - Repetitive overhead activity
  - Tendon degeneration
  - Glenohumeral instability/dislocation
  - Inflammatory disease
  - Scapulothoracic dysfunction
  - Normal aging

History

- Pain located over the anterior lateral shoulder, radiating to the deltoid muscle.
- Pain commonly occurs insidiously without a known traumatic event.
- Patient may have limited active motion and/or weakness.
- Nighttime pain is common.
- Pain radiating below the elbow can occur but should alert the physician to consider a cervical radiculopathy.
- In younger patients, higher-energy trauma is more likely to be the cause of symptoms.

Physical Examination (Video 34.1 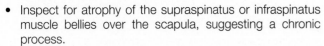)

- Inspect for atrophy of the supraspinatus or infraspinatus muscle bellies over the scapula, suggesting a chronic process.
- Passive range of motion is usually preserved in patients with a rotator cuff tear, although adhesive capsulitis can occur concomitantly.
- Active range of motion may be diminished due to pain or weakness.
- Weakness or pain to resistance with extended arm at 90 degrees of flexion and 30 degrees of abduction tests the supraspinatus tendon (empty can test or Jobe test).
- Weakness of external rotation with arm abducted to 90 degrees and elbow flexed to 90 degrees indicates involvement of teres minor and infraspinatus muscles (horn blower's test).
- With massive infraspinatus tears, the patient may not be able to maintain the arm in position after passive external rotation (lag sign).
- Abnormal liftoff or belly press test results indicate involvement of the subscapularis muscle.
- Examination for labral, biceps, and acromioclavicular joint pathology should be done to evaluate for associated pathology.
- Cervical spine examination is recommended.

Imaging

- Routine shoulder radiographs include anteroposterior, scapular Y, and axillary views.
- Radiographs of degenerative tears frequently show subacromial spurs, greater tuberosity sclerosis, cysts, or excrescence.
- The most important radiographic finding is elevation of the humeral head related to the glenoid. This is indicative of a massive chronic tear. Another common finding is erosion of the superior aspect of the glenoid (Fig. 34.1).
- Magnetic resonance imaging (MRI) is very effective for evaluating the rotator cuff (Fig. 34.2) but not necessary for diagnosis. An MRI can describe partial- or full-thickness tears, as well as size and location of tears.
- The degree of muscle atrophy on MRI offers clues to chronicity of the tear and whether repair is possible.
- Although operator dependent, ultrasound can be as effective as MRI in evaluating rotator cuff pathology (Fig. 34.3).

Additional Tests

- A diagnostic subacromial lidocaine injection may allow a better examination for range of motion and strength once pain is eliminated.

Differential Diagnosis

- Subacromial impingement
- Glenoid labrum tear

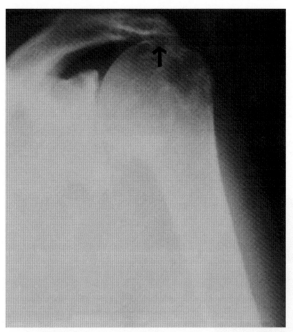

Fig 34.1 The most important radiographic finding is elevation of the humeral head *(arrow)* in relation to the glenoid.

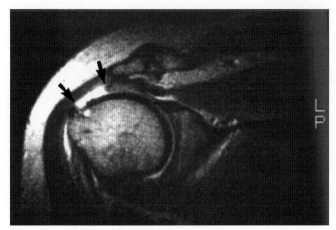

Fig 34.2 Magnetic resonance imaging is very effective for evaluating the rotator cuff. *Arrows* show the defect in the supraspinatus tendon.

- Acromioclavicular joint arthrosis
- Adhesive capsulitis
- Glenohumeral arthritis
- Inflammatory disorder
- Peritoneal pathology
- Cervical radiculopathy

Treatment
Partial-Thickness Tears
- Conservative treatment
  - Activity modification
  - Nonsteroidal antiinflammatory drugs
- Physical therapy
  - Rotator cuff and periscapular strengthening
  - Passive and active range of motion exercises

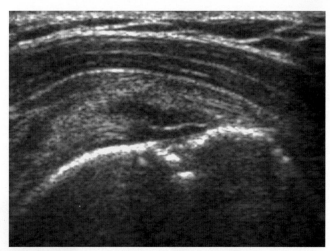

Fig 34.3 Ultrasound view of a supraspinatus tear.

- Subacromial steroid injection may be considered for recalcitrant pain or pain-limiting therapy.
- For persistent symptoms (>6 months), arthroscopy is considered.
  - Method of surgical intervention (i.e., irrigation and débridement vs. arthroscopic vs. open cuff repair) depends on severity of tear, patient age, and functional status (Fig. 34.4).
  - Arthroscopic subacromial decompression.

Full-Thickness Tears
- In older patients and/or chronic tears, conservative management as mentioned previously is often effective.
- Massive irreparable rotator cuff tears in older patients with low functional demand can be treated with arthroscopic débridement.
- Early surgery is indicated for acute, full-thickness traumatic tears because delay in treatment can result in muscle atrophy, tendon retraction, and surgical complications.
- Shoulder arthrodesis, hemiarthroplasty, or total shoulder arthroplasty may be indicated depending on the size of the tear, functional mobility of the shoulder, and general health of the patient.

When to Refer
- Partial-thickness tears not responding to conservative treatment.
- Full-thickness tears that are acute; occur in younger patients; or are refractory to conservative treatment.

Prognosis
- Surgical intervention is usually not indicated for patients without pain or limitations of activities of daily living.
- Resolution of partial-thickness tears have been reported to be between 33% and 90% with nonoperative measures.
- Surgery provides 76-88% good to excellent results in those with persistent pain after conservative treatment.
- Full-thickness tear prognosis is dependent on patient age, activity level, size, and chronicity of tear.

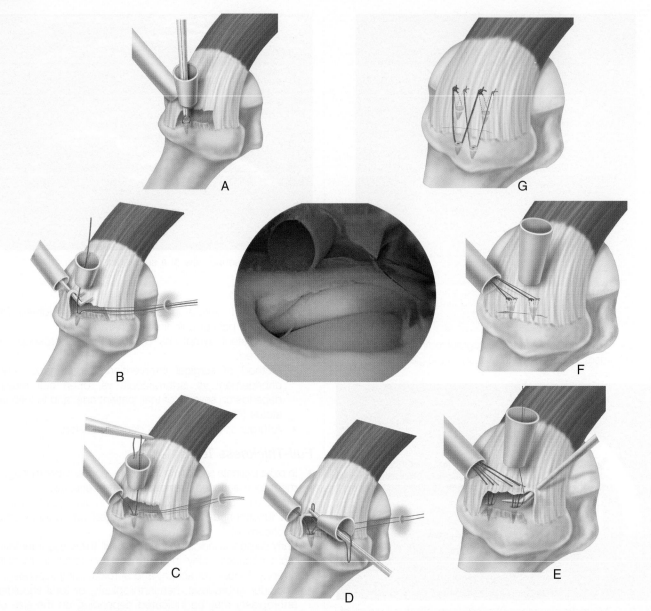

Fig 34.4 Arthroscopic rotator cuff repair. Rotator cuff footprint débridement not shown. **(A–G)** Anchors installed over footprint and horizontal mattress sutures placed, creating a double row repair.

- A successful repair of a chronic tear correlates to the degree of fatty infiltration and atrophy of muscles affected.
- Repairable tears provide more than 90% patient satisfaction in most studies.

Troubleshooting

- Rotator cuff disease can frequently be managed nonoperatively, and physical therapy is an essential part of this treatment course.
- Elevation of the humeral head on radiographs suggests a chronic rotator cuff tear.
- Patients should receive no more than three subacromial injections over the course of 1 year to minimize the risk of tendon rupture.

Patient Instructions

- Follow physician and physical therapy instructions with regard to exercises and limitations.
- Home-based exercises are vital to successful management and should be performed diligently and correctly.
- Increased pain or weakness after diagnosis of a partial-thickness or small full-thickness rotator cuff tear should be reevaluated because enlargement of the tear may have occurred, which could prompt a change in management.

Considerations in Special Populations

- Partial-thickness rotator cuff tears in young overhead athletes are frequently treated more aggressively with arthroscopic evaluation and management.

- Rotator cuff tears are common in geriatric patients and respond well to conservative treatment.
- Massive irreparable rotator cuff tears with significant symptoms can be treated surgically with tendon transfers or shoulder arthroplasty (reverse shoulder prosthesis).

Suggested Readings

Ainsworth R, Lewis JS. Exercise therapy for the conservative management of full thickness tears of the rotator cuff: a systematic review. *Br J Sports Med*. 2007;41:200–210.

Feeley BT, Gallo RA, Craig EV. Cuff tear arthropathy: current trends in diagnosis and surgical management. *J Shoulder Elbow Surg*. 2009;18(3):484–494.

Kuhn JE, Dunn WR, Sanders R, et al. Effectiveness of physical therapy in treating atraumatic full-thickness rotator cuff tears: a multicenter prospective cohort study. *J Shoulder Elbow Surg*. 2013;22(10):1371–1379.

Kukkonen J, Joukainen A, Lehtinen J, et al. Treatment of nontraumatic rotator cuff tears: a randomized controlled trial with two years of clinical and imaging follow-up. *J Bone Joint Surg Am*. 2015;97(21):1729–1737.

Rutten MJ, Jager GJ, Blickman JG. From the RSNA refresher courses: US of the rotator cuff: pitfalls, limitations, and artifacts. *Radiographics*. 2006;26(2):589–603.

Somerville LE, Willits K, Johnson AM, et al. Clinical assessment of physical examination maneuvers for rotator cuff lesions. *Am J Sports Med*. 2014;42(8):1911–1919.

Tuite MJ, Small KM. Imaging evaluation of nonacute shoulder pain. *AJR Am J Roentgenol*. 2017;209(3):525–533.

Yamamoto A, Takagishi K, Osawa T, et al. Prevalence and risk factors of a rotator cuff tear I the general population. *J Shoulder Elbow Surg*. 2010;19(1):116–120.

Chapter 35 Glenohumeral Disorders

Kelley Anderson, Joel Himes, Melissa McLane

ICD-10-CM CODES
M19.019	*Glenohumeral arthritis, primary OA, unspecified shoulder*
M19.011	*Glenohumeral arthritis, primary OA, right shoulder*
M19.012	*Glenohumeral arthritis, primary OA, left shoulder*
M87.0	*Glenohumeral avascular necrosis*

Glenohumeral Arthritis

Key Concepts

- The glenohumeral joint is a ball-and-socket joint with smooth articular surfaces and synovial fluid within the joint space that allows for smooth multidirection range of motion with little resistance.
- Glenohumeral osteoarthritis develops gradually as the articular cartilage becomes damaged and/or lost, causing increased roughness, resistance in motion, and decreased joint space.
- Presentation is often in the fourth or fifth decade of life.
- Glenohumeral osteoarthritis can be primary or secondary.
  - Primary osteoarthritis is idiopathic, "wear and tear" over time
  - Secondary causes include but are not limited to:
    - Trauma
    - Infection
    - Previous joint surgery
    - Inflammatory
    - Osteonecrosis
    - Obesity
    - Genetics
    - Lifestyle/occupation
    - Rotator cuff tear arthropathy
    - Instability
    - Metabolic (gout, pseudogout, sickle cell)

History

- Patients will present with gradually increasing pain that is not focal and often vague.
- As the disease progresses, patients will report limited function and range of motion with a varying degree of crepitus.
- Patients may state they have stiffness in the morning that improves with activity.
- It is important to obtain a thorough medical history including onset of symptoms, alleviating/worsening factors, duration and timing of symptoms, prior surgeries and/or trauma, medications, systemic illness, occupation and lifestyle activities, and family history.

Physical Examination

- Inspect the cervical spine and bilateral shoulders for atrophy, ecchymosis, deformity, erythema, or swelling.
- Palpate the acromioclavicular joint, sternoclavicular joint, clavicle, humeral head, and scapula to assess for deformity or pain bilaterally.
- Assess range of motion both actively and passively and compare to normal degrees of motion:
  - Flexion 0 to 180 degrees
  - Extension 0 to 60 degrees
  - Abduction 0 to 180 degrees
  - External rotation 0 to 90 degrees
  - Internal rotation 0 to 70 degrees
  - Adduction 0 to 45 degrees
- Assess abduction bilaterally to evaluate scapulothoracic rhythm.
- Complete strength testing, motor, and sensory exam.
- Special tests: Spurling maneuver, rotator cuff testing (Jobe, external rotation, horn blower test, lift off, and belly press test), instability testing (apprehension/Jobe's relocation, load and shift test, Kim test), biceps testing (Speed and Yergason), acromioclavicular (AC) joint (Scarf), impingement testing (Hawkin and Neer).

Imaging

- Plain radiographs are diagnostic.
  - An anteroposterior (AP) view (Fig. 35.1) is used to evaluate the humeral head and presence of osteophytes. It is also important to check for glenoid bone loss and loss of space between the acromion and humeral head.
  - An axillary view is used to evaluate the status of the posterior glenoid because osteoarthritis of the glenohumeral joint generally causes posterior glenoid erosions and overall malalignment of the shoulder joint.
- Computed tomography
  - May be needed to assess glenoid bone loss in anticipation of possible shoulder replacement or reverse shoulder arthroplasties.

Differential Diagnosis

- Rotator cuff disease
- Acromioclavicular osteoarthritis
- Inflammatory arthritis
- Cervical radiculopathy
- Osteonecrosis
- Shoulder dislocation

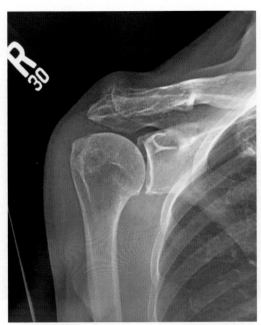

Fig 35.1 Anteroposterior view of the right shoulder showing glenohumeral osteoarthritis.

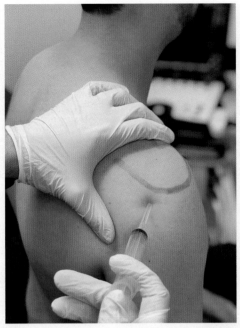

Fig 35.2 Demonstrating clinical landmark for the posterolateral approach to glenohumeral joint injection.

Treatment

- Early stages
  - Modalities including ice, heat, transcutaneous electrical nerve stimulation (TENS) unit.
  - Medications including nonsteroidal antiinflammatory drugs, acetaminophen.
  - Nutritional supplements including glucosamine and chondroitin sulfate.
  - Activity modifications aimed at decreasing repetitive activities.
  - Physical therapy focusing on strengthening and improving range of motion.
- Late stages
  - Intra-articular corticosteroid injections may be tried for pain control (Fig. 35.2).
  - Patients failing conservative medical treatment should be evaluated for potential surgical options such as debridement and synovectomy, glenoid or humeral osteotomies, arthrodesis, and/or arthroplasty.

Patient Instructions

- Discuss benefits and risks of nonsteroidal antiinflammatories.
- Encourage daily activities and home exercises to help prolong function.
- Avoid use of narcotics.

Glenohumeral Avascular Necrosis

Key Concepts

- Osteonecrosis or avascular necrosis refers to the disruption of blood flow to the humeral head, causing cell death and eventual subchondral bone collapse.

- Can involve the anterior humeral circumflex artery, arcuate artery, or posterior humeral circumflex artery.
- Second most common site for osteonecrosis (femoral head is most common).
- Avascular necrosis has been divided into four causes:
  - Mechanical vascular interruption
  - Thrombosis and embolism
  - Injury to or pressure on a vessel wall
  - Venous occlusion
  There are multiple causes of this vascular disruption.
  - Trauma: fracture, dislocation, surgery
  - Corticosteroid use
  - Alcohol use
  - Dysbarism (changes in ambient pressure)
  - Idiopathic
  - Radiation
  - Systemic diseases: sickle cell, Gaucher, systemic lupus erythematosus, rheumatoid arthritis

History

- Patients usually present with generalized shoulder pain without an obvious inciting event.
- May then progress to loss of range of motion, weakness and occasionally crepitus.
- Obtaining a thorough history may help ascertain the cause.

Physical Examination

- Please see physical exam for osteoarthritis

Classification

- Stage I: no changes on radiographs, changes may be present on magnetic resonance imaging (MRI)

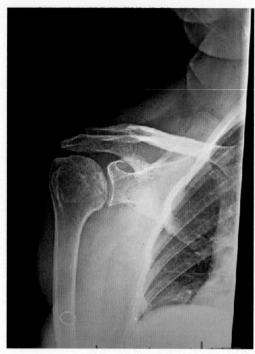

Fig 35.3 Anteroposterior view of the right shoulder demonstrating osteonecrosis with early crescent sign.

- Stage II: humeral head remains spherical but has increased sclerosis
- Stage III: subchondral collapse, crescent sign (Fig. 35.3)
- Stage IV: collapse of articular surface
- Stage V: osteoarthritis that includes the glenoid

Imaging

- Radiographs are usually obtained with multiple views (AP, lateral, scapular Y view) but usually best appreciated on AP
- Magnetic resonance is usually the preferred imaging modality due to its sensitivity (Fig. 35.4)

Differential Diagnosis

- Same as for osteoarthritis

Treatment

- Treatment of underlying cause is the ideal primary intervention as this may significantly modify the progression of osteonecrosis.

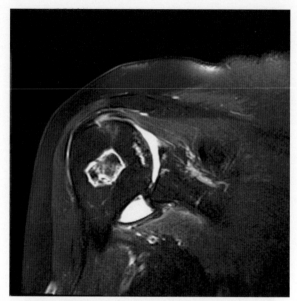

Fig 35.4 Magnetic resonance imaging without contrast demonstrating osteonecrosis with subchondral collapse.

- Educate on possible offending agents (i.e., corticosteroids, alcohol).
- Nonsurgical options such as pain medication, activity modification, and physical therapy can be effective in stage I and II disease.
- Surgical options include core decompression and arthroscopy, humeral head resurfacing, hemiarthroplasty, and total arthroplasty.

Suggested Readings

Boileau R, Sinnerton R, Chuinard C, Walch G. Arthroplasty of the shoulder. *J Bone Joint Surg Br*. 2006;88B:562–575.

Boselli K, Ahmad C, Levine W. Treatment of glenohumeral arthrosis. *Am J Sports Med*. 2010;38(12):2558–2572.

Brems J. *Management of Osteoarthritis of the Shoulder. Oku Shoulder and Elbow 2*. Rosemont, IL: American Academy of Orthopaedic Surgeons; 2002:257–266.

Cusher M, Friedman R. Osteonecrosis of the humeral head. *J Am Acad Orthop Surg*. 1997;5:339–346.

Hasan S, Romeo A. Nontraumatic osteonecrosis of the humeral head. *J Shoulder Elbow Surg*. 2002;11(3):281–298.

Johnson L III, Galatz L. *Osteonecrosis and Other Noninflammatory Degenerative Diseases of the Glenohumeral Joint. Oku Shoulder and Elbow 2*. Rosemont, IL: American Academy of Orthopaedic Surgeons; 2002:267–274.

Sperling J, Steinmann S, Cordasco F, et al. Shoulder arthritis in the young adult: arthroscopy to arthroplasty. *Instr Course Lect*. 2006;55:67–74.

Thomas M, Bidwai A, Rangan A, et al. Glenohumeral osteoarthritis. *Shoulder Elbow*. 2016;8(3):203–214.

Chapter 36 Adhesive Capsulitis (Frozen Shoulder)

John M. MacKnight

ICD-10-CM CODES
M75.00 *Adhesive capsulitis of shoulder*
M75.01 *Adhesive capsulitis of right shoulder*
M75.02 *Adhesive capsulitis of left shoulder*

Key Concepts

- Progressive loss of active and passive glenohumeral motion resulting from contraction of the glenohumeral synovial capsule (Fig. 36.1)
- Commonly referred to as "frozen shoulder," or arthrofibrosis
- Pathophysiology is poorly understood but likely inflammatory. Recent data have implicated cytokines and matrix metalloproteases in the development of pathologic changes in the synovium.
- "Primary" adhesive capsulitis is idiopathic. Insidious onset of shoulder pain leads to avoidance of use and a slowly progressive decline in shoulder motion and functional ability.
- "Secondary" adhesive capsulitis may be associated with a number of underlying conditions or genetic predispositions (Box 36.1).
- Prevalence in the general population is 3-5%; as high as 20% in diabetics.
- 70% of patients are female; there is a 20-30% incidence of future involvement of the opposite shoulder.
- Peak incidence between ages 40 and 59

History

- Stages 1 and 2 ("Painful freezing phase")
  - Symptoms present for weeks up to 9 months.
  - Aching shoulder pain at rest and sharp at the extremes of range of motion (ROM). Pain generally precedes ROM loss.
  - External rotation is often lost first, with progressive loss of motion in internal rotation, forward flexion, and abduction thereafter.
  - Majority of motion loss in first 3 months is secondary to painful synovitis; beyond 3 months is primarily due to capsular contraction and loss of capsular volume.
  - Histologically, inflammatory cell infiltration of the synovium followed by synovial proliferation
- Stage 3 ("Adhesive phase")
  - Symptoms present for 9 to 14 months.
  - Prominent stiffening of the shoulder with significant loss of ROM.

- Patients often report a history of an extremely painful phase that has resolved, resulting in a relatively pain-free but stiff shoulder.
- Histologically, dense collagenous tissue within the joint capsule
- Stage 4 ("Resolution or thawing phase")
  - Occurs spontaneously, generally after a minimum of 2 years
  - Characterized by slow, steady recovery of ROM resulting from capsular remodeling in response to use of the arm and shoulder

Physical Examination

- Patients in stages 1 and 2 have pain on palpation of the anterior and posterior capsule with radiating pain to the deltoid insertion.
- Evaluation of active *and* passive ROM should be performed:
  - Active and passive forward flexion, abduction, internal rotation, and external rotation are measured and recorded with the patient standing.
  - Passive glenohumeral motion is measured with the patient supine; scapulothoracic motion is constrained by manual pressure on the acromion.
- As able, a complete general shoulder exam should be attempted to evaluate for additional pathologies.
- Cervical spine examination should be performed as well.

Imaging

- Radiographs are typically negative but should be obtained to evaluate for significant rotator cuff disease, glenohumeral arthritis, or calcific tendinitis.
  - Routine radiographic evaluation should include anteroposterior (AP) views in internal and external rotation, axillary, and outlet views.
  - Disuse osteopenia may be seen.
- Dynamic ultrasonography may reveal thickening of the joint capsule and limited sliding movement of the supraspinatus tendon.
- MRI should not be pursued routinely in the adhesive capsulitis patient, but if the diagnosis of adhesive capsulitis remains in question, an MRI to evaluate for significant rotator cuff or labral cartilage pathology may be obtained.
  - Characteristic MRI findings for adhesive capsulitis include coracohumeral ligament (CHL) thickening and contraction.

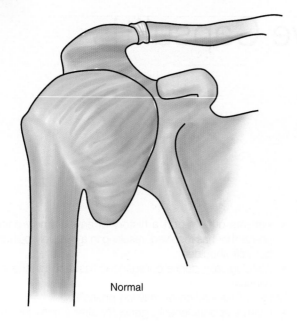

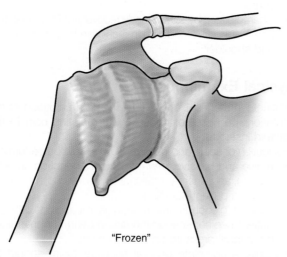

Fig 36.1 Fibrosis and contraction of the glenohumeral synovium.

Differential Diagnosis

- Significant rotator cuff impingement or tear
- Labral tear
- Acromioclavicular osteoarthritis
- Cervical radiculopathy

Treatment

- Early Stages
  - Primary early goal is relief of pain
  - Nonsteroidal antiinflammatory drugs (NSAIDs)
    - Non-NSAID analgesics
    - Oral corticosteroids
  - Activity modification/relative rest
  - Formal physical therapy
    - Gentle joint mobilization
    - Modalities to assist with pain control and inflammation including transcutaneous electrical nerve stimulation

(TENS), iontophoresis, phonophoresis, cryotherapy, moist heat, ultrasound, hydrotherapy, low-level laser, and short-wave therapy
- Glenohumeral corticosteroid injection (stages 1 and 2 only):
  - May be performed under fluoroscopic guidance
  - Multiple studies demonstrate efficacy, particularly when initiated early in the treatment course
  - Decrease fibromatosis and myofibroblasts in adhesive shoulders
- Sodium hyaluronate intra-articular injection (non–US Food and Drug Administration (FDA) approved)
- Suprascapular nerve block
- Hydrodilatation
- Collagenase injections (a future potential option, not adequately studied at present)
- Late Stage
  - Once pain-free
  - Aggressive physical therapy for passive and active restoration of ROM
  - Graded return to full function as symptoms allow

When to Refer

- Patients failing to restore full ROM despite multiple injections and a completed course of aggressive physical therapy
- Treatment considerations for refractory cases:
  - Closed manipulation of glenohumeral joint under regional or general anesthesia; efficacy remains under debate.
  - Arthroscopic or open capsulotomy

Prognosis

- 5- to 10-year follow-up: 39% full recovery, 54% clinical limitation without functional disability, and 7% had functional limitation.

- 50% of patients with frozen shoulder may have some degree of pain and stiffness an average of 7 years after onset of the disease.
- Outcome is generally favorable even if requiring surgical manipulation.
- Spontaneous remission and restoration of ROM takes an average of 30 months.

Troubleshooting

- Only pain-free shoulders should undergo aggressive physical therapy; attempts to aggressively restore ROM in patients with painful shoulders will generally fail.
- Close follow-up is essential to ensure compliance with management program and to limit the overall time of shoulder dysfunction.
- Counsel the patient regarding chronic nature of this condition and expected time frame to recovery.
- Counsel that surgery, if necessary, carries a risk of fracture and neurologic injury.
- The patient should receive no more than three glenohumeral corticosteroid injections over the course of 1 year.

Patient Instructions

- Follow physician and physical therapist instructions closely with respect to the type and quantity of shoulder activities which are acceptable.
- Home-based exercises are vital to overall management and should be performed diligently and regularly.
- Aggressively manage pain per physician direction.

Considerations in Special Populations

- Those caring for geriatric patients will encounter this condition commonly and should be vigilant for its potential presence in any geriatric patient with shoulder pain.
- Treatment principles will be the same as outlined previously, although special care should be taken to place the patient in a physical therapy setting appropriate for their physical abilities/limitations.
- Appreciate that any manipulative or surgical management carries a greater risk for morbidity in the geriatric population.

Suggested Readings

Dias R, Cutts S, Massoud S. Frozen shoulder. *BMJ*. 2005;331(7530): 1453–1456.

D'Orsi GM, Via AG, Frizziero A, Oliva A. Treatment of adhesive capsulitis: a review. *Muscles Ligaments Tendons J*. 2012;2:70–78.

Iannotti JP, Kwon YW. Management of persistent shoulder pain: a treatment algorithm. *Am J Orthop*. 2005;34(12 suppl):16–23.

Le HV, Lee SJ, Nazarian A, Rodriguez EK. Adhesive capsulitis of the shoulder: review of pathophysiology and current clinical treatments. *Shoulder Elbow*. 2017;9(2):75–84.

Manske RC, Prohaska D. Diagnosis and management of adhesive capsulitis. *Curr Rev Musculoskelet Med*. 2008;1:180–189.

Meislin RJ, Sperling JW, Stitik TP. Persistent shoulder pain: epidemiology, pathophysiology, and diagnosis. *Am J Orthop*. 2005;34(12 suppl): 5–9.

Neviaser AS, Neviaser RJ. Adhesive capsulitis of the shoulder. *J Am Acad Orthop Surg*. 2011;19:536–542.

Sheridan MA, Hannafin JA. Upper extremity: emphasis on frozen shoulder. *Orthop Clin North Am*. 2006;37(4):531–539.

Chapter 37 Acromioclavicular Joint Injuries

Adam C. Fletcher

ICD-10-CM CODE
S43.50 *Sprain of unspecified acromioclavicular joint*

Key Concepts

- The clavicle links the upper extremity to the axial skeleton via the acromioclavicular (AC) joint and sternoclavicular joint.
- The AC joint is composed of the distal clavicle and its articulation with the acromion of the scapula. The joint contains a cartilaginous disc surrounded by a joint capsule.
- The AC joint is stabilized via two major ligament complexes (Fig. 37.1).
  - The AC ligament along with the joint capsule provide anteroposterior (AP) stability.
  - The coracoclavicular (CC) ligaments, composed of the conoid and trapezoid ligaments, provide vertical stability.
- The AC ligament is typically injured first, followed by the CC ligaments.
- A common term for injury to the AC joint is a "separated shoulder."

History

- The most frequent cause of AC joint injury is a fall or blow to the shoulder with the arm adducted, which forces the acromion inferiorly in relation to the clavicle.
- Additional injury modes include a fall on an outstretched hand and forced adduction of the arm across the body.
- Pain typically develops immediately after injury and is well localized to the AC joint.
- With more severe injuries, symptoms may radiate over the trapezius and deltoid muscles.
- Injury classification (Rockwood) (Fig. 37.2)
  - Type I: sprain or partial tear of AC ligaments, no injury to CC ligaments
  - Type II: complete tear of AC ligaments, sprain or partial tear of CC ligaments
  - Type III: complete tear of both AC and CC ligaments
  - Type IV: complete tear of both AC and CC ligaments with associated posterior displacement of clavicle into the trapezius
  - Type V: complete tear of both AC and CC ligaments with more than 100% superior displacement of distal clavicle

- Type VI: complete tear of both AC and CC ligaments with clavicle displacement under the acromion or coracoid (very rare)

Physical Examination

- Tenderness is present directly at the AC joint, often with localized swelling.
- Type III through VI injuries involve tenderness at the coracoid as well as deformity at the AC joint.
- Passive cross-body adduction of arm (crossover or scarf test) can elicit pain at the AC joint in equivocal cases.
- Shoulder weakness and reduced active range of motion (ROM) may occur secondary to pain.
- Careful neurovascular examination in the upper extremity should be included due to close proximity of neurovascular structures to the clavicle.
- Pertinent findings by classification type:
  - I: AC tenderness, no deformity, minimal or no swelling
  - II: AC tenderness, mild deformity, minimal swelling
  - III: AC and coracoid tenderness, the distal clavicle is superiorly displaced and can often times be reduced with gentle downward pressure
  - IV: findings similar to those for type III, with posterior displacement of the clavicle
  - V: severe deformity, the clavicle often not manually reducible due to penetration of deltotrapezial fascia (Fig. 37.3)
  - VI: very rare, severe deformity, may present with neurovascular injury

Imaging

- Plain radiographs are very helpful in determining the type of AC injury and ruling out fracture.
- A single AP view should contain both AC joints, or two separate AP views can be used to compare the affected and unaffected sides.
- Additional helpful views include axillary and Zanca.
- Radiographic findings by type:
  - I: No radiographic findings.
  - II: Widening of the AC joint relative to the unaffected side. A Zanca view may reveal widening not noted on standard AP views.
  - III: Widening of the CC distance by 25-50% compared with unaffected side on AP view (Fig. 37.4).
  - IV: Axillary view will show posterior displacement of clavicle.

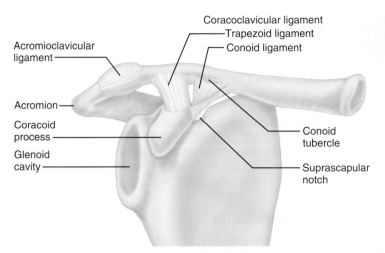

Fig 37.1 Anatomy of acromioclavicular joint with ligamental attachments.

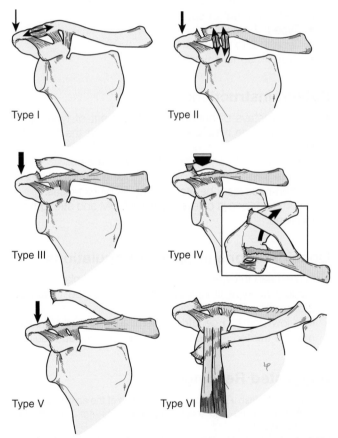

Fig 37.2 Rockwood classification of distal clavical injuries. (From Rockwood CA, Green DP [Eds]. *Fractures*. 2nd ed. Philadelphia: JB Lippincott; 1984.)

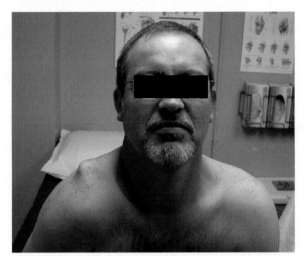

Fig 37.3 Patient with a chronic type V acromioclavicular injury with obvious deformity of the right shoulder.

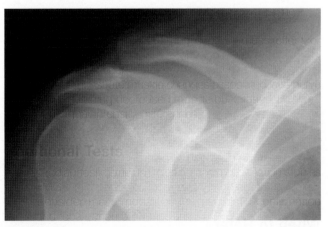

Fig 37.4 Anteroposterior view showing a type III acromioclavicular separation.

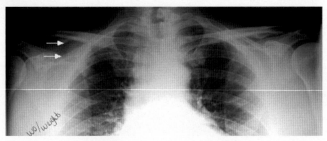

Fig 37.5 Anteroposterior view of both shoulders with a greater than 100% increase in the coracoclavicular distance of the affected shoulder with a type V injury *(arrows).*

- V: The CC distance is more than doubled (>100%) compared with unaffected side on AP view (Fig. 37.5).
- VI: The distal clavicle is located under the acromion or coracoid on AP view.
- Weighted x-ray views of the AC joint are no longer recommended.
- Advanced imaging with computed tomography (CT) or magnetic resonance imaging (MRI) is typically not required unless injury to other structures is suspected.

Differential Diagnosis

- Superior labral injury
- Distal clavicle fracture
- Brachial plexus injury ("stinger"/"burner")
- AC joint degenerative arthritis
- Distal clavicular osteolysis

Treatment

- Treatment is dictated by the injury classification.
- Type 1 and II injuries are managed nonoperatively.
  - Ice
  - Nonsteroidal antiinflammatory medications
  - Rest from sports activities
  - Consider sling for comfort
  - Taping techniques for stabilization may be beneficial
  - Advance range of motion activities as tolerated with eventual progression to strengthening of the rotator cuff and periscapular musculature
- Type III injuries tend to be managed nonoperatively in the majority of cases, although surgical intervention is considered if pain persists longer than 3 months or if injury occurs in an overhead thrower.
- Types IV, V, and VI injuries are treated with early surgery to reduce deformity and reconstruct the CC ligaments.

When to Refer

- Type IV, V, and VI injuries
- Consider referral for type III injuries in overhead throwers
- Patients with symptoms that persist longer than 3 to 4 months

Prognosis

- It has been reported that 9% of type I injuries and 23% of type II injuries will have some persistent symptoms with nonoperative management.
- Type III injuries result in an average 17% deficit in bench press strength compared with the uninvolved extremity.
- Approximately 10% of type III injuries eventually need surgery.
- Surgical results are predictably good (>90%) if reduction is maintained for the first few months. Various surgical methods have been described with variable failure rates.

Troubleshooting

- Careful radiographic evaluation for posterior displacement (type IV) or greater than 100% displacement (type V) is crucial in determining appropriate management.
- Average time out of sports is:
  - Type I: 1 week
  - Type II: 2 to 4 weeks
  - Type III: up to 6 weeks

Patient Instructions

- The mainstays of nonoperative treatment of type I to III injuries include rest, ice, and protection in the form of a sling.
- Shoulder ROM can be advanced as tolerated.
- In more severe injury, a period in a sling for 2 to 3 weeks is often necessary before initiating ROM exercises.
- Return to sports is delayed until full ROM and strength are regained.

Considerations in Special Populations

- In overhead throwers (quarterbacks, baseball players), early surgery for type III injuries is often performed to restore proper throwing mechanics.
- In a low-demand geriatric patient, type IV and V injuries may be treated nonoperatively, often with good results.

Suggested Readings

Bergfeld JA, Andrish JT, Clancy WG. Evaluation of the acromioclavicular joint following first- and second-degree sprains. *Am J Sports Med.* 1978;6:153–159.

Bradley JP, Elkousy H. Decision making: operative versus nonoperative treatment of acromioclavicular joint injuries. *Clin Sports Med.* 2003;22:277–290.

Schlegel TF, Burks RT, Marcus RL, Dunn HK. A prospective evaluation of untreated acute grade III acromioclavicular separations. *Am J Sports Med.* 2001;29:699–703.

Spencer EE Jr. Treatment of grade III acromioclavicular joint injuries: a systematic review. *Clin Orthop Relat Res.* 2007;455:38–44.

Taft TN, Wilson FC, Oglesby JW. Dislocation of the acromioclavicular joint: an end-result study. *J Bone Joint Surg Am.* 1987;69A:1045–1051.

Tibone J, Sellers R, Tonino P. Strength testing after third-degree acromioclavicular dislocations. *Am J Sports Med.* 1992;20:328–331.

Chapter 38 Acromioclavicular Degenerative Joint Disease

Thomas M. Howard

ICD-10-CM CODE
M19.019 *Primary osteoarthritis, unspecified shoulder*

CPT CODE
20605 *Arthrocentesis, aspiration and/or injection; intermediate joint or bursa- acromioclavicular*

Key Concepts

- Acromioclavicular (AC) joint osteoarthritis is the most common cause of AC pain.
- The AC joint is a small, diarthrodial joint that is formed by the acromion (part of the scapula) and the distal end of the clavicle (collar bone).
- The joint has a small surface area that is at risk of arthritis (wearing of the cartilage in the AC joint) due to significant forces acting across it.
- Osteoarthritis of the AC joint can be an isolated cause of anterosuperior shoulder pain, or it can be a contributor to the development of subacromial impingement.
- AC arthritis results from an acute or chronic repetitive injury due to:
  - Long-term overhead activities
  - Sports such as tennis, swimming, pitching, volleyball, and weightlifting
  - Heavy labor
  - Complication of an AC joint injury such as AC separation
- AC osteoarthritis is commonly seen on radiographs or magnetic resonance imaging studies in asymptomatic patients.
- AC arthritis is more common in patients older than 60 years, and the incidence doubles after age 80.

History

- Pain in the superior or anterior part of the shoulder
- Pain is worse with overhead, flexed, or adducted positions of the shoulder.
- Lifting activities exacerbate the pain.
- Patients may note audible crepitus in the shoulder area.
- The patient may have a history of AC separation or frequent trauma to the shoulder.
- Unrelenting pain with continued activity
- History of chronic repetitive activity and/or recent increase in use of the affected shoulder

Physical Examination

- Pain and/or crepitus of AC joint with passive or active overhead activity
- Positive cross-arm adduction test with pain at AC joint
  - This test is done with the arm elevated forward to 90 degrees with hyperadduction applied across the sternum while the examiner palpates the AC joint (Fig. 38.1).
- A diagnostic injection using 1 mL lidocaine with a 25-gauge needle into the AC joint can be helpful to isolate pain to the AC joint. These injections are easier performed with image guidance using ultrasound.
- A complete shoulder examination should be performed to rule out impingement syndrome, adhesive capsulitis, and glenohumeral arthritis.

Imaging

- Typical findings on a radiograph of the AC joint include joint narrowing, osteophyte formation, sclerosis, and subchondral cysts (Fig. 38.2).
- If the diagnosis is in doubt, magnetic resonance imaging or diagnostic sonography can be helpful to rule out other causes of shoulder pain.
- Studies show little correlation between radiographic studies and physical examination findings for the AC joint.
- Recent data have shown that the presence of bone marrow edema in the medial acromion, lateral clavicle, or both on T2-weighted magnetic resonance images did correlate with a symptomatic AC joint.

Differential Diagnosis

- See Table 38.1.

Treatment

- Symptomatic/pain relief with nonsteroidal antiinflammatory drugs and/or hot and cold compresses
- Activity modification when symptomatic to avoid overhead activities and weightlifting, such as bench press, dips, and push-ups
- Physical therapy to correct muscle imbalance and maintain range of motion
- Corticosteroid injection into the AC joint from a superoanterior approach and directed inferiorly (Fig. 38.3). Ultrasound-guided injection can improve accuracy and reduce patient discomfort for these procedures.

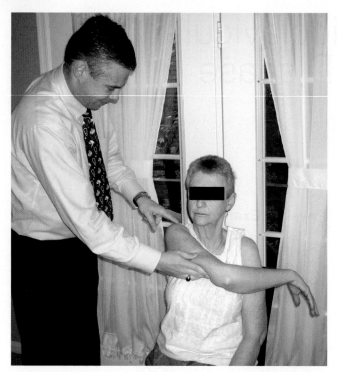

Fig 38.1 Positive cross-arm adduction test with pain at acromioclavicular joint.

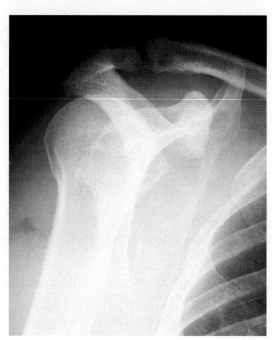

Fig 38.2 Typical radiographic findings of the acromioclavicular joint include joint narrowing, osteophyte formation, sclerosis, and subchondral cysts.

- Surgery can be considered if conservative management fails.
  - This includes the Mumford procedure with open resection of the distal clavicle.
  - A quicker recovery can be achieved if this is done arthroscopically with preservation of the superior capsule and overlying fascia, which are important stabilizing structures of the AC joint.

When to Refer

- Refer patients with refractory pain, those unwilling to accept activity modifications, and those with a poor response to steroid injections.

Troubleshooting

- Counsel regarding the chronic nature of this condition and expected time frame to recovery or deterioration.
- Patient should receive no more than three AC joint corticosteroid injections over the course of 1 year.
- Risks of steroid injection into the joint include atrophy of the fat pad, discoloration of the overlying skin, and steroid flare.

Patient Instructions

- AC arthritis is often due to constant overhead lifting. This activity should be avoided while the patient is symptomatic.
- Most cases of AC arthritis can be managed conservatively with rest, nonsteroidal antiinflammatory drugs, physical therapy, and avoidance of overhead activities.

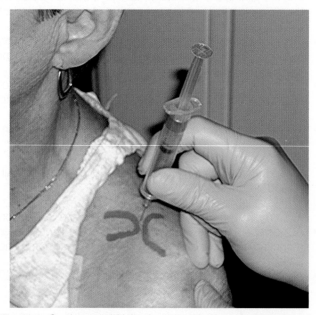

Fig 38.3 Corticosteroid injection into the acromioclavicular joint from a superoanterior approach and directed inferiorly.

Considerations in Special Populations

- Sports involving arm loading, such as gymnastics, weightlifting, and swimming, increase the risk of AC arthritis.
- Workers performing tasks involving static loading of the arms and vibration, such as foremen, bricklayers, and jackhammer operators, have an even greater risk of AC arthritis compared with athletes in sports cited previously.

TABLE 38.1 Differential Diagnosis of Acromioclavicular Pain

Condition	Location of Pain	Differentiating Feature
Rotator cuff tendinosis/ strain/tear	Superolateral	Pain with abducting shoulder at 70–120 degrees (painful arc) with weakness
Biceps tendon injury	Anterior	Pain with resisted elbow flexion and supination; tenderness in bicipital groove
Glenohumeral instability	Anterior	Often as a result of shoulder subluxation or dislocation; positive apprehension sign
Primary and secondary impingement	Superolateral	Positive Neer and/or Hawkins sign; pain with overhead activity
Calcific tendinosis	Superolateral	Seen on radiograph or magnetic resonance imaging as a result of rotator cuff injury
Glenohumeral arthritis	Superolateral and/or posterior	Rest pain, stiffness, and crepitus on movement
Acromion or distal clavicle fracture	Superior	Seen on radiograph as a result of trauma
Glenohumeral labral tear	Anterior	Seen in throwers or overhead motion athletes; positive O'Brien test
Acromioclavicular osteolysis	Superior	Pain in acromioclavicular joint; most common in weightlifters
Cervical spine disease	Variable	Neck pain; positive Spurling test
Thoracic outlet syndrome	Generalized	Intermittent pain, weakness, and neurovascular symptoms; positive Roos test
Adhesive capsulitis	Anterior	Active and passive range of motion of the glenohumeral joint is greatly restricted
Suprascapular neuropathy	Posterior	Pain and weakness with wasting of infraspinatus muscle
Referred pain (angina, Pancoast tumor, gallbladder)	Variable; axillary pain is usually not from the shoulder	Constant pain not associated with shoulder movement; systemic symptoms; pain aggravated by deep inspiration

Acknowledgment

The author acknowledges Dr. Michael Simpson for his contributions to the previous edition of this chapter.

Suggested Readings

Bonsell S, Pearsall AW IV, Heitman RJ, et al. The relationship of age, gender, and degenerative changes observed on radiographs of the shoulder in asymptomatic individuals. *J Bone Joint Surg Br*. 2000;82B:1135–1139.

Cadet E, Ahmad C, Levine W. The management of acromioclavicular joint osteoarthrosis: debride, resect, or leave it alone. *Instr Course Lect*. 2006;55:75–83.

Charron K, Schepsis A, Voloshin I. Arthroscopic distal clavicle resection in athletes. *Am J Sports Med*. 2006;35:53–58.

Ernberg LA, Potter HG. Radiographic evaluation of the acromioclavicular and sternoclavicular joints. *Clin Sports Med*. 2003;22:255–275.

Menge TJ, Boykin RE, Bushnell BD, Byram IR. Acromioclavicular osteoarthritis: a common cause of shoulder pain. *South Med J*. 2014;107(5):324–329.

Rabalais RD, McCarty E. Surgical treatment of symptomatic acromioclavicular joint problems: a systematic review. *Clin Orthop Relat Res*. 2007;455:30–37.

Stein BE, Wiater JM, Pfaff HC, et al. Detection of acromioclavicular joint pathology in asymptomatic shoulders with magnetic resonance imaging. *J Shoulder Elbow Surg*. 2001;10:204–208.

Tallia AF, Cardone DA. Diagnostic and therapeutic injection of the shoulder region. *Am Fam Physician*. 2003;67:1271–1278.

Chapter 39 Acromioclavicular Osteolysis

Thomas M. Howard

ICD-10-CM CODE
M89.519 *Distal clavicle osteolysis*

Key Concepts

- Acromioclavicular (AC) osteolysis of the shoulder can be traumatic; however, atraumatic causes are more common.
- Systemic disease should always be considered in the differential diagnosis.
- Repetitive loading of the AC joint is thought to be the precipitating factor leading to inadequate bone formation and remodeling; normal bone remodeling cannot occur due to continued stress on the joint.
- Atraumatic osteolysis has become more common because of the increased popularity of weightlifting.
- Early diagnosis and treatment can increase the chance of success with conservative measures. This approach has been shown to reverse the osteolysis process and result in varying degrees of healing.
- A delayed diagnosis usually results in a permanently widened AC joint with varying degrees of pain and mechanical dysfunction.

History

- Most commonly seen in males with a long history of strength training
- Weightlifting, football, swimming, and throwing activities are other causes of overuse.
- Osteolysis can also result from acute trauma or repetitive minor trauma to the AC joint.
- Pain in the AC joint begins insidiously and may occur only with the precipitating activity, most notably with bench presses, military presses, and dips.
- Most commonly unilateral but can also be bilateral
- As osteolysis progresses, the pain may persist for several days after the activity.

Physical Examination

- Pain and/or crepitus of the AC joint with passive or active overhead activity
- Positive cross-arm adduction test with pain at AC joint
  - This test is done with the arm elevated forward to 90 degrees with hyperadduction applied across the sternum while the examiner palpates the AC joint.

- A diagnostic injection using 1 mL lidocaine with a 25-gauge needle into the AC joint can be helpful to isolate pain to the AC joint.
- A complete shoulder examination should be performed to rule out impingement syndrome, adhesive capsulitis, and glenohumeral arthritis.
- Range of motion and strength are normal.

Imaging

- Diagnosis can be confirmed with radiographs or a bone scan.
- Radiographs show lucency, osteopenia, and osteophytes at the distal clavicle (Fig. 39.1).
- In later stages, tapering down of the distal clavicle and widening of the AC joint may be seen.
- A bone scan will show increased uptake at the distal clavicle and may precede radiographic findings.
- Magnetic resonance imaging of the shoulder can be helpful for ruling out other causes of shoulder pain and is effective at revealing soft-tissue swelling, subchondral cysts, cortical thinning, bone marrow edema, and synovial hypertrophy.

Differential Diagnosis

- Acromioclavicular arthritis
- Undiagnosed clavicle fracture
- Osteoid osteoma
- Other etiologies showing lysis or erosion of the distal clavicle: multiple myeloma, metastasis, scleroderma, hyperparathyroidism, infection, rheumatoid arthritis, rickets, spinal cord injury, and progeria

Treatment

- Symptomatic pain relief with nonsteroidal antiinflammatory drugs and/or hot and cold compresses
- Activity modification to eliminate lifting exercises and aggravating activities can alleviate symptoms and prevent progression.
- Physical therapy does not offer any proven benefit but is helpful to maintain the range of motion and strengthen the surrounding musculature.
- Resumption of activity even after 1 year may exacerbate symptoms.
- Corticosteroid injection from a superior approach with or without ultrasound guidance. Ultrasound guidance improves accuracy and patient discomfort with this procedure.

- Risks of steroid injection into the joint include atrophy of the fat pad, discoloration of the overlying skin, and steroid flare.

Patient Instructions

- Avoid exacerbating activities, especially bench presses, military presses, and dips.
- Pain in the AC joint may persist as long as 1 year after cessation of activities that stress the AC joint.
- To prevent osteolysis, limit upper extremity weightlifting and avoid lifting very heavy weights.

Acknowledgment

The author acknowledges Dr. Michael Simpson for his contributions to the previous edition of this chapter.

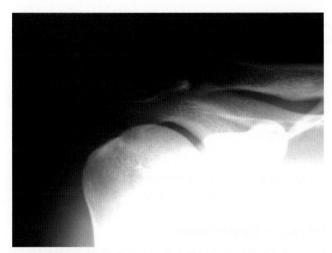

Fig 39.1 Radiograph of acromioclavicular osteolysis.

- Distal clavicle excision (Mumford procedure [open] or arthroscopic) may be performed if conservative therapy fails.
- Arthroscopic distal clavicle excision can allow patients to return to activities more rapidly and is the preferred method.

When to Refer

- Refer patients with refractory pain who are not improving despite several months of conservative treatment.

Troubleshooting

- Counsel regarding the chronic nature of this condition and expected time frame to recovery.
- Patient should receive no more than three AC corticosteroid injections over the course of 1 year.

Suggested Readings

Auge WK, Fischer RA. Arthroscopic distal clavicle resection for isolated atraumatic osteolysis in weight lifters. *Am J Sports Med*. 1998;26: 189–192.

Cahill BR. Atraumatic osteolysis of the distal clavicle: a review. *Sports Med*. 1992;13:214–222.

Charron KM, Schepsis AA, Voloshin I. Arthroscopic distal clavicle resection in athletes. *Am J Sports Med*. 2006;35:53–58.

Gajeski BL, Kettner NW. Osteolysis of the distal clavicle: serial improvement and normalization of acromioclavicular joint space with conservative care. *J Manipulative Physiol Ther*. 2004;27:480–488.

Hawkins BJ, Covey DC, Thiel BG. Distal clavicle osteolysis unrelated to trauma, overuse, or metabolic disease. *Clin Orthop Relat Res*. 2000;370: 208–211.

Kassarjian A, Llopis E, Palmer WE. Distal clavicular osteolysis: MR evidence for subchondral fracture. *Skeletal Radiol*. 2007;36:17–22.

Scavenius M, Iversen BF. Nontraumatic clavicular osteolysis in weight lifters. *Am J Sports Med*. 1992;20:463–467.

Chapter 40 Sternoclavicular Injuries

Thomas E. Brickner

ICD-10-CM CODES
S43.60XA *Sternoclavicular joint sprain*
M25.519 *Sternoclavicular joint pain*

Key Concepts

- Pathophysiology may be acute traumatic injury or arthritic condition.
- Mechanism of injury is either a direct blow to the medial clavicle or an indirectly transmitted force from posterolateral shoulder compression.
- Motor vehicle accidents and sports injuries are most common causes.
- Sternoclavicular (SC) dislocations represent less than 1% of all joint dislocations and only 3% of all upper extremity dislocations.
- Anterior dislocations are more common than posterior dislocations (10 to 20:1).
- Posterior dislocations are associated with intrathoracic or superior mediastinal injuries in up to 30% of cases.

Anatomy

- Diarthrodial, saddle-type joint with less than half the clavicular end plate articulating with the sternum (Fig. 40.1)
  - High degree of motion during the first 90 degrees of arm elevation
- Inherently unstable and depends on ligamentous structures, both periarticular and extra-articular, for support (Fig. 40.2)
- Periarticular ligaments include the intra-articular disc ligament, the interclavicular ligament, and the capsular ligaments
  - Posterior capsular ligament is the most important anterior-posterior stabilizer
- Extra-articular ligament is the costoclavicular ligament and connects the first rib and medial clavicle
  - Resists cephalad and caudal displacement of the clavicle
- SCJ contains a fibrocartilaginous, intra-articular disc

History

- Pain at the SC joint, especially with shoulder motion, arm elevation, or lateral compression.
- Patients with posterior dislocations may complain of dysphagia, dyspnea, dysphonia, or paresthesias if posteriorly located structures are injured.
- Late compression of vital structures may still occur if posterior dislocations are left unreduced.
- Mechanical symptoms with pain and clicking may occur if intra-articular disc is torn.

- High degree of recurrent instability following anterior dislocations but typically well tolerated.

Physical Examination

- Swelling, pain, and possible palpable defect overlying the SC joint
- Increased translation compared to uninjured side with manual stressing
- Paresthesias and decreased peripheral pulses of upper extremity, if associated with retroclavicular arterial damage
- Vascular engorgement of upper extremity, if venous structures compromised
- Dysphagia, if esophagus is compressed
- Dyspnea and stridor, if lungs and/or trachea damaged

Imaging

- X-rays for routine surveillance but limited diagnostically
  - Serendipity view with radiograph beam projected 40 degrees cephalad
  - Raised clavicular end indicative of anterior displacement
  - Depressed clavicular end indicative of posterior displacement
- Computed tomography scan recommended for definitive diagnosis of dislocations and evaluation of mediastinal and thoracic structures
- Ultrasound imaging may show dislocation when compared to contralateral side
- Magnetic resonance imaging indicated for evaluation of intra-articular disc pathology

Differential Diagnosis

- Contusion or fracture of sternum or clavicle
- Sternocleidomastoid strain

Treatment
Anterior Dislocations

- At diagnosis
  - Ice, analgesia
  - Grade I: Immobilize with figure-of-eight bandage or sling for 1 to 2 weeks
  - Grade II: Immobilize for 3 to 6 weeks
  - Grade III: Closed reduction followed by immobilization for 4 to 6 weeks
- Later
  - Grade III injuries often remain unstable after initial treatment but have little long-term functional impairment.

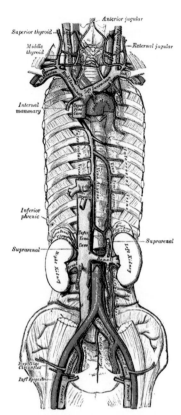

Fig 40.1 Vascular anatomy of the superior mediastinum. (From Gray H. *Gray's Anatomy of the Human Body*. 20th ed. Philadelphia: Lea & Febiger; 1918, Image 577.)

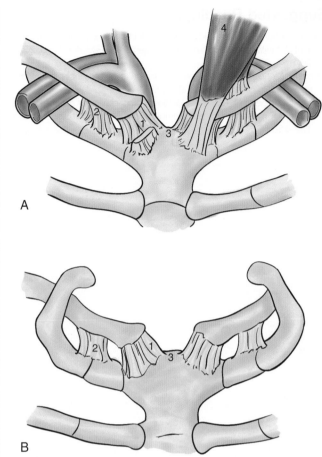

Fig 40.2 Anatomy of the sternoclavicular joint from anterior (A) to posterior (B) views. The structures are (1) anterior capsule (in part A) and posterior capsule (in part B), (2) costoclavicular ligament, (3) interclavicular ligament, and (4) the sternocleidomastoid tendon. (Adapted from Spencer EE, Kuhn JE, Huston LJ, et al. Ligamentous restraints to anterior and posterior translation of the sternoclavicular joint. *J Shoulder Elbow Surg*. 2002;11:43–47, with permission.)

- Open reduction with stabilization and possible medial clavicular resection reserved for chronic symptoms with instability or cosmetic concerns.

Posterior Dislocations

- Closed reduction as soon as possible
- General anesthesia or heavy sedation may be needed
- Abduction-traction technique is primary method
  - Rolled towel between scapula in supine position
  - Abduct arm to 90 degrees; apply traction and gently extend
  - Pull medial clavicle forward, if necessary
- Adduction-traction technique
  - Position as previously described
  - Adduct arm and apply downward traction and downward pressure on shoulder
- After reduction, immobilize in figure-of-eight bandage or sling and swathe for 4 to 6 weeks
- Physical therapy and active shoulder exercises after 3 weeks
- Open reduction indicated if closed reduction is unsuccessful

Troubleshooting

- Numerous surgical techniques described for chronic, symptomatic instability, including tendinous grafts, suture anchors, and mesh devices

- Strongly advised to avoid hardware across the SC joint for fixation due to the risk of migration and potential damage to mediastinal structures
- If resection of the medial clavicle is necessary, then it is recommended to either preserve or reconstruct the costoclavicular and capsular ligaments
- Open or arthroscopic excision of disc is option for chronic, symptomatic tears
- Intra-articular corticosteroid injection may provide temporary relief of SCJ pain

Considerations in Special Populations

- Physeal injury is more likely than a true SC dislocation in younger age groups.
- Medial clavicular epiphysis is last to ossify (18 to 20 years old) and does not fuse to shaft of clavicle until 23 to 25 years old.

Suggested Readings

Bae D, Kocher M, Waters P, et al. Chronic recurrent anterior sternoclavicular joint instability: results of surgical management. *J Pediatr Orthop*. 2006; 26(1):71–75.

Bicos J, Nicholson G. Treatment and results of sternoclavicular joint injuries. *Clin Sports Med*. 2003;22:359–370.

Gove N, Ebraheim N, Glass E. Posterior sternoclavicular dislocations: a review of management and complications. *Am J Orthop*. 2006;35: 132–136.

Morell D, Thyagarajan D. Sternoclavicular joint dislocation and its management: a review of the literature. *World J Orthop*. 2016;7(4):244–250.

Renfree K, Wright T. Anatomy and biomechanics of the acromioclavicular and sternoclavicular joints. *Clin Sports Med*. 2003;22:219–237.

Tytherleigh-Strong G, Rashid A, Lawrence C, Morrissey D. Arthroscopic intra-articular disk excision of the sternoclavicular joint. *Arthrosc Tech*. 2017;6(3):599–605.

Chapter 41 Scapulothoracic Problems

Michael Argyle, Jon Umlauf, Anthony Beutler

ICD 10-CM CODES

M25.51	*Shoulder pain (meant for joint)*
M75.80	*Other shoulder lesions, unspecified shoulder (scapular bursitis)*
M79.62	*Pain in limb, upper arm (meant for region)*
M89.8X1	*Other specified disorders of bone, shoulder (scapular dyskinesis)*
S44.90X	*Injury of unspecified nerve at shoulder and upper arm level, unspecified arm (nerve injury)*
G54.0	*Brachial plexus disorders (Parsonage-Turner syndrome)*

Scapular Dyskinesis

Key Concepts

- Appropriate scapular function is essential in transferring power from the core to the upper extremity by maintaining optimal glenohumeral surface contact throughout shoulder range of motion.
- Abnormal scapular positioning and/or movement is called scapular dyskinesis.
- Scapular dyskinesis should be considered a potential contributor for most shoulder conditions.
- Direct scapular trauma may result in nerve injuries and subsequent dyskinesis (Fig. 41.1).
- Rehabilitation consisting of progressive strengthening and coordinating specific muscle groups improves scapular function.
- Scapular stabilizers include trapezius, serratus anterior, levator scapulae, rhomboids, and pectoralis minor.

History

- Presents clinically as asymmetry in motion of the scapula compared to the contralateral side; patient may or may not complain of pain in scapular region.
- May be due to previous trauma.
- Dyskinesis is divided into three types:
  - Type I—excessive anterior tilt with inferior angle prominence
  - Type II—excessive lateral rotation with medial border prominence

- Type III—lack of acromial elevation with superior medial border prominence. Combination patterns are also common.
- Dyskinesis is typically due to changes in flexibility, strength imbalance, or altered muscle activation patterns.

Physical Examination

- Visual inspection should be completed at rest and during motion.
- Scapular dyskinesis at rest is often termed "SICK" scapula characterized by:
  - **S**capular malposition
  - **I**nferior medial border prominence
  - **C**orcacoid pain
  - Scapular dys**k**inesias.
- Dynamic exam may elicit early scapular elevation or medial border prominence with arm raising and lowering when compared to the contralateral side.
- The scapular assistance and scapular retraction test are useful special tests to determine if correction of the dyskinesis will reduce pain.
- Evaluate potential causative factors with an appropriate physical exam including rotator cuff, labrum, acromioclavicular (AC) joint, and impingement tests.

Imaging

- X-rays can identify clavicle or AC joint injury.
- Magnetic resonance imaging (MRI) may identify rotator cuff injury or labral injury.

Additional Tests

- Nerve conduction tests (NCT) and electromyelography (EMG) studies can be useful if dyskinesis occurs after traumatic injury to determine if there is an injury to the long thoracic, dorsal scapular, or spinal accessory nerves (see Fig. 41.1).

Differential Diagnosis

- Please see Table 41.1.

Treatment

- Treatment is directed at the etiology for dyskinesis.
- Neuropraxia affecting the serratus anterior and trapezius often resolve spontaneously.

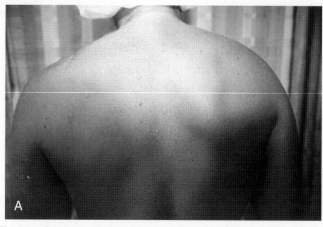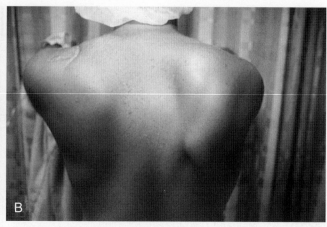

Fig 41.1 Scapular winging associated with long thoracic nerve injury and serratus muscle palsy. **(A)** The scapula assumes a superomedial position at rest. **(B)** Winging is accentuated with elevation of the arms. (From Kuhn JE. Scapulothoracic crepitus and bursitis in athletes. In: DeLee JC, Drez D Jr, Miller MD, eds. *DeLee and Drez's Orthopaedic Sports Medicine*. 2nd ed. Philadelphia: Saunders; 2003:1009.)

TABLE 41.1 Differential Diagnosis

Etiology	Findings
Serratus anterior weakness/palsy (long thoracic nerve injury, avulsion, or congenital absence of serratus anterior)	Winging accentuated with push-up against wall (see Fig. 41.1)
Trapezius weakness/palsy (spinal accessory nerve injury, congenital absence of trapezius)	Causes scapular winging and elevation; winging accentuated by arm abduction at shoulder level
Rhomboid weakness (dorsal scapular nerve or C5 nerve root injury)	Winging accentuated with slow lowering of the arm from forward elevation
Amyotrophic brachial neuralgia (Parsonage-Aldren-Turner syndrome)	Spontaneous onset of severe shoulder girdle pain with onset of weakness and winging of the scapula after a few days
Facioscapulohumeral dystrophy	Onset of weakness in the second decade of life; weakness of multiple muscle groups causes severe winging and inability to elevate arm >90°; asymmetry of facial muscles
Skeletal deformity (scoliosis) or solitary, localized lesion of the scapula, rib, or clavicle	Static winging, deformity noted on physical examination or imaging studies
Congenital or postinjection fibrosis of the deltoid	Abduction or flexion contracture and static winging
Degenerative or inflammatory joint disease of the shoulder	Abduction or internal rotation contracture; evidence of joint disease on imaging studies

- Early well-tolerated range of motion exercises help restore function and decrease pain.
- Consideration of scapular muscle balance is key; selective activation and strengthening of weaker muscles with less focus on the overactive muscles can improve muscle balance (Fig. 41.2).
- Taping or bracing may be considered in patients with difficulty in maintaining corrective posture or who are unable to exercise without pain.
- Deficits due to neurologic injury should be evaluated and followed with NCS/EMG.
- Surgical referral should be made for bony lesions, complete deficits caused by penetrating trauma or surgery, congenital abnormalities, or for patients with neurologic deficits that continue after 1 year of injury.

Troubleshooting

- Early surgical referral is advised for patients with traumatic causes of muscle paralysis for evaluation of and possible repair of a transected nerve.

Prognosis

- Most cases of scapular dyskinesis are secondary to other shoulder pathologies and respond to muscle strengthening and retraining programs. Three to 6 months of appropriate rehabilitation may be required in cases of long-standing shoulder pain/injury before significant improvement is seen.
- Majority of primary nerve injuries are neuropraxias that resolve spontaneously but may require 6 months to 2 years for complete resolution of symptoms.

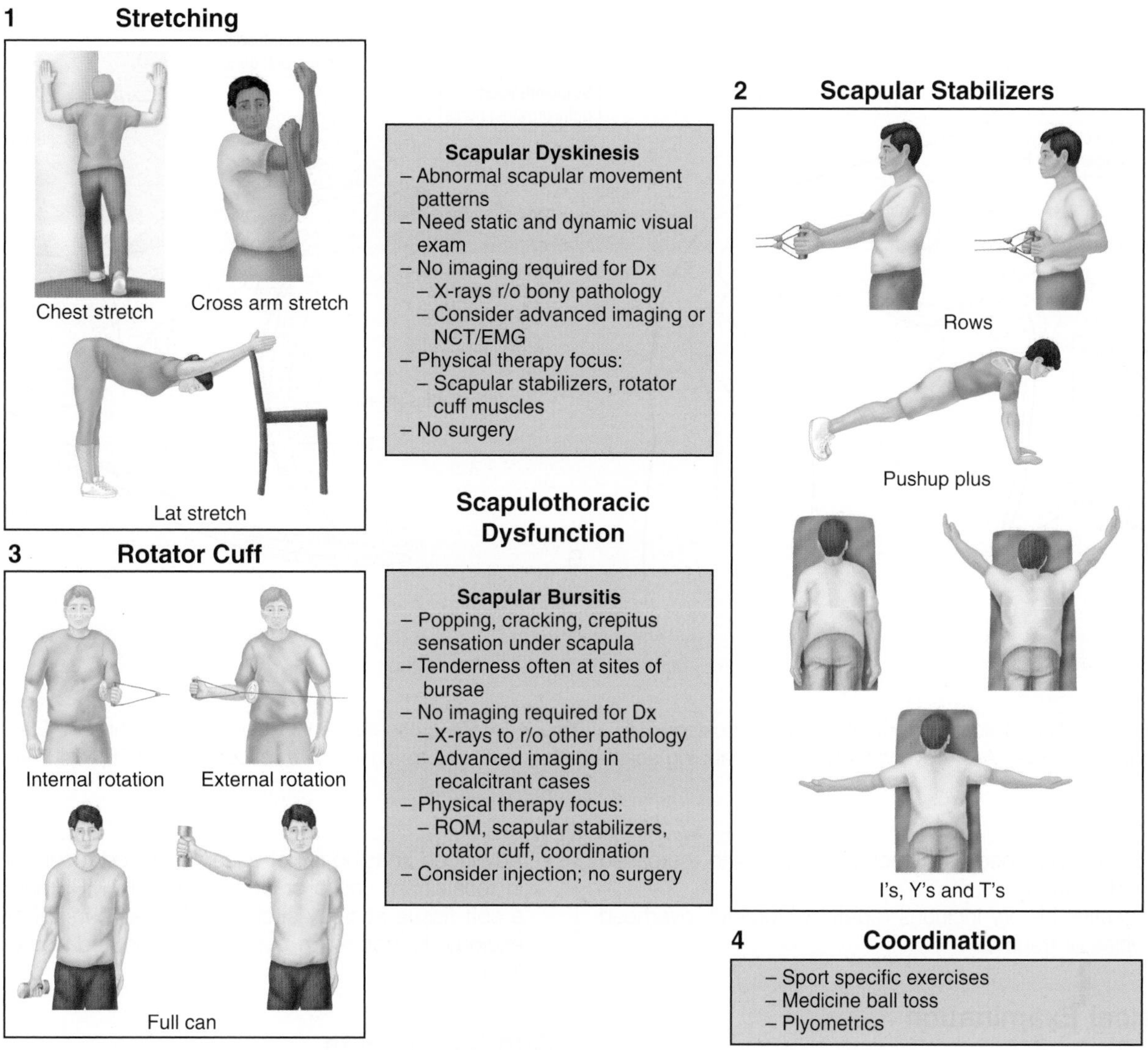

1 Stretching

Chest stretch

Cross arm stretch

Lat stretch

Scapular Dyskinesis
– Abnormal scapular movement patterns
– Need static and dynamic visual exam
– No imaging required for Dx
  – X-rays r/o bony pathology
  – Consider advanced imaging or NCT/EMG
– Physical therapy focus:
  – Scapular stabilizers, rotator cuff muscles
– No surgery

Scapulothoracic Dysfunction

Scapular Bursitis
– Popping, cracking, crepitus sensation under scapula
– Tenderness often at sites of bursae
– No imaging required for Dx
  – X-rays to r/o other pathology
  – Advanced imaging in recalcitrant cases
– Physical therapy focus:
  – ROM, scapular stabilizers, rotator cuff, coordination
– Consider injection; no surgery

3 Rotator Cuff

Internal rotation

External rotation

Full can

2 Scapular Stabilizers

Rows

Pushup plus

I's, Y's and T's

4 Coordination

– Sport specific exercises
– Medicine ball toss
– Plyometrics

Fig 41.2 Scapulothoracic dysfunction presentation and treatment guide.

Patient Instructions

- Compliance with physical therapy and recommended bracing will help maintain current function and prevent future disability.
- Avoid repetitive activities that may have caused or continue to aggravate the condition.

Considerations in Special Populations

- Wheelchair athletes are at especially high risk of shoulder injuries, as >50% of reported injuries involve the shoulder/arm/elbow.
- Demands of training and daily use of arms as a means of propulsion increase the risk of overuse injuries and abnormal muscle mechanics in this population.

Scapular Bursitis ("Snapping Scapula")

Key Concepts

- Etiology is not well understood but thought to be the result of abnormal motions between the scapula and posterior chest wall and/or anomalous anatomy.
- Weakness or imbalances of shoulder and scapular muscles may lead to abnormal joint mechanics of the shoulder complex.

History

- Patients complain of popping, snapping, or cracking sensation and occasionally frank crepitus between the scapula and thoracic wall with movement of the arm.

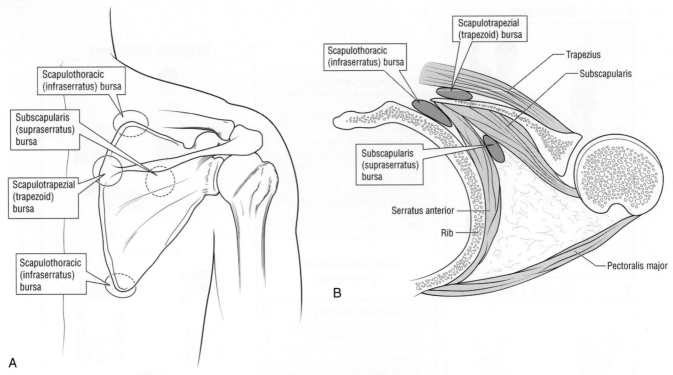

Fig 41.3 Location of scapular bursal spaces in posterior **(A)** and superior **(B)** cross-sectional views. (From Kuhne M, Boniquit N, Ghodadra N, Romeo AA, Provencher MT. The snapping scapula: diagnosis and treatment. *Arthroscopy.* 2009;25[11]:1298–1311.)

- May have nonspecific subscapular pain with increased shoulder activity
- Suggestive history includes repetitive, forceful, overhead activities or trauma.

Physical Examination

- Visual inspection may reveal static and/or dynamic asymmetry of scapulae or scapular winging.
- Poor posture with anteriorly rounded shoulders is evidence of poor balance of scapular stabilization strength and is a classic finding in this condition.
- Palpation may reveal hypertonic upper trapezius with weakness, pectoralis minor or levator scapulae tightness. Palpation may produce pain at the superomedial and inferomedial borders of the scapula near commonly affected bursae (Fig. 41.3).
- Range-of-motion abnormalities may include decreased glenohumeral internal and external rotation.
- Strength testing may find weakness of trapezius, serratus anterior, levator scapulae, rhomboids, pectoralis minor, and rotator cuff.
- Evaluate for long thoracic nerve or suprascapular nerve impairment especially after trauma.
- Evaluate for cervical radiculopathy with Spurling test.
- Evaluate for glenohumeral impingement and instability.

Imaging

- Radiographs are rarely useful other than ruling out more severe etiology.

- Advanced imaging is not usually required/recommended. In recalcitrant cases or persistent pain, MRI may isolate a soft-tissue etiology such as inflamed bursa if no bony etiology is noted on x-ray or computed tomography (CT).

Additional Tests

- NCT and EMG are appropriate in evaluation of patients with a winging scapula on exam to evaluate for long thoracic nerve dysfunction causing serratus anterior weakness.

Differential Diagnosis

- Abnormalities of bone, muscle, or bursae involved in scapulothoracic movement can all be causes of snapping scapula syndrome (Box 41.1).
- Underlying problems with the cervical spine or glenohumeral joint may be the precipitating cause of pain/symptoms.

Treatment

- After serious pathology has been appropriately excluded, conservative treatment is usually curative.
- Initial care includes therapeutic exercises to improve range of motion, strengthen rotator cuff and scapular stabilizers (see Fig. 41.2), improve scapulothoracic-rotator cuff coordination, and correct posture.
- A short course of nonsteroidal antiinflammatory drugs (3 to 7 days) at pain management dosing (400 to 600 mg ibuprofen q8h) may be helpful.

BOX 41.1 **Causes of Snapping Scapula Syndrome**

Bony Abnormalities

Scapula
  Exostoses or spurs
  Osteochondromas
  Scapular tubercle of Luschka (bony or fibrocartilaginous protrusion at the superior angle of the scapula)
  Anterior angulation of the superior angle of the scapula
  Fractures (acute or healed)
  Sprengel deformity (congenital undescended scapula)
Rib
  Tumors
  Abnormal angulations
  Fractures (acute or healed)
Vertebrae
  Omovertebral bone (abnormal cervical transverse process)
  Scoliosis or thoracic kyphosis

Soft-Tissue Abnormalities

Superomedial, inferomedial, or subscapular bursitis
Shoulder muscle atrophy
  Serratus anterior atrophy secondary to long thoracic nerve palsy
  Subscapularis atrophy secondary to glenohumeral fusion
Skeletal muscle intrafascicular fibrosis due to chronic inflammation
Subscapular elastofibroma

Other

After first rib resection for thoracic outlet syndrome
Tuberculosis or syphilitic lesions

Adapted from Carlson HL, Haig AJ, Stewart DC. Snapping scapula syndrome: three case reports and an analysis of the literature. *Arch Phys Med Rehabil*. 1997;78:506–511.

- Corticosteroid injection to the superomedial or inferomedial border of the scapula is a useful diagnostic and/or therapeutic option for more severe symptoms or failure of physical therapy (Fig. 41.4).
- Refer to sports medicine, orthopaedic surgery, or physiatry specialty care for failure of conservative treatment or distinct anatomic abnormalities.

Troubleshooting

- Nerve injuries may present as an inability to recruit scapulothoracic stabilization muscles and continued weakness throughout rehabilitation exercises; consider further investigation with electromyography and nerve conduction studies.
- Nonpainful crepitus is not always pathologic, but patients are at a relatively higher risk of developing pain over time.

Patient Instructions

- Most cases will resolve or improve over the course of 3 to 6 months of physical therapy.

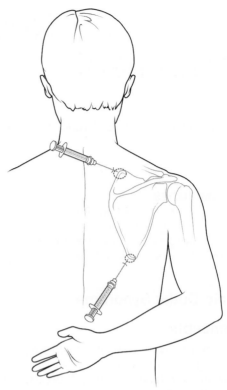

Fig 41.4 The two common locations of scapular bursal injections are at the superomedial border and at the inferior tip. (From Kuhne M, Boniquit N, Ghodadra N, Romeo AA, Provencher MT. The snapping scapula: diagnosis and treatment. *Arthroscopy*. 2009;25[11]:1298–1311.)

- Avoid repetitive activities that create or reproduce snapping, as this may cause or aggravate pain.

Suggested Readings

Cricchio M, Frazer C. Scapulothoracic and scapulohumeral exercises: a narrative review of electromyographic studies. *J Hand Ther*. 2011;24(4):322–334.

Kibler WB, Ludewig PM, Mcclure PW, et al. Clinical implications of scapular dyskinesis in shoulder injury: the 2013 consensus statement from the 'scapular summit'. *Br J Sports Med*. 2013;47(14):877–885.

Kibler WB, Sciascia A. Current concepts: scapular dyskinesis. *Br J Sports Med*. 2009;44(5):300–305.

Kuhne M, Boniquit N, Ghodadra N, et al. The snapping scapula: diagnosis and treatment. *Arthroscopy*. 2009;25(11):1298–1311.

Reinold MM, Escamilla R, Wilk KE. Current concepts in the scientific and clinical rationale behind exercises for glenohumeral and scapulothoracic musculature. *J Orthop Sports Phys Ther*. 2009;39(2):105–117.

Roche SJ, Funk L, Sciascia A, Kibler WB. Scapular dyskinesis: the surgeon's perspective. *Shoulder Elbow*. 2015;7(4):289–297.

Tate A, McClure P. Examination and management of scapular dysfunction. In: Skirven TM, Osterman AL, Fedorczyk JM, Amadio PC, eds. *Rehabilitation of the Hand and Upper Extremity*. 6th ed. Philadelphia: Elsevier; 2011:1209–1226.

Chapter 42 Neurovascular Entrapment

Kate Quinn, James Alex, William Dexter

ICD-10-CM CODES
G54.0	*Thoracic outlet syndrome*
G56.8	*Suprascapular nerve entrapment*
G58.9	*Long thoracic nerve entrapment*
S44.30XA	*Quadrilateral space syndrome*

Thoracic Outlet Syndrome

Key Concepts

- Thoracic outlet syndrome (TOS) refers to symptoms related to neurologic and/or vascular compression involving the brachial plexus and subclavian vessels between the thoracic aperture and axilla.
- Types of TOS include neurogenic, arterial, and venous.
- Affected structures are vulnerable to compression at the following areas:
  - The interscalene triangle containing the subclavian artery and three trunks of the brachial plexus. Bordered by the anterior, middle, and posterior scalenes and first rib.
  - The costoclavicular space contains the entire neurovascular bundle and is the most frequent site of arterial compression. Bordered by the clavicle, subclavius muscle, first rib, anterior and middle scalenes.
  - The rectopectoralis minor space is bordered by the pectoralis minor tendon, subscapularis, and anterior chest wall.
- Anatomic and other risk factors for development include:
  - Cervical rib, elongated C7 transverse processes, first rib anomaly, fibrous bands, malunion of clavicle or first rib fracture, cervical muscle spasm or hypertonicity, space-occupying lesion
  - History of neck trauma, postural changes with sagging of the shoulders, repetitive overhead arm motion

History

- Typically presents with pain, paresthesia, dysesthesia, weakness, edema, or skin changes in the affected arm and hand
- Paresthesias can involve entire arm without dermatomal preference or more prominent in fourth and fifth digits and ulnar aspect of the forearm
- Symptoms are exacerbated by arm exertion and elevation

Physical Exam

- Complete cervical, shoulder, and neurovascular exam

- Frequently tender over the scalenes, trapezius, or anterior chest wall
- Positive response to provocative maneuvers affecting the neurovascular structures
  - Elevated arm stress test (EAST)/Roos test
    - Arms placed in 90 degree abduction and external rotation
    - Open and close hands repeatedly over 3-minute period
    - Positive test reproduces symptoms
  - Wright test
    - Bring shoulder overhead in hyperabduction and external rotation
    - Positive if have diminished radial pulse or reproduced symptoms
  - Costoclavicular/military brace/Eden maneuver
    - Thrust shoulders posteriorly and inferiorly, lift chest
    - Positive if have diminished radial pulse or reproduced symptoms
  - Adson maneuver
    - Arm abducted, neck extended, turn head toward the affected side
    - Positive if have diminished radial pulse or reproduced symptoms with inhalation

Imaging

- Anteroposterior chest radiograph
- Magnetic resonance imaging (MRI) chest without contrast

Additional Tests

- Cervical and/or shoulder plain radiographs
- Electromyography (EMG) and nerve conduction velocity (NCV) often normal
- If vascular cause suspected, consider magnetic resonance angiography chest with and without contrast or computed tomography (CT) angiography chest with contrast, or ultrasound of the subclavian vessels
- Magnetic resonance, CT, and ultrasound protocols should include neutral and abduction positions of the upper limb to evaluate dynamic compression of neurovascular structures

Differential Diagnosis

- Cervical radiculopathy
- Brachial plexus injury

- Carpal tunnel syndrome
- Cubital tunnel syndrome
- Space-occupying lesion of the costoclavicular space, tumor (Pancoast)
- Peripheral neuropathy
- Complex regional pain syndrome
- Parsonage-Turner syndrome
- Cervical spinal cord tumor

Treatment
- Conservative Measures
  - Behavior modification, ergonomic and postural correction, relaxation techniques, biofeedback, manual therapy, physical therapy, home exercise program, shoulder girdle strengthening, cervical traction, job modifications, and work restrictions
- Medications
  - Muscle relaxants
  - Nonsteroidal antiinflammatory drugs (NSAIDs)
  - Tricyclic antidepressants
  - Serotonin-norepinephrine reuptake inhibitors
  - Anticonvulsants
- Trigger point injections
- Intramuscular anterior scalene block
- Botulinum toxin injection into the scalene(s)

When to Refer
- In emergency cases associated with arterial or venous thrombus
- Surgical indications include three months of failed conservative treatment, disability with activities of daily living, uncontrolled pain, progressive weakness
- Surgical approaches include first or cervical rib resection with or without scalenectomy or neurolysis

Prognosis
- Conservative measures often provide relief in 50-90% of patients, typically within 6 weeks
- Surgical complication rate exceeds 30%, including pleural effusion, pneumothorax, chylothorax
- One year after surgery, 60% of patients have persistent disability

Troubleshooting
- Carefully exclude proximal or distal disorders including cervical disc lesion and nerve entrapment at the elbow or the hand
- Encourage adherence to home exercise program

Suprascapular Nerve Entrapment

Key Concepts
- The suprascapular nerve originates from the upper trunk of the brachial plexus and innervates the supraspinatus and infraspinatus muscles.

- Suprascapular nerve entrapment often occurs at the site of the suprascapular notch where the nerve passes beneath the superior transverse scapular ligament.
- Another potential site of entrapment is at the level of the spinoglenoid ligament where the nerve courses beneath the scapular spine.
- Previous shoulder injury, repetitive overuse, or posterior labral tear may lead to the development of a posterior ganglion cyst and nerve impingement via mass effect.
- Associated with direct blows to the superior shoulder or prolonged compression, repetitive overhead activities, including volleyball, tennis, baseball, basketball, and weightlifting

History
- Patient presents with insidious or traumatic onset of posterior shoulder pain, dull ache, or shoulder weakness in abduction and external rotation.
- Pain is exacerbated by overhead activity or reaching across the body.

Physical Examination
- Complete general shoulder and cervical spine examination including neurovascular exam
- Tinel sign or pain with palpation of the suprascapular notch may be present.
- Weakness with resisted shoulder abduction suggests supraspinatus muscle involvement; weakness with resisted external rotation of the shoulder suggests infraspinatus involvement.
- Cross-arm adduction test
  - The examiner adducts the affected arm across the patient's chest eliciting reproduction of the pain.

Imaging
- Plain radiography of the shoulder and cervical spine
- Musculoskeletal ultrasound
  - May be helpful in identifying sites of mass effect or neuritis
- MRI of the shoulder
  - May demonstrate muscle changes associated with nerve injury including decreased muscle bulk, fatty infiltration, and signal intensity differences

Additional Tests
- Electrodiagnostic studies including nerve conduction studies or EMG
  - Consider these modalities for diagnostic confirmation and localization of the lesion.

Differential Diagnosis
- Cervical radiculopathy of the C5 and C6 nerve roots
- Glenohumeral or acromioclavicular joint disorder
- Ganglion cyst associated with glenoid labral tear
- Supraspinatus and/or infraspinatus tear
- Complex regional pain syndrome

Treatment

- At diagnosis
  - Conservative measures include
    - Overhead activity restrictions
    - Physical therapy
    - Scapular stabilization program
    - Flexibility program for surrounding muscles of glenohumeral joint
  - Injection of local anesthetic into the suprascapular notch to manage pain symptoms
- Later
  - Introduction of rotator cuff strengthening program
  - Graded return to activity once symptoms resolve

When to Refer

- Surgical consultation is warranted if the entrapment is associated with trauma.
- Consider surgical consultation if there is no improvement after 6 months of conservative treatment.

Prognosis

- Most patients will improve with conservative measures alone; however, the prognosis is not well known.
- Operative treatment improves functional impairments and relief of pain for most patients.

Troubleshooting

- Overhead activity restriction is vital to improvement.
- Counsel the patient that resolution may take 6 to 12 months.
- Counsel the patient that surgery, if necessary, carries a risk of nerve or vascular injury.
- Close follow-up is warranted to ensure compliance with a management program and to limit the duration of activity restrictions.

Long Thoracic Nerve Entrapment

Key Concepts

- The long thoracic nerve arises from C5, C6, and C7 nerve roots and innervates the serratus anterior muscle.
- Entrapment can occur after repetitive exercise or trauma when the shoulder girdle compresses the long thoracic nerve against the second rib.
- Middle scalene entrapment is also a common etiology.
- Particular populations affected include weightlifters, new military recruits carrying heavy backpacks, backstroke swimmers, and football players.

History

- Patients may present without symptoms or with a unilateral winged scapula.

Physical Examination

- Complete shoulder examination including neurovascular exam
- Scapular winging may be noted during shoulder flexion or with wall push-up.
- There are no associated sensory changes with this condition.

Imaging

- Usually not indicated unless coincident trauma

Additional Tests

- EMG is helpful in confirming the diagnosis or localizing entrapment.

Differential Diagnosis

- C5 to C7 radiculopathy
- Trapezius muscle dysfunction
- Brachial plexus neuropathy

Treatment

- At diagnosis
  - No overhead or exacerbating activity
  - A sling may provide support
  - Physical therapy
  - General shoulder strengthening program
  - Resistance exercises for serratus anterior muscle
- Later
  - Graded return to activity once symptoms and scapular winging resolve

When to Refer

- Neurologic consultation warranted if no improvement with 6 weeks of conservative treatment

Prognosis

- Prognosis for recovery is good unless the nerve has been completely severed by trauma.

Troubleshooting

- Avoidance of exacerbating activity is vital to improvement.
- Refractory cases may respond well to surgical microneurolysis and decompression, particularly when middle scalene entrapment is involved.

Quadrilateral Space Syndrome

Key Concepts

- The quadrilateral space is bordered by the teres major inferiorly, the long head of the triceps medially, the surgical neck of the humerus laterally, and the teres minor superiorly.

- The axillary nerve and posterior humeral circumflex artery pass through this space.
- The axillary nerve provides motor innervation to the teres minor and deltoid muscles and sensation to the "regimental badge" area of the inferior deltoid as the superior lateral cutaneous branch.
- Anatomic entrapment of the nerve or mechanical injury of the artery can occur due to space-occupying lesions such as glenoid labral cyst, ganglion, bony fracture fragment, or fibrous bands, as well as muscle hypertrophy.
- Repetitive overhead activity can result in mechanical trauma to the posterior humeral circumflex artery and in aneurysmal dilation with thrombosis.
- Common predisposing activities include volleyball, baseball, swimming, yoga, and window cleaning.

History

- Neurogenic symptoms include nondermatomal pain, numbness, fasciculations, or weakness of the shoulder and arm.
- Vascular symptoms include pain of the shoulder, forearm, digits; discolored, pale or blue digits; cold digits; absent pulses.
- Athletes can exhibit early arm fatigue or less endurance with activity.
- Symptoms are typically exacerbated by overhead activity with forward flexion, abduction, and external rotation positions of the humerus.

Physical Examination

- Perform complete shoulder and cervical spine exam including neurovascular exam
- Point tenderness may be noted overlying the quadrilateral space.
- Patients may exhibit paresthesias over the lateral shoulder.
- Deficits with active range of motion testing of the first 30 degrees of shoulder abduction and forward flexion associated with weakened or denervated deltoid muscle
- Reduced strength with resisted external rotation of the shoulder may be associated with weakened or denervated teres minor muscle.
- Weakness can be seen with the shoulder in forward flexion and abduction positions.
- Examination may reveal cool, pale hand and digits and delayed capillary refill, as well as splinter hemorrhages of the digits.

Imaging

- Plain radiographs of the shoulder including internal and external rotation views
- Angiography including digital subtraction angiography, computed tomography angiography, or magnetic resonance angiography
  - Perform with the arm in abduction and external rotation position
- MRI of the shoulder
  - May show signs of teres minor and/or deltoid denervation including fatty infiltration and decreased muscle bulk

Additional Tests

- Ultrasonography
- EMG
  - Can be used to rule out other diagnoses

Differential Diagnosis

- Cervical radiculopathy including C5 and/or C6
- Suprascapular nerve entrapment
- Raynaud phenomenon
- Complex regional pain syndrome
- TOS
- Rotator cuff or labral tear
- Hypothenar hammer hand syndrome

Treatment

- Empiric injection of local anesthetic into quadrilateral space
- At diagnosis
  - Conservative treatment including
    - Rest and restriction from exacerbating activity
    - Oral antiinflammatories
- Later
  - Physical therapy
  - Range of motion exercises for deltoid, rotator cuff
  - Progressive strengthening for deltoid, rotator cuff
  - Graded return to activity once asymptomatic and full function returns

When to Refer

- Surgical consultation warranted if no improvement over 3- to 6-month period of conservative treatment
- Overhead athletes may benefit from prompt referral for surgical decompression at time of diagnosis.
- If vascular etiology present
  - Surgical ligation of the posterior circumflex humeral artery with or without thrombolysis
  - Consider anticoagulation
- If neurogenic etiology present
  - Surgical neurolysis, excision of fibrous bands or space-occupying lesion

Prognosis

- 1.5:1 prevalence of neurogenic etiology compared to vascular etiology of quadrilateral space syndrome
- Most patients respond well to conservative treatment in setting of neurogenic etiology
- Expected recovery with conservative treatment is 3 to 6 months but can be longer in high-demand overhead athletes.
- Return to play following surgical intervention can vary from 3 to 6 months.

Troubleshooting

- Close interval follow-up important to assess recovery and grade the return to activity recommendations

- Limit progression to unrestricted activities until full nerve function recovered
- Return to play for patients who require anticoagulation for vascular etiologies should be addressed on a case by case basis.

Patient Instructions

- Follow physician and physical therapist instructions closely regarding activity restrictions
- Home exercise program as established by physical therapist must be completed regularly as instructed.
- Surgery may be indicated if conservative measures do not improve symptoms or vascular etiology responsible.

Suggested Readings

Brown SA, Doolittle DA, Bohanon CJ, et al. Quadrilateral space syndrome: the Mayo Clinic experience with a new classification system and case series. *Mayo Clinic Proc*. 2015;90(3):382–394.

Cummins C, Messer T, Nuber G. Suprascapular nerve entrapment. *J Bone Joint Surg Am*. 2000;82A:415–424.

Nath RK, Somasundaram C. Meta-analysis of long thoracic nerve decompression and neurolysis versus muscle and tendon transfer operative treatments of winging scapula. *Plast Reconstr Surg Glob Open*. 2017;5(8):e1481.

Povlsen B, Hansson T, Povlsen SD. Treatment for thoracic outlet syndrome. *Cochrane Database Syst Rev*. 2014;(11):CD007218.

Waldman S. Suprascapular nerve entrapment. In: *Atlas of Uncommon Pain Syndromes*. Philadelphia: Elsevier; 2013:96–98.

Chapter 43 Proximal Humerus Fractures

Seth R. Yarboro, Michelle E. Kew

ICD-10-CM CODES
S42.20*A   *Closed fracture of upper end of humerus*
S42.20*B   *Open fracture of upper end of humerus*
S42.21*A   *Closed displaced fracture of surgical neck of humerus*
S42.21*B   *Open displaced fracture of surgical neck of humerus*

Key Concepts

- In patients older than 65 years, proximal humerus fracture is the third most common fracture after hip and distal radius fractures.
- Females older than 50 years are at the highest risk.
- These fractures are often managed nonoperatively in the elderly population with good functional results.
- Isolated greater tuberosity fractures are more common in younger individuals and may be associated with shoulder dislocation.
- The degree of fracture displacement predicts the risk of injury to the blood supply of the humeral head (>2 mm medial hinge displacement and <8 mm medial metaphyseal extension predict head ischemia).

History

- Proximal humerus fractures primarily result from indirect force (fall on an outstretched arm) or a direct blow to the shoulder.
- Factors contributing to fracture include: age, poor bone quality (as seen in osteoporotic/elderly), fall risks such as syncope, and medical comorbidities.
- Patients usually report pain with movement of extremity/shoulder.
- Numbness or tingling in the extremity is usually self-limited, benign, and not found in any anatomic pattern.
- Elderly patients often require a workup for the reason for their fall, which may include syncope, heart disease, stroke, and metabolic abnormalities.

Physical Examination

- Patients typically guard the upper extremity by holding it close to the chest, supported by the contralateral hand.
- Painful range of motion and pseudoparalysis (restriction of motion due to pain) may obscure the motor examination.
- Swelling and thick soft-tissue coverings usually obscure bony deformity, but it may be more apparent in very thin patients.
- Ecchymosis can last as long as 2 to 4 weeks and often moves into a dependent position.
- Injuries to the neck, chest, and head must be excluded, especially in the setting of high-energy trauma.
- Perform a careful neurovascular examination with particular attention to axillary nerve function (sensation in the lateral "sergeant's patch" distribution and active motor function of the deltoid muscle), as well as function of the distal extremity.

Pathomechanics

- Fracture fragments are displaced by the pull of surrounding muscles, including pectoralis major, supraspinatus, infraspinatus, and subscapularis
- Younger patients tend to have minimally displaced fractures or more comminution of dense bone due to higher-energy trauma.
- Older patients, with decreased bone density, typically have greater fracture displacement even with lower-energy trauma.

Imaging

- Adequate imaging is essential for a complete evaluation.
- True anteroposterior (Grashey) view of the shoulder with internal and external rotation views if tolerated
- Scapular Y view
- Axillary lateral view (or Velpeau axillary view): Important to rule out associated shoulder dislocation
- A computed tomography (CT) scan can be performed to further characterize the fracture and should be obtained if glenoid involvement or a possible split of the humeral head is suspected.

Classification

- Neer classification (Figs. 43.1 and 43.2) is based on the number of parts, where each part is defined as a fragment with displacement of more than 1 cm and/or angulation of more than 45 degrees
- A valgus-impaction pattern is associated with a better prognosis than the classic four-part fracture due to a better chance of maintenance of the vascular supply; less than 2 mm medial hinge displacement and greater than 8 mm medial metaphyseal extension predicts head ischemia.

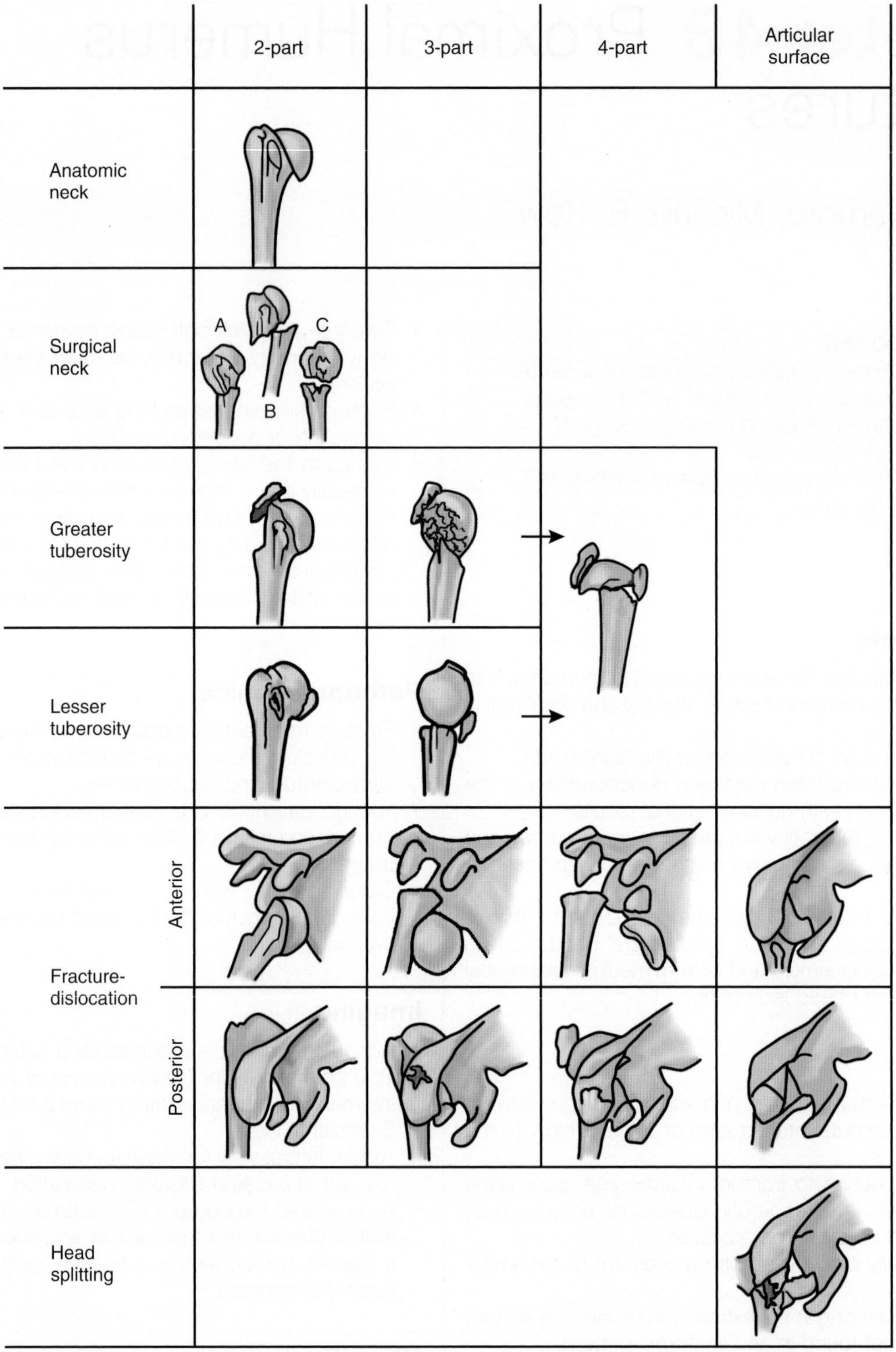

	2-part	3-part	4-part	Articular surface
Anatomic neck				
Surgical neck				
Greater tuberosity				
Lesser tuberosity				
Fracture-dislocation — Anterior				
Fracture-dislocation — Posterior				
Head splitting				

Fig 43.1 Neer classification: accepted method for the classification of proximal humerus fractures, based on the number of parts displaced more than 1 cm or more than 45 degrees.

Neer Classification of Proximal Humerus Fractures

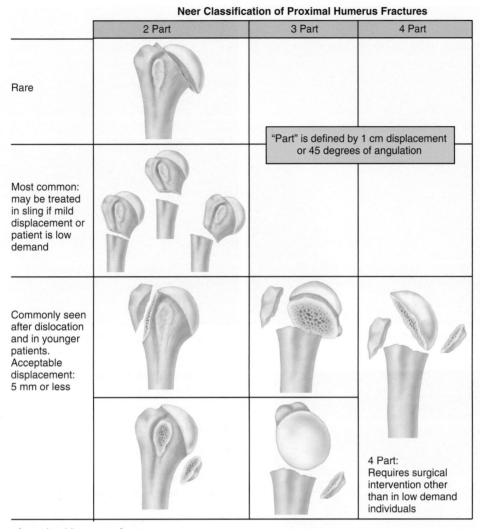

	2 Part	3 Part	4 Part
Rare			
		"Part" is defined by 1 cm displacement or 45 degrees of angulation	
Most common: may be treated in sling if mild displacement or patient is low demand			
Commonly seen after dislocation and in younger patients. Acceptable displacement: 5 mm or less			4 Part: Requires surgical intervention other than in low demand individuals

Fig 43.2 Overview of proximal humerus fractures.

Treatment

- Nonoperative
  - Nonoperative is the mainstay of treatment for most geriatric or low-demand proximal humerus fractures with generally good results.
  - Acceptable for minimally displaced fractures not meeting Neer criteria of less than 1 cm of displacement and 45 degrees of angulation
  - Initial closed treatment: non-weightbearing in a sling, encouraging active elbow and hand motion
  - At 2 weeks: Obtain a radiograph to ensure that the fracture has not displaced, and begin passive motion as tolerated as well as active pendulum exercises
  - At 4 to 6 weeks: If radiographs demonstrate maintenance of alignment, begin active motion as tolerated
  - At 2 to 3 months: Confirm radiographic and clinical healing, and then begin more aggressive range of motion exercises, capsular stretching, and periscapular muscle stretching and active strengthening
- Operative
  - Operative indications are dependent on fracture displacement; bone quality; patient's age, work, and functional demands; overall medical condition; and the presence of other fractures in the multitrauma patient.
  - Younger or higher-functioning patients may benefit from open reduction internal fixation (ORIF) for displaced proximal humerus fractures (Fig. 43.3).
  - Greater tuberosity fractures may benefit from fixation if displaced greater than 5 mm.
  - Goals of surgery are to restore alignment and rotator cuff function and to allow early range of motion (ROM) and rehabilitation.
  - Surgical procedure options can include closed reduction and percutaneous pinning, open reduction and internal fixation, shoulder hemiarthroplasty (Fig. 43.4), and total shoulder arthroplasty.

Differential Diagnosis

- Acute rotator cuff tear: Magnetic resonance imaging (MRI) confirms examination findings.
- Clavicle fracture: Deformity seen over clavicle, confirmed radiographically
- Acromioclavicular separation: Deformity at the acromioclavicular joint, confirmed radiographically

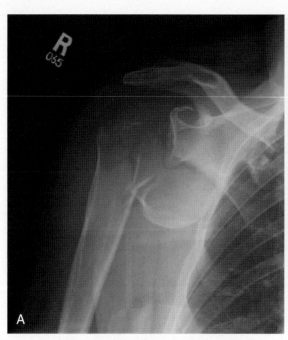

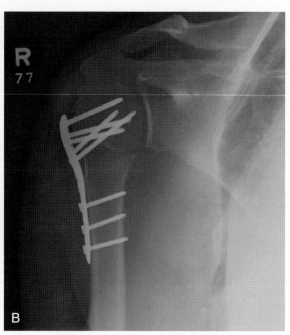

Fig 43.3 (A) Four-part proximal humerus fracture-dislocation. **(B)** Appearance after open reduction and internal fixation.

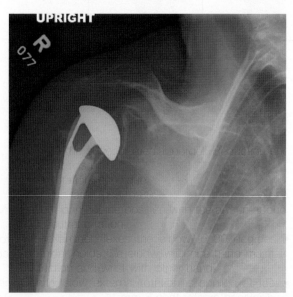

Fig 43.4 Proximal humerus fracture treated with hemiarthroplasty.

- Calcific tendinitis: acute exacerbation, rotator cuff calcification seen radiographically, relieved with nonsteroidal antiinflammatory drugs ± aspiration.

Additional Tests

- Not routinely required
- MRI: most effective method for evaluating soft-tissue injuries, such as rotator cuff tear

When to Refer

- If the fracture is displaced to a significant degree (5 mm for greater tuberosity, 1 cm or 45 degrees for other fragments)

and the patient is a surgical candidate, orthopaedic referral is most appropriate.

Troubleshooting

- The patient should be counseled on benefits and risks of surgery.
- Benefits
  - Fracture stabilization and decreased pain allow for early joint mobilization.
  - Anatomic reduction restores rotator cuff dynamics and articular congruity.
- Risks
  - Bleeding, infection, and neurovascular injury (axillary nerve is at risk in most approaches to the proximal humerus)
  - Failure of fixation, malunion, nonunion, and avascular necrosis of the humeral head
  - Shoulder stiffness can be seen after surgical management (prevented by early mobilization and appropriate physical therapy postoperatively).

Suggested Readings

Hodgson S. Proximal humerus fracture rehabilitation. *Clin Orthop Relat Res*. 2006;442:131–138.

Kancherla VK, Singh A, Anakwenze OA. Management of acute proximal humeral fracture. *J Am Acad Orthop Surg*. 2017;25:45–52.

Neer CS. Four-segment classification of displaced proximal humeral fractures. *AAOS Instr Lect*. 1975;24:160–168.

Nho SJ, Brophy RH, Barker JU, et al. Management of proximal humeral fractures based on current literature. *J Bone Joint Surg Am*. 2007;89A(suppl 3):44–58.

Rees J, Hicks J, Ribbans W. Assessment and management of three- and four-part proximal humeral fractures. *Clin Orthop Relat Res*. 1998;353:18–29.

Vallier HA. Treatment of proximal humerus fractures. *J Orthop Trauma*. 2007;21:469–476.

Chapter 44 Humeral Shaft Fractures

Anthony J. Bell, Michelle E. Kew, Seth R. Yarboro

ICD-10-CM CODES
S42.3A *Closed fracture of shaft of humerus*
S42.3B *Open fracture of shaft of humerus*

Key Concepts

- Humeral shaft fractures may be transverse, oblique, spiral, or segmental; the type of fracture depends on the mechanism and amount of energy imparted.
- Fragment displacement depends on the location of the fracture and the forces of the muscle attachments across the fracture site.
- Because union rates greater than 90% have been demonstrated with nonoperative methods alone, conservative treatment is generally preferred.
- Operative treatment results in a similar rate of ultimate healing but exposes the patient to greater risk of complications.
- When operative treatment is necessary, open reduction internal fixation with plate and screws is favored.
- Intramedullary nailing is generally reserved for pathologic fractures or other patients with special bone or soft-tissue considerations due to the higher reoperation rate and prevalence of postoperative shoulder dysfunction.
- Radial nerve palsy has markedly different potential for recovery in open versus closed fractures.
- The Holstein-Lewis fracture is located in the distal one third of the humeral shaft and has a relatively higher likelihood of radial nerve entrapment because it pierces the lateral intermuscular septum and is relatively tethered.
- See Fig. 44.1 for the AO (Arbeitsgemeinschaft für Osteosynthesefragen) classification of humeral shaft fractures.

Etiology

- The incidence of humeral shaft fractures is bimodal with a peak of young male patients in the 20 to 30 age bracket (25 per 100,000), and a second larger peak of older females in the 60 to 80 age bracket (100 per 100,000).
- As age increases, the etiology of fracture changes from high-energy trauma in the young to overwhelmingly low-impact trauma, such as ground-level falls, in the elderly.
- Humeral shaft fractures in the young are often part of multiple traumas as a result of their mechanisms. In the elderly they are often associated with osteoporosis.

Physical Examination

- Patients will usually present with pain, swelling, deformity, and a shortened extremity.

- It is important to perform a thorough neurovascular examination of the injured extremity before and after reduction attempts due to the vulnerability of the radial nerve.

Imaging

- Anteroposterior (AP) and lateral radiographs are often all that are necessary to diagnose the fracture.
- Scapular Y or transthoracic lateral may prevent patient discomfort and unnecessary rotation at the fracture site while obtaining lateral view.
- Reserve magnetic resonance imaging or computed tomography for suspected pathologic fracture.
- Contralateral humerus radiographs can be used for preoperative planning.

Treatment
Nonoperative

- Closed treatment can be successful in achieving satisfactory union for most fractures of the humeral shaft with union rates as high as 90-97% having been reported.
- Malunion of up to 20 degrees of anteroposterior angulation, 30 degrees of varus or valgus, 15 degrees of rotation, and 2 to 3 cm of shortening are generally well tolerated functionally and cosmetically (Fig. 44.2).
- Closed treatment generally begins with initial stabilization followed by transition to functional bracing.
- Coaptation splint (Fig. 44.3)
  - Most widely used method of initial stabilization for most fractures
  - Often uncomfortable given the bulkiness of the splint
  - The splint may slip down the arm; this can be prevented by placing an extension over the shoulder.
- Hanging arm cast (Fig. 44.4)
  - Uses gravity to effect fracture reduction and apply traction.
  - Cast arm from axilla to wrist with the elbow at 90 degrees.
  - The cast must hang free from the body to allow proper use of gravity to effect alignment.
    - The patient must also remain upright for 1 to 2 weeks for the cast to be effective.
  - Weight may cause over-distraction in some fractures.
- Velpeau or sling and swathe bandage
  - Can be used for initial stabilization of fractures in smaller children and the elderly.
  - Does not aid in fracture reduction; used for comfort rather than immobilization.
  - Should change to a functional brace or other method once acute pain subsides.

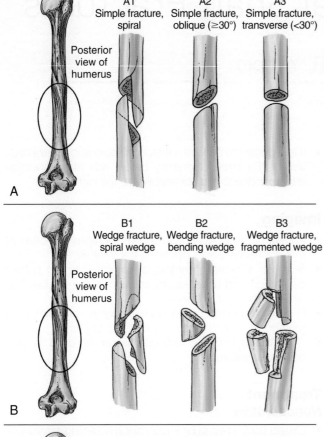

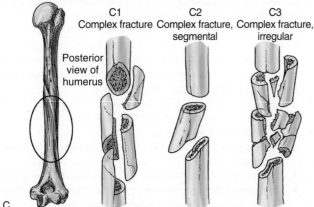

Fig 44.1 AO classification of humeral shaft fractures. **(A)** Simple fracture; **(B)** wedge fracture; **(C)** complex fracture. (From DeFranco MJ, Lawton JN. Radial nerve injuries associated with humeral fractures. *J Hand Surg Am.* 2006;31:655–663.)

- Functional brace (Fig. 44.5A and B)
  - The gold standard for closed treatment for humeral shaft fractures
  - Uses soft-tissue compression to effect fracture reduction
  - Cannot use if the patient has extensive soft-tissue injury, bone loss, distraction, or if acceptable alignment is unable to be maintained

- Typically applied 1 to 2 weeks after the injury when initial immobilization is removed
- Worn for longer than 8 weeks and periodically tightened as swelling subsides
- Care must be taken to promote elbow and shoulder motion to prevent stiffness.

Operative

- Indications for operative management include:
  - Open fracture, segmental or irreducible fractures
  - Associated brachial artery or brachial plexus or peripheral nerve injury
  - Ipsilateral radius and ulna fractures (floating elbow)
  - Fractures with intra-articular extension
  - Penetrating injury with radial nerve palsy
  - Pathologic fractures
  - Polytrauma
- Operative management options
- Open reduction internal fixation (Fig. 44.6)
  - Gold standard for operative fixation; studies report union in 92-98% of cases.
  - Most studies demonstrate a low rate (3-9%) of iatrogenic radial nerve palsy.
  - Preservation of soft tissues is emphasized with surgical technique; minimally invasive techniques have been described to address this concern; however, this may increase the risk to anatomic structures and the difficulty in achieving anatomic reduction.
- Intramedullary nailing
  - Promising union rates of 85-90% have been tempered in recent years due to concerns for other complications in comparison to plating.
  - Postoperative shoulder dysfunction associated with antegrade nailing, with occurrence rates up to 30% in some studies; risks of shoulder dysfunction may be lessened with attention to technique but it remains a concern.
  - Retrograde nailing has been associated with risk of elbow pain, fracture propagation, or iatrogenic fracture.
  - Malrotation has been shown to occur as frequently as 20% of cases in some studies.
  - Nailing may be preferred for select cases including pathologic fracture, severe soft-tissue injury, or osteoporotic bone.
- External fixation
  - Use with extensive soft-tissue injury, overlying burns, or compromise of the skin, or infected nonunion for temporary or definitive management.
- Postoperative course
  - Range of motion exercises in the hand and wrist should be started immediately, and active motion of the elbow encouraged as soon as possible after injury.
  - Range of motion exercises in the shoulder should begin as pain permits, starting with Codman exercises and progressing as pain allows.
  - Early weight bearing has been shown to be safe with large fragment (4.5 mm) plates; however smaller-caliber plates remain controversial, with many surgeons delaying weight bearing until radiographic evidence of healing. Intramedullary nails may be stable for weight bearing in some cases.

Humeral Shaft Fractures

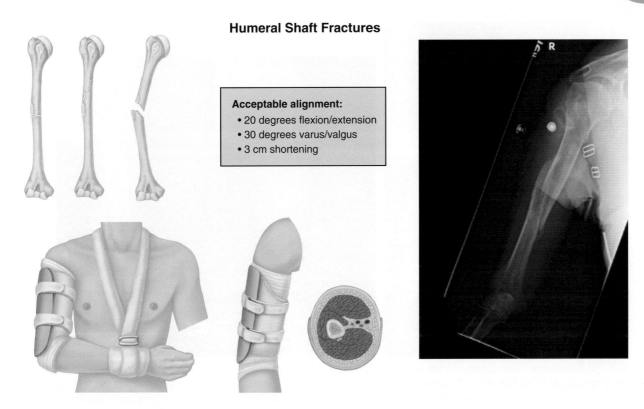

Acceptable alignment:
- 20 degrees flexion/extension
- 30 degrees varus/valgus
- 3 cm shortening

Isolated injuries are often treated in functional brace.
In polytrauma patients consider open reduction internal fixation to help early rehabilitation.

Fig 44.2 Overview of humeral shaft fractures.

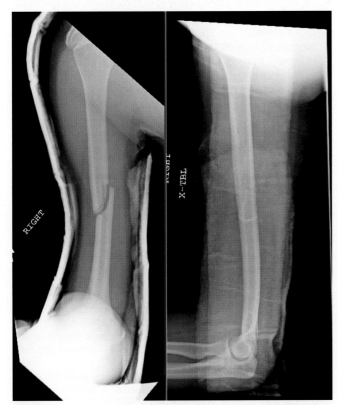

Fig 44.3 Well-aligned humeral shaft fracture in coaptation splint. Note valgus mold to prevent deformity.

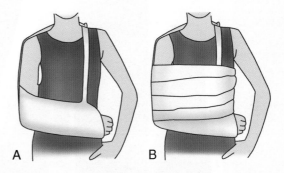

Fig 44.4 (A and B) Hanging arm cast. (With permission from Kronfol R. Splinting of musculoskeletal injuries. In: Rose BD, ed. *UpToDate*. Waltham, MA: UpToDate; 2007.)

Special Considerations

- Radial nerve palsy complicates approximately 12% of humeral shaft fracture injuries.
- Radial nerve injury occurs most commonly in middle third fractures (40-58%) versus distal third fractures (13-24%) and least common in the proximal third (3-11%).
- Distal third spiral (Holstein Lewis) fractures may have associated radial nerve palsy in approximately 18-22% of cases.
- Radial nerve palsy has been demonstrated to resolve in 70% of closed injuries without intervention, and nearly

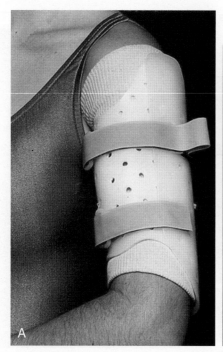

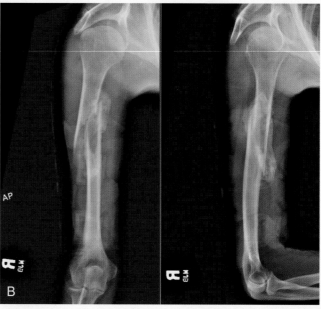

Fig 44.5 **(A)** Functional brace applied to left arm. **(B)** Well-healing humeral shaft fracture with satisfactory alignment maintained in functional brace. ([A] From Sarmiento A, Zagorski JB, Zych GA, et al. Functional bracing for the treatment of fractures of the humeral diaphysis. *J Bone Joint Surg Am*. 2000;82A:478–486, with permission from The Journal of Bone and Joint Surgery, Inc., 2000.)

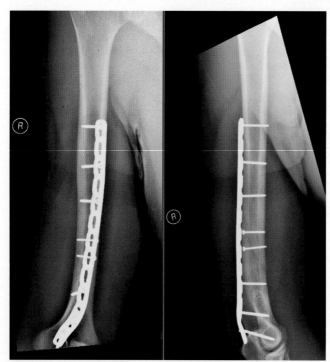

Fig 44.6 **Postoperative radiograph of plate-and-screw fixation of a well-reduced humeral shaft fracture.**

90% after delayed exploration. Early exploration does not appear to have benefit.

- Radial nerve palsy associated with open fracture in contrast has markedly poor outcomes, with less than 40% resolving without intervention. Early exploration does appear to have benefit in these cases.

- Radial nerve palsy is generally followed with detailed and graded motor and sensory exams and progression of Tinel sign over the course of the nerve.
- Timing of electromyography is controversial, but generally recommended if no signs of recovery have occurred at 6 to 12 weeks.
- Vascular injury is often a clinical diagnosis with a cold, pulseless extremity. If present, the patient should be emergently taken to the operating room, the fracture stabilized, and the brachial artery repaired in coordination with a vascular surgeon.

Suggested Readings

Attum B, Obremskey W. Treatment of humeral shaft fractures. *JBJS Rev*. 2015;3(9).

Carroll E, Schweppe M, Langfitt M, et al. Management of humeral shaft fractures. *J Am Acad Orthop Surg*. 2012;20(7):423–433.

Ekholm R, Adami J, Tidermark J, et al. Fractures of the shaft of the humerus. An epidemiological study of 401 fractures. *J Bone Joint Surg Br*. 2006;88B:1469–1473.

Gottschalk M, Carpenter W, Hiza E, et al. Humeral shaft fracture fixation: incidence rates and complications as reported by American Board of Orthopaedic Surgery Part II Candidates. *J Bone Joint Surg Am*. 2016;98(17):e71.

McKee MD, Larsson S. Humeral shaft fractures. In: Bucholz RW, Heckman JD, Court-Brown CM, Tornetta P, eds. *Rockwood and Green's Fractures in Adults*. 7th ed. Philadelphia: Lippincott; 2010:999–1038.

Sarmiento A, Zagorski JB, Zych GA, et al. Functional bracing for the treatment of fractures of the humeral diaphysis. *J Bone Joint Surg Am*. 2000;82A:478–486.

Shao YC, Harwood P, Grotz MR, et al. Radial nerve palsy associated with fractures of the shaft of the humerus, a systematic review. *J Bone Joint Surg Br*. 2005;87B:1647–1652.

Templeman DC, Sems SA. Humeral shaft fractures. In: Stannard JP, Schmidt AH, Kregor PJ, eds. *Surgical Treatment of Orthopaedic Trauma*. New York: Thieme; 2007:263–284.

Chapter 45 Scapula Fractures

Seth R. Yarboro, Michelle E. Kew

ICD-10-CM CODES
S42.11*A *Closed scapular body fracture*
S42.11*B *Open scapular body fracture*
S42.12*A *Closed acromial process fracture*
S42.12*B *Open acromial process fracture*
S42.13*A *Closed fracture of coracoid process*
S42.13*B *Open fracture of coracoid process*
S42.14*A *Closed fracture of glenoid cavity*
S42.14*B *Open fracture of glenoid cavity*
S42.10*A *Unspecified closed scapula fracture*
S42.10*B *Unspecified open scapula fracture*

Key Concepts

- Scapula fractures are a rare injury and comprise only 3-5% of shoulder girdle injuries and 0.4-1% of all fractures.
- Often seen in younger patients involved in high-energy trauma
- Associated injuries are common, especially with traumatic mechanism, leading to a delayed diagnosis of the scapular fracture
- Injuries associated with scapula fractures can include pneumothorax, pulmonary contusion, rib fractures, clavicle fracture, closed head injury, peripheral neurovascular injury (brachial plexus, brachial artery), and spinal cord injury.

History

- Usually caused by high-energy trauma, with as many as 50% resulting from motor vehicle accidents
- Mechanisms of injury and associated patterns
  - Blunt trauma to posterior chest wall: Scapular body fracture
  - Blunt trauma to shoulder: Acromion or coracoid fracture
  - Axial loading through outstretched arm: Scapular neck or intra-articular glenoid fracture
  - Glenohumeral dislocation: Glenoid rim fracture
  - Traction injuries: Avulsion fractures

Physical Examination

- Patient typically presents with the arm held adducted against the chest.
- The shoulder may have asymmetric appearance with a displaced scapular neck or acromion fractures.
- Swelling, abrasions, ecchymosis, tenderness, or crepitus over the scapular region are common.
- Painful shoulder range of motion in all directions, particularly with abduction

- Perform a complete trauma evaluation with careful assessment for associated pulmonary or neurovascular injuries

Imaging

- Multiple radiographic views are needed for accurate radiographic diagnosis of scapula fractures (Fig. 45.1).
- True anteroposterior view of shoulder (Grashey view, tangential to glenoid)
- Axillary lateral view to evaluate acromial and glenoid rim fractures; Scapular Y
- Stryker notch (45-degree cephalic tilt) to evaluate coracoid fractures
- Apical oblique view (Garth view) to evaluate anterior/inferior glenoid rim
- Standing bilateral weight-bearing views can evaluate injuries of the acromioclavicular joint and coracoclavicular ligaments
- Chest radiographs are usually obtained as part of the trauma evaluation and can identify rib fractures or other associated injuries.
- Computed tomography can be useful to aid in evaluating intra-articular glenoid or coracoid fractures, humeral head position, and associated injuries (see Fig. 45.1D and E).
- Full chest and cervical spine computed tomography scans are often performed as part of a complete multitrauma workup and may include relevant portions of the scapula.

Classification

- Scapular fractures are described by anatomic location (Zdravkovic and Damholt):
- Type I: scapular body
- Type II: apophyseal fractures, including acromion and coracoid process
- Type III: fractures of the superolateral angle, including the scapular neck and glenoid (Fig. 45.2)
- Scapular body (49-89%) and scapular neck (10-60%) fractures are the most common.

Differential Diagnosis

- Posterior rib fractures, chest wall injury
- Pleuritic pain
- Rotator cuff impingement or tear
- Scapulothoracic dysfunction
- Scapulothoracic dissociation

Nonoperative Treatment

- Treatment is often affected by treatment of associated injuries.

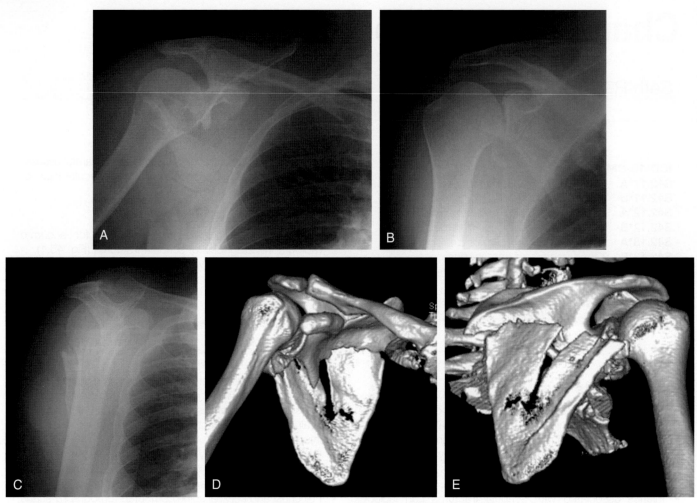

Fig 45.1 Anteroposterior (A), Grashey (B), and scapular Y (C) radiographs and three-dimensional reconstructions (D and E) of a computed tomography scan showing a scapular fracture involving the inferior glenoid.

- Most scapular fractures can be treated nonoperatively with supportive treatment for symptom relief, including a sling for comfort.
- Allow weight bearing as tolerated on the affected upper extremity with early gravity-assisted range of motion during the immediate posttrauma period
- Progressive range of motion and strengthening exercises
- Close radiographic follow-up of intra-articular fractures is required to monitor for displacement.

When to Refer

- Any patient who has an injury concerning for the previously mentioned surgical indications should be referred. Minimally displaced extra-articular scapular body fractures can be treated symptomatically and do not typically require referral.

Prognosis

- Nonunion is rare, and most fractures heal within 6 weeks.
- Uncomplicated scapula fractures have an excellent prognosis, though full functional recovery may take several months.

Operative Treatment

- General indications for surgical treatment
  - More than 25% of the glenoid articular surface
  - More than 10-mm displacement of articular fragment
  - More than 5-mm articular step-off
  - More than 40 degrees of angulation of scapular neck
  - Floating shoulder with concomitant clavicle and/or humeral fractures
  - Subacromial space impingement
  - Symptomatic nonunion/malunion
- The usual treatment involves open versus arthroscopic reduction and fixation with screws ± plates.
- Nonoperative management of comminuted intra-articular fractures is considered if the humeral head remains centered on the glenoid.
- Early gravity-assisted range of motion treatment may improve fracture alignment and overall outcome.

Troubleshooting

- Incomplete imaging is the most common diagnostic pitfall.

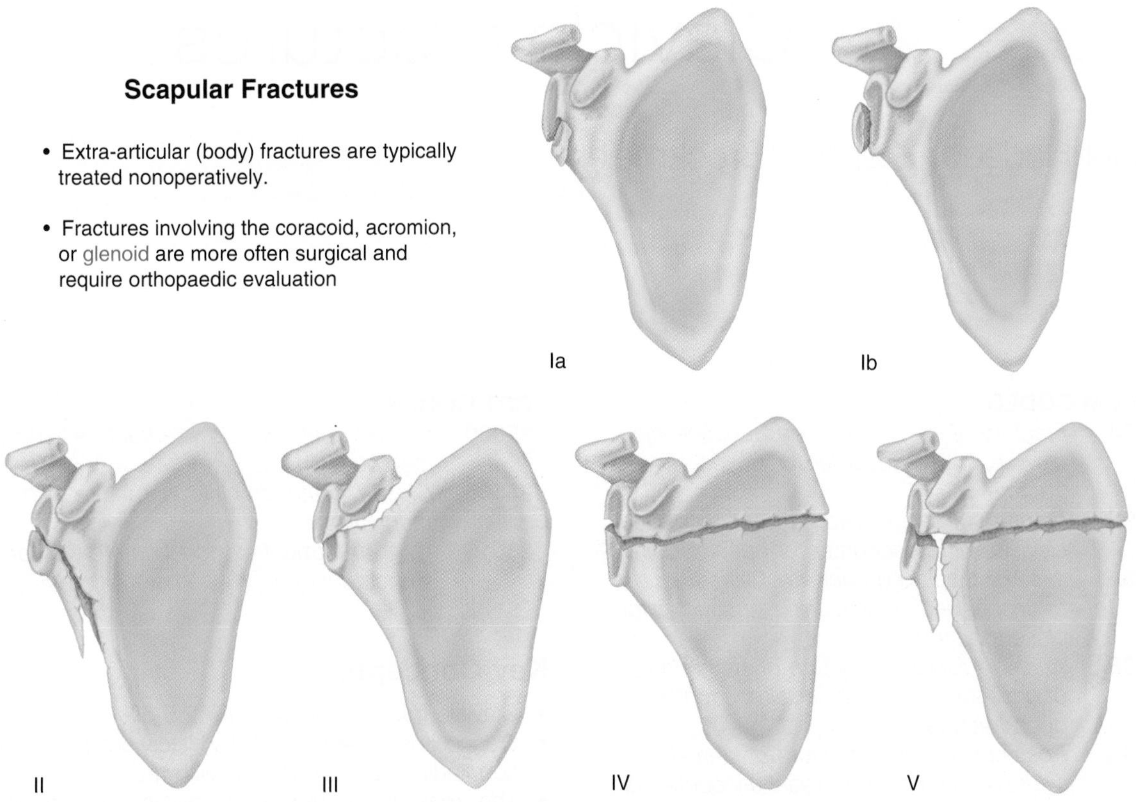

Scapular Fractures

- Extra-articular (body) fractures are typically treated nonoperatively.

- Fractures involving the coracoid, acromion, or glenoid are more often surgical and require orthopaedic evaluation

Ideberg classification of scapular fractures involving the glenoid

Fig 45.2 Overview of scapula fractures involving the glenoid.

- Os acromiale: Rounded, unfused apophysis that can resemble an acromial fracture is present in 2.7% of adults
- Glenoid hypoplasia can resemble an impaction fracture of the glenoid and is often associated with an acromial or humeral head abnormality.
- Pseudorupture of the rotator cuff will present with painful intramuscular swelling, rotator cuff weakness, and loss of active arm elevation; usually resolves within several weeks.

Patient Instructions

- Remind patients that use of a sling is for comfort only and encourage daily use of the upper extremity out of the sling as pain permits.
- Reinforce the importance of early range of motion therapy to prevent shoulder/elbow stiffness and loss of function.

Considerations in Special Populations

- Patients with high-energy mechanisms should receive a complete trauma evaluation to assess for associated injuries.

- Patients with low-energy mechanisms usually have scapula fracture patterns that are amenable to nonoperative treatment.

Suggested Readings

Bartonicek J. Scapular fractures. In: Bucholz RW, Heckman JD, Court-Brown CM, eds. *Rockwood and Green's Fractures in Adults*. 8th ed. Philadelphia: Wolters Kluwer; 2015:1475–1502.

Cole P, Gauger E, Schroder L. Management of scapula fractures. *J Am Acad Orthop Surg*. 2012;130–141.

DeFranco MJ, Patterson BM. The floating shoulder. *J Am Acad Orthop Surg*. 2006;14:499–509.

Goss TP. Fractures of the glenoid cavity. *J Bone Joint Surg Am*. 1992;74A:299–305.

Goss TP. Scapular fractures and dislocations: diagnosis and treatment. *J Am Acad Orthop Surg*. 1995;3:22–33.

Zdravkovic D, Damholt VV. Comminuted and severely displaced fractures of the scapula. *Acta Orthop Scand*. 1974;45(1):60–65.

Zlowodzki M, Bhandari M, Zelle BA, et al. Treatment of scapula fractures: systematic review of 520 fractures in 22 case series. *J Orthop Trauma*. 2006;20:230–233.

Chapter 46 Clavicle Fractures

Michael Hadeed, Stephen Brockmeier

ICD-10-CM CODES

S42.009A *Fracture of unspecified part of unspecified clavicle, initial encounter for closed fracture*

S42.009B *Fracture of unspecified part of unspecified clavicle, initial encounter for open fracture*

S42.013A *Anterior displaced fracture of sternal end of unspecified clavicle, initial encounter for closed fracture*

S42.013B *Anterior displaced fracture of sternal end of unspecified clavicle, initial encounter for open fracture*

S42.016A *Posterior displaced fracture of sternal end of unspecified clavicle, initial encounter for closed fracture*

S42.016B *Posterior displaced fracture of sternal end of unspecified clavicle, initial encounter for open fracture*

S42.019A *Nondisplaced fracture of sternal end of unspecified clavicle, initial encounter for closed fracture*

S42.019B *Nondisplaced fracture of sternal end of unspecified clavicle, initial encounter for open fracture*

S42.023A *Displaced fracture of shaft of unspecified clavicle, initial encounter for closed fracture*

S42.023B *Displaced fracture of shaft of unspecified clavicle, initial encounter for open fracture*

S42.026A *Nondisplaced fracture of the shaft of unspecified clavicle, initial encounter for closed fracture*

S42.026B *Nondisplaced fracture of the shaft of unspecified clavicle, initial encounter for open fracture*

S42.033A *Displaced fracture of lateral end of unspecified clavicle, initial encounter for closed fracture*

S42.033B *Displaced fracture of lateral end of unspecified clavicle, initial encounter for open fracture*

S42.036.A *Nondisplaced fracture of lateral end of unspecified clavicle, initial encounter for closed fracture*

S42.036.B *Nondisplaced fracture of lateral end of unspecified clavicle, initial encounter for open fracture*

CPT CODES

25000 *Closed treatment clavicle fracture without manipulation*

23505 *Closed treatment clavicle fracture with manipulation*

23515 *Open treatment clavicle fracture with or without internal or external fixation*

Key Concepts

- Clavicle fractures account for 2.5-5% of all fractures.
- Diagnosis is generally made by history and physical examination findings and confirmed with radiographs.
- The majority of clavicle fractures are appropriate for nonoperative treatment.
- Nonunion and symptomatic malunion were thought to be rare, but recent studies show rates to be higher than historically suspected, and operative treatment is becoming more common.
- If there is significant displacement or severe concomitant injury, operative intervention should be considered.

Function of the Clavicle

- Protects underlying brachial plexus, subclavian vessels, and apical pleura
- Provides the only bony link between the upper extremity and the axial skeleton
  - *Strut function*: It acts as a strut, preventing medial migration of the shoulder girdle, thus allowing the thoracohumeral muscles to maintain their optimal working length.
  - *Suspensory function*: With help from the trapezius muscle, the clavicle stabilizes the shoulder girdle against inferior displacement.

Classification of Fractures

- The most important features when determining treatment recommendations are the location, amount of comminution, shortening, and displacement (Fig. 46.1)
- Several systems exist, but the most commonly used is the Allman classification with subdivision by Neer and Craig
  - Group I: fracture of the middle third (70-80%)
  - Nondisplaced: less than 100% displacement
  - Displaced: at least 100% displacement
  - Group II: fracture of the distal third (10-20%)

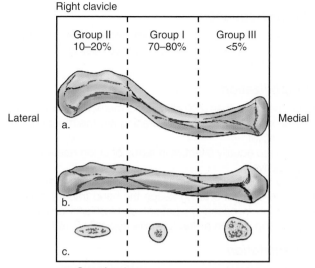

Right clavicle

| Group II 10–20% | Group I 70–80% | Group III <5% |

Lateral

Medial

a.

b.

c.

a. Superior view
b. Frontal view
c. Cross sections

Fig 46.1 Osteology and classification of clavicle fractures. The S-shaped bone resembles its namesake, the musical symbol the clavicula. The junction of the middle and lateral thirds is the thinnest portion of the bone and is the only section of bone not reinforced by muscular or ligamentous attachments. This explains why group I fractures are the most common. Group II fractures involve the lateral third. Group III fractures involve the medial third. (Modified with permission from Rockwood CA, Matsen FA, Wirth MA, et al. eds. *The Shoulder*. 5th ed. Philadelphia: Elsevier; 2017.)

- Type I: fracture is lateral to the coracoclavicular ligaments, and at least one of those ligaments remains intact; expect minimal displacement (STABLE)
- Type II:
- A: fracture is medial to the coracoclavicular ligaments and the ligaments are intact; expect significant medial displacement (UNSTABLE)
- B: either between or lateral to the coracoclavicular (CC) ligaments where the ligaments on the medial fragment are torn; expect medial displacement (UNSTABLE)
- Type III: intra-articular extension into acromioclavicular joint, CC ligaments are intact; expect minimal displacement (STABLE)
- Type IV: physeal fracture in the skeletally immature, ligaments are intact (STABLE)
- Type V: comminuted, with ligaments attached neither medially nor laterally, but rather to an inferior fragment of comminution; expect displacement (USUALLY UNSTABLE)
- Group III: fracture of the proximal third (<5%)

Fracture Biomechanics: Deforming Forces

- Medial segment
  - Displaced superiorly by sternocleidomastoid muscle
  - Displaced superiorly and posteriorly by trapezius muscle

- Lateral segment
  - Displaced anteriorly and rotated inferiorly by the weight of the arm
  - Displaced medially by the pectoralis major and latissimus dorsi muscles (acting through the humerus)
- Result of these forces is often shortening and overriding of segments

History

- Approximately 90% of the time, the clavicle fails in axial loading from blows to the point of the shoulder.
- Common mechanisms include motor vehicle collisions, falls from height, and sports injuries.
- Blunt or penetrating trauma along the shaft of the bone accounts for approximately 7% of clavicle fractures (i.e., seatbelt, lacrosse or hockey stick, blunt weapon, gunshot).
- Medial fractures are usually the result of high-energy mechanisms, are often accompanied by significant multisystem trauma, have a high associated mortality rate (from other injuries), and predominate in males.

Physical Examination

- Physical exam findings at the fracture site, which would indicate operative management include skin tenting, skin puckering, skin blanching, and an open fracture.
- A complete physical exam should be completed to include a distal neurovascular exam.
- Look for visible or palpable deformity; tenting of the skin; localized swelling, ecchymosis, abrasions, or tenderness; relative droop or shortening of the shoulder; scapular protraction; and motion or crepitus at the fracture site.
- Include peripheral pulses, distal motor strength, and sensation testing.
- A complete secondary survey should be performed in the setting of high-energy trauma. Examine for signs and symptoms of commonly associated injuries such as brachial plexopathy, hemothorax, pneumothorax, neurovascular injury, rib fractures, and scapular neck and body fractures.

Imaging

- Upright anteroposterior view of the shoulder and the clavicle (Fig. 46.2)
  - It is critical that the radiograph be taken with the patient upright before management decisions are finalized because this will often reveal increased displacement from supine imaging
- Cephalad and/or caudal oblique views can help to bring the image of the clavicle away from the thoracic cage
  - Serendipity view, 40-degree cephalic tilt
- Anteroposterior view of contralateral clavicle can help to assess relative length to evaluate shortening
- Axillary view or Zanca 15-degree oblique view of the shoulder can help to assess acromioclavicular joint involvement

Additional Tests

- Computed tomography scans can be helpful to provide detail in cases involving comminution, possible articular

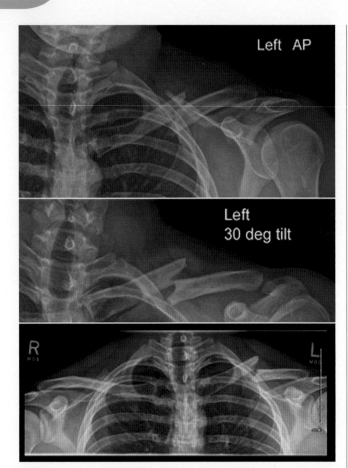

Fig 46.2 Midshaft clavicle fracture. *Top,* Note that on an antero-posterior *(AP)* view, the ipsilateral upper lung field, acromioclavicular joint, and sternoclavicular joint is visualized, but the fracture site is partially obscured by the rib cage and scapula. *Middle,* A cephalic tilt view brings the shadow of the clavicle fragments away from the rib cage and scapula, allowing a better view of the fracture pattern. *Bottom,* Anteroposterior view of both clavicles allows for measurement of relative shortening of the injured clavicle. Note the superiorly displaced medial fragment, inferiorly displaced lateral fragment, and overall shortening.

extension, medial fractures, and high-energy injury to the thorax
- Chest radiograph if pneumothorax is suspected
- Angiography if vascular injury is suspected

Differential Diagnosis
- The clavicle is the first bone to ossify (5th to 6th week of gestation) and the last bone to fuse (20 to 25 years); for young adults, physeal injuries must be considered
- Lateral third fracture: acromioclavicular separation
- Medial third fracture: sternoclavicular dislocation

Treatment
Goals
- Restoration of preinjury shoulder strength and motion
- Elimination of pain
- Minimization of deformity

Closed Reduction
- Closed reduction before immobilization is uncommon and has not been shown to improve healing or long-term alignment.

Immobilization
- Of the more than 200 described methods, sling immobilization and figure-of-eight bracing are the most common (Fig. 46.3).
- They are equally effective in terms of union rate and speed of recovery.
- Sling scores higher in patient comfort and satisfaction
- Figure-of-eight bracing keeps the hand free for activity.
- Duration is based on patient comfort and resolution of pain and motion at fracture site (typically 2 to 6 weeks).

Rehabilitation
- Usually simple home-based stretching exercises are sufficient after immobilization (or operative fixation); some cases may require formal physical therapy.
- Overhead activity should be avoided for 4 to 6 weeks to limit rotational stress on the fracture site during healing.
- Light duty work may begin when the patient is able to participate comfortably, depending on the job.
- Heavy labor and athletics may begin after radiographic and clinical union, anywhere from 6 to 12 weeks.

Operative Indications (Fig. 46.4)
- The majority are minimally displaced or nondisplaced and are treated successfully with immobilization (see Fig. 46.2)
- The decision to pursue operative intervention should be between both the surgeon and the patient and should include a thorough risk/benefit analysis of all treatment options
- Absolute surgical indications include an open fracture, concern for the overlying skin (tenting, blanching, puckering)
- Indications by fracture pattern
  - Middle third (most common)
    - Displacement >100%
    - Shortening >1.5 cm
    - Z fracture pattern
    - Significant fracture comminution
    - Special populations (see later)
  - Lateral third
    - Type IIA, type IIB, and most type V are operative (refer to previous explanations)
  - Medial third
    - Symptomatic malunion or nonunion

Surgical Complications
- Malunion, where the bone heals in a nonanatomic position
- Nonunion, where the bone does not heal; if symptomatic, can be treated with repeat open reduction and internal fixation
- Symptomatic hardware, particularly in thin individuals; often this is treated with removal of the hardware
- Infection, often treated with removal of hardware and irrigation and debridement, as well as a course of antibiotics

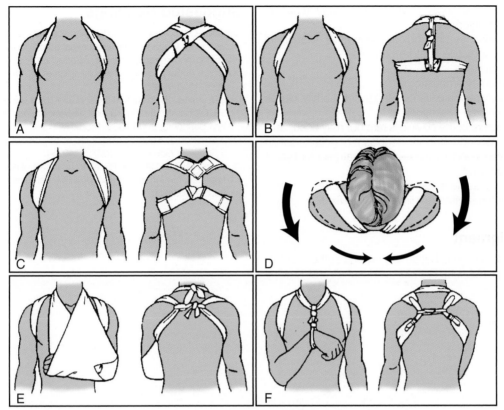

Fig 46.3 Midshaft clavicle fracture. Simple sling (not pictured) and figure-of-eight bracing are designed to maintain closed reduction of clavicle fractures. More than 200 combinations of sling and/or braces have been described. **(A)** Padded stockinette fastened with safety pins. **(B)** Stockinette not crossed in the back but secured with a second piece of stockinette that can be tightened daily to help maintain reduction. **(C)** Commercially available figure-of-eight brace. **(D)** The shoulders are pulled up and backward by the figure-of-eight brace, helping to maintain reduction. **(E)** A figure-of-eight brace with sling. **(F)** Figure-of-eight brace with cuff and collar. (Modified with permission from Rockwood CA, Matsen FA, Wirth MA, Lippitt SB, eds. *The Shoulder*. 3rd ed. Philadelphia: Saunders; 2004.)

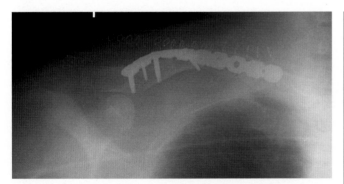

Fig 46.4 Open reduction with internal fixation using a clavicle plate. The plate is contoured to fit the shape of the clavicle.

When To Refer

- Group II or III fractures (far medial or far lateral)
- High-energy trauma or multiple additional injuries
- Group I fractures with possible surgical indications
- Nonunion or symptomatic malunion of fracture with closed treatment

Troubleshooting

- The overall nonunion rate for all clavicle fractures is approximately 7% for closed treatment, but increases to 15% or more with significant shortening, displacement, and comminution.
- Nonunion requires surgical referral.
- Malunion, if symptomatic with pain or functional disability, also merits referral.

Patient Instructions

- If nonoperative treatment is chosen, patients will be non-weightbearing in a sling for at least 4 to 6 weeks.
- Warn patients undergoing closed treatment to expect mild discomfort for as long as 3 months and some degree of permanent cosmetic deformity.

Considerations in Special Populations

- Children: Nearly all clavicular fractures in children are treated nonoperatively and heal with excellent results, even with poor patient compliance. Physeal injury may result in growth-related deformity.

- Certain populations may indicate operative fixation in traditional nonoperative fracture patterns.
  - Overhead athletes
  - Upper extremity ambulators
  - including polytrauma patients with lower extremity injuries
  - Contact athletes in season
- Pathologic fracture of the clavicle is rare but may occur as a result of a primary or metastatic neoplasm or postirradiation osteitis in patients undergoing radiation treatment for breast or neck carcinomas.
  - The medial clavicle is the most common site.
  - These fractures often require operative fixation.

Acknowledgment

We acknowledge the contribution of previous authors of this chapter: James H. Rubright, Brandon D. Bushnell, and Timothy N. Taft.

Suggested Readings

Canadian Orthopaedic Trauma Society. Nonoperative treatment compared with plate fixation of displaced midshaft clavicular fractures. A multicenter, randomized clinical trial. *J Bone Joint Surg Am*. 2007;89A:1–10.

Jeray KJ. Acute midshaft clavicular fracture. *J Am Acad Orthop Surg*. 2007;15:239–248.

Ring D, Jupiter JB. Injuries to the shoulder girdle. In: Browner BD, Jupiter JB, Levine AM, Trafton PG, eds. *Skeletal Trauma*. 3rd ed. Philadelphia: WB Saunders; 2003:1633–1653.

Throckmorton T, Kuhn JE. Fractures of the medial end of the clavicle. *J Shoulder Elbow Surg*. 2007;16:49–54.

Zlowodzki M, Zelle BA, Cole PA, et al. Treatment of acute midshaft clavicle fractures: systematic review of 2144 fractures. *J Orthop Trauma*. 2005;19:504–507.

Chapter 47 Anterior Shoulder Relocation Technique

Victor Anciano Granadillo, Stephen Brockmeier

ICD-10-CM CODES
S43.004 *Unspecified dislocation of right shoulder*
S43.005 *Unspecified dislocation of left shoulder joint*
S43.014 *Anterior dislocation of right humerus*
S43.015 *Anterior dislocation of left humerus*

CPT CODES
23650 *Closed treatment with manipulation of shoulder dislocation not requiring anesthesia*
23655 *Closed treatment with manipulation of shoulder dislocation requiring anesthesia*

Key Concepts

- Most commonly dislocated joint (45% of all joint dislocations)
- Ninety-seven percent of shoulder dislocations are anterior
- **T**raumatic **U**nilateral dislocations with a **B**ankart lesion requiring **S**urgery (TUBS) are common in anterior dislocations.
- High recurrence rate in teenagers and adults in their 20s (80-90%)
- Multiple associated injuries: labral and cartilage injuries (e.g., Bankart lesions), bony defects or fractures (e.g., Hill Sachs lesions, fractures of lesser and greater tuberosities), injury to axillary nerve, or rotator cuff injuries
- Multiple methods for closed reduction

History

- The majority of dislocations are trauma related, with sports injuries being the most prevalent.
- Anterior dislocation often results from the arm being forced into a position of abduction, external rotation, and extension.
- Posterior dislocation often results from a posteriorly directed blow with the arm in flexion and adduction.

Imaging

- Orthogonal views, usually an anteroposterior view of the shoulder (Grashey view) and a lateral axillary view, can help make the diagnosis (Fig. 47.1).
- If a patient cannot tolerate axillary view, Velpeau view can be a more comfortable alternative to evaluate shoulder dislocation (Fig. 47.2).
- Postreduction radiographs confirm the anatomic reduction and are critical in the evaluation of associated fractures or other bony abnormalities.

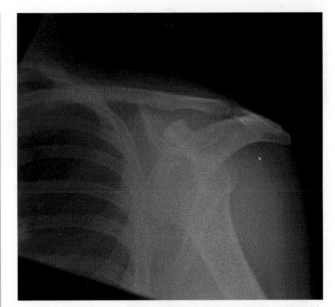

Fig 47.1 Anteroposterior radiograph of an anterior shoulder dislocation.

Anesthesia

- Reduction after intravenous sedation is the most common approach; however, this requires assistance by additional personnel to monitor airway and anesthesia.
- Intra-articular local anesthesia is also an option and has been found to shorten the emergency department stay and reduce complications with no change in success rates relative to intravenous sedation.
- Using 20 mL of 1% lidocaine or 4 mg/kg of 1% lidocaine is sufficient for adequate analgesia.
- Success without anesthesia has been advocated and documented by many authors, but patience is paramount when relying on time rather than medication to relax the patient and his or her muscles.

Reduction

There are many described reduction techniques with documented levels of success; however, no studies have provided sufficient evidence to establish a preferred method. The care provider should be familiar with many different options and apply them as appropriate in each individual case situation (Fig. 47.3).

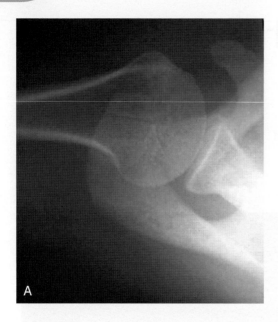

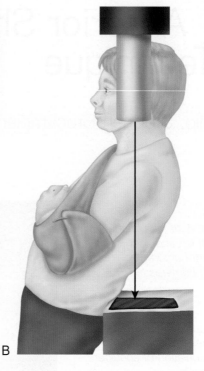

Fig 47.2 (A) X-ray of Velpeau view of shoulder. (B) Positioning of the patient for a Velpeau view.

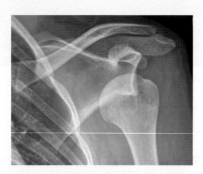

AP view of anterior shoulder dislocation

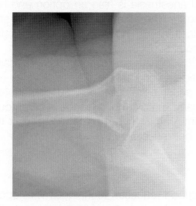

Axillary view of anterior shoulder dislocation

- Anterior shoulder dislocation is most common form of shoulder dislocation

- High recurrence rate in younger patients

- Conscious sedation vs. intra-articular analgesia are both viable options for reduction

- Multiple reduction techniques available.
  - Traction-counter traction
  - Kocher (Ext. Rot. + Flexion)
  - Milch (Abd + Ext Rot.)
  - External Rot. technique
  - Scapular manipulation technique

- Immobilize in adduction and internal rotation in sling post reduction.

- Refer to Orthopaedic Surgeon for evaluation

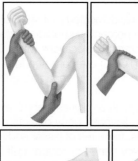
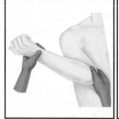
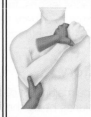

Kocher technique

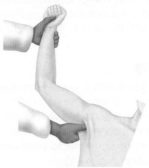

Milch technique

Fig 47.3 Anterior shoulder relocation pearls.

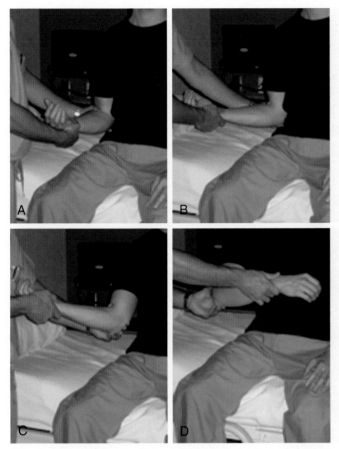

Fig 47.4 **(A)** Start with adduction at the shoulder and elbow flexion. **(B)** Externally rotate the arm at the shoulder. **(C)** Flex the arm forward at the shoulder until resistance is felt. **(D)** Internally rotate the arm at the shoulder.

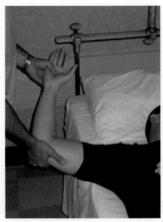

Fig 47.5 The shoulder approaches the zero position at 165 degrees of abduction, 45 degrees of forward flexion, and 90 degrees of external rotation.

- Traction, counter-traction methods
  - Traction on the arm with concurrent counter-traction on the rib cage has been established since the time of Hippocrates as a method of relocation.
  - Care should be taken to avoid too much pressure on vital neurovascular structures in the axillary recess.
  - Use of a partner providing counter-traction with a sheet wrapped around patient's rib cage is recommended instead of examiner's foot to diminish risk of damage to neurovascular structures.
- Kocher method
  - Often preferable in heavier patients, in patients older than the age of 40 years, and in dislocations older than 4 hours (Fig. 47.4)
  - Begin with arm adducted at shoulder.
    - Flex elbow to 90 degrees.
    - Externally rotate arm until resistance is felt.
    - Forward flex arm at shoulder as far as possible.
    - Internally rotate at shoulder for relocation.
- Milch method
  - May be performed with patient supine or prone. Involves abduction and external rotation of the shoulder.
  - Zero position maxim: At the zero position of 165 degrees of abduction, 45 degrees of forward flexion, and 90 degrees of external rotation, the scapula-humeral axis

and the rotator cuff axis align, which transforms any muscular pull of the rotator cuff into an axial pull favoring reduction.
- Supine
  - Slowly abduct the arm at the shoulder to a goal of 165 degrees.
  - While abducting the arm, externally rotate it.
  - At the zero position, the cuff muscles will be relaxed (Fig. 47.5).
  - The humeral head can be pushed gently back over the glenoid rim.
- Prone (better for patient relaxation and surgeon control of arm) (Fig. 47.6)
  - Position the patient lying prone with the affected arm hanging down.
  - Allow the patient time to relax, allowing the arm to swing freely. Some will spontaneously reduce at this point.
  - Flex the elbow to 90 degrees slowly, allowing adequate time for patient comfort. This relaxes the long head of the biceps muscle, preventing it from impeding reduction.
  - Place the patient's hand over the dorsal forearm of the care provider and grasp the elbow with the ipsilateral hand. Longitudinal traction may be gently applied at the arm with the care provider's contralateral hand.
  - Slowly abduct the patient's arm at the shoulder and concurrently externally rotate it.
  - A final lift over the rim of the glenoid may be necessary.
- Scapular manipulation method
  - Position the patient lying prone with the affected arm hanging free.
  - Apply traction weights to the affected arm and allow time for the patient's muscles to relax. Some will spontaneously reduce at this point. This maneuver of reduction without scapular manipulation is known as Stimson technique.
  - Grasp the superior-medial border of the scapula with one hand and with the other hand push the inferior tip of the scapula inferiorly and medially, creating a pivot

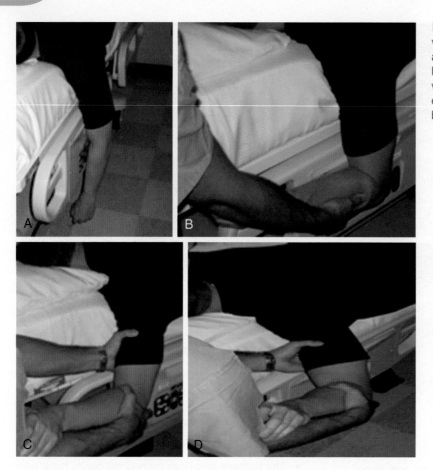

Fig 47.6 **(A)** Place the patient in a prone position with the affected arm hanging. **(B)** Slowly flex at the elbow to 90 degrees. **(C)** Grasp with one hand at the elbow while pulling with gentle traction with the other hand. **(D)** Abduct the arm and externally rotate it. A final lift into the glenoid may be necessary.

point at the superior-medial border. Reduction should occur at this point.

- External rotation technique
  - Success rate close to 80%
  - Patient is in supine position with the arm in adduction and neutral rotation.
  - The examiner flexes the elbow to 90 degrees. The examiner holds the elbow with one hand maintaining adduction and wrist with other hand.
  - Gentle, slow external rotation is applied at the wrist maintaining adduction.
  - Examiner may need to stop several times to allow patient's pain to decrease and muscles to fatigue. The examiner should not be applying significant force in external rotation.
  - Maneuver may require 5 to 10 minutes as patient's muscles fatigue and arm reaches the coronal plane.

Postreduction Immobilization

- Immobilization in adduction and internal rotation with a simple sling for 3 to 5 weeks followed by rehabilitation with physical therapy is commonly used.
- Recent data suggest that immobilization in slight abduction and external rotation with a "gunslinger"-type brace improves healing by tightening the anterior capsule and ligament support of the joint. This position is often not as well tolerated by patients.

- Return to heavy-duty work and athletics is permissible when the patient has regained full motion and strength relative to the uninjured side.

Recurrence

- Recurrence rates range from 30% to 100% after a primary dislocation.
- Younger male patients aged 15 to 35 years are at highest risk of recurrence.
- Be aware of recurrence in a small population of malingering patients. These patients may have secondary gains such work compensation claims or disability insurance.
- Older patients have a higher risk of associated rotator cuff tear.
- Open or arthroscopic surgery can decrease the risk of recurrence and a greater rate of return to play at preinjury level for athletes. Referral to an orthopaedic surgeon after initial successful reduction is mandatory.

Suggested Readings

Dala-Ali B, Penna M, McConnell J, et al. Management of acute anterior shoulder dislocation. *Br J Sports Med*. 2014;48(16):1209–1215.

Ianlenti MN, Mulvihill JD, Feinstein M, et al. Return to play following shoulder stabilization: a systematic review and meta-analysis. *Orthop J Sports Med*. 2017;5(9):2325967117726055.

Itoi E, Hatakeyama Y, Sato T, et al. Immobilization in external rotation after shoulder dislocation reduces the risk of recurrence. A randomized controlled trial. *J Bone Joint Surg Am*. 2007;89A:2124–2131.

Kuhn J. Treating the initial anterior shoulder dislocation: an evidence-based medicine approach. *Sports Med Arthrosc Rev*. 2006;14:192–198.

Marinelli M, de Palma L. The external rotation method for reduction of acute anterior shoulder dislocations. *J Orthop Traumatol*. 2009;10(1):17–20.

O'Connor D, Schwarze D, Fragomen A, Perdomo M. Painless reduction of acute anterior shoulder dislocations without anesthesia. *Orthopedics*. 2006;29:528–532.

Robinson M, Howes J, Murdoch H, et al. Functional outcome and risk of recurrent instability after primary anterior shoulder dislocation in young patients. *J Bone Joint Surg Am*. 2006;88A:2326–2336.

Youm T, Takemoto R, Park BK. Acute management of shoulder dislocations. *J Am Acad Orthop Surg*. 2014;12:761–771.

Chapter 48 Glenohumeral Joint Injection

Kelley Anderson, Joel Himes, Melissa McLane

CPT CODES
20610 *Aspiration and/or injection, large joint without ultrasound*
20611 *Aspiration and/or injection, large joint with ultrasound*

Equipment

- Sterile preparation: povidone-iodine, alcohol, chlorhexidine.
- Sterile gloves, sterile drapes, sterile ultrasound cover.
- Anesthetic agent: consider using skin pretreatment such as ethyl chloride during injection, lidocaine (1% or 2%), or bupivacaine (0.25% or 0.5%), which do not contain *p*-aminobenzoic acid (PABA), leading to fewer allergic reactions.
- Injection: syringe 10 to 20 mL, needle 20 to 22 gauge (1.5 inches or longer).
- Aspiration: syringe 20 mL or larger, needle 18 gauge (1.5 inches or longer).
- Steroids such as betamethasone, triamcinolone, methylprednisolone, and dexamethasone may be used as a single agent or in combination.
- Sterile gauze.
- Bandage.

Indications

- Injection
  - Osteoarthritis
  - Rheumatoid arthritis
  - Adhesive capsulitis
  - Internal impingement
  - Labral tears
  - Unknown diagnosis (diagnostic injection)
- Aspiration
  - Septic arthritis
  - Crystalline arthritis (gout, pseudogout)
  - Symptomatic effusion
  - Unknown diagnosis (diagnostic aspiration)

Contraindications

- Systemic sepsis
- Active cellulitis or overlying skin pathology
- Active osteomyelitis in the shoulder area
- Uncontrolled coagulopathy
- Allergy to anesthetic agents or injection agents
- Pregnancy (injection of steroid medications)

Technique (Video 48.1)

- The glenohumeral joint can be accessed through two approaches: anterior or posterior.
- Patient may be in a seated upright position with the arm in a neutral position resting in the lap or lateral recumbent/semiprone position with the affected shoulder up, forward flexed, and slightly internally rotated resting on a pillow.
- Anatomic landmarks for injection are identified and marked; if available, ultrasound may be used to identify the glenoid, humeral head, and glenohumeral joint space.
  - Anterior injection landmarks: coracoid process and humeral head.
  - Posterior injection landmarks: acromion and humeral head.
- The skin over the injection site is then cleaned with a sterile preparation technique.
- If desired, the injection site may be treated with ethyl chloride during initial needle advancement to aid in pain control.
- Using sterile precautions, a short-acting, local anesthetic is introduced subcutaneously. First creating a wheal and then advancing the needle and syringe on the planned track of injection (25 gauge, 1.5 inch or smaller, 5 mL or smaller).
- If injection only is performed, a needle and syringe (20 to 22 gauge, 1.5 inches or longer, 10 to 20 mL) are loaded with chosen medication(s). If aspiration only is performed, a larger-bore needle and syringe are used (18 gauge, 1.5 inches or longer, 20 mL or larger).
- Posterior approach: preferred approach with ultrasound.
  - Ultrasound guided: The patient should be in the semiprone/lateral recumbent position with affected shoulder up and facing the physician (Fig. 48.1). Position the probe in the long axis to the infraspinatus tendon. Then advance the needle in the long axis from superior-lateral to inferior-medial until the needle is visualized between the free edge of the labrum and the cartilage of the humeral head, deep to the infraspinatus tendon (Fig. 48.2).
  - Non-ultrasound guided: The patient should be placed in the seated upright position. The needle is inserted at a point 2 cm inferior and 1 cm medial to the posterolateral corner of the acromion (Fig. 48.3). The needle is then directed anterior-medial toward the coracoid process

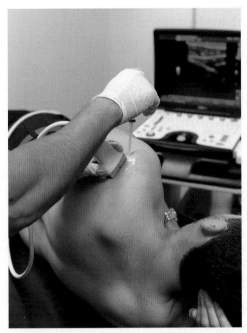

Fig 48.1 Posterior approach with ultrasound guidance: demonstrating a long-axis view of infraspinatus tendon and direction of needle advancement.

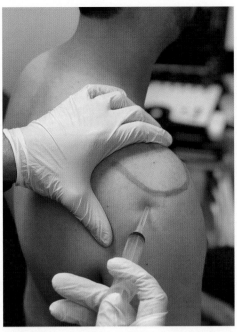

Fig 48.3 Posterior approach without ultrasound guidance: demonstrating the bony landmark of the posterior lateral acromion and direction of needle advancement toward the ipsilateral coracoid process.

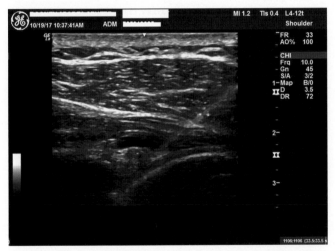

Fig 48.2 Posterior approach with ultrasound guidance demonstrating the glenoid, humeral head, labrum and visualization of the needle inferior to the infraspinatus in the glenohumeral joint space.

until the joint capsule is encountered. The index finger of the free hand may be used to palpate the coracoid process to assist with needle direction.

- Anterior approach
  - Ultrasound guided: The patient should be in the seated upright position. Position the probe in short axis view of the subscapularis. Then advance the needle in the long axis from lateral to medial until the needle is visualized between the labrum and insertion of the subscapularis tendon.
  - Non-ultrasound guided: The patient should be in the seated upright position. The needle is inserted at a point midway

between the coracoid process and the anterolateral corner of the acromion (Fig. 48.4). The needle is then directed posteriorly in a plane perpendicular to the body until the joint capsule is encountered.

- Prior to injection, gentle aspiration should be performed to confirm entry into the joint space rather than a vessel.
- Injection of the medication(s) should proceed with slow consistent pressure and readily flow into the joint space. If increased resistance is met, quickly reevaluate the location of the needle.
- After injection or aspiration, a small bandage is applied.
- Any intra-articular specimens are appropriately handled and sent to the laboratory for further evaluation.
- All materials are then properly disposed of.

Special Considerations

- If using ultrasound, it is important to prescan and mark locations with a sterile pen to assist in visualizing injection site/landmarks.
- Care should be taken when using an anterior approach, to avoid injury to the brachial plexus or axillary artery (using ultrasound will decrease these risks).
- Needle size should be dependent on patient size; larger patients will likely require longer needles (consider using a spinal needle).
- Many clinicians recommend at least a 3-month interval between steroid injections.
- Some patients may experience a vasovagal reaction from the injection, and care should be taken to allow patients feeling light-headed or dizzy to lie down for several moments, as needed.

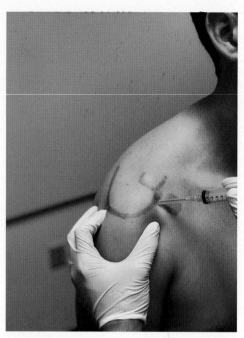

Fig 48.4 Anterior approach: demonstrating the bony landmarks of the anterior-lateral acromion and coracoid process and direction of needle advancement perpendicular to the body.

Complications

- Systemic effects of steroids such as hyperglycemia
- Tendon weakening or rupture
- Fat atrophy
- Muscle wasting
- Skin pigmentation changes
- Septic arthritis
- Nerve and vessel damage
- Steroid flare
- Steroid arthropathy

Patient Instructions

- The bandage may be removed within a few hours after aspiration or injection.
- Some soreness is expected for approximately 24 to 48 hours and may be addressed with ice, nonsteroidal antiinflammatory drugs, and/or acetaminophen.
- The postinjection site should not be submerged under water for 24 to 48 hours (e.g., hot tub, swimming pool, bath tubs).
- Observe relative rest from strenuous and repetitive maneuvers with the shoulder over the next 48 to 72 hours.
- Monitor the injection site for any redness, warmth, increased swelling, increase in pain, or development of systemic fever and/or chills.
- Diabetic patients should closely monitor blood glucose levels after injection of steroid medications and expect elevated levels for several days, which may require medical correction.

Suggested Readings

Chen CP, Lew HL, Hsu CC. Ultrasound-guided glenohumeral joint injection using the posterior approach. *Am J Phys Med Rehabil*. 2015;94(12):e117–e118.

DeLee JC, Drez D Jr, Miller MD, Thompson SR (eds): *DeLee and Drez's Orthopaedic Sports Medicine*, 2nd 4th ed. Philadelphia: Saunders Elsevier, 2015.

Dickson J. Shoulder injections in primary care. *Practitioner*. 2000;244: 259–265.

Gross C, Dhawan A, Harwood D, et al. Glenohumeral joint injections: a review. *Sports Health*. 2013;5(2):153–159.

Kerlan RK, Glousman RE. Injections and techniques in athletic medicine. *Clin Sports Med*. 1989;8:541–560.

Saunders S, Longworth S: *Injection Techniques in Orthopaedics and Sports Medicine*, 3rd ed. New York: Churchill Livingstone, 2006.

Tallia AF, Cardone DA. Diagnostic and therapeutic injection of the shoulder region. *Am Fam Physician*. 2003;67:1271–1278.

Zwar RB, Read JW, Noakes JB. Sonographically guided glenohumeral joint injection. *AJR Am J Roentgenol*. 2004;183:48–50.

Chapter 49 Subacromial Injection

Jeanne Doperak, Shane Hennessy

Equipment

- Choice of materials and exact procedure will vary by situation depending on indications for the procedure, patient/provider preferences, and materials available for use.
  - Sterile preparation solution: povidone-iodine, alcohol, chlorhexidine, others
  - Gloves: Sterile or standard
  - Skin pretreatments (optional): ethyl chloride (cold spray) or lidocaine cream
  - Aspiration needle and syringe: 18 or 16 gauge, 1.5 inch or larger, and 20 mL or larger
  - Injection needle and syringe: 20 to 22 gauge, 1.5 inch or larger, and 10 to 20 mL
  - Injection agent: Cocktail of corticosteroid (betamethasone, triamcinolone, methylprednisolone, etc.) ± anesthetic buffer (lidocaine 1% or 2%, bupivacaine 0.25% or 0.5%, etc.) based on provider preference
  - Sterile gauze: prepare for possible venous bleeder
  - Small bandage: coverage of procedure site

Indications

- Injection
  - Subacromial/subdeltoid bursitis
  - Rotator cuff impingement syndrome
  - Rotator cuff tendinosis
  - Rheumatoid arthritis
  - Calcific tendinosis
  - Diagnostic injection
- Aspiration
  - Septic bursitis
  - Subacromial/subdeltoid abscess
  - Crystalline deposition diseases
  - Diagnostic aspiration

Contraindications

- Septic arthritis
- Septic bursitis (injection only)
- Systemic sepsis
- Overlying skin pathology
- Active overlying cellulitis or osteomyelitis in the shoulder area
- Uncontrolled coagulopathy
- Allergy to anesthetic agents or injection agents

- Pregnancy (injection of steroid medications)
- Repairable rotator cuff tear
- Known interaction with chronic medications

Technique (Video 49.1)

- Informed consent is obtained and the correct shoulder is confirmed.
- Patient positioning: Seated with posterior shoulder adequately exposed. Arm should rest at patient's side in adduction, ± internal rotation.
- Anatomic landmarks for injection are identified and marked (Fig. 49.1).
- Superficial anesthetic (optional): Can apply EMLA cream prior to sterilization or treat injection site with ethyl chloride spray after sterilization and just prior to injection.
- The skin over and around the injection site is prepared with the chosen sterile preparation solution (Fig. 49.2). Gloves, sterile if desired, used for the remainder of the procedure.
- A larger needle and syringe (20 to 22 gauge, 1.5 inch or larger, 10 to 20 mL) are loaded with the chosen medication(s).
- The injection point is just inferior to the posterolateral corner of the acromion. The needle advances medially, anteriorly, and slightly superiorly into the subacromial space directed toward the coracoid process (Fig. 49.3).
- After entering the subacromial/subdeltoid space, the bursa may be aspirated. A larger syringe (20 mL or larger) provides adequate negative pressure for aspiration.
- If only injection is planned, gentle aspiration should still be performed to confirm that the needle has entered the bursa and not a vessel.
- Injection of the medication then proceeds with slow, consistent pressure and should flow readily into the space. Any increased resistance or pressure should prompt a reevaluation of location.
- After injection or aspiration, the needle is withdrawn and a small bandage is applied.
- All materials are appropriately disposed of, and any intra-articular specimens are appropriately handled and routed.

Considerations

- Subacromial space can communicate with the glenohumeral joint if a rotator cuff tear exists.
- Needle size depends on patient size; larger patients will likely require longer needles.
- Complications may include systemic effects, tendon weakening or rupture, fat atrophy, muscle wasting, skin pigment changes, septic arthritis, nerve and vessel damage, steroid flare, and steroid arthropathy.

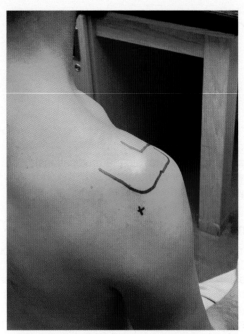

Fig 49.1 Patient positioning with anatomic landmarks highlighted.

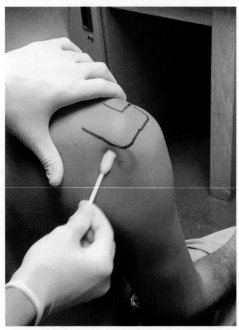

Fig 49.2 Sterile preparation of the injection site.

- Many clinicians recommend at least a 3-month interval between steroid injections.
- Some patients may experience a vasovagal reaction from the injection, and care should be taken to allow patients feeling light-headed or dizzy to lie down for several moments as needed.

Troubleshooting

- Difficult entry: Downward traction on the arm may help to open the subacromial space.

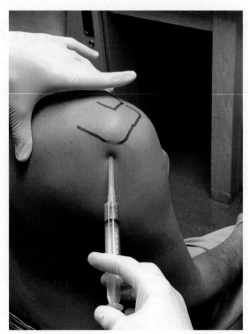

Fig 49.3 Needle positioning. Advance medially, anteriorly, and slightly superiorly toward coracoid process.

- "Hooked" acromion: Some patients have a lateral "hook" shape to their acromion, requiring a more exaggerated inferior starting point and more superiorly directed course of the needle.

Patient Instructions

- The bandage may be removed within a few hours after aspiration or injection.
- Some soreness may be expected for approximately 24 to 48 hours and may be addressed with ice, heat, nonsteroidal antiinflammatory drugs, and/or acetaminophen.
- Contact the physician immediately if any redness, warmth, increased swelling, severe increase in pain, fever, or chills develops.
- Diabetic patients should closely monitor blood glucose levels after injection of steroid medications and expect elevated levels for several days.
- Advise against excessive overhead activity, water submersion (pool, tub, etc.) for 48 hrs.

Ultrasound-Guided Approach

- The use of ultrasound (US) to perform guided injections and aspirations has grown in prevalence. This rise in use is likely due to the advantages US-guided injections provide, such as continuous and direct visualization providing high accuracy and less complications. A detailed discussion regarding US-guided technique remains out of the scope of this chapter; however, subacromial-subdeltoid bursal injections and aspirations are one of the more common examples. Please see the Suggested Reading section for more resources.

Suggested Readings

Dickson J. Shoulder injections in primary care. *Practitioner*. 2000;244: 259–265.

Jacobson JA. *Fundamentals of Musculoskeletal Ultrasound*. 3rd ed. Philadelphia: Elsevier; 2018.

Kerlan RK, Glousman RE. Injections and techniques in athletic medicine. *Clin Sports Med*. 1989;8:541–560.

Miller MD, Thompson SR, eds. *Delee and Drez's Orthopaedic Sports Medicine*. 4th ed. Philadelphia: Elsevier; 2015.

Saunders S, Longworth S. *Injection Techniques in Orthopaedics and Sports Medicine*. 3rd ed. New York: Churchill Livingstone; 2007.

Tallia AF, Cardone DA. Diagnostic and therapeutic injection of the shoulder region. *Am Fam Physician*. 2003;67:1271–1278.

Chapter 50 Acromioclavicular Injection

Tenley Murphy, Patrick Jenkins III, Christopher Miles

CPT CODES
20605 *Aspiration and/or injection, intermediate joint*
20606 *Aspiration and/or injection, intermediate joint, with ultrasound guidance, with permanent recording and reporting*

Equipment

- Sterile preparation solution: povidone-iodine, alcohol, chlorhexidine, etc.
- Gloves
- Ethyl chloride (cold spray), optional
- Aspiration/injection needle
  - 25 to 27 gauge, 1 inch needle if only injection is planned
  - 18 to 20 gauge, 1 inch needle if aspiration is planned
- Aspiration/injection syringe: 3 to 10 mL
- Injection agent(s)
  - Anesthetic options: lidocaine (1% or 2%), bupivacaine (0.25% or 0.5%), combinations
  - Steroid options: triamcinolone, betamethasone, methyl-prednisolone, others
- Sterile gauze: prepare to apply pressure for hemostasis
- Small bandage: to cover procedure site
- Ultrasound with high-frequency probe (linear array or small footprint/hockey stick probe)
- Assistant: to help with medication preparation, handoff of materials, patient positioning
- Choice of materials and procedure technique will vary depending on the indications for the procedure, patient's body habitus, provider preferences, and available materials

Indications

- Injection
  - Osteoarthritis
  - Posttraumatic arthritis
  - Inflammatory arthritis
  - Distal clavicle osteolysis
  - Unknown diagnosis (diagnostic injection)
- Aspiration
  - Septic arthritis
  - Crystalline deposition diseases
  - Unknown diagnosis (diagnostic aspiration)

Contraindications

- Septic arthritis (injection only)
- Septic bursitis (injection only)
- Cellulitis
- Osteomyelitis
- Bacteremia and sepsis
- Allergy to injection agents
- Pregnancy (injection of steroid medications)
- Fracture (injection only)
- Uncooperative patient
- Anticoagulation/antiplatelet therapy or bleeding diathesis (relative)
- Overlying skin pathology (relative)
- Osteoporosis adjacent to joint (relative)

Technique (Video 50.1)

- Obtain informed consent and confirm the correct side and procedure.
- Place the patient in a seated position to bring the shoulder to an easily accessible level with the humerus in adduction and internal rotation.
- Palpation-guided
  - Identify and mark the acromioclavicular (AC) joint by palpating the clavicle to its articulation with the acromion. A slight depression will be encountered.
  - With the chosen sterile preparation solution, prepare the skin over and around the marked injection site (Fig. 50.1).
  - If aspiration is planned, a larger-gauge needle with attached syringe should be prepared. If injection only is planned, a smaller-gauge needle with attached syringe containing appropriate medications should be prepared.
  - The injection site may be treated with ethyl chloride (cold spray) if desired. Since its effect is fleeting, it should be sprayed directly before injection/aspiration.
  - The needle is directed inferiorly into the joint with a medially directed tilt (Fig. 50.2).
  - A change in resistance or "pop" may be felt as the needle passes into the join capsule.
  - Negative pressure is then applied if aspiration is desired and to confirm needle placement extravascularly. Medicine is then administered slowly. Only 1 to 2 mL may enter the joint.
  - Apply a bandage over injection site and dispose of materials appropriately.
- Ultrasound-guided
  - The patient is positioned as described above with the ultrasound screen facing the provider who is positioned to visualize the AC joint and the monitor.
  - A high-frequency probe is used such as a linear array or small footprint probe.

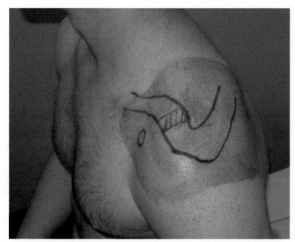

Fig 50.1 Properly positioned patient marked and prepped for injection.

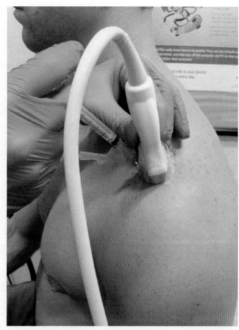

Fig 50.3 Ultrasound probe is positioned cephalad to the needle to visualize it entering the joint.

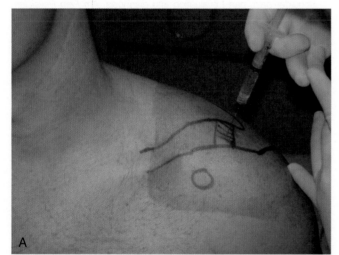

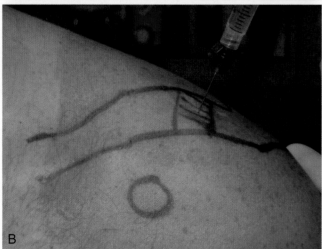

Fig 50.2 (A and B) For palpation-guided approach, the needle is directed inferiorly into the acromioclavicular joint with a medial tilt.

- Identify the joint space by walking the probe across the clavicle toward the acromion. Mark the skin directly over the joint space as well as the position of the ultrasound probe.
- Prep the skin as previously described.
- Place the sterile-covered probe over the marked area being careful not to contaminate the sterile field. Sterile gel is recommended.
- Introduce the needle into the joint under ultrasound visualization, which can be done in plane or out of plane in respect to the needle (Figs. 50.3 and 50.4).
- Apply a bandage over the injection site and dispose of materials appropriately.

Special Considerations

- The AC joint can prove very difficult to locate. More than 50% of palpation-guided AC joint injections are not in the joint. For this reason, direct visualization of the needle with ultrasound or fluoroscopy is helpful especially if the injection is being done for diagnostic purposes.
- Needle size depends on patient size; larger patients may require longer needles.
- Complications include systemic effects, fat atrophy, muscle wasting, skin hypopigmentation, septic arthritis, nerve and vessel damage, steroid flare, and steroid arthropathy.
- A 3-month interval between steroid injections is recommended.
- Patients may experience a vasovagal reaction from the injection. Patients feeling light-headed or dizzy may need to lie down for several minutes.

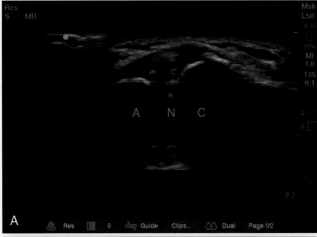

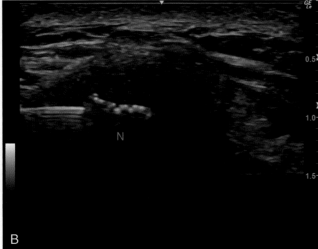

Fig 50.4 Ultrasound image of a needle in between that acromion "A" and clavicle "C" in the acromioclavicular joint out of plane with respect to the needle "N" (A) and in plane with respect to the needle "N" (B).

Troubleshooting

- Difficult entry
  - The needle can be "walked down the clavicle" medially to laterally until it drops into the joint. Extreme cases may require sonographic or fluoroscopic guidance.

Patient Instructions

- The bandage may be removed within a few hours after aspiration or injection.
- Soreness may be expected for 24 to 48 hours and can be treated with ice, nonsteroidal antiinflammatory drugs (NSAIDs), and/or acetaminophen.
- Contact the provider immediately if any redness, warmth, increased swelling, severe increase in pain, fever, or chills develop.
- Diabetic patients should closely monitor blood glucose levels after injection of steroid medications and expect elevated levels for several days.

Suggested Readings

Burbank KM, Stevenson JH, Czarnecki GR, Dorman J. Chronic shoulder pain: part I evaluation and diagnosis. *Am Fam Physician.* 2008;77(4):453–460.

Jacobson JA. Shoulder ultrasound. In: *Fundamentals of Musculoskeletal Ultrasound.* 3rd ed. Philadelphia: Elsevier; 2018:55–126.

Peck E, Lai JK, Pawlina W, Smith J. Accuracy of ultrasound-guided versus palpation-guided acromioclavicular joint injections: a cadaveric study. *PM R.* 2010;2(9):817–821.

Schaefer MP, Foorsov V. Shoulder injections. In: Agha M, Murphy D, eds. *Guide to Musculoskeletal Injections With Ultrasound.* New York: Springer; 2015:15–32.

Tallia AF, Cardone DA. Diagnostic and therapeutic injection of the shoulder region. *Am Fam Physician.* 2003;67(6):1271–1278.

Chapter 51 Ultrasound of the Shoulder Region

Jennifer Pierce

ICD-10-CM CODES
M25.519   *Shoulder pain*
M75.20   *Biceps tendinitis*
M75.102   *Rotator cuff tear*
M75.50   *Subacromial subdeltoid bursitis*

CPT CODES
76882   *Limited ultrasound extremity*
76942   *Ultrasound guidance for needle placement*

Overview

- A comprehensive ultrasound (US) evaluation of the shoulder can be performed in five steps to evaluate the long head of the biceps brachii, subscapularis, supraspinatus/infraspinatus, acromioclavicular joint/subacromial-subdeltoid bursa, and posterior shoulder joint/teres minor. In addition, a focused evaluation on specific patient symptoms can be addressed.
- Shoulder US can evaluate and diagnose tendon tears and tendinosis, joint effusions, bursitis, and dynamic testing for impingement.
- US is not the optimal imaging modality for intra-articular processes involving the labrum, cartilage, and osseous structures. Magnetic resonance imaging (MRI) or computed tomography (CT) is the better diagnostic tool for these entities.
- Like all musculoskeletal US examinations, correctly utilizing the appropriate transducer is important. Generally, a 9 to 12 MHz linear transducer is used. Lower-frequency transducers are utilized when evaluating larger body habitus patients and deeper structures such as the posterior shoulder joint.
- The US exam is performed with the patient seated and the sonographer sits on a stool, preferably with wheels to allow good maneuvering and access.

Equipment

- Ultrasound machine
- 9 to 12 MHz linear transducer
- 25-gauge 4-cm needle for acromioclavicular joint injections
- 22-gauge 10-cm spinal needle for shoulder joint injections

Technique

- Step 1: Long head of the biceps brachii
  - The patient lays their hand on their leg with the palm up (supinated), and the transducer is placed in the transverse plane to the anterior shoulder.
  - The bicipital groove is visualized along the anterior humeral cortex with the biceps tendon within the groove (Fig. 51.1). By turning the transducer 90 degrees, the longitudinal plane is also evaluated.
- Step 2: Subscapularis
  - In the same position as for the biceps tendon evaluation, the subscapularis is visualized inserting on the lesser tuberosity of the humeral head just medial to the bicipital groove.
  - Asking the patient to externally rotate the shoulder allows for better visualization of the subscapularis tendon fibers (Fig. 51.2).
- Step 3: Supraspinatus and infraspinatus
  - When the arm is in neutral position, much of the supraspinatus and infraspinatus is hidden under the acromion.
  - Placing the patient's palm along his or her posterolateral waist (along the "back pocket," called the modified Crass maneuver) with the elbow flexed and pointed posteriorly will rotate the humerus internally, and the supraspinatus tendon fibers and the greater tuberosity will be located more anteriorly. This will aid in visualizing much more of the proximal supraspinatus and infraspinatus tendons.
  - The transducer should be placed along the coronal and transverse plane to the tendons (Figs. 51.3–51.5).
- Step 4: Acromioclavicular (AC) joint/subacromial-subdeltoid (SA/SD) bursa
  - The AC joint can typically be palpated, and the US transducer is placed across the joint/distal clavicle.
  - In this plane, an AC joint steroid injection can be performed from a lateral to medial approach. With ultrasound, AC joint widening and joint effusion can be assessed (Fig. 51.6).
  - By moving the transducer lateral from the AC joint evaluation, the SA/SD bursa can be assessed subjacent to the deltoid and over the supraspinatus and infraspinatus tendons (Fig. 51.7).
- Step 5: Posterior shoulder joint
  - The evaluation of the posterior shoulder includes examining the infraspinatus, teres minor, and the posterior

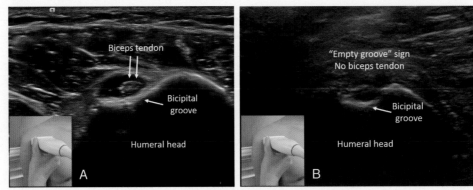

Fig 51.1 Transverse plane of the bicipital groove along the humeral head. **(A)** There is fluid surrounding the biceps tendon indicating tenosynovitis. The tendon is intact and located normally within the bicipital groove. **(B)** "Empty groove" sign is present due to a complete biceps tendon tear with retraction.

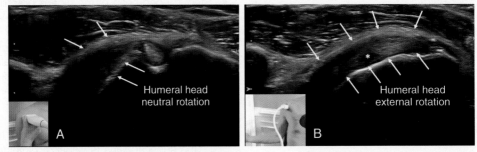

Fig 51.2 Longitudinal plane of the subscapularis. **(A)** When the arm is in neutral position or rotation, the subscapularis tendon is not completely visualized. **(B)** With external rotation of the arm, more of the subscapularis tendon can be seen and evaluated. Small intrasubstance tear is present. Asterisk *(*)* indicates hypoechoic *(darker region)* tear in subscapularis. *Arrows* indicate the subscapularis tendon.

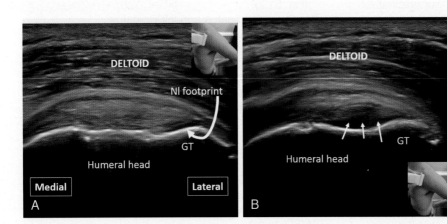

Fig 51.3 Longitudinal plane of the supraspinatus. **(A)** Intact supraspinatus fibers inserting onto the greater tuberosity (GT) with normal tendon linear, fibrillary, and hyperechoic architecture. **(B)** Focus of supraspinatus low-grade articular-sided partial tear at the greater GT footprint *(arrows)* where the tendon is hypoechoic with a small gap in the tendon.

glenohumeral joint for glenoid labral pathology and effusion.
- The arm is placed with the patient's hand reaching up and over to the contralateral anterior shoulder. This places the humerus in internal rotation for optimal visualization of the posterior tendons and shoulder joint capsule.
- The transducer is placed parallel to the spine of the scapula for a longitudinal plane evaluation of the tendons. Moving the transducer just below the spine, the infraspinatus muscle is visualized. Positioning the transducer more laterally will follow the infraspinatus tendon onto the greater tuberosity (Fig. 51.8).

- The glenohumeral articulation is also visualized subjacent to the infraspinatus.
- Further inferior positioning of the transducer will bring the teres minor muscle and tendon into view. Turning the transducer 90 degrees so that it is perpendicular to the spine of the scapula will provide a transverse plane evaluation of the infraspinatus and teres minor tendons.
- A shoulder joint steroid injection or aspiration can be performed from this posterior transducer placement paralleling the spine of the scapula with the glenohumeral articulation seen subjacent to the infraspinatus tendon.

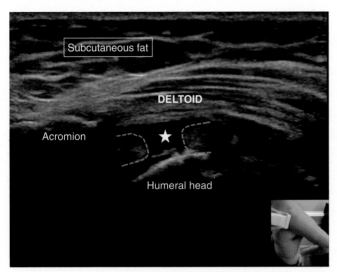

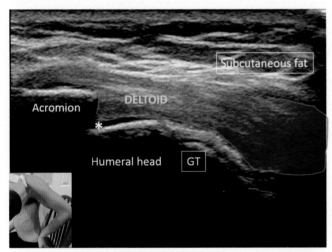

Fig 51.4 Longitudinal plane of the rotator cuff demonstrates a full-thickness infraspinatus tear. The torn margins of the tendon are outlined by *dashed lines*. A gap within the tendon fibers is present filled with fluid that communicates with the subacromial-subdeltoid bursa *(star)*.

Fig 51.5 Coronal oblique ultrasound image demonstrating a chronic, retracted full-thickness supraspinatus tear. The acromion-humeral interval is extremely narrowed. No supraspinatus tendon fibers are visualized inserting onto the greater tuberosity. The torn tendon fibers are retracted proximally, past the acromion. The only muscle fibers present are from the deltoid muscle inserting onto the lateral aspect of the acromion. *GT,* greater tuberosity; *asterisk (*)* indicates acromion-humeral interval.

The needle is placed from a lateral to medial approach (see Fig. 51.8).

Considerations in Special Populations

- Shoulder US has been proven to be diagnostically accurate and an effective modality for image-guided joint procedures. However, it can be challenging for the less experienced provider. A strong knowledge base of shoulder anatomy assists image interpretation. In cases where imaging is

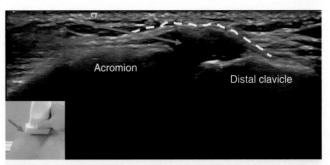

Fig 51.6 Longitudinal plane along the acromial clavicular (AC) joint demonstrates the joint capsule *(dashed line)* distended with a joint effusion *(star)*. Red arrow indicates orientation of needle when performing an AC joint injection or aspiration placed from a lateral to medial direction.

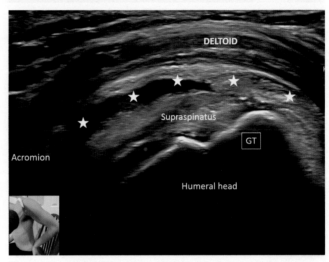

Fig 51.7 Longitudinal plane ultrasound along an intact supraspinatus inserting onto the greater tuberosity (GT). There is a distended subacromial subdeltoid bursa with fluid *(darker area)* and echogenic thickened bursal capsule and nodular synovitis *(whiter area)*. The star indicates area of subacromial subdeltoid bursa.

technically difficult, a skilled musculoskeletal radiologist should be consulted.

Troubleshooting

- Since most of musculoskeletal US involves imaging tendons, ligaments, or muscles, anisotropy (imaging artifact that results from viewing structures in a nonperpendicular angle) is a common challenge.
- When in longitudinal plane (transducer is parallel to the fibers) of the structure of interest, "heel-toe" the transducer by slightly lifting up one end and pressing down on the other.
- When imaging the structure of interest in the axial place (transducer is across the fibers), "toggle" the transducer by angling it forward and back.
- These subtle movements with the transducer direct the sound beams to reflect off the structures at true 90 degrees to eliminate the anisotropy artifact on US.

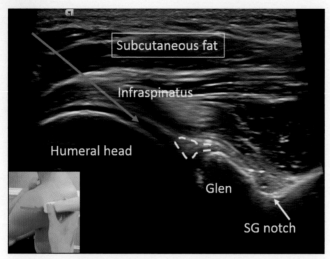

Fig 51.8 Transverse plane of the posterior glenohumeral joint below the level of the spine of the scapula shows a normal infraspinatus over the glenohumeral joint that has a small amount of physiologic fluid. The posterior superior labrum *(dash outlined)* is visualized along the glenoid rim. The *red arrow* points to the lateral to medial direction of needle for posterior shoulder injection or aspiration. *Glen,* Glenoid; *SG notch,* spinoglenoid notch.

Suggested Readings

Finnoff JT, Smith J, Peck ER. Ultrasonography of the shoulder. *Phys Med Rehabil Clin N Am*. 2010;21:481–507.

Jacobson JA. *Fundamentals of Musculoskeletal Ultrasound*. 3rd ed. Philadelphia: Elsevier; 2018.

Smith TO, Back T, Toms AP, Hing CB. Diagnostic accuracy of ultrasound for rotator cuff tears in adults: a systematic review and meta-analysis. *Clin Radiol*. 2011;66:1036–1048.

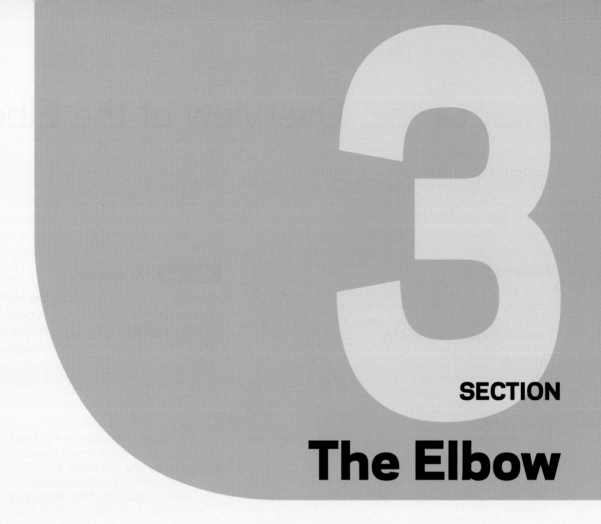

3

SECTION

The Elbow

Chapter 52 Overview of the Elbow

Jennifer A. Hart

Anatomy

- The elbow joint is made up of articulations between the distal humerus and the proximal radius and ulna (Fig. 52.1). These articulations allow two types of joint motion: flexion/extension and forearm rotation.

Humerus

- The articular surface of the distal humerus is composed of the trochlea and capitellum.
- The medial and lateral epicondyles are found just proximal to these structures.
- The medial epicondyle serves as an important attachment site for the ulnar collateral ligament, the common flexor tendons, and the pronator muscle.
- The lateral epicondyle serves as an attachment site for the radial collateral ligament and the common extensor tendon.

Ulna

- The proximal ulna articulates with the trochlea to form the medial aspect of the elbow joint and also articulates with the radial head via the radial notch.
- The olecranon process is the predominant posterior bony structure that serves at the insertion point for the common distal triceps tendon.

Radius

- The radial head articulates with the capitellum in the lateral elbow joint and is also responsible for allowing pronation and supination of the forearm via its articulation with the proximal ulna.

Muscles (Box 52.1)

- Neurovascular structures (Fig. 52.2)
  - The brachial artery divides into the radial and ulnar arteries at the elbow joint, each of which further divides into small branches at the wrist.
  - The ulnar artery passes through the medial aspect of the forearm, and the radial artery passes through the lateral forearm.
  - The primary nerves located around the elbow include the ulnar (C7-T1), median (C5-T1), and radial (C5-T1) nerves.
  - The ulnar nerve passes behind the medial epicondyle and runs between the two heads of the flexor carpi ulnaris muscle.
  - The medial nerve runs beneath the pronator teres muscle on its path to the carpal tunnel at the wrist. The radial nerve divides into superficial and deep branches

---

BOX 52.1 The Muscles

Flexion	**Supination**
Biceps brachii	Supinator
Coracobrachialis	Biceps brachii
Brachialis	
	Pronation
Extension	Pronator quadratus
Triceps brachii	Pronator teres
Anconeus	

---

to provide sensation to the posterior forearm and the majority of the extensor muscles there.
- Ligaments and soft tissue (Fig. 52.3)
  - The ulnar and radial collateral ligaments are important static stabilizers of the elbow joint.
  - The ulnar (medial) collateral ligament is composed of anterior and posterior bands and functions to resist excessive valgus load to the elbow.
  - The radial (lateral) collateral ligament similarly resists varus stress at the elbow joint and actually is made up of two separate structures: the radial collateral ligament and the lateral ulnar collateral ligament.
  - The olecranon bursa lies posteriorly over the olecranon process and is frequently inflamed from direct trauma to the "point" of the elbow.

History

- A thorough history can lead to the development of an accurate and complete list of differential diagnoses that can then be refined further with physical examination and diagnostic studies.
- At the basic level, the history should include the mechanism of injury, previous similar symptoms, and pain characteristics (location, quality, severity, and radiation) (Table 52.1).

Physical Examination (Video 52.1)

- Inspection and palpation (Fig. 52.4)
  - Anterior elbow: Observe and palpate the antecubital fossa for masses and the biceps tendons for rupture (loss of tendon continuity and focal tenderness).
  - Posterior elbow: Palpate the tip of the olecranon for fracture/avulsion and observe any swelling in the olecranon bursa. An enlarged and erythematous area over the posterior elbow may indicate an infected bursa.
  - Medial elbow: Deformity and/or tenderness over the medial epicondyle may indicate medial epicondylitis or

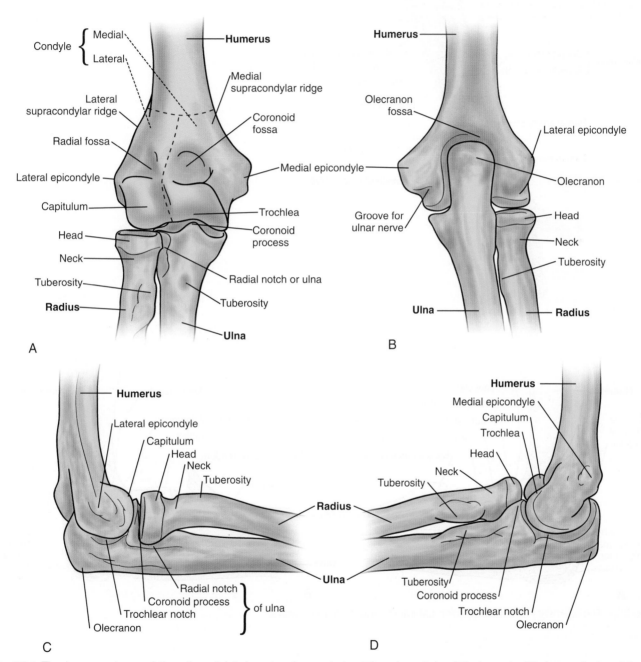

Fig 52.1 The bony anatomy of the elbow joint. In extension, anterior (A) and posterior (B) views. In 90-degree flexion, lateral (C) and medial (D) views.

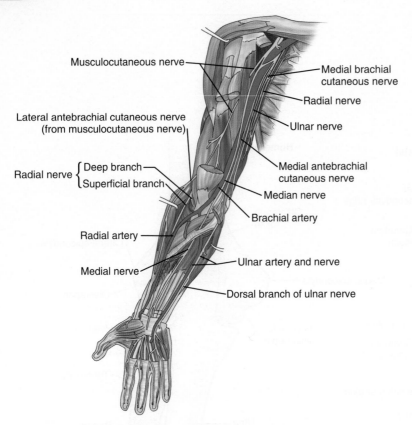

Musculocutaneous nerve

Medial brachial cutaneous nerve

Radial nerve

Ulnar nerve

Lateral antebrachial cutaneous nerve (from musculocutaneous nerve)

Medial antebrachial cutaneous nerve

Radial nerve { Deep branch / Superficial branch

Median nerve

Brachial artery

Radial artery

Ulnar artery and nerve

Medial nerve

Dorsal branch of ulnar nerve

Fig 52.2 The neurovascular structures of the elbow and arm (anterior view).

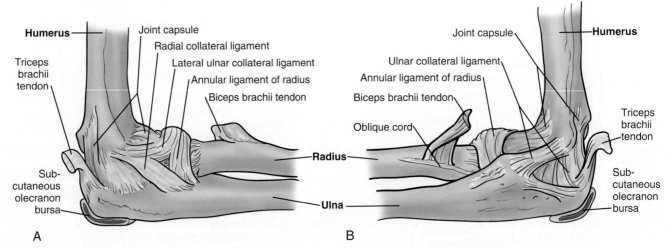

Humerus

Joint capsule

Radial collateral ligament

Lateral ulnar collateral ligament

Annular ligament of radius

Biceps brachii tendon

Triceps brachii tendon

Sub-cutaneous olecranon bursa

A

Joint capsule

Ulnar collateral ligament

Annular ligament of radius

Biceps brachii tendon

Oblique cord

Radius

Ulna

Humerus

Triceps brachii tendon

Sub-cutaneous olecranon bursa

B

Fig 52.3 The ligaments of the elbow joint. Lateral **(A)** and medial **(B)** views.

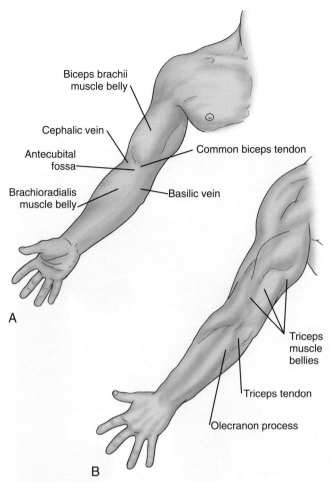

Biceps brachii
muscle belly

Cephalic vein

Antecubital
fossa

Common biceps tendon

Brachioradialis
muscle belly

Basilic vein

A

Triceps
muscle
bellies

Triceps tendon

Olecranon process

B

Fig 52.4 The surface anatomy of the elbow. Anterior (A) and posterior (B) views.

TABLE 52.1 History

Fall/Trauma	Fracture
Traction injury "pulled by hand"	Nursemaid's elbow/dislocation
Night pain	Tumor/infection
Lateral overuse pain	Tennis elbow
Medial overuse pain	Golfer's elbow
Posterior traumatic pain	Olecranon bursitis
Acute loss of strength	Biceps/triceps rupture/avulsion
Locking, younger patient	Osteochondritis dissecans
Locking, older patient	Degenerative joint disease
Neurologic symptoms	Nerve entrapment

ulnar collateral ligament injury. A quick tap posterior to the medial epicondyle may elicit a positive Tinel's sign indicating ulnar neuropathy.
- Lateral elbow: Deformity and/or tenderness over the lateral epicondyle may indicate tennis elbow, whereas tenderness over the radial head is suspicious for fracture.
- Range of motion
  - Flexion/extension: 0 to 145 degrees

BOX 52.2 Strength Testing

5: Full motion against gravity with maximum resistance
4: Full motion against gravity with moderate resistance
3: Full motion against gravity with no resistance
2: Full range of motion in gravity-eliminated position
1: No motion but muscle contraction is noted
0: No motion or muscle contraction

- Pronation: 80 to 90 degrees
- Supination: 85 to 90 degrees
- Strength testing (Fig. 52.5 and Box 52.2)
  - Flexion
  - Extension
  - Pronation
  - Supination
- Special tests
  - Reflexes: biceps (C5), triceps (C7) (Fig. 52.6)
  - Valgus and varus stress (Fig. 52.7)
    - Purpose: evaluation for integrity of the ulnar collateral or radial collateral ligaments
    - How to perform: stabilize the humerus and, with the elbow slightly flexed, exert pressure on the forearm first medially (varus) and then laterally (valgus)
    - Positive: indicated by laxity or "opening" of the joint medially or laterally
  - Tinel's sign (Fig. 52.8)
    - Purpose: evaluation for cubital tunnel syndrome (ulnar nerve entrapment)
    - How to perform: tap over the ulnar nerve as it passes by the medial epicondyle of the distal humerus
    - Positive: indicated by reproduction of paresthesia in the ulnar nerve distribution

Imaging

- Radiography
  - The most commonly ordered plain views of the elbow joint include anteroposterior, lateral, and oblique views. Stress views may be helpful when a collateral ligament injury is suspected (Fig. 52.9).
- Magnetic resonance imaging
  - Commonly used to evaluate the soft-tissue structures such as the ligaments (Fig. 52.10)
  - It is often the most helpful when combined with arthrography.
  - Other uses include evaluation of tumors, osteochondral lesions, and suspected biceps or triceps tendon ruptures.
- Computed tomography
  - Most helpful when evaluating bony problems such as complex intra-articular fractures
  - It can aid the surgeon in planning the approach and reduction of the fracture fragments.
  - It can also be useful in characterizing bony tumors seen on plain radiographs.
- Electromyography is a helpful adjunct when a patient is suspected of having a neurologic process. It can be combined with other imaging studies to localize and identify the source of the compression or injury.

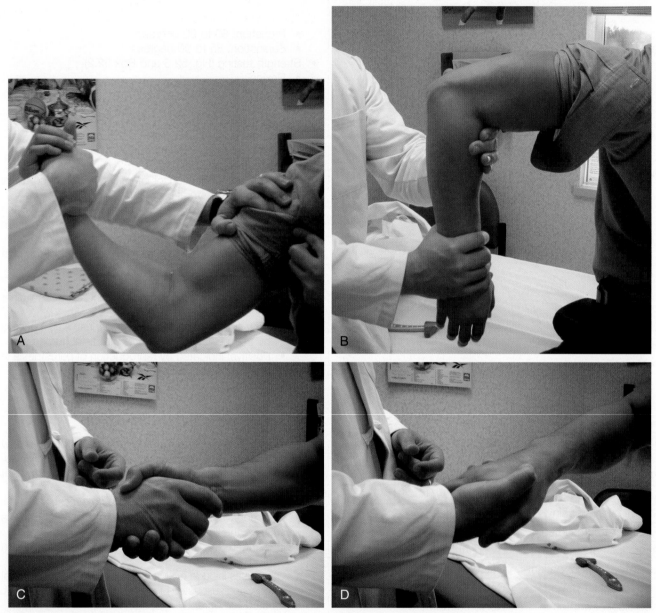

Fig 52.5 Manual muscle testing at the elbow joint. **(A)** Flexion. **(B)** Extension. **(C)** Pronation. **(D)** Supination.

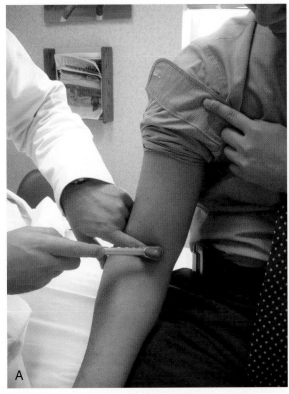

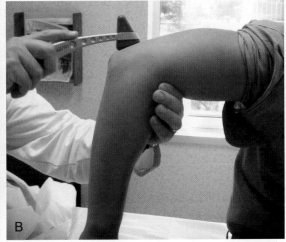

Fig 52.6 Reflex testing. (A) Biceps (C5). (B) Triceps (C7).

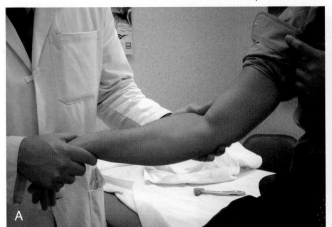

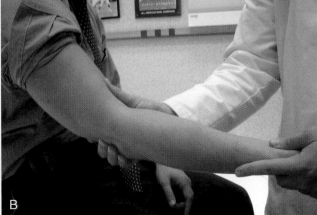

Fig 52.7 Stress testing for ligament integrity at the elbow. (A) Valgus. (B) Varus.

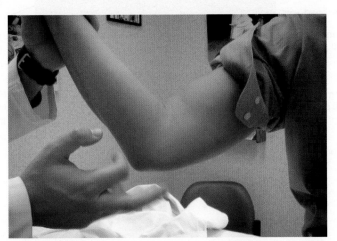

Fig 52.8 Tinel's sign for cubital tunnel syndrome (ulnar nerve entrapment).

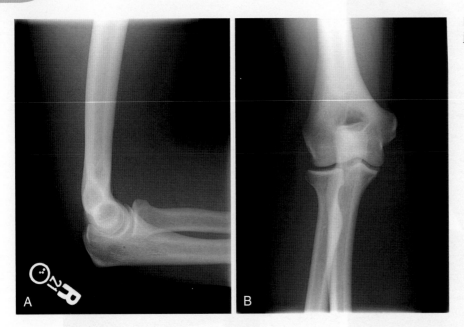

Fig 52.9 Standard radiographs of the elbow joint. (A) Anteroposterior. (B) Lateral.

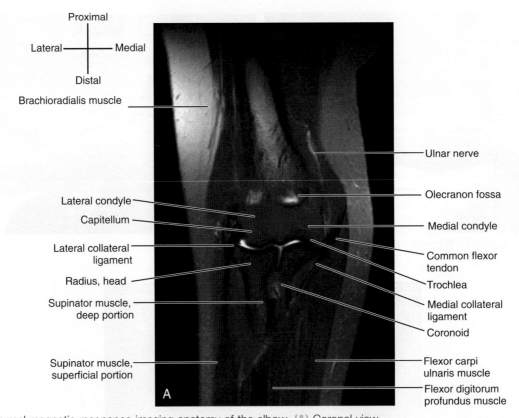

Proximal

Lateral ——— Medial

Distal

Brachioradialis muscle

Ulnar nerve

Lateral condyle

Olecranon fossa

Capitellum

Medial condyle

Lateral collateral ligament

Common flexor tendon

Radius, head

Trochlea

Supinator muscle, deep portion

Medial collateral ligament

Coronoid

Supinator muscle, superficial portion

Flexor carpi ulnaris muscle

Flexor digitorum profundus muscle

Fig 52.10 Normal magnetic resonance imaging anatomy of the elbow. (A) Coronal view.

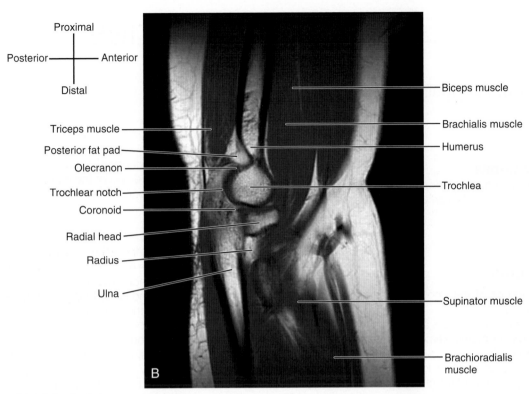

Proximal

Posterior——+——Anterior

Distal

Triceps muscle

Posterior fat pad

Olecranon

Trochlear notch

Coronoid

Radial head

Radius

Ulna

Biceps muscle

Brachialis muscle

Humerus

Trochlea

Supinator muscle

Brachioradialis muscle

B

Fig 52.10, cont'd (B) Sagittal view.

Suggested Readings

Alcid JG, Ahmad CS, Lee TQ. Elbow anatomy and structural biomechanics. *Clin Sports Med*. 2004;23:503–517.

Behr CT, Altchek DW. The elbow. *Clin Sports Med*. 1997;16:681–704.

Cain EL, Dugas JR. History and examination of the thrower's elbow. *Clin Sports Med*. 2004;23:553–566.

Chung CB, Chew FS, Steinbach L. MR imaging of tendon abnormalities of the elbow. *Magn Reson Imaging Clin N Am*. 2004;12:233–245.

Colman WW, Strauch RJ. Physical examination of the elbow. *Orthop Clin North Am*. 1999;31:15–20.

Fowler KAB, Chung CB. Normal MR imaging anatomy of the elbow. *Radiol Clin North Am*. 2006;44:553–567.

Frick MA. Imaging of the elbow: a review of imaging findings in acute and chronic traumatic disorders of the elbow. *J Hand Ther*. 2006;19:98–113.

Fritz FC, Breidahl WH. Radiographic and special studies: recent advances in imaging of the elbow. *Clin Sports Med*. 2004;23:567–580.

Hoppenfeld S. *Physical Examination of the Spine and Extremities*. Norwalk, CT: Appleton & Lange; 1976.

Miyasaka KC. Anatomy of the elbow. *Orthop Clin North Am*. 1999;30:1–13.

Chapter 53 Chondral Injuries

Anthony J. Archual, Aaron M. Freilich

ICD-10-CM CODES
M93.22   *Osteochondritis dissecans, elbow*
M24.10   *Other articular cartilage disorders, unspecified site*

Key Concepts

- Chondral lesions of the elbow may present as acute or repetitive injuries.
- Osteochondritis dissecans is a condition that may develop spontaneously or more commonly in juvenile athletes ("little leaguer's elbow").
- The pathology consists of localized avascular necrosis with subsequent loss of structural support for the adjacent cartilage.
- The cause is thought to be valgus overload of the radiocapitellar joint.
- This condition is commonly found in young throwing athletes (little leaguers) and gymnasts.
- Lateral elbow joint pathology may be caused by or associated with medial collateral ligament instability.
- The typical radiologic finding is a posteromedial osteophyte of the olecranon process.
- This condition commonly leads to the development of loose bodies.
- Osteochondrosis of the capitellum (Panner disease) is a related condition in children younger than the age of 10 years.

History

- Patients may present after acute injury.
  - Preceding injuries include elbow dislocation and periarticular fractures.
  - The mechanism most commonly reported is a fall onto the outstretched supinated hand.
- Chronic injuries leading to intra-articular pathology are commonly related to repetitive valgus stress, as seen in throwers and gymnasts.
- Patients typically report elbow pain with activity, decreased performance (throwing speed), stiffness, and swelling.
- Osteophytes and loose bodies may lead to mechanical symptoms with elbow range of motion such as locking and catching of the elbow.

Physical Examination

- Most commonly, the elbow will have lateral tenderness with crepitus over the radiocapitellar joint.

- Loss of terminal extension with a 15- to 20-degree flexion contracture may be one of the earliest findings.
- Swelling is commonly present.

Imaging

- Plain radiographs including anteroposterior, lateral, and oblique views of the elbow may show fragmented subchondral bone, subchondral lucencies, and irregular ossification.
  - Osteophytes and loose bodies may be appreciated at later stages of the disease.
- Magnetic resonance imaging of the elbow can be helpful to detect loose bodies not visible on plain radiographs, avascular necrosis, and associated ligament damage.
- Elbow arthroscopy allows direct visualization and grading of osteochondritis dissecans and at the same time allows treatment of certain conditions (Table 53.1).

Differential Diagnosis

- Lateral epicondylitis: lateral tenderness and pain with passive stretch of the common extensor mechanism (see Chapter 55)
- Panner disease: younger patients with avascular necrosis of the capitellum (see Chapter 220)
- Plica: mechanical symptoms, often a palpable catch, most commonly lateral (see Chapter 52)
- Posterolateral rotatory instability: pain with pushing up from a chair (see Chapter 59)
- Synovial osteochondromatosis: multiple loose bodies without evidence of chondral injury (see Chapter 15)

Treatment

- Nonoperative treatment should be attempted for grade I and II lesions with no detachment or loose bodies.
- Treatment consists of 4 weeks of complete activity restriction, with physical therapy for strengthening and range of motion, followed by a progressive throwing program.
  - Preinjury performance levels can be reached within 3 to 4 months.
- Operative treatment is indicated after failure of conservative treatment for grade I and II lesions.
  - Operative treatment is also indicated for any patient with higher-grade osteochondritis dissecans with evidence of unstable fragments or loose bodies and progressive or fixed joint contracture.
  - Surgical treatment options include elbow arthroscopy with removal of loose bodies and contracture release, drilling of the lesions, fixation of larger fragments, and osteochondral autografting transplant system (OATS).

TABLE 53.1 Grading of Osteochondrosis Lesions

Grade	Description	Treatment
I	Softening of cartilage	Drilling
II	Fibrillation and fissures	Drilling, removal of frayed portions to stable rim
III	Stable osteochondral fragment	Drilling and removal or fixation for larger fragments
IV	Loose but nondisplaced	Drilling or fixation of large fragments
V	Loose body	Drilling, mosaicplasty, or OATS for larger defects

OATS, Osteochondral autografting transplant system.

- In high-level athletes with defects >1 cm², OAT has been shown to achieve return to play at previous level.
- Subchondral bone and cartilage are transferred in a plug from the knee to the elbow.
- The prognosis varies with the grade of disease.
- Overall surgical treatment can improve elbow range of motion and eliminate mechanical symptoms.
- The best results are accomplished after removal of isolated loose bodies with minimal morbidity and early return to full function.
- Patients should be referred for surgical treatment in the presence of mechanical symptoms or failure to progress with conservative treatment.

Troubleshooting

- Little league pitchers with chondral injury secondary to valgus overload from repetitive throwing motions are a particularly challenging group of patients to treat.
- The majority of symptomatic elbows can be treated with activity modification and periods of rest followed by gradual return to throwing.
- Unfortunately, patients and their ambitious parents are often too impatient to comply with the suggested treatment course; close supervision and reinforcement of the treatment plan may be necessary.

Suggested Readings

Byrd JW, Jones KS. Arthroscopic surgery for isolated capitellar osteochondritis dissecans in adolescent baseball players: minimum three-year follow-up. *Am J Sports Med*. 2002;30:474–478.

DaSilva MF, Williams JS, Fadale PD, et al. Pediatric throwing injuries about the elbow. *Am J Orthop*. 1998;27:90–96.

Lyons ML, Werner BC, Gluck JS, et al. Osteochondral autograft plug transfer for treatment of osteochondritis dissecans of the capitellum in adolescent athletes. *J Shoulder Elbow Surg*. 2015;24:1098–1105.

Peterson RK, Savoie FH III, Field LD. Osteochondritis dissecans of the elbow. *Instr Course Lect*. 1999;48:393–398.

Pill SG, Ganley TJ, Flynn JM, Gregg JR. Osteochondritis dissecans of the capitellum: arthroscopic-assisted treatment of large, full-thickness defects in young patients. *Arthroscopy*. 2003;19:222–225.

Takahara M, Ogino T, Sasaki I, et al. Long term outcome of osteochondritis dissecans of the humeral capitellum. *Clin Orthop Relat Res*. 1999;363:108–115.

Woods GW, Tullos HS, King JW. The throwing arm: elbow joint injuries. *J Sports Med*. 1973;1:43–47.

Chapter 54 Osteoarthritis of the Elbow

Anthony J. Archual, Aaron M. Freilich

ICD-10-CM CODE
M19.02 *Primary osteoarthrosis, elbow*

Key Concepts

- The elbow positions the hand in space and stabilizes the limb for prehensile activities.
- Only 1-2% of patients with osteoarthritis will present with elbow involvement.
- Elbow arthritis occurs more commonly in male laborers.
- It is associated with progressive loss of range of motion and pain.
- Mechanical symptoms are common as a result of intra-articular loose bodies.
- Disease progression may result in increasing functional difficulties with use of hand for activities of daily living.

History

- Patients present with increasing pain and stiffness.
- Mechanical blocks to motion, clicking, and catching are also commonly reported.
- Pain with terminal extension is frequently seen in these patients.

- Decreased range of motion is often present early during the disease.

Physical Examination

- Inspection:
  - Swelling, deformity
  - Palpation of soft spot may allow detection of effusion.
  - Occasionally, loose bodies are palpable.
- Range of motion:
  - Flexion, extension, forearm pronation/supination
  - Loss of terminal extension early in disease
  - Range of motion of 30 to 130 degrees is necessary for activities of daily living.
- Neurovascular:
  - Check for ulnar neuropathy with elbow flexion test and Tinel sign over the cubital tunnel.

Imaging

- Plain radiographs should include anteroposterior (in extension), lateral (in 90 degrees of elbow flexion), and oblique views (Fig. 54.1).
- Findings associated with elbow osteoarthritis include
  - Posterior olecranon osteophyte

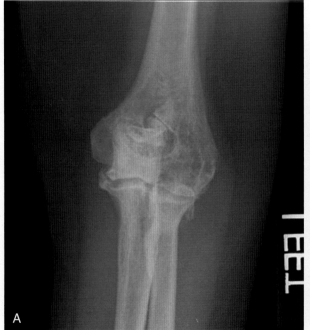
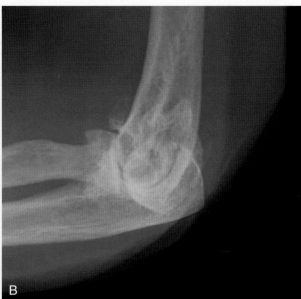

Fig 54.1 Anteroposterior (A) and lateral (B) 1radiographs of elbow arthritis.

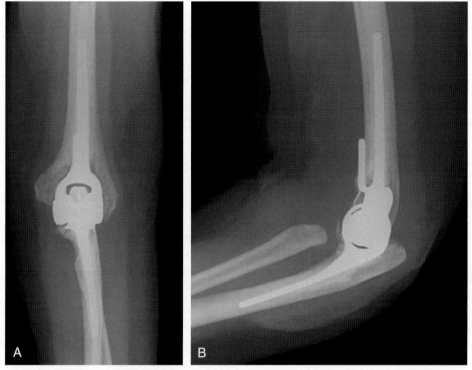

Fig 54.2 Anteroposterior (A) and lateral (B) radiographs of a total elbow arthroplasty.

- Radiocapitellar joint narrowing
- Osteophytes and loose bodies
- Computed tomography with three-dimensional reconstruction
  - Road map for preoperative planning
- Magnetic resonance imaging
  - If underlying instability is suspected
  - Assessment of ligamentous integrity

Treatment

- Nonoperative:
  - Activity modification
  - Nonsteroidal antiinflammatory drugs
  - Splinting
  - Ice/heat
  - Physical therapy
  - Intra-articular steroid injections
- Operative:
  - Removal of loose bodies
  - Ulnohumeral débridement, open or arthroscopic: This procedure can improve pain and range of motion and typically allows return to heavy manual labor.
  - Joint resurfacing with allograft tendon
- Preexisting ulnar nerve symptoms should be addressed by concurrent ulnar nerve release/transposition.
  - Ulnar nerve symptoms are the most common but transient complication of surgical treatment
  - Total elbow arthroplasty for older, low-demand patients (Fig. 54.2)
  - Will require a lifetime lifting restriction
  - Usually contraindicated in the younger osteoarthritic population

When To Refer

- Failure of nonoperative treatment
- Elbow stiffness interfering with activities of daily living (flexion less than 130 degrees); limited extension better tolerated
- Mechanical symptoms due to loose bodies

Suggested Readings

Adams JE, Wolff LH 3rd, Merten SM, Steinmann SP. Osteoarthritis of the elbow: results of arthroscopic osteophyte resection and capsulectomy. *J Shoulder Elbow Surg*. 2008;17:126–131.

Cheung EV, Adams R, Morrey BF. Primary osteoarthritis of the elbow: current treatment options. *J Am Acad Orthop Surg*. 2008;16:77–87.

Cohen AP, Redden JF, Stanley D. Treatment of osteoarthritis of the elbow: A comparison of open and arthroscopic debridement. *Arthroscopy*. 2000;16:701–706.

Gramstad GD, Galatz LM. Management of elbow osteoarthritis. *J Bone Joint Surg Am*. 2006;88A:421–430.

McAuliffe JA. Surgical alternatives for elbow arthritis in the young adult. *Hand Clin*. 2002;18:99–111.

Morrey BF. Primary degenerative arthritis of the elbow: treatment by ulnohumeral arthroplasty. *J Bone Joint Surg Br*. 1992;74B:409–413.

Rettig LA, Hastings H 2nd, Feinberg JR. Primary osteoarthritis of the elbow: lack of radiographic evidence for morphologic predisposition, results of operative debridement at intermediate follow-up, and basis for a new radiographic classification system. *J Shoulder Elbow Surg*. 2008;17:97–105.

Steinmann SP, King GJ, Savoie FH III. Arthroscopic treatment of the arthritic elbow. *J Bone Joint Surg Am*. 2005;87A:2114–2121.

Chapter 55 Tennis Elbow (Lateral Epicondylitis)

Matthew L. Lyons

ICD-10-CM CODES
M77.11 *Lateral epicondylitis, right*
M77.12 *Lateral epicondylitis, left*

Key Concepts

- Lateral epicondylitis, often referred to as tennis elbow, is a tendinosis of the common extensor origin (extensor carpi radialis brevis [ECRB] tendon), also termed angiofibroblastic tendinosis because of its histologic appearance.
- It often is associated with tendinosis at other sites.
- It frequently coexists with nerve compression neuropathy, most commonly carpal tunnel syndrome.
- The male-to-female ratio is approximately equal.
- It typically presents as an overuse condition related to activities increasing tension in finger and wrist extensors.
- Repetitive activities are thought to result in microtrauma at the tendon origin that fails to adequately heal, resulting in the tendinosis.
- Radial tunnel syndrome is a less commonly seen compression of the posterior interosseous nerve (PIN) that has a similar presentation, can be difficult to differentiate, and can coexist in up to 5% of cases.

History

- Most commonly seen in patients aged 35 to 50 years, with peak incidence at age 45.
- Patients present with pain at the origin of the ECRB, which is slightly anterior and distal to the lateral epicondyle at the elbow.
- Pain is most commonly sharp in nature and produced by activities requiring active wrist extension and passive wrist flexion with the elbow held in an extended position.
- Patients frequently describe a history of repetitive lifting or gripping and often deny any inciting event.
  - Inquire about racket sports and manual labor vocations with repetitive movements such as hammering or cleaning.

Physical Examination

- Tenderness is most common over the ECRB tendon origin just distal and anterior to the lateral epicondyle (Fig. 55.1).
  - Less frequently patients report pain directly over the bony lateral epicondyle and more posterior extensor digitorum communis (EDC) tendon origin.
- Decreased grip strength is frequently seen with the elbow held in an extended position.
  - A decrease in grip strength of 8% or greater with the elbow held in an extended position compared to a flexed position is strongly predictive of lateral epicondylitis.
- Provocative tests: useful in making the diagnosis, but can also be positive in other etiologies, such as radial tunnel syndrome
  - With the elbow held in an extended position:
    - Pain with resisted wrist extension/finger extension
    - Pain with passive wrist flexion (stretch of the common extensor origin)
- Examine for elbow instability, focusing on lateral ulnar collateral ligamentous injury and resulting posterolateral rotatory instability (PLRI).
  - Chair push-up test: Pain is indicative of lateral epicondylitis, posterolateral subluxation of radial head indicative of instability
  - PLRI test: supine position with arm overhead; with supination of forearm and valgus stress a visible clunk is witnessed when moving the elbow from a flexed to extended position.
- Elbow, shoulder and wrist range of motion: assess for crepitus and mechanical symptoms seen in arthritic conditions.
- Consider radial tunnel syndrome: pain is commonly located more anterior and distal in the forearm, over the proximal mobile wad.
- Examine for carpal tunnel symptoms.

Imaging

- Radiographic assessment is rarely helpful in making what is largely a clinical diagnosis, but can be useful in ruling out other diagnoses with a similar presentation.
- Anteroposterior and lateral plain radiographs of the elbow
  - Rarely show calcification in extensor origin
  - Will help to rule out other conditions with intra-articular pathology (arthritic conditions)
- Magnetic resonance imaging
  - Assess for complete rupture of the common extensor origin that may need to be repaired intraoperatively.
  - Rule out associated ligamentous injury (most important: PLRI from lateral ulnar collateral ligament [LUCL] disruption).
- Ultrasound
  - Variable sensitivity and specificity largely dependent on the skill and experience of the examiner.

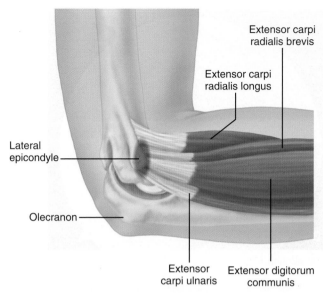

Extensor carpi
radialis brevis

Extensor carpi
radialis longus

Lateral
epicondyle

Olecranon

Extensor
carpi ulnaris

Extensor digitorum
communis

Fig 55.1 Anatomy of the lateral elbow.

Differential Diagnosis

- Radial tunnel syndrome: compression of the posterior interosseous branch of the radial nerve within the supinator muscle.
  - Pain located 3 to 4 cm distal and anterior to the lateral epicondyle over the mobile wad
  - May also present with pain with resisted supination and finger extension
- Other elbow tendinosis
  - Biceps: tenderness directly over the biceps tendon anteriorly
  - Triceps: tenderness directly over the triceps tendon posteriorly
- Carpal tunnel syndrome: numbness/tingling over median nerve distribution (thumb, index finger, and middle finger) Posterolateral rotatory elbow instability: instability with stress testing
- Intra-articular pathology
  - Arthritis: crepitus, loss of motion, radiographic changes
  - Loose bodies will often be accompanied by mechanical symptoms.
  - Posterolateral elbow plica: mechanical symptoms with painful clicking in maximal extension and supination and tenderness to palpation over the posterior radiocapitellar joint
  - Osteochondral radiocapitellar lesion: osteochondritis dissecans in teenage patients, particularly overhead athletes
- Cervical radiculopathy
- Shoulder pathology with referred pain

Treatment

- Observation: can be self-limiting, with symptoms resolving spontaneously
- Nonoperative treatment:
  - 3 Phase approach:
    1. Activity modification, rest, and antiinflammatory use
    2. Rehabilitation: therapy with stretching and isometric strengthening followed by sport-and activity-specific strengthening and work hardening
    3. Maintenance: equipment and technique modification (i.e., using a 2-handed backhand)
- Specific treatment options
  - Nonsteroidal antiinflammatory drugs: commonly used in the acute period, long-term benefit remains questionable
  - Bracing: no difference in efficacy between counterforce bracing and removable wrist splint
  - Physical therapy
  - Injection
- Corticosteroids have a short-term benefit that has not been shown to persist at 3 or 12 months.
- Recent studies showing worsened outcome at 12 months compared to placebo have raised caution and become contraindication for some.
  - Platelet-rich plasma has had mixed results with some studies showing improved long-term relief compared to corticosteroids and local anesthetic.
    - Cost may be a consideration.
  - Botulinum toxin has shown benefits in some but not all series, with potential side effect of weakness.
  - Needling of the tendon origin is recommended by some with hope of inducing a vascular healing response.
  - Less common modalities: Friction massage, iontophoresis, extracorporeal shock-wave therapy, pulsed electromagnetic field therapy—all with unclear long-term benefit.
- Operative treatment
  - Usually reserved for failure of conservative treatment after 6 to 12 months
  - While variability exists, surgical treatment commonly involves excision of the diseased ECRB tendon tissue, debridement of the wound bed, and repair of the tendon origin if indicated.
    - Accomplished through open or arthroscopic approach with similar outcome (Fig. 55.2)
  - Potential benefits to arthroscopic technique include faster recovery, including return to work, and ability to assess and address intra-articular pathology.
    - Percutaneous release of the tendon origin through a small incision has also been performed with results largely equivalent to debridement.
    - Secondary procedures such as lateral epicondyle denervation have been described with unclear benefit.
    - Revision surgery is reported to be 80% effective, with the most common finding being incomplete resection of the diseased tendon.
- Postoperative rehabilitation
  - Short period of immobilization with a splint with elbow at 90 degrees of flexion is most common.
  - Immediate range of motion in soft dressing more common in arthroscopic release.
  - Range of motion initiated at 2 weeks with return to light lifting and activities of daily living.
  - Strengthening initiated at 6 weeks postoperatively.
  - Return to sports between 3 and 6 months.

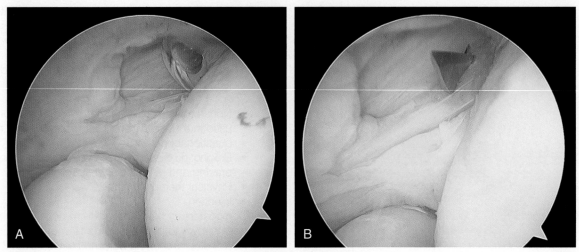

Fig 55.2 Arthroscopic appearance of lateral epicondylitis (A) and post release (B).

When to Refer

- Patients should be referred to a specialist for consideration of surgical treatment after failure of nonoperative treatment modalities for a minimum of 3 to 6 months.
- Elbow instability on exam or imaging is an indication for immediate referral.
- In patients with an atypical presentation and/or who fail to show any response to treatment, the diagnosis of radial tunnel syndrome should be considered and earlier consultation with an orthopaedic specialist may be warranted.

Prognosis

- Commonly improves with time. Only 4-11% of patients eventually require surgical intervention.
  - Poor prognosis: manual labor, involvement of dominant extremity, prolonged duration of symptoms, high analog pain scores, poor coping/life stressors.
- Nonoperative treatment:
  - Reported success rates of 85-90%.
  - Up to 40% may have residual or recurrent symptoms.
- Surgical treatment:
  - Decreased symptoms in 83-97% of patients.
  - Only 40% will be completely pain free.

Patient Instructions

- Patient reassurance is of paramount importance. While most patients will not require surgical intervention, improvement can be slow and prolonged, 12 to 18 months.
- Patients should be instructed and show good understanding of therapy modalities, including activity modification, icing, stretching, and the use of nonsteroidal antiinflammatory medications.
- Patients should be counseled on the potential benefits and risks for both nonoperative and operative treatment.

- Surgical benefits: decreased, but not necessarily resolved pain with the potential to return to previous activities
- Surgical risks: nerve injury (PIN), PLRI with overly aggressive debridement, heterotopic ossification (arthroscopy only), continued or recurrent symptoms.
- Following surgery, patients should be counseled on and demonstrate understanding of the postoperative therapy protocol.

Considerations in Special Populations

- Patients whose work activities appear to be the primary cause of their symptoms should be counseled that return to those activities may place them at risk for recurrent symptoms.
  - Infrequently, a permanent change in activities is required to achieve long-term relief.

Suggested Readings

Adams JE, Steinman SP. Elbow tendinopathies and tendon ruptures. In: Wolfe SW, Hotchkiss RN, Pederson WC, Kozin SH, Cohen MS, eds. *Green's Operative Hand Surgery*. Philadelphia: Elsevier; 2017:863–884.

Burn MB, Mitchell RJ, Liberman SR, et al. Open, arthroscopic, and percutaneous surgical treatment of lateral epicondylitis: a systematic review. *Hand*. 2017;Mar 1, [Epub ahead of print].

Calfee RP, Patel A, DaSilva MF, Akelman E. Management of lateral epicondylitis: current concepts. *J Am Acad Orthop Surg*. 2008;16:19–29.

Dorf ER, Chhabra AB, Golish SR, et al. Effect of elbow position on grip strength in the evaluation of lateral epicondylitis. *J Hand Surg Am*. 2007;32A:882–886.

Nirschl RP, Ashman ES. Elbow tendinopathy: tennis elbow. *Clin Sports Med*. 2003;22:813–836.

Sims SE, Miller K, Elfar JC, Hammert WC. Non-surgical treatment of lateral epicondylitis: a systematic review of randomized control trials. *Hand*. 2014;9:419–446.

Szabo SJ, Savoie FH, Field LD, et al. Tendinosis of the extensor carpi radialis brevis: an evaluation of three methods of operative treatment. *J Shoulder Elbow Surg*. 2006;15:721–727.

Chapter 56 Golfer's Elbow (Medial Epicondylitis)

Matthew L. Lyons

ICD-10-CM CODES
M77.01 *Medial epicondylitis, right*
M77.02 *Medial epicondylitis, left*

Key Concepts

- Medial epicondylitis is the most common cause of medial elbow pain.
- It is 5 to 10 times less frequent than lateral epicondylitis.
- Occurs as a result of microtrauma and degeneration affecting the common flexor tendon origin at the medial epicondyle.
- The pronator teres and flexor carpi radialis muscle origins are the most commonly involved (Fig. 56.1).
- Repetitive activities involving eccentric contracture of the wrist flexors and forearm pronators and valgus overload of the elbow, such as with throwing, have been implicated as precipitating factors.
- The most common cause is occupational.
- Although medial epicondylitis is referred to as golfer's elbow, only 10-20% of cases are due to recreational activities.
- Acute injury is much more common than in lateral epicondylitis (up to one-third of cases), but most patients do not describe an inciting event.
- It may be associated with ulnar neuropathy in as many as 50% of cases.

History

- Medial epicondylitis typically occurs between ages 30 and 50.
- Some studies suggest a female preponderance, while others indicate an equal distribution between men and women.
- Patients may present with either insidious or more acute onset of medial elbow pain that localizes to the medial epicondyle and radiates into the forearm.
- Symptoms are commonly activity related.
  - Occupations that require repetitive or constant forceful gripping, lifting of loads greater than 20 kg, and vibratory forces, such as construction workers, plumbers, and carpenters
  - Sports activities requiring repetitive wrist flexion and forearm pronation, such as golf, baseball, tennis, football, weight lifting, and bowling
  - Throwers and tennis players describe increased discomfort in the late cocking and early acceleration phases of throwing/serving.

- Concurrent diagnoses are common, especially in laborers.
  - Ulnar neuritis, carpal tunnel syndrome, lateral epicondylitis, rotator cuff tendinitis/tear.

Physical Examination

- Tenderness to palpation over the flexor-pronator origin at 5 to 10 mm distal/anterior to the medial epicondyle
- Range of motion is frequently normal, but patients may present with an elbow flexion contracture (throwers).
- Weakness with pronation compared to the contralateral side
- Provocative tests:
  - Increased pain with resisted wrist flexion and forearm pronation
  - Forceful grip may be decreased compared to the contralateral side or exacerbate medial elbow pain.
- Assess for concomitant conditions:
  - Ulnar neuritis: Inflammation may cause irritation of ulnar nerve.
  - Tinel sign over the cubital tunnel
    - Decreased sensation: 2 point discrimination in the ulnar nerve distribution of the hand.
    - Paresthesias with elbow hyperflexion for 30 to 60 seconds.
    - Motor weakness or atrophy in the hand: Wartenburg and Froment signs.
  - Ulnar nerve instability:
    - Subluxation/dislocation and paresthesias with elbow hyperflexion
    - Overdevelopment of the medial triceps head
  - Ulnar collateral ligament (UCL) injury: Overhead athlete
    - More distal apex of pain over sublime tubercle
    - Milking test: Forearm is held in supination and valgus stress is applied to thumb through full range of elbow flexion and extension.
      - Pain between 70 and 120 degrees of flexion indicates a positive test.
    - Valgus stress test: Pain with valgus stress applied to elbow in 30 degrees of flexion, forearm pronation, and wrist flexion

Imaging

- Radiographic assessment is rarely helpful in making what is largely a clinical diagnosis, but can be useful in ruling out other diagnoses with a similar presentation.

**Medial Epicondylitis
(Golfer's elbow)**

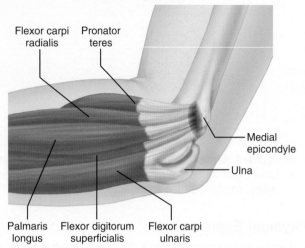

Flexor carpi radialis

Pronator teres

Medial epicondyle

Ulna

Palmaris longus

Flexor digitorum superficialis

Flexor carpi ulnaris

Fig 56.1 Anatomy of the medial elbow with tendinosis of the flexor-pronator origin.

- Radiographs: Anteroposterior and lateral views of the elbow
  - Plain radiographs of the elbow may reveal calcification distal to the medial epicondyle (25% of cases).
  - Rule out arthritis or acute osseous injury of the elbow.
- Magnetic resonance imaging:
  - Considered gold standard, indicated in unclear source of pain.
  - May show degenerative changes in the flexor pronator mass.
  - Assess integrity of the UCL.
  - Rule out other soft-tissue pathology.
- Ultrasound:
  - Can be effective in experienced hands.
  - Evaluate dynamically for complete disruption of tendon origin.

Differential Diagnosis

- Cubital tunnel syndrome
  - Positive Tinel sign, positive elbow hyperflexion test
- Ulnar nerve subluxation
  - Paresthesias and palpable anterior subluxation/dislocation of the ulnar nerve
- UCL insufficiency: most common in overhead athletes.
  - Common late finding in patients with chronic medial epicondylitis, as the intact common flexor tendon origin protects the underlying anterior bundle of the UCL.
- Elbow arthritis
  - Radiographic changes, crepitus, and/or mechanical symptoms with range of motion
- Intra-articular elbow fracture
- Triceps tendonitis
- Snapping medial head of the triceps
  - Mechanical snapping palpable with elbow range of motion; pain more posterior.
- Cervical radiculopathy

Treatment

- Nonoperative treatment
  - Goals: relieve acute pain, rehabilitate the injured tendon, prevent recurrence
  - Activity modification/rest: first line of treatment
    - Avoid throwing/precipitating factors for 6 to 12 weeks in athletes.
    - Passive stretching and icing
    - Oral antiinflammatories: short 1- to 2-week course
    - Bracing: counterforce bracing, nighttime splinting
      - Kinesio tape effective in throwers.
      - Nighttime extension bracing in patients with concomitant ulnar neuritis
  - Extracorporeal shockwave therapy (ESWT)
    - Thought to promote angiogenesis and healing while providing some analgesia.
    - Some studies have shown long-term effectiveness, but inadequate data exists for definitive treatment recommendations.
  - Cortisone injection
    - Short-term benefit that has not been shown to persist at 3 or 12 months.
    - Potential side effects: iatrogenic ulnar nerve injury, tendon degeneration, fat atrophy, skin pigmentation
  - Platelet-rich plasma
    - Has not been well studied in medial epicondylitis
    - Same potential for iatrogenic nerve injury
  - Ultrasound
  - Physical therapy and rehabilitation
    - Typically initiated once acute pain has subsided.
    - Initial goal of restoring range of motion, followed by concentric and then eccentric strengthening
    - Focus on prevention of recurrence
      - Core and lower body strengthening in throwers
      - Correct technique and equipment
- Operative treatment
  - Typically reserved for compliant patients who have not responded from 6 to 12 months of conservative treatment.
  - Less success than surgery for lateral epicondylitis
  - Open approach with resection of the diseased tendon and side-to-side or direct repair of the tendon origin is technique of choice.
  - Mini open approach has been described with successful outcome, but may limit safe visualization of ulnar nerve.
  - Arthroscopic debridement contraindicated due to potential for iatrogenic injury to the UCL and ulnar nerve.
  - Ulnar nerve symptoms addressed by concurrent cubital tunnel release with or without ulnar nerve transposition.
- Postoperative rehabilitation
  - Short period of immobilization in a splint with elbow at 90 degrees of flexion is most common.
  - Range of motion initiated at 2 weeks with return to light lifting and activities of daily living.
  - Strengthening initiated at 6 weeks.
  - Return to sports between 3 and 6 months.

When to Refer

- Patients should be referred to a specialist for consideration of surgical treatment after failure of nonoperative treatment modalities for a minimum of 6 and 12 months.

- UCL insufficiency or ulnar nerve symptoms on exam or imaging are an indication for referral.

Prognosis

- Nonoperative treatment is successful in 90-95% of patients within 3 to 6 months.
- Surgery is thought to be less successful than for lateral epicondylitis, with success rates reported between 83-96%.
- Results are worse when ulnar nerve symptoms are present prior to surgery.

Troubleshooting

- Younger patients, particularly overhead athletes, may present with subtle medial elbow instability that is difficult to distinguish clinically from medial epicondylitis. Magnetic resonance imaging may help to distinguish between these two entities.

Patient Instructions

- Patient reassurance is of paramount importance. While most patients will not require surgical intervention, improvement can be slow and prolonged.
- Patients should be instructed and show good understanding of therapy modalities, including activity modification, icing, stretching, and the use of nonsteroidal antiinflammatory medications.

- Patients should be counseled on the potential benefits and risks for both nonoperative and operative treatment.
  - Surgical benefits: decreased, but not necessarily resolved pain with the potential to return to previous activities
  - Surgical risks: iatrogenic injury to the UCL, ulnar nerve, medial antebrachial cutaneous nerve (painful neuroma or patchy numbness in medial elbow), continued or recurrent symptoms
- Following surgery, patients should be counseled on and demonstrate understanding of the postoperative therapy protocol.

Suggested Readings

Adams JE, Steinman SP, et al. Elbow tendinopathies and tendon ruptures. In: Wolfe SW, Hotchkiss RN, Pederson WC, eds. *Green's Operative Hand Surgery*. Philadelphia: Elsevier; 2017:863–884.

Amin NH, Kumar NS, Schickendantz MS. Medial epicondylitis: evaluation and management. *J Am Acad Orthop Surg*. 2015;23:348–355.

Badia A, Stennett C. Sports-related injuries of the elbow. *J Hand Ther*. 2006;19:206–226.

Eygendaal D, Safran MR. Postero-medial elbow problems in the adult athlete. *Br J Sports Med*. 2006;40:430–434.

Field LD, Savoie FH. Common elbow injuries in sport. *Sports Med*. 1998;26:193–205.

Hume PA, Reid D, Edwards T. Epicondylar injury in sport: epidemiology, type, mechanisms, assessment, management and prevention. *Sports Med*. 2006;36:151–170.

Vinod AV, Ross G. An effective approach to diagnosis and surgical repair of refractory medial epicondylitis. *J Shoulder Elbow Surg*. 2015;24(8):1172–1177.

Chapter 57 Distal Biceps Tendon Rupture

Matthew L. Lyons

ICD-10-CM CODES
S46.211A *Rupture of distal biceps tendon, initial encounter, right*
S46.212A *Rupture of distal biceps tendon, initial encounter, left*
S53.401A *Sprain of elbow, initial encounter, right*
S53.402A *Sprain of elbow, initial encounter, left*
M25.521 *Elbow pain, right*
M25.522 *Elbow pain, left*

Key Concepts

- Rupture of the distal biceps tendon is most commonly seen in the dominant extremity of men aged 40 to 49 and is the result of sudden eccentric contraction of the tendon against an excessive extension load applied to the flexed elbow.
- Tears are considered rare in woman and only single case studies exist.
- The rupture typically occurs at the tendon insertion onto the radial tuberosity in an area of preexisting tendon degeneration; however, injury at the musculotendinous junction is also reported.
- Physical examination demonstrates a palpable and visible deformity of the distal biceps muscle belly with weakness in supination and flexion.
- Risk factors include the dominant extremity, male gender, middle age, tobacco use, vocational activities involving high load or repetitive supination and flexion (e.g., plumber, laborer), sports (e.g., bodybuilder), and medical comorbidity (e.g., anabolic steroid use).
- The biceps brachii muscle is a supinator of the forearm and flexor of the elbow.
- The distal tendon of the biceps brachii muscle crosses the antecubital fossa to insert on the radial tuberosity. The footprint and geometry of the insertion are variable.
- The tendon passes near critical structures as it crosses the fossa, including the lacertus fibrosus, the radial nerve motor and sensory branches, lateral antebrachial cutaneous nerve, median nerve, brachial artery and branches, and venous structures (Fig. 57.1).
  - The lacertus fibrosus or bicipital aponeurosis is a division of the tendon that runs distally and medially at the antecubital fossa broadly expanding into the antebrachial fascia that attaches to the medial epicondyle.
- In complete ruptures, early surgical reattachment to the radial tuberosity is recommended for optimal results, which means expedient orthopaedic referral.

History

- Patients present with a history of an acute event involving an extension/pronation load.
  - Frequently but not always followed by a painful pop or tearing sensation in the antecubital region
- The event may be followed by pain, swelling, and ecchymosis that subside over a few days.
  - Visible deformity may be immediately present or appreciated as swelling subsides.
- After the acute inflammation subsides, patients may report weakness in vocational activities or sports but rarely in activities of daily living.
- Patients may report a history consistent with repetitive microtrauma from work or sporting activities before the acute event, although a history of activity-related pain is not expected.
- Vocational and recreational activities may predispose to rupture, including high load or repetitive supination and flexion (e.g., plumber, laborer) and sports (e.g., bodybuilder).
- Medical comorbidities such as rheumatoid arthritis, renal failure, and tobacco and anabolic steroid use may be a factor.
- In delayed or chronic presenters, weakness is more common than pain around the elbow/forearm.
- Weakness may be insignificant for the sedentary or average patient engaged in activities of daily living and desk work. However, the patient at risk of the injury is often more active and therefore more likely to be symptomatic.
- Cosmetic issues may also precipitate presentation.

Physical Examination

- Patients present with variable swelling and ecchymoses over the medial distal arm, elbow, and proximal forearm, and tenderness to palpation in the antecubital fossa.
- The ability to palpate the tendon in the antecubital fossa may be indicative of a partial tear.
- Deformity presents as accentuated upper arm anterior musculature in flexion ("Popeye" deformity), although this may be obscured by swelling.
- In comparison to the contralateral side, weakness should be present, greater with supination than with flexion.
- Combining specific provocative maneuvers increases the sensitivity and specificity of the examination.
  - Hook test
    - Examiner attempts to "hook" their index finger underneath the tendon from the lateral side as the patient contracts the tendon with the elbow in 90 degrees of flexion and full supination.

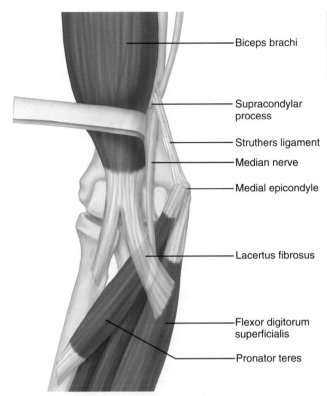

Biceps brachi

Supracondylar process

Struthers ligament

Median nerve

Medial epicondyle

Lacertus fibrosus

Flexor digitorum superficialis

Pronator teres

Fig 57.1 Anatomy of anterior elbow.

TABLE 57.1 Differential Diagnosis

Pathology	Differentiating Examination/ Clinical Scenario
Cubital bursitis[a] (with and without bicipital tendinosis); biceps partial tear or degeneration	Examination, MRI
Ligament or tendon injury other than biceps (e.g., ulnar collateral ligament or lateral ulnar collateral ligament)	Examination, MRI
Intra-articular injury (e.g., osteochondral fracture)	Examination, MRI
Bony fracture about the elbow	Radiographic analysis
Infectious or crystalline arthropathy	Lab work

[a]Cubital bursitis is enlargement of the bursal sac that lies between the biceps tendon and the anterior aspect of the radial tuberosity. This condition may exist in isolation or in association with a distal biceps tendon lesion. Tendon degeneration (bicipital tendinosis) without rupture may occur in isolation or in association with cubital bursitis or partial rupture.

MRI, Magnetic resonance imaging.

- Must distinguish the intact tendon from the lacertus fibrosus or underlying brachialis.
- Ruland biceps squeeze test (similar to Thompson squeeze test for Achilles tendon ruptures)
  - Examiner holds elbow in 70 degrees of flexion and slight pronation with one arm while squeezing the mid-arm biceps muscle with the other.
  - Failure to observe forearm supination is indicative of a positive test.
- Passive forearm rotation test
  - Involves inspection of the biceps muscle belly as the forearm is passively rotated from a supinated to pronated position with the elbow held in 90 degrees of flexion.
  - Loss of the normal proximal to distal motion of the muscle belly with this maneuver is indicative of a positive test.

Imaging

- Imaging studies are of debatable benefit, especially in the setting of clear physical exam findings.
- Plain radiographs: anteroposterior, lateral, and oblique views of elbow
  - Infrequently reveal a small avulsion fracture or hypertrophic bone formation at the radial tuberosity
- Magnetic resonance imaging (MRI)
  - Useful when diagnosis is unclear.
  - False negative read is possible.
  - Distinguish between partial and complete tears, tears at the myotendinous junction injury, and other elbow pathology.

- Positioning: flexion, abduction, supination (FABS) view: elbow flexion, forearm supination, shoulder abduction improves reliability
- Ultrasonography
  - Accurate in experienced hands.
  - Cost-effective relative to MRI.

Differential Diagnosis

See Table 57.1

Treatment

- Acute complete tears
  - Nonoperative management: Most commonly results in painless but significant loss of supination and flexion strength and potential for functional limitation.
    - Some studies report continued pain with activities.
    - Some potential for improvement in discomfort and strength over time.
    - Typically reserved for sedentary patients and those with medical comorbidities precluding surgical intervention.
  - Surgical management:
    - Historically: Performed through an extensile anterior approach of Henry, which resulted in a significant risk of neurologic injury.
    - Modified to 2-incision approach of Boyd and Anderson utilizing a transosseous tunnel.
      - Decreased chance of neurologic injury.
      - Increased risk of radioulnar synostosis and loss of forearm rotation.
      - Newer fixation options (button, interference screw, sutures anchors) have allowed limited-exposure single- and dual-incision techniques (Fig. 57.2).

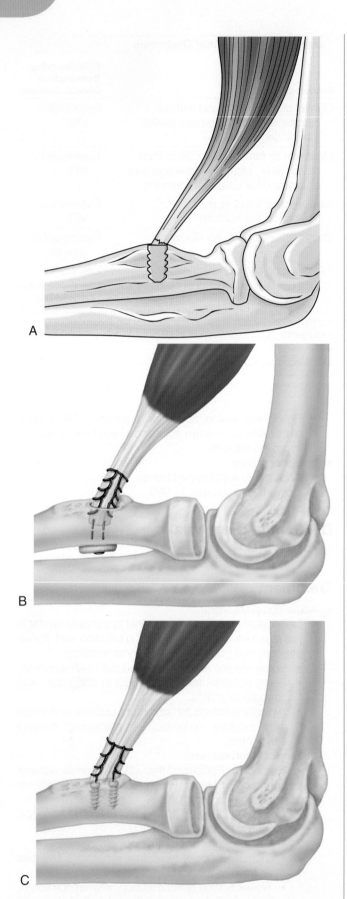

- Single incision
  - Increased risk of PIN or lateral antebrachial cutaneous nerve injury.
- Dual incision
  - Increased risk of heterotopic ossification or radio-ulnar synostosis.
- Outcome studies do not favor one technique over another, but advocate use of minimally invasive technique, clear understanding of anatomy, and careful retractor placement to minimize complications.
- While bone tunnel fixation has the strongest fixation strength of all techniques, it also carries an increased risk of loss of elbow motion compared to the modern fixation options.
- Of the modern fixation techniques, buttons have the highest load to failure in biomechanical studies.
  - Clinical outcomes appear to be largely equivocal regardless of fixation device.
- Partial tears:
  - Represent a distinct clinical entity and may be managed conservatively or operatively, depending on the severity of the tear and chronicity of symptoms.
  - Nonoperative treatment options: physical therapy, nonsteroidal antiinflammatory medications, cortisone injection, and platelet-rich plasma (PRP) injection.
    - Cortisone injections are contraindicated for some due to potential for tendon rupture and close proximity of neurovascular structures.
    - PRP has been successful in treating painful low-grade partial tears and tendinopathy.
      - Significant cost associated with the procedure should be taken into consideration.
  - Patients with a tear involving greater than 50% of the width of the tendon show improved outcomes with repair and repair has been shown to be favorable to debridement alone.
    - Laparoscopic-assisted repair has been described.
- Chronic ruptures:
  - Tears older than 4 to 6 weeks may have scarring, retraction, and tendon degeneration that precludes primary repair.
  - Intact lacertus fibrosus can prevent tendon retraction and allow primary repair of a more chronic injury.
  - When primary repair is not possible, tendon augmentation with a more extensile approach is often necessary.
    - May negatively impact final outcome, including strength and cosmetic appearance.
- Postoperative rehabilitation
  - Postoperative rehabilitation is variable, depending on the provider.
  - Patients are commonly immobilized in a long-arm plaster splint for the first 10 to 14 days, followed by transition to a hinged elbow brace and progressive motion.
    - Extension block starting at 60 degrees is common, with 20-degree advancement every 2 weeks to full extension at 6 weeks.
  - Recent studies have shown adequate healing with immediate progressive motion.
  - Light strength rehabilitation typically begins at 8 to 12 weeks.

Fig 57.2 Fixation of the distal biceps tendon with **(A)** interference screw, **(B)** biceps button, **(C)** suture anchors.

- Full-strength activities and return to sports at 5 to 6 months.

When to Refer

- If suspicion is high, consultation with an orthopaedist should be obtained urgently (within 1 week).
  - Advanced imaging need not be obtained prior to referral. For experienced providers, the diagnosis is largely clinical, and waiting for MRI may engender needless delay.
- If clinical suspicion is lower, an experienced nonoperative sports medicine or musculoskeletal provider may pursue further diagnosis or management.
  - MRI may be performed to narrow the differential.
- Late presentation of chronic tears represents a challenging variant, in which referral to a specialist should still be performed in an expedited manner.

Prognosis

- Surgical repair commonly results in full return of flexion and supination strength with low risk of recurrent rupture and improved function compared to nonoperative management.
- Loss of elbow extension and forearm rotation is a possible long-term side effect of surgery.
- While the overall incidence of complications is comparable for single- and 2-incision approaches, the 2-incision approach has a higher risk of loss of forearm rotation and rotational strength.

Troubleshooting

- When the initial diagnosis is unclear, clinicians should consider involving an orthopaedist rather than ordering and waiting for advanced imaging to be completed.
- In the eventuality that the primary mode of fixation does not prove stable, the surgeon needs to be prepared and capable of utilizing the full array of tendon fixation techniques.

Patient Instructions

- At the time of acute diagnosis, dorsal splinting with the elbow in 90 degrees of flexion and the forearm in neutral rotation is initiated.
  - Patients should understand the necessity for urgent evaluation by a surgeon, with the understanding that delay in diagnosis can have a detrimental effect on outcome.

- Patients should be counseled on the potential risks of surgery, including loss of motion, radioulnar synostosis or heterotopic ossification, failure to heal, recurrent rupture, weakness with forearm supination and elbow flexion, neurologic injury, and infection.
- Postoperatively:
  - Parameters for emergent return for evaluation should be given (e.g., pain out of proportion, pain to passive stretch, progressive tingling/numbness or weakness).
  - The importance of adherence to the rehabilitative protocol is paramount to avoid reinjury and need for revision surgery.
  - The postoperative protocol can appear complex to the patient, and the protocol should be provided in writing with appropriate time points for advancement of hinged bracing, extension blocks, weight-bearing status, formal occupational therapy, strength training, and return to work or sport.

Suggested Readings

Adams JE, Steinman SP. Elbow tendinopathies and tendon ruptures. In: Wolfe SW, Hotchkiss RN, Pederson WC, et al., eds. *Green's Operative Hand Surgery*. Philadelphia: Elsevier; 2017:863–884.

Barker SL, Bell SN, Connell D, Coghlan JA. Ultrasound-guided platelet-rich plasma injection for distal biceps tendinopathy. *Shoulder Elbow*. 2015;7(2):110–114.

Chavan PR, Duquin TR, Bisson LJ. Repair of the ruptured distal biceps tendon: a systematic review. *Am J Sports Med*. 2008;36(8): 1618–1624.

Darlis NA, Sotereanos DG. Distal biceps tendon reconstruction in chronic ruptures. *J Shoulder Elbow Surg*. 2006;15:614–619.

Devereaux MW, ElMaraghy AW. Improving the rapid and reliable diagnosis of complete distal biceps tendon rupture. *Am J Sports Med*. 2013;41(9):1998–2004.

John CK, Field LD, Weiss KS, Savoie FH. Single-incision repair of acute distal biceps ruptures by use of suture anchors. *J Shoulder Elbow Surg*. 2007;16:78–83.

Mazzocca AD, Burton KJ, Romeo AA, et al. Biomechanical evaluation of 4 techniques of distal biceps brachii tendon repair. *Am J Sports Med*. 2007;35:252–258.

Mazzocca AD, Spang JT, Arciero RA. Distal biceps rupture. *Orthop Clin North Am*. 2008;39:237–249.

O'Driscoll SW, Goncalves LB, Dietz P. The hook test for distal biceps tendon avulsion. *Am J Sports Med*. 2007;35:1865–1869.

Schamblin ML, Safran MR. Injury of the distal biceps at the musculotendinous junction. *J Shoulder Elbow Surg*. 2007;16:208–212.

Sutton KM, Dodds SD, Ahmad CS, Sethi PM. Surgical treatment of distal biceps rupture. *J Am Acad Orthop Surg*. 2010;18:139–148.

Chapter 58 Elbow Ligament Injuries

Jeffrey D. Boatright, D. Nicole Deal

ICD-10-CM CODES
S53.449A *Traumatic tear of UCL elbow*
S53.20XA *Traumatic rupture of radial collateral*
ligament of elbow radial collateral

Key Concepts

- The elbow is a highly constrained joint with intrinsic stability provided by both osseous and capsuloligamentous structures.
- It is composed of dynamic and static stabilizers.
  - Dynamic stabilizers include muscles that produce compressive forces across the elbow joint, such as the anconeus, brachialis, and triceps muscles.
  - Static stabilizers include the lateral collateral ligament complex (LCLC), medial collateral ligament (MCL), and ulnohumeral articulation.
    - The ulnohumeral articulation is the cornerstone of osseous stability and mobility in the flexion-extension plane.
      - The coronoid process resists posterior subluxation in flexion.
        - The medial facet of the coronoid imparts osseous stability to varus stress.
  - Secondary constraints include the radial head, common flexor and extensor origins, and elbow capsule.
    - The radial head is a secondary stabilizer to valgus loads. If the coronoid is fractured or insufficient with a concomitant MCL injury, the radial head becomes a primary stabilizer to valgus load.
- Ligamentous complex of the elbow (Fig. 58.1)
- Ligamentous constraints of the elbow contribute significantly to the stability of the joint.
- The collateral ligaments are anatomically contiguous with the joint capsule.
- The medial and lateral collateral ligaments have distinct functions.
  - The MCL is the primary stabilizer to valgus stress.
  - The LCL is an important restraint to posterolateral rotatory instability of the elbow.
- MCL (some authors refer to the MCL as the ulnar collateral ligament [UCL])
  - Originates on the medial epicondyle of the humerus, courses posterior to the axis of rotation, and inserts onto the sublime tubercle of the ulna
  - Full resection of the MCL leads to 6 to 8 degrees of valgus laxity and complete destabilization when the radial head is removed.

- Composed of three major bundles
  - Anterior band
  - Primary restraint to valgus stress between 30 and 120 degrees of flexion)
  - Nearly isometric
  - Posterior band
  - Tightest in flexion (less isometric)
  - Transverse band
    - Provides no contribution to elbow stability
- Lateral collateral ligamentous complex (LCLC)
  - The LCLC provides rotational and varus stability to the elbow.
  - Composed of three subunits
    - Radial collateral ligament
      - Originates on the anterior lateral epicondyle and inserts onto the annular ligament and supinator fascia
      - Provides varus stability
    - Annular ligament
      - Forms a sling around the radial head attaching to the sigmoid notch and supinator crest of the ulna
    - Lateral ulnar collateral ligament (LUCL)
      - Originates on the lateral epicondyle and inserts onto the supinator crest of the ulna
      - Primary stabilizer to varus and external rotation
        - A cadaveric study has shown that resection of both the radial collateral ligament and the LUCL is necessary to create instability. Full instability is recreated when the extensor mass is also transected.
- Two different forms of elbow instability exist with associated ligament injuries.
  - Simple instability
    - Injury to the MCL or LCLC, specifically the LUCL
  - Complex instability
    - Involves both ligamentous and osseous injury
      - Radial head fracture and complex instability
      - Coronoid fracture and complex instability
      - Terrible triad injury
        - Coronoid fracture, radial head fracture, and posterior ulnohumeral dislocation
      - Monteggia's fracture dislocation
        - Proximal one-third ulna fracture with radial head dislocation
      - Transolecranon fracture dislocation
        - Fracture through the olecranon with elbow dislocation

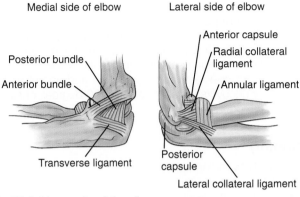

Medial side of elbow   Lateral side of elbow

Anterior capsule

Radial collateral
ligament

Posterior bundle

Annular ligament

Anterior bundle

Transverse ligament

Posterior
capsule

Lateral collateral ligament

Fig 58.1 Ligaments of the elbow.

History

- Should document hand dominance, occupation, as well as mechanism and chronicity of injury.
- Other history items directed specifically at the complaint should include:
  - What is the character of the pain?
    - Consider cervical spine or double crush neurologic injury with radicular pain.
  - Where is the pain?
    - Lateral elbow pain
      - LUCL instability
      - Lateral epicondylitis
      - Radiocapitellar arthritis
      - Radial tunnel syndrome
    - Medial elbow pain
      - MCL injury
      - Flexor-pronator origin disruption
      - Ulnar nerve compression/subluxation
      - Snapping triceps tendon
      - Medial epicondylitis
    - Posterior elbow pain
      - Triceps tendinopathy
      - Posterior impingement of olecranon osteophytes
    - Anterior elbow pain
      - Distal biceps pathology
      - Anterior capsular strain
      - Median nerve entrapment (pronator syndrome)
      - Primary osteoarthritis
  - Are there any exacerbating activities?
    - Medial elbow pain during the late cocking or acceleration phase of throwing is classic for MCL pathology in overhead throwing athletes.
    - Repetitive wrist extension exacerbates lateral epicondylitis.
  - Are there associated symptoms?
    - Valgus laxity from MCL insufficiency may cause traction of the ulnar nerve resulting in pain and/or paresthesias in an ulnar nerve distribution.
  - Severity and duration of symptoms?
  - Mechanism and chronicity of injury?
  - Mechanical complaints?
    - Loss of motion, catching, or locking?
- Mechanical complaints?
- Loss of motion, locking, and catching
- Instability

- Patients with MCL deficiency usually present with increasing pain along the medial elbow after repetitive throwing; this is a condition typically of the overhead throwing athlete.
- Common presentations
  - Throwing athletes with MCL injury will describe a sudden onset of symptoms including medial elbow pain, loss of velocity, and control.
    - May report hearing an audible "pop" at the time of injury, or may be insidious with gradually increasing symptoms over time.
    - Pain is greatest during the late cocking and early acceleration phase of the throwing cycle.
  - Chronic MCL insufficiency allows the medial olecranon to impinge on the olecranon fossa during terminal extension or the follow-through phase of throwing.
    - Valgus extension overload syndrome is a spectrum of conditions occurring with progressing MCL deficiency.
      - Posteromedial impingement of the elbow
      - Ulnar neuropathy
      - Increased radiocapitellar loading
  - Leads to radiocapitellar arthritis
- LUCL instability is usually seen as the result of elbow dislocation or iatrogenic injury after lateral elbow surgery and can lead to posterolateral rotatory instability. (See Chapter 59 for more information.)
  - Posterolateral rotatory instability of the elbow results from chronic insufficiency of the lateral ligamentous and muscular support of the elbow.
  - Typically presents with pain and subjective instability of the elbow with supination and axial loading (such as when pushing up from a seated position out of a chair).
  - Symptoms include locking, catching, and snapping when the elbow is extended with the forearm supinated.

Physical Examination

- Document motion of elbow, ligament laxity, or tenderness.
- The neck, shoulder, and wrist should be examined carefully in the patient with elbow pain.
- It is important to document the status of the ulnar nerve in patients with medial elbow pain.
- Medial and lateral ligamentous stability is assessed with the patient's forearm flexed at 30 degrees to unlock the olecranon from its fossa. The physician alternately applies valgus force and varus force to evaluate the area for medial or lateral laxity, pain, decreased mobility, and apprehension (i.e., sensation of impending dislocation).
- Key examination maneuver for MCL injury is the moving valgus stress test (Fig. 58.2).
  - With the patient seated and the shoulder abducted to 90 degrees, the elbow is maximally flexed while the examiner applies valgus stress to the elbow. The elbow is then quickly extended to 30 degrees while maintaining the valgus stress imparted at the elbow until the shoulder has reached maximum external rotation.
  - A positive test reproduces medial sided elbow pain and/or creates apprehension or guarding during the maneuver.
    - Frank instability can sometimes be appreciated as well.

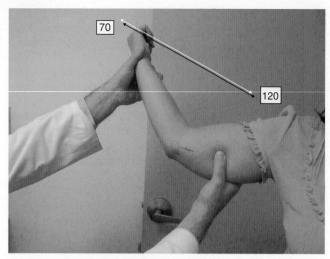

Fig 58.2 Moving valgus stress test. As described by O'Driscoll and colleagues, a valgus load is applied as the elbow is flexed and extended. A positive test is one in which pain is elicited at an elbow flexion/extension arc of 70 to 120 degrees.

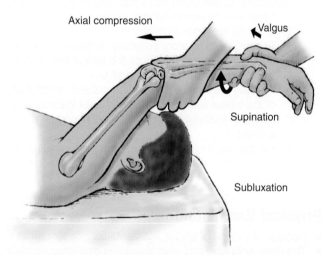

Fig 58.3 Lateral pivot shift test for posterolateral rotatory instability of the elbow. A supination valgus moment is applied during flexion, causing the elbow to subluxate maximally at approximately 40 degrees of flexion. Additional flexion causes reduction (with a palpable, visible "clunk," if successful). This test creates apprehension as the patient senses instability. (Modified from O'Driscoll SW, Jupiter JB, King GJW, et al. The unstable elbow. *Instr Course Lect.* 2001;50:89–102.)

- Key examination maneuvers for LCL injury or posterolateral rotatory instability (PLRI) are as follows:
  - Chair push-up test
    - The patient is asked to push up from a seated position in a chair with the hands on the arm rests and the forearms supinated.
    - Pain or apprehension with this maneuver is considered positive for PLRI.
  - Lateral pivot shift test (Fig. 58.3)
    - With the patient supine and the arm extended overhead and shoulder in external rotation, the examiner

stands above the patient's and grasps the lateral forearm just distal the elbow.
- The forearm is put in maximal supination and the elbow is slowly flexed while a valgus force and axial compression is applied across the elbow.
- A positive test reproduces pain and apprehension or uncovers instability at 40 to 50 degrees of elbow flexion.

Imaging

- Plain elbow radiographs
  - Valgus stress views
  - Varus stress views
- Magnetic resonance imaging of the elbow
  - Magnetic resonance imaging arthrography
    - Increases detection of partial MCL tears to 86% sensitivity
    - Better visualization of the undersurface of elbow ligaments
- Additional tests
  - Computed tomography arthrography
    - Eighty-six percent sensitive and 91% specific for complete MCL tears
  - Dynamic ultrasonography

Differential Diagnosis

- See the History section under "Where is the pain?"

Treatment

- At diagnosis
- Treatment principles are protection, rest, ice, compression, elevation, medication, and modalities (physical therapy).
- MCL injury
  - Refrain from throwing for 6 weeks
    - +/− nighttime splinting
  - Progressive physical therapy (PT) for guided range of motion and flexor-pronator mass strengthening
  - NSAIDs
  - Progressive throwing program
- LCL injury
  - See Chapter 59 on elbow dislocations.

When to Refer

- Patients with suspected elbow ligament injury should be seen early by an orthopaedic surgeon who can guide care, provide recommendations, and monitor response to treatment.

Prognosis

- Variable depending upon specifics of the injury, chronicity of injury, and occupation/sport

Patient Instructions

- Many partial injuries, even in high-level athletes, can be treated conservatively with a regimented treatment pathway that includes a well-described throwing protocol.

- Overhead athletes with a complete injury and a desire to return to play are typically treated surgically.

Considerations in Special Populations

- Throwing athletes with valgus elbow laxity should be educated about the unpredictable impact of this injury.
- Patients considering surgery (MCL reconstruction) should be educated about the risks associated with surgery, relatively involved and long postoperative rehabilitation program, and the possibility of being unable to return to his or her previous level of play.

Suggested Readings

Chumbley EM, O'Connor FG, Nirschl RP. Evaluation of overuse elbow injuries. *Am Fam Physician*. 2000;61:691–700.

Cohen MS. Lateral collateral ligament instability of the elbow. *Hand Clin*. 2008;24:69–77.

Dipaola M, Geissler WB, Osterman AL. Complex elbow instability. *Hand Clin*. 2008;24:39–52.

Hoppenfeld S, Hutton R. *Physical Examination of the Spine and Extremities*. New York: Appleton-Century-Crofts; 1976:35–57.

Lyons RP, Armstrong A. Chronically unreduced elbow dislocations. *Hand Clin*. 2008;24:91–103.

O'Driscoll SW, Bell DF, Morrey BF. Posterolateral rotatory instability of the elbow. *J Bone Joint Surg Am*. 1991;73A:440–446.

O'Driscoll SW, Lawton RL, Smith AM. The moving valgus stress test for medial collateral tears of the elbow. *Am J Sports Med*. 2005;33:231–239.

Safran MR, Caldwell GL III, Fu FH. Chronic instability of the elbow. In: Peimer CA, eds. *Surgery of the Hand and Upper Extremity*. New York: McGraw-Hill; 1996:467–490.

Vennix MJ, Wertsch JJ. Entrapment neuropathies about the elbow. *J Back Musculoskelet Rehabil*. 1994;4:31–43.

Wilder RP, Guidi E. Anatomy and examination of the elbow. *J Back Musculoskelet Rehabil*. 1994;4:7–16.

Chapter 59 Elbow Dislocations

Jeffrey D. Boatright, D. Nicole Deal

Key Concepts

- The elbow is a highly constrained joint. Dislocation is typically the result of a high-energy mechanism or fall.
  - For details on elbow constraint and stabilizers, see Chapter 58.
- Second most commonly dislocated joint (after shoulder)
- More frequent in males and in the nondominant extremity
- Two basic types of dislocations:
  - Simple elbow dislocation: dislocation without fracture (typically involves ligamentous injury)
  - Complex elbow dislocation: dislocation with fracture (+/− ligamentous injury)
- Descriptive classification is based on the direction of displacement of the olecranon relative to the humerus (e.g., posterolateral, posteromedial, lateral, medial, anterior; Figs. 59.1 and 59.2).
- Other variants include:
  - Monteggia fracture/dislocation—radial head dislocation associated with a proximal ulna fracture
  - Trans-olecranon fracture/dislocation—elbow dislocation through a displaced olecranon fracture
  - Terrible triad elbow injury—posterolateral elbow dislocation, radial head/neck fracture, and coronoid fracture
- Cadaveric studies have shown that most elbow dislocations occur as a valgus + extension + external rotation + axial load force is imparted on the elbow. This results in progressive disruption of capsuloligamentous structures in a lateral to medial direction.
- The lateral collateral ligament is disrupted first. As the rotatory force transmission continues, the anterior and posterior capsules are disrupted, followed finally by the medial collateral ligament.
  - This progression is known as the Horii circle.
- Elbow dislocations are the end stage of a spectrum of instability, from subluxation to dislocation. The three stages correspond with the pathoanatomic stages of the capsuloligamentous disruption. A perched dislocation is one in which the elbow is subluxed but the coronoid is impinged upon the trochlea (Figs. 59.3 to 59.6).

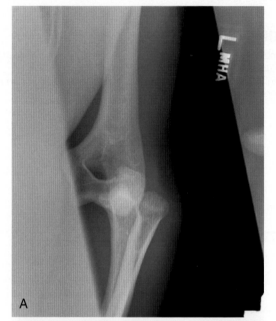

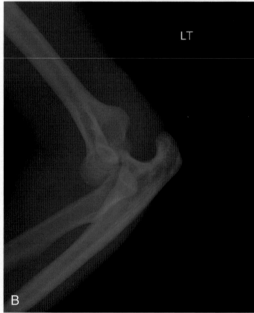

Fig 59.1 (A) Anteroposterior view of a posterolateral dislocation. (B) Lateral view of a posterolateral dislocation.

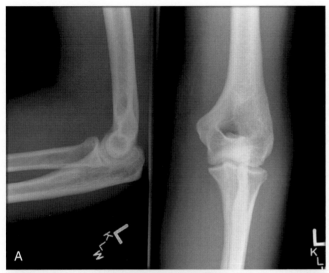

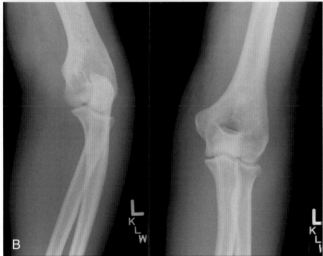

Fig 59.2 **(A)** Anteroposterior and lateral views after reduction. **(B)** Medial and lateral oblique views after reduction.

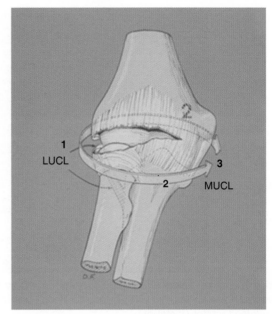

Fig 59.3 Illustration depicting the stages (*1*, *2*, and *3*) and the direction of soft-tissue injury seen with most elbow dislocations. *LUCL*, Lateral ulnar collateral ligament; *MUCL*, medial ulnar collateral ligament.

History

- The patient usually presents with a painful extremity that is shortened, deformed, and held in slight flexion after a fall on an outstretched arm.
- Important components of the history include documenting the mechanism of injury, hand dominance, occupation, and history of prior elbow trauma.

Physical Examination

- Diagnosis is made by clinical examination and verified with radiographs (Table 59.1).
- Assessment of the neurovascular status of the extremity pre- and postreduction is imperative.
- Assess for wounds about the elbow that could indicate an open injury.
- Postreduction, prior to splinting, typically while still sedated, the stable passive arc of motion should be assessed and documented.

TABLE 59.1 Diagnosis Made by Clinical Examination and Verified With Radiographs

Type of Dislocation	Clinical Presentation
Posterior elbow dislocations (see Figs. 59.1 and 59.2)	The elbow is flexed with an exaggerated olecranon; condyles of the elbow are not palpable
Anterior elbow dislocations	The elbow is held in extension and supination; the arm appears shortened; soft-tissue injury usually is severe
Lateral elbow dislocations/medial elbow dislocations	Some motion may still be maintained at the elbow joint; this is more common in lateral dislocations; motion takes place between the groove of the trochlea and capitellum (see Figs. 59.5 and 59.6)
Isolated ulnar dislocations	Cubitus varus deformity of the forearm is seen clinically; takes place when the humerus pivots around the radial head; the coronoid process may be displaced posteriorly to the humerus or the olecranon anteriorly to the humerus

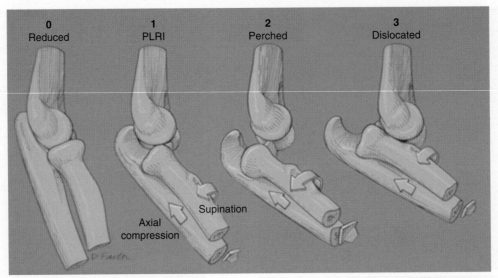

Fig 59.4 Illustration demonstrating the spectrum of elbow instability from subluxation to dislocation. The *arrows* indicate the forces responsible for displacements. Stages 1 to 3 demonstrate the stages of capsuloligamentous disruption (see Fig. 59.1). *PLRI*, posterolateral rotatory instability.

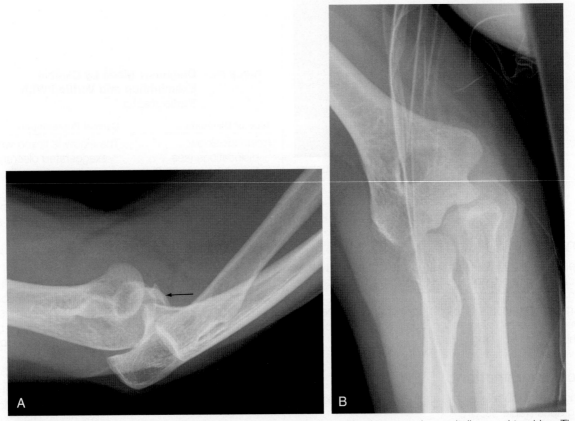

Fig 59.5 (A and B) Posterior dislocation of radial head with "perching" of the ulna between the capitellum and trochlea. The patient had a coronoid fracture *(arrow)*. On clinical examination, the patient was able to move the elbow. The patient was articulating within the groove between the trochlea and capitellum with the portion of the coronoid that was not fractured.

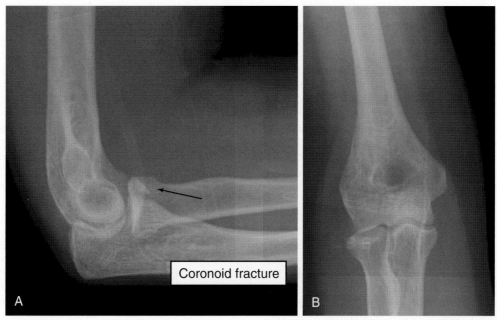

Coronoid fracture

A

B

Fig 59.6 (A) Anteroposterior postreduction radiographs of the patient in Fig. 59.5. (B) Lateral postreduction radiograph of the same patient.

- This information is crucial for clinical decision making in terms of follow-up and short- to mid-term treatment options (see the following).

Imaging

- Radiographic images include anteroposterior and lateral views of the elbow, both before and after reduction.
- Postreduction radiographs assess for associated fractures and concentric reduction.
  - Nonconcentric reduction could suggest soft-tissue interposition.
- On follow-up, we recommend oblique views of the elbow to assess for coronoid fractures, radial head fracture, and shear injuries of the capitellum that may not be recognized in anteroposterior and lateral views.

Additional Tests

- Arteriogram if suspected vascular injury
- Computed tomography is recommended when associated fractures are noted and referral to a specialist is anticipated.

Differential Diagnosis

- Please see Box 59.1.

Treatment

- Emergent referral should be made to an orthopaedic surgeon or more likely an emergency department (with orthopaedic consultation).
  - Vascular surgery consultation may be needed in patients with possible vascular injury.
- Urgent reduction and splinting of the joint (typically under conscious sedation) is indicated in all cases.

BOX 59.1 Differential Diagnosis

Chronic elbow injury
Congenital dislocation of the radial head
Distal humerus fracture
Radial head/neck fracture
Olecranon fracture
Elbow ligamentous sprain

- Techniques for reduction of elbow dislocations
- Posterior elbow dislocations
  - Axial traction on the extremity with correction of medial or lateral displacement and progressive flexion of the elbow usually produces an audible "clunk," which typically indicates a successful reduction.
  - It is helpful to have bedside fluoroscopy for immediate confirmation of reduction (while the patient is still sedated).
  - Another method (the Parvin method) involves placing the patient in the prone position with the humerus resting on the table and the forearm hanging perpendicular to the plane of the table. The humerus should be supported by the table, with padding or rolled towels, just proximal to the elbow joint. Five to 10 pounds of weight are applied to the wrist. Reduction should occur over a period of minutes as the muscles relax. The physician may push the olecranon into place if necessary.
- Anterior dislocation (rare)
  - Reduced with traction on the wrist and posterior pressure on the forearm. Take care to avoid hyperextension at the elbow, which may cause traction and potential injury to neurovascular structures around the elbow.
    - Interposition of the brachial artery and the median and ulnar nerves is possible.
    - Postreduction neurovascular exam is imperative.
  - Then assess the stable passive arc of motion.

- A failed closed reduction is indicative of an entrapped fracture fragment, inverted cartilaginous flap, or other interposed tissue.
- The elbow is splinted in a position of stability (based on postreduction range of motion and stability testing).
- For simple elbow dislocations that are stable on post reduction examination, full unprotected motion should be started no later than 1 week. The patient is instructed to work with pronation and supination with the elbow at 90 degrees of flexion. Varus/valgus stress to the elbow is also avoided for the first 6 weeks postinjury. The patient is also instructed to avoid full extension and supination early in the rehabilitation process. Elbow extension is permitted in a gradual and progressive manner.
  - If forearm pronation was required to prevent extension instability, a full range of motion is allowed in a hinged brace with the forearm fully pronated. The patient may only come out of the brace for motion exercises in full pronation under the guidance of a skilled therapist. The brace is worn for 4 weeks.
  - If an extension block was required, it is reduced gradually over 4 weeks. Extension blocks greater than 45 degrees typically require surgical intervention and early referral.
- Loss of extension between 5 and 10 degrees compared with the unaffected elbow is typically seen after this injury.
- Subacute or chronic elbow dislocations seen after 1 week require open reduction and early referral.
- Complex elbow dislocations often require surgical intervention.

Prognosis

- Highly dependent on type of dislocation, associated injuries, and appropriate postreduction aftercare.

Troubleshooting

- Fractures of the coronoid and radial head and elbow dislocation are known as the "terrible triad." Early referral is indicated for ligament reconstruction and fracture repair.
- Late instability after closed management of an elbow dislocation is usually in the form of posterolateral rotatory instability (PLRI).
  - Indicative of injury/attenuation of the lateral ligamentous complex
  - Typically presents with pain and subjective instability of the elbow with supination and axial loading (such as when pushing up from a seated position out of a chair)

Suggested Readings

Beingessner DM, Pollock JW, King GJW. Elbow fractures and dislocations. In: Court-Brown CM, Heckman JD, McQueen MM, et al, eds. *Rockwood and Green's Fractures in Adults*. 8th ed. Philadelphia: Wolters Kluwer; 2015:1179–1228.

Cohen MS, Hastings H. Acute elbow dislocation: evaluation and management. *J Am Acad Orthop Surg*. 1998;6:15–23.

Hobgood ER, Khan SO, Field LD. Acute dislocations of the adult elbow. *Hand Clin*. 2008;24:1–7.

Josefsson PO, Johnell O, Gentz CF. Long-term sequelae of simple dislocations of the elbow. *J Bone Joint Surg Br*. 1984;69B:605–608.

Mehta J, Bain G. Posterolateal rotatory instability of the elbow. *J Am Acad Orthop Surg*. 2004;12:404–415.

O'Driscoll SW, Jupiter JB, King GJ, et al. The unstable elbow. *Instr Course Lect*. 2001;50:89–102.

Tashjian RZ, Katarincic JA. Complex elbow instability. *J Am Acad Orthop Surg*. 2006;14:278–286.

Chapter 60 Olecranon Bursitis

Anthony J. Archual, Aaron M. Freilich

ICD-10-CM CODES
M70.2 *Olecranon bursitis*
M25.52 *Elbow pain*

Key Concepts

- The olecranon process is the most proximal posterior eminence of the ulna located on the dorsal aspect of the elbow.
  - Overlying this posterior eminence is the olecranon bursa.
  - The olecranon process contains broad attachments for the triceps tendon posteriorly.
  - The olecranon forms the greater sigmoid notch of the ulna, which articulates with the trochlea of the distal humerus.
- The olecranon bursa is a smooth sac between the loose skin and the bones of the elbow.
  - The bursa allows the skin to move without restraint over the underlying olecranon, preventing tissue tears by providing a mechanism for the skin to glide freely over the olecranon process.
  - Olecranon bursitis occurs when the bursa becomes inflamed (Fig. 60.1).
- Because of its superficial location, the bursa can become inflamed secondary to acute trauma, infection, inflammatory arthropathy, or repetitive shear forces across this area (i.e., student's or miner's elbow).

History

- Patients present with a swollen, painful enlargement of the posterior aspect of the elbow (e.g., golf ball/goose egg appearance).
- Patients may have chronic recurrent swelling over the posterior aspect of the elbow, which is usually not tender.
- Frequent trauma of the swollen elbow may occur because the olecranon process protrudes more than normal.
- Patients may report a history of isolated trauma or repetitive microtrauma (e.g., due to constant rubbing of the elbow against the table while writing).
- Onset may be sudden if the condition is secondary to infection or acute trauma.
- Onset may be gradual if olecranon bursitis is secondary to chronic irritation.
- A history of fever, marked tenderness, and overlying cellulitis suggests septic bursitis.
- Swelling is often the first symptom. The skin on the back of the elbow is loose, so a small amount of swelling may not be noticed right away. As the bursa grows, the swelling worsens causing pain as the bursa is stretched. The swelling may grow large enough to restrict motion of the elbow.
- A history of trauma or lacerating/puncture wound should be documented.
- The patient's hand dominance and field of work should be documented (i.e., student's or miner's elbow).
- Pain is located at the olecranon process, and traction osteophytes (olecranon spurs) can be seen on radiographic views, which indicate a chronic process (seen in patients with recurring bursitis).
- Reasons for olecranon bursitis
  - Trauma: A blow to the tip of the elbow could cause the bursa to produce excess fluid.
  - Prolonged pressure: Leaning on the tip of the elbow for long periods on hard surfaces, such as a tabletop, may cause the bursa to swell. Typically this type of bursitis would develop over several months.
  - Infection: If the tip of the elbow has an injury that breaks the skin, such as an insect bite or an abrasion, bacteria may enter the bursa and cause an infection. The infected bursa produces purulent fluid, redness, and swelling.
  - Medical conditions: Certain conditions such as rheumatoid arthritis and gout are associated with development of elbow bursitis.

Physical Examination

- Swollen and painful mass on the posterior aspect of the elbow
- Pain with flexion and stretch of inflamed bursa.
- Open wounds that could indicate a portal of entry for bacteria.
- Patients with systemic inflammatory processes (e.g., rheumatoid arthritis) or crystal deposition disease (e.g., gout, pseudogout) may reveal evidence of focal inflammation at other sites.
- Patients with rheumatoid arthritis may have rheumatoid nodules.
  - Elbow pain during active or passive motion should increase the clinician's suspicion of fracture of the olecranon process in the setting of recent trauma.
  - Loss of elbow extension against gravity would lead one to suspect a triceps rupture.
  - Intra-articular pathology (e.g., septic elbow, fractures, arthritis) coincides with a painful arc of motion not usually seen in olecranon bursitis.
  - It is important to try to identify the cause of the bursitis as early as possible, as chronic bursitis is likely to cause formation of scar tissue, which may lead to more regular flare-ups and possibly further complications.

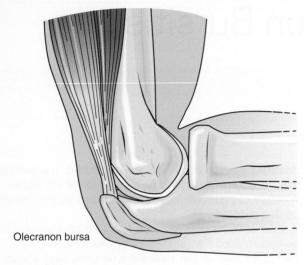

Olecranon bursa

Fig 60.1 Olecranon bursa.

TABLE 60.1 Differential Diagnosis

Pathology	Clinical Scenario/ Differentiating Examination
Triceps tendon rupture	Clinical examination by loss of elbow extension against gravity (partial rupture; magnetic resonance imaging)
Fracture of the olecranon process, radial head	Radiographic analysis
Crystalline inflammatory arthropathy (e.g., gout, pseudogout)	Pertinent laboratory work ordered
Synovial cyst of the elbow joint	Radiographic analysis

Imaging

- Radiographic anteroposterior and lateral views of the elbow
- Magnetic resonance imaging is recommended when triceps insufficiency is suspected. It also evaluates for underlying abscess or bone infection (osteomyelitis) with chronic septic bursitis.

Additional Tests

- Complete blood count and differential, erythrocyte sedimentation rate, and C-reactive protein level when suspecting a septic process followed by aspiration (see the section on aspiration of olecranon bursa).
- Check for rheumatoid factor to assess for rheumatoid arthritis and the uric acid level to assess for gout.

Differential Diagnosis

- Please see Table 60.1.

Treatment

- At diagnosis
  - A nonseptic bursa can usually be treated symptomatically and the patient advised to avoid rubbing the elbow. The RICE (rest, ice, compression, elevation) protocol should be followed. Small and moderate bursae can be treated by aspiration with or without injections of steroids followed by a compressive dressing (neoprene sleeve or elastic bandage).
  - The elbow is elevated and ice is applied. An elbow pad may be used to cushion the elbow (heelbow pad). Direct pressure to the swollen elbow should be avoided. Oral medications such as antiinflammatories may be used.
  - If swelling and pain do not respond to these measures, then removing fluid from the bursa and injecting corticosteroid medication into the bursa may be indicated.

- Later
  - Chronic bursitis, when it is recurrent and symptomatic, should be treated with an open or arthroscopic bursectomy.

When to Refer

- Consultation with an orthopaedist
  - Septic bursitis that deteriorates and does not respond to initial treatment of aspiration and culture-directed antibiotics
  - Chronic recurrent bursitis that is symptomatic
  - Suspected intra-articular elbow pathology or triceps tendon rupture
- Consultation with a physiatrist (physical medicine and rehabilitation physician) or with another qualified musculoskeletal specialist may be considered by physicians without the training, comfort, or procedural office supplies necessary for aspiration.
- Consultation with a rheumatologist may be helpful if findings are consistent with inflammatory arthropathy.

Prognosis

- Prognosis is typically good, and recovery is usually complete. Most of the patients with olecranon bursitis respond well to treatment unless there is a persistent infection. Corticosteroid injection is usually effective in nonseptic bursitis, and long-term sequelae are unusual.
- Some residual soft-tissue prominence is common.

Troubleshooting

- See olecranon bursa aspiration/injection section.

Patient Instructions

- The first approach in treating olecranon bursitis should be to eliminate mechanical stress from the affected area, such as avoiding leaning on the elbow. If a repetitive activity is the cause, this activity should be stopped until the bursitis has completely resolved.

- Olecranon bursitis that does not resolve from rest alone or that is causing pain may need medical intervention such as oral or topical nonsteroidal antiinflammatory drugs or corticosteroid injections.

Considerations in Special Populations

- Patients with end-stage renal disease are more likely to develop chronic recalcitrant olecranon bursitis due to their altered immune system.
- Patients with gout and tophi on their elbows, as well as patients with rheumatoid arthritis with rheumatoid nodules on their elbows, are more likely to have recurrences of olecranon bursitis.

Suggested Readings

Salzman KL, Lillegard WA, Butcher JD. Upper extremity bursitis. *Am Fam Physician*. 1997;56:1797–1806, 1811–1812.

Shell D, Perkins R, Cosgarea A. Septic olecranon bursitis: recognition and treatment. *J Am Board Fam Pract*. 1995;8:217–220.

Stewart NJ, Manzanares JB, Morrey BF. Surgical treatment of aseptic olecranon bursitis. *J Shoulder Elbow Surg*. 1997;6:49–54.

Wasserman AR, Melville LD, Birkhahn RH. Septic bursitis: a case report and primer for the emergency clinician. *J Emerg Med*. 2009;37(3):269–272.

Weinstein PS, Canoso JJ, Wohlgethan JR. Long-term follow-up of corticosteroid injection for traumatic olecranon bursitis. *Ann Rheum Dis*. 1984;43:44–46.

Chapter 61 Ulnar Nerve Entrapment

Jeffrey D. Boatright, D. Nicole Deal

ICD-10-CM CODES
G56.20-G56.23	*Cubital tunnel syndrome*
G58.7	*Mononeuritis multiplex (e.g., ulnar tunnel at the wrist and cubital tunnel in the elbow)*
For Differential	
M54.12	*Cervical radiculopathy*
M77.00	*Medial epicondylitis*

Key Concepts

- Cubital tunnel syndrome is compression of the ulnar nerve around the elbow.
- It is the second-most common site of nerve compression in the upper extremity.
  - Carpal tunnel syndrome (median nerve compression at the wrist) is the most common.
- The ulnar nerve can be compressed in any location along its path around the elbow but is most commonly entrapped in the cubital tunnel (Fig. 61.1).
- Patients typically present with numbness or paresthesias in the small finger and ulnar half of the ring finger.
  - Other symptoms include pain about the medial elbow, and patients with severe or chronic compression may have weakness and atrophy of the ulnar nerve innervated intrinsic muscles of the hand.
  - Symptoms are reproduced with percussion of the nerve (Tinel's sign) and/or with hyperflexion of the elbow combined with applied pressure along the course of the ulnar nerve at this level.
- Other signs of motor involvement include an ulnar claw hand (late finding) and/or positive Wartenberg, Froment, Masse, and Jeanne signs (described in the following).
- Intrinsic and extrinsic factors can compress the ulnar nerve around the elbow.
  - Intrinsic factors (e.g., perineuroma, hamartoma of the ulnar nerve)
  - Extrinsic factors (e.g., hypertrophic fibrous bands, tendons or other surrounding tissue, hypertrophic muscles, accessory muscles, and vascular lesions)
- Acute and chronic compression of ulnar nerve around the elbow (Table 61.1)

History

- Patients may present with ill-defined symptoms and pain about the medial elbow and/or ulnar side of the forearm.
- Sensory symptoms can include paresthesias, hyperesthesias, dense numbness, and/or tingling.

- Classically this involves the small finger and ulnar half of the ring finger.
- The first sensory deficits are light touch, pressure, and vibration.
- Pain and temperature sensation are the last to be impaired.
- Motor symptoms range from weakness to paralysis of the ulnar nerve innervated muscles.
  - Patients may report clumsiness with fine motor activities, difficulty grasping objects, and hand fatigue secondary to weak intrinsic hand musculature.
- Patients should be asked about the onset, duration, and progression of symptoms.
- Alleviating and exacerbating factors
- Changes in skin color, temperature, texture, and moisture may result from sympathetic nervous system dysfunction.
- Comorbidities (e.g., diabetes, hemophilia, gout, and generalized peripheral neuropathy, thyroid disease, and vitamin deficiency)
- Documentation of patient's handedness, occupation, prior trauma, and specific activities that produce symptoms
  - Symptoms with overhead elevation?
  - Thoracic outlet syndrome
  - Symptoms with elbow flexion?
  - Cubital tunnel syndrome
  - Symptoms with wrist flexion?
  - Ulnar tunnel syndrome (entrapment of the ulnar nerve at Guyon's canal)
  - Symptoms at night?
  - Worsening of symptoms at night is common in cubital tunnel syndrome due to the propensity to sleep with elbows in a flexed position.
  - Cubitus varus or valgus deformities, medial epicondylitis, and repetitive elbow flexion/valgus stress during occupational or athletic activities may lead to compression of the ulnar nerve at the elbow.

Physical Examination

- Cubital tunnel syndrome is primarily a clinical diagnosis, thus the physical examination is extremely important.
- This evaluation should include a cervical spine examination as well as a comparison to the contralateral upper extremity.
- Inspection:
  - Atrophy and wasting of the first webspace and interossei muscles
  - Clawing of the ulnar two digits (late finding)
  - Hyperextension of ring and small finger metacarpophalangeal joints with hyperflexion of proximal interphalangeal joints

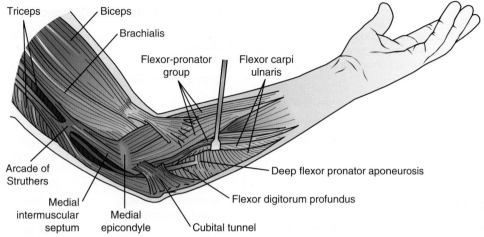

Fig 61.1 Potential sites of ulnar nerve entrapment around the elbow. Arcade of Struthers (fascial hiatus in the medial intermuscular septum, 8 cm proximal to the medial epicondyle), medial intermuscular septum, medial head of the triceps muscle, medial epicondyle, Osborne's ligament (cubital tunnel roof or retinaculum), anconeus epitrochlearis (anomalous muscle originating from the medial olecranon and inserting on the medial epicondyle), and flexor carpi ulnaris aponeurosis. Other sources of compression include tumors, cysts, osteophytes, heterotopic ossification, and medial epicondyle nonunion.

TABLE 61.1 Acute and Chronic Ulnar Nerve Entrapment

Condition	Causes
Acute ulnar nerve entrapment	Fractures/dislocations of the elbow; errant placement of retractors during surgery; malpositioning of patient during surgery; open injury (knife, gunshot wound)
Chronic ulnar nerve entrapment	Cubitus valgus (late presentation of distal physeal elbow injury in children); hypertrophic callus formation of previous elbow fracture/dislocation; ganglion cysts/tumors

- Ulnar claw deformity of the hand is seen with motor involvement (late presentation).
- Alignment of the elbow (cubitus valgus or varus)
- Surgical or traumatic scars
- Masse sign (see the following)
- Palpation
  - The ulnar nerve should be palpated while bringing the elbow through a full range of motion to evaluate for subluxation of the nerve over the medial epicondyle.
- Sensory examination:
  - Symptoms may include paresthesias, hyperesthesias, and/or numbness in the two ulnar digits (ring and small fingers) and dorso-ulnar aspect of the hand.
  - Symptoms may worsen with the use of the hand requiring elbow flexion (see elbow flexion compression test below).
  - Neurosensory testing should be performed in the context of both dermatomal and peripheral nerve distributions.
  - Semmes-Weinstein monofilaments measure cutaneous pressure threshold, a function of large nerve fibers (the first to be affected in compression neuropathy).

- Two-point discrimination should be measured on the fingertip pulp of each digit.
- The inability to perceive a difference of less than 5 mm is abnormal and constitutes a late finding in compression neuropathy.
- Motor examination
  - Examine individual muscle strength (grades 0 to 5), pinch strength, and grip strength.
  - Ulnar nerve innervated muscles in the hand include: adductor pollicis, flexor pollicis brevis, dorsal and palmar interossei, and fourth and fifth lumbricals.
  - Weakness with resisted abduction of the index finger is a sensitive test for dorsal interosseous muscle weakness when compared to the contralateral side.
- Classic signs associated with ulnar neuropathy:
  - Froment sign: Excessive flexion of the thumb interphalangeal (IP) joint (median nerve function) during key pinch results as compensation for a weakened adductor pollicis (ulnar nerve function).
  - Wartenberg sign: Inability to adduct (or maintain adduction of) the small finger due to weak third palmar interossei and fifth lumbrical
  - Jeanne sign: Excessive thumb metacarpophalangeal (MP) joint hyperextension during key pinch as a result of a weakened flexor pollicis brevis
  - Masse sign: Loss of the normal palmar curvature of the hand and hypothenar elevation due to opponens digiti quinti wasting
- Provocative tests
  - Elbow flexion/compression test
  - Most sensitive test
  - Patient's elbow is maximally flexed (flexion decreases the volume and increases the pressure within the cubital tunnel) while the examiner applies pressure to the ulnar nerve just posterior to the medial epicondyle.
  - Position is held for 30 to 60 seconds.
  - Worsening paresthesias or pain in an ulnar nerve distribution is considered a positive test.

- Percussion test (Tinel's sign)
- Examiner gently taps on the ulnar nerve as it travels just posterior to the medial epicondyle.
- Increased paresthesias or a radicular shooting pain in an ulnar nerve distribution is considered a positive test.

Imaging

- Not routinely indicated for cubital tunnel syndrome
- Radiographic views of elbow (anteroposterior and lateral views)
- Magnetic resonance imaging of the elbow

Additional Tests

- Electromyography/nerve conduction velocity studies
- Helpful in confirming the clinical diagnosis or occasionally in distinguishing from another diagnosis in the differential such as cervical radiculopathy or ulnar nerve compression within Guyon's canal at the wrist
  - Also of prognostic value when considering surgical decompression
- Exam is operator dependent and has high false-negative rate (20-45%).
- May be enhanced by using an "inching" technique across the elbow

Differential Diagnosis

- See Table 61.2.

Treatment

- Nonoperative treatment
  - Activity modification by avoiding sustained and repetitive elbow flexion beyond 30 to 45 degrees
  - A night splint or a towel wrapped around the elbow (to prevent extreme elbow flexion) is recommended.
  - Nonsteroidal antiinflammatory drugs
  - Eighty percent of patients with mild compression and 30% with severe compression see at least partial improvement in their sensory-related symptoms with these modalities.
- Operative treatment
  - Patients with symptoms of cubital tunnel syndrome after 3 months of nonoperative treatment or those with motor involvement are best treated with surgical decompression.
  - Referral at this time is appropriate.
  - Numerous surgical techniques have been described, such as in situ cubital tunnel decompression, medial epicondylectomy, and anterior ulnar nerve transposition (subcutaneous, adipofascial flap, subfascial, intramuscular, or submuscular).
  - Anterior submuscular transposition by musculofascial lengthening produces the best results, according to some meta-analyses.

When to Refer

- See "Treatment" section.

TABLE 61.2 Differential Diagnosis

Pathology	Clinical Scenario/Differentiating Features on Examination
Cervical root impingement (C8, T1)	Magnetic resonance imaging and radicular type pain; hypoactive deep tendon reflexes
Brachial plexus impingement (lower trunk and branches)/thoracic outlet syndrome (see section on thoracic outlet syndrome)	Chest and cervical oblique view radiographs to determine pulmonary cause of symptoms (e.g., Pancoast tumor, presence of cervical rib); patient may present with facial pain as well as temporomandibular joint pain
Wrist ulnar nerve entrapment/ulnar tunnel syndrome (see section on ulnar tunnel syndrome)	Intact sensation at dorso-ulnar side of the hand is a distinguishing feature
Pronator syndrome	Proximal arm nerve entrapment of the median nerve, not ulnar nerve; volar forearm pain and sensory disturbances in the distribution of the palmar cutaneous branch of the median nerve

Prognosis

- For patients with mild compression of the ulnar nerve, Dellon (2005b) found that 50% achieved excellent results with nonsurgical management and almost 100% achieved excellent results with surgical intervention. For patients with moderate compression, the anterior submuscular technique yielded the best results with the least recurrence; the intramuscular technique yielded the worst results with the most recurrence.
- Those with severe motor involvement and muscular atrophy should not expect full recovery of function but may still benefit from surgery in an attempt to halt progression.

Troubleshooting

- Congenital anomalies: The anconeus epitrochlearis muscle is an accessory muscle seen on the lateral aspect of the elbow that may lead to compression of the ulnar nerve.
  - Can only be seen during surgical decompression
- Examine patient for a subluxating ulnar nerve or prominent medial head of the triceps muscle, both of which can cause ulnar neuritis.
- Double crush phenomenon is seen when cervical radiculopathy or proximal nerve entrapment coexists with distal nerve compression.

Patient Instructions

- Patients treated early typically have excellent relief of symptoms.
- Late presentation with progressive motor or sensory deficits decreases the likelihood of full recovery and good clinical outcome.
- Persistent symptoms after surgery can be due to irreversible nerve damage from long-standing compression, incomplete decompression, other sites of compression (cervical spine), or perineural scarring.
- Injury to the posterior branch of the medial antebrachial cutaneous nerve can lead to hyperesthesia, hyperalgesia in the forearm, and a painful surgical scar.
- Subluxation of the ulnar nerve may occur with simple decompression alone.
  - This can lead to ongoing ulnar neuritis.
- Injury to the medial collateral ligament of the elbow resulting in elbow instability may occur as a complication of a submuscular transposition procedure.
- Individuals involved in high-level upper-extremity activities, such as a throwing sport or physically demanding occupation, may require a slightly extended rehabilitation period postoperatively.

Considerations in Special Populations

- Musicians may present with complaints of decreased finger dexterity and/or endurance compared to their baseline.
  - Violin, guitar, flute, and piano players
  - Symptoms can sometimes improve with relaxation techniques (e.g., Pilates) and changes in technique and/or practice schedule.

- Patients with tophaceous gout
  - Uric acid crystal deposits in or around the nerve can cause compressive symptoms.
- Rheumatoid arthritis
  - Caused by proliferation of synovium and tenosynovium
  - Compression of the posterior interosseous nerve can also be seen.
- Hemophiliacs
  - Predisposed to intramuscular, perineural, and intraneural bleeding

Suggested Readings

Davis GA, Bulluss KJ. Submuscular transposition of the ulnar nerve: review of safety, efficacy and correlation with neurophysiological outcome. *J Clin Neurosci*. 2005a;12:524–528.

Dellon AL. Compression neuropathy. In: Trumble T, Cornwall R, Budoff J, eds. *Core Knowledge in Orthopaedics: Hand, Elbow, and Shoulder*. Philadelphia: Mosby; 2005b:234–254.

Dellon AL. Review of treatment results for ulnar nerve entrapment at the elbow. *J Hand Surg Am*. 1989;14(4):688–700.

Elhassan B, Steinmann SP. Entrapment neuropathy of the ulnar nerve. *J Am Acad Orthop Surg*. 2007;15:672–681.

Henry M. Modified intramuscular transposition of the ulnar nerve. *J Hand Surg Am*. 2006;31:1535–1542.

Ruchelsman DE, Lee SK, Posner MA. Failed surgery for ulnar nerve compression at the elbow. *Hand Clin*. 2007;23:359–371, vi–vii.

Szabo RM, Kwak C. Natural history and conservative management of cubital tunnel syndrome. *Hand Clin*. 2007;23:311–318, v–vi.

Zlowodzki M, Chan S, Bhandari M, et al. Anterior transposition compared with simple decompression for treatment of cubital tunnel syndrome: A meta-analysis of randomized, controlled trials. *J Bone Joint Surg Am*. 2007;89:2591–2598.

Chapter 62 Fractures of the Distal Humerus

Rashard Dacus, Seth Bowman

ICD-10-CM CODES
S42.4	*Fracture of lower end of humerus*
S42.41	*Simple supracondylar fracture without intercondylar fracture of humerus*
S42.42	*Comminuted supracondylar fracture without intercondylar fracture of humerus*
S42.43	*Fracture (avulsion) of lateral epicondyle of humerus*
S42.44	*Fracture (avulsion) of medial epicondyle of humerus*
S42.45	*Fracture of lateral condyle of humerus*
S42.46	*Fracture of medial condyle of humerus*
S42.47	*Transcondylar fracture of humerus*

Key Concepts

- Epidemiology
  - Distal humerus fractures are relatively uncommon, with an incidence of approximately 6 cases per 100,000 people in the population per year.
  - Male/female distribution is nearly equal.
  - Most common in young males and elderly females
- Anatomy
  - The trochlea and capitellum constitute the distal articular humerus.
  - The humeral shaft divides into longitudinal medial and lateral columns.
  - The trochlea connects the columns distally at the joint.
  - The olecranon fossa is a triangular depression posteriorly.
  - The intramedullary canal tapers to end 2 to 3 cm proximal to the fossa.
  - The capitellum is part of the lateral column.
- Classification
  - Intra-articular: single column, both columns (T pattern, Y pattern, H pattern)
  - Extra-articular intracapsular: transcolumnar, high, low
  - Extracapsular: medial epicondyle, lateral epicondyle
  - Muller: type A, extra-articular; type B, single column; type C, both columns
- Goals of treatment
  - Restore articular surface, stabilize range of motion (ROM)
  - Stabilize the articular surface to the humeral shaft
- Additional findings
  - Humeral shaft fracture, olecranon or radial head fracture

History

- Symptoms: pain, inability to move elbow
- Mechanism of injury
  - Transcolumnar: axial load through forearm with elbow flexed
  - Intercondylar: axial load on olecranon with elbow flexed beyond 90 degrees

Physical Examination

- Visual inspection: edema, deformity, laceration/puncture, or ecchymosis
- Palpation: crepitus
- Range of motion: limited due to pain at elbow; always assess joints proximally and distally
- Neurologic: assess radial, median/anterior interosseous nerve, and ulnar nerve function
- Vascular: assess radial and ulnar arterial pulses; Allen test

Imaging

- Anteroposterior and lateral elbow
- Anteroposterior and lateral humerus
- Traction views and internal/external oblique views may help define fragments.
- Computed tomography helpful for surgical planning or for occult fracture (Fig. 62.1)

Differential Diagnosis

- Please see Table 62.1.

Treatment

- At diagnosis
  - There is a limited role for nonoperative management of these fractures.
  - Only nondisplaced fractures may be treated nonoperatively with a long-arm posterior elbow splint with the elbow in 90 degrees of flexion and the wrist in a neutral position.
  - Splint for 2 weeks.
- Later
  - After 2 to 3 weeks of immobilization, recheck radiographs to monitor for displacement.

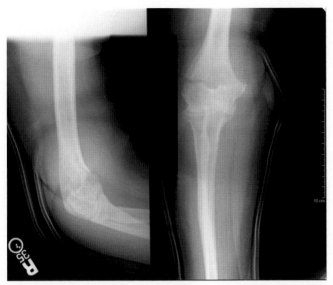

Fig 62.1 Anteroposterior and lateral radiographs of a low transverse distal humerus fracture.

TABLE 62.1 **Differential Diagnosis**

Differential Diagnosis	Differentiating Features	Chapter Reference
Elbow dislocation	Evidence of dislocation on radiographs	59, 66
Olecranon fracture	Fracture of proximal ulna evident on radiographs	64
Triceps avulsion	Radiographs are either negative for fracture or demonstrate an avulsion fracture from the proximal ulna; inability to perform elbow extension	58

- If reduction is maintained, transition to a hinged elbow brace and begin gentle ROM.

When to Refer

- All displaced and comminuted fractures should be placed into a long-arm posterior splint as described previously and the patient referred to an orthopaedic surgeon for surgical management within 1 week of injury.
- Evidence of nerve or vascular injury requires emergent referral or consultation.
- Surgical interventions may include the following:
  - Closed reduction and percutaneous pinning
  - Open reduction and internal fixation (Fig. 62.2)
  - Total elbow arthroplasty may be an option in the appropriate patient.
  - Comminuted fractures in osteoporotic bone specifically in elderly patients
  - Preexisting elbow pathology in a low-demand patient (Fig. 62.3)

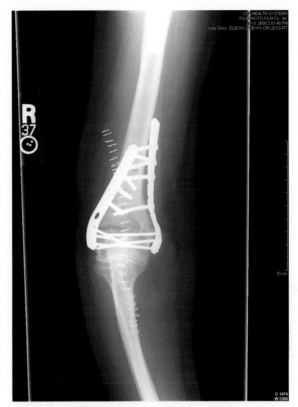

Fig 62.2 Plate fixation of a distal humerus fracture.

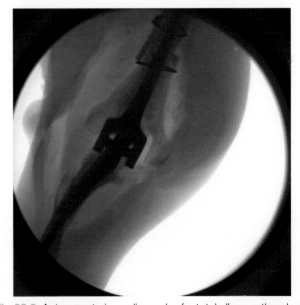

Fig 62.3 Anteroposterior radiograph of a total elbow arthroplasty.

Prognosis

- Inadequate or delayed reduction, intra-articular step-offs, and prolonged immobilization can result in significant elbow stiffness and disability.
- Regardless of the treatment modality, the full elbow ROM may never be equal to the uninjured elbow, but it should be functional (30 to 130 degrees of flexion).

- Heterotopic ossification is commonly associated with distal humerus fractures that are treated with open reduction and internal fixation. The incidence of heterotopic ossification may be decreased by early continuous passive ROM, the use of nonsteroidal antiinflammatory drugs (indomethacin), or radiation therapy.
- It has been recently shown in a prospective, randomized, control trial that total elbow arthroplasty has shorter surgical times and improved outcome scores up to 6 months compared to open reduction and internal fixation of distal humerus fractures in the elderly population.
- Ulnar nerve dysfunction may occur after this injury and is minimized by an ulnar nerve transposition at the time of the initial surgery.
  - Persistent ulnar nerve symptoms after open reduction and internal fixation may require secondary surgery for nerve mobilization or excision of heterotopic ossification.

Patient Instructions

- Keep splint on at all times until evaluated by orthopaedic surgeon.
- Pain medication is to be provided as indicated by presentation.
- Encourage elevation, rest, and finger ROM to decrease edema.

- Referral to an occupational or physical therapist may be necessary to promote the ROM.
- The patient may always have some elbow stiffness even after appropriate medical, surgical, and therapeutic modalities.

Suggested Readings

Anglen J. Distal humerus fractures. *J Am Acad Orthop Surg*. 2005;13: 291297.

Doornberg J, Lindenhovius A, Kloen P, et al. Two- and three-dimensional computed tomography for the classification and management of distal humeral fractures. Evaluation of reliability and diagnostic accuracy. *J Bone Joint Surg Am*. 2006;88A:1795–1801.

Gabel GT, Hanson G, Bennett JB, et al. Intraarticular fractures of the distal humerus in the adult. *Clin Orthop Relat Res*. 1987;216:99–108.

Jawa A, McCarty P, Doornberg J, et al. Extra-articular distal-third diaphyseal fractures of the humerus. A comparison of functional bracing and plate fixation. *J Bone Joint Surg Am*. 2006;88A:2343–2347.

McKee MD, Jupiter JB, Division of Orthopaedics, St. Michael's Hospital, University of Toronto. A contemporary approach to the management of complex fractures of the distal humerus and their seguelae. *Hand Clin*. 1994;10:479–494.

Varecka TF, Myeroff C. Distal humerus fractures in the elderly population. *J Am Acad Orthop Surg*. 2017;25:673–683.

Watts AC, Morris A, Robinson CM. Fractures of the distal humeral articular surface. *J Bone Joint Surg Br*. 2007;89B:510–515.

Chapter 63 Radial Head or Neck Fractures

Rashard Dacus, Seth Bowman

ICD-10-CM CODES
S52.12 *Fracture of head of radius*
S52.13 *Fracture of neck of radius*
S52.18 *Other fracture of upper end of radius*

Key Concepts

- Epidemiology
  - Radial head fractures account for approximately one-third of all elbow fractures.
  - 15-20% of the time radial head and neck fractures occur simultaneously.
- Classification
  - Radial head fractures
  - Mason classification: type I, nondisplaced; type II, marginal fracture with displacement; type III, comminuted fracture of the entire radial head (Fig. 63.1)
  - Radial neck fractures
  - Acceptable alignment for radial neck fractures: 30 degrees or less of angulation and 3 mm or less of translocation
  - In adults, 45 degrees is acceptable if passive supination and pronation are 60 degrees in both directions.
- Goals of treatment
  - Pain reduction, restoration of normal forearm rotation
  - Slow the progression of arthritic change
- Additional findings
  - Evaluate for Essex-Lopresti lesion (fracture of the proximal radius causes proximal migration of the radius and subsequent ulnar positive variance resulting in wrist pain).
  - Lateral collateral ligament disruption if associated with dislocation
  - Medial collateral ligament injury
  - Chondral injury to the capitellum (osteochondral defect)

History

- Symptoms: pain, limitation in elbow/forearm motion, weak grip
- Mechanism of injury
  - Radial head: fall onto outstretched upper extremity with axial load of radial head against capitellum
  - Radial neck: fall on an extended and supinated outstretched hand

Physical Examination

- Visual inspection: edema, ecchymosis
- Palpation: tenderness over the radial head; crepitus with fracture
- Range of motion: Evaluate supination/pronation; aspiration of hematoma and injection of local anesthesia aid in evaluation of mechanical block
- Neurologic: Assess radial nerve function.
- Vascular: Check distal perfusion if it is associated with a dislocation.

Imaging

- Anterior and lateral views of elbow; oblique views may aid in diagnosis
- Greenspan: allows view of radiocapitellar joint
- Radiocapitellar (forearm neutral, beam 45 degrees cephalad)
- Computed tomography for confirmation of occult fracture or surgical planning

Differential Diagnosis

- Please see Table 63.1.

Treatment
Radial Head Fracture

- At diagnosis
  - Nondisplaced fractures with no block to motion: sling for comfort, elevation, pain control

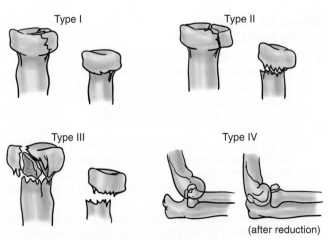

Type I   **Type II**

Type III   **Type IV**

(after reduction)

Fig 63.1 Modified Mason classification.

TABLE 63.1 Differential Diagnosis

Differential Diagnosis	Differentiating Features	Chapter Reference
Lateral epicondylitis	Tenderness to palpation directly over the lateral epicondyle and pain that is exacerbated by resisted wrist extension; normal radiographs	55
Posterolateral rotatory instability	Patient may report a history of dislocation or feeling of instability, clicking, or locking; positive lateral pivot shift test; magnetic resonance imaging helpful to identify injury of collateral ligaments	58
Insertional biceps tendinitis	Tenderness to palpation over distal biceps tendon at antecubital fossa; pain with resisted elbow flexion; normal radiographs	57
Radial tunnel syndrome	Tenderness to palpation over the mobile wad; normal radiographs	52, 68

- Later
  - Recheck radiographs at 1- or 2-week intervals to evaluate for displacement.
  - Begin early range of motion exercises (within 2 weeks of injury)
  - Radial neck fracture
- At diagnosis
  - Minimally displaced fracture: Splint in 90 degrees of flexion and neutral rotation.
- Later
  - Recheck radiographs to monitor for fracture displacement at 1- or 2-week intervals.
  - After 2 weeks, begin active range of motion.

When to Refer
Radial Head Fracture

- The following require operative management
  - Partial radial head fracture with block to motion
  - Partial radial head fracture with complex injury to the elbow and ligamentous instability
  - Comminuted fractures of radial head
- Operative methods
  - Open reduction and internal fixation of the radial head (for three or fewer fragments) or younger patients
  - Radial head excision (for more than three fragments) in a delayed fashion; usually only considered for low-demand, sedentary patients
  - Prosthetic replacement (for more than three fragments and longitudinal disruption of the forearm interosseous membrane) (Figs. 63.2 to 63.4)

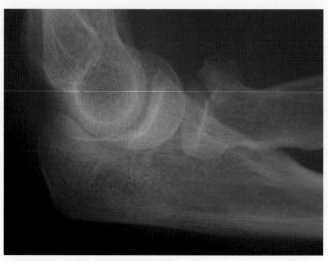

Fig 63.2 Lateral radiograph of radial head fracture.

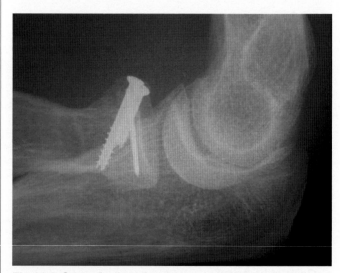

Fig 63.3 Screw fixation of radial head fracture.

Radial Neck Fracture

- Between 30 and 60 degrees of angulation or displaced: treatment can range from closed reduction under anesthesia to percutaneous Kirschner-wire fixation or open reduction and internal fixation.

Prognosis

- Patients with nondisplaced radial head and neck fractures can expect complete recovery and return of nearly full range of motion. Minimal loss of elbow extension can occur.
- Surgical treatment of displaced or comminuted fractures can significantly decrease morbidity related to range of motion. Most common complications after surgical reduction are instability, traumatic arthritis, and heterotopic ossification.
- High rate of avascular necrosis with open reduction and internal fixation in pediatric population

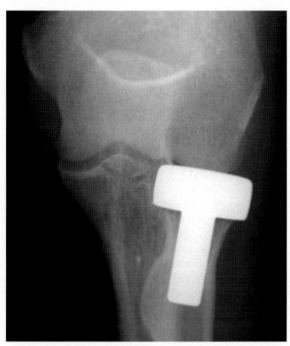

Fig 63.4 Anteroposterior radiograph of radial head replacement.

Troubleshooting

- Pain control is important in patients with acute nondisplaced fractures so that they may begin early range of motion exercises.
- If patient is too painful to accurately physically examine, consider hematoma block for pain control and then reevaluate.

- It is important to recheck radiographs after a nondisplaced fracture to monitor for displacement.
- Patients presenting with a displaced radial head or neck fracture should always have a wrist evaluation to check for an Essex-Lopresti lesion. This should also be considered in patients who present with late-onset wrist pain after open reduction and internal fixation of the radial head, radial head excision, or arthroplasty.
- Chondral injuries can predispose a patient to the development of traumatic elbow arthritis.

Patient Instructions

- Encourage elevation, rest, and early motion.
- Avoid longitudinal pressure on the forearm for 6 to 8 weeks for both operative and nonoperative management.

Suggested Readings

Goldberg I, Peylan J, Yosipovitch Z. Late results of excision of the radial head for isolated closed radial head fractures. *J Bone Joint Surg Am*. 1986;68A:675–679.

Koslowsky TC, Mader K, Gausepohl T, Pennig D. Reconstruction of mason type-III and type-IV radial head fractures with a new fixation device: 23 patients followed 1-4 years. *Acta Orthop*. 2007;78:151–156.

Steele JA, Graham HK. Angulated radial neck fractures in children. A prospective study of percutaneous reduction. *J Bone Joint Surg Br*. 1992;74B:760–764.

Tejwani NC, Mehta H. Fractures of the radial head and neck: current concepts in management. *J Am Acad Orthop Surg*. 2007;15:380–387.

Chapter 64 Proximal Ulna Fractures

Rashard Dacus, Seth Bowman

ICD-10-CM CODES

S52.01	*Torus fracture of upper end of ulna*
S52.02	*Fracture of olecranon process without intraarticular extension of ulna*
S52.03	*Fracture of olecranon process with intraarticular extension of ulna*
S52.04	*Fracture of coronoid process of ulna*
S52.09	*Other fracture of upper end of ulna*
S52.27	*Monteggia fracture*

Key Concepts

- Epidemiology
  - Coronoid fractures are identified in 10-15% of elbow dislocations.
  - As many as 30% of olecranon fractures are open.
  - Three percent to 5% have been associated ulnar neuropraxia.
- Classification
  - Olecranon fractures
  - Mayo: type I, nondisplaced or minimally displaced (<2 mm); type II, displacement of proximal fragment with stable elbow; type III, displacement of proximal fragment with instability of the ulnohumeral joint due to injury to ulnar collateral ligament; often there is an associated radial head fracture.
  - Shatzker (fracture pattern): transverse; transverse, impacted; oblique; oblique/distal; comminuted; fracture/dislocation
  - Coronoid process fractures (usually occur in conjunction with elbow dislocation with or without radial head fracture; termed "terrible triad" if all three are present)
  - Type I: coronoid tip fracture
  - Type II: 50% or less may be single fragment or comminuted
  - Type III: greater than 50% of process
  - Monteggia fracture: fracture of the proximal or middle third ulna with dislocation of the radial head
  - Type I (most common): anterior dislocation of radial head; fracture of ulnar diaphysis
  - Type II: posterior or posterolateral dislocation of radial head; fracture of ulnar diaphysis
  - Type III: lateral or anterolateral dislocation of radial head; ulnar metaphysis fracture
  - Type IV (rare): anterior dislocation of radial head; fracture of both forearm bones
- Goals of treatment
  - Articular restoration, stability, preservation of range of motion (ROM)

- Associated findings
  - Have a high suspicion for associated fractures or ligamentous injuries: Monteggia fracture, distal humerus fracture, elbow dislocation, coronoid process fracture, radial head or neck fracture, collateral ligament injury.
  - Transverse fractures of the tip of the coronoid are most commonly seen with terrible triad injuries and are associated with posterolateral rotatory instability.
  - Anteromedial coronoid fractures are most commonly seen with varus posteromedial instability.

History

- Symptoms: pain, inability to extend arm at the elbow, instability
- Mechanism of injury: direct blow to posterior elbow, fall on outstretched hand, or direct fall on flexed elbow

Physical Examination

- Visual inspection: edema, deformity, inspect skin for laceration/puncture
- Palpation: crepitus along posterior elbow
- ROM may be limited due to pain; active motion can be limited by separation of the triceps insertion from the ulnar shaft.
  - Important to assess integrity of collateral ligaments in varus and valgus stress in flexion and extension
- Neurologic: Assess motor and sensory function distal with special attention to median, ulnar, and radial nerve (posterior interosseous nerve).
- Vascular: Assess pulses and capillary refill.

Imaging

- Radiographs: anteroposterior, lateral, and oblique views of the elbow
- Lateral radiograph may show displacement of coronoid process or olecranon; assess for articular involvement and comminution in this view (Fig. 64.1).

Additional Tests

- Computed tomography to assess coronoid fragment or associated distal humerus fracture

Differential Diagnosis

- Please see Table 64.1.

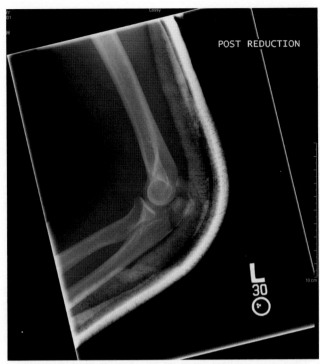

Fig 64.1 Lateral radiograph of olecranon fracture.

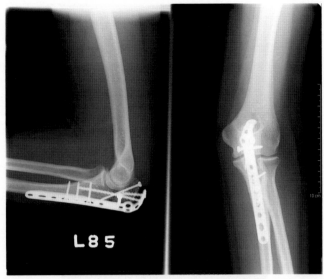

Fig 64.2 Anteroposterior and lateral radiographs of olecranon plating.

TABLE 64.1 Differential Diagnosis

Differential Diagnosis	Differentiating Feature	Chapter Reference
Olecranon bursitis	Normal radiographs; large soft-tissue swelling over posterior aspect of olecranon process	60
Bony contusion	Normal radiographs; may confirm on more advanced imaging such as magnetic resonance imaging	52
Elbow dislocation	Evidence of dislocation on radiographs or computed tomography scan; chronic dislocations may present with history of popping or clicking; perform lateral pivot shift test	59

Treatment
Olecranon Fractures
- At diagnosis
  - Nonoperative management: place into long-arm posterior splint or cast with the elbow in 60 degrees of flexion, forearm neutral
- Later
  - Obtain radiographs at 2-week intervals to monitor for displacement.

- Begin gentle ROM therapy at 3 weeks and avoid flexing the elbow past 90 degrees with the use of a hinged elbow brace.
- May progress to full active ROM at 6 to 8 weeks

When to Refer
- Types II and III or evidence of disruption of extensor mechanism; open fractures
  - Refer to orthopaedic surgeon for operative management.

Operative Methods
- Intramedullary fixation with cancellous lag screw fixation (6.5 vs. 7 mm)
- Tension band wiring with two parallel Kirschner wires
- Plating: 3.5 mm dynamic compression plating (Fig. 64.2)

Coronoid Process Fractures
- At diagnosis
  - Nonoperative as long as the elbow is stable and there is no block to motion
  - Reduce elbow dislocation if present.
  - Splint elbow in approximately 90 degrees of flexion for 2 to 3 weeks.
- Later
  - Recheck radiographs for fracture displacement and maintenance of elbow reduction.
  - Reassess elbow for stability. If unstable, continue splinting for an additional 1 to 2 weeks. If stable, begin protected active ROM in a hinged elbow brace.

When to Refer
- Type II: Assess elbow stability; if stable, fracture may be managed as a type I; if unstable, refer for surgical management.
- Type III: All fractures considered unstable; refer for operative management which most commonly consists of plate and screw fixation (Fig. 64.3).

253

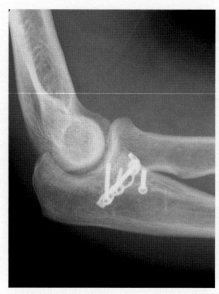

Fig 64.3 Lateral radiograph of anteromedial facet coronoid fracture plating. (From Park SM, Lee JS, Jung JY, et al. How should anteromedial coronoid facet fracture be managed? A surgical strategy based on O'Driscoll classification and ligament injury. *J Shoulder Elbow Surg.* 2015;24(1):74–82.)

Monteggia Fractures

- Now
  - Attempt reduction of radial head under conscious sedation and splint in long-arm posterior elbow splint.
  - In general, the radial head will normally reduce once the ulna is out to length.

When to Refer

- Nearly all Monteggia fractures will require open reduction and internal fixation. Refer all fractures to an orthopaedic surgeon.

Prognosis

- Olecranon fractures: Types I and II fractures have a good prognosis and minimal loss of motion. Type III fractures have less favorable results, with the most common complication being loss of ROM.
- Coronoid process fractures: Type I fractures have an excellent prognosis. Type II and III fractures frequently are associated with some loss of ROM.
- Monteggia fractures: High incidence of injury to posterior interosseous nerve in acute setting, but this usually resolves after reduction of radial head.

Troubleshooting

- When treating these fractures nonoperatively, it is important to recheck radiographs on a weekly or biweekly basis to monitor for late displacement, which can cause significant morbidity.
- Early protected ROM is essential to limit motion loss.

Patient Instructions

- Injured extremity is to be non-weightbearing for 4 to 6 weeks.
- Patients may require therapy or bracing to regain ROM.
- Potential for as much as 15 degrees of loss of extension
- Operative patients may begin ROM after suture removal.
- Olecranon process fractures may require hardware removal due to prominence (after 4 to 6 months).

Suggested Readings

Hak DJ, Golladay GJ. Olecranon fractures: treatment options. *J Am Acad Orthop Surg.* 2000;8:266–275.

Horner SR, Sadasivan KK, Lipka JM, Saha S. Analysis of mechanical factors affecting fixation of olecranon fractures. *Orthopedics.* 1989;12:1469–1472.

Murphy DF, Greene WB, Gilbert JA, Dameron TB Jr. Displaced olecranon fractures in adults. Biomechanical analysis of fixation methods. *Clin Orthop Relat Res.* 1987;224:210–214.

Rouleau DM, Sandman E, Van Riet R, Galatz LM. Management of fractures of the proximal ulna. *J Am Acad Orthop Surg.* 2013;21:149–160.

Chapter 65 Radial and Ulnar Shaft Fractures

Rashard Dacus, Seth Bowman

ICD-10-CM CODES
S52.20 *Fracture of ulnar shaft, closed*
S52.21 *Fracture of ulnar shaft, open*
S52.30 *Fracture of shaft of radius, closed*
S52.31 *Fracture of shaft of radius, open*
S52.37 *Galeazzi fracture*
S52.40 *Fracture of shafts of both ulna and radius, closed*
S52.41 *Fracture of shafts of both ulna and radius, open*

Key Concepts

- Fractures may occur as isolated single-bone fractures of the radius or ulna, both-bone fractures, or fracture-dislocations (Galeazzi fracture).
- Deforming forces on radius
  - Proximal one-third: The proximal fragment is supinated and flexed due to the biceps and supinator muscles; the distal fragment is pronated due to the pronator teres and quadratus muscles.
  - Middle one-third: The proximal fragment is held in a neutral position due to the balance between the supinator and pronator teres muscles; the distal fragment is pronated by the pronator quadratus muscles.
  - Distal one-third: The distal fragment of the radius is pronated and pulled toward the ulna.
- Classification
  - Transverse, oblique, spiral
  - Comminuted
  - Closed versus open
  - Proximal, diaphyseal, distal
  - Piedmont (fracture of the junction of the middle one-third and distal one-third of the radius)
- Galeazzi fracture is defined as a distal third radial shaft fracture with distal radioulnar joint dislocation.
- Goals of treatment: restore alignment, maintain forearm rotation
- Additional findings: Be aware of the potential for compartment syndrome. If suspected, compartment pressure evaluation is imperative

History

- Symptoms: pain, edema, difficulty with motion of the wrist/fingers, pronation/supination

- Mechanism of injury: direct blow to forearm, Galeazzi fracture, fall on outstretched hand with forearm in pronation

Physical Examination

- Visual inspection: deformity, skin integrity (closed vs. open fracture)
- Palpation: crepitus
- Physical inspection: Assess joints proximal and distal to the injury including the elbow and distal radioulnar joint for instability. Pain with passive stretch of fingers may indicate compartment syndrome
- Range of motion: limited due to pain
- Neurologic: Assess motor and sensory function distal to site of injury
- Vascular: palpation of radial and ulnar pulses, Allen's test, cap refill, Doppler if unable to palpate pulse

Imaging

- Radial and ulnar fractures
  - Anteroposterior, lateral, oblique forearm (Fig. 65.1)
- Radial shaft fractures (Galeazzi variant)
  - Anteroposterior, lateral, oblique forearm (Figs. 65.2 and 65.3)
- Ulnar shaft fractures
  - Anteroposterior, lateral, oblique forearm (Fig. 65.4)
  - Always image elbow and wrist to rule out concomitant injuries

Differential Diagnosis

- Please see Table 65.1.

Treatment
Radial and Ulnar Fractures

- At diagnosis
  - Only nondisplaced fractures may be managed nonoperatively and must be monitored closely for displacement due to deforming forces.
  - Nonoperative management is generally not recommended in the adult population.
  - Apply long-arm posterior splint with elbow in 90 degrees of flexion and refer to orthopaedist for monitoring.

When to Refer

- All displaced and/or open fractures should be referred to an orthopaedic surgeon for operative management.

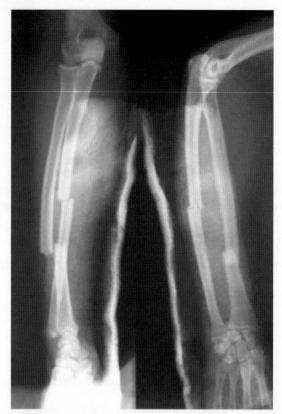

Fig 65.1 Anteroposterior *(left)* and lateral *(right)* radiographs of right both-bone forearm fracture.

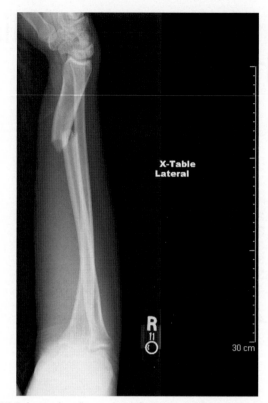

Fig 65.3 Lateral radiograph of Galeazzi fracture.

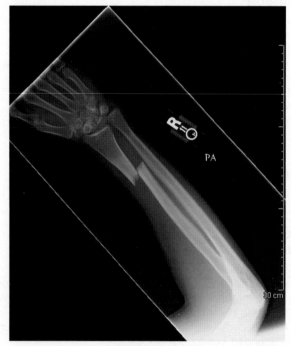

Fig 65.2 Anteroposterior radiograph of Galeazzi fracture.

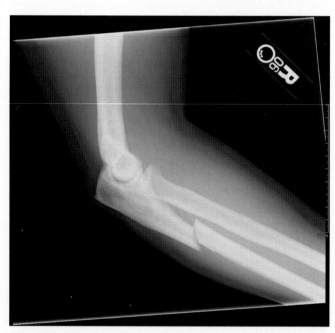

Fig 65.4 Lateral radiograph of proximal third ulnar shaft fracture.

TABLE 65.1 Differential Diagnosis

Differential Diagnosis	Differentiating Features	Chapter Reference
Both-bone forearm fracture	Radiographic evaluation	65
Isolated radius or ulna fracture	Radiographic evaluation	63–65, 97

- Operative methods
  - Internal fixation, plate fixation (3.5-mm dynamic compression plate)
  - External fixation: for open injuries with gross contamination, severe soft-tissue loss, infected nonunion, or open elbow fracture-dislocation
  - Intramedullary nailing (more common in pediatric population)

Radial Shaft Fractures

- At diagnosis
  - Nondisplaced fractures may be managed nonoperatively. Apply a sugar tong splint or Muenster cast if there is minimal edema.
- Later
  - Recheck radiographs every week for 3 weeks to monitor for displacement. Apply a Muenster cast for 4 weeks.
  - Recheck radiographs to evaluate for healing. If the fracture has healed, transition the patient into a brace for protection and begin gentle range of motion therapy.

When to Refer

- Displaced, angulated, or open fractures require open reduction and internal fixation.
- Operative methods: plating (3.5-mm dynamic compression plate) (Fig. 65.5)

Ulnar Shaft Fractures

- At diagnosis
  - Nondisplaced fractures with less than 10 degrees of angulation and less than 50% displacement of the ulnar shaft in any plane may be treated nonoperatively. Apply a sugar tong splint if edema is present or a short arm cast for 10 days.
- Later
  - Recheck radiographs at 10 days and transition the patient to a short-arm cast or a functional forearm brace for 4 to 6 weeks. Recheck radiographs every week for 3 weeks to monitor for displacement.

When to Refer

- Displaced fractures with more than 10 degrees of angulation or more than 50% of ulnar shaft displacement; apply a sugar tong splint and refer to an orthopaedic surgeon within 1 week of injury.
- Operative methods: plating (3.5-mm dynamic compression plate) (Fig. 65.6)

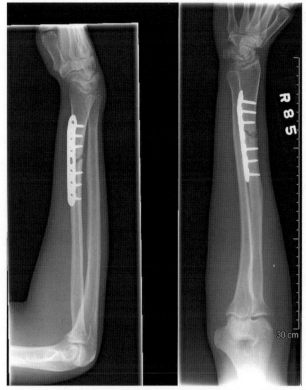

Fig 65.5 Oblique *(left)* and lateral *(right)* radiographs of plating of right distal third radial shaft.

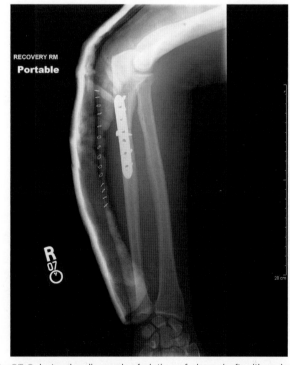

Fig 65.6 Lateral radiograph of plating of ulnar shaft with reduced radial head.

Galeazzi Fractures

- At diagnosis
  - Attempt reduction of the distal radioulnar joint and apply a sugar tong splint. Refer to an orthopaedic surgeon for surgical reduction and fixation.

Prognosis

- Early range of motion therapy in both-bone forearm fractures results in a good functional outcome.

Troubleshooting

- Always assess the wrist to ensure that the radius is not shortened and the distal radioulnar joint is not disrupted.
- Always assess the elbow for instability or associated fracture.
- Always assess for compartment syndrome in the acute setting.
- Forearm fractures with apex volar angulation will likely be more stable with forearm in pronation, while apex dorsal fractures will likely be more stable with forearm in supination. When in doubt, it is never wrong to splint the forearm in a neutral position.

Considerations in Special Populations

- Athletes: Refer to an orthopaedic surgeon because operative interventions can sometimes allow earlier return to play.

Patient Instructions

- Elevate arm.
- Alert someone if there is loss of sensation, perfusion, or excessive pain.
- No weightbearing for 4 to 6 weeks

Suggested Readings

Dymond IW. Treatment of isolated fractures of the distal ulna. *J Bone Joint Surg Br*. 1984;66B:408–410.

Grace TG, Eversmann WW Jr. Forearm fractures: treatment by rigid fixation with early motion. *J Bone Joint Surg Am*. 1980;62A:433–438.

Mekhail AO, Ebraheim NA, Jackson WT, Yeasting RA. Anatomic consideration for the anterior exposure of the proximal portion of the radius. *J Hand Surg Am*. 1996;21:794–801.

Mih AD, Cooney WP, Idler RS, Lewallen DG. Long-term follow-up of forearm bone diaphyseal plating. *Clin Orthop Relat Res*. 1994;299:256–258.

Shulte LM, Meals CG, Neviaser RJ. Management of adult diaphyseal both-bone forearm fractures. *J Am Acad Orthop Surg*. 2014;22:437–446.

Szabo RM, Skinner M. Isolated ulnar shaft fractures. A retrospective study of 46 cases. *Acta Orthop Scand*. 1990;61:350–352.

Chapter 66 Reduction of Elbow Dislocations

Rashard Dacus, Seth Bowman

CPT CODES
24600 *Closed reduction of elbow dislocation without anesthesia*
24605 *Closed reduction of elbow dislocation with anesthesia*

Equipment

- Conscious sedation, IV analgesia, or intra-articular hematoma block (see Chapter 67)
- Stretcher or examining table
- 2- to 5-kg weight for traction is optional and may replace manual traction.
- An assistant may be used to provide brachial countertraction, but this is not always necessary.
- Plaster or fiberglass splint material
- Cotton webril and/or stocking net
- 4-inch elastic bandage (Ace wrap or similar) or bias wrap
- Mini c-arm

Indications

- Simple (without fracture) and complex (with fracture) elbow dislocations

Contraindications

- None

Technique

- A thorough neurovascular examination should be performed and documented before reduction.
- Once the patient is sedated or the analgesic agent has taken effect, position the patient prone on the examining table with the afflicted extremity hanging over the edge.
- Parvin method (Fig. 66.1A)
  - With the arm hanging over the edge of the table from the shoulder, apply manual downward traction (or use a 2- to 5-kg weight) from the wrist for a few minutes.
  - Place one hand on the patient's wrist and provide downward traction; place the other hand under the patient's elbow on the antecubital fossa.
  - While applying downward traction, gently push up on the antecubital fossa, lifting the elbow, and allow the olecranon to reduce into the fossa.
- Alternate method (see Fig. 66.1B)

- Position the patient supine so that the arm is able to be brought over the side of the bed.
- Apply inline traction to improve coronal displacement with the forearm supinated to bring the coronoid under the trochlea.
- While applying counter-traction to the patient's arm just proximal to antecubital fossa, flex the elbow up while applying direct pressure to olecranon.
- Reduction is achieved when a "clunk" is palpated.
- Passive range of motion to within 20 degrees of full extension implies stability; apply a posterior long-arm splint with the elbow in 90 degrees of flexion and the forearm neutral.
- If the elbow is unstable through passive range of motion, re-reduce and apply a posterior long-arm splint with the elbow in 90 degrees of flexion and the forearm in pronation if the LCL is disrupted and supination if the MCL is disrupted. If unsure, splinting in neutral is never the wrong answer.
- Perform postreduction neurovascular examination and document it.
- Obtain postreduction anteroposterior and lateral view radiographs.

Troubleshooting

- Ensure that the patient is adequately sedated.
- Multiple attempts or techniques may need to be used to achieve reduction.
- Having a second person available to apply counter-traction and help with splinting is often helpful.
- Always obtain postreduction radiographs.
- Avoid lateral splinting until after the lateral radiographs have been taken to better see the coronoid.
- If one cannot achieve reduction, there may be superimposed tissue or loose bodies, which may require open reduction.
- If the elbow is unstable at 90 degrees, admit the patient for operative stabilization.
- If the neurovascular examination is worsening after reduction or if unable to achieve reduction, obtain immediate orthopaedic consult.

Complications

- Median nerve or brachial artery injury

Postreduction Management

- Observe the patient for 2 to 3 hours and recheck the neurovascular examination before discharge.

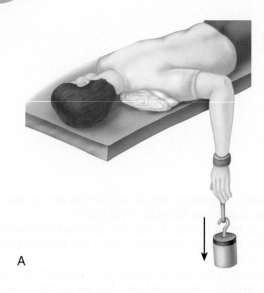

A

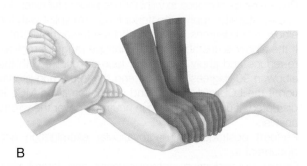

B

Fig 66.1 Posterior elbow dislocation illustrating both prone (A) and supine (B) maneuvers for reduction.

- Follow up at 1 to 2 weeks after injury and begin gentle range of motion therapy for simple elbow dislocations.
- For complex elbow dislocations, follow up within 1 week of injury. Further management depends on the fracture pattern.

Patient Instructions

- Keep the splint clean and dry.
- Do not remove the splint until the return appointment.
- Alert someone if there is loss of perfusion or sensation or if excessive pain develops.
- Loss of terminal extension after elbow dislocation is common.
- May require formal therapy or bracing to optimize range of motion

Suggested Readings

Dürig M, Müller W, Rüedi TP, Gauer EF. The operative treatment of elbow dislocation in the adult. *J Bone Joint Surg Am*. 1979;61A:239–244.

Hotchkiss RN. Fractures and dislocations of the elbow. In: Rockwood CA Jr, Green DP, Bucholz RW, Heckman JD, eds. *Rockwood and Green's Fractures in Adults*. Vol. 1. 4th ed. Philadelphia: Lippincott-Raven; 1996: 929–1024.

Josefsson PO, Johnell O, Gentz CF. Long-term sequelae of simple dislocation of the elbow. *J Bone Joint Surg Am*. 1984;66A:927–930.

O'Driscoll SW. Elbow dislocations. In: Morrey B, eds. *The Elbow and Its Disorders*. 3rd ed. Philadelphia: Saunders; 2000:409–420.

Ross G, McDevitt ER, Chronister R. The treatment of simple elbow dislocations using an immediate motion protocol. *Am J Sports Med*. 1999;27:308–311.

Chapter 67 Injection or Aspiration of the Elbow Joint

Anthony J. Archual, Aaron M. Freilich

CPT CODE
20610 *Aspiration and/or injection of a major joint or bursa*

Key Concepts

- Aspiration of the elbow joint allows examination of intra-articular effusions and aids in the diagnosis of multiple conditions affecting the elbow.
- Injection of the elbow allows the instillation of medication that can aid in the treatment of diseases affecting the elbow.
- The most common injection performed consists of corticosteroid for arthritic conditions.

Equipment (Fig. 67.1)

- 21-gauge needle for aspiration, 25-gauge for injection
- 1% lidocaine
- 10 to 40 mg triamcinolone acetonide or similar agent
- Disinfectant
- Sterile gloves
- Gauze
- Bandage

Contraindications

- Skin ulcerations
- Rash or overlying cellulitis
- Adverse reaction to either medication
- Brittle diabetes mellitus

Instructions/Technique (Video 67.1 ▶)

- The preferred access to the elbow joint is through the so-called soft spot, which can be palpated posterior to the radiocapitellar joint, anterior to the olecranon.
- Use sterile technique.
- Prepare the skin of the posterolateral aspect of the elbow and consider drape as a sterile field.
- Rest the elbow on the table in flexion with the forearm in neutral rotation and the shoulder in internal rotation while the patient is sitting on a chair.
- Palpate the lateral epicondyle and radiocapitellar joint.
- Gentle forearm rotation will aid in the identification of the radial head.
- Move the palpating finger posteriorly toward the olecranon and identify the soft spot. Effusions are commonly palpable in this area.
- Inject local anesthetic into the skin overlying this area if desired.
- Aiming the needle medially and anteriorly, enter the joint through the center of the soft spot.
- Joint fluid can then be aspirated and/or injection performed as indicated.

Considerations in Special Populations

- Advanced arthritic changes may make it difficult to enter the elbow joint. Fluoroscopic or ultrasound guidance may be helpful.
- In very obese patients, landmarks may be difficult to identify and a fluoroscope-assisted injection may be preferable.
- Diabetic patients often react with a transient increase in the blood sugar level that may last several days. It is important to make the patients aware of this and ask them to closely monitor their blood sugar levels.

Troubleshooting

- Patients with a history of vasovagal reactions may prefer a supine position. The elbow is positioned on a pillow with the shoulder in full external rotation and abduction.

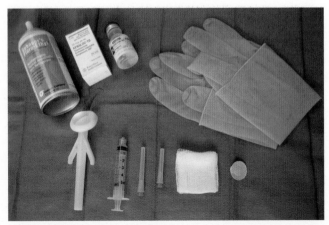

Fig 67.1 Equipment needed for injection or aspiration of the elbow joint.

- Injection should not encounter any resistance. If resistance is encountered, it indicates the extra-articular location of the needle tip.

Patient Instructions

- The patient needs to be informed about the risks and complications of the procedure, and verbal or written consent should be obtained.
- Tell the patient to expect some soreness after the local anesthetic wears off. Recommend the use of an over-the-counter pain medication to treat this, preferably a nonsteroidal antiinflammatory drug.

- The patient should resume stretching exercises and the use of any ancillary braces.
- Symptoms should be monitored for 4 to 6 weeks, followed by re-examination.

Suggested Readings

McNabb JW. Elbow joint. In: *A Practical Guide to Joint and Soft Tissue Injection and Aspiration*. 2nd ed. Philadelphia: Wolters Kluwer; 2010:66–68.

Chapter 68 Lateral Epicondylitis (Tennis Elbow) Injection

Matthew L. Lyons

CPT CODE
20550 *Injection of a tendon sheath, ligament, trigger point, or cyst*

Key Concepts
- Also called tennis elbow injection, the procedure is performed into the common extensor tendon, just distal to the lateral epicondyle.
- Long-term effectiveness of cortisone injection in lateral epicondylitis remains debatable.
- Potential side effects include common extensor tendon or lateral ulnar collateral ligament tear, skin hypopigmentation, fat atrophy, and increased blood glucose levels.

Equipment (Fig. 68.1)
- 3 or 5 mL syringe
- 18-gauge 1-inch needle
- 25-gauge 1-inch needle
- 1% lidocaine
- Injectable corticosteroid agent of choice (author's preference: betamethasone 6 mg/mL)
- Disinfectant: alcohol, chlorhexidine, or iodine
- Sterile gloves
- 4 × 4 gauze
- Bandage

Indications
- Symptomatic lateral epicondylitis by history and exam that has failed to respond to initial conservative treatment
  - The author recommends 3 months of conservative treatment prior to consideration of injection.

Contraindications
- Unclear diagnosis
- Multiple previous injections (author's limit is 3)
- Concern for lateral ulnar collateral ligament insufficiency
- Concern for infection
- Overlying skin ulceration or rash
- History of adverse reaction to injectable agents
- Poorly controlled diabetes mellitus

Instructions/Technique (Video 68.1)
- Prior to performing the procedure, the site is verified and verbal consent is obtained from the patient.
- Draw 2 mL of 1% lidocaine and desired dosage of corticosteroid into a syringe using an 18-gauge needle.
- With the patient seated in a chair, the elbow is rested on the table in 60 degrees of flexion, with the forearm in neutral rotation and the shoulder in slight abduction.
- Palpate the lateral epicondyle and locate and demarcate the point of maximal tenderness, typically slightly distal and anterior to the epicondyle.
- The overlying skin is widely disinfected, beginning over the injection site and moving peripherally in a circular motion.
- May use ethyl chloride spray for patient comfort; re-disinfect after using.
- Insert the 25-gauge needle at a 45-degree angle in a distal to proximal direction aiming toward the lateral epicondyle (Fig. 68.2). The radial nerve is at risk if you aim too far anteriorly.
- The injection is placed deep to the subcutaneous space, within the tendon. Subcutaneous injection can increase the risk of fat atrophy and skin hypopigmentation.
- Contact with bone confirms the correct depth of the needle; slightly withdraw the needle and begin injecting.
- As the solution is injected, the needle can be used to trephinate the lateral epicondyle.

Considerations in Special Populations
- In obese patients, landmarks may be difficult to identify and injection can be challenging.
- Diabetic patients often react with a transient increase in blood glucose levels that can last several days.

Troubleshooting
- If the solution does not inject smoothly, gently and minimally withdraw the needle from the bone or reposition until it injects without resistance.
- Patients with a history of vasovagal reactions may prefer a supine position.
  - The elbow can be rested on a pillow next to the patient with the forearm across the patient and the shoulder in internal rotation.

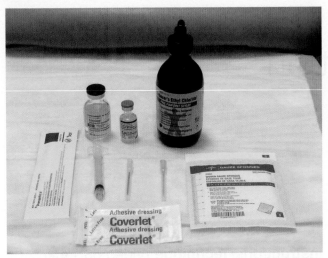

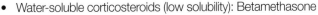

Fig 68.1 Setup for lateral epicondyle injection: local anesthetic agent, corticosteroid, ethyl chloride, chlorhexidine swab, needles, band-aid, and a syringe.

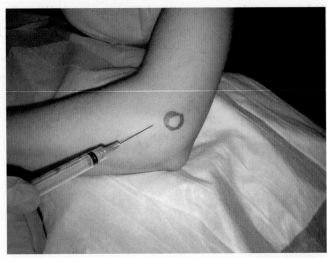

Fig 68.2 With the elbow in 90 degrees of flexion, the needle is inserted at a 45-degree angle just anterior and distal to the lateral epicondyle (demarcated by a purple circle).

- Water-soluble corticosteroids (low solubility): Betamethasone
  - Less tissue uptake, more rapid systemic absorption
  - May result in shorter duration of effect but less potential tissue damage, greater potential for side effects (i.e., increase in blood glucose levels)
- Fat-soluble corticosteroids (high solubility): Triamcinolone
  - Increased tissue uptake, slower absorption
  - Potential for increased duration of effect, but may increase risk of tendon/ligament degeneration

Patient Instructions

- The patient needs to be informed of the potential risks of the injection.
  - In particular, caution darker-complexion individuals of the risk of skin hypopigmentation and diabetic patients to monitor for increase in blood glucose levels.

- Advise patients that it may take 1 to 2 weeks for the steroid to take effect.
- Patients should limit heavy lifting and high-impact activities for 2 days following the procedure.
- Increased discomfort following the injection is normal for up to 48 hours.
  - If symptoms persist beyond this point or are accompanied by significant warmth, redness, or fevers and chills, immediate evaluation is necessary.
- Patients may resume stretching exercises and the use of any ancillary braces.
- Evaluation in clinic in 4 to 6 weeks to assess response to injection

Chapter 69 Medial Epicondylitis (Golfer's Elbow) Injection

Matthew L. Lyons

CPT CODE
20550 *Injection of tendon sheath, ligament, trigger point, or cyst*

Key Concepts
- Also termed golfer's elbow injection, the procedure is performed into the flexor-pronator muscle origin just distal to the medial epicondyle.
- Long-term effectiveness of cortisone injection in lateral epicondylitis remains debatable.
- Potential side effects include ulnar nerve injury, flexor-pronator tendon or ulnar collateral ligament tear, skin hypopigmentation, fat atrophy, and increased blood glucose levels.

Equipment (Fig. 69.1)
- 3 or 5 mL syringe
- 18-gauge 1-inch needle
- 25-gauge 1-inch needle
- 1% lidocaine
- Injectable corticosteroid agent of choice (author's preference: betamethasone 6 mg/mL)
- Disinfectant: alcohol, chlorhexidine, or iodine
- Sterile gloves
- 4 × 4 gauze
- Bandage

Indications
- Symptomatic medial epicondylitis by history and exam that has failed to respond to initial conservative treatment
  - The author recommends 3 months of conservative treatment prior to consideration of injection.

Contraindications
- Unclear diagnosis
- Multiple previous injections (author's limit is 3)
- Concern for ulnar collateral ligament insufficiency
- Concern for infection
- Overlying skin ulceration or rash
- History of adverse reaction to injectable agents
- Poorly controlled diabetes mellitus
- Previous ulnar nerve transposition

Instructions/Technique (Video 69.1)
- Prior to performing the procedure, the site is verified and verbal consent is obtained from the patient.
- Draw 2 mL of 1% lidocaine and desired dosage of corticosteroid into a syringe using an 18-gauge needle.
- With the patient seated in a chair, the elbow is rested on the table in 30 to 45 degrees of flexion, with the forearm supinated and the shoulder in slight abduction.
- Palpate the medial epicondyle and flexor-pronator tendon and locate and demarcate the point of maximal tenderness, typically slightly distal and anterior to the epicondyle.
- Palpate the ulnar nerve, ensure that there is no anterior subluxation and that it will not be in the path of the needle.
- The overlying skin is widely disinfected, beginning over the injection site and moving peripherally in a circular motion.
- May use ethyl chloride spray for patient comfort; re-disinfect after using.
- Insert the 25-gauge needle at a 45-degree angle in a distal to proximal direction aiming toward the medial epicondyle (Fig. 69.2).
  - Avoid the median nerve anteriorly and the ulnar nerve posteriorly.
- The injection is placed deep to the subcutaneous space, within the tendon. Subcutaneous injection can increase the risk of fat atrophy and skin hypopigmentation.
- Contact with bone confirms the correct depth of the needle; slightly withdraw the needle and begin injecting.
- As the solution is injected, the needle can be used to trephinate the medial epicondyle.

Considerations in Special Populations
- In obese patients, landmarks may be difficult to identify and injection can be challenging.
- Diabetic patients often react with a transient increase in blood glucose levels that can last several days.

Troubleshooting
- If the solution does not inject smoothly, gently and minimally withdraw the needle from the bone or reposition until it injects without resistance.
- Patients with a history of vasovagal reactions may prefer a supine position.
  - The elbow is positioned on a pillow with the shoulder in full external rotation and abduction.

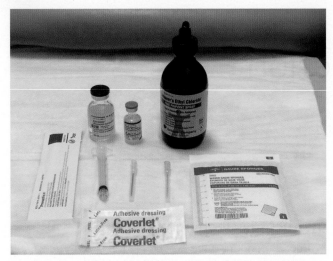

Fig 69.1 Setup for medial epicondyle injection: local anesthetic agent, corticosteroid, ethyl chloride, chlorhexidine swab, needles, bandage, and a syringe.

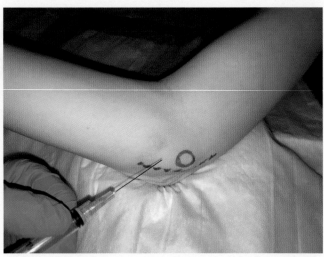

Fig 69.2 With the elbow in 45 degrees of flexion, the needle is inserted at a 45-degree angle just anterior and distal to the medial epicondyle (demarcated by a *purple circle*) (*dashed line,* course of ulnar nerve.)

- Water-soluble corticosteroids (low solubility): Betamethasone
  - Less tissue uptake, more rapid systemic absorption
  - May result in shorter duration of effect but less potential tissue damage, greater potential for side effects (i.e., increase in blood glucose levels)
- Fat-soluble corticosteroids (high solubility): Triamcinolone
  - Increased tissue uptake, slower absorption
  - Potential for increased duration of effect, but may increase risk of tendon/ligament degeneration

Patient Instructions

- The patient needs to be informed of the potential risks of the injection.
  - In particular, caution darker-complexion individuals of the risk of skin hypopigmentation and diabetic patients to monitor for increase in blood glucose levels.

- Advise patients that it may take 1 to 2 weeks for the steroid to take effect.
- Patients should limit heavy lifting and high-impact activities for 2 days following the procedure.
- Increased discomfort following the injection is normal for up to 48 hours.
  - If symptoms persist beyond this point or are accompanied by significant warmth, redness, or fevers and chills, immediate evaluation is necessary.
- Patients may resume stretching exercises and the use of any ancillary braces.
- Evaluation in clinic in 4 to 6 weeks to assess response to injection.

Chapter 70 Olecranon Bursa Aspiration/Injection

Anthony J. Archual, Aaron M. Freilich

CPT CODE
20605 *Aspiration and/or injection of intermediate bursa*

Key Concepts

- Olecranon bursa may become inflamed or septic, and aspiration may be indicated.
  - This is a technically reproducible technique secondary to the superficial location of the olecranon bursa.
- The bursa may become inflamed secondary to trauma, repetitive shear forces across the olecranon process, or excessive pressure along this area.
- The fluid may consist of blood in acute trauma, purulent material if infected, or thick proteinaceous fluid after repetitive injury.
- Therapeutic corticosteroid injection can be carried out once septic bursitis has been excluded.

Equipment (Fig. 70.1)

- 20-mL syringe
- 3-mL syringe for additional injection
- 18-gauge, 1.5-inch needle
- 25-gauge, 1.5-inch needle
- 1 mL of 1% lidocaine without epinephrine
- 1 mL of steroid solution of choice (we use 40 mg triamcinolone acetonide)
- Alcohol pads
- 3-mL ChloraPrep skin applicator (chlorhexidine gluconate, 2% wt/vol; isopropyl alcohol, 70% wt/vol)
- Sterile gauze pads
- Sterile adhesive bandage
- Nonsterile, clean chuck pads
- Topical anesthetic skin refrigerant, optional (we use Gebauer's Fluro-Ethyl spray [75% wt/vol; dichlorotetrafluoroethane, 25% vol/vol ethyl chloride])

Contraindications

- Open wound with exposed olecranon
- Uncooperative patient

Instructions/Technique
(Fig. 70.2 and Video 70.1)

- Patient position
  - Sitting if examining the patient on a hand table
  - The affected elbow is flexed to 45 degrees without maximal flexion to gain adequate access to the bursa. Too much flexion may shift fluid within the bursa, making aspiration difficult.
- Landmarks
  - Point of maximum fluid fluctuance is noted at this position.
  - Usually this point is in line with the olecranon process.
- Establish sterile field
  - Have the patient wash his or her hand and elbow with soap and water before injection.
  - Use ChloraPrep to establish sterile field once elbow is positioned over a nonsterile chuck pad (alcohol and povidone-iodine pads can be used to establish sterile field as alternative options).
- Anesthesia
  - Infiltrate 3 mL of 1% lidocaine into the planned area of aspiration.
  - Local anesthesia of the skin with topical vapocoolant spray before infiltration of area
- Technique
  - With sterile gloves and local anesthetic agent in place, introduce an 18-gauge needle in the center of the bursa.
  - Aspiration with a 20-mL syringe is performed. If a large collection of fluid is suspected, do not overtighten the needle to the syringe so that the syringe can easily be exchanged when full, leaving the needle in place.
  - If injection is planned after aspiration, grasp the hub of the needle with a hemostat or a free finger if it is not placed too tightly. Then attach the 3-mL syringe with steroid solution.
  - If resistance is met, advance or withdraw the needle slightly before attempting further injection.
- Aftercare
  - Apply a sterile adhesive bandage followed by a compressive tube dressing (if compressive tube dressing is not available, an elastic bandage may also be used).
  - Reexamine the elbow after 5 minutes to confirm pain relief and no active bleeding or drainage sites.

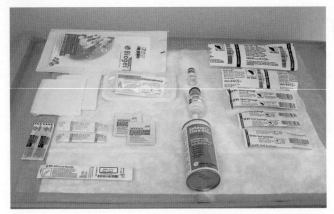

Fig 70.1 Equipment needed for olecranon bursa aspiration/injection.

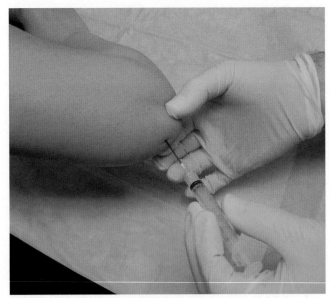

Fig 70.2 Olecranon bursa aspiration.

- Instruct the patient to avoid excessive use or heavy lifting of the elbow for the next 2 weeks.
- Consider using a neoprene elbow sleeve or elastic compressive bandage (e.g., heel bow pad).
- Consider reevaluation at 2 weeks for examination and documentation of effective aspiration/injection and to be certain that no complications have arisen.

Considerations in Special Populations

- People with an active skin lesion (e.g., psoriasis, eczema) are not ideal candidates for aspiration because of increased risk of infection.
- If acute hemorrhage or septic bursitis is suspected, do not follow aspiration with a corticosteroid injection.
- Inform diabetic patients of a possible glycemic rise secondary to corticosteroid injection (usually transient and minimal).

- In dark-skinned individuals, skin hypopigmentation is more noticeable and patients should be informed of this.

Troubleshooting

- To diminish skin hypopigmentation and skin atrophy, we recommend pinching up tissue to avoid subcutaneous corticosteroid injection. This creates greater distance between the skin and actual injection site.
- Corticosteroid is used mainly for recurrent olecranon bursitis.
- Patients with gouty arthritis may have a high recurrence of bursitis and increased risk of infection secondary to multiple aspirations. These patients benefit from early referral to a specialist for open elbow bursectomy and tophi removal.
- When aspiration is done for suspected septic bursitis, send aspirate for culture and sensitivity; cell counts (white blood cell [WBC] and red blood cell); aerobic, anaerobic, fungal, and mycobacterial organisms; and crystal evaluation.
  - The leukocyte count can help determine whether the fluid is infectious or inflammatory.
  - Within synovial aspirates, WBC counts are assessed as follows:
    - A WBC count less than 200/mL is considered normal.
    - A WBC count of 200 to 2000/mL is considered noninflammatory.
    - A WBC count in the range of 2000 to 100,000/mL is considered an indication of inflammation.
    - A WBC count greater than 100,000/mL is considered an indication of a septic condition.
- Gram stain also is helpful to determine quickly whether bacterial infection is present.
- If the Gram stain results are positive, antibiotics should be started immediately and bursal corticosteroid injection should be avoided.
- If the Gram stain results are negative or initially unavailable, antibiotics may be indicated based on the mechanism of injury, physical examination findings suggestive of infection, or the gross appearance of the aspirate.
- Gram stain can be followed by culture and sensitivity testing. The culture and sensitivity results should guide the use of antibiotics in cases of bacterial infection.
- Crystal analysis may reveal monosodium urate crystals in a patient with gout, calcium pyrophosphate crystals in a patient with pseudogout, or hydroxyapatite crystals.

Patient Instructions

- The patient is to keep the dressing in place for 48 hours.
- Some patients with corticosteroid injections may experience a flare, which improves in 48 to 72 hours and is managed with nonsteroidal antiinflammatory drugs.
- If a patient experiences fever, chills, or exquisite pain, he or she should contact a physician immediately to rule out a septic process.

Suggested Readings (see also Chapter 60)

McNabb JW. *A Practical Guide to Joint and Soft Tissue Injection and Aspiration*. Philadelphia: Lippincott Williams & Wilkins; 2005:133.

SECTION 4

The Wrist and Hand

Chapter 71 Overview of the Wrist and Hand

Jennifer A. Hart

Anatomy

- The wrist is made up of several articulations including the distal radioulnar joint, the ulnocarpal joint, the radiocarpal joint, and the carpometacarpal joints (Fig. 71.1).
- The hand is made up of five metacarpal bones. Each metacarpal articulates with the corresponding proximal phalanx (metacarpophalangeal [MCP] joint), which in turn articulates with the middle phalanx (proximal interphalangeal [PIP] joint), and finally the distal phalanx (distal interphalangeal joint) (Fig. 71.2).
- Of note, the thumb has no middle phalanx and, therefore, no PIP joint.
- Radius
  - The distal radius provides the majority of the proximal articular surface of the wrist joint, with the scaphoid and lunate providing the distal articular surface.
  - The styloid process forms the most lateral and distal point of the radius.
- Ulna
  - The distal ulna has a smaller distal articular surface than the proximal ulna does at the elbow.
  - The styloid process forms its most medial distal projection.
- Carpal bones
  - There are eight carpal bones that are arranged in two rows.
  - The proximal row contains the scaphoid, lunate, triquetrum, and pisiform. The distal row contains the trapezium, trapezoid, capitate, and hamate.
- Metacarpals and phalanges
  - The five metacarpal bones are triangular in cross section. Each triangle provides an important surface area for muscle attachment.
  - They articulate proximally with the distal row of carpal bones and distally with the proximal phalanx (MCP joint).
  - There are five corresponding proximal phalanges, four middle phalanges (the thumb does not include this bone), and five distal phalanges.
  - The palmar surfaces of these bones are flatter, the proximal and distal ends have a slight flare to form the articular surfaces, and the distal phalanges have a "tufted" distal end.
- Muscles (Box 71.1)
- Vascular structures
  - The wrist and hand receive their blood supply from the radial and ulnar arteries.
  - The radial artery passes through the anatomic snuff-box at the wrist and divides into the palmar carpal, dorsal carpal, and superficial palmar branches in the hand.
  - The ulnar artery is larger than the radial artery and also divides at the wrist to form the palmar carpal branch, dorsal palmar branch, dorsal carpal branch, deep palmar branch, and superficial palmar arch. The ulnar and radial arteries have an anastomosis at the wrist.
- Nerves
  - The ulnar, radial, and median nerves provide sensory and motor input to the distal upper extremity.
  - The ulnar nerve provides sensation to the ulnar side of the wrist and hand including the fifth finger and the ulnar half of the fourth finger (Fig. 71.3).
  - The median nerve innervates the majority of the palmar surface and includes the distal half of the thumb, the second finger, the third finger, and the radial half of the fourth finger (Fig. 71.4).
  - The radial nerve innervates the radial aspect of the dorsal hand (Fig. 71.5).
- Ligaments and soft tissue
  - The wrist has extensive ligamentous structures to support the joint and act as shock absorbers.
  - The triangular fibrocartilage complex is one of the more clinically significant structures and supports the radioulnar joint.
    - This complex is formed by the dorsal and volar radioulnar ligaments, the triangular fibrocartilage disc, and the ulnar collateral ligament.

History

- A thorough and accurate history is the first step to defining the differential diagnosis list for each individual patient encounter.
- The history must provide accurate information regarding any trauma to the wrist or hand as well as the location, severity, and frequency of the pain and any history of similar symptoms (Table 71.1).

Physical Examination (Video 71.1)

- Inspection and palpation (Fig. 71.6)
  - Anterior wrist and hand
    - The anterior wrist and hand should be carefully evaluated for any changes in skin color, deformity, atrophy of the thenar or hypothenar muscles, and bony tenderness along the bony structures.
  - Posterior wrist and hand
    - The posterior wrist and hand should also be evaluated for skin changes, deformity, and bony tenderness.

Anterior (palmar) view

Fig 71.1 The bony anatomy of the wrist joint.

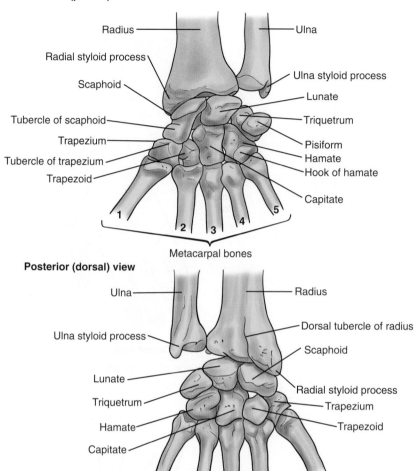

Radius — — Ulna

Radial styloid process —

Scaphoid —

Tubercle of scaphoid —

Trapezium —

Tubercle of trapezium —

Trapezoid —

Ulna styloid process

Lunate

Triquetrum

Pisiform

Hamate

Hook of hamate

Capitate

1 2 3 4 5

Metacarpal bones

Posterior (dorsal) view

Ulna — — Radius

Ulna styloid process —

Lunate —

Triquetrum —

Hamate —

Capitate —

Dorsal tubercle of radius

Scaphoid

Radial styloid process

Trapezium

Trapezoid

5 4 3 2 1

Metacarpal bones

Fig 71.2 Anterior (palmar) view of the bony anatomy of the right hand.

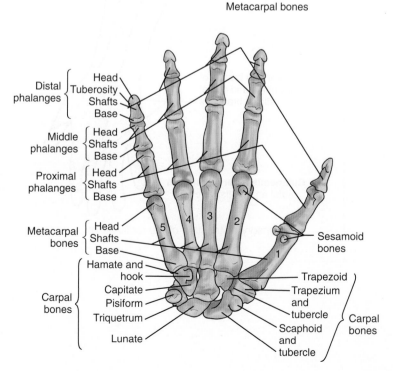

Distal phalanges — Head, Tuberosity, Shafts, Base

Middle phalanges — Head, Shafts, Base

Proximal phalanges — Head, Shafts, Base

Metacarpal bones — Head, Shafts, Base

5 4 3 2 1

Carpal bones — Hamate and hook, Capitate, Pisiform, Triquetrum, Lunate

Sesamoid bones

Trapezoid

Trapezium and tubercle

Scaphoid and tubercle

Carpal bones

BOX 71.1 Muscles

Wrist Flexors

Flexor carpi radialis
Palmaris longus
Flexor carpi ulnaris

Wrist Extensors

Extensor carpi radialis longus
Extensor carpi radialis brevis
Extensor carpi ulnaris

Finger Flexors

Flexor digitorum superficialis
Flexor digitorum profundus

Finger Extensors

Extensor digitorum
Extensor digiti minimi
Extensor indicis proprius

Thumb

Flexor pollicis longus
Abductor pollicis longus
Extensor pollicis brevis
Extensor pollicis longus

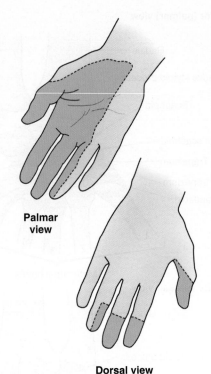

Palmar view

Dorsal view

Fig 71.4 Sensory distribution of the median nerve.

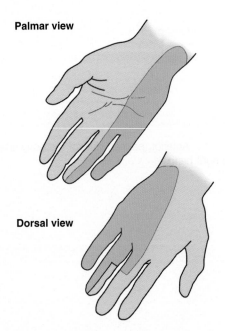

Palmar view

Dorsal view

Fig 71.3 Sensory distribution of the ulnar nerve.

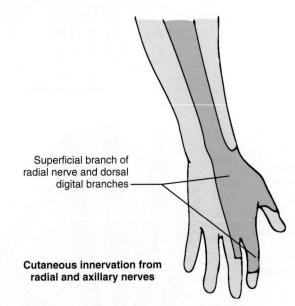

Superficial branch of radial nerve and dorsal digital branches

Cutaneous innervation from radial and axillary nerves

Fig 71.5 Sensory distribution of the radial nerve.

- In addition, special note should be taken here for rotational deformity of the fingers (often best noted by making a clenched fist) and nail bed abnormalities.
- Range of motion
  - Wrist flexion: 80 degrees
  - Wrist extension: 70 degrees
  - Radial deviation: 20 degrees
  - Ulnar deviation: 30 to 45 degrees
  - Finger (MCP) flexion: 90 degrees
  - Finger (MCP) extension: 30 to 45 degrees
  - Thumb (MCP) flexion: 50 degrees

TABLE 71.1 Pertinent History Points

History	Possible Diagnosis
Fall/trauma	Fracture
Numbness/paresthesia	Nerve entrapment
Night pain	Tumor/infection
Cold intolerance/skin color change	Raynaud phenomenon
Smoking history	Buerger disease
Developing mass osteoarthritis	Depuytren contracture, ganglion cyst

- Thumb (MCP) extension: 0 degrees
- Thumb abduction: 70 degrees
- Thumb adduction: 0 degrees
- Strength testing
  - Wrist flexion (Fig. 71.7A)
  - Wrist extension (see Fig. 71.7B)
  - Finger flexion (see Fig. 71.7C)
  - Finger extension (see Fig. 71.7D)
  - Finger abduction (see Fig. 71.7E)
  - Finger adduction (see Fig. 71.7F)
  - Opposition (see Fig. 71.7G)
- Special tests
  - Phalen test (Fig. 71.8)
    - Purpose: evaluation for carpal tunnel syndrome
    - How to perform: Passively flex the patient's wrist and hold it in that flexed position to try to reproduce the symptoms of numbness and paresthesia in the thumb and index finger.
    - Positive: reproduction of numbness and paresthesia in the thumb and index finger
  - Tinel's sign (Fig. 71.9)
    - Purpose: evaluation for carpal tunnel syndrome
    - How to perform: Tap over the anterior aspect of the wrist.
    - Positive: indicated by reproduction of numbness and paresthesia in the thumb and index finger

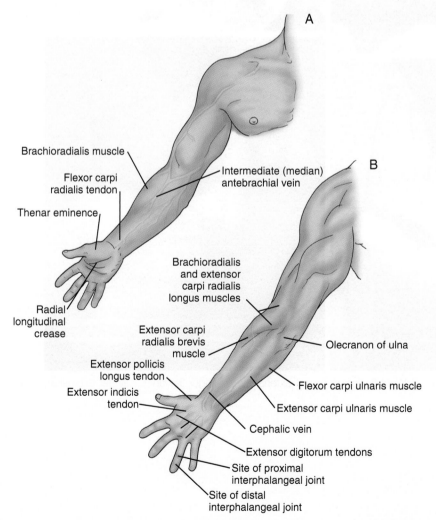

Fig 71.6 Surface anatomy of the wrist and hand. (A) Anterior; (B) posterior.

A

B

Brachioradialis muscle

Flexor carpi radialis tendon

Thenar eminence

Intermediate (median) antebrachial vein

Radial longitudinal crease

Brachioradialis and extensor carpi radialis longus muscles

Extensor carpi radialis brevis muscle

Extensor pollicis longus tendon

Extensor indicis tendon

Olecranon of ulna

Flexor carpi ulnaris muscle

Extensor carpi ulnaris muscle

Cephalic vein

Extensor digitorum tendons

Site of proximal interphalangeal joint

Site of distal interphalangeal joint

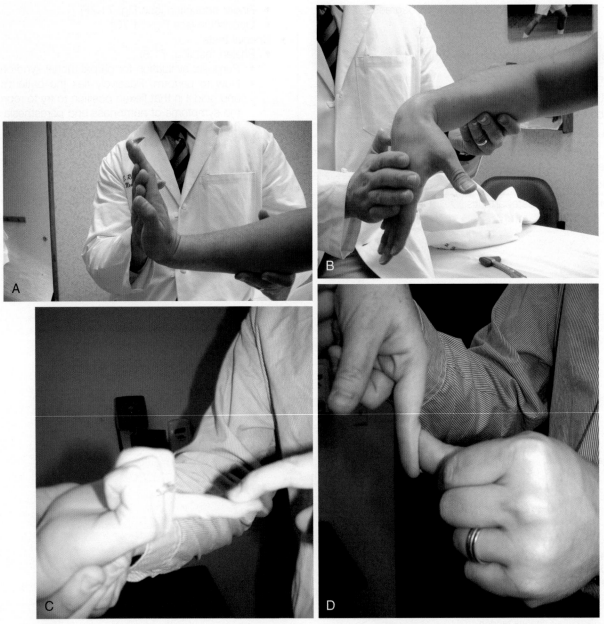

Fig 71.7 Strength testing of the wrist and hand. **(A)** Wrist flexion; **(B)** wrist extension; **(C)** finger flexion; **(D)** finger extension;

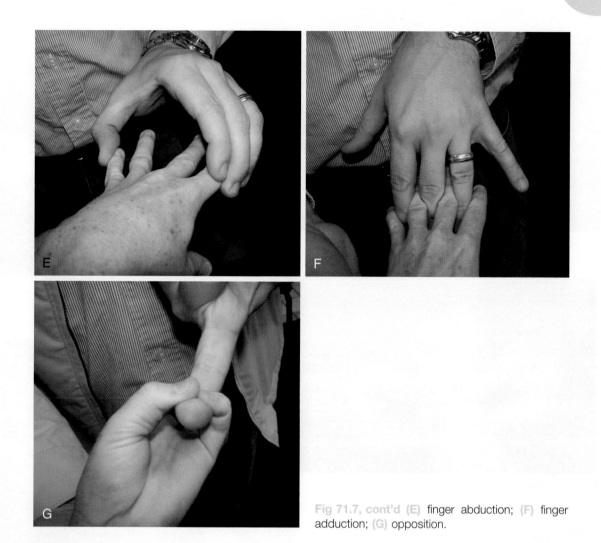

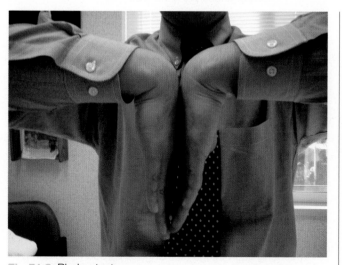

Fig 71.7, cont'd (E) finger abduction; (F) finger adduction; (G) opposition.

Fig 71.8 Phalen test.

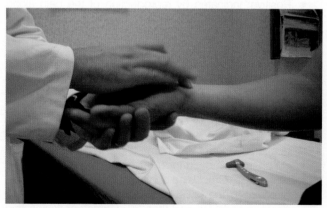

Fig 71.9 Tinel's sign.

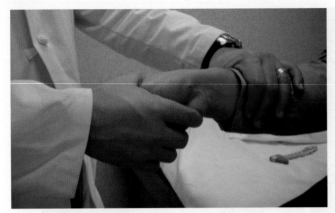

Fig 71.10 Finkelstein test.

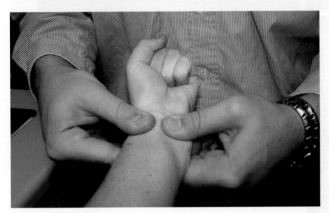

Fig 71.11 Allen test.

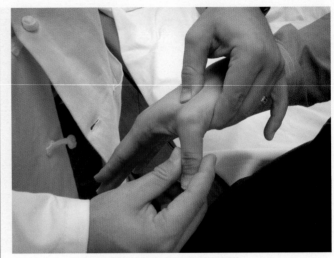

Fig 71.12 Valgus stress test of the thumb.

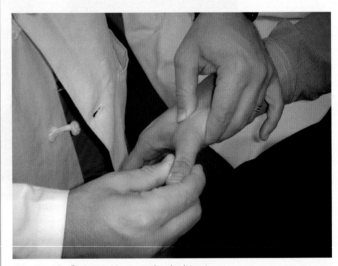

Fig 71.13 Carpometacarpal grind test.

- Finkelstein test (Fig. 71.10)
  - Purpose: evaluation for de Quervain tenosynovitis
  - How to perform: Ask the patient to make a fist, tucking the thumb under the other fingers and then placing the wrist in ulnar deviation.
  - Positive: indicated by reproduction of the pain along the side of the thumb
- Allen test (Fig. 71.11 and Video 71.2)
  - Purpose: evaluation for a patent radial artery
  - How to perform: With the patient's hand in a fist and elevated, occlude both the ulnar and radial arteries. Ask the patient to open his or her hand, which will appear blanched. Release the pressure on the ulnar artery.
  - Positive: Return of color within 7 seconds indicates a patent radial artery.
- Valgus stress test of the thumb (Fig. 71.12)
  - Purpose: evaluation for ulnar collateral ligament injury
  - How to perform: Using one hand to stabilize the thumb proximal to the MCP joint, place the thumb first in 0 degrees of flexion and then 30 degrees of flexion and apply gentle valgus stress to the MCP joint.
  - Positive: Opening of the MCP joint indicates rupture of the ulnar collateral ligament of the thumb.
- Carpometacarpal grind test (Fig. 71.13)
  - Purpose: evaluation for carpometacarpal arthritis
  - How to perform: Using one hand to stabilize the thumb proximal to the carpometacarpal joint, hold the thumb in the other hand and move it in a circular pattern.
  - Positive: Reproduction of pain at the carpometacarpal joint is indicative of arthritis there.

Imaging

- Radiography
  - Standard radiographic views of the wrist and hand include anteroposterior, lateral, and oblique views (Figs. 71.14 and 71.15). Special images are useful when evaluating for certain injuries, such as the carpal tunnel view or clenched-fist view (Fig. 71.16).
- Magnetic resonance imaging of the wrist is helpful when evaluating such things as triangular fibrocartilage complex tears.
- Computed tomography is most helpful when evaluating comminuted or severely displaced fractures to aid in preoperative planning.

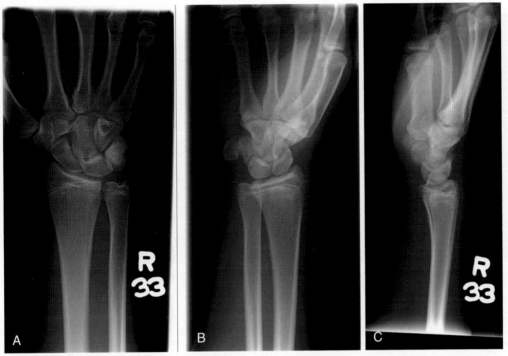

Fig 71.14 Standard radiographic views of the wrist. Anteroposterior (A); oblique (B); and lateral (C) views.

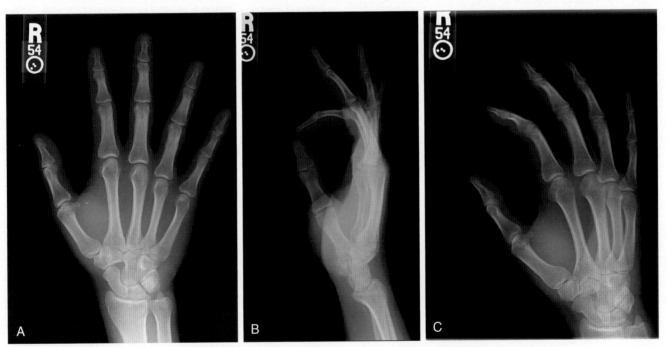

Fig 71.15 Standard radiographic views of the hand. (A) Anteroposterior; (B) lateral; (C) oblique.

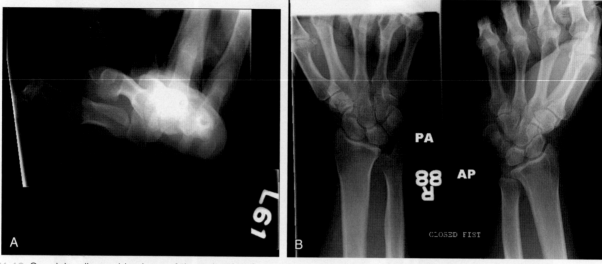

Fig 71.16 Special radiographic views of the wrist. (A) Carpal tunnel view; (B) clenched-fist view.

- Electromyography is a commonly used test in evaluating the wrist and hand because it can help to distinguish various upper-extremity nerve entrapments such as carpal tunnel syndrome, cubital tunnel syndrome, and cervical stenosis.

Suggested Readings

Green D, Hotchkiss R, Pederson W, Wolfe S, eds. *Green's Operative Hand Surgery*. Philadelphia: Churchill Livingstone; 2005.

Hoppenfeld S. *Physical Examination of the Spine and Extremities*. Norwalk, CT: Appleton & Lange; 1976.

Loreda RA, Sorge DG, Garcia G. Radiographic evaluation of the wrist: a vanishing art. *Semin Roentgenol*. 2005;40:248–289.

Reddy RS, Compson J. Examination of the wrist-surface anatomy of the carpal bones. *Curr Orthop*. 2005;19:171–179.

Schreibman KL, Freeland A, Gilula LA, Yin Y. Imaging of the hand and wrist. *Orthop Clin North Am*. 1997;28:537–582.

Watson HK, Weinzweig J. Physical examination of the wrist. *Hand Clin*. 1997;13:17–34.

Young D, Papp S, Giachino A. Physical examination of the wrist. *Orthop Clin North Am*. 2007;38:149–165.

Chapter 72 Scapholunate Ligament Injury

Jeffrey D. Boatright

ICD-10-CM CODES

S69.90XA	*Scapholunate ligament injury with no instability*
M25.339	*Scapholunate instability*
S63.8X1A	*Tear of right scapholunate ligament*
S63.8X2A	*Tear of left scapholunate ligament*
S63.599A	*Partial scapholunate tear*

Key Concepts

- The scapholunate ligament (SLL) is an interosseous ligament between the scaphoid and lunate that functions as a major stabilizer of the wrist.
  - It is a C-shaped structure.
  - It is strongest at its dorsal attachment with thinner and weaker volar and proximal portions.
- There is a wide spectrum of disorders that can result from injury to the SLL.
  - Classified based on the type of instability that is present (static versus dynamic) and the acuity of the injury (acute, subacute, and chronic).
- In an uninjured wrist, the lunate is held in a neutral position by the opposing flexion moment arm of the SLL and extension moment arm of the lunotriquetral ligament.
  - If the SLL is compromised, the lunate is subject to an unopposed extension force created by the intact lunotriquetral ligament
  - The result is a lunate extension deformity known as dorsal intercalated segment instability (DISI).
- Chronic, untreated scapholunate (SL) instability will result in a predictable pattern of degenerative changes in the wrist known as scapholunate advanced collapse (SLAC).
- The gold standard of diagnosis is wrist arthroscopy, although magnetic resonance imaging may be helpful in some settings.

History

- The patient may or may not report a history of a wrist sprain, typically from a fall on an outstretched hand or an axial load on the wrist.
- The patient may describe wrist pain or weakness, particularly with wrist extension and axial load (push-up position), or power grip.
- Other complaints may include intermittent swelling or mechanical symptoms within the wrist.
- Chronic SL instability, typically presents with pain and decreased wrist range of motion.

Physical Examination

- Inspection may reveal dorsal wrist edema.
- Examiner should evaluate wrist range of motion in all planes (flexion, extension, radial, and ulnar deviation).
- Palpate the SL interval with the wrist in slight flexion. Identify the soft spot on the dorsum of the wrist just distal to the Lister tubercle. Pain here may indicate an SLL injury (Fig. 72.1).
- The key examination maneuver for SL instability is the Watson maneuver (Fig. 72.2).
  - The examiner places four fingers on the dorsum of the distal radius, and the thumb applies a dorsally directed pressure to the scaphoid tubercle volarly.
  - The examiner's other hand passively brings the wrist from ulnar to radial deviation.
    - The pressure from the examiner's thumb on the scaphoid tubercle prevents the scaphoid from flexing as it is moved into radial deviation.
    - This causes the proximal pole to subluxate over the dorsal lip of the radius.
  - The examiner's thumb is then removed, which produces palpable clunk as the scaphoid reduces back into the scaphoid fossa.
    - A painful, palpable clunk is considered a positive test.

  This test must be compared to the contralateral wrist, as some patients will have a painless palpable clunk bilaterally, which is not considered abnormal but rather a sign of generalized ligamentous laxity.
- A thorough examination of the wrist should be performed to identify other areas of tenderness and possible injury. A thorough neurovascular examination and examination of the cervical spine, shoulder, and elbow should also be performed.

Imaging

- There are four stages of SL instability.
  - Predynamic instability
    - Partially ruptured or attenuated ligament that allows abnormal movement between the scaphoid and lunate and creates wrist synovitis
    - Radiographs appear normal.
  - Dynamic instability (Fig. 72.3)
    - The volar or dorsal portions of the SLL are disrupted.
    - Identified on clenched-fist PA radiograph as SL interval widening. Nonstress (standard PA) view of the wrist is normal.

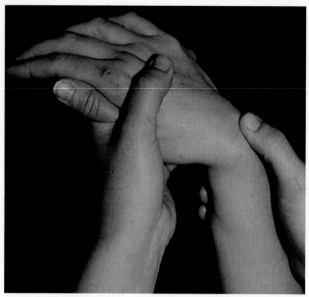

Fig 72.1 Palpation of the scapholunate interval. (From Green D, Hotchkiss R, Pederson W, Wolfe S, eds. *Green's Operative Hand Surgery*, Vol. 1, 5th ed. Philadelphia: Churchill Livingstone; 2005:492.)

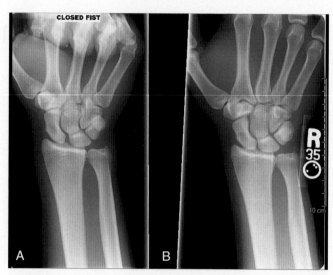

Fig 72.3 (A) Stress view ("clinched-fist view") of the wrist shows widening of the scapholunate (SL) interval. (B) Normal, nonstress view demonstrating normal SL interval.

- Static instability (Fig. 72.4)
  - Injury to the SLL and the secondary stabilizers of the wrist (volar carpal ligaments and dorsal wrist capsule)
  - Evidence of SL widening and DISI deformity on nonstress views
- SLAC wrist (SLAC)
  - Final stage of SL instability leading to a predictable pattern of degenerative arthritis (Fig. 72.5)
    - See Table 72.1 for progression and stages of SLAC wrist.
- The following should be evaluated on radiographs:
  - Scaphoid ring sign: produced when the SLL has been disrupted and the scaphoid falls into flexion
    - A distance of less than 7 mm from the ring to the scaphoid proximal pole indicates a rotatory subluxation of the scaphoid (Fig. 72.6).
  - Terry Thomas sign: widening of the SL interval by more than 5 mm (see Fig. 72.6)
    - Must compare with contralateral side, as there is significant variability between individuals.
      - Patients with generalized ligamentous laxity may have benign SL interval widening in the absence of injury.
    - If present on nonstress view, a static instability of the wrist is demonstrated.
  - Late stages of SLL instability result in a SLAC wrist with the following degenerative changes seen on posteroanterior radiographs (see Table 72.1 and Fig. 72.7).
- Lateral view
  - DISI deformity and increased SL angle (Fig. 72.8)
    - The normal SL angle is 30 to 60 degrees.
    - DISI deformity creates an angle greater than 70 degrees and is indicative of instability of the SLL.
- Posteroanterior clenched-fist view (Fig. 72.9)
  - An increase in the SL interval by more than 5 mm indicates a dynamic instability of the SLL.
  - Compare the affected side with the contralateral side.

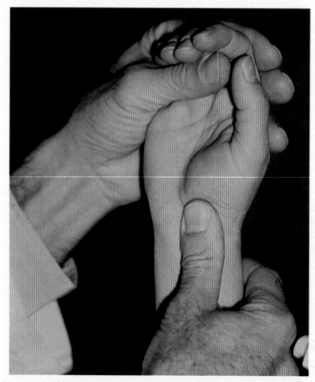

Fig 72.2 Watson maneuver. (From Green D, Hotchkiss R, Pederson W, Wolfe S, eds. *Green's Operative Hand Surgery*. Vol. 1. 5th ed. Philadelphia: Churchill Livingstone, 2005:493.)

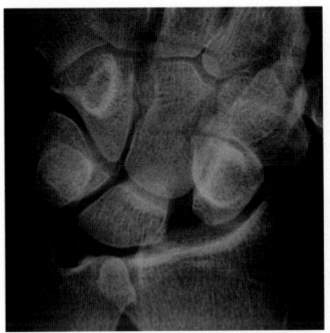

Fig 72.4 Static instability and dorsal intercalated segment instability deformity. (From Green D, Hotchkiss R, Pederson W, Wolfe S, eds. *Green's Operative Hand Surgery.* Vol. 1. 5th ed. Philadelphia: Churchill Livingstone, 2005:569.)

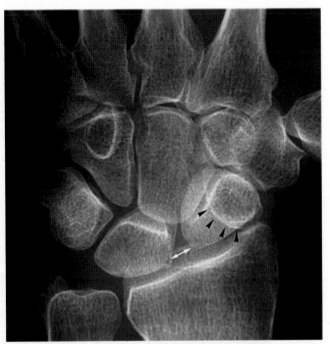

Fig 72.6 Scaphoid ring sign *(black arrowheads)* and Terry Thomas sign *(white arrow).* (From Wolfe S, Hotchkiss R, Pederson W, et al., eds. *Green's Operative Hand Surgery.* Vol. 1. 7th ed. Philadelphia: Elsevier, 2017:437.)

TABLE 72.1 Stages of Scapholunate Advanced Collapse Wrist

Stage	Joint Degeneration
I	Radial styloid-scaphoid articulation; radial styloid beaking
II	Stage I + radioscaphoid joint
III	Stage II + capitolunate joint and proximal migration of capitate
IV	Panarthritis including radiolunate joint

- 3.0-T magnetic resonance imaging (MRI) has a specificity of 70-85% for SLL ligament tear.
- Wrist arthroscopy remains the gold standard for diagnosis and treatment.

Differential Diagnosis

- Please see Table 72.2.

Treatment

- At diagnosis
  - Predynamic instability (mild wrist pain and with radiographs are normal, including stress views)
    - Nonsteroidal antiinflammatory drugs
    - Splint or short arm cast immobilization for 4 to 6 weeks
  - Dynamic instability, static instability
    - Splint immobilization and referral to specialist within 7 to 10 days for an acute injury

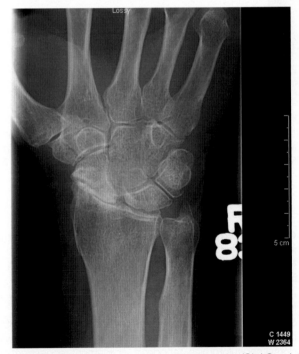

Fig 72.5 Scapholunate advanced collapse wrist (SLAC wrist).

Additional Tests

- Magnetic resonance imaging with gadolinium (Fig. 72.10)
  - Specificity varies dramatically depending on magnet strength, quality of images, radiologist experience, and technique.

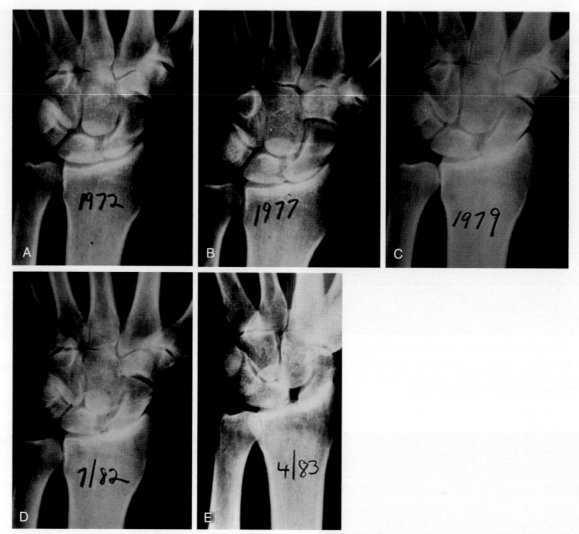

Fig 72.7 Stages of scapholunate (SL) advanced collapse. (A) No radiographic changes after SL ligament surgery. (B) Early extension of lunate and narrowing of radioscaphoid joint. (C) Radioscaphoid arthritis and proximal migration of capitate. (D) Radiocarpal arthritis and proximal migration of capitate. (E) Static instability with radiocarpal arthritis, SL interval widening on nonstress view, and proximal migration of capitate. (From Green D, Hotchkiss R, Pederson W, Wolfe S, eds. *Green's Operative Hand Surgery*. Vol. 1. 5th ed. Philadelphia: Churchill Livingstone, 2005:507.)

- SLAC wrist
  - Nonsteroidal antiinflammatory drugs
  - Splint or cast immobilization
  - Avoidance of provocative activity
  - Radiocarpal corticosteroid injection
- Later
  - Predynamic instability
    - Repeat radiographs. If asymptomatic, begin range of motion exercises and gradual return to activity. If symptomatic, refer to a specialist.
  - SLAC wrist: If conservative management fails, refer the patient to a specialist.

When to Refer

- When there are physical examination findings suggestive of an SLL injury or there is evidence of SL interval widening

or DISI deformity on plain radiographs (static or dynamic instability)
- If conservative management of a predynamic pattern of instability or SLAC wrist fails
- A patient may require a diagnostic wrist arthroscopy to identify, stage, and repair damage to the SLL.
- Surgical repair options include debridement of the SLL, pinning of the SLL with Kirschner wires, reconstruction with dorsal capsulotomies, tenodesis, or ligament reconstruction.
- Late stages of SLL instability resulting in SLAC wrist may require more involved surgical procedures such as proximal row carpectomy, limited arthrodesis, or total wrist fusion.

Prognosis

- All patients with complete SLL disruptions will develop degenerative changes (SLAC wrist) if left untreated.

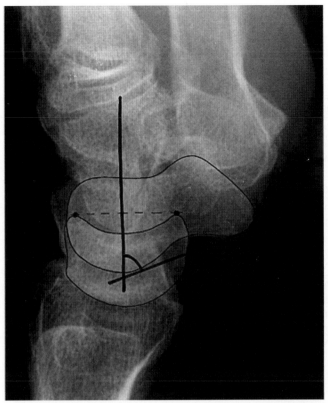

Fig 72.8 Dorsal intercalated segment instability (DISI) deformity and scapholunate (SL) angle. DISI deformity is described as SL angle greater than 70 degrees. (From Green D, Hotchkiss R, Pederson W, Wolfe S, eds. *Green's Operative Hand Surgery*. Vol. 1. 5th ed. Philadelphia: Churchill Livingstone, 2005:558.)

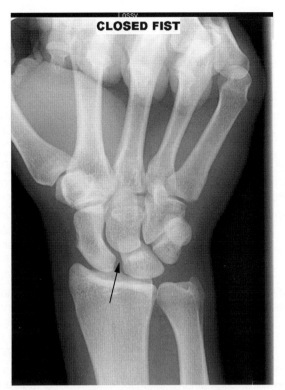

Fig 72.9 Posteroanterior clenched-fist view *(arrow)*.

- Patients whose injuries are recognized early and undergo early ligamentous repair can have an excellent outcome. Injuries that are recognized late or in the presence of degenerative changes are more difficult to treat and often have suboptimal outcomes.

Patient Instructions

- Evaluation by a specialist is important to prevent the development of progressive degenerative changes.

Considerations in Special Populations

- Athletes involved in contact sports are particularly prone to this injury.
- They often present with a remote history of a wrist sprain with a failure to seek treatment, and there should be a high suspicion for a missed SLL injury.
- Referral to a specialist is important to prevent long-term sequelae.

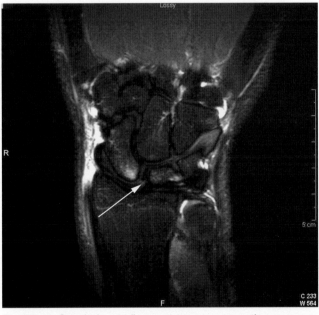

Fig 72.10 Scapholunate ligament tear on magnetic resonance imaging *(arrow)*.

TABLE 72.2 Differential Diagnosis

Condition	Differentiating Features	Chapter Reference
Acute fracture or wrist sprain	History of recent fall or trauma; no evidence of chronic degenerative changes on plain radiographs	92, 93, 75
de Quervain tenosynovitis	Positive Finkelstein sign	76
Rheumatoid arthritis	Evidence of erosive arthritis on radiographs; hand and finger deformities such as metacarpophalangeal dislocations; swan neck and boutonnière deformities of fingers	15
Gout	Punch-out lesions on radiographs	18
Calcium pyrophosphate dihydrate deposition or pseudogout	Calcium pyrophosphate dihydrate deposits visible in triangular fibrocartilage complex on plain radiographs	15
Carpal tunnel syndrome	History of numbness, tingling, and pain in the median nerve distribution; pain worse at night; positive provocative maneuvers for carpal tunnel syndrome; normal radiographs; evidence of carpal tunnel syndrome on electromyography/nerve conduction studies	79
Cubital tunnel syndrome or ulnar neuropathy at Guyon canal	Paresthesias and pain in the ulnar nerve distribution; positive provocative maneuvers for cubital tunnel syndrome at the elbow or in Guyon canal; normal radiographs; evidence of cubital tunnel syndrome or distal ulnar neuropathy on electromyography/nerve conduction studies	61
Tendonitis of common extensors (extensor carpi ulnaris, extensor radialis carpi brevis, extensor carpi radialis longus, flexor carpi ulnaris, or flexor carpi radialis)	Tenderness to palpation directly over the affected tendon; normal radiographs	77
Triangular fibrocartilage complex injury	Tender to palpation over the triangular fibrocartilage complex; normal radiographs if occurs as isolated injury; magnetic resonance imaging may help identify triangular fibrocartilage complex tear	75
Ganglion cysts, occult	May have evidence of a palpable, firm, slightly mobile mass; normal radiographs; magnetic resonance imaging can help to identify ganglion cysts	78

Suggested Readings

Garcia-Elias M, Lluch AL. Wrist instabilities, misalignments, and dislocations. In: Wolfe S, Hotchkiss R, Pederson W, et al, eds. *Green's Operative Hand Surgery*. 7th ed. Philadelphia: Elsevier; 2017:418–478.

Linscheid RL, Dobyns JH, Beaubout JW, et al. Traumatic instability of the wrist: diagnosis, classification, and pathomechanics. *J Bone Joint Surg Am*. 1972;54A:1612–1632.

Manuel J, Moran S. The diagnosis and treatment of scapholunate instability. *Orthop Clin North Am*. 2007;38:261–277.

Walsh J, Berger R, Cooney W. Current status of scapholunate interosseous ligament injuries. *J Am Acad Orthop Surg*. 2002;10:32–42.

Watson HK, Ballet FL. The SLAC wrist: scapholunate advanced collapse pattern of degenerative arthritis. *J Hand Surg Am*. 1984;5:320–327.

Watson HK, Winzweig J, Zeppieri J. Physical examination of the wrist. *Hand Clin*. 1997;13:17–34.

Watson HK, Winzweig J, Zeppieri J. The natural progression of scaphoid instability. *Hand Clin*. 1997;13:39–49.

Chapter 73 Wrist Osteoarthritis

Jeffrey D. Boatright

ICD-10-CM CODES
M19.039 *Wrist arthritis*
M12.539 *Traumatic arthritis of wrist*

Key Concepts

- Causes of wrist osteoarthritis (OA) may be primary-degenerative, secondary to inflammatory arthropathy (see Chapter 15), or posttraumatic in nature.
  - Posttraumatic wrist OA typically begins as a local injury and frequently develops into a predictable pattern of degenerative changes.
  - The most common cause of wrist posttraumatic OA is chronic scapholunate instability (SLAC wrist) (see Chapter 72).
- Frequent patterns/specific locations of wrist OA
  - Scapholunate advanced collapse wrist (SLAC wrist) (Fig. 73.1)
  - Scaphoid nonunion advanced collapse wrist (SNAC wrist) (Fig. 73.2)
  - Radiocarpal arthritis (Fig. 73.3)
  - Midcarpal arthritis
  - Distal radioulnar joint arthritis (Fig. 73.4)
  - Pisotriquetral OA
  - Scaphotrapezoid-trapezium (STT) arthritis (or triscaphe arthritis) (Fig. 73.5)
  - Avascular necrosis
  - Kienböck disease (avascular necrosis of the lunate) (Fig. 73.6)
  - Preiser disease (idiopathic scaphoid avascular necrosis)
- Physical examination is essential to identify and localize the area of tenderness.
- Must obtain radiographs (anteroposterior, lateral, and oblique views) to identify affected joints
- Maintain a high suspicion for SLAC wrist or SNAC wrist in a patient who reports a remote history of wrist injury or scaphoid fracture

History

- There may be a history of wrist injury or fracture.
  - Often this is reported as a prior "wrist sprain" for which the patient never sought medical evaluation.
- Wrist pain, morning stiffness, decreased motion, and decreased strength especially with grip may be reported.
- Pain is described as an underlying dull ache that becomes sharp with certain movements of the wrist and may fluctuate with activity, weather changes, or temperature changes.
- The patient may or may not have an underlying diagnosis of OA in other weight-bearing joints or the hands.
  - Absence of OA in other joints does not exclude the possibility of wrist OA.

- The patient may describe symptoms of carpal tunnel syndrome due to compression of the median nerve from generalized wrist synovitis.

Physical Examination

- Inspection of the wrist may reveal anything from normal appearance to severe deformity.
- Palpation is essential to identify the point of maximal tenderness.
  - A thorough examination of the wrist should be performed with an emphasis on palpating the following sites.
  - Anatomic snuffbox: Tenderness may indicate scaphoid fracture or nonunion, SNAC wrist, scaphoid avascular necrosis, STT OA, radioscaphoid arthritis, radial styloid OA.
  - Scaphoid tubercle tenderness may indicate OA involving the scaphoid.
  - Scapholunate interval tenderness may indicate chronic scapholunate ligament injury with SLAC wrist, SNAC wrist, or Kienböck disease.
  - STT joint, located just proximal to the base of the second metacarpal: pain may indicate STT arthritis (Fig. 73.7).
  - Pisotriquetral joint: pain may indicate pisotriquetral arthritis.
  - Diffuse tenderness may represent panarthritis.
- The following tests should be performed.
  - Piano key test or distal radioulnar joint (DRUJ) shuck test: The distal radius is stabilized with one hand while applying alternating dorsal and volar pressure over the ulnar head to produce translation of the distal ulna.
  - Pain may indicate distal radioulnar joint OA.
  - Perform Watson's maneuver to assess for scapholunate ligament disruption, a precursor to arthritis (see Chapter 72).
- Assess active wrist range of motion. Normal values are listed and any deficiencies or pain should be noted (should compare to the contralateral wrist).
  - Flexion: 70 degrees
  - Extension: 80 degrees
  - Radial deviation: 20 degrees
  - Ulnar deviation: 30 degrees
- A thorough neurovascular examination of the cervical spine, shoulder, elbow, and wrist should be performed to evaluate for additional pathology.

Imaging

- Obtain anteroposterior, lateral, and oblique views of the wrist as baseline radiographs.
  - Staging of specific pathology such as SNAC and SLAC wrist (Table 73.1; see also Table 72.1 in Chapter 72)

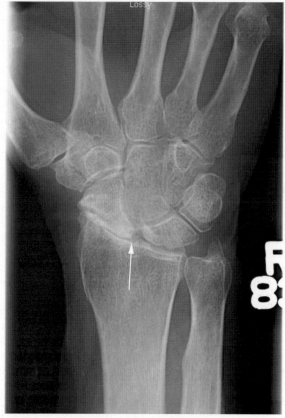

Fig 73.1 Scapholunate advanced collapse *(arrow)*.

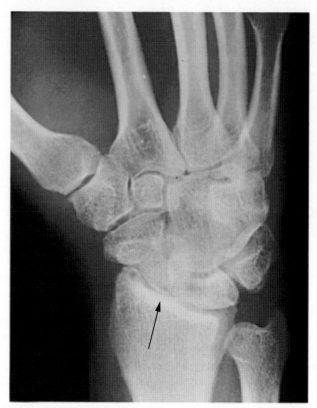

Fig 73.3 Radiocarpal arthritis *(arrow)*. (From Green D, Hotchkiss R, Pederson W, Wolfe S, eds. *Green's Operative Hand Surgery*. Vol. 1, 5th ed. Philadelphia: Churchill Livingstone; 2005:523.)

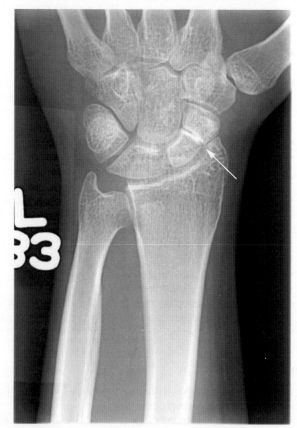

Fig 73.2 Scaphoid nonunion advanced collapse *(arrow)*.

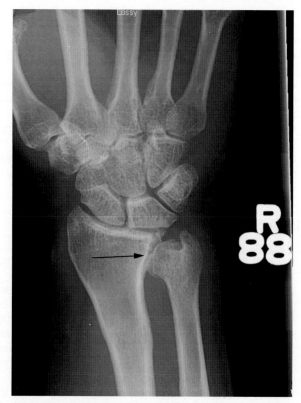

Fig 73.4 Distal radioulnar joint arthritis *(arrow)*.

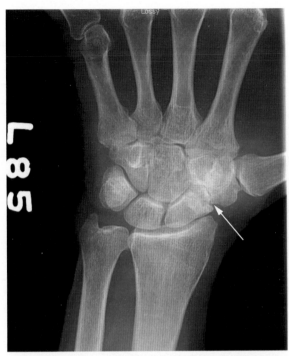

Fig 73.5 Scaphotrapezoid-trapezium arthritis *(arrow)*.

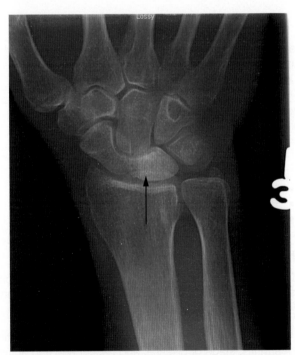

Fig 73.6 Avascular necrosis of the lunate *(arrow)*.

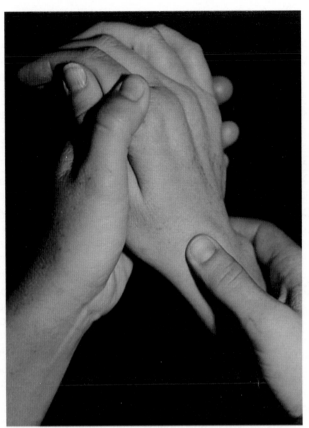

Fig 73.7 Palpation of scaphotrapezoid-trapezium joint. (From Green D, Hotchkiss R, Pederson W, Wolfe S, eds. *Green's Operative Hand Surgery*. Vol. 1, 5th ed. Philadelphia: Churchill Livingstone; 2005:492.)

TABLE 73.1	Stages of Scapholunate Advanced Collapse and Scaphoid Nonunion Advanced Collapse (SNAC) Wrist
Stage	**Joint Degeneration**
I	Radial styloid-scaphoid articulation; radial styloid beaking
II	Stage I + radioscaphoid joint (+ scaphocapitate in SNAC)
III	Stage II + capitolunate joint and proximal migration of capitate
IV	Panarthritis including radiolunate joint

- Additional views:
  - Navicular or scaphoid view to identify scaphoid nonunion or STT arthritis
  - A posteroanterior neutral clenched-fist view to evaluate for scapholunate ligament disruption, which appears as a widening of the scapholunate interval with a clenched fist

- May need to obtain contralateral clenched-fist view for comparison (see Chapter 72)
- Pisiform oblique view to evaluate the pisotriquetral joint

Additional Tests

- Typically not indicated
- Computed tomography can evaluate for arthritic changes if none can be identified on plain radiographs (rarely indicated).
- Three-phase bone scan to identify area of bone reactivity, which may indicate OA (rarely indicated)

TABLE 73.2 Differential Diagnosis

Condition	Differentiating Features	Chapter Reference
Acute fracture or wrist sprain	History of recent fall or trauma; no evidence of chronic degenerative changes on plain radiographs	72, 75
de Quervain tenosynovitis	Positive Finkelstein sign	76
Rheumatoid arthritis	Evidence of erosive arthritis on radiographs; hand and finger deformities such as metacarpophalangeal dislocations; swan neck and boutonnière deformities of fingers	15
Gout	Punch-out lesions on radiographs	15
Calcium pyrophosphate dihydrate deposition or pseudogout	Calcium pyrophosphate dihydrate deposits visible in triangular fibrocartilage complex on plain radiographs	15
Carpal tunnel syndrome	History of numbness, tingling, and pain in the median nerve distribution; pain worse at night; positive provocative maneuvers for carpal tunnel syndrome; normal radiographs; evidence of carpal tunnel syndrome on electromyography/nerve conduction studies	79
Cubital tunnel syndrome or ulnar neuropathy at Guyon's canal	Paresthesias and pain in the ulnar nerve distribution; positive provocative maneuvers for cubital tunnel syndrome at the elbow or in Guyon's canal; normal radiographs; evidence of cubital tunnel syndrome or distal ulnar neuropathy on electromyography/nerve conduction studies	61
Tendonitis of common extensors (extensor carpi ulnaris, extensor radialis carpi brevis, extensor carpi radialis longus, flexor carpi ulnaris, or flexor carpi radialis)	Tenderness to palpation directly over the affected tendon; normal radiographs	77
Triangular fibrocartilage complex injury	Tender to palpation over the triangular fibrocartilage complex; normal radiographs if occurs as isolated injury; magnetic resonance imaging may help to identify triangular fibrocartilage complex tear	75
Ganglion cysts, occult	May have evidence of a palpable, firm, slightly mobile mass; normal radiographs; magnetic resonance imaging can help to identify ganglion cysts	78

- MRI can be useful to identify a discrete chondral lesion, evaluate for avascular necrosis, or rule out other pathology if radiographs and physical exam are equivocal.

Differential Diagnosis
- Please see Table 73.2.

Treatment
- At diagnosis
  - Nonsteroidal antiinflammatory drugs, if tolerated; lifestyle and activity modifications; wrist brace; local modalities such as paraffin baths; and supplements such as glucosamine and chondroitin sulfate may be helpful if not contraindicated.
  - Counseling on the natural history of OA for realistic treatment goals
- Later (if nonsteroidal antiinflammatory drugs fail)
  - Ultrasound or fluoroscopically guided corticosteroid injection into affected joint; common injection sites are
  - Radiocarpal joint (fluoroscopy not necessary)

- Distal radioulnar joint
- STT joint
- Pisotriquetral joint

When to Refer
- Diagnosis of scaphoid nonunion, scaphoid avascular necrosis, Kienböck disease, or concern for acute scapholunate ligament injury or acute scaphoid fracture
- When conservative measures fail
- A variety of surgical options are available based on location of arthritis, stage of disease, and patient age and activity level. Options may include proximal row carpectomy, limited versus total wrist arthrodesis, total wrist arthroplasty, and tendon-interposition arthroplasty.

Prognosis
- OA is a chronic progressive disease.
- All patients with a complete scapholunate ligament disruption or an untreated scaphoid nonunion will develop a predictable pattern of progressive arthritis if left untreated.

Troubleshooting

- Radiocarpal joint corticosteroid injection (see Chapter 101)
  - Useful from a diagnostic standpoint in helping to differentiate between intra- and extra-articular pathology.
  - Can also be therapeutic from a symptomatic management standpoint.

Patient Instructions

- OA is a chronic degenerative condition that does not have a cure, and treatment goals are directed toward symptomatic management.
- Corticosteroid injections can take several weeks to become effective.

Considerations in Special Populations

- Young patients who present with wrist pain after traumatic injury should be monitored for occult scaphoid fractures and evidence of scapholunate ligament injury because identification and treatment of these injuries are the key to the prevention of OA.
- Treatment of laborers and young, active patients with wrist arthritis should be geared toward preserving strength and motion for as long as possible.

Suggested Readings

Cooney WP. Post-traumatic arthritis of the wrist. In: Cooney WP, Linscheid RL, Dobyns JH, eds. *The Wrist: Diagnosis and Operative Treatment*. Vol. 1. St. Louis: Mosby; 1998:588–629.

Ghazi R. Pisiform ligament complex syndrome and pisotriquetral arthrosis. *Hand Clin*. 2005;21:507–517.

Parmalee-Peters K, Eathorne S. The wrist: common injuries and management. *Prim Care*. 2005;32:35–70.

Peterson B, Szabo R. Carpal osteoarthritis. *Hand Clin*. 2006;22:517–528.

Rizzo M. Wrist arthrodesis and arthroplasty. In: Wolfe SW, Hotchkiss RN, Pederson WC, et al, eds. *Green's Operative Hand Surgery*. Vol. 1. 7th ed. Philadelphia: Elsevier; 2017:373–417.

Weiss K, Rodner C. Osteoarthritis of the wrist. *J Hand Surg Am*. 2007; 32A:725–746.

Chapter 74 Kienböck Disease

John B. Thaller, Mary C. Iaculli

ICD-10-CM CODES
M92.21   *Juvenile Kienböck disease*
M93.1   *Adult Kienböck disease*

Key Concepts

- Kienböck disease is a condition of avascular necrosis of the lunate.
- The exact etiology of Kienböck disease remains unknown.
- It is often related to a relative difference in the length of the radius and ulna bones. Specifically it is most common when the ulna is significantly shorter than the radius, causing an imbalance of pressure on the wrist.
- Other factors associated with the development of Kienböck disease include:
  - History of trauma
  - Horizontal slope of the distal radius
  - Ligamentous instability of the wrist
- Cadaver studies have demonstrated that a high percentage of lunate bones have only a single blood vessel responsible for nutritional blood flow. This tenuous blood supply is thought to predispose the lunate to avascular necrosis.
- It appears to be more common in men than in women and younger patients.

History

- Signs and symptoms of Kienböck disease are often vague and insidious in onset. They often include:
  - Dorsal or diffuse wrist pain
  - Swelling
  - Stiffness
- A history of trauma is present in nearly 50% of patients. However, sometimes the trauma is quite minor.

Physical Examination

- Examination findings are often nonspecific, including:
- Dorsal wrist tenderness over the lunate bone
- Decreased active and passive wrist range of motion, with or without crepitation
- Dorsal wrist effusion
- Decreased grip strength
- No physical examination finding is specific for Kienböck disease.

Imaging

- Plain radiographs
  - The Lichtman classification, which is useful for stratification, prognostication, and choosing treatment, is based on plain posteroanterior and lateral radiographs.
    - Stage I: Plain radiographs may be normal, or there may be a subtle lunate fracture noted. There is no sclerosis and no collapse (Fig. 74.1A).
    - Stage II: Increased density and sclerosis of the lunate (Fig. 74.2)
    - Stage IIIa: Lunate collapse with maintained carpal relationships (Fig. 74.3)
    - Stage IIIb: Lunate collapse with fixed scaphoid rotatory collapse
    - Stage IV: Extensive pancarpal osteoarthritis
- Magnetic resonance imaging (MRI)
  - In early disease, MRI may be the only radiographic abnormality. If plain radiographs are normal, then MRI may be necessary to establish the correct diagnosis.
  - Decreased signal on T1-weighted images (see Fig. 74.1B)
  - Increased signal on T2-weighted images
  - Fracture or collapse may also be evident on MRI.
- Computed tomography (CT)
  - Often the diagnosis may be confirmed on plain radiographs, but CT is necessary for proper staging of the disease.
  - Fig. 74.4 demonstrates a case in which the CT scan significantly altered the staging of the disease and subsequently affected the treatment choice. Plain radiographs appear to be stage I to II, and treatment would be aimed at lunate salvage, such as a joint leveling procedure or revascularization of the lunate. However, the CT scan revealed advanced collapse and fragmentation, which would prevent success with lunate salvage (see Fig. 74.4).

Differential Diagnosis

- Please see Table 74.1.

Treatment

- At the time of diagnosis:
  - Initial treatment depends entirely on proper radiographic staging.

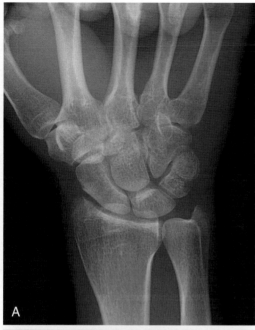

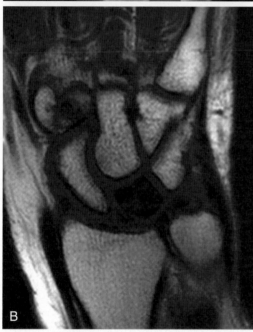

Fig 74.1 (A) Routine posteroanterior radiograph of a patient with wrist pain with no abnormal radiographic findings. (B) Coronal magnetic resonance imaging of the same patient with decreased signal on T1, consistent with poor vascularity of the lunate.

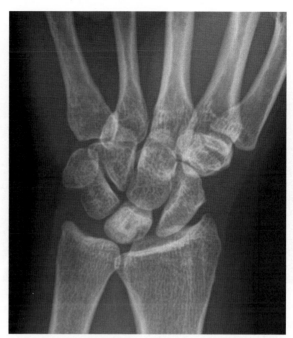

Fig 74.2 Routine posteroanterior radiograph of patient with stage II Kienböck disease. The lunate shows increased density and sclerosis but no collapse, loss of height, or fracture.

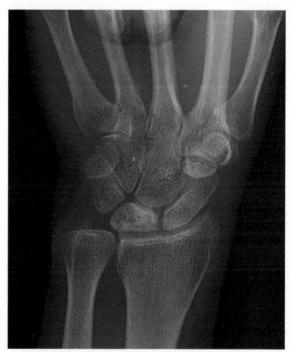

Fig 74.3 Routine posteroanterior radiograph of patient with stage IIIa Kienböck disease. The lunate shows increased sclerosis as well as collapse and some loss of height more radially than ulnarly.

- All patients should have plain radiographs and a CT scan to accurately assess for sclerosis, collapse, and fragmentation.
- Although MRI may be necessary to establish the early diagnosis of Kienböck disease, a CT scan is necessary for accurate staging.
- The role of nonoperative treatment in adults with an established diagnosis of Kienböck disease remains somewhat controversial.

- In patients with completely normal plain radiographs but a positive MRI, some authors advocate for a period of immobilization as the initial treatment. Others, however, feel that surgical treatment is indicated for all adults with the diagnosis of Kienböck disease.

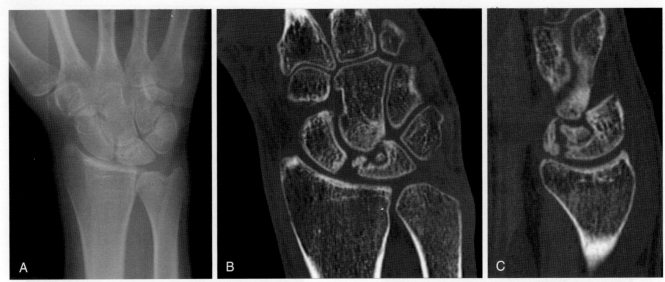

Fig 74.4 (A) Routine posteroanterior plain radiograph of patient with what appears to be an early stage of Kienböck disease. Coronal (B) and sagittal (C) computed tomography scan of the same patient revealing much more advanced collapse and fragmentation than are evident on the plain radiographs. (Used with permission of May Foundation for Medical Education and Research. All rights reserved.)

TABLE 74.1 Differential Diagnosis

Differential Diagnosis	Differentiating Feature
Lunate fracture	A simple lunate fracture may look similar to Kienböck fragmentation on plain radiographs and computed tomography scans. However, magnetic resonance imaging will be diagnostic in demonstrating avascularity of the lunate in Kienböck disease
Wrist sprain	Plain radiography and computed tomography scan may be normal in both conditions, but magnetic resonance imaging will be diagnostic of avascular necrosis, where it should be normal in a wrist sprain

- Later
  - Patients with more advanced radiographic disease or patients in whom nonoperative treatment has failed require surgical intervention.
  - There is no one universally accepted surgical procedure.
  - In patients with an ulnar negative variant, a radial shortening osteotomy has proven successful.
  - In more advanced stages, a vascularized bone graft procedure may be necessary to reintroduce blood supply to the lunate.
  - Patients with Kienböck stage IIIb and beyond will need a salvage procedure.
    - In these patients, the fragmentation of the lunate and the associated degenerative changes prevent successful reconstruction unless the lunate is removed or mechanically bypassed with a partial wrist fusion.

- A proximal row carpectomy, partial wrist fusion, or total wrist fusion may often be necessary to provide good pain relief in these advanced cases.

When to Refer
- Any patient with an MRI demonstrating avascular necrosis of the lunate should be referred to a hand surgeon for discussion of treatment options.
- Any patient who initially presents with collapse, fragmentation, or other advanced radiographic changes should also be referred immediately to a hand surgeon.

Prognosis
- Patients who present early and respond to nonoperative treatment can expect an excellent outcome with eventual resolution of symptoms.
- Patients who either present with or progress to further radiographic changes have a much more guarded prognosis.
- Natural history studies seem to demonstrate that the majority of patients will demonstrate progressive radiographic collapse, fragmentation, and arthrosis of the lunate, so the key to a good prognosis remains early recognition and early treatment.

Troubleshooting
- In patients with early disease, the diagnosis may be difficult to make.
- All patients who present with chronic diffuse wrist pain should have plain radiographs.
- If plain radiographs are normal and the patient fails to respond to routine appropriate nonoperative treatment, then MRI is warranted.
- MRI should be diagnostic in the majority of cases.

- CT should then be ordered for accurate staging to evaluate for fracture and fragmentation.

Considerations in Special Populations

- Younger patients have shown a more favorable outcome after both nonoperative and operative treatments for Kienböck disease.
- When avascular necrosis without fragmentation is diagnosed in a teenage patient, the initial treatment should always be immobilization.
- Patients being treated nonoperatively should be monitored closely. Progression of sclerosis, collapse, or fracture will often indicated that surgical intervention is necessary.

Suggested Readings

Beckenbaugh RD, Shives TC, Dobyns JH, Linscheid RL. Kienbock's disease: the natural history of Kienbock's disease and consideration of lunate fractures. *Clin Orthop Relat Res*. 1980;149:98–106.

Gelberman RH, Bauman TD, Menon J, Akeson WH. The vascularity of the lunate bone and kienböck disease. *J Hand Surg Am*. 1980;5:272–278.

Iwasaki N, Minami A, Oizumi N, et al. Predictors of clinical results of radial osteotomies for Kienbock's disease. *Clin Orthop Relat Res*. 2003;415:157–162.

Lichtman DM, Degnan GG. Staging and its use in the determination of treatment modalities for Kienbock's disease. *Hand Clin*. 1993;9:409–416.

Raven E, Haverkamp D, Marti RK. Outcome of Kienbock's disease 22 years after distal radius shortening osteotomy. *Clin Orthop Relat Res*. 2007;460:137–141.

Salmon J, Stanley JK, Trail IA. Kienbock's disease: conservative management versus radial shortening. *J Bone Joint Surg Br*. 2000;82B:820–823.

Shin A, Bishop A. Vascular anatomy of the distal radius: implications for vascularized bone grafts. *Clin Orthop Relat Res*. 2001;38:60–67.

Chapter 75 Triangular Fibrocartilage Complex Injuries

Jeffrey D. Boatright

ICD-10-CM CODES
S63.599A   *TFCC tear*
S63.509A   *Wrist sprain*

Key Concepts

- The triangular fibrocartilage complex (TFCC) is located on the ulnar aspect of the wrist and functions as a major stabilizer of the distal radioulnar joint (DRUJ).
- It is composed of (Fig. 75.1):
  - Fibrocartilage disc
  - Volar and dorsal distal radioulnar ligaments
  - Meniscus homologue
  - Volar ulnocarpal ligaments: ulnolunate and ulnotriquetral ligaments
  - Floor of the extensor carpi ulnaris tendon sheath
- The TFCC carries 18-20% of the axial load of the wrist.
  - Any factor that increases the axial load on the ulnar aspect of the wrist puts the TFCC at risk of injury.
  - Patients with ulnar positive variance (due to anatomic variation, distal radius malunion, growth arrest, or radial head resection) are at greater risk of developing central TFCC pathology.
  - 2 mm of positive ulnar variance changes the axial load distribution of the wrist dramatically.
    - Normal wrist: 20% load goes to the ulna, 80% to the radius.
    - +2 mm ulnar variance: 40% ulna, 60% radius
- TFCC injury classification (Fig. 75.2)
  - Type 1: traumatic lesions
  - Type 1A: central TFCC perforation (most common)
  - Type 1B: base of the ulnar styloid with or without ulnar styloid fracture
  - Type 1C: carpal detachment (volar ulnolunate ligaments)
  - Type 1D: radial detachment with or without radial avulsion fracture
  - Type 2: degenerative lesions
  - Type 2A: thinning of the articular disc
  - Type 2B: thinning of the articular disc and lunate chondromalacia
  - Type 2C: central perforation of the TFCC and lunate chondromalacia
  - Type 2D: central perforation of the TFCC, lunate chondromalacia, and lunotriquetral ligament perforation
  - Type 2E: central perforation of the TFCC, lunate chondromalacia, lunotriquetral ligament perforation, ulnocarpal arthritis

- Vascular supply
  - The ulnar peripheral TFCC is vascularized, whereas the central aspect of the TFCC is avascular; this principle guides treatment options.
  - Peripheral lesions can usually be repaired as they have a high healing potential.
  - Central lesions may be treated conservatively or require arthroscopic debridement because poor vascularity lends a poor healing potential.
- Posteroanterior neutral view radiographs of the wrist must be obtained to assess for ulnar positive variance.
- Lateral radiographs may show DRUJ instability with dorsal subluxation of the ulnar head relative to the radius.
- Arthroscopy remains the gold standard for diagnosis; however, MRI arthrogram is a noninvasive diagnostic tool with improving sensitivity in detecting TFCC pathology.

History

- The patient typically reports ulnar-sided wrist pain that may increase with power grip or ulnar deviation.
- May report "clicking," "catching," or other mechanical symptoms in the wrist.
- May report a recent or remote history of a fall on an outstretched hand, sudden rotational force, axial loading with distraction, or repetitive loading.
- May have a history of distal radius malunion with radial shortening.

Physical Examination

- Inspection may reveal a prominent ulnar styloid if the DRUJ is significantly disrupted or there is edema on the ulnar aspect of the wrist.
- Palpate the TFCC on the ulnar aspect of the wrist.
  - Distal to the ulnar styloid in the soft spot between the extensor carpi ulnaris and flexor carpi ulnaris tendons (fovea)
  - Dorso-ulnar wrist, just distal to the ulnar head and just radial to the fifth compartment
  - Tenderness may indicate a peripheral TFCC tear.
- Ulnar grind test:
  - The examiner extends, axially loads, and ulnarly deviates the wrist.
  - Reproducible pain may indicate a TFCC tear.
- Palpate the DRUJ with the wrist in pronation and perform the piano key test.

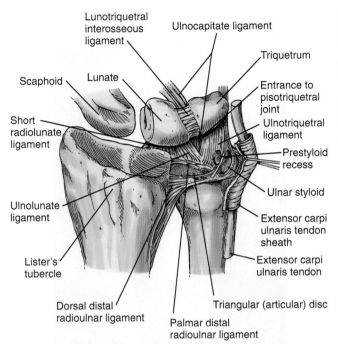

Fig 75.1 Anatomy of the triangular fibrocartilage complex. (Modified from Cooney WP, Linscheid RL, Dobyns JH, eds. *The Wrist: Diagnosis and Operative Treatment*. St Louis: Mosby; 1998.)

- The distal radius is stabilized with one hand while applying alternating dorsal and volar pressure over the ulnar head to produce translation of the distal ulna.
- Compare to the contralateral side.
- Increased motion or pain with motion can indicate DRUJ instability and/or TFCC pathology.
- A thorough examination of all wrist structures should be performed, taking care to isolate the area of tenderness.
- A thorough neurovascular examination of the upper extremity should also be performed.

Imaging

- Posteroanterior and lateral radiographs of the wrist are standard.
  - Posteroanterior neutral position: the arm is abducted to 90 degrees at the shoulder, the elbow is flexed to 90 degrees, and the forearm is in a neutral pronation (Fig. 75.3).
  - Assess for ulnar positive variance defined as more than 4 mm (Figs. 75.4 and 75.5).
  - Assess for DRUJ widening compared to the contralateral wrist.
  - Assess for DRUJ dislocation on lateral radiographs.
  - Note that radiographs may be normal in the setting of even severe TFCC pathology.
- Additional views
  - Pronated posteroanterior grip view: obtain if a degenerative TFCC lesion is suspected because this view may demonstrate ulnocarpal abutment.

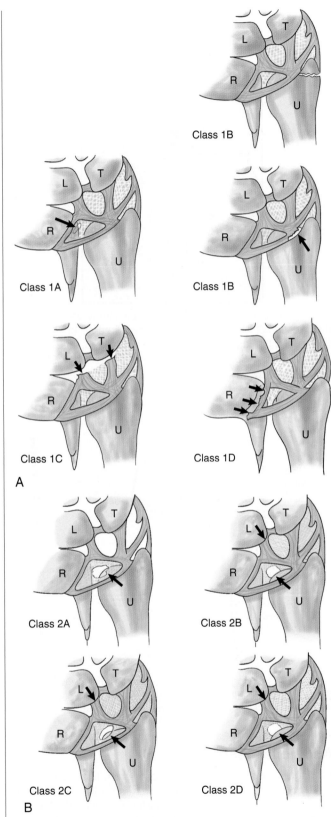

Fig 75.2 (A and B) Classification of triangular fibrocartilage complex injuries. *L*, lunate; *R*, radius; *T*, triquetrum; *U*, ulna. (Modified from Palmer AK. Triangular fibrocartilage complex lesions: a classification. *J Hand Surg Am*. 1989;14:594–606.)

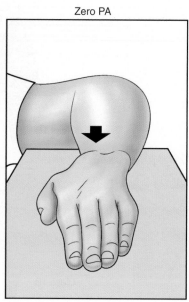

Fig 75.3 Posteroanterior *(PA)* neutral view. *Arrow* demonstrates the direction of x-ray beam from posterior to anterior. (Modified from Green D, Hotchkiss R, Pederson W, Wolfe S, eds. *Green's Operative Hand Surgery*. Vol. 1, 5th ed. Philadelphia: Churchill Livingstone; 2005.)

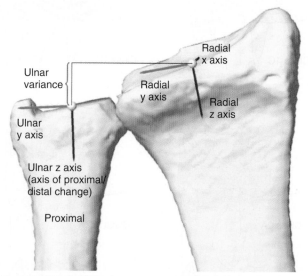

Fig 75.4 Measuring ulnar positive variance. (From Fu E, Li G, Souer JS, et al: Elbow position affects distal radioulnar joint kinematics. *J Hand Surg* 34(7):1261-1268, 2009.)

Additional Tests

- Magnetic resonance imaging arthrogram (Fig. 75.6)
  - Improved techniques and high-resolution MRI have greatly increased the sensitivity for detecting TFCC tears.
  - May reveal other related pathology such as chondral lesions or bone signal changes within the ulnar aspect of the lunate or the triquetrum, which is consistent with ulnocarpal abutment syndrome
- Arthroscopy remains the gold standard for diagnosis and treatment.

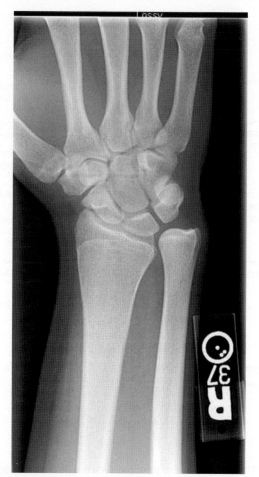

Fig 75.5 Ulnar positive variance.

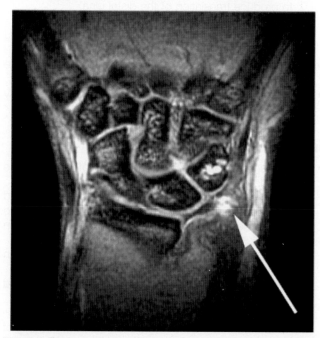

Fig 75.6 Triangular fibrocartilage complex tear *(arrow)* on magnetic resonance imaging. (From Adams B. Distal radioulnar joint. In: Trumble TE, ed. *Hand Surgery Update 3: Hand, Elbow, and Shoulder*. Rosemont, IL: American Society for Surgery of the Hand; 2003, pp 147–157.)

Differential Diagnosis

- Please see Table 75.1.

Treatment

- At diagnosis
  - If a TFCC tear is suspected in the presence of normal radiographs and no DRUJ instability, 4 to 6 weeks of wrist immobilization and nonsteroidal antiinflammatory drugs (NSAIDs) for pain relief should be initiated.

- Later
  - Once the patient is pain free, occupational therapy may help facilitate weaning from the splint, progressive wrist range of motion protocol, and finally a guided strengthening program with a graduated return to activities.

When to Refer

- Persistent symptoms after 4 to 6 weeks of conservative management

TABLE 75.1 Differential Diagnosis

Condition	Differentiating Features	Chapter Reference
Extensor carpi ulnar tendonitis	Tenderness to palpation over extensor carpi ulnar tendon sheath; pain with resisted wrist extension	77
Flexor carpi ulnar tendonitis	Tenderness to palpation over flexor carpi ulnar tendon sheath; pain with resisted wrist flexion	77
Pisotriquetral osteoarthritis	Pain over pisotriquetral joint; evidence of pisotriquetral arthritis on radiograph, pisiform oblique view	73
Distal radioulnar joint osteoarthritis	Pain with distal radioulnar joint ballottement; evidence of arthritis at distal radioulnar joint on radiograph	73
Occult ganglion cysts	May have history of wrist mass that increases and decreases in size; visualized on magnetic resonance imaging	78
Cubital tunnel syndrome	Paresthesias in ulnar nerve distribution, worse with elbow flexion or leaning on the elbow; positive provocative maneuvers for cubital tunnel syndrome; electromyography/nerve conduction studies show evidence of cubital tunnel syndrome	61
Ulnar nerve compression at Guyon canal	Paresthesias in the fourth and fifth digits; tenderness to palpation over Guyon canal with positive Tinel sign; electromyography/nerve conduction studies show evidence of ulnar neuropathy at Guyon canal	61
Hook of hamate fracture	Tenderness over the hook of the hamate; carpal tunnel view shows hook of hamate fracture on radiograph; may require computed tomography scan to diagnose fracture	
Ulnar artery thrombosis	May or may not have color and temperature changes in the fingers; Allen test reveals radial artery dominant flow; computed tomography angiography helpful to visualize occult hook of hamate fractures and evidence of thrombosis	17
Essex-Lopresti lesion	History of elbow injury or pain or radial head excision; posteroanterior and lateral views of elbow reveal fracture malunion or resected radial head; must also obtain views of wrist to identify ulnar positive variance	63
Scapholunate ligament disruption	Pain over scapholunate interval; may have a positive Watson's maneuver; posteroanterior clenched-fist radiograph reveals scapholunate widening greater than 5 mm[a] compared with contralateral side; magnetic resonance imaging shows ligament disruption	72
Lunotriquetral ligament disruption	Positive lunotriquetral shuck test; evidence of volar intercalated segment instability deformity on lateral radiographs; magnetic resonance imaging shows ligament disruption	72
Calcium pyrophosphate dihydrate deposition syndrome or pseudogout	Calcium pyrophosphate dihydrate deposits visible in the triangular fibrocartilage complex on plain radiographs	15

[a]There is some controversy surrounding this value. A wide interval may be defined as more than 3 mm if there are correlating physical examination findings and widening of the interval compared with the uninjured wrist.

- If patient has positive physical examination findings and any of the following:
  - Positive ulnar variance
  - Evidence of DRUJ instability
  - Distal radius or ulna fracture
- If surgery is indicated, there are many different options based on the location and type of injury.
- The gold standard of diagnosis and treatment is wrist arthroscopy; some injuries may be repaired or debrided arthroscopically, whereas others may require ulnar shortening osteotomy or other more complex open procedures.

Prognosis

- Variable depending upon specifics of the injury and associated pathology.
- A large percentage of these injuries can be treated non-operatively with good outcomes.
- Surgical results in those with appropriate indications are typically good to excellent but can be impacted by other concurrent pathology.

Patient Instructions

- Conservative management of this injury can be a slow process typically involving 4 to 6 weeks of immobilization followed by the above-described hand therapy program. Return to full pain-free activity can range from 3 to 6 months. Patience with this protocol must be exhibited. Initially, the patient should wear the wrist brace at all times except for hygiene, and avoidance of high-impact and other symptom-provoking activities is paramount. Work accommodations may be required, including allowance for brace wear, avoiding heavy lifting, etc.

Considerations in Special Populations

- If a TFCC injury is suspected in a high-level athlete, immobilize the wrist in a splint and perform magnetic resonance imaging. Refer to a hand specialist within 7 days for evaluation and treatment.

Suggested Readings

Adams BD, Leversedge FJ, et al. Distal radioulnar joint. In: Wolfe SW, Hotchkiss RN, Pederson WC, eds. *Green's Operative Hand Surgery*. Vol. 1. 7th ed. Philadelphia: Elsevier; 2017:479–515.

Ahn A, Chang D, Plate A. Triangular fibrocartilage complex tears—a review. *Bull Hosp Jt Dis*. 2006;64(3–4):114–118.

Elkowitz SJ, Posner MA. Wrist arthroscopy. *Bull Hosp Jt Dis*. 2006;64(3–4):156–165.

Palmer AK. Triangular fibrocartilage complex lesions: a classification. *J Hand Surg Am*. 1989;14:594–606.

Palmer AK, Bille B, Anderson A. Acute injuries of the distal radioulnar joint: tears by the triangular fibrocartilage. In: Cooney WP, eds. *The Wrist: Diagnosis and Operative Treatment*. Philadelphia: Wolters Kluwer; 2010:[Chapter 42].

Palmer AK, Werner FW. The triangular fibrocartilage complex of the wrist—anatomy and function. *J Hand Surg Am*. 1981;6:153–162.

Parmalee-Peters K, Eathorne S. The wrist: common injuries and management. *Prim Care Clin Office Pract*. 2005;32:35–70.

Rettig AC. Athletic injuries of the wrist and hand. Part i: traumatic injuries of the wrist. *Am J Sports Med*. 2003;31:1028–1048.

Chapter 76 de Quervain Tenosynovitis

David Schnur

ICD-10-CM CODE
M65.4 *Radial styloid tenosynovitis*

Key Concepts

- Tenosynovitis of the first dorsal compartment of the wrist
  - The abductor pollicis longus and extensor pollicis brevis tendons occupy the first dorsal compartment (Fig. 76.1).
- Fritz de Quervain first described the condition in 1895.
- Attributed to and exacerbated by activities involving thumb abduction with ulnar deviation of the wrist
- Anatomy of the first dorsal compartment can have significant variation.
  - The extensor pollicis brevis tendon is absent in 5-7% of extremities.
  - The compartment has a longitudinal septum in 24-34% of extremities.
  - The abductor pollicis longus muscle often has two or more slips with various insertions.
- Anatomic variation can lead to failure of nonoperative treatment.

History

- Several weeks or months of pain over the radial styloid
- Exacerbated with movement of the thumb
- Can have associated swelling over the radial styloid
- Can have pseudotriggering
- Most common in fourth and fifth decades
- Much more common in women
  - Can occur after childbirth

Physical Examination

- Tenderness on palpation over the first dorsal compartment
  - 1 to 2 cm proximal to the radial styloid
- Finkelstein's test (Fig. 76.2 and Video 76.1)
  - With the thumb grasped in the palm, ulnar deviation of the wrist causes sharp pain.
- Can have pain with resisted abduction of thumb
- Occasionally associated with a ganglion over the first dorsal compartment

Imaging

- Radiographs
  - Useful to differentiate from carpometacarpal arthritis of the thumb
  - Can rule out radial styloid fracture as the cause of pain

- Occasionally see localized osteopenia or spurring of the radius
- Not typically necessary to make the diagnosis
- Magnetic resonance imaging can assist in diagnosis if diagnosis is difficult.

Differential Diagnosis

- Please see Table 76.1.

Treatment

- At diagnosis
  - Splinting or casting can relieve symptoms but is often not curative as a single therapy.
  - Corticosteroid injection should be considered a first-line treatment and can be combined with immobilization.
    - Occasionally a second injection is necessary.
    - For details and proper injection technique, refer to Chapter 100.
- Later
  - Surgical release of the first dorsal compartment is typically reserved for patients in whom conservative treatment failed.
    - A 2-cm transverse incision is made over the first dorsal compartment just proximal to the radial styloid.
    - Longitudinal dissection is performed down to the level of the first dorsal compartment with care to protect cutaneous nerves.
    - The compartment is released, and care is taken to ensure that intracompartmental septa are divided if present (Fig. 76.3).

When to Refer

- Once the diagnosis is made, timing of the referral is dependent on the comfort of the provider in rendering conservative treatment.
  - If the provider is experienced in corticosteroid injection of the first dorsal compartment, then referral should be made if this therapy fails and operative treatment is necessary.
  - If the provider is not comfortable with giving the injection, then referral should be made at the time of diagnosis.

Prognosis

- Good with conservative measures alone and excellent with surgical intervention

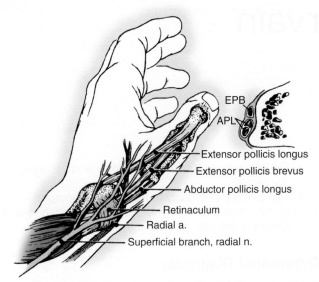

Fig 76.1 Anatomic relationship of the first dorsal compartment. *APL*, Abductor pollicis longus; *EPB*, extensor pollicis brevis. (From Budoff JE: Tendinopathies of the hand, wrist, and elbow. In Trumbel TE, Rayan GM, Budoff JE, et al (eds): *Principles of Hand Surgery and Therapy*. 3rd ed. Philadelphia, Elsevier, 2017.)

EPB
APL
Extensor pollicis longus
Extensor pollicis brevus
Abductor pollicis longus
Retinaculum
Radial a.
Superficial branch, radial n.

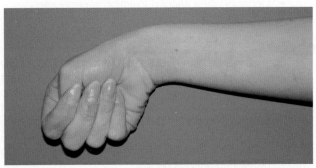

Fig 76.2 Demonstration of Finkelstein test with the thumb in the palm and the wrist ulnarly deviated.

Troubleshooting

- Failure of conservative treatment may indicate anatomic variation or tenosynovitis at the intersection of the first and second compartments.
- The patient should be counseled on the risks of conservative and surgical treatment.
  - Corticosteroid injection can cause hypopigmentation and fat atrophy; this may occur more often than with other types of injections because of the superficial nature of the injection.
  - The most serious complication of surgical intervention is injury to the superficial sensory branch of the radial nerve, which can cause numbness or significant pain. Failure of relief of symptoms is also possible.

Patient Instructions

- Patients should be given details of the disease process.
- In addition, they should be instructed not to lift objects with the hands vertical to the ground using an ulnar to radial deviation motion.

TABLE 76.1 Differential Diagnosis

Diagnosis	Differentiating Features	Chapter Reference
Carpometacarpal arthritis of the thumb	Pain typically more distal, negative Finkelstein test, positive carpometacarpal grind	80
Radial styloid fracture	History of trauma with positive radiographs, pain over dorsal radial styloid on palpation	92
Radiocarpal arthritis	Pain more dorsal over radiocarpal joint on palpation, radiographs with arthritic changes	73

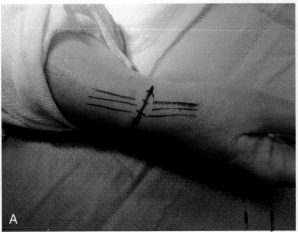
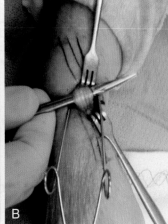

Fig 76.3 Surgical treatment of de Quervain tenosynovitis. (A) The first dorsal compartment is approached through a short transverse incision. (B) The extensor retinaculum is divided longitudinally. (From Ingari JV: Wrist tendinopathies. In: Miller MD, Thompson SR (eds): *DeLee & Drez's Orthopaedic Sports Medicine: Principles and Practice*, 3th ed. Philadelphia, Elsevier, 2015.)

A   B

- This is especially important for mothers of young children with this condition because they tend to lift their children in this fashion.

Considerations in Special Populations

- Conservative treatment in the diabetic population may be less effective.

Suggested Readings

de Quervain F. On a form of chronic tendovaginitis by Dr. Fritz de Quervain in la Chaux-de-Fonds 1895. *Am J Orthop*. 1997;26:641–644.

Gundes H, Tosun B. Longitudinal incision in surgical release of de Quervain disease. *Tech Hand Up Extrem Surg*. 2005;9:149–152.

Kulthanan T, Chareonwat B. Variations in abductor pollicis longus and extensor pollicis brevis tendons in de Quervain syndrome: A surgical and anatomical study. *Scand J Plast Reconstr Surg Hand Surg*. 2007;41:36–38.

Witt J, Pess G, Gelberman RH. Treatment of de Quervain tenosynovitis. A prospective study of the results of injection of steroids and immobilization in a splint. *J Bone Joint Surg Am*. 1991;73:219–222.

Wolfe SW. Tenosynovitis. In: Green DP, Hotchkiss RN, Pederson WC, Wolfe SW, eds. *Operative Hand Surgery*. 5th ed. Philadelphia: Churchill Livingstone; 2005:2150–2154.

Chapter 77 Tendinitis of the Wrist

David Schnur

ICD-10-CM CODES
M65.841 *Synovitis and other tenosynovitis, right hand*
M65.842 *Synovitis and other tenosynovitis, left hand*
M65.849 *Synovitis and other tenosynovitis, unspecified hand*

Key Concepts

- Tenosynovitis of the wrist can affect the following tendons (Fig. 77.1):
  - Extensor pollicis longus (EPL)
  - Extensor carpi ulnaris (ECU)
  - Flexor carpi radialis (FCR)
  - Muscle bellies of the abductor pollicis longus and the extensor pollicis brevis (intersection syndrome)
  - Fourth extensor compartment (extensor digitorum communis and extensor indicis proprius)
  - Extensor digiti minimi
- Intersection syndrome describes pain and swelling about the muscle bellies of the abductor pollicis longus and the extensor pollicis brevis at the point in which they cross the radial wrist extensors (Fig. 77.2).
  - Anatomically located 4 cm proximal to the wrist on the dorsoradial aspect
  - Originally thought to occur as a result of friction between the muscle bellies of the abductor pollicis longus and extensor pollicis brevis tendons and the radial wrist extensors; now believed to be entrapment of the second dorsal compartment (extensor carpi radialis longus and extensor carpi radialis brevis)
- EPL tenosynovitis is rare and occurs on the dorsal wrist at the Lister tubercle (the location at which the EPL wraps around and heads for the thumb).
  - If undiagnosed, can lead to tendon rupture
  - Can occur with blunt trauma or fractures of the distal radius
- ECU tenosynovitis is a more common problem and occurs on the dorsoulnar aspect of the wrist.
  - Common cause of ulnar-side wrist pain
  - Can be initiated by a twisting injury of the wrist
  - Can cause dysesthesias along the distribution of the dorsal sensory branch of the ulnar nerve
  - Can cause pain at night
- FCR tendinitis can occur at the point where the tendon crosses the ridge of the trapezium on the volar radial aspect of the wrist.
  - Uncommon
  - Can lead to rupture of the FCR tendon
- Fourth extensor compartment tendinitis most commonly affects the tendons of the ECU to the small and index fingers because of the more acute angle that these tendons take from the compartment to their respective insertions.
  - Uncommon except in rheumatoid arthritis
  - Can occur after a distal radius fracture and has been associated with dorsal hardware on the dorsal distal radius
- Extensor digiti minimi tendinitis is uncommon, except in rheumatoid arthritis.

History

- Pain and swelling around the wrist
- Pain with certain motions and activities
- Most commonly worse with activity but can occur at night (especially ECU tendinitis)
- Prolonged pain after blunt trauma or distal radius fracture
- Crepitus with certain conditions may be reported.

Physical Examination

- Intersection syndrome
  - Can have swelling and even redness
  - Tenderness to palpation 4 cm proximal to the radial styloid (Fig. 77.3)
  - Pain with wrist extension and radial deviation
  - Occasionally palpable crepitus
- EPL
  - Pain with resisted thumb extension
  - Pain on palpation over Lister tubercle
  - Swelling at Lister tubercle
- ECU
  - Pain on palpation of tendon with resisted wrist extension and ulnar deviation
  - Can have palpable crepitus
- Flexor carpi ulnaris (FCU)
  - Can have swelling over volar wrist
  - Pain on palpation of tendon with resisted wrist flexion
- Fourth dorsal compartment and extensor digiti minimi
  - Swelling and pain on palpation over central dorsal wrist
  - Pain with resisted finger extension

Imaging

- Plain radiographs do not tend to be helpful in the diagnosis except in a rare case of calcific tendinitis.
- Magnetic resonance imaging can be used to confirm or assist with diagnosis and will show inflammation around the tendon.

Additional Tests

- Injection of a local anesthetic agent into the respective tendon sheath should give substantial or complete relief of symptoms and can be used for diagnostic purposes.

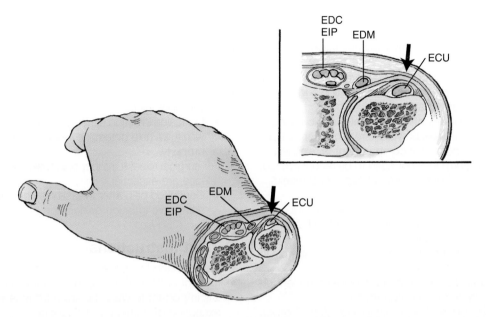

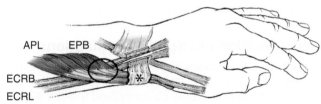

Fig 77.1 Location of the six dorsal compartments of the wrist. Note the contribution of the extensor carpi ulnaris *(ECU)* tendon sheath to the triangular fibrocartilage complex *(arrow)*. *EDC*, Extensor digitorum communis; *EDM*, extensor digiti minimi; *EIP*, extensor indicis proprius. (Modified with permission from Green DP, Hotchkiss RN, Pederson WC, Wolfe SW, eds. *Operative Hand Surgery*. 5th ed. Philadelphia: Churchill Livingstone, 2005:2151, Fig. 60.13.)

Fig 77.2 Location of the intersection syndrome where the extensor pollicis brevis *(EPB)* and the abductor pollicis longus *(APL)* cross the radial wrist extensors *(circled area)*. The second dorsal compartment has been released in the manner recommended for the treatment of intersection syndrome. *ECRB*, Extensor carpi radialis brevis; *ECRL*, extensor carpi radialis longus. (Modified with permission from Green DP, Hotchkiss RN, Pederson WC, Wolfe SW, eds. *Operative Hand Surgery*. 5th ed. Philadelphia: Churchill Livingstone, 2005:2155, Fig. 60.19.)

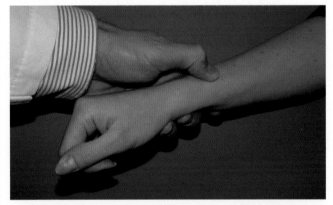

Fig 77.3 Location of pain in patient with intersection syndrome. The extensor pollicis brevis and the abductor pollicis longus cross the radial wrist extensors approximately 4 cm proximal to the radial styloid.

Differential Diagnosis

- Most other causes of wrist pain are included in the differential diagnosis for tendinitis.
- ECU tendinitis is typically the most difficult diagnosis of the different types of tendinitis.
  - Symptoms may mimic those from both triangular fibrocartilage complex pathology as well as distal radioulnar joint pathology.
- FCR tendinitis can be difficult to diagnose also because its symptoms can mimic those of basal joint arthritis, scaphoid fractures and nonunions, and volar ganglion cysts.

Treatment

- At diagnosis
  - First-line therapies for the stenotic conditions of the wrist are modification of activity, nonsteroidal antiinflammatory drugs, and splinting.
  - Immobilization is best accomplished with a well-formed thermoplastic splint with the wrist in approximately 20 degrees of extension.
  - Steroid injection into the tendon sheath can be considered as first-line therapy with immobilization, or in cases in which immobilization alone has failed.

- Later
  - Surgical release of the affected tendon should be performed if nonoperative therapy has failed.
  - Intersection syndrome
    - A longitudinal incision is made over the radial wrist extensors from the level of their insertion and carried proximally approximately 4 cm.
    - The muscle bellies of the abductor pollicis longus and extensor pollicis brevis are retracted proximally, and the second dorsal compartment is released.
    - The retinaculum does not need to be reconstructed, and the wrist should be immobilized for 2 weeks.
  - EPL tendinitis
    - A longitudinal incision is made over the Lister tubercle.
    - The third dorsal compartment is identified, and the EPL tendon is completely released.
    - It is translocated to the radial side of the tubercle in a subcutaneous plane.
    - The compartment is reclosed to prevent the tendon from re-entering the compartment.
    - After a short period of immobilization (5 to 7 days), unrestricted activity is allowed.
  - Fourth and fifth compartment tendinitis (extensor digitorum communis, extensor indicis proprius, extensor digiti minimi)
    - The need for surgical release of these compartments is very rare.
  - ECU tendinitis
    - A longitudinal incision is made over the ECU tendon.
    - Care is taken to preserve and protect the dorsal sensory branches of the ulnar nerve.
    - The entire fibro-osseous canal is released.
    - Surgical reconstruction of the canal is not necessary.
  - FCR tendinitis
    - A longitudinal incision is made over the FCR tendon volarly.
    - Care is taken to protect the palmar cutaneous branch of the median nerve.
    - The sheath of the tendon is released past the level of the trapezial tubercle.
    - Any osteophytes on the trapezium should be removed, and any frayed portion of the tendon should be debrided.

When to Refer

- The patient should be referred to a hand specialist if conservative measures have not brought about improvement in 4 to 6 weeks.
- Many of the steroid injections for these conditions are difficult and should be performed only by those with previous experience or by a hand surgeon.

Prognosis

- Good with conservative measures and excellent with operative intervention

Troubleshooting

- With splint immobilization, patients need to wear a splint continually.
  - Try to assess and ensure patient compliance.
- Steroid injections most commonly are not effective because of improper injection location.
  - Lidocaine injection either preceding the steroid or mixed with it will help determine whether the injection is located properly.
- For surgical release, proper diagnosis and adequate tendon release are essential.
  - Continued pain after release may be caused by cutaneous nerve irritation or damage.

Patient Instructions

- Patients need to be educated on the disease process.
- Instruct patients that if splint immobilization is prescribed, it is important to wear the splint full time with the possible exception of bathing and sleeping.
- If a nonsteroidal antiinflammatory drug is prescribed, the patient should take it regularly for the period prescribed and not only as needed for pain.
- If a steroid injection is used, instruct patients that pain may increase for 24 to 48 hours and that the effect of the steroid will not be experienced for 5 to 7 days.
- Have patients return in 2 weeks if there is no pain relief.
- When surgery is recommended, patients should be educated on the risks and benefits of the procedure.

Considerations in Special Populations

- Patients with diabetes should be instructed to monitor their blood sugar level after a steroid injection.
- A steroid injection should be considered first-line therapy in patients who cannot tolerate immobilization.

Suggested Readings

Brown J, Helms CA. Intersection syndrome of the forearm. *Arthritis Rheum*. 2006;54:2038.

Costa CR, Morrison WB, Carrino JA. MRI features of intersection syndrome of the forearm. *AJR Am J Roentgenol*. 2003;181:1245–1249.

Grundberg AB, Reagan DS. Pathologic anatomy of the forearm: intersection syndrome. *J Hand Surg Am*. 1985;10:299–302.

Ostric SA, Martin WJ, Derman GH. Intersecting the intersection: a reliable incision for the treatment of de Quervain's and second dorsal compartment tenosynovitis. *Plast Reconstr Surg*. 2007;119:2341–2342.

Wolfe SW. Tenosynovitis. In: Green DP, Hotchkiss RN, Pederson WC, Wolfe SW, eds. *Operative Hand Surgery*. 5th ed. Philadelphia: Churchill Livingstone; 2005:2137–2158.

Chapter 78 Ganglion Cysts

David Schnur, Jerrod Keith

ICD-10-CM CODES
M67.431 *Ganglion, right wrist*
M67.432 *Ganglion, left wrist*

Key Concepts

- Most common soft-tissue masses of the hand and wrist, accounting for 50-70%
- Most prevalent in women and in second through fourth decades of life
- Not true cysts because they lack an epithelial lining and etiology is not well defined.
- Mucin-filled cyst; communicates through a stalk to the adjacent joint capsule, tendon, or tendon sheath
- Aspiration and injection can be curative, but surgical resection reduces the rate of recurrence.
- Dorsal wrist ganglion cysts (60-70%)
  - Usually over the dorsal radial aspect of the wrist, between the third and fourth extensor compartments (Fig. 78.1)
  - Arise from the dorsal scapholunate ligament
- Volar wrist ganglion cysts (18-20%)
  - Usually occur under the volar wrist crease, just radial to the flexor carpi radialis tendon; these can be quite extensive (Fig. 78.2).
  - Two-thirds arise from the radiocarpal joint and one-third from the scaphotrapezial joint.
- Volar retinacular cysts (10-12%)
  - Arise from the palmar digital sheath in the region of the A1 and A2 pulleys
- Other ganglions
  - Degenerative mucous cysts in the dorsal distal interphalangeal joint of elderly patients
  - Proximal interphalangeal joint
  - Extensor tendons
  - Over first dorsal compartment with de Quervain disease

History

- Can occur suddenly or develop over several months
- Pain, weakness, and poor cosmetic appearance are the most common reasons for presentation.
- At least 10% of patients report antecedent traumatic events.
- Repetitive minor trauma believed to be a factor in development.
- Often enlarge with increased activity and subside with rest

Physical Examination

- Thorough examination of the hand and wrist, including provocative maneuvers to rule out carpal instability
- Firm or rubbery, mobile, 1 to 3 cm in size, often nontender
- Smaller cysts may be more painful because they compress the posterior interosseous nerve during emergence through the fourth extensor compartment.
- Carpal tunnel symptoms
  - Compression of the median nerve due to ganglions from the volar carpus within the carpal canal
- Ulnar nerve palsy
  - Compression in Guyon canal due to ganglions from joints around the hamate
- Longitudinal grooving of the nail may be an early indication of a mucous cyst.
- Heberden's nodes and osteoarthritic changes of the distal interphalangeal joint are often associated with mucous cysts.
- Ganglion cysts remain stationary with flexion and extension, whereas proliferative tenosynovitis does not.
- May transilluminate

Imaging

- Begin with plain radiographs if there is suspicion of an underlying bony abnormality
  - Intraosseous ganglion cysts appear as radiolucent lesions with well-defined sclerotic borders.
- Ultrasonography and magnetic resonance imaging can be used to diagnose occult ganglion cysts.
  - Ultrasonography shows a well-defined anechoic structure close to a joint with posterior acoustic enhancement.
  - Magnetic resonance imaging shows a homogeneous signal with well-defined margins, which is hyperintense on T2-weighted sequences.

Additional Tests

- Physical examination is usually sufficient.
- Aspiration can be diagnostic and therapeutic.
  - Contents are highly viscous, clear, sticky, jelly-like mucin composed of glucosamine, albumin, globulin, and high concentrations of hyaluronic acid.

Differential Diagnosis

- Dorsal wrist ganglions
  - Giant cell tumor of the tendon sheath, lipoma, a true synovial cyst, tenosynovitis of the extensor tendons, anomalous muscles
- Volar wrist ganglions
  - Similar to dorsal, except anomalous muscles are rare in this area
- Volar retinacular cysts
  - Giant cell tumor of the tendon sheath, epidermoid inclusion cysts, foreign body granuloma, fibroma, lipoma, neurilemoma

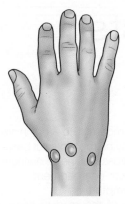

Fig 78.1 Common locations of dorsal wrist ganglion cysts.

Dorsal wrist ganglions
(3 locations)

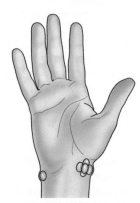

Volar wrist ganglions
(2 locations)

Fig 78.2 Typical locations of volar wrist ganglions.

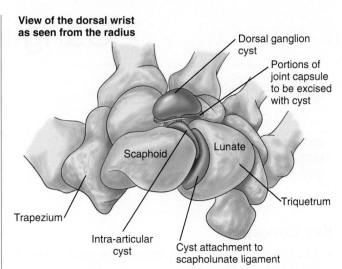

View of the dorsal wrist
as seen from the radius

Fig 78.3 Representation of a ganglion cyst with its pedicle attachment to the scapholunate ligament.

Labels: Dorsal ganglion cyst; Portions of joint capsule to be excised with cyst; Scaphoid; Lunate; Triquetrum; Trapezium; Intra-articular cyst; Cyst attachment to scapholunate ligament

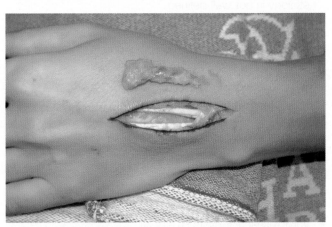

Fig 78.4 Intraoperative view of excised dorsal ganglion cyst and stalk.

- In general, the differential diagnosis includes solid tumors and proliferative tenosynovitis.

Treatment

- Indications for treatment include pain, weakness, and disfigurement.
- Initial conservative management includes supportive splinting, nonsteroidal antiinflammatory drugs, and aspiration, with or without injection.
  - Injections of steroids or hyaluronidase are often performed.
  - Injection of sclerosing agents is not recommended.
  - At least temporary resolution in as many as 80% of patients with dorsal wrist ganglion cyst aspiration; high rate of recurrence
  - Recurrence rates of volar wrist ganglions after aspiration are much higher.
- Surgical excision should be offered for patients in whom nonoperative treatment fails or who remain symptomatic. Avoid cyst rupture and include the entire stalk.
- Dorsal wrist ganglion excision
  - Transverse incision over the cyst
  - The stalk typically arises from the dorsal aspect of the scapholunate ligament, and the cyst is excised at the base of the stalk along with a portion of the joint capsule (Figs. 78.3 and 78.4).
- Dorsal wrist ganglion can be treated arthroscopically by stalk excision at its origin along the level of the dorsal scapholunate ligament.
- Volar wrist ganglion excision
  - A longitudinal incision curving around the radial aspect of the cyst allows for extension if needed.
  - Often located between the first extensor compartment tendons and the flexor carpi radialis sheath
  - The radial artery is usually intimately involved, and a small portion of the cyst may be left behind.
- Volar retinacular cyst
  - Good success with aspiration and injection; surgery is recommended only after several attempts at conservative management have failed.
  - A small window of tendon sheath is excised along with the cyst.
- Degenerative mucous cysts
  - Surgical excision for pain, open wound, or draining

Troubleshooting

- Complete excision of the cyst and stalk at the base reduces the recurrence rate.
- Surgical dissection should be done under magnification to avoid small arterial or nerve branches, as well as to identify the cyst stalk and ligamentous attachments.
- Aspiration of volar wrist ganglions is not often recommended due to the close proximity of the radial artery.
- Allen test should be performed prior to excision of volar wrist ganglion due to potential radial artery injury.
- Do not close the joint capsule after cyst excision, as it can result in joint stiffness.
- Occult wrist ganglions can be a cause of unexplained wrist pain, and excision is often curative.

Patient Instructions

- Reassure patients that this is not a malignant condition.
- If patients are asymptomatic, treatment can be delayed because the cyst may spontaneously regress.
- Postoperatively the wrist is immobilized in a splint for 7 to 10 days, after which the splint is removed, and the patient should begin wrist motion. Early finger motion is encouraged.

Considerations in Special Populations

- Degenerative mucous cysts usually occur between the fifth and seventh decades of life.

Suggested Readings

Angelides AC. Ganglions of the hand and wrist. In: Green DP, Hotchkiss RN, Pederson WC, Wolfe SW, eds. *Green's Operative Hand Surgery*. 5th ed. Philadelphia: Churchill Livingstone; 2005.

Minotti P, Taras J. Ganglion cysts of the wrist. *J Am Soc Surg Hand*. 2002; 2:102–107.

Nahra M, Bucchieri J. Ganglion cysts and other tumor related conditions of the hand and wrist. *Hand Clin*. 2004;20:249–260.

Nguyen V, Choi J, Davis K. Imaging of wrist masses. *Curr Probl Diagn Radiol*. 2004;33:147–160.

Young L, Bartell T, Logan S. Ganglions of the hand and wrist. *South Med J*. 1988;81:751–760.

Chapter 79 Carpal Tunnel Syndrome

David Schnur

ICD-10-CM CODES
G56.00 *Carpal tunnel syndrome, unspecified upper limb*
G56.01 *Carpal tunnel syndrome, right upper limb*
G56.02 *Carpal tunnel syndrome, left upper limb*

Key Concepts

- Group of symptoms associated with compression of the median nerve as it passes through the carpal canal
- Most common compression neuropathy of the upper extremity, present in approximately 4% of adults
- Clinical diagnosis but can be further confirmed with electrodiagnostic testing, although no more sensitive or specific than clinical diagnosis
- Imaging studies may be of benefit, including ultrasound or MRI.
- The volar surface of the carpal canal is the flexor retinaculum, which attaches to the hamate and triquetrum on the ulnar side and the scaphoid and trapezium on the radial side.
- The carpal bones account for the dorsal confines of the canal.
- The median nerve travels through the carpal canal. It gives off the recurrent motor branch at the distal end of the flexor retinaculum. It then divides into the digital nerves and gives sensation to the thumb and index finger and the long and radial sides of the ring finger (Fig. 79.1).
- There may be anatomic variations at the level of the takeoff of the motor branch, as well as which fingers are innervated by the nerve.
- Intrinsic muscles innervated by the median nerve include the abductor pollicis brevis muscle, superficial head of the flexor pollicis muscle, opponens pollicis muscle, and lumbrical muscles of the index and long fingers.

History

- Paresthesia in the thumb and index and long fingers and radial aspect of the ring finger
- Pain, typically in the same distribution or in the thenar eminence
- Symptoms often worse at night
- Symptoms may be exacerbated with repetitive motion
- May report weakness and dropping objects

Physical Examination (Video 79.1)

- Direct compression test (Durkan test)
  - The thumb is used to place compression over the median nerve at or just distal to the distal wrist crease for 60 seconds.
  - Paresthesia or replication of symptoms in the median nerve distribution indicates a positive test result.
- Tinel sign
  - Firm percussion over the median nerve at the level of the carpal canal causing electric shock sensation in the thumb or index, long, or ring finger is considered a positive result.
- Phalen maneuver
  - Wrist flexed maximally for at least 60 seconds
  - Paresthesia or replication of symptoms indicates a positive result
- Scratch Collapse Test
  - With the elbows bent at 90 degrees and the wrists neutral, medial pressure is placed on the dorsum or outside of the hands as a baseline. The patient should be able to resist.
  - Using a fingernail, a gentle scratch is performed over the median nerve at the carpal canal and the test is repeated
  - If the patient is unable to resist the medial pressure, the test is positive
- Two-point discrimination
  - 5 mm considered normal
- Visual inspection for atrophy of the thenar eminence (Fig. 79.2)
- Strength testing for opposition of the thumb, key pinch, and grip strength

Imaging

Ultrasound may be useful in the diagnosis. In patients with carpal tunnel syndrome (CTS) the nerve may be hypoechoic and the cross-sectional area may be greater than 10 mm². MRI can be used if the diagnosis is in question but is expensive and typically not necessary.

Additional Tests

- Electrodiagnostic studies
  - Electromyography
  - Evaluates either spontaneous or volitional electrical activity in the muscle
  - Fibrillation potentials at rest are the earliest signs of muscle denervation.
  - Nerve conduction velocity studies
  - Can be used to study motor and sensory portions of the nerve
  - Median motor distal latency considered abnormal if more than 4.5 ms
  - Sensory latencies wrist to digit II more than 3.5 ms or palm to wrist more than 2.2 ms
  - Also compare median and ulnar sensory latencies, with a difference of more than 0.5 ms abnormal with wrist

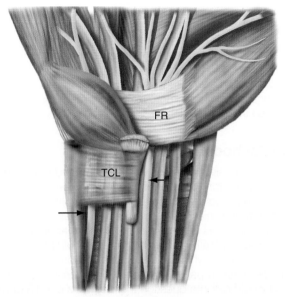

Fig 79.1 Anatomy of the carpal canal. The median nerve gives off the palmar cutaneous branch before entering the canal *(short arrow)*. The median nerve then travels through the canal and gives off the motor branch. The *long arrow* indicates the ulnar nerve as it enters the Guyon canal. *FR,* Flexor retinaculum; *TCL,* transverse carpal ligament. (From Ma C, Beltran LS, Bencardino JT, Beltran J: Compressive and entrapment neuropathies of the upper extremities. In Pope TL, Bloem HL, Beltran J, et al (eds). *Musculoskeletal Imaging*, 2nd ed. Philadelphia, Elsevier; 2015.)

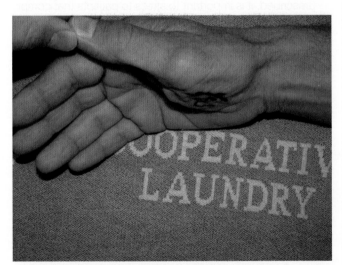

Fig 79.2 Severe atrophy of the thenar musculature.

to digit II and a difference of more than 0.3 ms in the palm to wrist
- Sensitivity and specificity are not necessarily greater than physical exam

Differential Diagnosis (Table 79.1)

- Median nerve compressions at higher levels can mimic CTS symptoms or can coexist as a double crush.

TABLE 79.1 Differential Diagnosis

Differential Diagnosis	Differentiating Feature(s)
Proximal median nerve compression	Resisted pronation test replicates symptoms, provocative tests over carpal tunnel negative with pure pronator syndrome
Ulnar nerve compression	Symptoms on ulnar side of the hand, Tinel sign, and direct compression over cubital tunnel positive

- Compression points of the median nerve proximal to the wrist should always be evaluated when examining patients suspected of having CTS.
- Ulnar nerve compression at the cubital tunnel or through Guyon canal should be evaluated because it can coexist with or mimic CTS.

Treatment

- At diagnosis
  - First-line treatment of mild to moderate CTS is splinting, oral nonsteroidal antiinflammatory drugs, and corticosteroid injection.
  - For splinting, the wrist should be placed in a neutral position (most over-the-counter splints put the wrist in 30 degrees of extension, which can increase pressure in the carpal canal). Because of the nonfunctional position of the wrist in a neutral position, most patients will not tolerate the splint during normal daily activities; therefore nighttime splinting should be recommended.
  - Nonsteroidal antiinflammatory drug use has variable effects on CTS but can be tried as a first-line therapy.
  - Corticosteroid injection should be considered once the diagnosis of CTS is made. Corticosteroid injection is useful as both a diagnostic tool and a therapeutic modality. Relief from carpal tunnel injection has also been proven to be a good prognostic indicator of relief after surgical intervention. In addition, approximately 30% of patients may get long-term therapeutic results from the injection and not need further treatment. For specifics on steroid injection of the carpal canal, refer to Chapter 102.
- Later
  - Surgical release of the carpal tunnel should be considered if conservative measures have failed or there is severe disease with significant and worsening of numbness of the fingers rather than just paresthesias.
  - To release the carpal tunnel, an incision is made in the proximal palm along the radial border of the fourth ray under tourniquet control or with local anesthesia with epinephrine (Fig. 79.3).
  - The dissection is performed through the flexor retinaculum to the carpal canal.
  - The distal end of the retinaculum is identified and divided distally to proximally, taking care to protect the median nerve (Fig. 79.4).
  - Dissection is performed in the forearm, and the antebrachial fascia is divided.

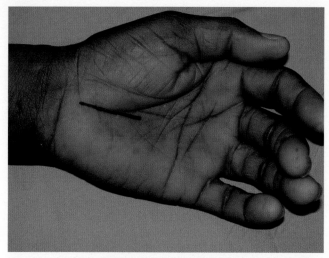

Fig 79.3 Incision placement for release of the carpal tunnel in line with the radial side of the fourth ray.

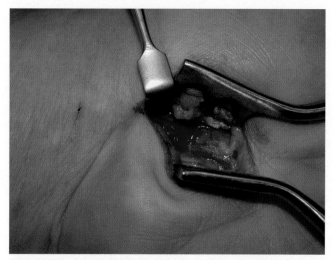

Fig 79.4 The median nerve is seen in the carpal canal. This nerve has significant hyperemia, which is indicative of long-standing compression.

- The tourniquet (if used) is released, hemostasis is obtained, and the incision is closed at the level of the skin. The tourniquet may also be released after closure.
- Release of the flexor retinaculum can also be done using endoscopic techniques.

When to Refer

- Referral is dependent on the comfort of the practitioner treating CTS.
- After 1 to 3 months with no improvement of symptoms, splinting and nonsteroidal antiinflammatory drugs should be augmented with steroid injection or surgery should be considered. At this time, the patient should be referred to a hand specialist. Some hand surgeons appreciate when patients are referred after electrodiagnostic testing, whereas others believe that these tests are not indicated until after failure of carpal tunnel injections or not at all. In addition, patients should be referred if they have a decrease in two-point discrimination or any thenar atrophy.

Prognosis

- The prognosis is excellent.
- Many patients will respond at least temporarily to first-line treatment of CTS.
- Those patients who require surgery will have an excellent chance of significant improvement of symptoms if they are treated in a timely fashion.

Troubleshooting

- If a patient fails treatment with splinting and nonsteroidal antiinflammatory drugs, compliance may be an issue.
- With failure to decrease or eliminate symptoms after carpal tunnel injection, it is important to assess whether the injection was properly placed. With the addition of local anesthetic to the injection, the patient should be instructed to take note of which, if any, fingers become numb.
- No decrease in pain after surgical intervention is unusual and would call into question the diagnosis of CTS or may indicate that there is another location of compression (double crush).
- Long-standing paresthesia in the fingers may not be improved with surgery, and this should be explained to patients before intervention.

Patient Instructions

- After a diagnosis is made, patients should be educated on the disease process.
- If splinting and nonsteroidal antiinflammatory drugs are prescribed, it is important to stress to patients that compliance is paramount to improvement.
- With steroid injection, patients are instructed to take note of which, if any, fingers become numb. Patients should also be instructed that symptoms will not improve for 5 to 7 days and that they may increase for 24 to 48 hours.
- Surgical patients should be instructed on the risks of surgery, especially the possibility of permanent nerve damage (a rare complication). They should also be instructed that pain in the palm (pillar pain) can last many months and that in rare cases this pain may be permanent.

Considerations in Special Populations

- When performing steroid injection on diabetic patients, instruct them to monitor and treat elevated blood sugars.
- Pregnant patients have a higher incidence of CTS. These patients can be treated with splinting and a steroid injection. Surgery should only be considered in extreme cases. Although these patients often improve after delivery, those who have significant symptoms should be considered for surgical decompression if further pregnancies are likely.
- Patients with significant loss of two-point discrimination or thenar atrophy and no pain should be considered for surgery to halt progression of their symptoms, although improvement may not be expected.
- Pediatric patients with CTS should have a work-up for other pathologic conditions that may cause secondary compression of the median nerve. The diagnosis of lipofibromatous

hamartoma of the median nerve should also be entertained. The work-up for these patients should include magnetic resonance imaging.

- People who work with frozen foods have a higher incidence of CTS.

Suggested Readings

Bland JD. Carpal tunnel syndrome. *BMJ*. 2007;335:343–346.

Braun RM, Rechnic M, Fowler E. Complications related to carpal tunnel release. *Hand Clin*. 2002;18:347–357.

Cranford CS, Ho JY, Kalainov DM, Hartigan BJ. Carpal tunnel syndrome. *J Am Acad Orthop Surg*. 2007;15:537–548.

Gannon C, Muffly M, Rubright RT, Baratz ME. Aberrant nerve in limited open carpal tunnel release. *J Hand Surg Am*. 2006;31:1407–1408.

Green DP. Diagnostic and therapeutic value of carpal tunnel injection. *J Hand Surg Am*. 1984;9:850–854.

Hermiz SJ, Kalliainen LK. Evidence-based medicine: current evidence in the diagnosis and management of carpal tunnel syndrome. *Plast Reconstr Surg*. 2017;140:120e–129e.

Mackinnon SE, Novak CB. Compression neuropathy. In: Green D, Hotchkiss R, Pederson W, Wolfe S, eds. *Operative Hand Surgery*. Vol. 1. 5th ed. Philadelphia: Churchill Livingstone; 2005:999–1046.

Thoma A, Veltri K, Haines T, Duku E. A systematic review of reviews comparing the effectiveness of endoscopic and open carpal tunnel decompression. *Plast Reconstr Surg*. 2004;113:1184–1191.

Chapter 80 Thumb Basal Joint Arthritis

David Schnur

ICD-10-CM CODES
M18.10 *Unilateral primary osteoarthritis of first carpometacarpal joint, unspecified hand*
M18.11 *Unilateral primary osteoarthritis of first carpometacarpal joint, right hand*
M18.12 *Unilateral primary osteoarthritis of first carpometacarpal joint, left hand*
M18.0 *Bilateral primary osteoarthritis of first carpometacarpal joints*

Key Concepts

- Type of osteoarthritis that most commonly affects the trapeziometacarpal (TM) joint of the thumb but can affect all five articulations of the thumb basal joint
- The TM joint is a biconcave saddle joint with minimal bony constraints.
- Ligamentous stability is very important for the TM joint.
- The anterior oblique ligament or "beak" ligament is a primary stabilizer of the TM joint, but recent studies suggest that the dorsoradial ligament may be more important.
- Degeneration and weakening of these ligaments result in laxity of the TM joint, which, in turn, results in abnormal translation of the metacarpal on the trapezium, which leads to excessive shear forces on the joint.
- Women have a greater predilection for the disease, with a female-to-male ratio of 10:1.
- Commonly presents in fifth and sixth decades of life
- Because of adduction of the thumb, there may be compensatory hyperextension of the metacarpophalangeal joint and laxity of the volar plate.
- Left TM joint often exhibits symptoms related to osteoarthritis first possibly because stronger thenar muscles in right handed individuals may have a protective effect on the basilar joint.

History

- Pain at the base of the thumb, particularly during pinch and grasp
- Difficulty turning keys in doors or other pinch and twist motions
- Pain and weakness with opening jars
- Occasionally pain that is not well localized and pain in entire thumb reported
- May report the appearance of the thumb "zigzag"

Physical Examination

- Observation of the thumb may reveal prominence of the base of the thumb metacarpal.
- Hyperextension of the metacarpophalangeal (MP) joint may be visible with motion or pinch.
- Tenderness at TM joint on palpation
- Grind test
  - Axial load on the thumb combined with circumduction elicits pain and often crepitance in the joint.
  - It is very sensitive (97%) but not very specific (30%).
- Traction-shift test
  - The metacarpal is passively subluxed and then relocated, causing pain.
  - This test is very specific.

Imaging

- Plain radiographs should be adequate to confirm the diagnosis (Fig. 80.1).
- Radiographic staging according to Eaton and Littler
  - Stage 1: normal joint with possible widening
  - Stage 2: joint space narrowing with debris and osteophytes less than 2 mm
  - Stage 3: joint space narrowing with debris and osteophytes greater than 2 mm
  - Stage 4: scaphotrapezial joint space narrowing in addition to TM joint involvement
  - Stage 5: pantrapezial arthritis
- Bone scan may be useful if diagnosis is in question (Fig. 80.2).

Additional Tests

- A local anesthetic agent can be injected into the TM joint and should alleviate most of the pain (Fig. 80.3).

Differential Diagnosis

- Please see Table 80.1.

Treatment

- At diagnosis
  - First-line treatment for this disease involves nonsteroidal antiinflammatory drugs, topical diclophenac gel, intra-articular steroid injections (see Chapter 103), thenar

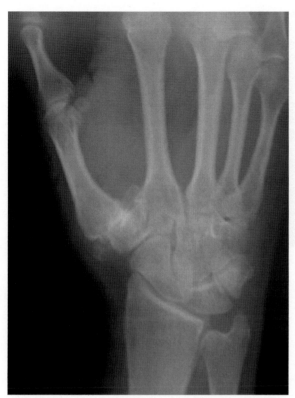

Fig 80.1 Radiographic appearance of basal joint arthritis. Note the narrowing of the joint space and osteophyte formation.

TABLE 80.1 Differential Diagnosis

Differential Diagnosis	Differentiating Feature	Chapter Reference
de Quervain tenosynovitis	Pain and tenderness more proximal; positive Finkelstein test	76
Carpal tunnel syndrome	Often associated with numbness of the fingers; not acutely exacerbated with specific activities	79
Trigger thumb	Pain over A1 pulley and often associated with triggering	81
MCP joint osteoarthritis	Pain at MCP joint and tenderness on palpation of MCP joint; radiographs with arthritic changes at MCP joint	—
Sesamoiditis and subsesamoid arthritis	Pain typically volar over MCP joint	—

MCP, Metacarpophalangeal.

cone strengthening therapy, and immobilization with a thumb spica or neoprene splint.
- These treatments, although not curative, may improve symptoms and delay the need for operative intervention.
- These therapies may be tried sequentially or may be done in combination.
- Later
  - Once patients have failed nonoperative treatment, surgery should be considered.
  - Many surgical procedures have been described for this disease process, which include TM arthrodesis, trapezium excision with or without ligament reconstruction and tendon interposition (LRTI) arthroplasty, implant arthroplasty, and arthroplasty with the Arthrex TightRope.
  - TM arthrodesis is indicated when the arthropathy is limited to the TM joint and the patient has a high-demand hand (i.e., laborer).
  - This procedure trades motion for retention of power and strength and long-term durability.
  - Soft-tissue arthroplasties have gained increasing popularity, and of these procedures the LRTI described by Burton and Pellegrini is probably the most common surgery performed.
  - This involves excision of the trapezium followed by harvest of the flexor carpi radialis tendon (Fig. 80.4).
  - The tendon is used to reconstruct the beak ligament and then formed into an "anchovy" and used as a soft-tissue spacer between the base of the metacarpal and the scaphoid (Figs. 80.5 and 80.6).

- Examination of the scaphotrapezoid joint is essential, and if arthritis is present at this location, it must be addressed simultaneously.
- Simple trapeziectomy has also gained more favor recently and has been shown to be as beneficial as the LRTI, with fewer complications.

When to Refer

- Referral to a hand specialist for this condition, like many conditions in the hand, depends on the practitioner's comfort with diagnosing TM arthritis and executing nonoperative therapy.
- Certainly once the nonoperative therapies have been instituted and the patient still has significant functional impairment from the disease, the patient should be referred to the hand surgeon for consideration for surgical treatment.

Prognosis

- TM arthritis is a progressive disease and only definitively treated with surgery.
- Nonoperative modalities often alleviate symptoms but only temporarily.
- The prognosis for pain relief and good function is very good after surgical treatment. Approximately 80% of patients have significant improvement in pain and retain good functional range of motion.

Troubleshooting

- The degree of arthritis on radiographs and the severity of symptoms may not correlate.

313

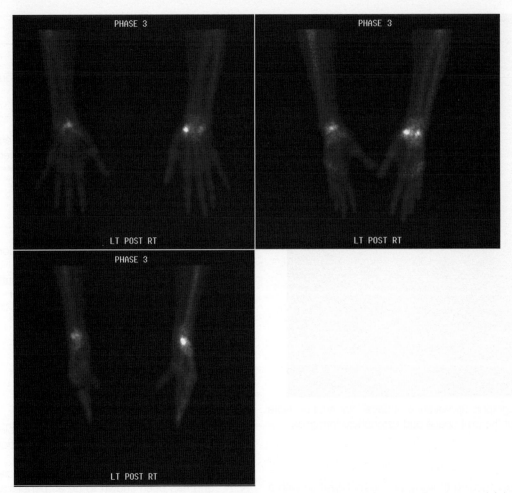

Fig 80.2 Bone scan of patient with basal joint arthritis. Note increased uptake of the trapeziometacarpal joint on phase 3. *LT,* Left; *RT,* right.

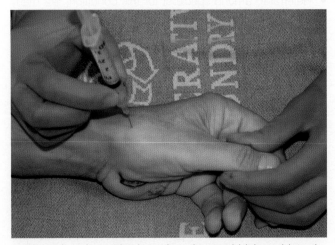

Fig 80.3 Local anesthesia and corticosteroid injected into the trapeziometacarpal joint can help to diagnose basal joint arthritis and give relief of symptoms.

- Patients with little change on radiographs may have significant symptoms, and, conversely, patients with severe disease radiographically may have surprisingly mild symptoms.
- Patients who do not respond to nonsteroidal antiinflammatory drugs, splinting, and therapy should have a corticosteroid injection in the TM joint, if indicated.
- No response or partial response to the steroid injection may indicate scaphotrapezoid trapezium or pantrapezial involvement.
- Continued pain after surgical treatment may indicate unrecognized scaphotrapezoid joint involvement.

Patient Instructions

- Patients should be instructed about the progressive nature of the process once the diagnosis is made.
- Hand therapists are often an excellent source for patient information and instruction; this is one of the reasons that referral to the therapist for splinting and thenar cone strengthening is helpful.
- For patients undergoing surgery, the entire postoperative course needs to be explained to the patient.

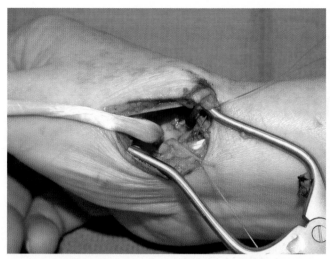

Fig 80.4 Intraoperative appearance after the trapezium has been excised and the flexor carpi radialis tendon has been harvested and kept attached to the base of the index metacarpal.

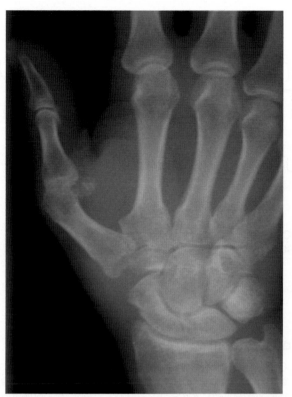

Fig 80.6 Radiographic appearance of the clear space with the flexor carpi radialis "anchovy" between the scaphoid and the base of the thumb metacarpal.

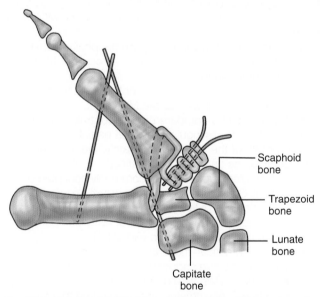

Scaphoid bone

Trapezoid bone

Lunate bone

Capitate bone

Fig 80.5 Drawing of the ligament reconstruction and tendon interposition once the flexor carpi radialis tendon has been made into an "anchovy" and inserted into the space where the trapezium was before resection. (Modified with permission from Green DP, Hotchkiss RN, Pederson WC, et al., eds. *Operative Hand Surgery*. 5th ed. Philadelphia: Churchill Livingstone; 2005.)

Considerations in Special Populations

- Young patients with high-demand hands should be considered for TM arthrodesis.
- Patients undergoing surgical treatment who have developed more than 30 degrees of hyperextension of the MP joint should have either a capsulodesis or an arthrodesis of this joint.
- Patients with concomitant carpal tunnel syndrome should have carpal tunnel release if the basilar joint arthritis is treated surgically.

Suggested Readings

Baker RH, Al-Shukri J, David TR. Evidence based medicine: thumb basal joint arthritis. *Plast Recontr Surg*. 2017;139:256e–266e.

Burton R, Pellegrini VD. Surgical management of basal joint arthritis of the thumb: part II. Ligament reconstruction with tendon interposition arthroplasty. *J Hand Surg Am*. 1986;11:325–332.

Damen A, van der Lei B, Robinson PH. Carpometacarpal arthritis of the thumb. *J Hand Surg Am*. 1996;21:807–812.

Luria S, Waitayawinya T, Nemechek N, et al. Biomechanical analysis of trapeziectomy, ligament reconstruction with tendon interposition, and tie-in trapezium implant arthroplasty for thumb carpometacarpal arthritis: A cadaver study. *J Hand Surg Am*. 2007;32:697–706.

Tomaino MM, King J, Leit M. Thumb basal joint arthritis. In: Green DP, Hotchkiss RN, Pederson WC, Wolfe SW, eds. *Operative Hand Surgery*. 5th ed. Philadelphia: Churchill Livingstone; 2005:461–485.

- In addition, it needs to be stressed to patients undergoing surgery that complete pain relief may not be accomplished until 3 to 6 months postoperatively.
- It also needs to be explained that patients will have some loss of strength compared with the precondition strength.
- Patients typically have loss of strength with basilar joint arthritis and are grateful for the return of power after surgery.

Chapter 81 Ulnar Collateral Ligament Injuries of the Thumb (Gamekeeper's Thumb, Skier's Thumb)

Jeffrey D. Boatright

ICD-10-CM CODE
S63.649A *Rupture of ulnar collateral ligament (UCL) of thumb*

Key Concepts

- Common acute injury among ball-sport athletes, cyclists, and skiers resulting from an acute radially directed and hyperextension force to thumb metacarpophalangeal (MCP) joint
  - Acute injury is commonly referred to as skier's thumb.
- Instability can also be chronic, typically resulting from inadequate treatment of an acute tear or treatment of an unrecognized Stener lesion (see the following).
  - Chronic injury is commonly referred to as gamekeeper's thumb.
  - Stener lesion: Interposition of the adductor aponeurosis between the torn UCL and the thumb proximal phalanx base at the time of a complete tear. This will prevent adequate healing with closed management.
- May be associated with a fracture, most commonly an avulsion fracture at the base of the proximal phalanx
- The thumb UCL has two components:
  - Proper UCL is a more dorsal structure and is tightest in flexion.
  - Accessory UCL is a more volar structure and is tightest in extension.

History

- Acute injury
  - Typically results from a fall on an outstretched hand with the thumb abducted, causing a sudden radially directed force to the thumb MCP joint and injury to the ulnar collateral ligament (Fig. 81.1).
  - Patients will present with a painful, swollen thumb MCP joint, particularly along the ulnar side.
- Chronic injury
  - Attenuation over time due to occupational use (classic gamekeeper's thumb) is less common.
  - Presentation more than 6 weeks after injury
  - Patients present with pain, swelling, weakness, and instability, particularly with activities requiring pinch.

Physical Examination

- Swelling, ecchymosis, and localized tenderness to the ulnar aspect of the MCP joint
- May be able to diagnose a Stener lesion by palpation of a mass just proximal to the MCP joint.
  - This physical exam finding has a low sensitivity, but a Stener lesion is likely if present.
- The key physical exam maneuver is determining the degree of instability to a radially directed stress at the MCP joint.
- The examiner stabilizes the thumb metacarpal shaft with one hand while grasping the proximal phalanx shaft and exerting a radially directed stress across the MCP joint with the other hand.
  - This should be performed in both full extension and in 30 degrees of flexion at the MCP joint.
  - This should be compared to the contralateral thumb.
  - Important to distinguish between partial and complete ruptures of the UCL. Unfortunately, there is significant controversy on how this is defined.
    - Complete rupture (most commonly accepted definition): Greater than 30 degrees of laxity in full extension, 40 degrees of laxity in 30 degrees of flexion, as well as greater than 15 degrees of laxity compared with the contralateral thumb (Fig. 81.2)
  - A more practical measure may be the presence or absence of a firm endpoint with radially directed stress.
    - Grade 1: Pain with no instability
    - Grade 2: Asymmetric laxity (compared to the contralateral thumb) but with a firm endpoint
      - The degree of laxity does not reach the previously mentioned thresholds.
    - Grade 3: Complete rupture. Frank joint instability with no firm endpoint, exceeding the above-mentioned thresholds
- Note that in the acute setting, guarding secondary to pain and muscle spasm is common and may produce an unreliable examination. Therefore consider performing the exam after injection of local anesthetic either in the form of an intra-articular injection or local infiltration around the ligament.

Imaging

- Radiographs
  - Posterolateral, lateral, and oblique views of the thumb
  - Observe for fracture (avulsion or intra-articular) and/or joint subluxation in either the coronal or sagittal plane.

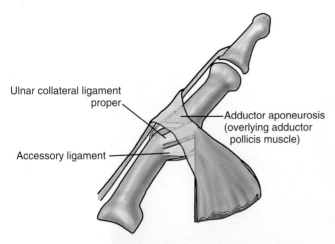

Ulnar collateral ligament
proper

Adductor aponeurosis
(overlying adductor
pollicis muscle)

Accessory ligament

Fig 81.1 Ulnar collateral ligament.

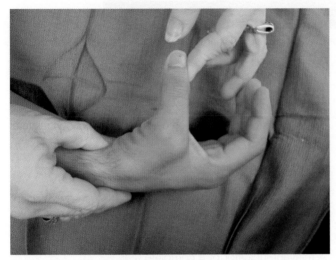

Fig 81.2 Complete rupture of ulnar collateral ligament with angulation of greater than 30 degrees found on radial stress exam.

- Observe for the presence of MCP joint arthritic changes, particularly in the setting of a chronic injury.
- Stress radiographs are controversial. Falling out of favor due to concern for iatrogenic conversion of a partial or minimally displaced complete rupture into a complete or Stener lesion type injury.
  - Never perform in the setting of a fracture, thus nonstress radiographs should always be obtained first.
- Ultrasonography
  - Noninvasive
  - Relatively inexpensive
  - Sensitivity and specificity high (75-95%) for Stener and non-Stener lesions, but may decrease if the procedure is delayed
  - Highly operator dependent
- Magnetic resonance imaging
  - May be more accurate than ultrasonography, especially when magnetic resonance arthrography is performed
  - Sensitivity is dependent upon quality of imaging and radiologist experience.
  - Higher cost

Differential Diagnosis

- Generalized laxity: Compare with contralateral side and examine multiple joints.
- Proximal phalanx fracture: Can occur in isolation or in conjunction with injury to the UCL.

Treatment

- At diagnosis
  - Acute, partial tears
    - Treatment is generally nonoperative in a thumb spica splint or cast for 4 to 6 weeks (see the following protocol).
    - May consider a thermoplastic thumb spica splint in compliant patients.
      - Similar outcomes and higher patient satisfaction with splint compared to cast.
  - Acute, complete tears
    - Theoretically, complete tears without a Stener lesion can be treated with cast immobilization; however, after completion of closed management and appropriate therapy, some will remain symptomatic and may require surgery.
      - As such, some argue the most predictable result is with operative exploration and repair, which can be done with a variety of techniques (Fig. 81.3); dependent on location of tear.
    - Associated fractures are also indications for operative management.
      - Displaced intra-articular fractures involving more than 25% of the base of the proximal phalanx
      - Avulsion fracture with greater than 5 mm of displacement
  - Chronic, partial tears
    - Consider intra-articular corticosteroid injection followed by cast or splint immobilization and nonsteroidal antiinflammatory drugs for 3 weeks.
  - Chronic, complete tears
    - Can be treated like partial tears as a temporizing measure or in sedentary patients
    - Most patients are candidates for operative exploration and repair versus ligament reconstruction, particularly those desiring to return to athletic or other high-demand activities.
    - MCP fusion may be required in cases of advanced joint degeneration.
- Later
  - Acute, partial tears
    - Four weeks of full-time thumb spica cast or splint immobilization with the thumb interphalangeal (IP) joint left free and the MCP joint in slight flexion.
    - Followed by 2 additional weeks in a thumb spica splint for part-time wear coming out 4 to 6 times/day for thumb range of motion therapy.
    - Avoid pinch or grasp for 6 weeks total, then graduated return to activities as comfort allows, wearing splint for contact sport or other high-demand activities.
  - Acute, complete tears
    - Surgically repaired tears will also be immobilized for 3 to 4 weeks in a thumb spica cast or splint.

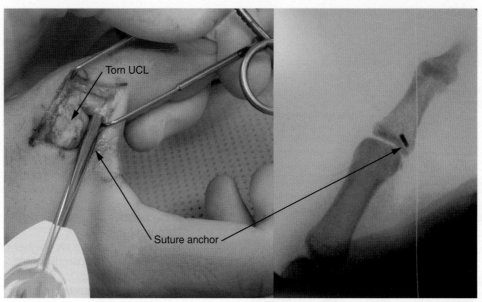

Fig 81.3 Operative exploration and repair techniques for acute, complete tears. *UCL,* Ulnar collateral ligament.

- This is followed by use of a removable splint for 2 to 3 weeks, during which time range of motion exercises of the thumb MCP joint are initiated.
- Full, unrestricted activity can be allowed at 12 weeks, assuming return of near-normal range of motion and strength.
- Athletes returning to contact sports should protect the thumb with splinting or tape for an additional 4 weeks.
  - Chronic tears
    - After ligament reconstruction, the initial cast is left on for 6 weeks rather than 4, and unrestricted activity is delayed for 16 to 18 weeks.

When to Refer

- All acute, complete tears, with and without fractures
- All chronic tears
- Cases in which differentiating between partial and complete tears is deemed difficult (frequent)
- Suspected tear in a high-level athlete

Prognosis

- Operative treatment
  - Complete tears
    - When treated operatively within 3 weeks, can expect greater than 90% good to excellent results
    - Pain and stiffness are typically minimal after appropriate therapy.
    - Return to athletic activities is as high as 95%.
    - Traction injury to the crossing branches of the sensory branch of the radial nerve is the most common complication.
  - Chronic tears
    - Overall satisfaction is very high.
    - Consistent restoration of thumb stability

- Mild, occasional pain may be seen in as many as 33% of patients.
- Restoration of motion usually 80-90% of contralateral side

Troubleshooting

- Although physical examination alone is usually sufficient to make the diagnosis, do not hesitate to refer when distinguishing between partial and complete tears is difficult.
- Absence of a firm endpoint may be the most clinically relevant indicator of a complete tear.
- All patients with pain on the ulnar side of the thumb MCP joint and a typical history should have a radiograph first.

Patient Instructions

- Early treatment of acute partial (nonoperative) and complete (operative) tears is best.
- Counsel patients that although results of acute repairs and chronic reconstructions are favorable, optimal results require a 4-month commitment to rehabilitation.
  - Loss of 6 to 10 degrees of MCP joint motion is expected.
  - Can have intermittent ulnar-sided soreness for up to a year post operation.

Considerations in Special Populations

- Acute injuries to the thumb MCP joint ulnar collateral ligament are typically seen in the younger, athletic population.
- Older, sedentary patients with chronic instability can typically be treated symptomatically; should osteoarthritis develop, there are favorable results with MCP fusion.

Suggested Readings

Campbell CS. Gamekeeper's thumb. *J Bone Joint Surg Br.* 1995;37B: 148–149.

4

Henry MH. Hand fractures and dislocations. In: Court-Brown CM, Heckman JD, McQueen MM, et al, eds. *Rockwood and Green's Fractures in Adults*. 8th ed. Philadelphia: Wolters Kluwer; 2015:915–990.

Heyman P. Injuries to the ulnar collateral ligament of the thumb metacarpophalangeal joint. *J Am Acad Orthop Surg*. 1997;5:224–229.

Merrell G, Hastings H. Dislocations and ligament injuries in the digits. In: Wolfe SW, Hotchkiss RN, Pederson WC, et al, eds. *Green's Operative Hand Surgery*. Vol. 1. 7th ed. Philadelphia: Elsevier; 2017:278–317.

Richard JR. Gamekeeper's thumb: ulnar collateral ligament injury. *Am Fam Physician*. 1996;53:1775–1780.

Stener B. Displacement of the ruptured ulnar collateral ligament of the metacarpophalangeal joint of the thumb: a clinical and anatomical study. *J Bone Joint Surg Br*. 1962;44B:869–879.

Chapter 82 Trigger Finger

Trent Gause II

ICD-10-CM CODES

M65.30	*Trigger finger, unspecified finger*
M65.311, M65.312, M65319	*Trigger finger, right, left, unspecified thumb*
M65.321, M65.322, M65329	*Trigger finger, right, left, unspecified index finger*
M65.331, M65.332, M65339	*Trigger finger, right, left, unspecified middle finger*
M65.341, M65.342, M65349	*Trigger finger, right, left, unspecified ringer finger*
M65.351, M65.352, M65359	*Trigger finger, right, left, unspecified small finger*

Key Concepts

- Stenosing tenosynovitis, commonly known as trigger finger.
- Mechanical symptoms of locking, catching, or popping when inflamed flexor tendons pass through a narrowed and restricted pulley in the hand, most commonly A1, but it has been reported to occur in A2, A3, and palmar aponeurosis.
- Normal gliding of flexor digitorum superficialis and flexor digitorum profundus tendons is disrupted, leading to increased resistance as tendons pull through the A1 pulley. Tendon entrapment creates a cycle of further inflammation and constriction at the pulley and ultimately worsening of symptoms (Fig. 82.1).
- The A1 pulley becomes grossly thickened with the histologic response of an increase in collagen and hyperplasia. Microscopic examination reveals fibrocartilaginous metaplasia of the inner layer of the surface of the pulley.
- The digits affected in order of prevalence: ring, thumb, long, index, small.
- Lifetime incidence of 2% after the age of 30 years; 10% incidence with diabetes.
- Affects women two to six times more than men.
- Peak incidence at 55 to 60 years of age.
- Idiopathic trigger finger most common.
- Systemic risk factors include
  - Diabetes
  - Rheumatoid arthritis
  - Collagen vascular disorders
  - Dupuytren disease
  - Gout
  - Renal disease
  - Amyloidosis
- Local trauma as risk factor
  - Activities with power grip cause shearing at the edges of the A1 pulley
  - Recent surgery

History

- Grade 0: mild crepitus without triggering of digit
- Grade I: pretriggering
  - Early symptoms consist of generalized dull ache and pain in the area of the A1 pulley located over the metacarpal head in the palm of the hand; there may not be reproducible catching.
  - Pain can be referred to the entire digit of the affected hand; patients may incorrectly localize pain to the proximal interphalangeal joint of the affected finger.
  - Feelings of morning stiffness and swelling of finger also reported.
- Grade II: active
  - Later symptoms of reproducible locking or catching during flexion and extension of fingers; the patient can actively extend the digit.
- Grade III: passive
  - With increasing severity, the involved digit becomes locked and passive extension is necessary to unlock the digit.
- Grade IV: contracture
  - Most severe trigger fingers still have reproducible catching, but also have a fixed flexion contracture at the proximal interphalangeal joint.
  - In extreme cases, the patient may present with a permanently locked finger.

Physical Examination

- Tenderness over the A1 pulley; in palmar flexion, a crease over the metacarpal head
- Palpable nodule in the flexor digitorum superficialis tendon moves with flexion
- Popping sensation over the A1 pulley with flexion or extension of the digit
- Triggering may not be reproducible by the examiner, but the patient is usually able to reproduce the offending click with maximal active flexion (Fig. 82.2).

Imaging

- No imaging is necessary.
- The diagnosis of trigger finger is overtly clinical, based on history and examination.
- Plain radiographs are obtained only if suspicion of other pathology exists.

Differential Diagnosis

- Please see Table 82.1.

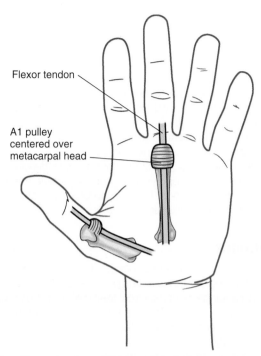

Flexor tendon

A1 pulley
centered over
metacarpal head

Fig 82.1 Flexor tendon with the pulley system.

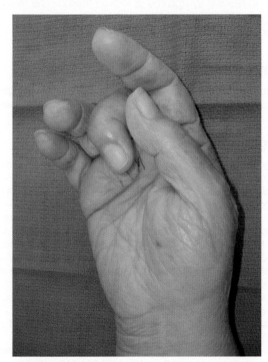

Fig 82.2 Example of locked trigger finger.

Treatment

- Activity modification
- Splinting of metacarpophalangeal (MCP joint)
  - Useful for grades 0 to 3, must allow for proximal and distal interphalangeal joint movement and immobilize for 6 weeks, may take up to 4 months for relief.
  - Some authors advocate 0 degrees of MCP flexion, others suggest 10 to 15 degrees.

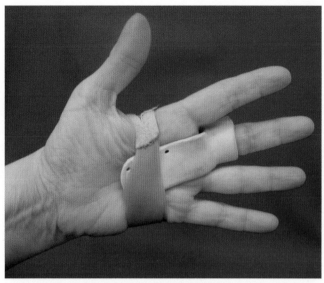

Fig 82.3 Example of splinting for trigger finger.

TABLE 82.1 Differential Diagnosis

Condition	Differentiating Feature
Dupuytren disease (see Chapter 88)	Nodular cords do not move with tendons with flexion and extension
Metacarpophalangeal joint locking	Locked metacarpophalangeal joint but proximal and distal phalangeal joints flex normally; often associated with collateral ligament impingement on metacarpal head osteophyte; rarely caused by abnormal sesamoids

- At diagnosis
  - Patients with symptoms of pretriggering without reproducible locking can be treated with nonsteroidal antiinflammatory drugs, splinting in extension, or stretching (Fig. 82.3).
- Later
  - Patients with palpable mechanical symptoms of triggering should be treated with corticosteroid injection as the first-line treatment (see Chapter 104 for technique); a series of up to three injections may be given. Less efficacious if symptoms are present for >6 months.

When to Refer

- Patients in whom conservative measures, including steroid injections, have failed or those who have a locked finger should be referred to a hand surgeon for evaluation of operative treatment.
- Only actively triggering fingers should be considered for operative intervention.
- Surgical treatment includes either a day surgery procedure with release of the A1 pulley or some experienced hand

surgeons may perform an office-based procedure of percutaneous release of the A1 pulley.

Prognosis

- As many as 80% of patients have resolution of symptoms after one steroid injection.
- After three injections, the success rate varies but is reported as high as 93%.
- Surgical treatment will relieve mechanical symptoms with few complications.
- Patients may complain of prolonged soreness after surgical release, but mechanical symptoms resolve immediately after surgical treatment.

Troubleshooting

- Multiple steroid injections can theoretically cause rupture of tendons despite only one report in the literature. However, most series of steroid injections are limited to three.
- Diabetics should be counseled that they may have a transient increase in blood sugar levels after corticosteroid injection.
- Steroid injections are proven to be more effective in nondiabetic patients compared with those with diabetes, and patients without diabetes are significantly less likely to require surgical release than diabetics.

Patient Instructions

- Steroid injection may cause a painful postinjection flare that can be treated with a few days of oral antiinflammatory medication.
- Patients with previous trigger fingers are at increased risk of developing triggering in other digits.
- Active use of fingers is encouraged after injection and surgical release.
- Formal hand therapy is rarely needed to improve hand function.

Considerations in Special Populations

- Although diabetic patients are less likely to respond as well as patients with idiopathic trigger finger, a steroid injection should still be initially attempted.

Pediatric Triggering

- True triggering is rare in children. The incidence is 1 to 3 in 1000. It most commonly occurs in the thumb with the middle finger the next most affected digit.
- Most commonly, children have "congenital trigger thumb," although this is not truly a congenital condition because it

does not occur at birth. It develops later and more properly is a "developmental trigger thumb."
- Develops at approximately 2 years of age.
- Mechanical symptoms may be noted, but at presentation the thumb is locked in fixed flexion at the interphalangeal joint; however, fingers classically present with triggering.
- A nodule or Notta node is commonly palpated at the A1 pulley.
- Flexor tendon thickening is seen without constriction or hyperplasia of the A1 pulley in congenital trigger thumb.
- Trigger fingers may present secondary to underlying conditions such as mucopolysaccharidosis, juvenile rheumatoid arthritis, Elhers-Danos, Down syndrome, and other central nervous system disorders.

Treatment

- Trigger thumb especially locked digits and trigger finger are generally treated with surgical release; however, recent literature suggests nonsurgical treatment may be an option. Nonsurgical options include observation, stretching programs, casting, and orthoses.
- Trigger finger
- Children do not tolerate injections.
- Surgical treatment of release of the A1 pulley is most effective to resolve symptoms of locked thumb. The release of trigger fingers has a higher rate of recurrence.
- Nodule dissipates with time.

Acknowledgment

The author thanks Drs. Megan M. Wood and Jack Ingari for their contributions to the previous edition of this chapter.

Suggested Readings

Baumgarten KM, Gerlach D, Boyer MI. Corticosteroid injection in diabetic patients with trigger finger. *J Bone Joint Surg Am*. 2007;89A:2604–2611.

Eastwood DM, Gupta KJ, Johnson DP. Percutaneous release of the trigger finger: an office procedure. *J Hand Surg Am*. 1992;17A:114–117.

Makkouk AH, Oetgen ME, Swigart CR, Dodds SD. Trigger finger: etiology, evaluation, and treatment. *Curr Rev Musculoskelet Med*. 2008;2:92–96.

Marks MR, Gunther SF. Efficacy of cortisone injection in treatment of trigger fingers and thumbs. *J Hand Surg Am*. 1989;14A:722–727.

Newport ML, Lane LB, Stuchin SA. Treatment of trigger finger by steroid injection. *J Hand Surg Am*. 1990;15A:748–750.

Saldana MJ. Trigger digits: diagnosis and treatment. *J Am Acad Orthop Surg*. 2001;9:246–252.

Shah AS, Bae DS. Management of pediatric trigger thumb and trigger finger. *J Am Acad Orthop Surg*. 2012;4:206–213.

Turowski GA, Zdankiewicz TD, Thompson JG. Results of surgical treatment of trigger finger. *J Hand Surg Am*. 1997;22A:145–149.

Chapter 83 Flexor Tendon Injuries

Adam R. Cochran, Jonathan E. Isaacs

ICD-10-CM CODES
S66   *Injury of muscle, fascia, and tendon at wrist and hand level*
S66.0 *Injury of long flexor muscle, fascia, and tendon of the thumb at wrist and hand level*
S66.1 *Injury of flexor muscle, fascia, and tendon of other and unspecified finger at wrist and hand level*

Key Concepts

- Flexor tendon injuries usually result in significant functional deficits if they are not properly treated.
- Timely surgical treatment is based on anatomic location of injury.
- Specific treatment recommendations vary based on the anatomic locations (zones) of ruptures/lacerations and the time from injury.
- Injuries can involve the flexor digitorum superficialis (FDS), flexor digitorum profundus (FDP), or both.
- Frequently associated with adjacent nerve/vessel injuries (which often require surgical repair).
- Postoperative peritendinous adhesions are a major concern and can result in poor tendon gliding, stiffness, and functional disability.
- Appropriate rehabilitation is critical (balance between decreasing adhesion formation while protecting the repair).

Anatomy

- There are two flexor tendons to each digit extending from the FDS muscle bellies and the FDP muscle belly, and one flexor tendon to the thumb extending from the flexor pollicis longus muscle belly.
- The FDS and FDP muscle bellies are in the volar forearm and the tendons, which form in the distal forearm, go through the carpal tunnel, and continue to insert on the base of the proximal phalanges and distal phalanges, respectively.
- The flexor pollicis longus tendon also traverses the carpal tunnel and inserts on the base of the distal phalanx of the thumb.
- The FDS is superficial (volar) to the FDP until approximately the metacarpophalangeal (MCP) joint, where it splits (Camper chiasma); the FDP tendon continues through the chiasm to become the more superficial tendon, and the two slips of the FDS insert on the palmar surface at the base of the middle phalanx (Fig. 83.1B).
- Just proximal to the MCP joint, the FDS, and FDP are enclosed by a common flexor tendon sheath (see Fig. 83.1C).

- The sheath contains synovial fluid and facilitates gliding and nutritional supply of tendons.
- The sheath is composed of several annular and cruciate pulleys that stabilize the tendons and act as a mechanical fulcrum for flexion.
- Flexor tendons are divided into five anatomic zones (see Fig. 83.1A).
  - Zone I: the portion of the FDP distal to the insertion of the FDS
  - Zone II ("no man's land"): the area within the tendon sheath containing both tendons
  - Zone III: origin of the lumbricals (the intrinsic hand muscles), between the carpal tunnel and the flexor tendon sheaths
  - Zone IV: carpal tunnel
  - Zone V: proximal to the carpal tunnel
- The FDS flexes the proximal interphalangeal (PIP) joint.
- The FDP flexes the distal interphalangeal (DIP) and PIP joints.
- The lumbricals originate in the palm from the tendons of the FDP, run under the transverse metacarpal ligaments (volar to the axis of rotation of the MCP joints), and insert distally and dorsally to the extensor mechanism at the level of the proximal phalanx.
  - Four lumbricals, one to each digit except the thumb.
  - The action of the lumbrical is simultaneous flexion of the MCP joint and extension of the PIP and DIP joints.
  - Intrinsic and extrinsic muscles must function together for normal finger motion.
- The blood supply to the tendons is a combination of diffusion (via synovial fluid bathing the tendon) and perfusion (via vincula, which are interval soft-tissue attachments between the phalanges and the dorsal surface of the FDP and FDS).
- The digital neurovascular bundles lie just radial and ulnar to the flexor tendons and are susceptible to concurrent injury.

History

- Usually the result of an acute event, usually a laceration/open wound, but can be seen in closed avulsion injuries, or rupture.
- Obvious loss of finger flexion (PIP, DIP, or both, depending on level of injury)
  - Abnormal posturing
  - Inability to flex the involved finger(s) (Fig. 83.2)
- Lacerations frequently will involve injury to adjacent nerves resulting in numbness distal to the injury.
- Ruptures typically occur in the setting of chronic attrition (rheumatoid arthritis or in association with retained internal fixations such as plates or screws).

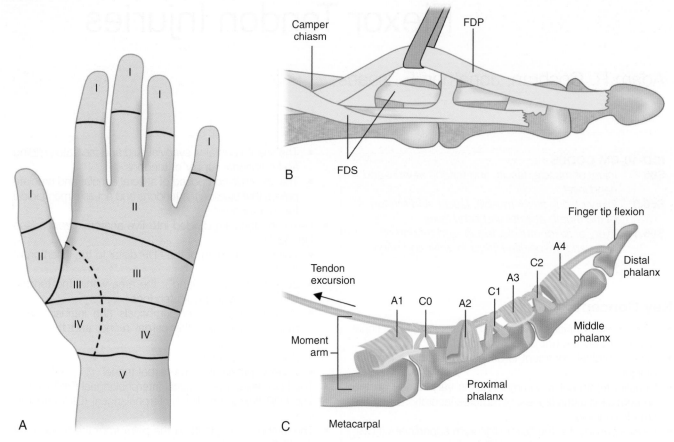

Fig 83.1 (A to C) Flexor zones in relation to pulleys and decussation of the flexor digitorum profundus (FDP) through camper chiasma. Care should be taken to preserve pulleys during flexor tendon repair, but not at the expense of the repair itself. FDS, flexor digitorum superficialis. (From Sud A, Ranjan R. *Textbook of Orthopaedics*. Philadelphia, Elsevier, 2018.)

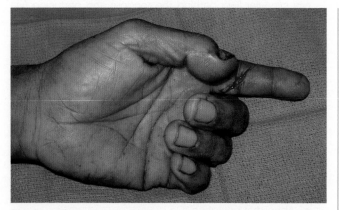

Fig 83.2 Example of a tendon laceration. Note the loss of the normal cascade and the patient's inability to flex the injured finger.

Physical Examination

- Observation
  - Posture of fingers: With the hand in a resting position, the fingers are normally held in a slightly flexed posture, with flexion increasing in a cascading fashion from the index finger to the small finger.
  - The injured tendon will cause its finger to assume a more extended posture.
  - If only the FDP tendon is injured, then flexion of the MCP and PIP joints may be normal and the DIP joint will be abnormally extended.
  - If the FDS and FDP tendons are both disrupted, the entire finger will fall into a resting extended position, clearly disrupting the arcade.
- Neurovascular examination
  - Assess capillary refill in the affected digit(s): sluggish or absent refill may indicate a devascularized digit, which requires *emergent* surgical intervention.
  - Assess sensation to light touch on both the ulnar and radial sides of the digit(s): sensation that is absent or

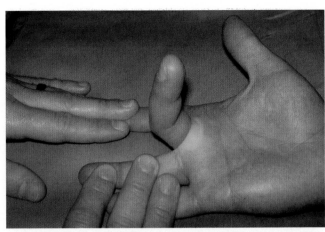

Fig 83.3 To test the integrity of the flexor digitorum superficialis, keep all other fingers extended, including the distal interphalangeal joints, and ask the patient to flex the affected finger. If the tendon is intact, the finger will flex at the proximal interphalangeal and metacarpophalangeal joints.

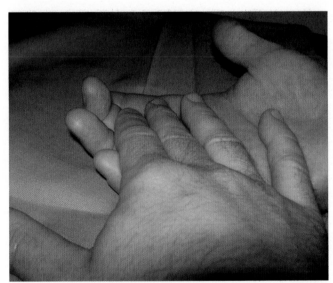

Fig 83.4 To test the integrity of the flexor digitorum profundus, isolate the distal interphalangeal joint by holding the metacarpophalangeal and proximal interphalangeal joints extended, and ask the patient to flex the finger.

altered compared with noninjured fingers indicates likely digital nerve damage.
- Check the integrity of the tendons
  - Do not probe or try to retrieve lacerated flexor tendons.
  - Independently examine the FDP and FDS tendons.
  - FDS: Keep all other fingers extended, including the DIP joints, and ask the patient to flex the affected finger; if the tendon is intact, it will flex at the PIP and MCP joints (Fig. 83.3).
  - FDP: Isolate the DIP joint by holding the MCP and PIP joints extended and ask the patient to flex the finger (Fig. 83.4).
  - Alternative techniques

- Passively extend the patient's wrist, and the tenodesis effect should cause all fingers with intact tendons to flex accordingly.
- Squeeze the volar forearm musculature. If tendons are intact all digits should slightly flex.
- With partial transections, a normal arcade may be present, and the patient may still have intact function.
- Pain with flexion against resistance may indicate partial injury.
- Clicking or catching may occur during motion.

Imaging

- If the mechanism of injury also may have caused injury to the phalanges or joints, plain radiographs of the hand/finger are appropriate.
- Other modalities are typically not indicated in a primary injury.
- Magnetic resonance imaging or ultrasonography can be used to differentiate between postrepair tendon adhesions and rerupture.

Treatment

- At diagnosis
  - If the injury is caused by a laceration, administer intravenous antibiotics and assess the need for a tetanus update.
  - Irrigate the wound, apply a clean dressing, and apply a splint (dorsal splint with the wrist in neutral flexion and the MCP joints in 60 to 70 degrees of flexion).
  - Consult with a hand surgeon, who may ask to close the skin wound with sutures before applying a dressing or splint.
  - Chronic ruptures from attrition (i.e., rheumatoid arthritis) can be splinted for comfort.
- Later
  - Complete disruption of a flexor tendon will typically require surgical repair (typically within 7 to 10 days), as will many partial tendon injuries.
  - This may be accompanied by repair of the digital neurovascular structures.
  - Surgical options are based on the level of injury, the degree of contamination, the soft-tissue damage, and the time from injury.

Surgical Repair
Acute Repair

- In clean wounds, primary end-to-end repair can usually be performed within 1 to 2 weeks of injury (Fig. 83.5).
  - Zone I: similar to repair of avulsion injuries (Jersey finger) (see Chapter 86)
  - Zone II: FDP tendon typically repaired end-to-end with four deep core sutures and a running superficial epitenon suture
  - FDS tendons are usually repaired separately with simple suture techniques
  - Repair of pulleys/tendon sheath is done as necessary
  - Zones III to V: FDS and FDP are repaired independently with core sutures with or without a running epitenon suture

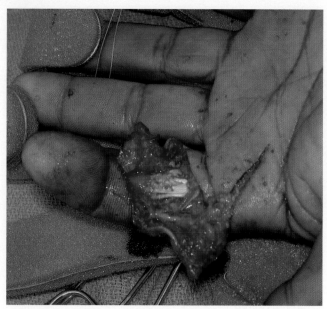

Fig 83.5 Intraoperative view of an acute zone II flexor digitorum profundus and flexor digitorum superficialis tendon repair. Note the tight sheath above and below the repair, which is one reason why adhesions and loss of motion are so problematic.

- Repair or excision of a damaged lumbrical in zone III depending on injury

Delayed/Staged Repair

- In delayed presentations (more than 3 to 4 weeks), cases of rerupture, excessive scarring of repair, dirty wounds, and some acute zone II injuries, staged repair is indicated.
  - Stage I: the FDS and/or FDP are excised, and a prosthetic (i.e., silicone) rod is placed
  - Pulley system is reconstructed as needed at this time
  - Range of motion preserved with therapy
  - Stage II (at 3 months): the prosthetic graft is removed, and the tendon graft is placed within the sheath and sutured to the proximal and distal stumps

Basics of Rehabilitation

- Multiple protocols have been described for different injuries.
- Initial postoperative immobilization with the MCP joints in flexion and interphalangeal joints in extension to avoid contractures
- Regular follow-up with a hand therapist is imperative to optimal outcome.

- In general, motion is started within a few days to decrease tendon adhesions and to improve excursion/motion.
- Initially, passive flexion (or carefully controlled/protected active flexion) and active extension are performed within the confines of a dorsal extension block splint.
- Gradual supervised progression over 3 months of increased extension, active flexion, and active flexion against resistance until full activity is allowed.

When to Refer

- If the examiner is confident that the patient has a complete or partial tendon injury, with or without concomitant neurovascular injury, he or she should refer the patient to a surgeon for repair.
  - Surgery preferably occurs within 1 to 2 weeks of an injury.
  - Repairs after 2 weeks are complicated by tendon retraction and scarring.

Prognosis

- Dependent on anatomic location(s) of injury, mechanism of injury, time until surgery, coexisting injuries, quality of repair, and patient compliance with postoperative rehabilitation.
- The most common complication is postoperative tendon adhesions, which can lead to a decreased range of motion and stiffness.
- Another complication is rerupture of the repaired tendon (most commonly 1 to 2 weeks postoperatively), often requiring two-stage repair as described previously.

Considerations in Special Populations

- Children do not require the same postoperative protocols; they are unable to comply with the complex instructions. However, this population does quite well with 4 weeks of immobilization and then unrestricted activity.

Suggested Readings

Carty M, Blazar P. Complex flexor and extensor tendon injuries. *Hand Clin*. 2013;29:283–293.

Chauhan A, Palmer BA, Merrell GA. Flexor tendon repairs: techniques, eponyms, and evidence. *J Hand Surg Am*. 2014;39(9):1846–1853.

Lutsky KF, Giang EL, Matzon JL. Flexor tendon injury, repair and rehabilitation. *Orthop Clin North Am*. 2015;46:67–76.

Netscher DT, Badal JJ. Closed flexor tendon ruptures. *J Hand Surg Am*. 2014;39(11):2315–2323.

Pulos N, Bozentka DJ. Management of complications of flexor tendon injuries. *Hand Clin*. 2015;31(2):293–299.

Chapter 84 Boutonniere Deformity

Trent Gause II

ICD-10-CM CODES
M20.021 *Boutonniere deformity of right finger(s)*
M20.022 *Boutonniere deformity of left finger(s)*
M20.029 *Boutonniere deformity of unspecified finger(s)*

Key Concepts

- Also known as buttonhole deformity
- Deformity of the finger involving flexion of the proximal interphalangeal (PIP) joint and hyperextension of the distal interphalangeal (DIP) joint (Fig. 84.1)
- Caused by disruption or attenuation of the central slip and triangular ligament of the extensor expansion on the dorsal finger (Fig. 84.2)
- Traumatic, infectious, or inflammatory etiology
- The balance of the finger extensor mechanism is altered, which over time leads to fixed volar subluxation of the lateral bands and focus of extension force exclusively on the distal joint. This causes loss of active PIP joint extension and hyperextension of the DIP joint, respectively.
- If left untreated, fixed flexion occurs at the PIP joint secondary to volar plate and oblique retinacular ligament contracture.

History

- Closed injury
- Forced flexion of an actively extended PIP joint ("jammed" finger)
- Crush injury
- Volar dislocation of the PIP joint
- Open injury
- Laceration over the PIP joint
- Open wound at the level of the PIP joint with tendon necrosis
- Burns
- Infection
- Subcutaneous infection
- Intra-articular infection of the PIP joint
- Inflammatory
- Rheumatoid and other inflammatory arthritides
- Gout

Physical Examination

- Acute
  - The examiner must have a high index of suspicion because the deformity may evolve over the course of 1 week after the initial injury
  - PIP joint effusion
  - Localized tenderness over the dorsal aspect of the PIP joint at the insertion of the central tendon
  - Elson test (Fig. 84.3)
  - A positive test result is demonstrated when the patient bends the PIP joint 90 degrees over the edge of a table and, with resisted middle phalanx extension, the DIP joint goes into rigid extension (all the forces are distributed to the terminal tendon through the intact lateral bands)
  - A negative test result is demonstrated when the DIP joint remains floppy with this maneuver
- Boyes test
  - Assess ability to actively flex DIP with the PIP held in extension
  - Fix the PIP joint and ask patient to flex the DIP joint
  - Intact extensor mechanism should demonstrate full DIP flexion motion
  - Patients with contracted lateral bands will have decreased active flexion
  - May not be positive in an acute setting
- Chronic
  - Assess the PIP and DIP joints for flexibility and evidence of arthritis
- True boutonniere deformity should not be confused with a pseudo deformity
  - Pseudo deformity: flexion contracture of PIP joint in which the triangular ligament is competent, thus allowing for the DIP to retain mobility
  - Flexion contracture caused by scarring of the volar plate
  - Distinguish by using the Elson and Boyes test as described previously

Imaging

- Radiographs of acute and chronic injuries are imperative in determining the mode of treatment. Look for bony fragments and subtle DIP extensions.
- Standard views of the affected digit should include antero-posterior, lateral, and oblique views.
- Acute: Fractures and volar subluxations are often seen (Fig. 84.4).
  - Chronic: Arthritic changes may be present from infection or inflammatory arthritis. Classified according to Burton boutonniere deformity, which also guides treatment
  - Type I: passively correctable deformity
  - Type II: fixed contracture with contracted lateral bands, no joint involvement
  - Type III: volar plate and collateral ligament contractures, intra-articular fibrosis
  - Type IV: Type III plus PIP joint arthritis

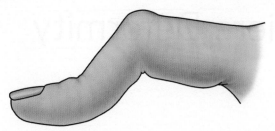

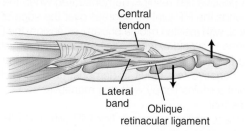

Fig 84.1 Extensor tenotomy for supple boutonniere deformity. The deformity is characteristic of the chronic boutonniere deformity. (Adapted from Green DP, Hotchkiss RN, Pederson WC, Wolfe SW, eds. *Green's Operative Hand Surgery*. 5th ed. Philadelphia: Churchill Livingstone; 2005, Fig. 6.22A.)

Central tendon

Lateral band

Oblique retinacular ligament

Fig 84.2 Pathomechanics of the boutonniere deformity. Attenuation of the central slip results in unopposed flexion at the proximal interphalangeal joint. (Adapted from Strauch RJ. Extensor tendon injury. In: Wolfe SW, Hotchkiss RN, Pederson WC, et al, eds. *Green's Operative Hand Surgery*. 7th ed. Philadelphia: Elsevier; 2017, Fig. 5.20A.)

Differential Diagnosis

- Pseudo-boutonniere deformity
  - Flexion contracture of the PIP joint but without restriction if DIP joint mobility
  - Extensor mechanism is unaffected
  - Caused by PIP joint hyperextension injury that results in fibrosis of the volar ligamentous complex
  - Treated with aggressive motion as opposed to true boutonniere, which requires a period of immobilization
  - Radiographs often demonstrate avulsion fractures of the PIP volar plate and calcification about the volar mechanism of the proximal phalanx.

Treatment

- Depends on the chronicity of the injury and the flexibility of the digit
- Acute injuries (0 to 2 weeks)
  - Lacerations require exploration and anatomic reapproximation of the central slip
  - Closed injuries not involving a fracture require 6 weeks of immobilization of the PIP joint in extension, leaving the DIP joint free (Fig. 84.5)
  - Flexion of the DIP joint draws the extensor mechanism distally and facilitates dorsal translation of the lateral bands
  - Closed injuries involving a fracture or dislocation require reduction followed by an assessment of joint stability

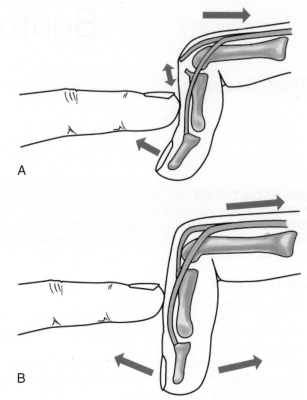

A

B

Fig 84.3 Elson test. (A) With a disrupted central slip, attempted active extension of the proximal interphalangeal joint against resistance allows proximal movement of the origin of the lateral bands holding the distal joint in extension. (B) With an intact central slip, attempted active extension of the proximal interphalangeal joint against resistance affects the middle phalanx but leaves the distal joint flail.

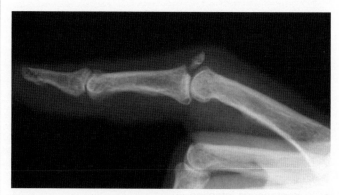

Fig 84.4 An avulsed bone fragment at the insertion of the central slip. (From Green DP, Hotchkiss RN, Pederson WC, Wolfe SW, eds. *Green's Operative Hand Surgery*. 5th ed. Philadelphia: Churchill Livingstone; 2005, Fig. 6.17B.)

- If the reduction is adequate and the joint is stable, immobilize the PIP joint with the DIP joint free for 6 weeks
- If the reduction cannot be obtained or the joint is unstable, open reduction and internal fixation are required
- Subacute injuries (2 to 8 weeks)
  - Treat supple PIP joints like acute closed injuries without fractures, except leave the splint on for 8 weeks

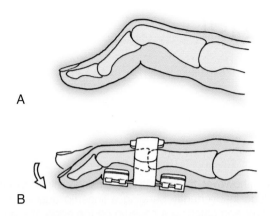

A

B

Fig 84.5 **(A)** Schematic representation of a boutonniere deformity. **(B)** A Bunnell splint is applied to maintain extension at the proximal interphalangeal (PIP) joint. The strap over the PIP joint is progressively tightened until the PIP joint is fully extended. The patient is encouraged to actively and passively flex the distal interphalangeal joint. The splint is worn until the patient can maintain active extension of the PIP joint. (From Piper SL, Lattanza L: Extensor tendon injuries. In Trumble TE, Rayan GM, Budoff JE, et al. *Principles of Hand Surgery and Therapy*. 3rd ed. Philadelphia: Elsevier; 2017.)

- Stiff PIP joints require treatment to regain full mobility
- Dynamic or progressive static splints can be used
- If full motion is restored, leave the splint on for an additional 8 weeks
- If motion cannot be restored, treat the injury like a chronic stiff boutonniere deformity (see the following)
- Chronic injuries (>8 weeks)
  - Probably will not be amenable to splint therapy
  - The status of the PIP and DIP joints determines the treatment protocol in these long-standing injuries
  - Flexible PIP joints require operative rebalancing of the extensor mechanism through anatomic repair, reconstruction using local tissue, or tendon grafting
  - Treatment of stiff PIP joints requires staged treatment
  - The first priority is to reestablish joint motion through splinting or surgery
  - Once full motion is established, an extensor tendon reconstruction is typically required
  - Arthritic PIP joints require arthroplasty or fusion depending on whether the extensor mechanism is intact or disrupted, respectively

When to Refer

- Open injuries
- Fractures or irreducible dislocations requiring open reduction and internal fixation

- Residual deformity after failure of splinting program
- Flexion contracture unresponsive to conservative treatment

Troubleshooting

- Early diagnosis is essential for successful treatment.
- The examiner must have a high index of suspicion of central slip injury during the acute phase because a boutonniere deformity may be delayed.
- In a stiff deformity, full extension must be obtained either through splinting or surgical release before definitive treatment can be performed.
- It is important to differentiate between boutonniere and pseudo-boutonniere deformities because surgery for either condition when the other is actually the problem will have poor results.
- The most common complication encountered in treating acute closed deformities is incomplete correction.
- Full flexion of the PIP and DIP joints with an extension lag of 20 degrees or less produces a finger with few functional limitations.

Patient Instructions

- The splint for acute injury must be worn full time for a minimum of 6 weeks.
- An additional 6 weeks of night splinting follows for protection.
- Concomitant active and passive flexion of the DIP joint must be done during splint wear.

Considerations in Special Populations

- Rheumatoid arthritis patients can be treated with a similar algorithm.
- It is important to address the wrist pathology before surgical treatment of boutonniere deformity in these patients.
- Severe rheumatoid boutonniere deformities often require joint fusion.

Acknowledgment

The author thanks Drs. Jack Ingari and Daniel T. Fletcher, Jr. for their contributions to the previous edition of this chapter.

Suggested Readings

Baratz ME, Schmidt CC, Hughes TB. Extensor tendon injuries. In: Green DP, Hotchkiss RN, Pederson WC, Wolfe SW, eds. *Green's Operative Hand Surgery*. 5th ed. Philadelphia: Churchill Livingstone; 2005:199–205.

Coons MS, Green SG. Boutonniere deformity. *Hand Clin*. 1995;11:387–402.

Elson RA. Rupture of the central slip of the extensor hood of the finger, a test for early diagnosis. *J Bone Joint Surg Br*. 1986;68B:229–231.

Massengill JB. The boutonniere deformity. *Hand Clin*. 1992;8:787–801.

McKeon KE, Lee DH. Posttraumatic boutonnière and swan neck deformities. *J Am Acad Orthop Surg*. 2015;23(10):623–632.

Souter WA. The problem of boutonniere deformity. *Clin Orthop Relat Res*. 1974;104:116–133.

Chapter 85 Mallet Finger

Trent Gause II

Key Concepts

- A mallet finger (also known as *drop finger* or *baseball finger*) is a finger that droops at the tip due to an injury to the terminal extensor mechanism.
- The terminal extensor mechanism is composed of a broad, flat terminal tendon that spans the distal interphalangeal (DIP) joint to insert at the dorsal base of the distal phalanx (Fig. 85.1).
- An isolated injury to the terminal extensor mechanism will cause an extensor lag (i.e., loss of active extension) at the DIP joint.
- Specific injuries to the terminal extensor mechanism include
  - Rupture of the terminal tendon
  - Laceration of the terminal tendon
  - Fracture of the distal phalanx at the terminal tendon's insertion
- As the more proximal joints are typically uninjured, the finger acquires the classic mallet posture, a drooping tip on an otherwise normal digit (Fig. 85.2).
- When the terminal tendon is disrupted, forces on the extensor mechanism are no longer transmitted across the DIP joint, but rather are concentrated at the proximal interphalangeal (PIP) joint.
  - Thus, in addition to an extensor lag at the DIP joint (i.e., a mallet deformity), a terminal tendon injury can also produce a hyperextension deformity at the PIP joint.
  - This condition, called a compensatory swan neck deformity (Fig. 85.3), is particularly common in patients with naturally hyperextensible PIP joints.
- Over time, mallet and swan neck deformities can become fixed; for this reason, it is desirable that treatment for a mallet finger be initiated reasonably promptly.

History

- The typical chief symptom is an inability to extend the DIP joint.
- Many patients present with a history of a sports-related injury (e.g., jammed finger) or a traumatic event such as a knife accident.
  - These patients will likely have significant pain at the site of injury.

- Often, however, the trauma is surprisingly minor; examples include inadvertently banging a fingertip against a desk drawer and catching a fingertip on the edge of a pocket.
  - These patients may have little or no pain.
  - Such scenarios are typical in older patients and are probably indicative of an attritional tendon rupture from arthritic changes at the DIP joint.

Physical Examination

- Often there is edema and erythema over the dorsal DIP joint region.
- There may be a laceration or abrasion over the dorsal middle phalanx or DIP joint regions.
- Usually (but not always) there is mild to moderate tenderness at the site of injury.
- An extensor lag at the DIP joint is usually immediately evident, but occasionally the lag takes time to develop.
  - This presentation is more typical of attritional ruptures, in which a few wispy fibers of tendon or scar tissue remain in continuity.
  - In these early cases, a lag will become evident if the patient is asked to make a tight fist (stretching the remaining fibers) and then extend the fingers.
- Flexor function is typically not affected.
- Passive extension is usually intact, unless the injury is chronic, in which case a fixed flexion contracture may develop.
- Hyperextension may be present at the PIP joint (i.e., compensatory swan neck deformity).

Imaging

- Radiographs should be obtained for all mallet fingers.
  - Order three views (posteroanterior, lateral, and oblique) of the individual digit.
  - It is important to get a true lateral view, which is most likely to reveal dorsal fractures.
  - Attempts to image all digits simultaneously rarely result in true lateral views.
  - Many mallet injuries involve a small fracture of the dorsal lip of the distal phalanx, where the tendon insertion is avulsed along with a small piece of bone (Fig. 85.4).
  - If the fracture fragment is large (i.e., >30% of the articular surface), volar subluxation of the distal phalanx can occur (Fig. 85.5).
- Additional imaging tests, such as computed tomography or magnetic resonance imaging, are usually not indicated.

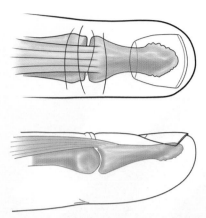

Fig 85.1 The thin, flat terminal tendon *(blue)* inserts at the dorsal lip of the base of the distal phalanx, just distal to the distal interphalangeal joint. Note that the tendon is immediately subcutaneous, the joint is immediately deep to the tendon, and the nail bed begins just distal to the tendon insertion.

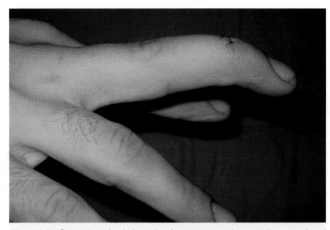

Fig 85.3 Swan neck deformity (hyperextension at the proximal interphalangeal joint and flexion at the distal interphalangeal joint) can be seen with mallet injuries, especially in people with naturally hyperextensible proximal interphalangeal joints.

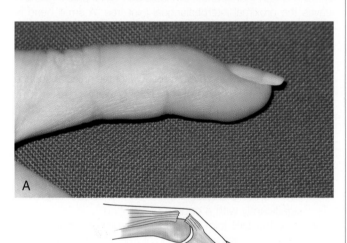

Fig 85.2 The mallet posture is due to discontinuity of the extensor mechanism across the distal interphalangeal joint. In this case, the discontinuity was due to closed rupture of the terminal tendon. Lacerations/abrasions of the tendon and fractures of the distal phalanx at the tendon's insertion can also create the mallet posture. (A) Depicts the clinical deformity of flexion at the DIP that may be seen, while (B) depicts the underlying anatomic injury, including rupture of the terminal slip at the DIP.

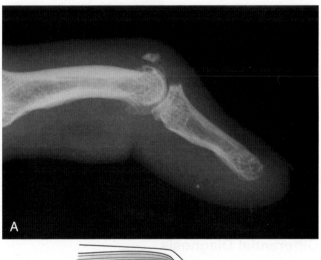

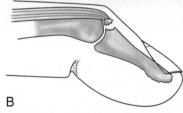

Fig 85.4 Many mallet injuries involve fractures of the distal phalanx. In most cases, the fragment is small and represents an avulsion of the tendon insertion. The distal phalanx remains properly located at the distal interphalangeal joint. These injuries usually heal well with splinting. (A) Depicts the radiographic findings that may occur with a mallet finger including flexion of the distal phalanx at the DIP joint and an bony avulsion from the dorsal cortex of the distal phalanx base. (B) Depicts the underlying anatomy in which the extensor tendon is attached to the bony fragment that has been avulsed.

Classification

- Acute mallet fingers are defined as occurring within 4 weeks; chronic deformities present later than 4 weeks
- Doyle Classification—divides mallet injuries into four types
  - Type I: Closed injury—with or without small dorsal avulsion injury
  - Type II: Open injury—laceration near or at DIP
  - Type III: Open injury—deep abrasion that involves skin loss and tendon surface injury
  - Type IV: Mallet fracture—subdivided into A, B, C
  - A: Distal phalanx physeal injury (pediatric)
  - B: Fracture fragment involving 20-50% of the articular surface
  - C: arise from hyperextension. Associated with volar subluxation and involve more than 50% of the articular surface

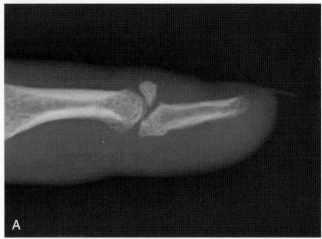

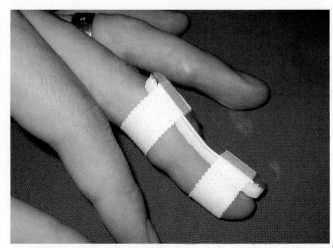

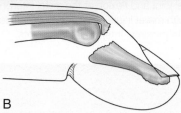

Fig 85.5 Distal phalanx fractures that encompass a large portion of the articular surface may lead to incongruity of the distal interphalangeal joint and volar subluxation of the distal phalanx. These cases may require surgery. (A) Depicts the radiographic findings of a mallet finger in which a larger articular portion of the distal phalanx has been fractured, with volar subluxation of the distal phalanx at the joint. (B) Illustrates that the extensor tendon is attached to the dorsal fragment and the distal phalanx is subluxed volar and unstable.

Fig 85.6 A piece of aluminum-foam splint material can be fashioned into an effective mallet splint. The material should be cut to a length that spans the middle and distal phalanges and leaves the proximal interphalangeal joint free. A small bend in the aluminum keeps the distal interphalangeal joint in mild (5 degrees) of hyperextension.

Differential Diagnosis

- An isolated extensor lag at the DIP joint is virtually pathognomonic for an injury of the terminal extensor tendon or its bony insertion.
- Some patients with arthritis can develop primary hyperextension at the PIP joint with secondary drooping of the distal phalanx; this is called a primary swan neck deformity.
  - The feature distinguishing a primary swan neck deformity from a compensatory one is the presence of (typically long-standing) pain and swelling at the PIP joint before the development of the deformity.
- A fixed flexion contracture of the DIP joint can be seen with both long-standing mallet injuries and unrelated disorders of the joint or flexor mechanism; the distinction is usually evident from the history.
- Rarely an exostosis (bony growth) of the dorsal DIP joint region can create the appearance of a mallet deformity; such a pseudo-mallet can be distinguished with radiographs.

Treatment

- Relatively few mallet injuries require surgical intervention; the exceptions are
  - Lacerations or abrasions of the terminal tendon

- Fractures involving more than 30% of the articular surface or volar subluxation of the distal phalanx
- Otherwise nonoperative injuries in patients who cannot perform their work duties while wearing a splint
- The remainder (and majority) of mallet injuries, including those involving tendon ruptures or small avulsion fractures, can be treated with splinting of the DIP joint in slight hyperextension.
  - Even chronic mallet fingers can often be improved significantly with a course of splinting.
  - Only the DIP joint needs to be splinted; in fact, it is desirable to leave the PIP joint free, not only to prevent stiffness but also because flexion at this joint relieves tension on the terminal extensor tendon.
- The standard splinting protocol calls for full-time extension splinting for 6 to 8 weeks (counted from the date splinting was initiated, not the date of injury) followed by splinting only at night for 2 weeks.
  - If the DIP joint needs to be flexed at any time during the full-time splinting period, the 6-week time frame starts over.
  - If during the 2-week nighttime splinting period, the extensor lag begins to return, the patient resumes full-time splinting for another 2 weeks, again followed by 2 weeks of nighttime splinting.
- Types of splints
  - Aluminum–foam splint (Fig. 85.6)
  - This is preferably placed dorsally to facilitate continued use of the digit.
  - A slight bend is created in the aluminum to maintain the DIP joint in approximately 5 degrees of hyperextension.
  - More aggressive hyperextension can cause ischemia of the skin dorsal to the DIP joint and must therefore be avoided.
  - Stack splint (Fig. 85.7)
  - This is a prefabricated plastic splint designed specifically for mallet fingers.

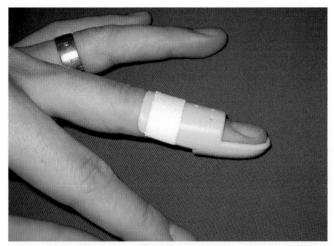

Fig 85.7 A stack splint is designed to hold the distal interphalangeal joint in extension while permitting full motion at the proximal interphalangeal joint. These splints come in multiple sizes and should be selected to provide a snug but comfortable fit.

- It is available in various sizes and should be selected to provide a snug but comfortable fit.
- It may be necessary to use a larger size initially to accommodate wound dressings or edema and then downsize as the finger heals.
- Occasionally these splints do not provide the proper degree of hyperextension at the DIP joint; a trick is to apply moleskin to the inside of the splint on the surface in contact with the volar fingertip to push the joint into the desired 5 degrees of hyperextension.
- Customized thermoplastic splint constructed by an occupational therapist
- The patient should be given the following instructions
  - During the period of full-time splinting, the splint should be removed only to cleanse the finger and splint.
  - To avoid inadvertent flexion of the DIP joint, the splint should be worn in the shower; afterward, the splint may be removed to wash and dry the finger and splint, taking great care not to flex the DIP joint. The splint is then immediately replaced.
  - Use of the splinted digit is encouraged, although strenuous gripping should be avoided to prevent unintentional flexing of the DIP joint.
- With this splinting protocol, the majority of patients will achieve a satisfactory outcome, although a slight (and usually inconsequential) residual extensor lag is common, as is a persistent prominence over the dorsal DIP joint region.
- Some hand surgeons recommend operative repair of mallet injuries in an effort to obviate a residual extensor lag, which in some cases is significant enough to create a functional and/or cosmetic impairment.
  - Outcomes for operative repair are usually good as well, although stiffness preventing full flexion, rather than an extensor lag, is a risk; the argument hinges on whether it is better to lose terminal extension or terminal flexion and whether the patient wishes to avoid surgery.
- Lacerations of the terminal tendon should be repaired at the time of skin closure.

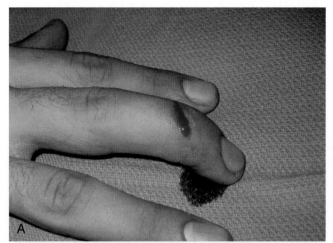

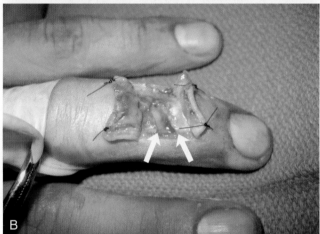

Fig 85.8 Tendon lacerations can be repaired at the time of skin repair. (A) In this case, an oblique laceration was present across the dorsum of the middle phalanx. (B) Flaps of dorsal skin have been created proximally and distally to facilitate exposure of the tendon edges *(arrows)*. A 1-inch Penrose drain has been wrapped around the digit proximally as a tourniquet. The tendon will be repaired with multiple figure-of-eight stitches using 3-0 Vicryl.

- These repairs can often be achieved in the clinic or emergency department settings, assuming the wound is clean and fresh.
- The repair technique is a matter of personal preference, but an acceptable method would be to place figure-of-eight or horizontal mattress stitches using a permanent (e.g., Ethibond) or long-lasting absorbable (e.g., Vicryl) suture, size 3-0 or 4-0 (Fig. 85.8).
- Very distal lacerations, where the tendon is extremely thin, can be very difficult or impossible to repair directly, and simultaneous approximation of the skin and tendon in a single layer (tenodermodesis) is an effective alternative (Fig. 85.9).
- In these cases, a nonabsorbable monofilament suture (nylon or Prolene, size 3-0 or 4-0), as would be used for skin closure, is preferred.
- All terminal tendon repairs should be protected postoperatively with the splinting protocol described previously.

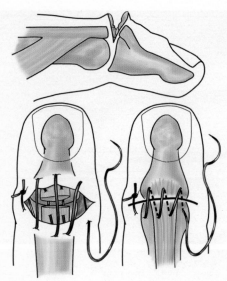

Fig 85.9 Lacerations of the terminal tendon very near its insertion where the tendon is extremely thin can be repaired with a single suture that simultaneously approximates the skin and tendon.

When to Refer

- Abrasion injuries in which there is a segmental loss of tendon substance, as might be seen with a power tool or motorcycle accident.
- Distal phalanx fractures that encompass more than one-third of the articular surface may lead to volar subluxation of the distal phalanx and/or posttraumatic arthritis of the DIP joint.
  - Although many hand surgeons contend that even these injuries can be treated with splinting alone, many others believe that operative reduction and fixation with a pin or screw is necessary.
- Those who could otherwise be treated nonoperatively but who cannot wear a splint at work (such as surgical personnel or food preparers) can be treated with a pin across the DIP joint.
- Those in whom a prolonged course of splinting failed.
- Those with a fixed DIP and/or PIP deformity.
- Children in whom treatment can be difficult due to poor compliance with splinting.

Acknowledgment

The author thanks Drs. Steven L. Henry and Jack Ingari for their contributions to this chapter in the previous edition.

Suggested Readings

Bendre AA, Hartigan BJ, Kalainov DM. Mallet finger. *J Am Acad Orthop Surg*. 2005;13(5):336–344.

Garberman SF, Diao W, Peimer CA. Mallet finger: results of early versus delayed closed treatment. *J Hand Surg Am*. 1994;19A:850–852.

Handoll HH, Vaghela MV. Interventions for treating mallet finger injuries. *Cochrane Database Syst Rev*. 2004;(3):CD004574.

Kalainov DM, Hoepfner PE, Hartigan BJ, et al. Nonsurgical treatment of closed mallet finger fractures. *J Hand Surg Am*. 2005;30A:580–586.

Katzman BM, Klein DM, Mesa J, et al. Immobilization of the mallet finger: effects on the extensor tendon. *J Hand Surg [Br]*. 1999;24B:80–84.

Kronlage SC, Faust D. Open reduction and screw fixation of mallet fractures. *J Hand Surg [Br]*. 2004;29B:135–138.

Nakamura K, Nanjyo B. Reassessment of surgery for mallet finger. *Plast Reconstr Surg*. 1994;93:141–149.

Okafor B, Mbubaegbu C, Munshi I, et al. Mallet deformity of the finger: five-year follow-up of conservative treatment. *J Bone Joint Surg Br*. 1997;79B:544–547.

Rayan GM, Mullins PT. Skin necrosis complicating mallet finger splinting and vascularity of the distal interphalangeal joint overlying skin. *J Hand Surg Am*. 1987;12A:548–552.

Strauch RJ. Extensor tendon injury. In: Wolfe SW, Hotchkiss RN, Pederson WC, et al, eds. *Green's Operative Hand Surgery*. 7th ed. Philadelphia: Elsevier; 2017:152–182.

Takami H, Takahashi S, Ando M. Operative treatment of mallet finger due to intra-articular fracture of the distal phalanx. *Arch Orthop Trauma Surg*. 2000;120:9–13.

Chapter 86 Jersey Finger (Flexor Digitorum Profundus Avulsion)

Trent Gause II

ICD-10-CM CODES

S63.621A	*Sprain of interphalangeal joint of right thumb—initial encounter*
S63.622A	*Sprain of interphalangeal joint of left thumb—initial encounter*
S63.629A	*Sprain of interphalangeal joint of unspecified thumb—initial encounter*
S63.630A	*Sprain of interphalangeal joint of right index finger—initial encounter*
S63.631A	*Sprain of interphalangeal joint of left index finger—initial encounter*
S63.632A	*Sprain of interphalangeal joint of right middle finger—initial encounter*
S63.633A	*Sprain of interphalangeal joint of left middle finger—initial encounter*
S63.634A	*Sprain of interphalangeal joint of right ring finger—initial encounter*
S63.635A	*Sprain of interphalangeal joint of left ring finger—initial encounter*
S63.636A	*Sprain of interphalangeal joint of right little finger—initial encounter*
S63.637A	*Sprain of interphalangeal joint of left little finger—initial encounter*
S63.638A	*Sprain of interphalangeal joint of other finger—initial encounter*
S63.639A	*Sprain of interphalangeal joint of unspecified finger—initial encounter*

*****A –** initial encounter
*****B –** subsequent encounter
*****S –** sequela

Key Concepts

- Flexor tendon ruptures from insertion onto the distal phalanx of a digit from a forceful extension on a flexed digit, typically in an athlete grabbing a jersey (Fig. 86.1)
- Occurs most commonly in the ring finger (~75%), but can occur in any finger
  - Ring finger most prominent and longest finger during gripping motion
- Can occur with or without fracture
  - On radiographs, may be a small bony avulsion or large intra-articular fragment
- If seen early, operative repair is indicated
- If missed and patient asymptomatic, no treatment needed

- If missed and a tender palmar mass develops, the tendon stump can be excised
- If missed and the distal interphalangeal (DIP) joint is unstable, it can be fused
- Early referral of suspected jersey finger leads to the best results

History

- The player feels a "pop" in the finger after grabbing another player's jersey.
- Ring finger is involved 75% of the time
- Unable to flex at DIP after injury
  - Injury finger lacks flexion at DIP, therefore it will appear extended relative to the other fingers when a fist is made.
- May describe finger was "jammed" or twisted
- The mechanism is forced extension on the tip of the clenched, flexed digit.
- Often missed acutely and presents late with inability to flex at the DIP joint

Physical Examination

- Largely a clinical diagnosis.
- The resting posture of the hand is disrupted with the injured finger held extended (Fig. 86.2).
- Tender at the insertion of the flexor tendon at the base of the distal phalanx.
- Also tender at the location of the tendon stump.
- Leddy-Packer classification system frequently used:
  - Type I: The tendon retracts into the palm. The tendon is devoid of nourishment from the vincular blood supply or from fluid diffusion from the tendon sheath. Has the most shortening of the tendon
  - Type II: The tendon retracts to the level of PIP (A3 pulley). Vincular blood supply remains intact, tendon is not severely retracted
  - Type III: The tendon retracts to A4 pulley, usually with a large bony piece. Vincular blood supply intact
  - Type IV: The least common type, similar to a type III injury but the tendon is also avulsed from the displaced large bony fragment. Can be seen as a small bony fleck that retracts from the large bony avulsion. Can retract to the palm as in a type I injury
- Unable to actively flex the distal phalanx against resistance

335

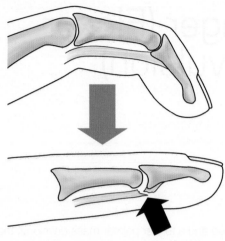

Fig 86.1 When a flexed digit is "jerked" into extension, rupture of the flexor digitorum profundus tendon (jersey finger) can occur.

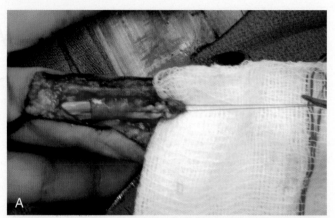

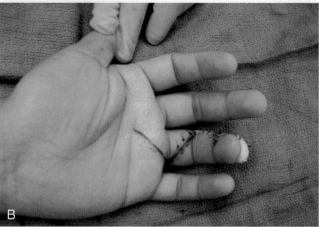

Fig 86.3 (A) Intraoperative photograph of ruptured flexor tendon before final repair. (B) Resting, flexed posture of ring finger restored after surgical repair of flexor digitorum profundus avulsion (jersey finger).

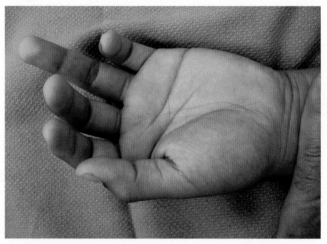

Fig 86.2 Loss of normal flexion posture with ring finger (injured) held in extension.

Imaging

- Plain radiographs of the involved digit will reveal fractures, if present.
- Magnetic resonance imaging can reveal the level of tendon retraction.
  - Magnetic resonance imaging is not needed to make a diagnosis
  - May be useful if the level of tendon is uncertain
  - Can consider ultrasound as well to aid in determining the amount of retraction

Differential Diagnosis

- Phalangeal fractures can cause pain and mimic flexor digitorum profundus avulsion.
  - The patient is unable to flex the DIP joint due to pain
  - Radiographs help make the diagnosis of fracture
  - Fracture can accompany tendon rupture

Treatment

- Tendon retraction and time from injury are key
  - Type I: The tendon is retracted into the palm, and surgical repair is needed within 7 to 10 days due to a compromised blood supply to the tendon
  - Type II: The tendon retracts to the A3 pulley and can be repaired up to 3 months later because the tendon blood supply is largely intact. Typically, it is recommended that the tendon is repaired within 3 weeks
  - Type III: The tendon retracts to the A4 pulley with a bone fragment; the bone fragment should be surgically fixed within 6 weeks
  - Type IV: Largely treated in the same manner as type I
- Early referral to an orthopaedic hand surgeon for surgical repair is the best option (Fig. 86.3).
- Chronic injuries: largely depends on patient's symptoms and functional impairment. Fusion of the joint or excision of the painful tendon stump can be considered. Tendon reconstruction is also an option for patients who required DIP motion.

Patient Instructions

- To restore active DIP flexion, early surgical repair is needed.
- If missed or left untreated, a painful mass (tendon stump) in the palm or a "floppy" DIP joint can develop.
- If a painful palmar mass develops late, it can be excised.
- If a late, unstable DIP joint is bothersome, fusion can help.

Acknowledgment

The author thanks Dr. Jack Ingari for his contribution to this chapter in the last edition.

Suggested Readings

Freilich AM. Evaluation and treatment of Jersey finger and pulley injuries in athletes. *Clin Sports Med.* 2015;34(1):151–166.

Leddy JP. Avulsions of the flexor digitorum profundus. *Hand Clin.* 1985;1: 77–83.

Murphy BA, Mass DP. Zone I flexor tendon injuries. *Hand Clin.* 2005;21: 167–171.

Pannunzio ME. Rugger Jersey finger. *Am J Orthop.* 2004;33:596.

Peterson JJ, Bancroft LW. Injuries of the fingers and thumb in the athlete. *Clin Sports Med.* 2006;25:527–542, vii–viii.

Ruchelsman DE, Christoforou D, Wasserman B, et al. Avulsion injuries of the flexor digitorum profundus tendon. *J Am Acad Orthop Surg.* 2011;19(3):152–162.

Tuttle HG, Olvey SP, Stern PJ. Tendon avulsion injuries of the distal phalanx. *Clin Orthop Relat Res.* 2006;445:157–168.

Chapter 87 Nail Bed Injuries

Monika Debkowska, Jonathan E. Isaacs

ICD-10-CM CODES
S61.3 *Open wound of other finger with damage to nail*
S68.6 *Traumatic transphalangeal amputation of other and unspecified finger*
S62.6 *Fracture of other and unspecified finger(s)*
S60.1 *Contusion of finger with damage to nail*
S60.4 *Other superficial injuries of other fingers*
S60.9 *Unspecified superficial injury of wrist, hand, and fingers*

Key Concepts

- The goal of treatment of nail bed injuries is to restore anatomy which will allow return of function and maximize cosmetic result.
- Anatomy and physiology (Fig. 87.1)
  - The germinal matrix, sterile matrix, and dorsal nail bed make up the nail bed.
    - Germinal matrix: specialized cells that generate the majority of the nail plate; located proximal to the lunula
    - Sterile matrix: contributes to the nail bed; located distal to the germinal matrix, acts to promote nail plate adherence to the nail bed
    - Dorsal nail bed: gives the nail plate its hard, shiny coat
- Nail plate: the "nail"
- Lunula: curved white portion of the proximal nail plate; overlies the distal portion of the germinal matrix
- Eponychium: thin layer of skin that extends over the dorsal nail bed and nail plate, forms the nail fold
- Perionychium: the folds of skin alongside of the nail plate
- Hyponychium: the area between the distal nail plate and skin of the fingertip that acts as a barrier to infection
- Nerve supply to perionychium via dorsal branches of the volar digital nerves
- Arterial supply to the nail via two dorsal branches of the volar digital arteries
- Four primary functions of the fingernail
  - Protection of the fingertip
  - Improved tactile sensation (counterforce)
  - Regulation of peripheral circulation
  - Assist in picking up objects
- The nail plate grows an average of 0.1 mm/day or 100 days for complete growth, but distal growth is halted for 3 weeks as the proximal nail thickens.

History

- Most nail bed injuries occur in children and adolescence.
- Long finger is the most commonly involved digit.

- Mechanism of injury: usually result of a crush or pinching type mechanism.
  - Crush injury to the fingertip results in a compression of the nail bed between the nail and underlying bone, often creating a linear, stellate, or tearing laceration or avulsion injuries of the nail bed.
  - Penetrating injuries through the nail plate result in linear lacerations of the nail bed at the same level.
- Determine when the injury occurred.
- Record comorbidities that may interfere with wound healing.
  - Advise against smoking or use of nicotine products.

Physical Examination

- Look for an obvious (open) or more subtle (closed) injury in which the patient has pain/swelling and hematoma under an intact and adherent nail plate.
- If injury involves more than the nail bed, assess for tissue viability and loss of sensation.
  - The finger should be examined prior to injecting a local block to obtain an accurate neurovascular exam
- May or may not involve the bone (radiograph necessary)

Treatment
Closed Nail Bed Injuries

- Can treat symptomatically or can remove nail plate and repair nail bed
- Regardless of subungual hematoma size and/or fracture, trephination leads to similar cosmetic and functional outcomes with low infection rates and decreased health costs
- Pressure from hematoma under nail plate often very painful
  - Trephination (creation of hematoma drainage hole) with an electrocautery device or a large-bore needle may alleviate discomfort.
    - Heat dissipated by underlying blood
    - 18-Gauge large-bore needle spun like a drill tip until it has gone through the nail plate

Open Nail Bed Injuries

- Nail partially or completely avulsed from nail bed
- If underlying fracture, treat as open fracture with irrigation/débridement and antibiotics (though can be done in emergency room).
- Usually repair of soft tissue is enough to align bone fragments.
- A displaced distal shaft fracture may require pinning (with Kirschner wire or percutaneously placed 20-gauge needle "drilled" across tip of finger by hand).
- Injuries are often intimidating, but after hemostasis is obtained and adequate irrigation performed, the "pieces" will often come together.

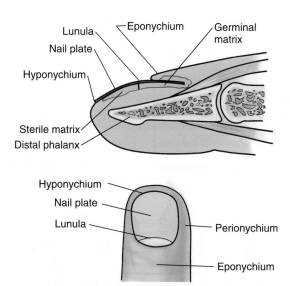

Fig 87.1 Fingertip anatomy.

- Steps to repair
  - Digital block
  - Copious irrigation with saline
  - Prep and drape hand (sterile procedure)
  - Tourniquet control is obtained with a finger Tournicot or a sterile Penrose drain wrapped around the base of the finger.
  - Remove any partially avulsed or remaining nail plate with a hemostat or by separating its connection with the nail bed using a Freer elevator (be careful not to avulse more of the nail bed).
  - Repair the skin surrounding the nail bed with 5-0 nylon sutures first.
  - Repair the nailbed:
    - Meticulously reapproximate the wound edges of the nail bed with a 6-0 tapered chromic suture under loupe magnification.
    - Alternatively, use Histoacryl Blue (monomeric n-butyl-2-cyanoacrylate) or octylcyanoacrylate (Dermabond). Octylcyanoacrylate has superior tensile strength.
      - No differences in cosmetic and functional outcomes exist at 1 year after treatment with suture repair and octylcyanoacrylate tissue adhesive.
      - Using octylcyanoacrylate tissue adhesive heals nailbed wounds significantly faster than suture repair.
  - Place a new "nail plate" to act as a spacer under the nail fold and to splint the nail bed.
    - If the nail plate is mostly intact, it can be cleaned and replaced.
      - Prior to replacing the native nail, create several holes to allow for drainage to prevent infection
    - Other options include:
      - Silicone sheet
      - A piece of the foil packaging from the suture
      - Dry Nu Gauze or Xeroform with the petroleum scraped off (this will absorb some of the blood, dry out, and harden into a protective "nail plate")

- The nail/foil/silicone sheet is held in place with a 5-0 nylon suture that should be removed in 2 weeks (Fig. 87.2).
  - Simple sutures from spacer to eponychium and paronychia
- The wound is dressed with nonadherent gauze (Xeroform or Adaptec) followed by a 2 × 2 gauze patch and a protective aluminum splint held in place with Coban.
- Any injury that involves the germinal matrix (extends proximal to the eponychial fold) will require appropriate exposure of the injured area. The eponychial fold must be incised (45 degrees angle to long axis at the proximal corners) and raised as a proximally based flap. The incisions can be repaired with simple interrupted 5-0 nylon (see Fig. 87.2).
- Treatment of more extensive injury may require referral to a hand specialist.
- In cases of severe crush injury or partial tip amputation with an avulsed nail bed, the nail bed may be protected with a nail plate to allow spontaneous regeneration or reconstructed with:
  - Full- or split-thickness nail bed graft
  - Integra secured with octylcyanoacrylate
  - split thickness skin graft if entire nail bed is avulsed
  - reverse cross finger flap
- Loss of more than 50% of supporting bone (partial amputation) is an indication for nail ablation, which requires the excision of the germinal matrix.

Prognosis

- The final functional and cosmetic outcome depends on the amount of nail bed that remains intact, the severity of the injury, and the patient's comorbidities.
- The patient may, on average, expect full nail growth in approximately 2 to 5 months. There is normally a lag in nail growth after this type of injury. The new nail may have temporary divots, a "hump," or stripes that will usually improve with time.

Complications

- If scar is present due to inappropriate alignment of lacerated edges, nail deformities are likely to occur.
- If the eponychium is damaged, the nail may look dull.
- Eponychium fusing with germinal matrix can lead to fissured nail and tender scar.
- Scarring of the germinal matrix can lead to split nail or absence of the nail.
- Sterile matrix damage can lead to nonadherence (onycholysis) of the nail.
- Bone spur or uneven nail bed can lead to nail ridge.
- If the lateral skin groove is not maintained it can lead to ingrown nails.

Considerations in Special Populations

- Pediatric nail bed injuries typically require the involvement of a hand surgeon.
  - More likely to need conscious sedation or a trip to the operating room for repair.

4

Nail Bed Injuries

Closed Injuries:
- Treat symptomatically, with trephination or as an open injury

Open Injuries:
- If underlying fracture, treat as open fracture with I&D and antibiotics
- Irrigate, remove nail plate, repair nail bed
  - Chromic suture or octylcyanoacrylate
- Secure new "nail plate"
- Evaluate germinal matrix if involved

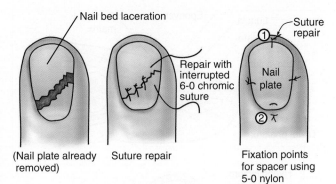

(Nail plate already removed)   Suture repair   Fixation points for spacer using 5-0 nylon

Nail bed laceration · Repair with interrupted 6-0 chromic suture · Suture repair · Nail plate

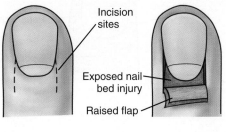

Incision sites · Exposed nail bed injury · Raised flap

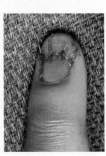

Remove nail plate.   Evaluate nail bed injury.   Use chromic suture to repair nail bed.

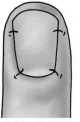 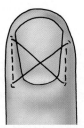 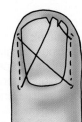

Secure nail plate with either simple sutures, X-shaped suture, or transverse figure of eight suture.

Fig 87.2 Treating nail bed injuries.

- Consider a more restrictive dressing (such as a cast) to prevent disruption or contamination of the repair.
- Seymour fractures—suspected with proximal nail avulsion or widening of physis. Nail must be removed with adequate irrigation and debridement, splinting, or possible pinning for reduction and stability.
- Acrylic nails/ultraviolet (UV) gel nail polish
  - Harbor pathogens.
  - Mask nail bed injury.
  - If pain/swelling over the fingertip with concerning mechanism treat with high suspicion. Remove acrylic nail/gel nail polish to adequately assess the fingertip.

Patient Instructions

- Hand elevation to decrease swelling and pain
- Leave the dressing intact until return appointment to minimize disruption to the repair.

- Avoid getting the repaired site dirty or wet; avoid using the injured extremity until cleared to do so by the physician.

Suggested Readings

Brown R, Zook E, Russell R. Fingertip reconstruction with flaps and nail bed grafts. *J Hand Surg Am*. 1999;24A:345–351.

Dean B, Becker G, Little C. The management of the acute traumatic subungual haematoma: a systematic review. *Hand Surg*. 2012;17:151–154.

Meek S, White M. Subungual hematomas: is simple trephining enough? *J Accid Emerg Med*. 1998;l5:269–271.

Richards A, Crick A, Cole R. A novel method of securing the nail following nail bed repair. *Plast Reconstr Surg*. 1999;103:1983–1985.

Roser S, Gellman H. Comparison of nail bed repair versus nail trephination for subungual hematomas in children. *J Hand Surg Am*. 1999;24A:1166–1170.

Chapter 88 Dupuytren Contracture

Blane Kelly, Jonathan E. Isaacs

ICD-10-CM CODE
M72.0 *Contracture of palmer fascia*

Key Concepts

- Slowly progressive fibroproliferative disease of the palmar fascia (Fig. 88.1)
- Results in characteristic cord and nodule formation in the palm and fingers
- Usually painless but can result in digital flexion contractures, which may inhibit function
- The only current treatment (not cure) is surgical.
- Demographics
  - More prevalent in persons of Northern European descent
  - 5-15% of men in the United States older than 50 are affected.
  - More common in males (80%)
  - Males often have an earlier onset and more aggressive disease progression.
  - Bilateral involvement 65% of the time
- Etiology
  - Multifaceted and not completely understood
    - Genetic predisposition: positive family history in 27-68% of patients
    - Immunologic or benign neoplastic changes in the palmar fascia
    - Trauma
    - The palmar subdermal fat pads undergo age-related thinning in the populations most prone to Dupuytren contracture. This may expose the underlying fascia to repetitive traumatic shear and compression forces that may trigger an excessive reparative process in the palmar fascia leading to Dupuytren-type changes.
- Associated conditions
  - Diabetes mellitus
  - Alcoholism
  - Human immunodeficiency virus infection
  - Epilepsy (antiseizure medication)
  - Trauma
  - Manual labor
  - Cigarette smoking
  - Previous myocardial infarction

History

- Insidious onset and progression
- Painless cord and nodule-like thickenings in the palm that may extend into the digits
- Nodules are occasionally tender.
- Flexion contractures of the involved fingers progress with time and cord formation.

- In nondiabetic patients, the ring and little fingers are most commonly affected and the thumb and index finger are least involved.
- Diabetic patients usually have more predominant involvement of the radial side of the hand.

Physical Examination (Fig. 88.2)

- Firm palpable nodules in the distal palm and fingers. Palpable painless cords extending from the midpalm toward and into the fingers.
- Palmar skin in the diseased area blanches on finger extension.
- Grooves or pits in the palmar skin denoting adherence to the underlying diseased fascia.
- Tender knuckle pads (Garrod pads) over the dorsal aspect of the proximal interphalangeal joints may be seen in more aggressive disease.
- Metacarpophalangeal or proximal interphalangeal joint flexion contractures with possible compensatory distal interphalangeal joint hyperextension contracture; alternatively, the distal interphalangeal joints may not be involved or are rarely part of flexion contracture.
- Other manifestations
  - Plantar fascia: Ledderhose disease
  - Darto fascia: Peyronie disease

Stages of Dupuytren Contracture

- Proliferative: The most biologically active stage characterized by the development of nodules composed of fibroblasts and type III collagen
- Involutional: Cords and skin pits develop as normal palmar fibroblasts transform into myofibroblasts. These cells deposit collagen, which thickens the cords and has contractile components that draw the tissue tightly together and pull the fingers down.
- Residual: The most biologically quiescent phase is characterized by nodular regression but also metacarpophalangeal joint and proximal interphalangeal joint contractures. Tendon-like cords are visible underlying the palmar skin and contain densely packed inelastic, longitudinally oriented, predominantly type I collagen fibers. At this stage, relatively few cells remain.

Surgical Anatomy of the Diseased Palmar Fascia

- A normal anatomic structure, the central aponeurosis, is the core of Dupuytren disease activity.
  - Triangular fascial layer with its apex proximal.
  - Fibers are oriented longitudinally, transversely, and vertically.

- The longitudinal fibers fan out as pretendinous bands toward the digits, and each bifurcates distally.
- Each bifurcation has three layers: A superficial layer inserts into the dermis; a middle layer continues to the digit as the spiral band; and a deep layer passes almost vertically and dorsally.
- Transverse fibers make up the natatory ligament located in the distal part of the palm and the transverse ligament of the palmar aponeurosis.
- In Dupuytren disease, normal fascial structures (referred to as bands) become thickened and contracted and are referred to as cords (Fig. 88.3).

Types of Cords and Their Relationship to Neurovascular Anatomy

- Central cord
  - Direct extension of the pretendinous band in the palm that remains directly subcutaneous.
  - Lies between the neurovascular bundles.
  - Distally, the cord usually (but not always) attaches asymmetrically to the tendon sheath and periosteum of the middle phalanx.
- Spiral cord (Fig. 88.4)
  - Arises from the pretendinous fibers of the palmar fascia.
  - Runs behind the neurovascular bundles just distal to the metacarpophalangeal joint and joins the lateral digital sheet to insert on the flexor sheath of the middle phalanx.
  - Spirals around the neurovascular bundle displacing it medially, centrally, and superficially (rendering it at risk during surgery).
  - Usually causes severe proximal interphalangeal joint contracture.
- Lateral cord
  - Involves the lateral digital sheet and natatory ligament.
  - Attaches primarily to the skin and generally does not cause severe proximal interphalangeal joint contracture.

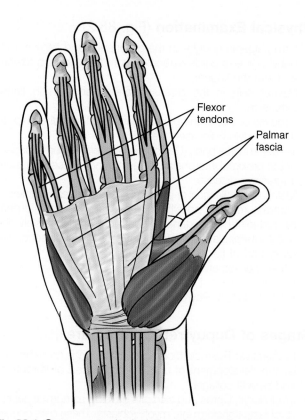

Fig 88.1 Gross anatomic depiction of palmar fascia.

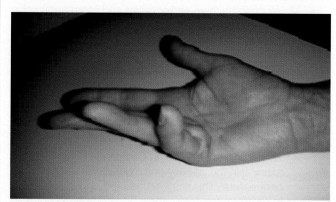

Fig 88.2 Nodule-like and cordlike changes in the ring and little fingers resulting in characteristic flexion contractures of the involved digits. (Courtesy of Bobby Chhabra, MD.)

Fig 88.3 Normal palmar and digital fascial structures become nodular and contractile, resulting in characteristic finger contractures and palpable cords.

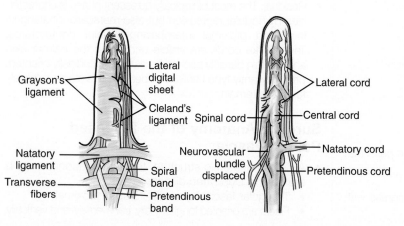

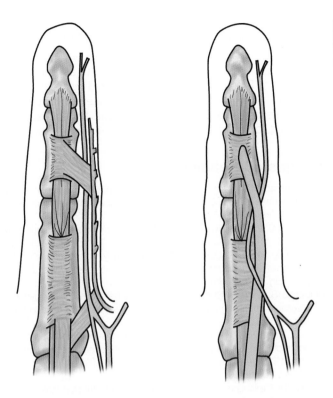

Fig 88.4 The spiral cord wraps around the digital neurovascular bundle and pulls it superficial and midline. This puts the bundle at risk during surgical dissection.

- Does not disturb the neurovascular bundle except that its bulk can push the bundle toward the midline.
- A distal extension of the lateral cord can rarely cause distal interphalangeal joint contracture.
- Abductor cord
  - In the little finger, a cord coming off the abductor digiti minimi muscle is often found on the ulnar border of the finger.
  - This may lead to contracture of the distal interphalangeal joint of the little finger.

Treatment

- Nonsurgical
  - There is no consistently successful nonsurgical/nonprocedural treatment option.
- Surgical
  - The goal of surgical treatment is to excise or incise the diseased fascia to relieve contractures—not to cure the disease.
  - Surgery is indicated with metacarpophalangeal joint contracture of 30 degrees or more (patient is unable to place the hand flat onto the tabletop [table test]) or when any proximal interphalangeal joint contractures are observed (and functionally inhibitive).
- Procedures
  - Fasciotomy involves incising (not excising) the involved fascia.

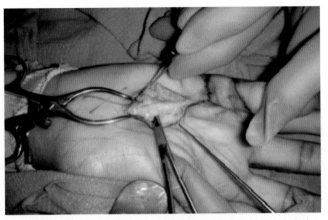

Fig 88.5 Intraoperative view of the diseased palmar fascia being excised. (Courtesy of Bobby Chhabra, MD.)

- Provides more temporary relief but with less surgical morbidity.
- Needle fasciotomy involves percutaneous release of Dupuytren cords using the bevel of a needle through the skin.
  - 80% good short-term relief
  - recurrence rate of 50% at 3 to 5 years
- Collagenase is a metalloprotease enzyme isolated from clostridium histolyticum.
  - Two-step process: (1) injection of collagenase directly into cord; (2) manipulation (into extension) 24 to 72 hours later.
  - Recurrence rate of 19% at 2 to 5 years.
  - Collagenase injections and percutaneous needle fasciotomy have similar short-term outcomes.
- Dermofasciectomy: radical excision of diseased fascia and overlying skin. The wound is either left open to heal secondarily (open palm technique) or resurfaced with a full-thickness skin graft. Usually reserved for recurrent or severe disease but recurrence rates are lower.
- Regional fasciectomy (most widely used surgical procedure): excision of grossly involved fascia (Fig. 88.5).
  - Better at correcting metacarpophalangeal joint contractures then proximal interphalangeal joint contractures; carries an acceptably low morbidity rate.
- Dynamic external fixators may be used as an adjuvant to surgical release in a patient with severe contractures.
- Amputation of an absolutely nonfunctional digit that has failed to respond to previously mentioned therapies remains an option.
- Postoperative
  - Rehabilitation is a gradual process of increased activity and decreased splinting to achieve optimal restoration of movement.
    - Frequent visits to the occupational therapist help to restore preoperative flexion and to maintain extension gained at the time of surgery.
    - Patient motivation and severity of disease dictate the intensity and duration of therapy.
- Final results are realized in approximately 6 to 12 weeks.

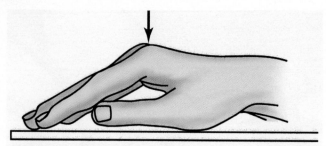

Fig 88.6 The table test. When the patient can no longer place his or her hand flat on a tabletop, it is time to refer the patient.

Complications

- The incidence of complications is 20%.
- The most common complications are postoperative joint stiffness and loss of preoperative flexion. Other complications include hematoma, skin loss, infection, nerve injury, vascular injury, prolonged edema, and reflex sympathetic dystrophy.
- Collagenase injection complications include injury to digital nerve or artery (higher in recurrent disease), hematoma, skin tears.

Prognosis

- The long-term overall recurrence rate is approximately 50% and can be in the same area of the hand or in a new area.
- Metacarpophalangeal joint contractures are readily corrected with surgery (80%).
- Proximal interphalangeal joint contractures are usually not completely corrected (20-56% are corrected).

When to Refer

- Observation is the mainstay of early treatment, and referral is not necessary until surgery is indicated by the inability to place the hand flat on a table (table test) (Fig. 88.6).

Considerations in Special Populations

- A subset of patients has a more aggressive and rapidly progressive form of the disease referred to as Dupuytren diathesis. These patients are characterized by onset before age 40, a positive family history, and bilateral involvement. These patients have a poor prognosis with limited response to surgical treatment and a high rate of recurrence.

Suggested Readings

Badalamente MA, Hurst LC. Efficacy and safety of injectable mixed collagenase subtypes in the treatment of Dupuytren's contracture. *J Hand Surg Am*. 2007;32A:767–774.

Black EM, Blazar PE. Dupuytren disease: an evolving understanding of an age-old disease. *J Am Acad Orthop Surg*. 2011;19(12):746–757.

Cordova A, Tripoli M, Corradino B, et al. Dupuytren's contracture: an update of biomolecular aspects and therapeutic perspectives. *J Hand Surg [Br]*. 2005;30B:557–562.

Hindocha S, John S, Stanley JK, et al. The heritability of Dupuytren's disease: familial aggregation and its clinical significance. *J Hand Surg Am*. 2006;31A:204–210.

Loos B, Puschkin V, Horch RE. 50 years experience with Dupuytren's contracture in the erlangen university Hospital—a retrospective analysis of 2919 operated hands from 1956 to 2006. *BMC Musculoskelet Disord*. 2007;8:60.

Rayan GM. Clinical presentation and types of Dupuytren's disease. *Hand Clin*. 1999;15:87–96, vii.

Rayan GM. Dupuytren's disease: anatomy, pathology, presentation, and treatment. *Instr Course Lect*. 2007;56:101–111.

Reilly RM, Stern PJ, Goldfarb CA. A retrospective review of the management of Dupuytren's nodules. *J Hand Surg Am*. 2005;30A:1014–1018.

Shaw RB Jr, Chong AK, Zhang A, et al. Dupuytren's disease: history, diagnosis, and treatment. *Plast Reconstr Surg*. 2007;120:44e–54e.

Chapter 89 Hand Tumors

Dan A. Zlotolow

ICD-10-CM CODES

C40.10	*Chondrosarcoma*
C49.10	*Epithelioid sarcoma*
C43.60	*Melanoma*
D16.00	*Giant cell tumor of bone*
D16.10	*Osteochondroma*
D16.10	*Enchondroma*
D17.30	*Lipoma*
D18.01	*Glomus tumor*
D18.01	*Hemangioma*
M19.049	*Carpometacarpal boss*
D48.1	*Giant cell tumor of the tendon sheath*
M65.849	*Tenosynovitis*
M67.449	*Retinacular cyst*
R22.9	*Epidermal inclusion cyst*

Key Concepts

- Most tumors in the hand are benign.
- Painful or fast-growing tumors need an urgent workup.
- Intraosseous tumors are common and can lead to fracture with minor trauma.
- Expansile bone lesions, even if benign, can be aggressive.
- A dark streak in the fingernail of a light-skinned person is a subungual melanoma until proven otherwise.
- Most malignancies in the hand involve the skin.
- Solid tumors do not transilluminate.
- The diagnosis needs to be certain before the problem is treated with "observation."

History

- The growth rate of the tumor is important for identifying aggressive lesions.
- Previous trauma can cause deformity that can mimic a tumor.
- Minor injury resulting in a fracture is suspicious for an enchondroma.
- Inflammatory arthropathies with boggy synovitis or tenosynovitis can mimic periarticular or peritendinous tumors.
- History of tophaceous gout
- Northern European (Viking) ancestry, antiseizure medications, smoking, and alcohol abuse history consistent with Dupuytren disease

Physical Examination

- Overlying skin changes (lesions involving the skin are of concern for malignancy)
- Coloration (hemangiomas have a blue tint)

- Pulse/bruit (vascular malformations and aneurysms)
- Consistency (giant cell tumors of the tendon sheath and tenosynovitis are boggy, lipomas are firm in one direction and fluctuant in the other, cysts and bony masses are firm)
- Transillumination with a penlight (only positive in clear fluid-filled masses such as ganglia and early tenosynovitis)
- Adherence to underlying tissues (mobile discrete masses tend to be benign)
- Glomus tumors demonstrate pinpoint tenderness, are most common under the nail, have a slight bluish tint, and cause pain with exposure to ice-cold water (Fig. 89.1).
- Tinel sign (tapping over the mass creates shooting pain in the nerve distribution) indicates a neural tumor or neuroma.
- Look for signs of infection (blanching erythema, induration, warmth, fluctuance).

Imaging

- Enchondromas often present as incidental findings on radiographs (Fig. 89.2).
- Look for scalloping/expansion of the bone cortex (indicates an aggressive lesion).
- Expansile lesions of bone (enchondroma, aneurysmal bone cyst, giant cell tumor of bone, chondrosarcoma)
- Periarticular masses can be evaluated with radiographs, which typically demonstrate degenerative changes in a joint with large osteophytes in patients with osteoarthritis or joint erosions with a soft-tissue mass in patients with inflammatory arthropathies.
- Magnetic resonance imaging with or without contrast medium may demonstrate lesion if large enough; useful for glomus tumors, hemangiomas, tenosynovitis, and lipomas
- Angiography to identify aneurysms, hemangiomas, and arteriovenous malformations

Additional Tests

- White blood cell count, platelet count, erythrocyte sedimentation rate, and C-reactive protein to differentiate a tumor from an infection
- Uric acid levels and joint aspiration to rule out gout
- Rheumatoid panel to evaluate for rheumatoid arthritis

Differential Diagnosis

- Please see Table 89.1.

Treatment

- At diagnosis
  - If lesion is stable in size, does not cause pain, and is mobile, patient reassurance is indicated

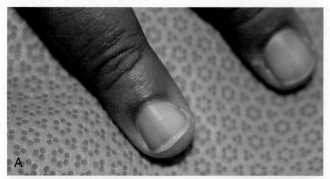

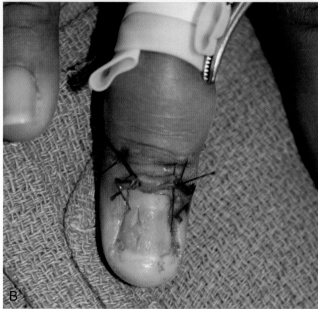

Fig 89.1 Glomus tumors are most common under the nail plate and classically present with a slight bluish tint, cold sensitivity, and severe point tenderness. Note the subtle appearance clinically (A) and the typical tumor size intraoperatively (B).

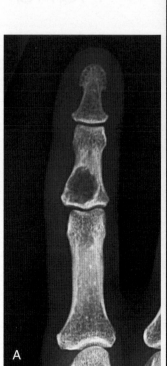

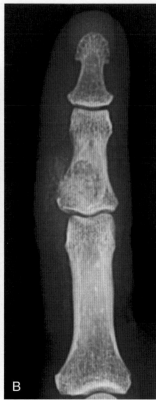

Fig 89.2 Enchondromas are either incidental findings on radiographs or present with pain (impending fracture) (A) or a pathologic fracture. Although these lesions meet many radiographic and histologic criteria for malignant lesions, they are overwhelmingly benign. Simple curettage and bone grafting are usually curative (B).

- Later
  - Regular periods of observation, initially every 3 to 6 months, are warranted, with eventual yearly checkups if the mass does not change.

When to Refer

- Any lesion involving the skin requires a referral to a dermatologist and/or a hand surgeon to rule out a malignancy.
- Any patient with a lesion that changes in character or size, causes pain, is rigidly fixed to underlying tissues, or does not transilluminate should be referred to a hand surgeon.

Prognosis

- Most masses in the hand are benign and have a good prognosis.
- Even malignant lesions, if caught early, can typically be cured with wide excision.

Patient Instructions

- Enchondroma
  - If the tumor is an incidental radiographic finding, explain to the patient that these benign tumors can be found in up to 30% of the population and that no treatment is necessary.
  - If the tumor is painful or associated with fracture, refer the patient to a hand surgeon urgently with reassurance that the prognosis is good.
- Retinacular cyst
  - If the cyst is small or painless, explain that the mass is a marker of a minor injury to the flexor sheath of the finger and that the mass may disappear on its own.
  - If the cyst is large or painful, refer the patient to a hand surgeon for aspiration or excision.
- Epidermal inclusion cyst
  - A benign mass composed of incarcerated skin keratin that may be self-limited or exhibit periodic episodes of worsening, then resolving, pain
  - It can be removed if symptomatic, and recurrence is rare.
- Extensor tenosynovitis
  - If the mass is painless or recent, reassure the patient that the mass will likely go away on its own but that

TABLE 89.1 Differential Diagnosis

Differential Diagnosis	Differentiating Feature	Chapter Reference
Chondrosarcoma	Firm mass, stippled calcification on radiograph, cartilage on magnetic resonance imaging	89
Epithelioid sarcoma	Can be confused with Dupuytren nodule; look for ulcerations	89
Melanoma	Pigmented skin lesion	89
Giant cell tumor of bone	Expansile epiphyseal lesion	89
Osteochondroma	Epiphyseal or metaphyseal lesion of cartilage and bone growing away from the physis	893
Enchondroma (see Fig. 89.2)	Expansile cartilaginous mass	89
Lipoma	Firm in one direction, fluctuant in the other	89
Glomus tumor (see Fig. 89.1)	Pinpoint tenderness, bluish, cold intolerance	89
Hemangioma	Bluish tint	89
Carpometacarpal boss (Fig. 89.3)	Firm mass over carpometacarpal joints	89
Giant cell tumor of the tendon sheath	Boggy, dark on all magnetic resonance imaging sequences, high hemosiderin content	89
Dupuytren nodule (Fig. 89.4)	Firm nonulcerating cord in palm or digit along fascial tracks	88
Tenosynovitis (Fig. 89.5)	Boggy, moves with the tendons, can transilluminate	77
Retinacular cyst	Firm, transilluminable mass over tendon sheath	77
Epidermal inclusion cyst	Pattern of enlarging and shrinking, filled with keratin	89
Traumatic nail bed deformity	Ridging or split of the nail associated with an injury to the nail bed	87
Neuroma	Positive Tinel sign over tumor	89
Arthritis	Pain with joint motion, osteophytes, and loss of joint space on radiograph	73
Gout	Uric acid crystal deposits, multiarticular, tophi	15

a persistent or painful mass can damage the extensor tendons and lead to delayed tendon rupture.
  - If the mass is painful or long-standing, refer the patient to a hand surgeon urgently to excise the mass before tendon rupture occurs.
- Hemangioma
  - If the lesion is painless, reassure the patient.
  - If the lesion is painful, refer the patient to a hand surgeon for excision.
- Chondrosarcoma
  - Most lesions are low grade and rarely metastasize.
  - An urgent referral to an oncologist and a hand surgeon is required.
- Giant cell tumor of the tendon sheath
  - Can degrade the tendon and should be removed if painful
- Giant cell tumor
  - Can be aggressive benign lesion and should be evaluated by an oncologist
  - Often requires a wide excision to effect a cure
- Osteochondroma
  - Benign lesions that can cause tendon or local tissue irritation
  - Can be removed if symptomatic, but malignant transformation uncommon in solitary lesion
- Melanoma
  - Inform the patient of the need for an urgent dermatologic evaluation.

- Epithelioid sarcoma
  - Despite its benign appearance, it can be a very aggressive malignancy.
  - Requires wide excision and lymph node biopsy
- Lipoma
  - Benign tumor that can be observed or removed if unsightly
- Carpometacarpal boss
  - An osteophyte at the carpometacarpal joint that can be removed if painful
- Glomus tumor
  - Removal is effective in relieving pain.
  - Recurrence is rare, but a second primary tumor may develop.

Considerations in Special Populations

- Gout
  - Tophaceous gout can cause large and sometimes ulcerating lesions filled with a white uric acid paste that is the consistency of toothpaste.
- Rheumatoid arthritis
  - Rheumatoid nodules can be firm and mimic soft-tissue tumors.
  - Periarticular synovitis can cause large, painful soft-tissue masses.
  - Tenosynovitis can be particularly aggressive and result in early tendon rupture.

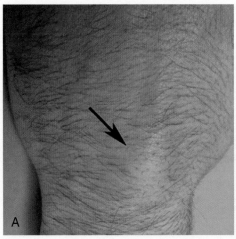
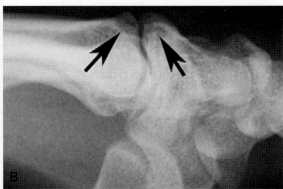

Fig 89.3 A carpometacarpal boss *(arrows)* is a benign exostosis at the second or third carpometacarpal joint and is often confused with a dorsal wrist ganglion. The differentiating features are its more distal location (A) and its more firm and immobile character on palpation. Radiographs will show the typical "volcano" appearance of the carpometacarpal joint (B). (From Park MJ, Namdari S, Weiss APC. The carpal boss: review of diagnosis and treatment. *J Hand Surg Am*. 2008;33A:446–449.)

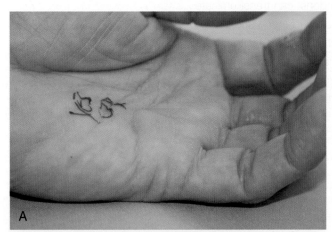
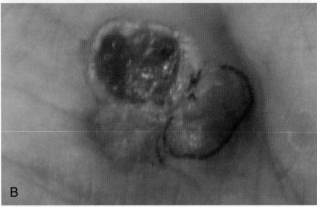

Fig 89.4 A Dupuytren nodule is often mistaken for a soft-tissue tumor (A). Be aware that epithelioid sarcomas can present with a similar appearance, although ulcerations and pain are differentiating factors (B). ([B] From Pai KK, Pai SB, Sripathi H, et al. Epithelioid sarcoma: a diagnostic challenge. *Indian J Dermatol Venereol Leprol*. 2006;72:446–448.)

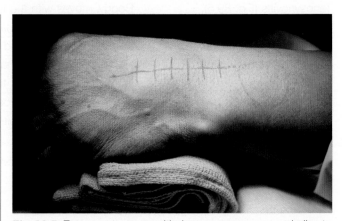

Fig 89.5 Extensor tenosynovitis has an appearance similar to that of dorsal wrist ganglia. However, tenosynovitis is marked by proximal termination at the extensor retinaculum, motion with extensor tendon motion, and a softer consistency on palpation.

- Osteoarthritis
  - Osteophytes can resemble firm, immobile tumors near joints.
  - Associated synovial cysts can develop as part of a degenerative process.
  - Radiographic evaluation to differentiate from other tumors

Suggested Readings

Bos GD, Pritchard DJ, Reiman HM, et al. Epithelioid sarcoma. An analysis of fifty-one cases. *J Bone Joint Surg Am*. 1988;70A: 862–870.

Buecker PJ, Villafuerte JE, Hornicek FJ, et al. Improved survival for sarcomas of the wrist and hand. *J Hand Surg Am*. 2006;31A: 452–455.

Harness NG, Mankin HJ. Giant-cell tumor of the distal forearm. *J Hand Surg Am*. 2004;29A:188–193.

Jewusiak EM, Spence KF, Sell KW. Solitary benign enchondroma of the long bones of the hand: results of curettage and packing with freeze-dried cancellous bone allograft. *J Bone Joint Surg Am*. 1971;53A: 1587–1590.

McDermott EM, Weiss APC. Glomus tumors. *J Hand Surg Am*. 2006;31A: 1397–1400.

O'Connor MI, Bancroft LW. Benign and malignant cartilage tumors of the hand. *Hand Clin*. 2004;20:317–323.

Park MJ, Namdari S, Weiss APC. The carpal boss: review of diagnosis and treatment. *J Hand Surg Am*. 2008;33A:446–449.

Rizzo M, Beckenbaugh RD. Treatment of mucous cysts of the fingers: review of 134 cases with minimum 2-year follow-up evaluation. *J Hand Surg Am*. 2003;28(3):519–524.

Simon M, Finn H. Diagnostic strategy for bone and soft tissue tumors. *J Bone Joint Surg Am*. 1993;75A:622–631.

Chapter 90 Hand Infections

Robert P. Waugh, Dan A. Zlotolow

ICD-10-CM CODES
L02.529	*Carbuncle and furuncle, hand (finger, thumb, wrist)*
L03.019	*Felon (pulp abscess or whitlow excluding herpetic whitlow)*
L03.019	*Onychia and paronychia of finger*
M65.849	*Other tenosynovitis of hand and wrist*

Key Concepts

- Acute infections of the hand can present as surgical emergencies.
- Common hand infections include those of the skin (cellulitis, soft-tissue abscesses), the nail (paronychia), or the fingertip pulp (felon).
- More serious but less common infections include those of the flexor tendon sheath (pyogenic flexor tenosynovitis) and necrotizing fasciitis.
- It is important and sometimes difficult to distinguish between inflammatory and infectious processes.
- Infections are influenced substantially by host factors contributing to immunocompromise, including diabetes, human immunodeficiency virus, alcoholism, malnutrition, and steroid use.
- Treatment of pyogenic infection is directed toward identifying the pathogen (holding antibiotics until a culture is taken), as well as decompressing and draining any infected fluid collections.
- More serious hand infections require emergent referral to a hand surgeon for definitive management; these include necrotizing fasciitis, pyogenic flexor tenosynovitis, deep space abscesses, and joint infections.
- Never culture an open wound because this will only grow the patient's colonizing skin flora. A true culture can only be obtained from a wound that you have created after the skin has been prepped.
- Persistent infections should be evaluated for osteomyelitis.

History

- Pertinent parts of the patient's medical history include identifying any risk factors for immunocompromise as well as the tetanus immunization status.
- Patients may be able to recall the precipitating factors leading to infection, which can be of help in planning operative management and directing antibiotic treatment (e.g., dog bites vs. intravenous (IV) drug injections vs. rusty nails).

- Patients with gout or other inflammatory arthritides may present similarly to those with infection and will usually improve with nonsteroidal antiinflammatory drugs.
- They should be monitored closely for the first 24 to 48 hours for improvement to ensure that the diagnosis is correct.
- Injuries in patients who present with a "fight bite" laceration on their metacarpophalangeal joint are very likely to be intra-articular given the proximity of the joint capsule to the skin in a clenched fist.
- These innocuous-looking wounds require surgical exploration (Fig. 90.1).

Physical Examination

- Infections present with erythema, pain, and tenderness in the affected area.
  - The examiner should evaluate the area for fluctuance or induration to distinguish cellulitis from an underlying abscess.
- Paronychia, the most common hand infection, presents with erythema and tenderness along the nail fold and can progress to an abscess in this space (Fig. 90.2A).
- The anatomy of a fingertip infection (felon) (Fig. 90.3) may obscure the diagnosis because these deep infections can present with pain and moderate swelling only, without evidence of underlying pus.
- Felons require incision and decompression (see Fig. 90.2B).
- Watch for Kanavel four cardinal signs of pyogenic flexor tenosynovitis; all four must be present to make the diagnosis (this is a surgical emergency!):
  - Fusiform swelling of the entire digit
  - Extreme tenderness along the course of the flexor tendon
  - Exquisite pain on passive extension of the finger
  - A resting position of the finger in a semiflexed position
- Deep space infections present with swelling of the entire hand, usually more pronounced dorsally. In addition, wide thumb abduction, semiflexed fingers, and isolated swelling of the hypothenar area suggest fluid collection in these spaces.

Imaging

- Plain radiographs are an important part of the evaluation of hand infections. It is vital to identify foreign objects such as hypodermic needles or tooth fragments, as well as gas collections in the wound. Plain radiographs can also reveal underlying fractures and osteomyelitis.
- Although a good history and physical examination usually obviate the need for advanced imaging studies, computed

tomography can be helpful in identifying deep fluid collections in some cases.

- Magnetic resonance imaging should be performed if radiographs do not show evidence of osteomyelitis, but the suspicion remains high.

Additional Tests

- Laboratory tests should include
  - Complete blood count with manual differentiation
  - C-reactive protein

- Erythrocyte sedimentation rate
- The white blood cell (WBC) count may be normal, especially in long-standing infections.
- C-reactive protein and erythrocyte sedimentation rate are nonspecific infection markers that help to establish a baseline value that the clinician can follow over time. Infection markers that do not decrease or begin to increase after treatment suggest a residual or recurrent infection.
- Erythrocyte sedimentation rate and C-reactive protein will also be increased in inflammatory conditions.
- A random glucose level may reveal previously undiagnosed diabetes, a condition that predisposes one to infection and complicates healing.

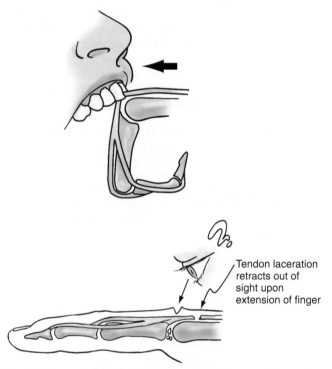

Fig 90.1 A punch to the mouth accompanied by a small laceration near the metacarpophalangeal joint should raise suspicion of a fight bite. This injury is characterized by its benign appearance and severe sequelae, which can include tendon rupture, septic arthritis, and osteomyelitis. (Modified from Carter PR. *Common Hand Injuries and Infections. A Practical Approach to Early Management.* Philadelphia: WB Saunders; 1983:206.)

Tendon laceration retracts out of sight upon extension of finger

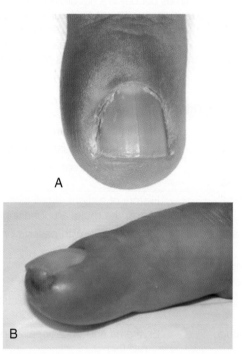

Fig 90.2 Clinical appearance of a paronychia (A) and a felon (B). ([A] From Rigopoulos D, Larios G, Gregoriou S, et al. Acute and chronic paronychia. *Am Fam Physician.* 2008;77:341; [B] from Clark D. Common acute hand infections. *Am Fam Physician.* 2003;68:2170.)

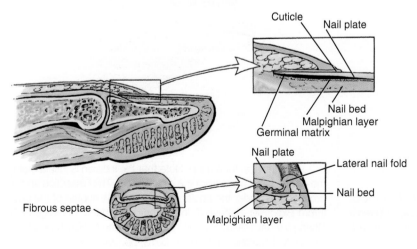

Cuticle
Nail plate
Nail bed
Malpighian layer
Germinal matrix
Nail plate
Lateral nail fold
Nail bed
Malpighian layer
Fibrous septae

Fig 90.3 Anatomy of the fingertip. Note the fibrous septae in the fingertip pulp that must be transected to decompress a felon. The nail is a modified hair that grows at the rate of 1 mm per week. Infections deep to the eponychium and the lateral nail fold (paronychia) can be drained by elevating the eponychial fold bluntly and the lateral fold sharply with a blade pointing away from the center of the nail. (Modified from Carter PR. *Common Hand Injuries and Infections. A Practical Approach to Early Management.* Philadelphia: WB Saunders; 1983:37.)

Differential Diagnosis

- Please see Table 90.1.

Treatment

- In the office or emergency department
  - Acute paronychia
    - Drain by using a blade pointing away from the center of the nail and opening the lateral nail fold and bluntly elevating the eponychial fold from the nail plate to evacuate the exudate. Obtain a sample for culture. Pack the nail fold open (Fig. 90.4).
    - After drainage, the patient should soak the finger two to three times per day in a hot diluted povidone-iodine solution and change the wet-to-dry dressings also two to three times daily. Once-daily dry dressings are appropriate after 3 or 4 days when the incision has stopped draining.
    - Place the patient on 7 to 10 days of oral antibiotics.

TABLE 90.1 Differential Diagnosis

Condition	Differentiating Feature
Local abscess	Demarcated fluctuance or induration
Deep space abscess	Swelling of the entire hand, especially dorsally
"Fight bite"	History of fistfight, small laceration over the metacarpophalangeal joint
Septic arthritis	Exquisite pain with passive or active motion of the joint
Pyogenic flexor tenosynovitis	Positive Kanavel signs
Felon	Swelling and tenderness distal to the distal interphalangeal joint
Paronychia	Erythema and occasionally pus at the nail fold
Gout	History of gout, improvement with nonsteroidal antiinflammatory drugs

- Felons
  - Under digital block, carry the incision down the side of the finger away from the thumb except for the small finger, where the incision should be made facing the thumb. Begin your incision 0.5 cm distal to the distal interphalangeal crease and stop just as the finger starts to curve toward the fingertip (Fig. 90.5A).
  - Open the incision bluntly; the palmar aspect of the distal phalanx is the roof of the incision deeply. Spread down into the pulp to break up the septae containing the infection (see Fig. 90.5B). Culture and then irrigate the wound.
  - Pack the wound open with iodoform gauze and have the patient change the dressing two to three times daily for 3 to 4 days and then convert to once-daily dry dressings.
  - Place the patient on 7 to 10 days of oral antibiotics.
  - Have the patient follow up in approximately 5 days for a wound check.
- Local abscesses
  - Treat these abscesses in a fashion similar to that for abscesses elsewhere in the body.
  - Carry the incision across the abscess through the skin sharply and expose the abscess space bluntly. Use an adequate incision to expose the entire abscess. Evacuate all infected contents and irrigate the wound. Do not attempt to drain volar hand abscesses in the office.
  - Pack the wound open with iodoform gauze and have the patient change the dressing two to three times daily for 3 to 4 days and then convert to once-daily dry dressings.

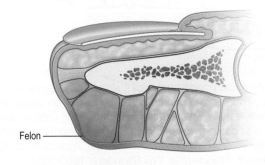

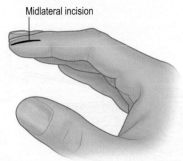

Felon

Midlateral incision

Fig 90.5 Incision for a felon. Note that the incision is just lateral to the nail fold and away from the digital nerve. The dissection should proceed just under the phalanx to open all the septae of the pulp. (From Bidic SM, Schaub T. Infections of the hand. In Neligan PC, Chang J (Eds). *Plastic Surgery*, 3rd ed. *Volume 6: Hand and Upper Extremity*. Philadelphia, Elsevier, 2013, pp. 333-345.)

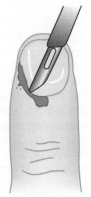

Fig 90.4 Incision for paronychia involving the lateral nail fold. (From Marx JA, Hockberger RS, Walls RM (Eds): *Rosen's Emergency Medicine: Concepts and Clinical Practice*. 8th ed. Philadelphia, Elsevier, 2014.)

- Place the patient on 7 to 10 days of oral antibiotics.
- Have the patient follow up in approximately 5 days for a wound check.

When to Refer

- Patients who exhibit Kanavel signs, show evidence of deep space infections, or have puncture wounds that enter joints are likely to require surgical exploration, débridement, and irrigation. These patients should be referred to a hand surgeon that day. Refrain from administering antibiotics unless the patient is septic because this will make it difficult to identify an organism at the time of surgery.

Prognosis

- Most patients with hand infections do well once the infection is controlled. However, inadequately treated infections can lead to serious consequences. The swelling and edema of an untreated infection causes increased tissue pressure and can result in tissue necrosis. Likewise, untreated pyogenic flexor tenosynovitis can lead to tendon rupture.

Troubleshooting

- The most common complication of a treated hand infection is recurrence. This is usually due to incomplete débridement or failure to allow the wound to stay open after evacuation of the abscess cavity. The tendency of inexperienced clinicians is to make the incision too small and be too timid in packing the wound.
- Recurrent exposure to the cause of the infection is also common (e.g., IV drug abusers, certain manual laborers, frequently manicured women). Counsel patients on the risk factors for hand infections to reduce recurrent infection.

Patient Instructions

- Patients should be meticulous about dressing changes. If they are not able to change their dressings by themselves or with the help of someone else, they may need home nursing assistance or in some cases inpatient admission.
- Be sure to instruct patients to complete their entire antibiotic regimen.
- Patients should keep their hand dry when showering and should absolutely avoid submerging it if bathing.

Considerations in Special Populations

- Be aware that patients with diabetes or those on long-term steroid treatment are likely to take longer to heal. Aggressive management of underlying medical problems as well as proper nutrition will optimize their recovery.

Suggested Readings

Boles D, Schmidt C. Pyogenic flexor tenosynovitis. *Hand Clin*. 1998;14: 567–578.

Infections. In: Boyes J, ed. *Bunnell's Surgery of the Hand*. Philadelphia: JB Lippincott; 1970:613–642.

Brook I. Paronychia: a mixed infection. *J Hand Surg [Br]*. 1993;18:358–359.

Connor R, Kimbrough R, Dabezies E. Hand infections in patients with diabetes mellitus. *Orthopedics*. 2001;24:1057–1060.

Glass K. Factors related to the resolution of treated hand infections. *J Hand Surg Am*. 1982;7:388–394.

Gonzalez M, Garst J, Nourbash P, et al. Abscesses of the upper extremity from drug abuse by injection. *J Hand Surg Am*. 1993;18:868–870.

Hausman M, Lisser S. Hand infections. *Orthop Clin North Am*. 1992;23: 171–185.

Jebsen P. Infections of the fingertip: paronychias and felons. *Hand Clin*. 1998;5:547–555.

Patzakis M, Wilkins J, Bassett R. Surgical findings in clenched-fist injuries. *Clin Orthop Relat Res*. 1987;220:237–240.

Zook E. Infection of the nail apparatus: paronychia. In: Krull EA, Zook EG, Baran R, Haneke E, eds. *Nail Surgery: A Text and Atlas*. Philadelphia: Lippincott Williams & Wilkins; 2001:195–200.

Chapter 91 Hand Dislocations

Dan A. Zlotolow

ICD-10-CM CODES
S63.016A *Dislocation radioulnar joint, distal*
S63.026A *Dislocation radiocarpal joint*
S63.036A *Dislocation midcarpal joint*
S63.056A *Dislocation carpometacarpal joint*
S63.116A *Dislocation metacarpophalangeal joint, thumb*
S63.269A *Dislocation metacarpophalangeal joint, finger*

Key Concepts

- A dislocation is a complete disruption of joint congruity.
- A subluxation implies that at least a portion of the articulating surfaces are still in contact.
- The progression of joint injury begins with a mild sprain with no joint laxity through ligament disruption, joint subluxation, and finally dislocation.
- Closed reduction is most often accomplished with traction, slight exaggeration of deformity, and correction of deformity.
- Soft-tissue interposition can block closed reductions in some dislocations.
- Be aware of associated fractures.
- Open dislocations are a surgical emergency.
- Dislocations are often missed, even by experienced practitioners.

History

- The mechanism of injury is very helpful for identifying associated injuries.
- Assess whether the dislocation is recurrent (has happened before) or chronic (has occurred in the past but was never reduced).
- Determine the energy that went into causing the dislocation.

Physical Examination

- High-energy injuries warrant a thorough secondary survey including the lower limbs, spine, and both upper limbs.
- Look for open wounds that may indicate an open dislocation (assume it is open until proven otherwise).
- Evaluate the compartments of the forearm and hand to make sure they are soft.
- Identify associated neurovascular compromise by checking sensation to light touch and capillary refill.
- Check for generalized ligamentous laxity.

Imaging

- Plain radiographs are essential for diagnosis.
- A good radiographic series usually obviates the need for advanced imaging studies and includes true anteroposterior and true lateral views.
- Computed tomography can be helpful if bony detail is obscured, as for carpometacarpal dislocations (Fig. 91.1) or distal radioulnar joint dislocations (Fig. 91.2).
- Magnetic resonance imaging is rarely needed and may be used to determine associated injuries preoperatively.

Additional Tests

- No additional tests are routinely necessary.

Differential Diagnosis

- Please see Table 91.1.

Treatment

- Radiocarpal or midcarpal dislocations (Fig. 91.3)
  - These are difficult reductions to accomplish and will likely require an orthopaedic consultation at the time of injury.
  - Traction, volar pressure on the lunate, and wrist flexion are typically effective.
- Distal radioulnar joint dislocations
  - Depending on the direction of the dislocation, these will reduce in either pronation or supination.
  - Use a sugar tong splint to hold the wrist and the forearm in the position of reduction.

TABLE 91.1 Differential Diagnosis

Differential Diagnosis	Differentiating Feature	Chapter Reference
Sprain, grade I	No joint laxity with stress testing	75
Sprain, grade II	Laxity present, but ligament is intact with firm endpoint	75
Sprain, grade III	Complete ligament injury with no endpoint on stress testing	75
Subluxation	Joint not concentrically reduced, but articular surfaces remain in contact	75

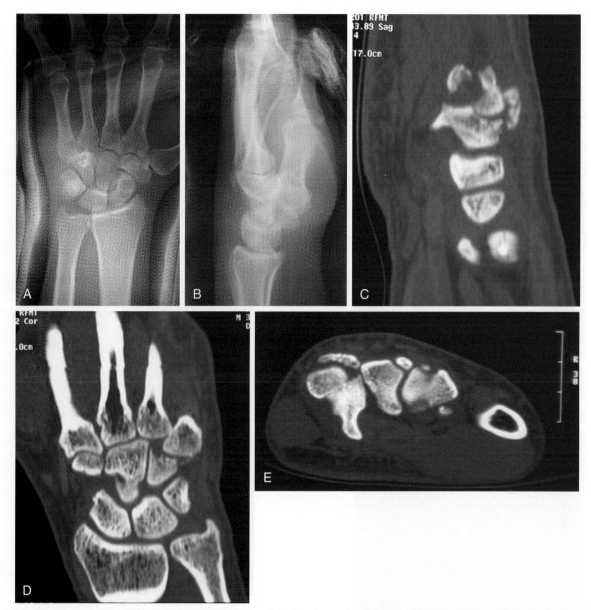

Fig 91.1 Many carpometacarpal dislocations are missed on initial radiographs. A high index of suspicion and computed tomography scanning may be necessary to make the diagnosis. Note the subtle findings on the anteroposterior (A) and lateral (B) radiographs compared with the computed tomography scan (C to E). Computed tomography in this case shows impaction of the fifth metacarpal base into the body of the hamate.

- Carpometacarpal dislocations
  - Closed reduction requires traction and direct pressure over the dislocated metacarpal joint.
  - These are inherently unstable injuries and difficult to assess on plain radiographs.
  - Postreduction computed tomography scans are necessary to assess the quality of the reduction.
  - Place in an ulnar gutter or clamshell splint with the wrist in neutral position, the metacarpophalangeal joints in flexion, and the interphalangeal joints free.
- Metacarpophalangeal dislocations
  - Soft-tissue interposition can prevent closed reduction.
  - Reduce by using traction, exaggeration of deformity, and translation.
  - Place in an ulnar gutter or clamshell splint with the wrist in extension, the metacarpophalangeal joints in flexion, and the proximal interphalangeal joints in extension.
- Interphalangeal dislocations
  - Soft-tissue interposition can prevent closed reduction
  - Reduce by using traction, exaggeration of deformity, and translation
- Dorsal dislocation (Fig. 91.4)
  - If the joint is stable in full extension, buddy tape to adjoining finger.

355

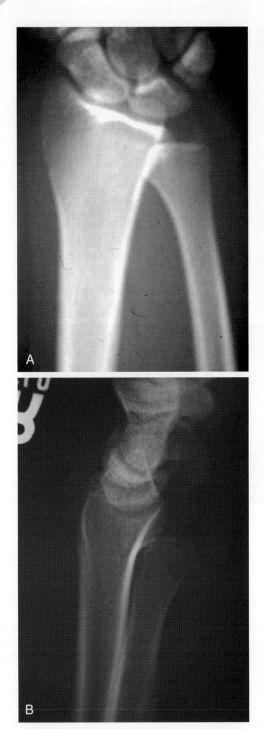

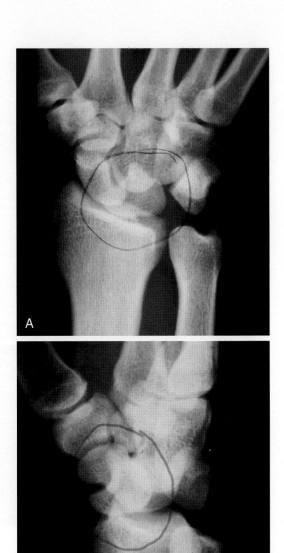

Fig 91.3 A perilunate dislocation is a high-energy injury with a fair long-term prognosis. Although the radiographic findings are well understood, this injury is underdiagnosed, resulting in complete loss of wrist function for the patient and legal entanglements for the physician. Note the triangular appearance of the lunate on the anteroposterior view (A), as well as the "empty cup" appearance of the lunate on the lateral view (B).

Fig 91.2 (A) Distal radioulnar joint dislocation. (B) A true lateral radiograph, identified by overlap of the distal pole of the scaphoid with the pisiform, is necessary to make the diagnosis. (From Szabo B. Distal radioulnar joint instability. *J Bone Joint Surg Am*. 2006;88A:884–894.)

When to Refer

- Any open dislocation
- Any suspicion of compartment syndrome
- Irreducible dislocations
- High-energy mechanism

- If the joint tends to redislocate, place in an extension block splint to allow a stable range of motion.
- Always place finger splints on the dorsum of the finger.
- Volar dislocation
  - More rare; splint the proximal interphalangeal joint in extension

Prognosis

- Most patients will have some residual loss of motion at the dislocated joint, even if optimal treatment is provided.

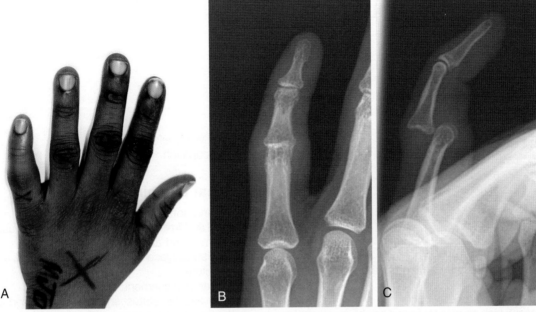

Fig 91.4 (A) Proximal interphalangeal dislocations can have a benign clinical appearance. (B) An anteroposterior radiograph will often not demonstrate the dislocation. (C) A good lateral radiograph is crucial.

- Outcome is principally dependent on patient compliance with their therapy protocol and on their propensity for scarring.

Troubleshooting

- Appropriate reduction maneuvers can avoid catastrophes such as soft-tissue interposition, neurovascular injury, and iatrogenic fracture.
- A well-made splint can make the difference between a good outcome and a recurrently dislocated or ankylosed/arthritic joint.

Patient Instructions

- Ice and elevation are critical to limit swelling.
- For radiocarpal or intercarpal dislocations, patients should be referred to a hand surgeon within a couple of days for definitive management as long as a closed reduction was achieved.

Considerations in Special Populations

- Children with unossified epiphyses may have complete Salter I fractures that can mimic dislocations.

- Patients with ligamentous laxity have a propensity for dislocation and should be counseled about their condition.

Suggested Readings

Adkinson JW, Chapman MW. Treatment of acute lunate and perilunate dislocations. *Clin Orthop Relat Res*. 1982;164:199–207.

Betz RR, Browne EZ, Perry GB, Resnick EJ. The complex volar metacarpophalangeal joint dislocation. A case report and review of the literature. *J Bone Joint Surg Am*. 1982;64A:1374–1375.

Bowers WH. The proximal interphalangeal joint volar plate. II. A clinical study of hyperextension injury. *J Hand Surg Am*. 1981;6A:77–81.

Deshmukh NV, Sonanis SV, Stothard J. Neglected volar dislocations of the interphalangeal joint. *Hand Surg*. 2004;9:71–75.

Dobyns JH, McElfresh EC. Extension block splinting. *Hand Clin*. 1994;10:229–237.

Mueller JJ. Carpometacarpal dislocations: report of five cases and review of the literature. *J Hand Surg Am*. 1986;11A:184–188.

Chapter 92 Distal Radius Fracture

Jennifer A. Hart

ICD-10-CM CODES
S52.509A *Distal radius fracture*
S52.502A *Distal radius fracture, left*
S52.501A *Distal radius fracture, right*

Key Concepts

- Distal radius fracture is a common fracture of the upper extremity
- There is a bimodal age distribution
  - Adolescent: high energy; fall from a height, motor vehicle accident, athletics
  - Elderly: low energy; fall from standing position
  - Osteoporosis is a critical risk factor.
- Mechanism: fall on outstretched hand
- Fracture on tension side (volar) and comminution on compression side (dorsal)
- Axial load in forearm is split 80% radius and 20% ulna

History

- It is important to obtain the following patient information
  - Age
  - Hand dominance
  - Mechanism of injury: high versus low energy
  - Comorbidities
  - Activity level
  - Occupation

Physical Examination

- Skin and soft-tissue swelling is common.
- Painful and limited range of motion of wrist is usually present.
- Deformity and angulation:
  - Dorsal displacement: Colles fracture (90% of distal radius fractures)
  - Volar displacement: Smith fracture
- Neurovascular status should be assessed with special attention to the median nerve.
  - Carpal tunnel compression symptoms are present in 13-23% of injuries.
- Palpate the anatomic snuffbox for tenderness, which may suggest a scaphoid fracture.
- Examine finger and thumb motion to confirm tendon continuity.
- Always examine the ipsilateral hand, elbow, and shoulder for associated injuries.

Imaging

- Posteroanterior and lateral radiographs
  - Normal values
    - Radial inclination: 22 degrees (range, 13 to 30 degrees) (Fig. 92.1)

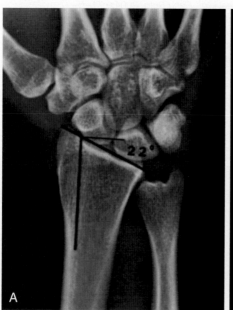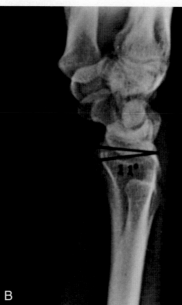

Fig 92.1 The anteroposterior radiograph (A) illustrates normal radial inclination of approximately 22 degrees. The lateral radiograph (B) illustrates normal volar tilt of the distal articular surface of approximately 11 degrees. (From Green DP, Hotchkiss RN, Pederson WC, et al., eds. *Green's Operative Hand Surgery*. 5th ed. Philadelphia: Churchill Livingstone; 2005, Fig. 16.7.)

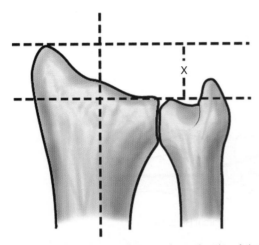

Fig 92.2 Radial length is the distance from the tip of the radial styloid to the ulnar articular surface on an anteroposterior radiograph (X). Radial length averages 11 to 12 mm, with a range of 8 to 18 mm.

- • Radial length: 11 to 12 mm (range, 8 to 18 mm) (Fig. 92.2)
- • Volar tilt: 11 degrees (range, 1 to 21 degrees) (see Fig. 92.1)
- • Evaluate the distal radioulnar joint.
- • Evaluate for associated carpal injuries.
- • Evaluate for associated ulnar fracture.
- • Navicular or scaphoid view
  - • Evaluate for scaphoid fracture.
- • Elbow anteroposterior and lateral views with any associated elbow pain
  - • Evaluate for associated injury.
  - • Monteggia fractures: proximal ulnar fracture with radial head dislocation
  - • Galeazzi fractures: radial diaphysis fracture at the junction of the middle and distal thirds with associated disruption of distal radioulnar joint
- • Fracture description
  - • Open versus closed
  - • Intra-articular versus extra-articular
  - • Comminution: dorsal versus volar
  - • Loss of radial height: radial shortening
  - • Displacement and angulation
  - • Look for an associated distal ulnar fracture.

Differential Diagnosis

- • Please see Table 92.1.

TABLE 92.1 Differential Diagnosis

Fracture Eponym	Differentiating Features
Colles fracture	Dorsal comminution, dorsal displacement, dorsal angulation (apex volar), radial shortening, silver fork deformity (Fig. 92.3)
Smith fracture	Volar displacement, volar angulation (apex dorsal), unstable fracture, garden spade deformity (Fig. 92.4)
Barton fracture	Dorsal rim displacement of distal radius, unstable articular fracture-subluxation with carpus displacement (see Fig. 92.4)
Volar Barton fracture	Volar rim displacement of distal radius, unstable articular fracture-subluxation with carpus displacement (see Fig. 92.4)
Chauffeur fracture	Radial styloid fracture with carpus displaced ulnarly (Fig. 92.5)
Die-punch fracture	Depression of lunate fossa with proximal migration of lunate (see Fig. 92.5)

Treatment

- • Initial treatment
  - • Radiographs to define injury
  - • Nondisplaced fracture (Fig. 92.6)
    - • Sugar tong splint
    - • Referral to orthopaedist to be seen in 5 to 7 days
  - • Displaced fracture (Fig. 92.7)
    - • Closed reduction and splinting (see Chapter 97)
    - • Hematoma block
    - • Finger traps and traction
    - • Sugar tong splint (Fig. 92.8)
    - • Referral to orthopaedist to be seen in 3 to 5 days
  - • Acceptable reduction (Fig. 92.9)
    - • Radial shortening less than 2 mm
    - • Neutral tilt
    - • Articular step-off less than 1 mm

When to Refer

- • Refer to orthopaedist for all distal radius fractures
- • Nonoperative
  - • Nondisplaced fractures
  - • Stable fracture patterns with acceptable reduction

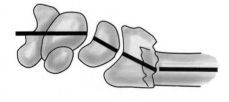
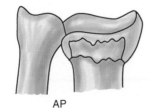

Lateral   AP

Fig 92.3 Representation of the typical deformity seen in a Colles fracture. Dorsal comminution and displacement with shortening of the radius relative to the ulna are present. *AP,* Anteroposterior. (Modified from Wolfe SW, Hotchkiss RN, Pederson WC, et al., eds. *Green's Operative Hand Surgery.* 7th ed. Philadelphia: Elsevier; 2017, Fig. 15.14.)

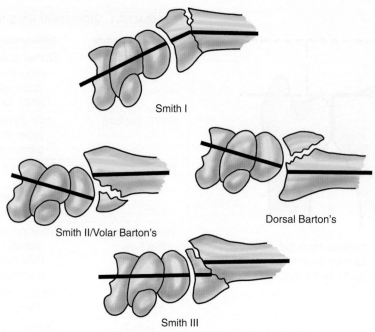

Fig 92.4 Thomas classification of Smith fractures. Type I Smith fracture: extra-articular fracture with palmar angulation and displacement of the distal fragment. Type II Smith fracture: intra-articular fracture with volar and proximal displacement of the distal fragment along with the carpus. Type III Smith fracture: extra-articular fracture with volar displacement of the distal fragment and carpus. (In type III, the fracture line is more oblique than in a type I fracture.) A type II Smith fracture is essentially a volar Barton fracture. A dorsal Barton fracture, illustrated for comparison, shows the dorsal and proximal displacement of the carpus and distal fragment on the radial shaft. (Modified from Wolfe SW, Hotchkiss RN, Pederson WC, et al., eds. *Green's Operative Hand Surgery*, 7th ed. Philadelphia: Elsevier; 2017, Fig. 15.15.)

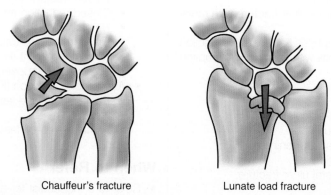

Fig 92.5 A chauffeur fracture is illustrated with the carpus displaced ulnarly by the radial styloid fracture. A lunate load (die-punch) fracture is shown with a depression of the lunate fossa of the radius that allows proximal migration of the lunate and/or proximal carpal row. *Arrows* represent deforming forces and displacement. (Modified from Wolfe SW, Hotchkiss RN, Pederson WC, et al., eds. *Green's Operative Hand Surgery*. 7th ed. Philadelphia: Elsevier; 2017, Fig. 15.16.)

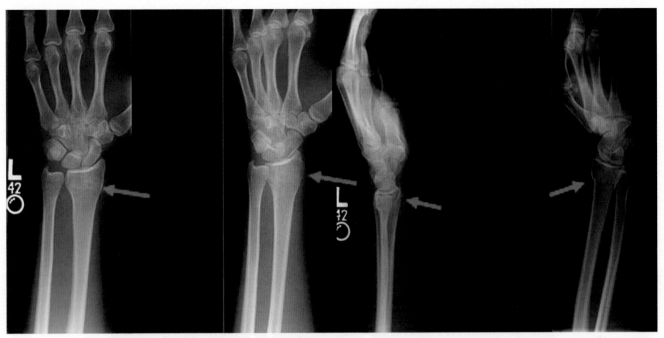

Fig 92.6 Nondisplaced distal radius fracture *(arrow)*. Treat in splint followed by cast. (From *left* to *right*, Posteroanterior, oblique, lateral, and oblique views of the left wrist are shown.)

- Elderly (older than 65 years) or low-demand patients with comorbidities with reasonable reduction
- Operative
  - Open fractures
  - Unstable fracture patterns: comminution or intra-articular
  - Associated neurovascular or tendon injuries
  - Unacceptable reduction
  - Young active patient
- Complications
  - Posttraumatic arthritis
  - Malunion
  - Nonunion
  - Median neuropathy
  - Finger and wrist stiffness
  - Tendon ruptures: extensor pollicis longus tendon
  - Chronic regional pain syndrome

Patient Instructions

- Keep the splint clean and dry.
- Elevate the arm above the heart for 48 hours to decrease swelling and pain.
- Take pain medications as prescribed.
- Follow up with orthopaedist as instructed

Considerations in Special Populations

- Pediatric patients
  - Salter-Harris classification (Fig. 92.10)
  - Only one reduction attempt should be made to prevent further damage to the physis.
  - High potential for remodeling
  - Referral to orthopaedist for all displaced and physeal fractures

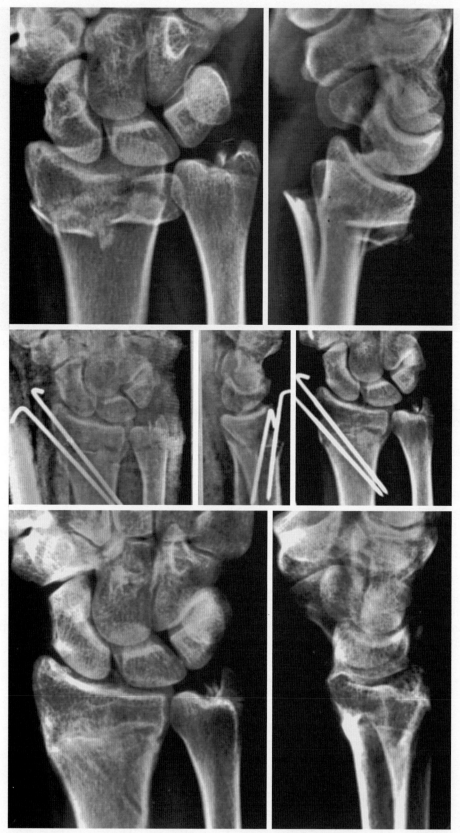

Fig 92.7 Unstable dorsally displaced fracture associated with a dorsal die-punch fragment treated by closed manipulation, intrafocal pinning, and cast fixation for 5 weeks. Follow-up radiographs at 6 months reveal an anatomic result. (From Green DP, Hotchkiss RN, Pederson WC, et al., eds. *Green's Operative Hand Surgery.* 5th ed. Philadelphia: Churchill Livingstone; 2005, Fig. 16.26.)

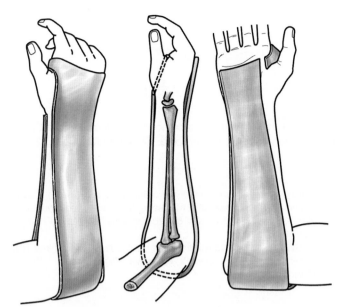

Fig 92.8 Sugar tong splint for a distal radius fracture. This splint controls forearm rotation while allowing for some elbow flexion. The palmar crease should be free to allow full metacarpophalangeal flexion. (From Wolfe SW, Hotchkiss RN, Pederson WC, et al., eds. *Green's Operative Hand Surgery*. 7th ed. Philadelphia: Elsevier; 2017, Fig. 15.24.)

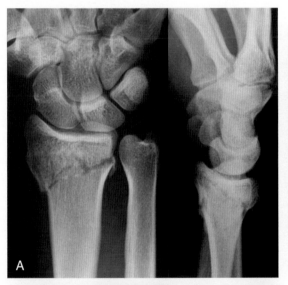

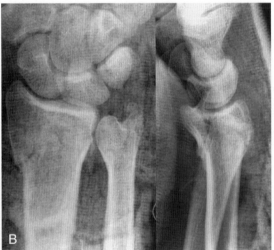

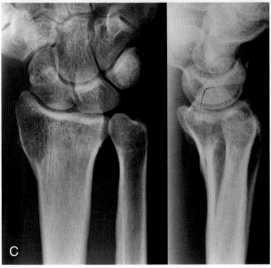

Fig 92.9 (A) Typical radiographic appearance of a Colles fracture in a young adult. (B) The fracture was manually reduced and held in slight flexion, ulnar deviation, and slight pronation in a sugar tong splint for 3 weeks, followed by a short-arm cast for another 3 weeks. (C) Follow-up radiographs at 1 year reveal loss of 2 mm of length but maintenance of normal volar and ulnar tilt. Notice the asymptomatic nonunion of the tip of the ulnar styloid. (From Wolfe SW, Hotchkiss RN, Pederson WC, et al., eds. *Green's Operative Hand Surgery*. 7th ed. Philadelphia: Elsevier; 2017, Fig. 15.25.)

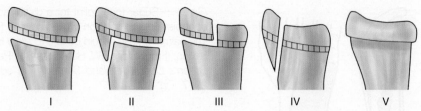

Fig 92.10 Salter-Harris classification of distal radial epiphyseal fractures in children. Type V is a crush injury. (Modified from Green DP, Hotchkiss RN, Pederson WC, et al., eds. *Green's Operative Hand Surgery*. 5th ed. Philadelphia: Churchill Livingstone; 2005, Fig. 16.63.)

Suggested Readings

Egol KA, Koval KJ, Zuckerman JD. Distal radius. In: *Handbook of Fractures*. 5th ed. Philadelphia: Wolters Kluwer; 2015:266–278.

Jiuliano JA, Jupiter J. Distal radius fractures. In: Trumble TE, Budoff JE, Cornwall R, eds. *Hand, Elbow, and Shoulder: Core Knowledge in Orthopaedics*. Philadelphia: Mosby; 2006:84–101.

McQueen MM, et al. Fractures of the distal radius and ulna. In: Court-Brown CM, Heckman JD, McQueen MM, eds. *Rockwood and Green's Fractures in Adults*. 8th ed. Philadelphia: Wolters Kluwer; 2015:1057–1120.

Wolfe SW, et al. Distal radius fractures. In: Wolfe SW, Hotchkiss RN, Pederson WC, eds. *Green's Operative Hand Surgery*. 7th ed. Philadelphia: Elsevier; 2017:516–587.

Chapter 93 Scaphoid Fracture

Jennifer A. Hart

ICD-10-CM CODE
S62.009A *Scaphoid fracture of the wrist*

Key Concepts

- The scaphoid is the most commonly fractured carpal bone.
- The typical mechanism of injury is a fall on the outstretched hand
- 80% of the scaphoid is covered with articular cartilage
- Vascular supply (Fig. 93.1)
  - Branches off radial artery
  - Enters dorsally and distally and courses proximally
  - Fractures through waist and proximal third render the proximal fragment at risk of avascular necrosis
- The scaphoid links the proximal and distal carpal rows.
- Carpal bones are connected by capsular and interosseous ligaments.

History

- It is important to obtain the following information:
  - History of sprain with persistent pain and swelling
  - Age
  - Hand dominance
  - Mechanism of injury
  - Comorbidities
  - Activity level
  - Occupation

Physical Examination

- Skin and soft-tissue swelling
- Painful and limited range of motion of wrist
  - Tenderness to deep palpation in anatomic snuff-box
  - Between extensor pollicis longus and extensor pollicis brevis muscles
  - Scaphoid shift test
  - Pain with dorsal to volar shifting of scaphoid
  - Watson test
  - Pain and dorsal scaphoid subluxation as wrist moves from ulnar to radial deviation with compression of scaphoid tuberosity
- Deformity and angulation
- Neurovascular status
- Examine finger and thumb motion to confirm tendon continuity.
- Always examine ipsilateral hand, elbow, and shoulder for associated injuries.

Imaging

- Posteroanterior view with hand in a fist and lateral view radiographs (Fig. 93.2)
  - Evaluate distal radius, ulna, and all carpal bones.
  - Evaluate lateral radiograph for perilunate dislocation (Fig. 93.3).
  - Evaluate distal radioulnar joint
- Scaphoid view
  - Evaluate scaphoid for fracture.
  - Ulnar deviation of wrist assists in fracture definition (Fig. 93.4).
- Scaphoid radial oblique view, supinated posteroanterior view
- Fracture description
  - Pattern (Fig. 93.5)
    - Horizontal oblique
    - Transverse
    - Vertical oblique
  - Stability
    - Stable, nondisplaced fracture with no step-off
    - Unstable
    - Displacement more than 1 mm
    - Scapholunate angle more than 60 degrees (Fig. 93.6)
    - Lunatocapitate angle more than 15 degrees (see Fig. 93.6)
  - Location (Fig. 93.7)
    - Tuberosity
    - Distal third
    - Middle third or waist (most common)
    - Proximal third
- Magnetic resonance imaging (MRI), bone scan, computed tomography (CT)
  - Initial radiographs nondiagnostic in 25% of cases
  - Studies to be used to evaluate for occult scaphoid fracture (Fig. 93.8)
- Elbow anteroposterior and lateral with any associated pain
  - Evaluate for associated injury.
  - Monteggia fractures: proximal ulnar fracture with radial head dislocation
  - Galeazzi fractures: radial diaphysis fracture at the junction of the middle and distal thirds with associated disruption of the distal radioulnar joint

Treatment

- At diagnosis
  - Radiographs to define injury
  - Thumb spica splint for all suspected and defined injuries
  - Injury with positive examination but normal radiographs

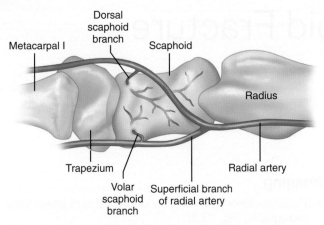

Fig 93.1 Dorsal and volar blood supply to the scaphoid from branches of the radial artery. (From Trumble TE, et al, editors: *Core Knowledge in Orthopaedics: Hand, Elbow, and Shoulder.* Philadelphia, Mosby, 2006, p 117.)

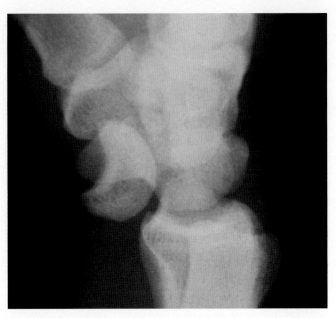

Fig 93.3 On a lateral radiograph, the lunate is displaced volarly while the capitate is articulating with the radius. (From Elhassan B, Waitayawinyu T, Bridgeman JT, et al. Fractures and dislocation of the carpus. In: Trumble TE, Rayan GM, Budoff JE, et al., eds. *Principles of Hand Surgery and Therapy.* 2nd ed. Philadelphia: Saunders; 2010, Fig. 5.90.)

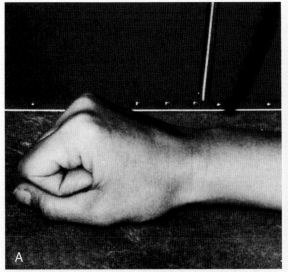

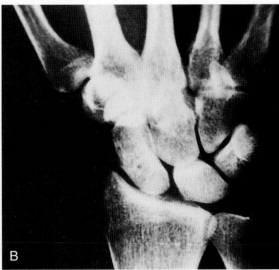

Fig 93.2 (A) Positioning for a posteroanterior radiograph obtained with the fingers flexed into a fist. (B) Slight dorsiflexion is produced to place the longitudinal axis of the scaphoid in a plane more nearly parallel to that of the film. (From Green DP, Hotchkiss RN, Pederson WC, et al., eds. *Green's Operative Hand Surgery*, 5th ed. Philadelphia: Churchill Livingstone; 2005, Fig. 17.5.)

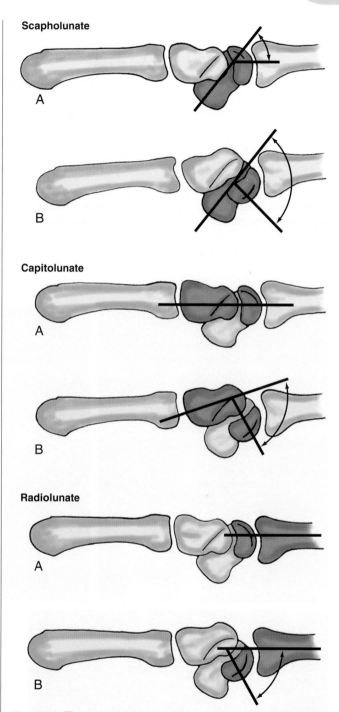

Scapholunate

A

B

Capitolunate

A

B

Radiolunate

A

B

Fig 93.6 The carpal bone angles are of considerable aid in identifying carpal instability patterns. In each illustration the normal angle (A) is shown in comparison with the abnormal angle (B) seen when there is dorsal intercalary segmental carpal instability. The scapholunate angle, when greater than 80 degrees, is definitive evidence of either a scapholunate dissociation or a palmarly displaced scaphoid fracture. The capitolunate angle should theoretically be 0 degrees with the wrist in neutral, but the normal range probably extends to as much as 15 degrees. The radiolunate angle is abnormal if it exceeds 15 degrees. (Modified from Green DP, Hotchkiss RN, Pederson WC, eds. *Green's Operative Hand Surgery*. 4th ed. New York: Churchill Livingstone; 1999, Fig. 28.13.)

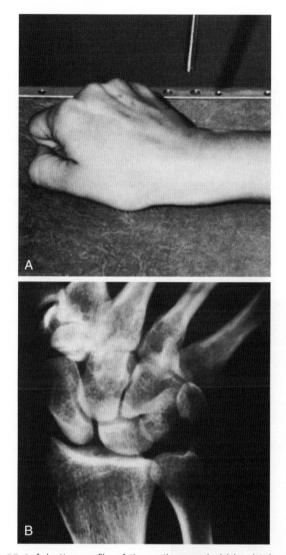

Fig 93.4 A better profile of the entire scaphoid is obtained in the posteroanterior view with the fingers flexed into a fist (A) and the wrist in ulnar deviation (B). (From Green DP, Hotchkiss RN, Pederson WC, et al., eds. *Green's Operative Hand Surgery*. 5th ed. Philadelphia: Churchill Livingstone; 2005, Fig. 17.6.)

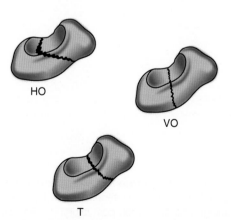

HO

VO

T

Fig 93.5 Russe separated fractures based on fracture plane orientation into transverse (T), horizontal oblique (HO), and vertical oblique (VO) fractures. (From Drijkoningen T, Ten Berg PW, Strackee SD, Buijze GA: Classification systems of scaphoid fractures. In Buijze GA, Jupiter JB: *Scaphoid Fractures: Evidence-Based Management*. Philadelphia, Elsevier, 2018.)

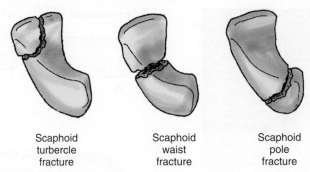

Scaphoid
turbercle
fracture

Scaphoid
waist
fracture

Scaphoid
pole
fracture

Fig 93.7 Scaphoid fractures can be simply described as involving the distal pole or tubercle, waist, or proximal pole. (Modified from Elhassan B, Waitayawinyu T, Bridgeman JT, et al. Fractures and dislocation of the carpus. In: Trumble TE, Rayan GM, Budoff JE, et al., eds. *Principles of Hand Surgery and Therapy*, 2nd ed. Philadelphia: Saunders, 2010, Fig. 5.9.)

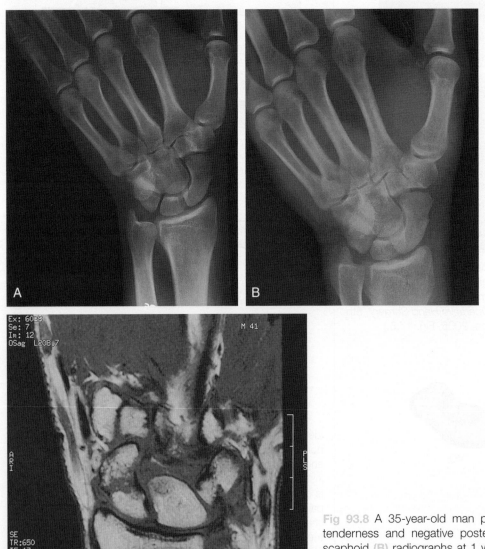

Fig 93.8 A 35-year-old man presented with persistent snuff-box tenderness and negative posteroanterior (A) and posteroanterior scaphoid (B) radiographs at 1 week post injury. (C) An occult non-displaced scaphoid fracture was detected with magnetic resonance imaging. (From Green DP, Hotchkiss RN, Pederson WC, et al., eds. *Green's Operative Hand Surgery*. 5th ed. Philadelphia: Churchill Livingstone; 2005, Fig. 17.10.)

- Immobilize for 12 to 14 days
- Repeat radiographs if still symptomatic
- If negative, consider MRI, CT, or bone scan, with MRI being the most diagnostic (see Fig. 93.8)
- If acute diagnosis necessary (athlete), consider MRI immediately to detect occult fractures
- Nonoperative
  - Stable, nondisplaced fractures
    - Short arm thumb spica cast with wrist in neutral position for 6 to 8 weeks
    - Then short arm spica cast for an additional 4 to 6 weeks until radiographic evidence of union
    - Follow up every 3 months for 1 year to confirm union.
  - Nonoperative union rates, based on blood supply
    - Distal third: 100% union
    - Middle third: 80-90% union
    - Proximal third: 60-70% union
  - Expected time to union
    - Tuberosity: 6 weeks
    - Distal third: 6 to 8 weeks
    - Middle third: 8 to 12 weeks
    - Proximal third: 12 to 24 weeks
- Operative
  - Unstable fractures with displacement
  - Proximal pole fractures
  - Nonunion after attempting nonoperative treatment

- Fractures associated with other injuries (perilunate dislocation)
- Open reduction with internal fixation
  - Compression screw (Fig. 93.9)
  - Open versus percutaneous techniques
  - With or without bone graft
  - Union rate of 93-97%
  - Begin aggressive range of motion when radiographic union is evident

Complications

- Delayed union, nonunion, and malunion are seen more often with proximal fractures.
- May require delayed open reduction and internal fixation with bone graft
- Osteonecrosis is more common with proximal pole fractures.
- Early wrist osteoarthritis is seen with untreated nonunion or malunion.

When to Refer

- All scaphoid fractures should be referred to an orthopaedic surgeon or hand specialist.
- Delay in diagnosis and treatment results in a high rate of nonunion and poor functional outcome.

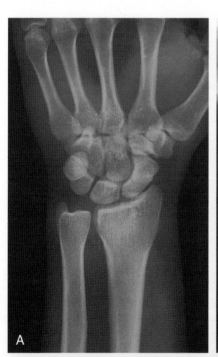
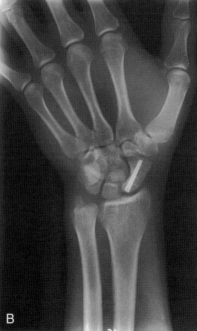
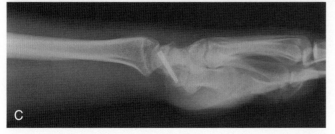

Fig 93.9 (A) A 24-year-old football player suffered a nondisplaced scaphoid fracture in midseason. Posteroanterior scaphoid (B) and lateral (C) radiographs showing a compression screw placed percutaneously. The patient returned to practice at 6 weeks. (From Green DP, Hotchkiss RN, Pederson WC, et al., eds. *Green's Operative Hand Surgery*. 5th ed. Philadelphia: Churchill Livingstone; 2005, Fig. 17.14.)

Patient Instructions

- Keep the splint clean and dry.
- Elevate the arm above the heart for 48 hours to decrease swelling and pain.
- Take pain medications as prescribed.
- Follow up with an orthopaedist as instructed.
- Good results are seen with cast immobilization for tuberosity and distal third fractures.
- Surgery is commonly performed for middle and proximal third fractures to improve union rates.
- Increased risk of osteonecrosis with proximal third fractures; early surgery is recommended to enhance healing rates (even in nondisplaced fractures).

Suggested Readings

Duckworth AD, Ring D. Carpus fractures and dislocations. In: Court-Brown CM, Heckman JD, McQueen MM, et al., eds. *Rockwood and Green's Fractures in Adults*. 8th ed. Philadelphia: Wolters Kluwer; 2015:991–1056.

Egol KA, Koval KJ, Zuckerman JD. *Handbook of Fractures*. 5th ed. Philadelphia: Wolters Kluwer; 2015.

Knoll VD, Trumble TE. Scaphoid fractures and nonunions. In: Trumble TE, Budoff JE, Cornwall R, eds. *Hand, Elbow, and Shoulder: Core Knowledge in Orthopaedics*. Philadelphia: Mosby; 2006:116–131.

Lee SK. Fractures of the carpal bones. In: Wolfe SW, Hotchkiss RN, Pederson WC, et al., eds. *Green's Operative Hand Surgery*. 7th ed. Philadelphia: Elsevier; 2017:588–652.

Chapter 94 Thumb Fractures

Jennifer A. Hart

ICD-10-CM CODES
S62.509A *Thumb fracture, closed*
S62.509B *Thumb fracture, open*

Key Concepts

- Injuries to the thumb commonly result from a fall, an industrial accident, or an athletic injury.
- The most common thumb fracture is Bennett fracture.
- Thumb metacarpal fractures are prone to displacement due to the deforming forces created by tendon attachments (Fig. 94.1).
- The key to an optimal outcome is a good reduction; all intra-articular fractures should be reduced with less than 1 mm step-off.
- Improperly treated Bennett or Rolando fractures can result in traumatic arthritis of the thumb carpometacarpal joint and cause severe impairment of thumb function.

Types of Fractures

- Bennett fracture (Fig. 94.2)
  - Intra-articular oblique fracture through the ulnar-volar metacarpal base; ulnar fracture fragment (Bennett fragment) varies in size and remains attached to the trapezium by the anterior oblique ligament.
  - There is subsequent proximal and radial subluxation of the remainder of the metacarpal base from the carpometacarpal joint due to the pull of the abductor pollicis longus tendon, which inserts on the radial side of the metacarpal base.
  - All require surgical fixation.
- Rolando fracture (Fig. 94.3)
  - Intra-articular Y- or T-shaped fracture with both a radial fragment and an ulnar fragment
  - Also includes comminuted intra-articular base fractures
  - All require surgical fixation.
- Extra-articular metacarpal shaft fractures (Fig. 94.4)
  - Uncommon and usually located transversely or obliquely just above the metacarpal base
  - This fracture has a tendency to dorsally angulate due to the forces of the various tendon attachments on the thumb. As much as 20 degrees of angulation may be accepted because the multiplanar motion of the thumb carpometacarpal joint is able to compensate.

History

- Patient may report a history of a fall or an injury to the thumb with a hyperflexion, hyperextension, or hyperabduction type of mechanism.
- Patient may report pain, edema, and loss of thumb range of motion.

Physical Examination

- Inspection may reveal edema or a deformity of the thumb or its metacarpal.
- Identify any open injuries.
- The fracture site will be exquisitely tender to palpation, and crepitus or gross instability may be present.
- Assess the patient's active range of motion in all planes and check for rotational deformity.
- Assess ligamentous stability by applying varus and valgus stress to all joints (this should be performed only after radiographs have confirmed no evidence of a ligament avulsion fracture).
- Sensation should be checked over the radial and ulnar borders of the thumb and any deficits should be noted.
- Capillary refill should be tested; normal is less than 2 seconds.
- Always assess for secondary injuries with a thorough wrist and hand examination. Be sure to palpate the anatomic snuffbox to assess for scaphoid tenderness, which may indicate a scaphoid fracture.

Imaging

- Anteroposterior, lateral, and oblique views of the thumb should be obtained, and the thumb carpometacarpal joint should be included in the views.
- Note the following
  - Displacement: displaced or nondisplaced
  - Articular involvement: intra-articular or extra-articular
  - Character of fracture: transverse, longitudinal, oblique, spiral, comminuted
  - Fracture location: distal or proximal phalanx, metacarpal head, shaft, or base
  - Deformity: angulation (volar/dorsal, radially/ulnarly, number of degrees), rotation

Differential Diagnosis

- Please see Table 94.1.

Treatment

- Bennett fracture
  - Fracture is considered unstable.
  - Place patient in a thumb spica splint and refer to a hand specialist to be seen within 7 days of injury.
  - Surgery is necessary for these fractures.

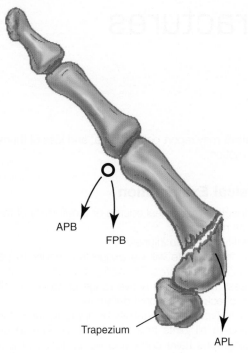

Fig 94.1 Thumb anatomy. Extensor tendon attachments. *APB,* Abductor pollicis brevis; *APL,* abductor pollicis longus; *FPB,* flexor pollicis brevis.

APB

FPB

Trapezium

APL

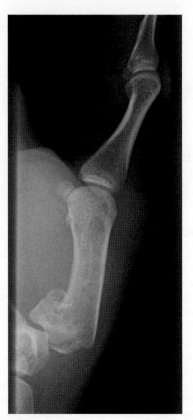

Fig 94.3 Rolando fracture.

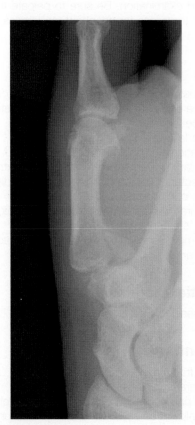

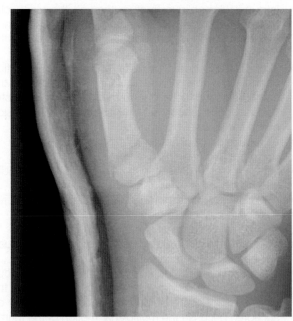

Fig 94.4 Extra-articular metacarpal fracture.

Fig 94.2 Bennett fracture.

TABLE 94.1 Differential Diagnosis

Condition	Differentiating Feature
Thumb carpometacarpal osteoarthritis (see Chapter 80)	No history of injury; tenderness to palpation at the thumb carpometacarpal joint; positive carpometacarpal grind test; radiographs: arthritis changes evident at thumb carpometacarpal joint
de Quervain tenosynovitis (see Chapter 76)	Tenderness to palpation over first extensor compartment; positive Finkelstein's sign; negative radiographs
Trigger finger (see Chapter 82)	Tenderness to palpation over thumb A1 pulley; palpable tender nodule or evidence of triggering at A1 pulley; negative radiographs
Ulnar collateral or radial collateral ligament sprain (see Chapter 81)	Tenderness to palpation over ulnar collateral or radial collateral ligament at thumb metacarpophalangeal joint; laxity of metacarpophalangeal joint with varus or valgus stress in flexion or extension; radiographs may reveal a small avulsion fracture
Scaphoid fracture (see Chapter 93)	Tenderness to palpation at anatomic snuffbox; scaphoid tubercle tenderness; radiographs may reveal a scaphoid fracture

- Rolando fracture
  - Fracture is considered unstable.
  - Place in a thumb spica splint and refer to a hand specialist to be seen within 7 days of injury.
  - Surgery is necessary for these fractures.
- Extra-articular base fractures
  - At diagnosis
    - Closed reduction under a local block should be attempted to minimize the amount of dorsal angulation.
    - May accept as much as 20 degrees of angulation
    - A thumb spica splint should be applied and worn for 1 week to allow the edema to subside.
    - Then a thumb spica cast with the interphalangeal joint free should be applied for 3 weeks.
    - Repeat radiographs once the cast has been applied to ensure that the fracture has maintained alignment.
  - Later
    - After 3 weeks of cast immobilization, repeat radiographs. If the fracture shows evidence of healing,

transition the patient into a removable thumb spica splint and begin range of motion therapy.

When to Refer

- More than 20 degrees of angulation
- More than 2 mm of shortening
- Rotation
- Open fracture

Prognosis

- All intra-articular fractures are at risk of developing traumatic arthritis. This risk is minimized by adequate articular reduction with a step-off of less than 1 mm.

Patient Instructions

- Patients may require a referral to a hand therapist to restore thumb range of motion after cast immobilization or surgery.
- If a fracture requires surgical treatment, there are several options that the surgeon may recommend, including closed reduction and percutaneous pinning, open reduction and internal fixation, or external fixation.

Considerations in Special Populations

- Athletes are prone to thumb injuries and should be referred to a hand specialist for early intervention and return to play.
- Manual laborers are also prone to thumb injuries. If adequate fracture reduction is not obtained, there may be a significant impact on their ability to perform their job duties.

Suggested Readings

Calandruccio JH. Fractures, dislocations, and ligamentous injuries. In: Azar FM, Beaty JH, Canale ST, eds. *Campbell's Operative Orthopaedics*. Vol. 4. 13th ed. Philadelphia: Elsevier; 2017:3403–3461.

Day CS. Fractures of the metacarpals and phalanges. In: Wolfe SW, Hotchkiss RN, Pederson WC, et al, eds. *Green's Operative Hand Surgery*. Vol. 1. 7th ed. Philadelphia: Elsevier; 2017:231–277.

Henry MH. Hand fractures and dislocations. In: Court-Brown CM, Heckman JD, McQueen MM, et al, eds. *Rockwood and Green's Fractures in Adults*. Vol. 1. 8th ed. Philadelphia: Wolters Kluwer; 2015:915–990.

Laub DR Jr. Thumb fractures and dislocations. *Medscape (website)*. 2017. Available at: https://emedicine.medscape.com/article/1287814-overview. Accessed April 20, 2018.

Rettig AC. Athletic injuries of the wrist and hand: part II: overuse injuries of the wrist and traumatic injuries to the hand. *Am J Sports Med*. 2004;2:262.

Soyer AD. Fractures of the base of the first metacarpal: current treatment options. *J Am Acad Orthop Surg*. 1999;7:403–412.

Chapter 95 Metacarpal Fractures

Jennifer A. Hart

ICD-10-CM CODES
S62.309A	Metacarpal bone fracture, closed
S62.309B	Metacarpal bone fracture, open
S62.339A	Neck of metacarpal bone fracture
S62.329A	Shaft of metacarpal bone fracture
S62.213A	Bennett's fracture of metacarpal base
S62.223A	Rolando's fracture

Key Concepts

- Along with phalangeal fractures, metacarpal fractures are the most common types of fracture in the upper extremity.
- "Hand fractures can be complicated by deformity from no treatment, stiffness from overtreatment, and both deformity and stiffness from poor treatment." (Swanson)
- Twenty-seven percent of finger fractures are treated inappropriately in the emergency department due to inaccurate reduction or improper splinting.

History

- It is important to obtain the following patient information
  - Age
  - Hand dominance
  - Mechanism of injury
  - Comorbidities
  - Occupation

Physical Examination

- Skin and soft-tissue swelling
- Painful and limited range of motion
- Neurovascular status
  - Capillary refill less than 2 seconds
  - Two-point discrimination
- Rotational and angulation deformity
  - Grip to evaluate rotation (Fig. 95.1)
- Always examine the ipsilateral hand, elbow, and shoulder for associated injuries.
- "Fight bite:" curved laceration over metacarpophalangeal joint = open fracture or open joint and should be thoroughly irrigated (Fig. 95.2)

Imaging

- Posteroanterior, lateral, and oblique radiographs of the affected digit
- Description of fracture
  - Open versus closed
  - Bone involved and location within bone
- Displacement and angulation
- Comminution
- Intra-articular versus extra-articular

Differential Diagnosis

- Metacarpal head fracture (Fig. 95.3)
  - Axial loading or direct trauma
  - Often intra-articular
- Metacarpal neck fracture (Fig. 95.4)
  - Boxer's fracture
  - Often involves ring and small fingers
- Metacarpal shaft fracture (Fig. 95.5)
  - Transverse: often apex dorsal angulation
  - Oblique or spiral: rotational malalignment
  - Comminuted: shortening
- Metacarpal base fracture (Fig. 95.6)
  - Rare injuries in index and long fingers
  - Intra-articular fracture of ring or small finger
    - Reverse Bennett fracture: fracture dislocation of small finger metacarpal: hamate joint
- Metacarpophalangeal joint dislocations (Fig. 95.7)
  - Dorsal dislocation
    - More common
    - Usually involve thumb and index finger
    - Simple (reducible) or complex (irreducible)
  - Volar dislocation
    - Less common
    - Usually complex (irreducible)

Treatment

- Metacarpal head
  - Radiographs to define injury
  - Closed reduction and splinting
    - Require anatomic reduction to establish joint congruity
    - Splint in intrinsic plus position (Fig. 95.8)
    - Early range of motion
  - Operative indications
    - Unstable fractures or if more than 1 mm step-off
    - Fight bite: open fracture with high incidence of infection; treat with antibiotics to cover human mouth organisms
    - Open reduction and internal fixation versus closed reduction and percutaneous pinning
- Metacarpal neck
  - Radiographs to define injury
    - Often volar comminution with dorsal angulation
  - Closed reduction and splinting in intrinsic plus position: Jahss maneuver (Fig. 95.9)
  - Acceptable reduction

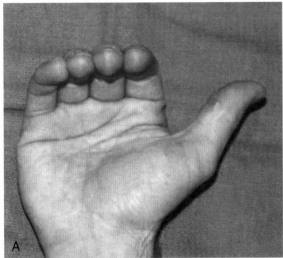

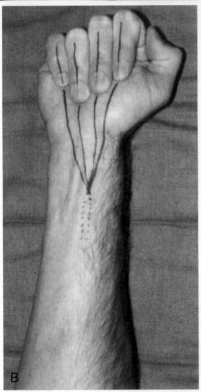

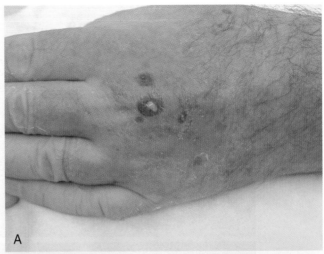

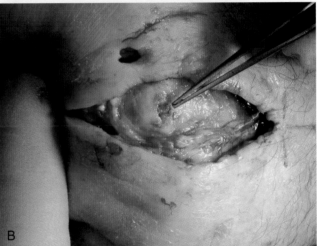

Fig 95.1 (A) Evaluation of rotational discrepancy in the digits has been described to include nail plate alignment, which is rather inaccurate. (B) Viewing axially along the segment of the ray in question to evaluate the parallelism of the next digital segment is most accurate. When the digits are flexed, both metacarpophalangeal and proximal interphalangeal joints align to converge at a point overlying the flexor carpi radialis tendon above the level of the wrist. (From Bucholz RW, Heckman JD, Court-Brown C, eds. *Rockwood and Green's Fractures in Adults*. 6th ed. Philadelphia: Lippincott Williams & Wilkins; 2006, Fig. 24.2.)

Fig 95.2 (A) Fight bite with laceration over metacarpophalangeal joint. (B) Open irrigation and débridement demonstrate tooth indentation in bone.

- Index and long fingers: less than 15 degrees of angulation
- Ring and small fingers: less than 45 degrees of angulation
- Unstable fractures require open reduction and internal fixation versus closed reduction and percutaneous pinning.
- Metacarpal shaft
  - Radiographs to define injury
  - Closed reduction and splinting in intrinsic plus position
  - Operative indications
    - Open fractures
    - Multiple metacarpal fractures
    - Associated neurovascular or tendon injuries
    - Failure of attempted closed reduction
    - Rotational deformity more than 10 degrees
    - Dorsal angulation more than 10 degrees for index and long fingers
    - Dorsal angulation more than 20 degrees for ring and small fingers
  - Open reduction and internal fixation with plate and screws or closed reduction and percutaneous pinning

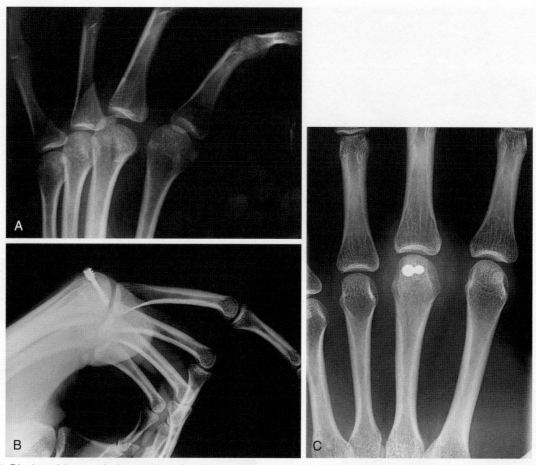

Fig 95.3 (A) Displaced intra-articular sagittal slice fracture of the middle finger metacarpal head. Postoperative posteroanterior (B) and lateral (C) views show anatomic reduction and fixation with a Herbert screw. Full metacarpophalangeal mobility was restored. (From Day CS. Fractures of the metacarpals and phalanges. In: Wolfe SW, Hotchkiss RN, Pederson WC, et al., eds. *Green's Operative Hand Surgery*. 7th ed. Philadelphia: Elsevier; 2017, Fig. 7.1.)

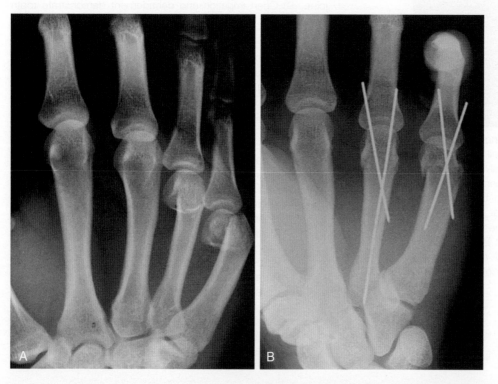

Fig 95.4 (A) Severely displaced neck fractures of the ring and small finger metacarpals. (B) Closed reduction using the Jahss maneuver and percutaneous crossed pins. (From Day CS. Fractures of the metacarpals and phalanges. In: Wolfe SW, Hotchkiss RN, Pederson WC, et al., eds. *Green's Operative Hand Surgery*. 7th ed. Philadelphia: Elsevier; 2017, Fig. 7.4.)

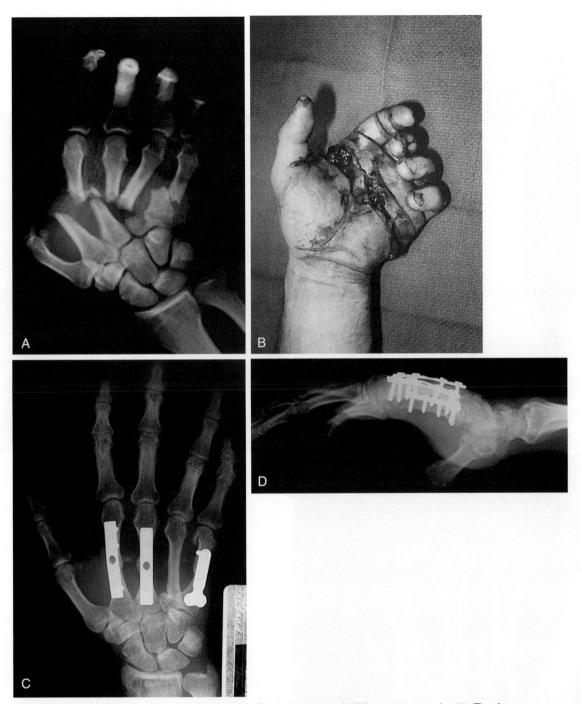

Fig 95.5 Plate fixation for metacarpal shaft fractures. **(A)** Shaft fractures of all four metacarpals. **(B)** The fractures were open and revascularization was required. **(C)** Anteroposterior radiograph showing healed fractures. Plate fixation provided a stable framework for microvascular repairs. **(D)** Lateral view. (From Day CS. Fractures of the metacarpals and phalanges. In: Wolfe SW, Hotchkiss RN, Pederson WC, et al., eds. *Green's Operative Hand Surgery*. 7th ed. Philadelphia: Elsevier; 2017, Fig. 7.12.)

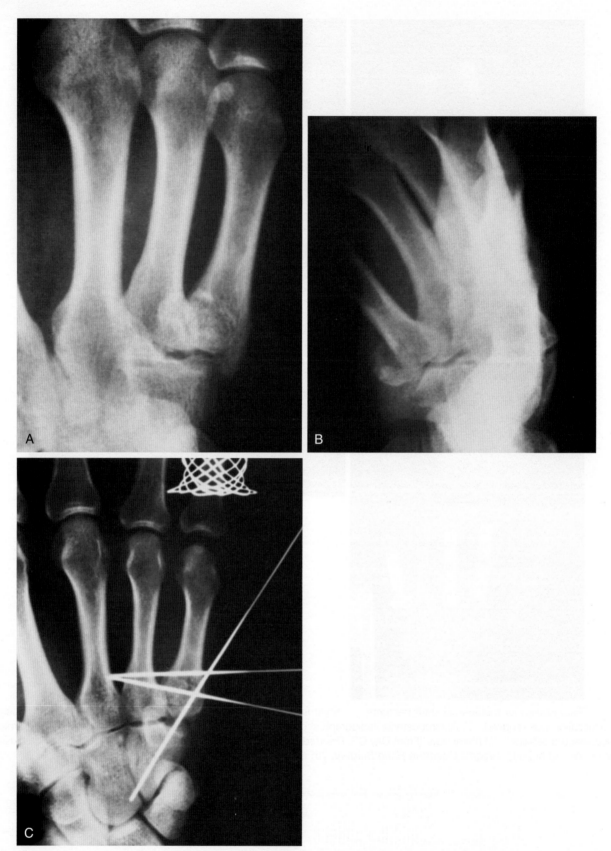

Fig 95.6 (A) An intra-articular fracture of the base of the fifth metacarpal with proximal and dorsal subluxation of the carpometacarpal joint. (B) An oblique view taken with the hand pronated 30 degrees from its fully supinated position shows the extent of the intra-articular injury. (C) Reduction was obtained by longitudinal traction and lateral pressure on the displaced bone. Firm fixation with a transarticular pin as well as transfixation pins into the adjacent metacarpal allowed early motion. (From Day CS. Fractures of the metacarpals and phalanges. In: Wolfe SW, Hotchkiss RN, Pederson WC, et al., eds. *Green's Operative Hand Surgery*. 7th ed. Philadelphia: Elsevier; 2017, Fig. 7.16.)

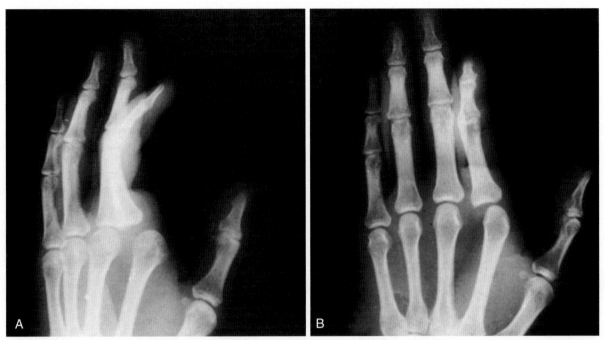

Fig 95.7 Radiographs of a dorsal irreducible (complex) dislocation. (A) An oblique view shows the dorsal dislocation and widened joint space caused by interposition of the volar plate. (B) The ulnar shift of the proximal phalanx suggests rupture of the radial collateral ligament. (From Green DP, Hotchkiss RN, Pederson WC, Wolfe SW, eds. *Green's Operative Hand Surgery*. 5th ed. Philadelphia: Churchill Livingstone; 2005, Fig. 9.13.)

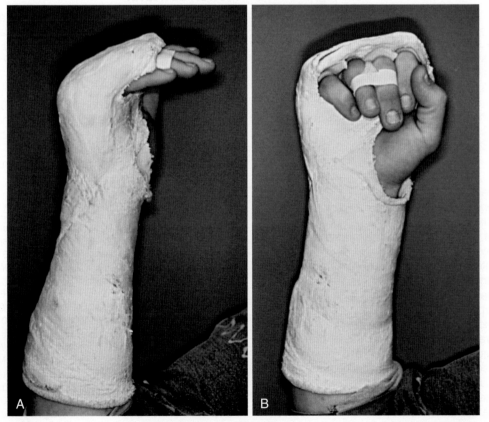

Fig 95.8 (A) Clam-digger cast for a metacarpal shaft fracture. The wrist is extended 30 degrees, the metacarpophalangeal joints are flexed 80 to 90 degrees, and the interphalangeal joints are extended. (B) Active range of motion is encouraged, and supplemental buddy taping can help control rotation. (From Day CS. Fractures of the metacarpals and phalanges. In: Wolfe SW, Hotchkiss RN, Pederson WC, et al., eds. *Green's Operative Hand Surgery*. 7th ed. Philadelphia: Elsevier; 2017, Fig. 7.7.)

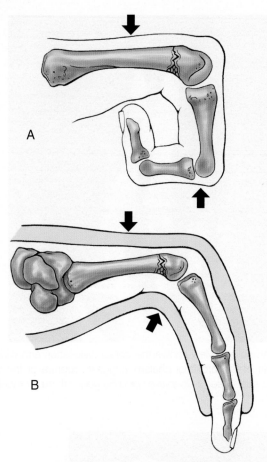

Fig 95.9 **(A)** The Jahss maneuver for reduction of a metacarpal neck fracture. *Arrows* indicate the direction of pressure application for fracture reduction. **(B)** After reduction, the fingers are held in an intrinsic-plus (safe) position in an ulnar gutter splint with molding as indicated by *arrows*. (Adapted from Day CS. Fractures of the metacarpals and phalanges. In: Wolfe SW, Hotchkiss RN, Pederson WC, et al., eds. *Green's Operative Hand Surgery*. 7th ed. Philadelphia: Elsevier; 2017, Fig. 7.2.)

- Metacarpal base
  - Radiographs to define injury
  - Closed reduction and splinting
    - Base of the index, long, and ring fingers; minimal displacement
    - Associated with ligament avulsion
    - Early range of motion
  - Reverse Bennett fracture
    - Metacarpal displaced by pull of extensor carpi ulnaris and flexor carpi ulnaris muscles
    - Radiograph of hand in 30 degrees of pronation
    - Often requires open reduction and internal fixation or closed reduction and percutaneous pinning to restore articular surface
    - A fracture diagnosed late can be treated conservatively with the option for fusion of the carpometacarpal joint if pain continues.

- Metacarpophalangeal joint dislocations
  - Dorsal dislocation
    - Reducible when phalanx is still in contact with metacarpal head
    - Dorsal pressure to base of proximal phalanx to maintain contact with metacarpal head and prevent volar plate entrapment
    - Traction is contraindicated.
    - Irreducible or complex dislocations occur when the volar plate is interposed in the metacarpophalangeal joint.
    - Complex dislocations require open reduction.
    - After reduction, place into a splint in the intrinsic plus position.
  - Volar dislocation
    - Often complex and irreducible by closed means
    - Require open reduction
    - After reduction, place into a splint in intrinsic plus position.
- Complications
  - Stiffness
  - Posttraumatic arthritis
  - Malunion: may cause weakness of grip or pain
  - Malrotation: may result in scissoring and overlap of digits
  - Nonunion
  - Tendon adhesions

When to Refer

- All metacarpal fractures or joint dislocations should be referred to an orthopaedist or hand specialist for evaluation and definitive treatment.

Patient Instructions

- Keep splint clean and dry.
- Elevate the arm above the heart for 48 hours to decrease swelling and pain.
- Take pain medications as prescribed.
- Follow up with the orthopaedist as instructed.

Suggested Readings

Day CS. Fractures of the metacarpals and phalanges. In: Wolfe SW, Hotchkiss RN, Pederson WC, et al, eds. *Green's Operative Hand Surgery*. 7th ed. Philadelphia: Elsevier; 2017:231–277.

Egol KA, Koval KJ, Zuckerman JD. *Handbook of Fractures*. 5th ed. Philadelphia: Wolters Kluwer; 2015.

Henry MH. Hand fractures and dislocations. In: Court-Brown CM, Heckman JD, McQueen MM, et al, eds. *Rockwood and Green's Fractures in Adults*. 8th ed. Philadelphia: Wolters Kluwer; 2015:915–990.

Markiewitz AD. Fractures and dislocations involving the metacarpal bone. In: Trumble TE, Budoff JE, Cornwall R, eds. *Hand, Elbow, and Shoulder: Core Knowledge in Orthopaedics*. Philadelphia: Mosby; 2006:38–55.

Merrell G, Hastings H. Dislocations and ligament injuries of the digits. In: Wolfe SW, Hotchkiss RN, Pederson WC, et al, eds. *Green's Operative Hand Surgery*. 7th ed. Philadelphia: Elsevier; 2017:278–317.

Swanson AB. Fractures involving the digits of the hand. *Orthop Clin North Am*. 1970;1:261–274.

Chapter 96 Phalangeal Fractures

Jennifer A. Hart

ICD-10-CM CODES
S62.609A *Fracture phalanges, hand, closed*
S62.609B *Fracture phalanges, hand, open*
S62639A *Closed fracture of distal phalanx or phalanges of hand*
S62.639B *Open fracture of distal phalanx or phalanges of hand*

Key Concepts

- Phalangeal fractures are the most common upper extremity fracture.
- The primary goal of treatment is to maintain joint motion and congruity.
- "Hand fractures can be complicated by deformity from no treatment, stiffness from overtreatment, and both deformity and stiffness from poor treatment." (Swanson)
- Twenty-seven percent of finger fractures are treated inappropriately in the emergency department by inaccurate reduction or improper splinting.
- The proximal interphalangeal (PIP) joint is the most unforgiving joint in the hand.
- Prolonged mobilization has a deleterious effect on the overall outcome.

History

- It is important to obtain the following patient information:
  - Age
  - Hand dominance
  - Mechanism of injury
  - Comorbidities
  - Occupation

Physical Examination

- Skin and soft-tissue swelling
- Nail bed injuries
- Painful and limited range of motion
  - Examine each joint for congruent range of motion
- Neurovascular status
  - Capillary refill less than 2 seconds
  - Two-point discrimination
- Rotational and angulation deformity
  - Grip to evaluate rotation
- Check tenodesis effect
  - Wrist flexion results in finger extension.
  - Wrist extension results in finger flexion.

- Abnormality of the normal cascade of fingers suggests injury.
- Possible tendon injury on fracture fragment
- Complete examination may require injection of a local anesthetic agent.
  - Check the nerve status before administering a local anesthetic agent.
- Always examine the ipsilateral hand, elbow, and shoulder for associated injuries.

Imaging

- Posteroanterior, lateral, and oblique radiographs of affected digit
- Description of fracture
  - Open versus closed
  - Bone involved and location within bone
  - Displacement and angulation
  - Comminution
  - Intra-articular versus extra-articular

Differential Diagnosis

- Proximal phalanx fracture
  - Intra-articular
    - Condyle fractures
      - Unicondylar (Fig. 96.1)
      - Bicondylar (Fig. 96.2)
  - Extra-articular
    - Transverse: stable fracture pattern (Fig. 96.3)
    - Oblique: unstable (Fig. 96.4)
    - Spiral: unstable (Fig. 96.5)
    - Comminuted: unstable (Fig. 96.6)
- PIP joint dislocation
  - Dorsal dislocation (Fig. 96.7)
    - Hyperextension of the PIP joint
    - Evaluate for associated fracture
    - Pilon fracture of the middle phalanx
  - Volar dislocation (Fig. 96.8)
    - Less common
    - Can disrupt extensor mechanism (central slip)
  - Volar rotary subluxation (Fig. 96.9)
    - Condyle buttonholes in the tear of the central tendon
- Middle phalanx fracture
  - Intra-articular
    - Condyle fractures
      - Unicondylar
      - Bicondylar
  - Extra-articular
    - Transverse: stable fracture pattern
    - Oblique: unstable

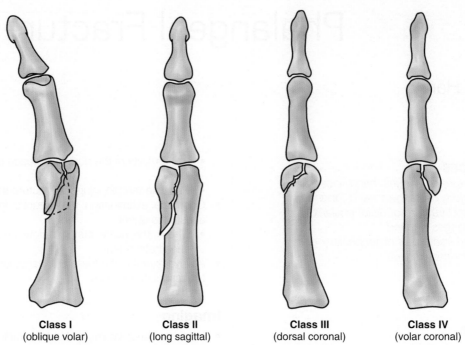

Class I	Class II	Class III	Class IV
(oblique volar)	(long sagittal)	(dorsal coronal)	(volar coronal)

Fig 96.1 Weiss-Hastings classification of unicondylar fractures of the proximal phalanx. These fractures are nearly all unstable and nearly always require operative fixation. (Adapted from Weiss APC, Hastings HH. Distal unicondylar fractures of the proximal phalanx. *J Hand Surg [Am]*. 1993;18A:594–599.)

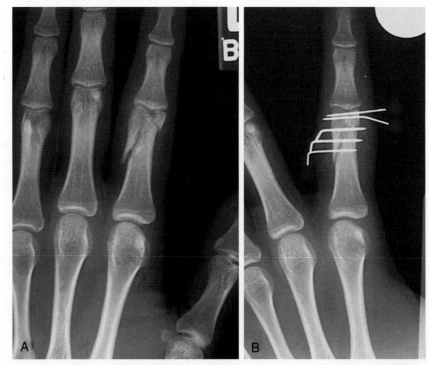

Fig 96.2 (A) Fragmented and displaced bicondylar proximal phalangeal fracture. (B) Percutaneous fixation. (From Day S. Fractures of the metacarpals and phalanges. In Wolfe SW, Hotchkiss RN, Pederson WC et al. (eds). *Green's Operative Hand Surgery*, 7th ed. Philadelphia, Elsevier, 2017.)

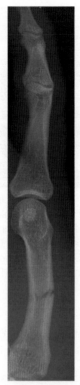

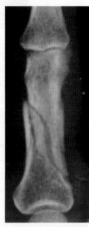

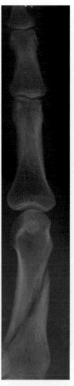

Fig 96.3 Transverse phalangeal shaft fracture. (From White TO, Mackenzie SP, Gray AJ: *McRae's Orthopaedic Trauma and Emergency Fracture Management, 3rd ed. Philadelphia, Elsevier, 2016.*)

Fig 96.4 Oblique unstable phalangeal shaft fractures. (From Rogers LF, West OC: *Imaging Skeletal Trauma*, 4th ed. Philadelphia, Elsevier, 2015.)

Fig 96.5 Spiral fracture of the phalanx. (From White TO, Mackenzie SP, Gray AJ: *Orthopaedic Trauma and Emergency Fracture Management*, 3rd ed. Philadelphia, Elsevier, 2016.)

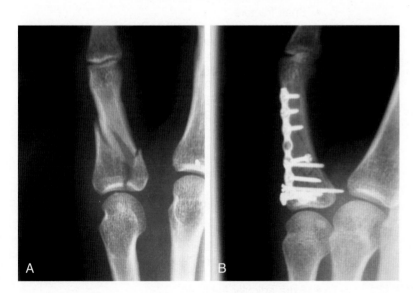

Fig 96.6 Comminuted fracture of the phalangeal shaft (A) can be stabilized for early motion with a condylar blade plate (B) placed laterally in the mid-axial plane. (From Green JB, Deveikas C, Ranger HE, et al: Hand, wrist, and digit injuries. In Magee DJ, Zachazewski JE, Quillen WS, Manske RC (eds): *Pathology and Intervention in Musculoskeletal Rehabilitation,* 2nd ed. Philadelphia, Elsevier, 2016.)

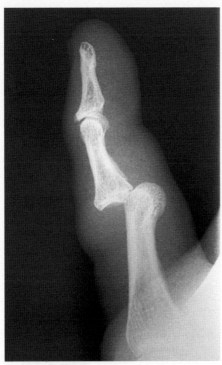

Fig 96.7 Dorsal dislocation of the proximal interphalangeal (PIP) joint. (From Eiff MP, Hatch R: *Fracture Management for Primary Care*, 3rd ed. Philadelphia, Elsevier, 2018.)

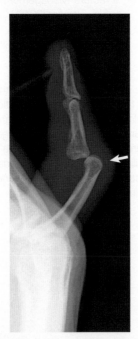

Fig 96.8 Volar dislocation with a small avulsion indicating extensor mechanism injury, which is a less common variant. (From Chew FS, Gerson RF. Upper extremity. Hand and Wrist. In: Mirvis SE, Kubal WS, Shanmuganathan K, et al (eds): *Problem Solving in Emergency Radiology,* Philadelphia, Elsevier, 2015.)

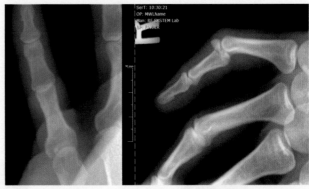

Fig 96.9 Large displaced central slip avulsion fracture with resultant volar rotatory subluxation of the proximal interphalangeal joint. (From Ruchelsman DE, Bindra RR. Fractures and dislocations of the hand. In: Browner BD, Jupiter JB, Krettek C, Anderson PA (eds): *Skeletal Trauma: Basic Science, Management, and Reconstruction*, 5th ed. Philadelphia, Elsevier, 2015.)

- • Spiral: unstable
  - • Comminuted: unstable
- • Distal interphalangeal (DIP) joint dislocation (Fig. 96.10)
  - • Injury due to hyperextension, hyperflexion, or impaction
  - • Most often dorsal or lateral
  - • Hinge joint with strong collateral ligaments
- • Distal phalanx fractures (Fig. 96.11)
  - • Most common hand fracture
  - • Thumb and middle finger most common
  - • Tuft fracture (see Fig. 96.11C)
    - • Crush injury
    - • Often seen with a nail matrix injury or laceration = open fracture
    - • Painful subungual hematoma
  - • Shaft fracture
    - • Transverse (see Fig. 96.11B)
    - • Longitudinal (see Fig. 96.11A)
- • Intra-articular fracture (see Fig. 96.11G)
  - • Bony mallet: avulsion of extensor tendon from the distal phalanx (see Fig. 96.11D)
  - • Flexor digitorum profundus avulsion from the distal phalanx (see Fig. 96.11F)

Treatment

- • Early motion after adequate initial healing is the key to prevent stiffness.
- • Splint the injured joint only and avoid crossing surrounding joints.
- • If there is associated tendon or neurovascular injury requiring surgery, then also stabilize the bone injury at the same operative intervention.
- • Proximal phalanx
  - • Extra-articular fractures
    - • Stable (transverse) and nondisplaced
      - • Closed reduction with axial traction
      - • Buddy taping for 3 to 4 weeks
      - • Monitor closely for displacement.
    - • Unstable (spiral, oblique, comminuted)
      - • Closed reduction and splinting in intrinsic plus position

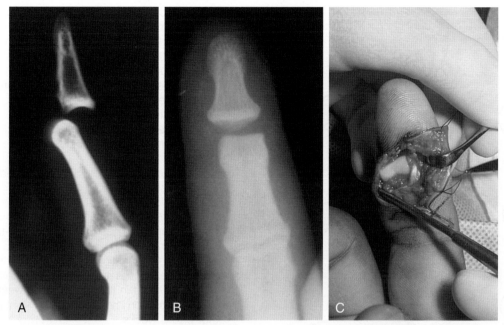

Fig 96.10 **(A)** Irreducible dorsal dislocation of an index distal interphalangeal joint. **(B)** The posteroanterior view shows a wide gap between the middle and distal phalanges suggestive of soft-tissue interposition. This appearance is typical of an irreducible dislocation in which the interposed soft tissue prevents reduction of the joint. These injuries are commonly open, and, at exploration **(C)**, the head of the middle phalanx was seen ulnar to the displaced flexor tendon. The volar plate was interposed between the base of the distal phalanx and the head of the middle phalanx. (From Merrell G, Hastings H. Dislocations and ligament injuries of the digits. In: Wolfe SW, Hotchkiss RN, Pederson WC, et al., eds. *Green's Operative Hand Surgery*. 7th ed. Philadelphia: Elsevier; 2017.)

- Often requires closed reduction and percutaneous pinning or open reduction and internal fixation (see Figs. 96.3, 96.5, and 96.6)
  - Refer to a hand specialist.
- Intra-articular fractures
  - Unstable or displaced
  - Condylar fractures
  - Closed reduction to align fracture fragments via axial traction
  - Splint in intrinsic plus position with radial or ulnar gutter splints
  - Nonoperative
    - Closed minimally displaced fractures with acceptable alignment
    - Monitor closely for displacement.
  - Operative (see Fig. 96.2)
    - Open fractures
    - Significant shortening or malrotation
    - Articular step-off
    - Failed closed treatment: displaced extra-articular fractures
- PIP joint dislocation
  - Dorsal dislocation with no fracture
    - Longitudinal traction for reduction and buddy taping for several weeks until pain has resolved
    - Early motion is encouraged if the dislocation is stable after reduction.
  - Dorsal dislocation with fracture
    - The goal is a congruous articular surface and early motion.
- Extension block splinting (Fig. 96.12) or open reduction and internal fixation
  - Refer to a hand specialist.
- Volar dislocation with no fracture
  - Extensor mechanism (central slip) injury
  - Longitudinal traction for reduction
  - Extension splinting of proximal interphalangeal joint for 6 weeks to prevent boutonniere deformity
  - Refer to a hand specialist.
- Volar dislocation with fracture
  - Dorsal bony avulsion may require open reduction and internal fixation.
  - Refer to a hand specialist.
- Volar rotary subluxation
  - Difficult closed reduction often requires open reduction.
  - Refer to a hand specialist.
- Middle phalanx
  - Extra-articular fractures
    - Stable (transverse) and nondisplaced
      - Closed reduction with axial traction
      - Buddy taping for 3 to 4 weeks
      - Monitor closely for displacement.
    - Unstable (spiral, oblique, comminuted)
      - Closed reduction and splinting in intrinsic plus position
      - Often require closed reduction and percutaneous pinning or open reduction and internal fixation
      - Refer to a hand specialist.
  - Intra-articular fractures
    - Unstable or displaced

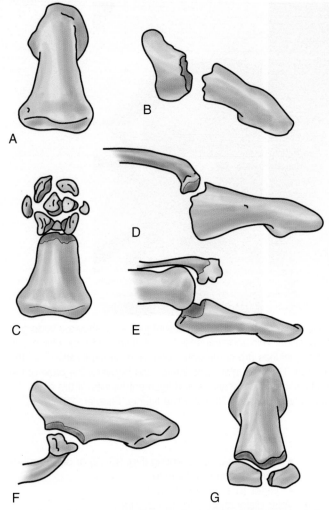

Fig 96.11 Fracture patterns seen in the distal phalanx include the longitudinal shaft (A), transverse shaft (B), tuft (C), dorsal base avulsion (D), dorsal base shear (E), volar base (F), and complete articular (G). (From Bucholz RW, Heckman JD, Court-Brown C, et al., eds. *Rockwood and Green's Fractures in Adults*. 6th ed. Philadelphia: Lippincott Williams & Wilkins; 2006.)

- Closed reduction to align fracture fragments via axial traction
- Splint in intrinsic plus position with radial or ulnar gutter splints
- Nonoperative
  - Closed minimally displaced fractures with acceptable alignment
- Operative
  - Open fractures
  - Significant shortening
  - Articular step-off
  - Failed closed treatment: displaced extra-articular fractures
- DIP joint dislocation
  - Reduce closed injuries with traction.
  - Open injuries are due to a minimal soft-tissue envelope 60% of the time.
    - Thorough irrigation, antibiotics, and reduction
    - Nail bed injuries require repair with absorbable suture.
  - Splint DIP joint in flexion for 2 to 3 weeks
  - Volar dislocation immobilized in DIP joint extension splint for 6 to 8 weeks
- Distal phalanx
  - Tuft fracture
    - Decompression of subungual hematoma with needle
    - Nail bed repair: repair all nail matrix lacerations with absorbable suture after thorough irrigation and antibiotics (see Chapter 87)
    - Immobilize with aluminum foam splint
  - Shaft fracture
    - Transverse
      - Nondisplaced: aluminum foam splint including DIP joint for 3 to 4 weeks
      - Displaced: closed reduction and percutaneous pinning (often requires nail bed repair); refer to a hand specialist
- Intra-articular fracture
  - Bony mallet
    - DIP joint extension splint for 6 to 8 weeks (see Chapter 85)
    - Refer to a hand specialist.

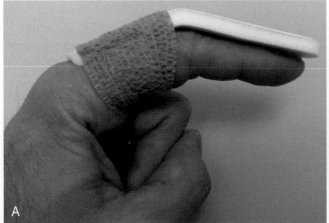
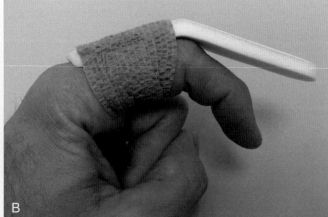

Fig 96.12 (A and B) Dorsal (extension block) splinting at 30-40 degrees of flexion at the PIP joint allowing freedom of flexion at the PIP joint while limiting extension. (From Porter AST: Common sports injuries. In: Kellerman RD, Bope ET (eds): *Conn's Current Therapy 2018*. Philadelphia, Elsevier, 2018.)

- Flexor digitorum profundus avulsion
  - Flexor tendon repair (see Chapter 83)
  - Refer to a hand specialist.
- Complications
  - Stiffness
  - Hyperesthesia, cold intolerance, or numbness
  - Post-traumatic arthritis
  - Malunion: may cause weakness of grip or pain
  - Malrotation: may result in scissoring and overlap of digits
  - Nonunion

When to Refer

- All phalangeal fractures and complicated interphalangeal dislocations should be referred to an orthopaedist or a hand specialist for evaluation.

Patient Instructions

- Keep the splint clean and dry.
- Elevate the arm above the heart for 48 hours to decrease swelling and pain.
- Take pain medications as prescribed.
- Follow up with an orthopaedist as instructed.
- Early motion and therapy are very important after adequate initial healing.

Suggested Readings

Day CS. Fractures of the metacarpals and phalanges. In: Wolfe SW, Hotchkiss RN, Pederson WC, et al, eds. *Green's Operative Hand Surgery*. 7th ed. Philadelphia: Elsevier; 2017:231–277.

Egol KA, Koval KJ, Zuckerman JD. *Handbook of Fractures*. 5th ed. Philadelphia: Wolters Kluwer; 2015.

Henry MH. Hand fractures and dislocations. In: Court-Brown CM, Heckman JD, McQueen MM, et al, eds. *Rockwood and Green's Fractures in Adults*. 8th ed. Philadelphia: Wolters Kluwer; 2015:915–990.

Merrell G, Hastings H. Dislocations and ligament injuries of the digits. In: Wolfe SW, Hotchkiss RN, Pederson WC, et al, eds. *Green's Operative Hand Surgery*. 7th ed. Philadelphia: Elsevier; 2017:278–317.

Slade JF, Magit DP. Phalangeal fractures and dislocations. In: Trumble TE, Budoff JE, Cornwall R, eds. *Hand, Elbow, and Shoulder: Core Knowledge in Orthopaedics*. Philadelphia: Mosby; 2006:22–37.

Swanson AB. Fractures involving the digits of the hand. *Orthop Clin North Am*. 1970;1:261–274.

Chapter 97 Distal Radius Fracture Reduction

Jennifer A. Hart

CPT CODES
25600 *Closed treatment of distal radial fracture (e.g., Colles' or Smith's type) or epiphyseal separation, includes closed treatment of fracture of ulnar styloid, when performed; without manipulation*
25605 *Closed treatment of distal radial fracture (e.g., Colles' or Smith's type) or epiphyseal separation, includes closed treatment of fracture of ulnar styloid, when performed; with manipulation*

Equipment

- Lidocaine for hematoma block
- Finger traps and an intravenous (IV) pole for traction
- Countertraction weight
- Soft roll padding
- Sugar tong splinting material (plaster or fiberglass)
- Ace bandage

Contraindications

- Nondisplaced fractures may worsen alignment.
- Stable fracture patterns with acceptable reduction
  - Radial shortening less than 2 mm
  - Neutral tilt
  - Articular step-off less than 1 mm
- Elderly (older than 65 years old) or low-demand patients with comorbidities with reasonable alignment and may not tolerate reduction

Technique and Tips

- Complete full physical examination before reduction
  - Skin and soft-tissue swelling
  - Painful and limited range of motion of wrist
  - Deformity and angulation
  - Dorsal displacement: Colles fracture (90% of distal radius fractures)
  - Volar displacement: Smith fracture
  - Neurovascular status, especially median nerve
  - Carpal tunnel compression symptoms are present in 13-23% of injuries.
  - Palpate anatomic snuffbox for tenderness that may suggest scaphoid fracture.
  - Examine finger and thumb motion to confirm tendon continuity.

- Always examine the ipsilateral hand, elbow, and shoulder for associated injuries.
- Provide adequate anesthesia.
- Hematoma block (Fig. 97.1)
  - 10 mL of 1% lidocaine without epinephrine
  - Prepare skin with povidone-iodine and alcohol.
  - Inject at the level of the fracture on the dorsal wrist in the middle of the radius.
  - Draw back after the needle is placed; you should see blood to confirm proper placement.
  - Inject 10 mL of lidocaine.
  - May provide fast-acting IV pain medication such as fentanyl

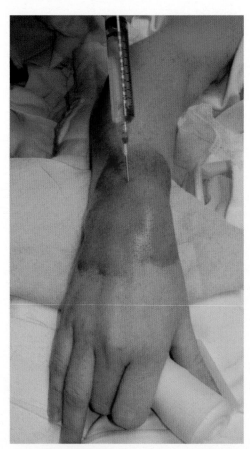

Fig 97.1 Hematoma block: 10 mL of 1% lidocaine without epinephrine injected at the level of the fracture on the dorsal wrist in the middle of the radius. Draw back after the needle is placed; you should see blood to confirm proper placement.

- Conscious IV sedation may be required in children and some adults.
- Place the thumb and index and middle fingers in finger traps, making sure that the fit is tight (Fig. 97.2).
  - Using only these digits provides the ulnar deviation often needed to aid in reduction.
  - Protect the skin, especially in the elderly, with tape.
- Hang the upper extremity in finger traps from an IV pole (see Fig. 97.2).
  - Patient placed supine on bed
  - Shoulder at 90 degrees abduction and neutral external rotation
  - The elbow should be at 90 degrees of flexion.
  - Hang 5 to 15 pounds of countertraction from the distal humerus.
  - Confirm patient comfort once positioned.
  - Allow the countertraction weight to work using ligamentotaxis for approximately 5 minutes.
- Closed manipulation of dorsally displaced fractures (Fig. 97.3)
  - Longitudinal traction to release the fracture fragments
  - Reproduce the fracture mechanism by hyperextending the wrist.
  - Pull longitudinal traction while flexing the wrist and placing direct pressure on the dorsal fracture fragment with your thumb.
  - Be careful not to tear fragile skin in the elderly.
  - Palpate the distal radius dorsally to confirm improvement in dorsal displacement.
  - May use fluoroscopy at this point to confirm reduction
  - Sometimes takes several attempts to completely unlock fragments and obtain adequate reduction

- Splint placement
  - Wrap the arm including the distal humerus, elbow, forearm, wrist, and proximal hand to the metacarpophalangeal joints with a soft roll.
  - May take the thumb out of the finger trap at this point to place the soft roll around the thumb in the first web space
  - Leave the index finger in the trap to make placement of the splint easier while the arm is hanging.
  - Confirm that padding is adequate, especially at the bony prominences at the elbow.
  - Place a sugar tong splint using plaster or fiberglass around the elbow and on the dorsal and volar surfaces of the forearm with the forearm in a neutral position (see Fig. 92.8 in Chapter 92).
  - Dorsally: Stop the splint at the metacarpophalangeal joints to allow finger motion.
  - Volarly: Stop at the proximal palmar skin crease to allow metacarpophalangeal flexion to 90 degrees.
  - Wrap the splinting material with an Ace bandage.
  - Three-point molding of the splint (Fig. 97.4)
  - Place one hand dorsally distal to the fracture.
  - Place the second hand volarly proximal to the fracture.
  - The third point is at the elbow dorsally.
  - Try to obtain a dorsal buttress to prevent collapse.
  - Avoid excessive wrist flexion, as it can cause median nerve compression symptoms.
  - Place in slight ulnar deviation and neutral forearm rotation.
  - Postreduction examination
  - Always obtain postreduction radiographs after the splint has been placed.
  - Always perform a complete postreduction examination including sensation, motor, and vascular examination.

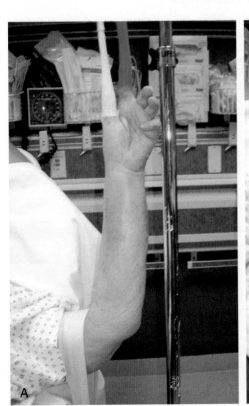
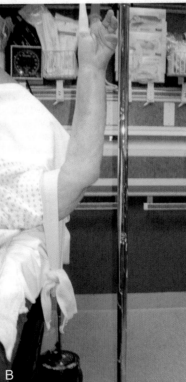

Fig 97.2 (A) The upper extremity is hung in finger traps from an IV pole. (B) Five to 15 pounds of countertraction is hung from the distal humerus. Confirm patient comfort once the patient is positioned. Allow the countertraction weight to work using ligamentotaxis for approximately 5 minutes.

A   B

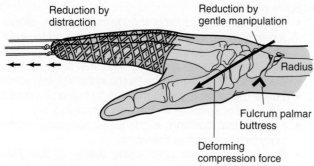

Reduction by distraction

Reduction by gentle manipulation

Radius

Fulcrum palmar buttress

Deforming compression force

Fig 97.3 Treatment of Colles' fracture to effect reduction. (From Kalb RL, Fowler GC: Fracture care. In Pfenninger JL, Fowler GC: *Pfenninger & Fowler's Procedures for Primary Care*. 3rd ed. Philadelphia, Elsevier, 2011.)

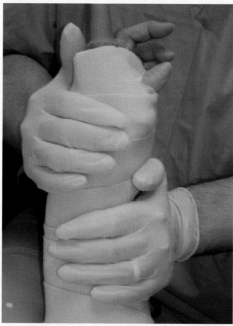

Fig 97.4 Three-point molding of the splint. Place one hand dorsally distal to the fracture and the other hand volarly proximal to the fracture. Your knee can be used as the third point at the elbow dorsally.

- Refer to an orthopaedist for all distal radius fractures.
  - New radiographs to be obtained within 1 week to confirm maintenance of reduction
  - May tighten the splint by rewrapping the bandage as swelling decreases
  - If definitive nonoperative therapy, orthopaedist will change the splint to a cast when the swelling has decreased.

Considerations in Special Populations

- Pediatrics
  - Often requires IV conscious sedation
  - Only one reduction attempt should be made to prevent further damage to the physis
  - High potential for remodeling
  - Refer to an orthopaedist for all displaced and physeal fractures

Troubleshooting

- Inadequate reduction may be secondary to inadequate pain control and anesthesia.
- Provide adequate pain control to allow for adequate traction.

Patient Instructions

- Keep the splint clean and dry.
- Elevate the arm above the heart for 48 hours to decrease swelling and pain.
- Take pain medications as prescribed.
- Follow up with an orthopaedist as instructed.

Suggested Readings

Egol KA, Koval KJ, Zuckerman JD. Distal radius. In: *Handbook of Fractures*. 5th ed. Philadelphia: Wolters Kluwer; 2015:266–278.

Jiuliano JA, Jupiter J. Distal radius fractures. In: Trumble TE, Budoff JE, Cornwall R, eds. *Core Knowledge in Orthopaedics: Hand, Elbow, and Shoulder*. Philadelphia: Mosby; 2006:84–101.

McQueen MM, et al. Fractures of the distal radius and ulna. In: Court-Brown CM, Heckman JD, McQueen MM, eds. *Rockwood and Green's Fractures in Adults*. 8th ed. Philadelphia: Wolters Kluwer; 2015: 1057–1120.

Wolfe SW, et al. Distal radius fractures. In: Wolfe SW, Hotchkiss RN, Pederson WC, eds. *Green's Operative Hand Surgery*. 7th ed. Philadelphia: Elsevier; 2017:516–587.

Chapter 98 Finger Dislocations

Amy Kite, Jonathan E. Isaacs

ICD-10-CM CODES
S63 *Dislocation and sprain of joints and ligaments at wrist and hand level*
S63.0 *Subluxation and dislocation of wrist and hand joints*
S63.1 *Subluxation and dislocation of thumb*
S63.2 *Subluxation and dislocation of other finger(s)*

Key Concepts

- The proximal interphalangeal (PIP) joint is a commonly dislocated joint due to a relative lack of protection and a long lever arm.
- Dislocations of the distal interphalangeal (DIP) and metacarpophalangeal (MCP) joints are less common.
- DIP joint dislocations are often open injuries due to the thin, adherent soft-tissue envelope.
- MCP joint dislocations are more likely to require an open reduction.
- Dislocations are described by the direction of displacement of the distal aspect of the digit: dorsal, volar, and lateral. Dorsal dislocation is the most common injury pattern.
- Treatment depends on the degree of ligament and bony injury and the presence or absence of residual instability.

Anatomy

- The DIP and PIP joints share a similar anatomy in the basic form of a three-sided box. The floor is formed by the volar plate and the sides by collateral ligaments (Fig. 98.1A and B). The MCP joint has stout collateral ligaments but a less substantial volar capsule.
  - Volar plate (DIP and PIP joints)
    - A stout volar capsule thickening that inserts into the periosteum; it is more firmly attached proximally and is suspended by insertions of the collateral ligaments.
    - Primary function is to resist hyperextension.
    - Often avulsed in dislocations, the volar plate can block reduction if it becomes interposed within the joint.
  - Collateral ligaments (DIP, PIP, and MCP joints)
    - Stout lateral capsular thickenings that originate on the dorsolateral aspect of the more proximal bone; run obliquely to insert on the volar-lateral 40% of the distal articular rim
    - Primary restraints to radial and ulnar deviation
    - Depending on the specific dislocation mechanism, the collateral ligaments are often disrupted. This disruption can occur partially or in whole and can affect joint stability.

- Extensor mechanism
  - Two components: The central mechanism inserts just distal to the PIP joint (central slip) and again just distal to the DIP joint (terminal tendon).
  - The lateral band extends from the intrinsic muscles of the hand and inserts into the extensor hood.
  - This anatomy is important because both the central slip and terminal tendon are vulnerable to avulsion injury during volar dislocations.
  - Dislocations of MCP and PIP joints can become trapped between the lateral band and the central mechanism.

History

- Finger dislocations are generally referred after spontaneous reduction or reduction by the patient, trainer, or parent.
- Often describe a mechanism of jamming, hyperextension, or twisting
- May describe chronic instability, pain, or swelling

Physical Examination

- Swelling and ecchymosis are common. Unreduced dislocations are usually obvious, although may be obscured by swelling. Open dislocations are not uncommon, and skin integrity should be assessed.
- Neurovascular examination includes sensory testing and capillary refill documented before reduction or digital block.
- Palpate to localize points of tenderness to identify ligament, volar plate, bone, and tendon injuries both before and after reduction.
- Check range of motion and stability postreduction (may require digital block). Redislocation or subluxation during active range of motion indicates gross instability.
- Next, evaluate stability with gentle lateral stress and hyperextension; this may indicate subtle instability.
- Isolate the injured joint and test for active flexion and extension to identify associated tendon injuries.

Imaging

- Anteroposterior and lateral views of the affected joint pre- and postreduction to confirm reduction and to evaluate for associated bony injury (perform before testing for instability)
- Fluoroscopic stress views are often helpful to evaluate stability.
- Other imaging modalities (such as magnetic resonance imaging) are not usually necessary.

Classification

- In general, dislocations are described according to the location of the distal component relative to the proximal

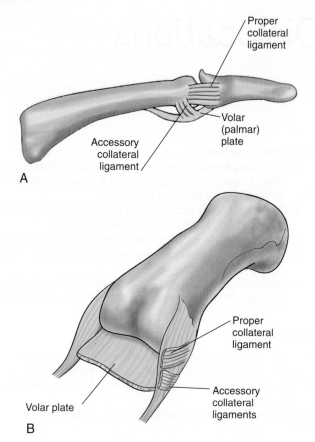

Fig 98.1 (A) and (B), The metacarpophalangeal, proximal interphalangeal, and distal interphalangeal joints share a basic three-sided box architecture. The volar plate forms the floor and resists hyperextension, whereas stout collateral ligaments protect from lateral forces.

component. Associated bone and soft-tissue injuries further stratify dislocations and help not only to communicate adequately the injury severity but also to guide treatment strategy and predict outcome.

- Dorsal, volar, lateral
- Associated with or without fracture
- Stable versus unstable
- Reducible (simple) versus irreducible (complex)
- Chronic or acute

Treatment

- Digital block or proper anesthesia is mandatory for reduction and stability testing.
- Complex (i.e., irreducible) dislocations require surgical exploration.
- Open injuries need appropriate irrigation/debridement and antibiotic treatment.
- Avoid prolonged immobilization; simple/stable injuries are generally conducive to brief periods of immobilization followed by protected range of motion.

DIP (and Thumb Interphalangeal) Joint Dislocations

- Reduction maneuver: slow, steady traction of the distal phalanx accompanied by direct pressure over the deformity

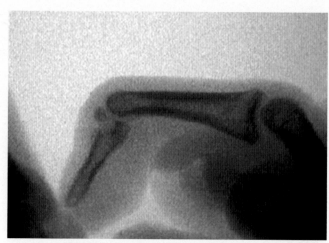

Fig 98.2 Distal interphalangeal bony mallet injury. Postreduction radiographs and active strength testing reveal associated injuries, such as this fracture involving the articular surface and insertion of the extensor tendon. This injury pattern necessitates referral to a hand surgeon for possible surgical stabilization (versus prolonged extension splinting). (From Green DP, Hotchkiss RN, Pederson WC, Wolfe SW, eds. *Green's Operative Hand Surgery.* 5th ed. Philadelphia: Churchill Livingstone; 2005.)

- Treatment depends on stability and associated tendon injury.
  - If grossly unstable, the DIP joint needs operative fixation. If instability is subtle, splint the joint in 20 degrees of flexion for 2 weeks and then reevaluate it. A stable joint can be treated symptomatically with temporary splinting (1 to 2 weeks), followed by early mobilization when tolerated.
  - Loss of active extension, with or without a small dorsal bone fragment, indicates extensor tendon avulsion or tear and requires prolonged (6 weeks) splinting in full extension (Fig. 98.2).
  - Avoid splinting across the PIP joint, which can cause stiffness and hyperextension of the DIP.
- Small fractures should be treated the same as a sprain (with treatment based on stability as previously described).
- Significant fractures (>40% of the joint surface) should be splinted and the patient referred to a hand specialist for possible fixation.

Proximal Interphalangeal Joint Dislocations

- Dorsal
  - Most dorsal dislocations are reduced with gentle distal traction while applying volarly directed pressure over the PIP joint (Fig. 98.3).
  - Treatment depends on stability.
    - If grossly unstable, the collateral ligaments need operative fixation.
    - If instability is subtle, splint in 20 degrees of flexion for 3 weeks and then reevaluate the joint.
    - A stable joint can be treated symptomatically with temporary splinting (1 to 2 weeks) followed by early mobilization (buddy taping) when tolerated.
  - In cases of fracture-dislocation, treatment may depend on the size of the articular fracture fragment.

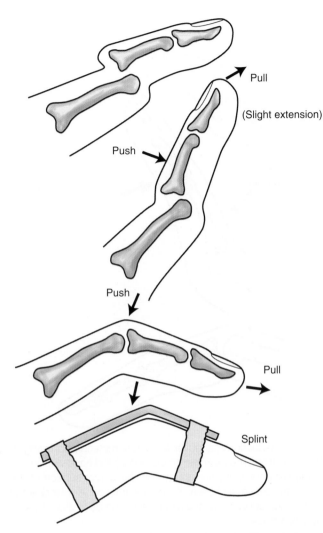

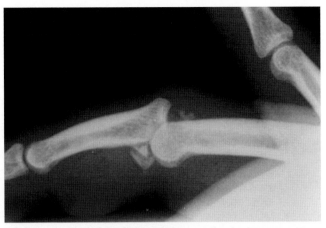

Fig 98.4 Fracture/dislocation of proximal interphalangeal joint involving approximately 40% of the volar articular surface of the middle phalanx. Fractures/dislocations involving less than 40% of the articular surface are amenable to extension block splinting. (From Green DP, Hotchkiss RN, Pederson WC, Wolfe SW, eds. *Green's Operative Hand Surgery.* 5th ed. Philadelphia: Churchill Livingstone; 2005.)

Fig 98.3 Reduction maneuver for dorsal proximal interphalangeal dislocation. Gentle traction and slight exaggeration of deformity, followed by volar pressure to slide the joint back into place.

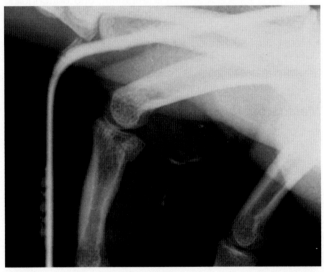

Fig 98.5 Extension block splinting of proximal interphalangeal (PIP) joint. Extension block splinting, as with this stable fracture dislocation, allows active flexion at the PIP joint. The splint is extended at weekly intervals. (From Green DP, Hotchkiss RN, Pederson WC, Wolfe SW, eds. *Green's Operative Hand Surgery.* 5th ed. Philadelphia: Churchill Livingstone; 2005.)

- Small fragments (<10% or volar lip avulsions) can be treated the same as dislocations based on the joint stability.
- Large fragments (>40% of the joint surface) are typically grossly unstable. These should be splinted for comfort and referred to a specialist for surgical fixation or application of a dynamic external fixation.
- Intermediate fragments (10-40%) can often be stable after reduction when kept in slight flexion (Fig. 98.4). These can be treated by extension block splinting in 30 degrees of flexion, followed by weekly reduction of the splint by 10 degrees until full extension is achieved. Maintenance of reduction must be verified weekly (Fig. 98.5). This can be difficult to judge and referral to a specialist would be appropriate.
- Volar
  - Rare and often unstable; easy to reduce but difficult to maintain; these injuries are often open.
  - Always involve a central slip tendon avulsion (boutonnière injury) and should be referred to a hand surgeon.

- A variant of volar dislocations, rotational subluxation poses a reduction dilemma. This pattern can be recognized on a lateral radiograph: the proximal phalanx will appear in profile as a true lateral and the middle phalanx as an oblique view (not a true lateral). The head of the proximal phalanx is incarcerated between the lateral band and extensor mechanism. Traction alone may result in a "Chinese finger trap" effect, in which increased longitudinal traction acts to tension the soft tissue and form a tightening noose around the proximal phalanx neck that blocks reduction.

- Reduction is attempted by gentle flexion of the PIP and MCP joints (to relax the lateral bands) followed by axial and rotational force to finesse the proximal phalanx to anatomic position. Exaggeration of the deformity often aids in the reduction. If it is unsuccessful, open reduction will be required.
- Splinting
  - Stable volar dislocations of the PIP joint should be placed in full extension of the PIP joint only (the same treatment as for an isolated boutonnière deformity) for 6 weeks; this will approximate the central slip to allow healing.
  - Motion of both the MCP and DIP joints is encouraged to avoid stiffness and actually aids in healing of the extensor tendon.

Lateral Dislocations

- Often spontaneously or easily reduced; they may be stable with buddy taping of simple splinting (in slight flexion).
- In general, involve partial or complete disruption of the collateral ligaments.
- Blocks to reduction can include an interposed collateral ligament, extensor tendon entrapment, and buttonholing through the dorsal apparatus; these typically require operative exploration.
- Most can be treated by conservative means, including buddy taping and active range of motion to prevent stiffness. Joints grossly unstable to lateral stress (>20 degrees of joint angulation) should be referred to a hand specialist.

Metacarpophalangeal Dislocations

- Dorsal
  - Dislocation may be simple (the proximal phalanx stays in contact with the head of the metacarpal) or complex (base of the proximal phalanx is bayoneted and dorsal to the head of the metacarpal). Simple dislocations present with the dislocated finger appearing to point straight in the air away from the joint. Complex dislocations are characterized by puckering of the palmar skin, shortening of the digit, and extensive swelling at the MCP joint.
  - Reduction for simple dislocations must be done in the following manner (to avoid converting to a complex dislocation).
    - Do not pull on the digit. Push or slide the base of the dislocated digit back into place without breaking contact between the articular surface of the proximal phalanx and the metacarpal (Fig. 98.6).
  - Complex dislocations are irreducible due to entrapment of the volar plate and require open treatment by a hand surgeon.
  - Splinting
    - Extension block splint, with fingers flexed enough to ensure a stable reduction
    - Encourage patients to fully flex the fingers.
    - Each week, the extension block is reduced 10 degrees until full extension is achieved.
    - Buddy taping alone is not adequate for initial treatment.

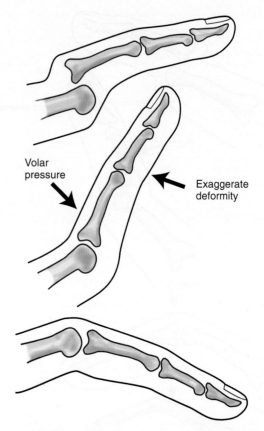

Volar pressure

Exaggerate deformity

Fig 98.6 Reduction maneuver for dorsal metacarpophalangeal joint dislocation. The examiner grasps the injured hand with fingers on the patient's palm and thumb on the dorsal surface of the base of the proximal phalanx. Avoid axial traction. A volar-directed force is then applied with the examiner's thumbs to slide the joint back into place.

Troubleshooting

- Attempts at reduction are generally always recommended; however, certain injuries render the joint irreducible under closed means. Prompt referral to a specialist is indicated.
- Meticulous pre- and postreduction examination of perfusion, sensation, and skin integrity is mandatory.
- Proper digital or regional anesthesia will often yield superior results in both the reduction maneuver and accurate stability testing.
- Associated significant bony or unstable ligamentous injuries warrant referral to a hand surgeon.
- Chronically unstable joints generally will not respond to prolonged immobilization and require ligamentous reconstruction.
- Overtreatment (prolonged splinting) often results in stiffness and flexion contractures (of the PIP joints) and extension contractures (of the MCP joints).
- Prolonged swelling and discomfort for several months even in a stable joint are not uncommon.
  - Fig. 98.7 reviews pertinent injuries associated with finger dislocations as well as when to refer to a hand surgeon for operative intervention.

Finger dislocations

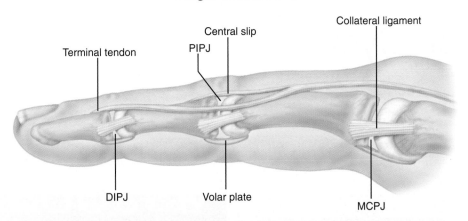

Terminal tendon

Central slip

PIPJ

Collateral ligament

DIPJ

Volar plate

MCPJ

Injury

- PIPJ Dislocations: most common joint dislocation, dorsal dislocations injure volar plate, volar dislocations injure central slip
- DIPJ Dislocations: often open
- MCPJ Dislocations: more difficult to reduce
- Operative Intervention: irreducible, unstable, fracture >40% joint surface

Fig 98.7 Overview of finger dislocations and treatment. *DIP,* Distal interphalangeal; *J,* joint; *MCP,* metacarpophalangeal; *PIP,* proximal interphalangeal.

Suggested Readings

Calfee RP, Sommerkamp TG. Fracture–dislocation about the finger joints. *J Hand Surg.* 2009;34A:1140–1147.

Chen F, Kalainov DM. Phalanx fractures and dislocations in athletes. *Curr Rev Musculoskelet Med.* 2017;10(1):10–16.

Daniels JM II, Zook EG, Lynch JM. Hand and wrist injuries: part II. Emergent evaluation. *Am Fam Physician.* 2004;69:1949–1956.

Freiberg A, Pollard BA, Macdonald MR, Duncan MJ. Management of proximal interphalangeal joint injuries. *Hand Clin.* 2006;22:235–242.

Gonzalez RM, Hammert WC. Dorsal fracture-dislocations of the proximal interphalangeal joint. *J Hand Surg Am.* 2015;40(12):2453–2455.

Haase SC, Chung KC. Current concepts in treatment of fracture-dislocations of the proximal interphalangeal joint. *Plast Reconstr Surg.* 2014;134(6):1246–1257.

Shah CM, Sommerkamp TG. Fracture dislocation of the finger joints. *J Hand Surg Am.* 2014;39(4):792–802.

Chapter 99 Aspiration of Ganglion Cyst

David Schnur

CPT CODE
20612 *Aspiration and/or injection of ganglion cyst any location*

Equipment
- Syringe (3 to 5 mL)
- 18-Gauge needle (to draw up medicine)
- 27-Gauge needle (inch)
- Local anesthetic (1-2% lidocaine plain)
- Corticosteroid (optional)
- Sterile prep solution (alcohol or povidone-iodine)
- Hemostat (if using injectable agent)
- Ethyl chloride, optional but suggested
- Sterile gauze and adhesive bandage

Indication
- Diagnosed ganglion cyst with pain or loss of function
- Mass with suspected diagnosis of a ganglion cyst

Contraindications
- Ganglion cyst of the volar wrist
- Volar retinacular ganglion less than 3 or 4 mm

Instructions/Technique
- Verbal consent is obtained and the correct side is verified.
- Have the patient wash the wrist with soap and water for 1 to 2 minutes.
- Place the patient in a semirecumbent or recumbent position.
- Place 1 mL of a local anesthetic agent in the syringe.
- Prep the area with alcohol or povidone-iodine.
- Use ethyl chloride for patient comfort (recommended).
- Using a 27-gauge needle, inject the skin overlying the ganglion.
- Use an 18-gauge needle to aspirate the ganglion (Fig. 99.1).
- Fluid in the ganglion is clear or clear yellow and viscous (Fig. 99.2).
- If injecting a corticosteroid, use a hemostat to remove the syringe and leave the needle in the cyst.
- Fill the syringe with the corticosteroid using an 18-gauge needle.

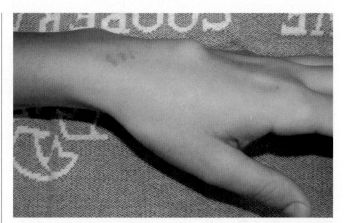

Fig 99.1 Typical appearance of a dorsal wrist ganglion. The needle is inserted directly into the ganglion, aiming slightly proximally until clear or clear yellow viscous fluid is aspirated.

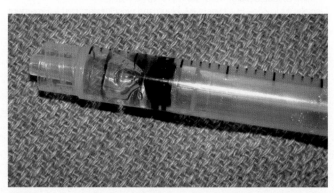

Fig 99.2 Appearance of viscous cyst fluid in the syringe after aspiration.

- Reattach the syringe and inject the agent into the cyst.
- Massage the area of the cyst in an attempt to express any additional fluid (not recommended if corticosteroid is injected into the cyst, because corticosteroids expressed into subcutaneous tissue may cause fat atrophy or hypopigmentation).
- Apply an adhesive bandage.
- With successful aspiration, immediate reduction in the size of the cyst or disappearance of the cyst should be observed and symptoms improved or resolved.

Considerations in Special Populations

- Diabetic patients may experience an increase in blood sugar level if corticosteroids are injected and should be instructed to check it and treat themselves appropriately.

Troubleshooting

- Unsuccessful aspiration of a mass may indicate that it is a solid mass.

Patient Instructions

- Aspiration should improve symptoms.
- Patients should be instructed about the possibility or probability of recurrence of the cyst.
- After one or two recurrences, patients should be considered for surgery if symptomatic.

Chapter 100 de Quervain/First Dorsal Compartment Injection

David Schnur

CPT CODE
20550 *Injection; single tendon sheath, or ligament, aponeurosis*

Equipment

- Injection syringe (3 to 5 mL)
- 18-Gauge needle (to draw up medicine)
- 25-Gauge needle
- Local anesthetic (1% to 2% lidocaine plain)
- Injectable agent (corticosteroid of choice)
- Sterile prep solution (alcohol or povidone-iodine)
- Hemostat
- Ethyl chloride, optional but suggested
- Sterile gauze and adhesive bandage

Indications

- Tenosynovitis of the first dorsal compartment
- Pain consistent with de Quervain tenosynovitis
- Loss of function of the thumb

Contraindications

- Fat atrophy or hypopigmentation with previous injection
- Multiple injections (more than three) without effect
- Brittle diabetics may experience an increase in the blood sugar level with injections.
- Allergy to commercial corticosteroid preparations

Instructions/Technique (Video 100.1 ▶)

- Verbal consent is obtained and the correct side is verified.
- Have the patient wash the wrist with soap and water for 1 to 2 minutes.
- Place the patient in a semirecumbent or recumbent position.
- Place 1 to 2 mL of a local anesthetic in the syringe.
- Identify the location of the first dorsal compartment while the patient abducts the thumb and mark it (Fig. 100.1).
- Prep the area with alcohol or povidone-iodine.
- Use ethyl chloride for patient comfort (recommended).
- Insert a 25-gauge needle with local anesthetic in the first dorsal compartment with the needle aimed slightly distally to proximally, entering the compartment just proximal to the radial styloid (Fig. 100.2).
- Inject approximately 1 mL of a local anesthetic agent into the compartment.

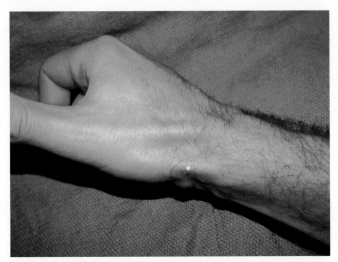

Fig 100.1 With the thumb extended and abducted from the hand, the tendons of the first dorsal compartment can be identified *(asterisk)*. Mark this location with a pen to the compartment when the thumb is relaxed.

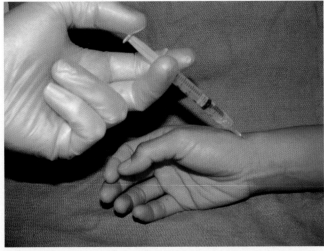

Fig 100.2 The first dorsal compartment is injected just proximal to the tip of the radial styloid with the needle aimed slightly proximally.

- May encounter resistance with injection that suddenly gives way as local anesthetic passes through the compartment
- Having the patient abduct the thumb at this point may confirm the correct location (the syringe will move with the thumb).

- Using a hemostat, remove the syringe and leave the needle in the first dorsal compartment.
- Fill the syringe with corticosteroid using an 18-gauge needle.
- Reattach the syringe and inject the steroid into the compartment.
- Remove the needle quickly to minimize steroid infiltration into subcutaneous tissue.
- Apply an adhesive bandage.
- If the local anesthetic agent is injected into the correct location, Finkelstein test should elicit significantly less pain.

Considerations in Special Populations

- Diabetic patients may experience an increase in the blood sugar level and should be instructed to check it and treat themselves appropriately.

Troubleshooting

- If the local anesthetic does not inject or is very difficult to inject, gently reposition the needle because it may be in the tendon.

- Minimize volumes of injection because the corticosteroid will pass into the subcutaneous tissue proximal to the compartment and may cause fat atrophy or hypopigmentation.
- Be sure to warn dark-skinned individuals about the possibility of hypopigmentation.
- Failure or partial relief of symptoms may indicate a septum within the compartment separating tendons.

Patient Instructions

- Explain to the patient that it will take several days to experience the effects of the corticosteroid.
- Occasionally patients will have increased pain in the 24 hours after the injection; consider giving a prescription for pain medication.
- Splinting is optional after injection but may aid in the short-term relief of symptoms.
- Tell the patient to return after 2 weeks for a second injection if symptoms persist.

Chapter 101 Radiocarpal Joint Injection

Dan A. Zlotolow, Bryan Sirmon

CPT CODES

20605 *Arthrocentesis, aspiration and/or injection; intermediate joint or bursa; without ultrasound guidance.*

Make sure to include a modifier 25 if also billing for the office visit under the same diagnosis code. One cannot bill for the office visit if the purpose of the visit is for the injection.

Radiocarpal Joint Injection

- Wrist injection/aspiration
- Triangular fibrocartilage complex injection

Equipment (Fig. 101.1)

- Two 3-mL syringes
- Two large-bore needles (18-gauge)
- One 25-gauge needle
- 2% lidocaine without epinephrine
- 0.5% bupivacaine without epinephrine
- 40 mg/mL triamcinolone acetonide (or other corticosteroid of your choice)
- Alcohol wipes or povidone-iodine prep sticks
- Ethyl chloride spray (optional)
- 2 × 2-inch gauze
- Small self-adhesive bandage

Indications

- Injection
  - Osteoarthritis
  - Rheumatoid arthritis
  - Posttraumatic joint stiffness/arthritis
  - Wrist pain that has failed splinting and activity modification
  - Diagnostic purposes
- Aspiration
  - Suspected joint infection
  - Gouty arthritis

Contraindications

- Injection
  - Suspected septic arthritis
  - Overlying skin compromise
- Aspiration
  - Overlying cellulitis or skin compromise

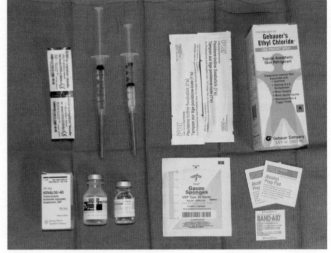

Fig 101.1 Recommended supplies.

Instructions/Technique
Injection

- Load one syringe with 1.5 mL of 2% lidocaine and 1.5 mL of 0.5% bupivacaine using a large-bore needle, and then change to the 25-gauge needle.
- Load the other syringe with 0.5 mL of 2% lidocaine and 1 mL of triamcinolone acetonide using the other large-bore needle.
- Obtain verbal or written consent for the procedure including risks, benefits, and alternatives.
- Identify the correct site and side for the injection. Perform time-out if mandated by your facility.
- Mark the soft spot 1 cm distal to Lister tubercle for a radiocarpal injection.
- Mark the soft spot just distal to the distal radioulnar joint for a triangular fibrocartilage complex injection (Fig. 101.2).
- Prep the skin with an antiseptic solution (Fig. 101.3).
- Use a short burst of ethyl chloride to numb the skin (optional).
- Inject a small wheel of local anesthetic from the first syringe, slowly infiltrating the area with local anesthetic until the joint is reached (Fig. 101.4).
- Keeping light thumb pressure on the plunger at all times facilitates identification of joint penetration (the resistance should ease after a slight pop is felt).
- While maintaining the needle in the joint, switch syringes and inject the contents of the second syringe into the joint (Fig. 101.5).

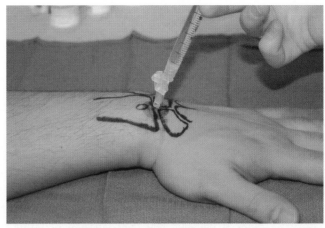

Fig 101.4 Provide a local infusion of the bupivacaine/lidocaine mix as you search for the joint (note that the thumb is always on the plunger to aid with proprioception).

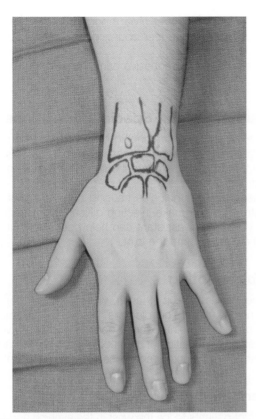

Fig 101.2 Identify the landmarks for the injection sites.

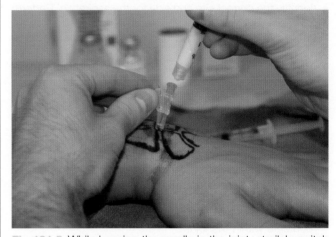

Fig 101.5 While keeping the needle in the joint, sterilely switch syringes.

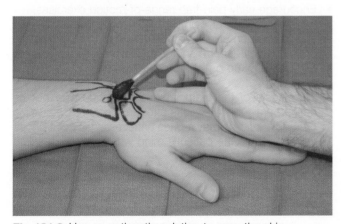

Fig 101.3 Use an antiseptic solution to prep the skin.

- If resistance is experienced, move the needle slightly in or out until the injectate goes in easily. Little to no resistance should be encountered if within the joint (Fig. 101.6).
- Remove the needle and apply pressure with the gauze bandage (Fig. 101.7).
- Place a sterile self-adhesive bandage over the injection site.

Aspiration

- Load one syringe with 1.5 mL of 2% lidocaine and 1.5 mL of 0.5% bupivacaine using a large-bore needle, and then change to the 25-gauge needle.
- Maintain the other syringe empty in close proximity.

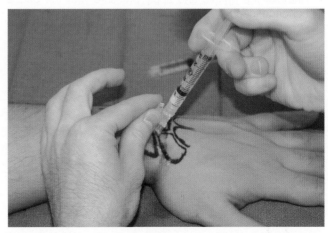

Fig 101.6 Inject the triamcinolone acetonide into the joint.

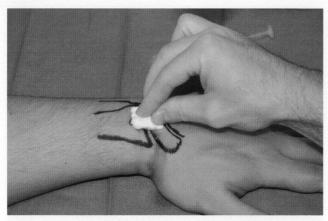

Fig 101.7 Apply a bandage and hold pressure to prevent bleeding.

- Obtain verbal or written consent for the procedure including risks, benefits, and alternatives.
- Identify the correct site and side for the aspiration. Perform time-out if mandated by your facility.
- Mark the soft spot 1 cm distal to Lister tubercle for a radiocarpal aspiration.
- Prep the skin with an antiseptic solution (see Fig. 101.3).
- Use a short burst of ethyl chloride to numb the skin (optional).
- Inject a small wheel of local anesthetic from the first syringe, slowly infiltrating the area with local anesthetic until the joint is reached (see Fig. 101.4).
- Keeping light thumb pressure on the plunger at all times facilitates identification of joint penetration (the resistance should ease after a slight pop is felt).
- While maintaining the needle in the joint, switch to the empty syringe and withdraw the plunger to aspirate the contents within the joint.
- If no aspirate returns through 25-gauge needle, ensure adequate analgesia and repeat above steps with larger-bore needle in same trajectory.
- Remove the needle and apply pressure with the gauze bandage (see Fig. 101.7).

- Label the syringe and order appropriate labs for micro-analysis of aspirate (cell count, gram stain, culture, and crystal analysis).
- Place a sterile self-adhesive bandage over the aspiration site.

Considerations in Special Populations

- Patients with diabetes should be cautioned that cortico-steroid injections may increase their blood sugar levels and that close monitoring should be performed over the next 1 to 2 days.
- Patients with pathologies causing complete joint space destruction can make injection difficult. Light traction on the digits by an assistant can help open the joint space and ease entry into the joint.

Troubleshooting

- If the joint is difficult to enter, walk along the bone with the needle until the needle "falls" into the joint. Remember, the radiocarpal joint extends dorsally and has a volar tilt proximally. Angulation of the needle slightly proximally may improve the trajectory and ease entry into the joint.

Patient Instructions

- Instruct patients to ice the wrist in the evening and to take whatever medication they take for a headache before going to bed.
- Encourage early pain-free range-of-motion exercises.
- Increasing levels of pain, an enlarging effusion, or fever should merit an urgent visit back to the physician's office or emergency department for evaluation of septic arthritis.
- Always follow up on labs ordered from aspirate and treat accordingly.
- The effects of the triamcinolone acetonide may not be noticed until up to 2 weeks after an injection. Counseling on this time frame may reduce unnecessary patient phone calls and ease the patient's mind when relief is transient or not immediate.

Chapter 102 Carpal Tunnel Injection

David Schnur

CPT CODE
20526 *Injection, therapeutic (e.g., local anesthetic,
corticosteroid), carpal tunnel*

Equipment

- Injection syringe (3 to 5 mL)
- 18-Gauge needle (to draw up medicine)
- 25-Gauge needle (1.5 inches)
- Local anesthetic (1-2% lidocaine plain)
- Injectable agent (corticosteroid of choice)
- Sterile prep solution (alcohol or povidone-iodine) (Fig. 102.1)
- Hemostat
- Ethyl chloride, optional but suggested
- Sterile gauze and adhesive bandage

Indications

- Diagnosed carpal tunnel syndrome
- Suspected carpal tunnel syndrome based on history and physical examination
- Pain
- Subjective numbness in the thumb and index and long fingers

Contraindications

- Marked increase in two-point discrimination or severe carpal tunnel syndrome based on electromyography/nerve conduction velocity (surgery should be considered as initial treatment)
- Anticoagulation with significant increase in prothrombin time or partial thromboplastin time
- Fat atrophy or hypopigmentation with previous injection
- Multiple injections (more than three) without effect
- Brittle diabetics may experience an increase in the blood sugar level with injections.
- Allergy to commercial corticosteroid preparations

Instructions/Technique (Video 102.1)

- Consent is obtained and the correct side is verified.
- Have the patient wash the wrist with soap and water for 1 to 2 minutes.
- Place the patient in a semirecumbent or recumbent position.
- Place 1 to 2 mL of a local anesthetic agent in a syringe.
- Prep the area with alcohol or povidone-iodine.
- Use ethyl chloride for patient comfort (recommended).

- Insert the 25-gauge needle with local anesthetic into the carpal canal.
  - The needle should be inserted into the skin at the level of the proximal wrist crease and aimed toward the metacarpophalangeal joints of the fingers.
  - The thumb or index finger is used to locate the hook of the hamate.
  - The needle is inserted just ulnar to the palmaris longus tendon and aimed just radial to the hook of the hamate (Figs. 102.2 and 102.3).
  - Once the needle is inserted to the level of the hub, the patient is asked to wiggle the fingers slightly.
  - If the needle is in the correct position, the syringe will move with the fingers.
  - If at any time during the insertion of the needle the patient experiences shooting pain or shock into the fingers, the needle should be pulled out and reinserted.
- Inject approximately 1 mL of local anesthetic into the carpal canal.
- Using a hemostat, remove the syringe and leave the needle in the carpal canal.
- Fill the syringe with a corticosteroid using an 18-gauge needle.
- Reattach the syringe and inject the corticosteroid into the carpal canal.
- Remove the needle quickly to minimize steroid infiltration into the subcutaneous tissue.
- Apply an adhesive bandage.
- Have the patient flex and extend the fingers multiple times.
- Numbness in the thumb or index, long, or radial ring finger indicates correct placement of the corticosteroid.
- Absence of numbness is not predictive of the location of the corticosteroid.
- Relief of symptoms strongly supports the diagnosis of carpal tunnel syndrome.
- Relief of symptoms has been shown to be predictive of relief of symptoms with surgical release.

Considerations in Special Populations

- Diabetic patients may experience an increase in the blood sugar level and should be instructed to check it and treat themselves appropriately.

Troubleshooting

- If the local anesthetic does not inject or is very difficult to inject, then gently reposition the needle because it may be in the tendon.

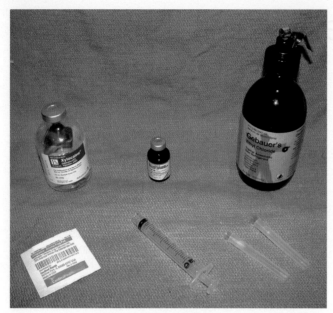

Fig 102.1 Set-up for carpal tunnel injection: local anesthetic agent, corticosteroid, ethyl chloride, alcohol swab, needles, and a syringe.

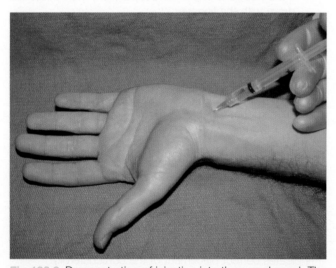

Fig 102.2 Demonstration of injection into the carpal canal. The needle is inserted just proximal to the wrist crease, directed distally, and inserted at an angle of approximately 30 degrees.

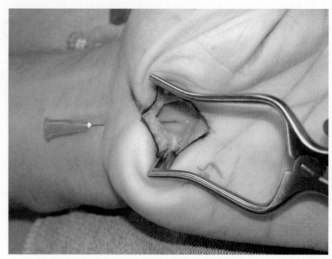

Fig 102.3 With the needle in the proper position for injection, the end of the needle is seen in the carpal canal.

- Be sure to warn dark-skinned individuals about the possibility of hypopigmentation.
- Water-soluble corticosteroids have a lower chance of nerve damage if they are accidentally injected into a nerve.
- If the patient has a sensation of electrical shock in the fingers or the needle does not move when the fingers are wiggled, then pull the needle tip out into the subcutaneous tissue and redirect it.

Patient Instructions

- Explain to the patient that it will take several days to experience the effects of the corticosteroid.
- Occasionally patients will have increased pain in the 24 hours after the injection; consider giving a prescription for pain medication.
- Splinting is optional after injection but may aid in the short-term relief of symptoms.
- Tell the patient to return after 2 weeks for a second injection if symptoms persist.
- Successful injection should relieve symptoms for at least 6 weeks but can give considerably longer relief.

Chapter 103 Carpometacarpal Injection

David Schnur

CPT CODE
20605 *Arthrocentesis, aspiration, and/or injection intermediate joint or bursa*

Equipment

- Injection syringe (3 to 5 mL)
- 18-Gauge needle (to draw up medicine)
- 25-Gauge needle (inches)
- Local anesthetic agent (1-2% lidocaine plain)
- Injectable agent (corticosteroid of choice)
- Sterile prep solution (alcohol or povidone-iodine)
- Hemostat
- Ethyl chloride, optional but suggested
- Sterile gauze and adhesive bandage

Indications

- Diagnosed carpometacarpal (CMC) arthritis
- Suspected CMC arthritis based on history, physical examination, and radiographs
- Pain
- Loss of function of the thumb
- Failed conservative treatment (splinting and therapy)

Contraindications

- Anticoagulation with significant increase in prothrombin time or partial thromboplastin time
- Fat atrophy or hypopigmentation with previous injection
- Multiple injections (more than three) without effect
- Brittle diabetics may experience an increase in the blood sugar level with injections.
- Allergy to commercial corticosteroid preparations

Instructions/Technique (Video 103.1 ▶)

- Verbal consent is obtained and the correct side is verified.
- Have the patient wash the wrist with soap and water for 1 to 2 minutes.
- Place the patient in a semirecumbent or recumbent position.
- Place 0.5 mL of local anesthetic agent in a syringe.
- Identify the location of the CMC joint and mark it (just proximal to the prominence of the base of the thumb metacarpal; Fig. 103.1).
- Prep the area with alcohol or povidone-iodine.
- Use ethyl chloride for patient comfort (recommended).

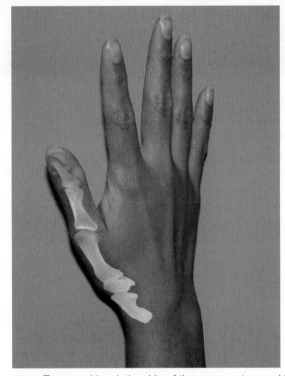

Fig 103.1 Topographic relationship of the carpometacarpal joint to the thumb.

- Place traction on the thumb to open the joint space.
- Insert a 25-gauge needle with the local anesthetic into the CMC joint (Fig. 103.2).
- Inject approximately 0.5 mL of local anesthetic into the joint.
- May encounter resistance with small joints; can put less than 0.5 mL into the joint.
- Using a hemostat, remove the syringe and leave the needle in the CMC joint.
- Fill the syringe with the corticosteroid using an 18-gauge needle (typically 1 mL of corticosteroid).
- Reattach the syringe and inject the corticosteroid into the joint.
- May not be able to get the full 1 mL of anesthetic into the joint
- Remove the needle quickly to minimize corticosteroid infiltration into subcutaneous tissue.
- Apply an adhesive bandage.
- If the local anesthetic is injected into the correct location, a grind test should elicit significantly less pain.

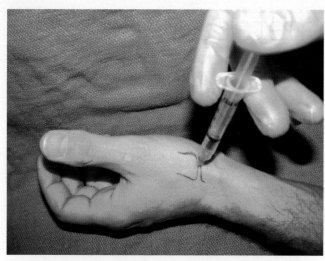

Fig 103.2 Needle inserted in the carpometacarpal joint of the thumb.

Considerations in Special Populations

- Diabetic patients may experience an increase in the blood sugar level and should be instructed to check it and treat themselves appropriately.

Troubleshooting

- If the local anesthetic does not inject or is very difficult to inject, then gently reposition the needle by "walking" the needle either proximally or distally as needed.
- Most joints will be slightly difficult to inject because of the small volume, but occasionally a very arthritic joint will easily accept larger volumes.
- Be sure to warn dark-skinned individuals about the possibility of hypopigmentation.
- Significant resistance to injection may not be encountered with patients with advanced disease; this can be due to the loss of integrity of the CMC joint.

Patient Instructions

- Explain to the patient that it will take several days to experience the effects of the corticosteroid.
- Occasionally patients will have increased pain in the 24 hours after the injection; consider giving a prescription for pain medication.
- Splinting is optional after injection but may aid in the short-term relief of symptoms.
- Tell the patient to return after 2 weeks for a second injection if symptoms persist.

Chapter 104 Trigger Finger Injection

Trent Gause II

Key Points
- >90% of trigger fingers may resolve after one to three corticosteroid injections.

Equipment (Fig. 104.1)
- 5 mL-syringe
- 18-Gauge needle
- 25-Gauge needle
- Alcohol prep pads
- Adhesive bandage
- Rubber surgical gloves (optional but recommended)
- 1% lidocaine, without epinephrine
- Corticosteroid (dexamethasone 8 mg/mL is author's preference; triamcinolone acetonide and betamethasone are acceptable alternatives)

Contraindications
- Known or suspected suppurative flexor tenosynovitis is a contraindication for corticosteroid injection.

Technique (Video 104.1 ▶)
- Place the patient's involved hand, palm facing up (supinated), on examination table or other flat surface.
- Prepare the syringe by using the 18-gauge needle to mix 1 mL of 1% lidocaine without epinephrine and 1 mL of corticosteroid (e.g., 1 mL of 8 mg/mL dexamethasone).
- Use alcohol prep pads to cleanse the top of each medication bottle before aspiration of the medication into the syringe.
- Discard the 18-gauge needle and place a 25-gauge needle on the syringe.
- Use a sterile alcohol prep to cleanse the involved digit in the area of the proposed injection.
- Inject the mixture of lidocaine and corticosteroid into the area of the A1 pulley (Fig. 104. 2).
- Penetrate the dermis (Fig. 104.3).
- The injection is efficacious whether it is in the tendon sheath or superficial to it.
- Place a bandage over the injection site.

Considerations in Special Populations
- Diabetics may experience a transient increase in serum glucose levels (75% higher than the preinjection level at postinjection day 1), lasting as long 5 days.

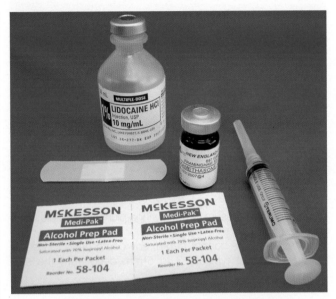

Fig 104.1 Equipment required for a trigger finger injection.

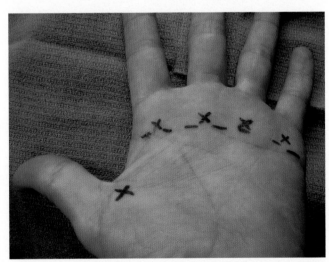

Fig 104.2 A line drawn from the proximal palmar crease radially to the distal palmar crease ulnarly provides a good landmark for trigger finger injections. *X* marks the spot for needle penetration of the skin.

- The efficacy of the injection is lessened in diabetics; resolution of triggering is still possible in approximately 50% of cases.

Troubleshooting
- If unable to inject, the needle may be embedded in the tendon; withdraw or advance it slightly and continue to

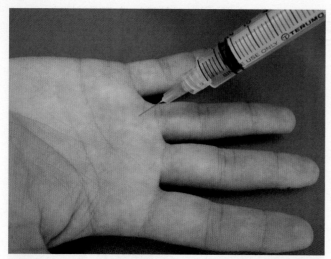

Fig 104.3 A 25-gauge needle is inserted through the skin in the area of the A1 pulley.

exert gentle pressure on the syringe plunger until fluid flows easily.
- If unsure of the correct depth, any depth deep to dermis is acceptable, typically 3 to 5 mm deep from the skin surface.

- If after one injection, symptoms are not relieved after 1 to 2 weeks, a second injection has been shown to be helpful in as many as 85-90% of patients.
- If symptomatic triggering persists or recurs after three injections, refer for consideration of surgical management.
- Avoid neurovascular bundles by staying in the midline of the digit.

Patient Instructions

- Counsel patients that injection may cause painful throbbing at the injection site (steroid flare) on the night of the injection, and pain medication (a nonsteroidal antiinflammatory drug or narcotic) can be used on the night of injection if needed.
- Counsel patients regarding anesthesia in the digit, which lasts as long as 2 hours after injection, due to lidocaine.
- The bandage can be removed 1 to 2 hours after injection.
- The corticosteroid may take several days to provide symptom relief.
- If symptoms are not relieved after 1 to 2 weeks, the patient should return for consideration of a second injection.
- Follow up as needed if symptoms recur.

Acknowledgment

The author would like to thank Dr. Jack Ingari for his contribution to much of this chapter in the previous edition.

Chapter 105 Digital Blocks

Obinna Ugwu-Oju, Jonathan E. Isaacs

CPT CODES
- Do not list a separate CPT code for digital block.
- Code for the procedure that is being performed (digital blocks are always included in this code).
- The CPT code 64450 (Injection, anesthetic agent; other peripheral nerve or branch) is billable in the event that it is being used for pain control alone.

Indications
- Digital block provides significant digital anesthesia with minimal morbidity.
- Examination of a painful digit.
- Perform surgical procedures confined to the digits.

Contraindications
- Avoid using epinephrine in fingers with a tenuous vascular supply (e.g., Raynaud's, peripheral vascular disease). Patients with previous surgery involving the digital arteries should not have epinephrine administered.
  - A definitive neurovascular examination should be performed before administration of local anesthetic.
- Do not inject into infected tissue.

Equipment (Fig. 105.1)
- Use a 10-mL syringe and a 25-gauge or 27-gauge needle.

Instructions/Technique (Video 105.1)
- Digital nerve block is possible because of predictable nerve anatomy (Fig. 105.2).
- Two digital nerves run parallel to the flexor tendon sheath.
- Each sends a main branch distally to the dorsal skin from approximately the proximal interphalangeal joint.
- The proximal dorsal skin of the digits receives innervation from separate cutaneous nerve fibers.
- To minimize discomfort, warm the injection solution, buffer with sodium bicarbonate (8.4% $NaHCO_3$), insert needle perpendicular to the skin, and slowly infiltrate anesthetic subdermally.
- Commercially available lidocaine, with or without epinephrine, is produced with preservatives at an acidic level (pH between 4 and 7). Adding 1 mL of 8.4% sodium bicarbonate to 9 mL of 1% or 2% lidocaine will bring the mixture closer to a physiologic pH and has been shown to reduce pain.
- Lidocaine warmed from 40°C to 43°C can reduce pain with subcutaneous injection. Vials can be warmed in an IV-solution warmer to reach satisfactory temperatures.
- Dorsal approach (Fig. 105.3)
  - Insert the needle at the base of the digit just proximal to the web and advance it until the needle can be felt tenting the skin of the palm just proximal to the web.
  - Inject while withdrawing the needle.
  - Before removing the needle completely, redirect it across the extensor surface of the finger and make a skin wheal (for dorsal nerve fibers).

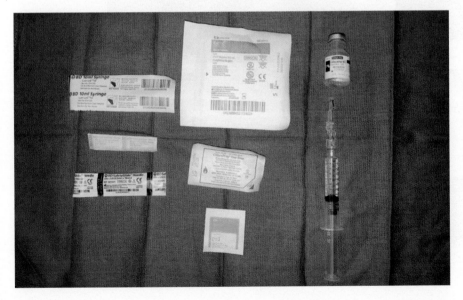

Fig 105.1 Equipment for digital blocks.

Digital Blocks

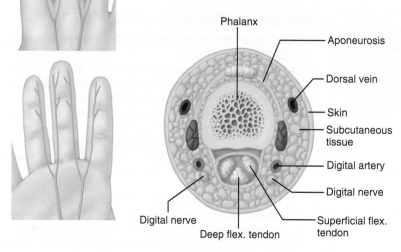

- Common method of anesthesia for procedures on digits
- Both dorsal and colar approaches require two injections, with dorsal supplementation for the proximal digit
- Epinephrine safe to use in most patients, and can decrease blood loss or need for a tourniquet

Fig 105.2 The course of the digital nerves from dorsal and volar approaches, along with an axial view of digit demonstrating the proximity of the digital nerves to the arteries and the flexor sheath.

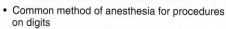

Phalanx
Aponeurosis
Dorsal vein
Skin
Subcutaneous tissue
Digital artery
Digital nerve
Superficial flex. tendon
Digital nerve
Deep flex. tendon

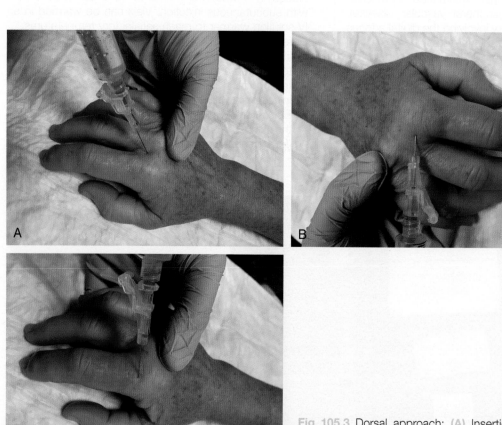

Fig 105.3 Dorsal approach: **(A)** Insertion of the needle into the web space for an index finger digital block. **(B)** Prior to removal of needle, needle redirected radially across extensor surface for dorsal nerve fibers. **(C)** Reinsertion of needle for radial digital nerve of the index finger.

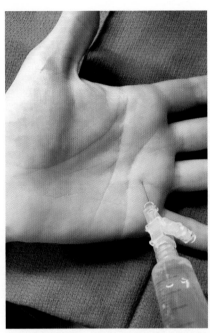

Fig 105.4 Volar approach: Needle insertion near distal palmar crease for ring finger block. Local anesthetic is directed slightly radial and ulnar from midline for both digital nerves.

- Remove the needle and inject again on the other side of the finger.
- Two to 3 mL of the local anesthetic should be injected on each side of the finger.
- Avoid inadvertent ring block by limiting the volume of anesthetic.
- Volar approach (Fig. 105.4)
  - Inject 2 to 3 mL of local anesthetic agent subcutaneously near the distal palmar crease.
  - Aim a few millimeters radially and then ulnar to the midline to inject anesthetic around both digital nerves.
  - This more direct approach to the digital nerve is effective but can be painful.
  - May require dorsal supplement for procedures involving the dorsum of the finger, though the volar approach usually covers the distal half of the proximal phalanx to the fingertip.

Considerations in Special Populations

- Severe scarring/burns may limit anesthetic infiltration.
- Doses:
  - Lidocaine: 4.5 mg/kg without epinephrine, 7 mg/kg with epinephrine
  - Bupivacaine/ropivacaine: 2.5 mg/kg without epinephrine, 3 mg/kg with epinephrine
- Type of local anesthetic:
  - Epinephrine decreases the amount of bleeding and increases the duration of the local anesthetic in the tissue. It is suitable to use with the exception of patients with compromised vascular supply.

- Lidocaine has a considerably shorter duration of effect compared to bupivacaine or ropivacaine. It should be considered when a shorter procedure is expected, including superficial lacerations, paronychia, or skin biopsies.
- Lidocaine can also be used in pediatric populations, where small total body weight limits the amount of local anesthetic that can be used safely. This is generally only an issue where multiple blocks are done.
- Bupivacaine and ropivacaine have longer durations of effect, with bupivacaine with epinephrine possibly having pain relief for 15 hours and touch/pressure numbness for 30 hours. These anesthetic agents are used when longer pain relief is needed. For digital blocks, onset of action is very similar to lidocaine. Adding lidocaine is not necessary to achieve a faster onset.
- Bupivacaine also provides hyperemia and temperature increases in digital blocks, making it an appropriate choice in the management of frostbite.

Troubleshooting

- Inadequate anesthesia may indicate that the injection did not properly infiltrate adjacent to the digital nerves. Make sure adequate time (approximately 4 minutes) is given for the block to set up before resorting to repeat injection.
- Local anesthetic can be injected as a field block if necessary.
- Ischemic injury after digital block is very rare.
- Addition of epinephrine does not seem to increase complications in current studies. More recent reports of digital necrosis are due to injections at significantly higher concentrations of epinephrine, as seen in accidental digital administration of an EpiPen.
- Phentolamine, a competitive α-receptor antagonist, is the medical reversal agent for epinephrine-induced vasospasm. If signs of digital ischemia are present, including discoloration or lack of capillary refill, injection of 1 mg/1 mL of phentolamine at the same site as the digital block can reverse the effects of epinephrine. Other signs of pain or paresthesias are reliable in the setting of local anesthetic administration.

Patient Instructions

- Patients should be warned not to expect sensation to return to their finger for at least several hours. Additionally, the sensation of pain may return sooner than normal sensation.

Suggested Readings

Lalonde DH, Wong A. Dosage of local anesthesia in wide awake hand surgery. J Hand Surg Am. 2013;38:2025–2028.

Nodwell T, Lalonde D. How long does it take phentolamine to reverse adrenaline-induced vasoconstriction in the finger and hand? A prospective, randomized, blinded study: the dalhousie project experimental phase. Can J Plast Surg. 2003;11:187–190.

Thompson CJ, Lalonde DH, Denkler KA, Feicht AJ. A critical look at the evidence for and against elective epinephrine use in the finger. Plast Reconstr Surg. 2007;1:260–266.

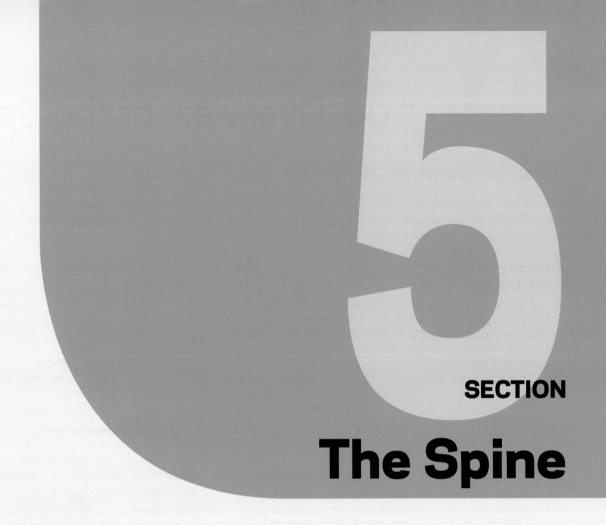

SECTION 5

The Spine

Chapter 106 Overview of the Spine

Uma Srikumaran, A. Jay Khanna

Anatomy
Spinal Column

- The spinal column is made up of 33 vertebrae: 7 cervical, 12 thoracic, 5 lumbar, 5 sacral, and 4 coccygeal vertebrae.
- Although each vertebra has a distinctive shape based on its location in the spine, with a few exceptions, they share a common structure.
- In general, a single vertebra is made up of the vertebral body, bilateral pedicles, bilateral superior and inferior facets, bilateral lamina, bilateral transverse processes, and the spinous process (Fig. 106.1).
- The intervertebral disc lies between two vertebral bodies and is made up of the annulus fibrosus and the nucleus pulposus (see Fig. 106.1).
- It is important to evaluate the overall alignment of the spine in both the sagittal and coronal planes (Fig. 106.2).
  - Coronal plane alignment is evaluated with anteroposterior standing radiographs, and sagittal plane alignment is evaluated with lateral standing radiographs.
- The normal range of cervical lordosis is approximately 30 to 50 degrees, normal thoracic kyphosis ranges from 20 to 50 degrees, and normal lumbar lordosis ranges from 30 to 80 degrees.

Ligaments

- Several important ligaments connect the vertebrae and provide strength and stability, including the anterior and posterior longitudinal ligaments, which attach to the anterior and posterior aspects of the vertebral body.
- The ligamentum flavum connects the lamina, and the interspinous and supraspinous ligaments connect the spinous processes (Fig. 106.3).

Muscles

- The spine is further stabilized by the musculature of the back and neck (Figs. 106.4 and 106.5).
- At the deepest level, the iliocostalis, longissimus, and spinalis muscles comprise the erector spinae muscle and lie between the transverse and spinous processes of adjacent segments.
  - Superficial to this layer are the rhomboids, serratus posterior, trapezius, and latissimus dorsi muscle groups.

Spinal Cord

- The spinal cord lies within the bony canal created by the vertebral column.
- Thirty-one pairs of nerve roots exit this column through the intervertebral foramina: 8 cervical, 12 thoracic, 5 lumbar, 5 sacral, and 1 coccygeal nerve roots (Fig. 106.6).

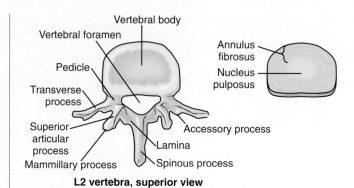

L2 vertebra, superior view

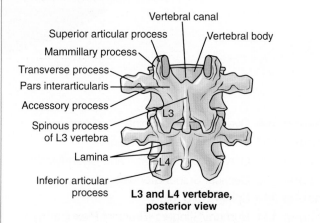

L3 and L4 vertebrae, posterior view

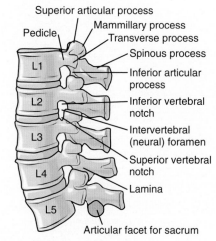

Lumbar vertebrae, assembled: left lateral view

Fig 106.1 The bony anatomy of the lumbar vertebrae and the intervertebral disc.

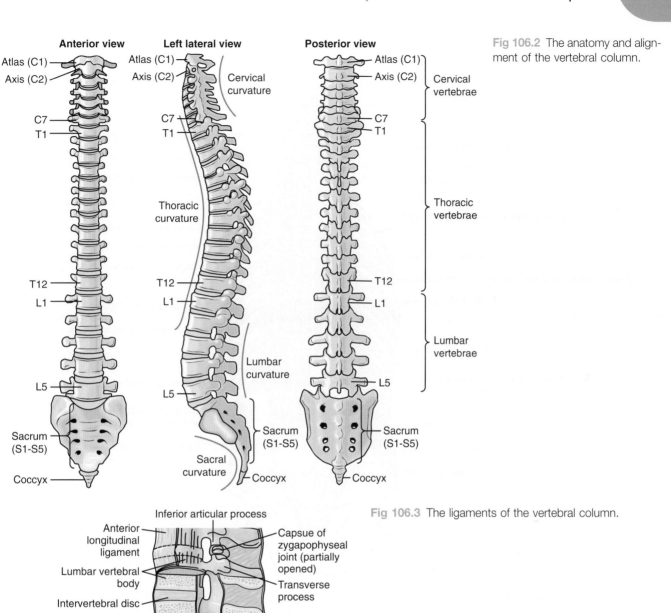

Anterior view

Atlas (C1)
Axis (C2)

C7
T1

T12
L1

L5

Sacrum
(S1-S5)

Coccyx

Left lateral view

Atlas (C1)
Axis (C2)

Cervical
curvature

C7
T1

Thoracic
curvature

T12
L1

Lumbar
curvature

L5

Sacrum
(S1-S5)

Sacral
curvature

Coccyx

Posterior view

Atlas (C1)
Axis (C2)

Cervical
vertebrae

C7
T1

Thoracic
vertebrae

T12
L1

Lumbar
vertebrae

L5

Sacrum
(S1-S5)

Coccyx

Fig 106.2 The anatomy and alignment of the vertebral column.

Fig 106.3 The ligaments of the vertebral column.

Inferior articular process

Anterior
longitudinal
ligament

Lumbar vertebral
body

Intervertebral disc

Anterior longitudinal
ligament

Posterior longitudinal
ligament

Intervertebral foramen

Capsue of
zygapophyseal
joint (partially
opened)

Transverse
process

Spinous process

Ligamentum
flavum

Supraspinous
ligament

**Left lateral view
(partially sectioned
in median plane)**

Pedicle
(cut surface)

Posterior
surface of
vertebral bodies

Posterior
longitudinal
ligament

Intervertebral
disc

**Anterior vertebral
segments:
posterior view
(pedicles sectioned)**

Pedicle
(cut surface)

Ligamentum
flavum

Lamina

Superior
articular
process

Transverse
process

Inferior
articular
facet

**Posterior vertebral
segments:
anterior view**

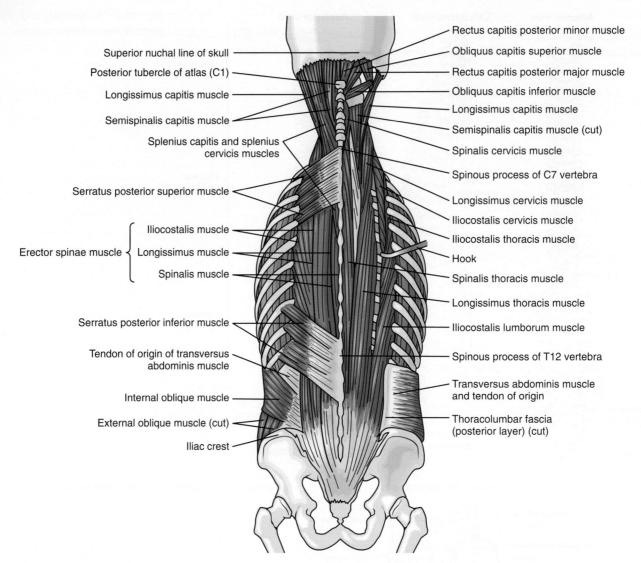

Rectus capitis posterior minor muscle
Obliquus capitis superior muscle
Rectus capitis posterior major muscle
Obliquus capitis inferior muscle
Longissimus capitis muscle
Semispinalis capitis muscle (cut)
Spinalis cervicis muscle
Spinous process of C7 vertebra
Longissimus cervicis muscle
Iliocostalis cervicis muscle
Iliocostalis thoracis muscle
Hook
Spinalis thoracis muscle
Longissimus thoracis muscle
Iliocostalis lumborum muscle
Spinous process of T12 vertebra
Transversus abdominis muscle and tendon of origin
Thoracolumbar fascia (posterior layer) (cut)

Superior nuchal line of skull
Posterior tubercle of atlas (C1)
Longissimus capitis muscle
Semispinalis capitis muscle
Splenius capitis and splenius cervicis muscles
Serratus posterior superior muscle
Iliocostalis muscle
Erector spinae muscle { Longissimus muscle
Spinalis muscle
Serratus posterior inferior muscle
Tendon of origin of transversus abdominis muscle
Internal oblique muscle
External oblique muscle (cut)
Iliac crest

Fig 106.4 The deep muscles of the back.

Patient Evaluation
History

- As with any patient, a comprehensive history and physical examination are essential components of the diagnosis and decision-making process.
- The complete history begins with the chief complaint and details of the patient's symptoms.
  - Important details include the duration of symptoms or pain, exacerbating and alleviating factors, the anatomic distribution of symptoms, the onset of symptoms, and the quality and severity of the pain.
- For the spine patient, specific attention should be given to the precise distribution of the symptoms in an effort to determine whether the symptoms fit into a particular dermatome or neural pattern.
- A detailed history regarding the neurologic deficits should be documented.
  - For patients with a traumatic injury or a history of trauma, the clinician should note the mechanism of injury.

- A thorough description of previous evaluations and treatments, especially spine surgery, is also important.
- Finally, an occupational history should be obtained.
- It is important to use the history along with the physical examination to differentiate patients with myelopathy (dysfunction from spinal cord compression) and those with radiculopathy (dysfunction of nerve roots).
  - Patients with radiculopathy often present with pain in a specific distribution in the upper or lower extremity, weakness and atrophy of particular muscle groups, and decreased muscle tone.
  - Patients with myelopathy will present with the opposite spectrum of findings, including generalized weakness and no dermatomal pain. Patients with myelopathy also have a more nonspecific history, reporting frequent falls, gait and balance instability, paresthesias in a bilateral pattern, and difficulty with fine motor control, including buttoning a shirt, handwriting, or turning a doorknob.
- Attention should be given to determining the effect of various actions on the patient's symptoms.

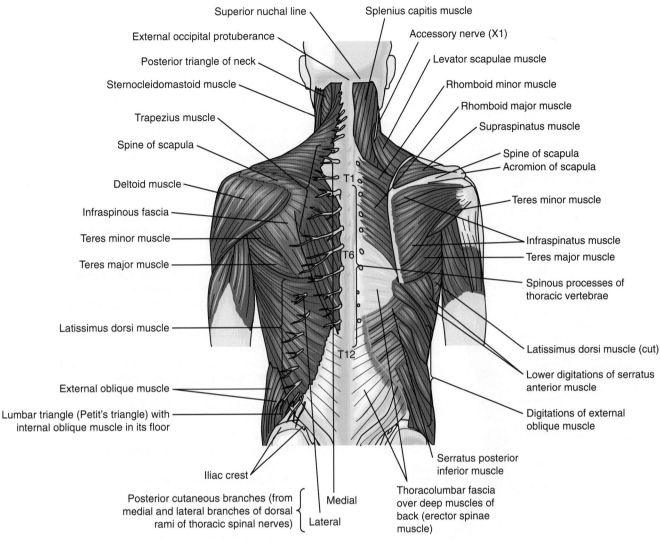

Fig 106.5 The superficial muscles of the back.

- Patients with neurogenic claudication often have improvement of their symptoms with leaning forward (e.g., on a grocery cart).
- Patients with discogenic pain often have improvement in and worsening of symptoms with extension and flexion, respectively, of the lumbar or cervical spine.
- Finally, it is important to ascertain the presence of any "red flags" that may suggest systemic illnesses and the need for more immediate imaging and aggressive evaluation.
  - These findings include fevers, chills, night sweats, unexpected weight loss, loss of appetite, and night pain.
  - Cauda equina syndrome, characterized by perineal or saddle paresthesia, lower extremity motor and sensory deficits, and bowel or bladder difficulties, also requires immediate imaging and evaluation for surgical intervention.

Physical Examination (Video 106.1 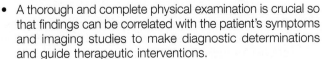)

- A thorough and complete physical examination is crucial so that findings can be correlated with the patient's symptoms and imaging studies to make diagnostic determinations and guide therapeutic interventions.

- The physical examination is divided into the following areas: inspection and palpation, range-of-motion evaluation, and neurologic examination.

Inspection and Palpation

- Inspection begins with a general evaluation of appearance, weight, posture, and gait.
- Determination of any deformity, such as scoliosis and excessive kyphosis/lordosis, is important.
- Evaluation of the skin involves looking for signs of infection or of underlying disease, such as café au lait marks and patches of hair.
- Palpation should include evaluation of the bony architecture and the paraspinal musculature; the extremities should be examined for associated or concurrent abnormalities.
- Careful palpation can reveal points of bony tenderness, areas of soft-tissue pain, or areas of swelling.

Range-of-Motion Evaluation

- Active range of motion is assessed for all areas of the spine.

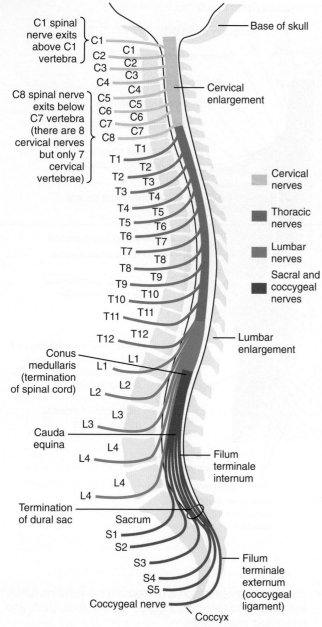

C1 spinal
nerve exits
above C1
vertebra

C1
C2
C3
C4
C5
C6
C7
C8

C1
C2
C3
C4
C5
C6
C7

Base of skull

Cervical
enlargement

C8 spinal nerve
exits below
C7 vertebra
(there are 8
cervical nerves
but only 7
cervical
vertebrae)

T1
T2
T3
T4
T5
T6
T7
T8
T9
T10
T11
T12

T1
T2
T3
T4
T5
T6
T7
T8
T9
T10
T11
T12

Cervical
nerves

Thoracic
nerves

Lumbar
nerves

Sacral and
coccygeal
nerves

Lumbar
enlargement

Conus
medullaris
(termination
of spinal cord)

L1
L2
L3
L4
L4

L1
L2
L3
L4

Cauda
equina

Filum
terminale
internum

Termination
of dural sac

Sacrum
S1
S2
S3
S4
S5
Coccygeal nerve

Coccyx

Filum
terminale
externum
(coccygeal
ligament)

Fig 106.6 The spinal cord and segmental nerves.

- Flexion, extension, rotation, and lateral bending can all be evaluated.
- Attention to positions that cause or alleviate symptoms can provide insight into the source of the abnormality.
  - However, in the emergency setting, as with a patient who has a history of trauma, range-of-motion evaluation may not be appropriate, and spinal precautions should be followed during the entire examination.

Neurologic Examination

- The neurologic examination includes evaluation of sensation, motor function, and reflexes.
  - The sensory examination should be documented with regard to the distribution of dermatomes (Fig. 106.7).

- Motor function is graded on a 0- to 5-point scale by testing motor groups that correlate with particular neurologic levels (Fig. 106.8 and Table 106.1).
  - 5: Full motion against gravity with maximum resistance
  - 4: Full motion against gravity with moderate resistance
  - 3: Full motion against gravity with no resistance
  - 2: Full motion in gravity-eliminated position
  - 1: No motion, but muscle contraction noted
  - 0: No motion or muscle contraction
- Abnormal reflexes should also be elicited.
  - Clonus: evaluates for upper motor neuron injury (Fig. 106.9)
  - Abruptly dorsiflex the ankle and count the beats of ankle motion.
  - Positive: more than four beats of flexion
  - Babinski sign: evaluates for upper motor neuron injury (Fig. 106.10)
  - Use the handle of a reflex hammer to rub along the plantar aspect of the foot from the heel to the toes.
  - Positive: great-toe extension
  - Hoffmann sign: evaluates for cervical myelopathy (Fig. 106.11)
  - Flick the distal phalanx of the middle finger in a palmar direction.
  - Positive: the fingers and thumb flex; additional tests performed to aid in diagnosis
  - Spurling maneuver: distinguishes shoulder pain from radicular pain (Fig. 106.12)
  - Ask the patient to rotate and laterally flex the head to the affected side.
  - Positive: maneuver exacerbates the patient's radicular pain
  - Adson test: evaluates for thoracic outlet syndrome/cervical rib (Fig. 106.13)
  - Feel for the radial pulse on the affected side and then abduct, extend, and externally rotate the arm. Ask the patient to take a deep breath and turn the head to the affected side.
  - Positive: diminished radial pulse with maneuver
  - Straight leg raise: evaluates for sciatica (Fig. 106.14)
  - With the patient supine, raise the leg on the affected side.
  - Positive: The maneuver produces or exacerbates radicular symptoms.
  - Waddell sign: identifies nonorganic symptoms, unlikely to improve with intervention
  - Gentle rolling of the skin over the back produces radicular symptoms.
  - Twisting the torso with motion through the knees produces back pain.
  - Slight axial compression to the head produces pain.
  - Supine and seated straight leg raise tests produce different responses.
  - Positive: Three or more positive responses indicate a likely nonorganic abnormality.
- During the physical examination, it is important to look for clues that would help further differentiate radiculopathic and myelopathic pain.
  - Such findings include weakness, diminished reflexes, decreased muscle tone, and a dermatomal distribution of pain for radicular pathology.

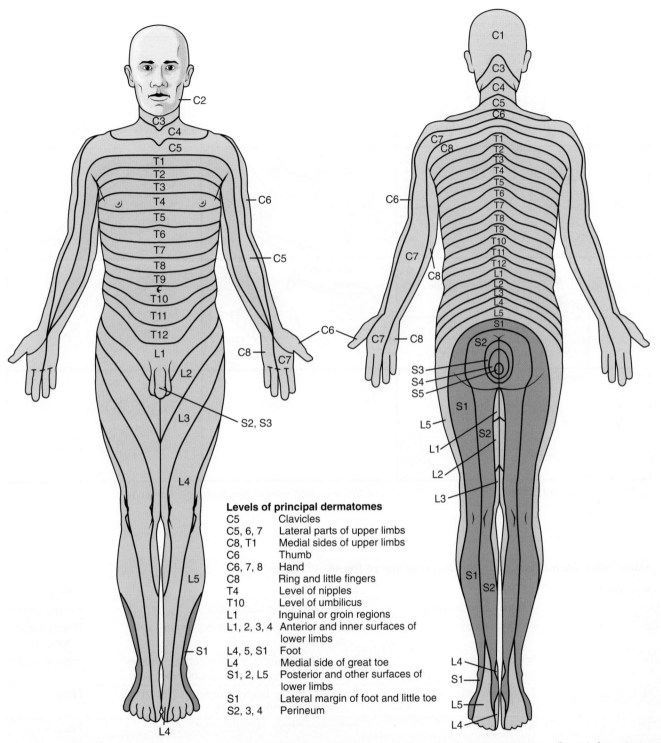

Levels of principal dermatomes

C5	Clavicles
C5, 6, 7	Lateral parts of upper limbs
C8, T1	Medial sides of upper limbs
C6	Thumb
C6, 7, 8	Hand
C8	Ring and little fingers
T4	Level of nipples
T10	Level of umbilicus
L1	Inguinal or groin regions
L1, 2, 3, 4	Anterior and inner surfaces of lower limbs
L4, 5, S1	Foot
L4	Medial side of great toe
S1, 2, L5	Posterior and other surfaces of lower limbs
S1	Lateral margin of foot and little toe
S2, 3, 4	Perineum

Fig 106.7 Schematic demarcation of dermatomes. There is actually considerable overlap between any two adjacent dermatomes.

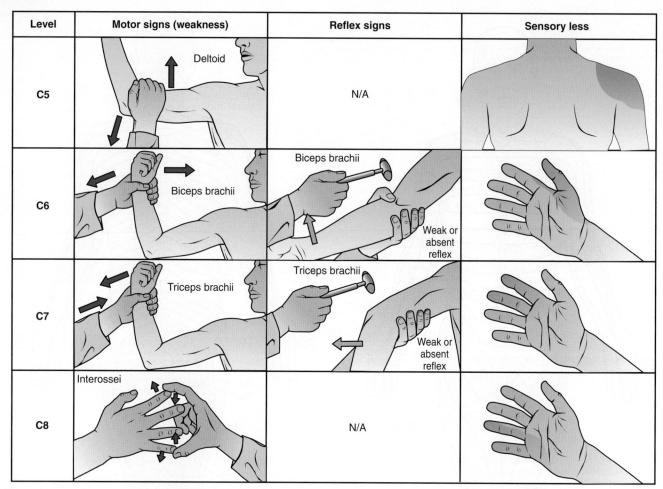

Level	Motor signs (weakness)	Reflex signs	Sensory less
C5	Deltoid	N/A	
C6	Biceps brachii	Biceps brachii — Weak or absent reflex	
C7	Triceps brachii	Triceps brachii — Weak or absent reflex	
C8	Interossei	N/A	

Fig 106.8 Assessment of the cervical nerves. Please note that the chart reflects only the upper extremity.

TABLE 106.1 Motor Function: Evaluation of Nerve Roots

Neurologic Level	Sensation	Motor	Reflex
C5	Lateral shoulder/arm	Deltoid (shoulder abduction)	Biceps tendon
C6	Radial forearm	Biceps/wrist extensors (elbow flexion, wrist extension)	Brachioradialis tendon
C7	Middle finger	Triceps/wrist flexors/finger extensors (elbow extension, wrist flexion, finger extension)	Triceps tendon
C8	Ulnar forearm	Interossei/finger flexors (finger abduction/adduction, finger flexion)	None
T1	Medial arm	Interossei (finger abduction/adduction)	None
T12, L1, L2, L3	Anterior thigh	Iliopsoas (hip flexion)	None
L2, L3, L4	Anterior thigh	Quadriceps/adductors (knee extension, leg adduction)	None
L4	Medial lower leg and foot	Tibialis anterior (foot dorsiflexion/inversion)	Patellar tendon
L5	Dorsum of foot and lateral lower leg	Extensor hallucis longus (great-toe dorsiflexion)	None
S1	Lateral/plantar aspect of foot	Peroneus longus/brevis (foot plantar flexion/eversion)	Achilles tendon
S2, S3, S4	Perianal	Bladder, intrinsic foot muscles	None

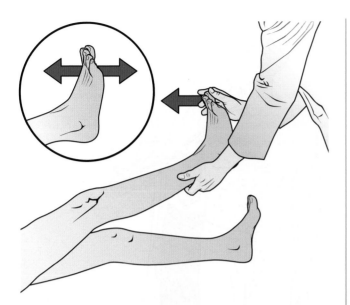

Fig 106.9 Evaluation of clonus.

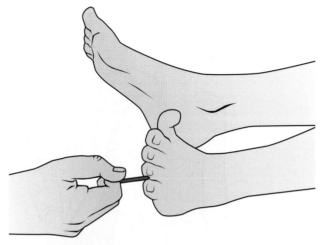

Fig 106.10 Babinski sign.

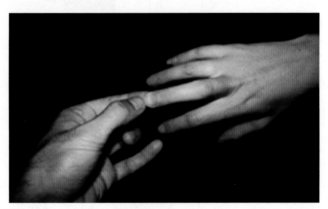

Fig 106.11 Hoffmann sign.

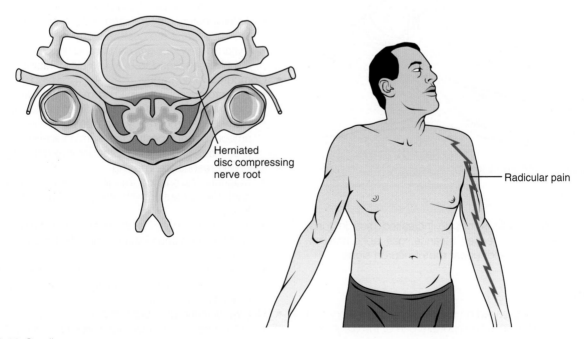

Herniated disc compressing nerve root

Radicular pain

Fig 106.12 Spurling maneuver.

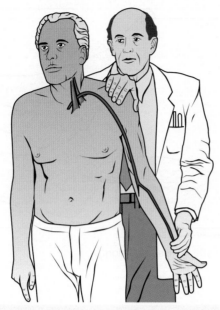

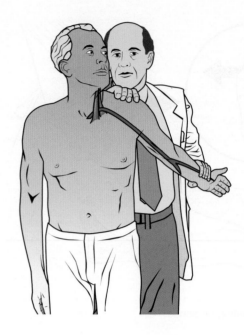

Fig 106.13 Adson test.

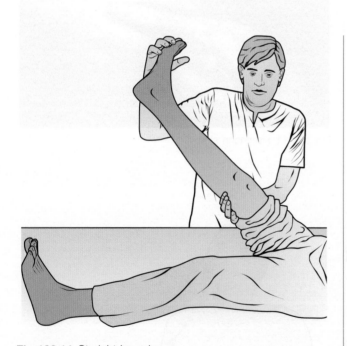

Fig 106.14 Straight leg raise.

- Myelopathic findings include increased muscle tone, hyperreflexia, decreased balance, gait abnormalities, and the presence of upper motor neuron signs.

Imaging

- Imaging the spine based on the results of the history and physical examination is an important part of the diagnostic and therapeutic protocol algorithm.

- There are multiple imaging modalities with which to evaluate spinal abnormalities, each of which has different strengths and weaknesses.
- An understanding of spinal anatomy, normal variations, and the incidence of degenerative changes is critical for the appropriate interpretation of imaging studies.
- In addition, reviewing the radiologist's reports and discussing the findings with the radiologist can be a valuable practice.
- Conventional radiography (Fig. 106.15)
  - This modality is often the initial imaging modality of choice because of its ease of acquisition and cost-effectiveness.
  - Anteroposterior, lateral, and oblique views of the spinal area of interest are customary.
  - Dynamic view radiographs, such as flexion and extension, are often obtained to evaluate for instability.
- Computed tomography
  - This cross-sectional imaging modality is well suited in the trauma setting for evaluation of fractures.
  - Computed tomography can also accurately assess the amount of bony destruction from a variety of pathologic processes and assist in preoperative planning.
- Magnetic resonance imaging
  - Magnetic resonance imaging provides high levels of anatomic resolution with respect to both bone and soft tissue.
  - It is commonly used for the evaluation of the degenerative spine, ligamentous injuries, and infectious or neoplastic processes.
  - Most clinicians consider magnetic resonance imaging to be the advanced imaging modality of choice for evaluation of the spine.
- Nuclear scintigraphy (bone scan)
  - Often used to evaluate for metastatic disease, stress fractures, and infection

Suggested Readings

Bono CM, Schoenfeld AJ, eds. *Spine*. 2nd ed. Philadelphia: Wolters Kluwer; 2017.

Emery SE. Cervical spondylotic myelopathy: diagnosis and treatment. *J Am Acad Orthop Surg*. 2001;9:376–388.

Fayad LM, Fishman EK. Computed tomography of musculoskeletal pathology. *Orthopedics*. 2006;29:1076–1082.

Hoppenfeld S, ed. *Physical Examination of the Spine and Extremities*. East Norwalk, CT: Appleton-Century-Crofts; 1976.

Khanna AJ, Carbone JJ, Kebaish KM, et al. Magnetic resonance imaging of the cervical spine: current techniques and spectrum of disease. *J Bone Joint Surg Am*. 2002;84A:70–80.

Khanna AJ, Shindle MK, Wasserman BA. Imaging of the spine. In: McLain RF, Markman M, Bukowski RM, et al, eds. *Cancer in the Spine: Comprehensive Care*. Totowa, NJ: Humana Press; 2006:73–81.

Rhee JM, Yoon T, Riew KD. Cervical radiculopathy. *J Am Acad Orthop Surg*. 2007;15:486–494.

Scoliosis Research Society: *White paper on sagittal alignment*. Available at: www.srs.org/professionals/resources/sagittal_plane_white_paper.pdf. Accessed February 3, 2009.

Waddell G, McCulloch JA, Kummel E, et al. Nonorganic physical signs in low-back pain. *Spine*. 1980;5:117–125.

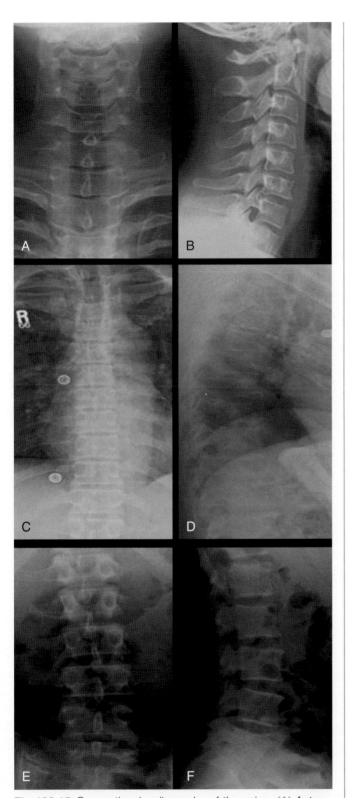

Fig 106.15 Conventional radiographs of the spine. (A) Anteroposterior cervical spine; (B) lateral cervical spine; (C) anteroposterior thoracic spine; (D) lateral thoracic spine; (E) anteroposterior lumbar spine; (F) lateral lumbar spine.

Chapter 107 Whiplash (Cervical Strain)

Dennis Q. Chen, Xudong Li

ICD-10-CM CODE
S13.4XXA *Sprain of ligaments of cervical spine*

Key Concepts

- "Whiplash" typically occurs following an abrupt flexion/extension movement to the cervical spine.
- "Whiplash" has been used to describe both the injury and resultant neck pain.
  - The syndrome can include neck pain and stiffness, occipital headache, upper back pain, shoulder girdle pain, dizziness, tinnitus, memory loss, visual disturbances, temporomandibular joint pain, dysphagia, hoarseness, and depression.
- More than 50% of patients are improved by 3 months and 75% by 12 months.
- Persistent pain after 6 months is classified as chronic whiplash.
- Prognostic factors for worse outcomes include psychosocial factors, litigation, female gender, radiating pain, and high initial intensity of pain.
- Common sources of neck pain after whiplash injury include the facet joints, nerve roots, cervical disks, and supporting soft-tissue structures.
- Cervical radiographs are obtained when a cervical spine fracture, instability, or neurologic deficits (paresthesias, numbness, weakness) are suspected.
- Magnetic resonance imaging is not warranted in the acute or subacute setting after whiplash injury without neurologic abnormalities detected on examination.
- Initial treatment should consist of patient education, reassurance, symptomatic treatment, and discontinuing any cervical orthosis as soon as possible.
- Surgery for axial neck pain is controversial and is indicated in a very small subset of patients.

History

- Acceleration-deceleration injury: rear-end collision or block/tackle during contact sports (e.g., football, ice hockey)
- Women have twice the risk of whiplash injury as men.
- Headache and neck pain at rest or with motion
- May have numbness, tingling, or weakness in the extremities
- May report loss of consciousness or amnesia of the event
- Inquire about duration and intensity of symptoms, employment status, psychiatric illness, and desire to pursue legal recourse.

Physical Examination

- Observation
  - Neck stiffness
- Palpation
  - Midline and paraspinal cervical tenderness/muscle spasm
- Range of motion
  - Assess only after fracture and instability have been ruled out.
  - Cervical flexion/extension, rotation, and lateral bending
- Special tests
  - Complete neurologic examination, including upper and lower extremity sensation, strength, and reflexes

Imaging

- Radiographs: Anteroposterior, lateral, and open-mouth views are necessary in the setting of trauma with pain or neurologic deficit.
  - Adequate imaging must include top of T1 vertebra; obtain swimmer's view, if necessary (Fig. 107.1).
- Assess alignment by looking at the anterior vertebral line, posterior vertebral line, spinolaminar line, and posterior spinous line. These lines should follow a slight lordotic curve without any step-offs. Any malalignment should be considered evidence of ligamentous injury and instability
  - Flexion-extension views are best performed in a delayed fashion when acute spasm has subsided in the awake and alert patient without neurologic deficit to confirm ligamentous stability.
- Computed tomography
  - May be obtained to rule out fractures; more sensitive than radiographs
- Magnetic resonance imaging
  - Performed if ligamentous injury is suspected or neurologic deficits are present
  - Should not be used as a screening tool; high rate of false positives
  - May be used to identify the cause of persistent arm pain or other signs of nerve root compression

Differential Diagnosis

- Cervical disc herniation
- Cervical stenosis
- Cervical spine tumor or infection
- Dislocation or subluxation of the spine ("jumped facet")
- Spinal fracture
- Ligamentous injury/instability

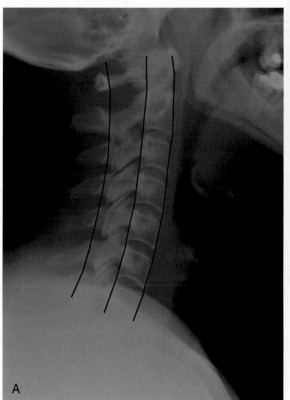

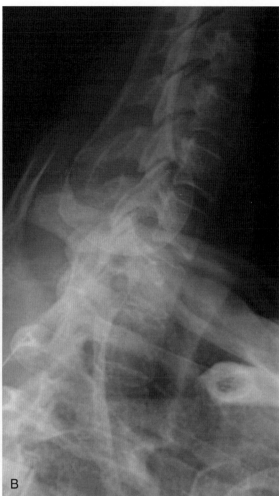

Fig 107.1 Cervical spine radiographs. **(A)** Lateral view. **(B)** Swimmer's view.

- Exacerbation of degenerative or inflammatory arthritis (degenerative disc disease, facet arthritis)

Treatment

- At diagnosis
  - Patients may return to full activity as tolerated and discontinue cervical orthoses once they are clinically or radiographically cleared to do so.
  - Refrain from contact sports until full range of motion returns.
  - Clinical follow-up for symptom reassessment
  - Medications: Acetaminophen, nonsteroidal antiinflammatory drugs (NSAIDs), and/or muscle relaxant for symptomatic relief. Short course of narcotic pain medication may be helpful. Chronic pain following whiplash may require referral to pain management specialist.
  - Physical therapy: range of motion/stretching/strengthening, focus on body mechanics/ergonomics/posture, and overcoming fear-based avoidance of activity
  - Spinal injections and percutaneous radiofrequency neurotomy may relieve chronic pain after whiplash injury.

- Later
  - Surgery to address disc herniation, instability, or canal/foraminal stenosis may be necessary for persistent radicular pain, numbness, or weakness (Fig. 107.2).

When to Refer

- Patients with instability, numbness, weakness, radicular pain, or pain refractory to initial treatment should undergo cervical spine magnetic resonance imaging and referral to a spine surgeon.

Prognosis

- Approximately 50% of individuals will recover from pain and disability within 3 to 6 months of injury, but the remainder will continue to report symptoms up to 1 to 2 years or longer after the motor vehicle crash.
- Of those who do not recover, between 30% and 40% are likely to have persistent mild to moderate levels of pain, and between 10% and 20% will have moderate to severe pain syndromes.

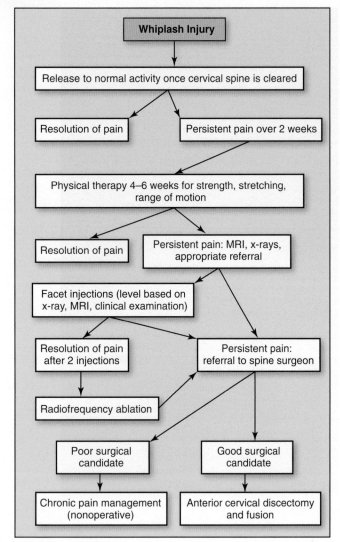

Fig 107.2 Treatment algorithm for whiplash injuries. *MRI,* Magnetic resonance imaging.

Troubleshooting

- Patients should be counseled on the warning signs of worsening weakness, numbness, or bowel/bladder incontinence.
- Should neurologic symptoms or pain persist, further workup and invasive treatment may be indicated.

Patient Instructions

- Educate patients on the prognosis and the importance of returning to full activity and employment.

Considerations in Special Populations

- Patients with prior cervical spine surgery and/or hardware placement should have their implants evaluated for position change or damage.
- Litigant patients appear to do as well as nonlitigant patients when undergoing radiofrequency neurotomy for chronic neck pain or headache.
- Patients with rheumatoid arthritis are at increased risk of ligamentous cervical spine injury from trauma.

Suggested Readings

Bannister G, Amirfeyz R, Kelley S, Gargan M. Whiplash injury. *J Bone Joint Surg.* 2009;91:845–850.

Côté P, Soklaridis S. Does early management of whiplash-associated disorders assist or impede recovery? *Spine.* 2011;36(25 suppl): S275–S279.

Cusick JF, Pintar FA, Yoganandan N. Whiplash syndrome: kinematic factors influencing pain patterns. *Spine.* 2001;26(11):1252–1258.

Gun RT, Osti OL, O'Riordan A, et al. Risk factors for prolonged disability after whiplash injury: a prospective study. *Spine.* 2005;30(4): 386–391.

Hartling L, Brison RJ, Ardern C, Pickett W. Prognostic value of the Quebec classification of whiplash-associated disorders. *Spine.* 2001;26(1): 36–41.

Jull G, Söderlund A, Stemper B, et al. Toward optimal early management after whiplash injury to lessen the rate of transition to chronicity: discussion paper 5. *Spine.* 2011;36(25 suppl):S335–S342.

Panjabi MM, Shigeki I, Pearson AM, Ivancic PC. Injury mechanisms of the cervical intervertebral disc during simulated whiplash. *Spine.* 2004;29(11): 1217–1225.

Pierre C, Cassidy JD, Carroll L, et al. A systematic review of the prognosis of acute whiplash and a new conceptual framework to synthesize the literature. *Spine.* 2001;26:E445–E458.

Rosenfeld M, Gunnarsson R, Borenstein P. Early intervention in whiplash-associated disorders: a comparison of two treatment protocols. *Spine.* 2000;25(14):1782–1787.

Sapir DA, Gorup JM. Radiofrequency medial branch neurotomy in litigant and nonlitigant patients with cervical whiplash: a prospective study. *Spine.* 2001;26(12):E268–E273.

Schofferman J, Bogduk N, Slosar P. Chronic whiplash and whiplash-associated disorders: an evidence-based approach. *J Am Acad Orthop Surg.* 2007;15(10):596–606.

Chapter 108 Cervical Disc Disease and Spondylosis

Rabia Qureshi, Jason A. Horowitz, Hamid Hassanzadeh

ICD-10-CM CODES

M43.02	*Spondylosis, cervical region*
M50.0	*Cervical disc disorder with myelopathy*
M50.1	*Cervical disc disorder with radiculopathy*
M50.2	*Other cervical disc displacement*
M50.3	*Other cervical disc degeneration*
M54.12	*Radiculopathy, cervical region*
M99.61	*Osseous and subluxation stenosis of intervertebral foramina, cervical region*
M99.71	*Connective tissue and disc stenosis of intervertebral foramina, cervical region*

Key Concepts

- Cervical spondylosis is degeneration affecting the intervertebral bodies and intervertebral discs of the cervical spine, usually in older adult patients (Fig. 108.1).
- Cervical spondylosis is the result of wear and tear with aging, but can be affected by various external factors.
- Symptoms of cervical degeneration can result from nerve root and/or cord compression due to intervertebral disk (IVD) degeneration, osteophyte formation, spinal instability, or spinal malalignment.
- The outer portion of the IVD is the annulus fibrosis, while the inner portion is the gelatinous nucleus pulposus. Both components undergo degenerative changes over time that can lead to disk space narrowing and/or disk protrusion/herniation (see Fig. 108.1B).
- The clinical symptoms/neurological deficits in cervical spondylosis vary greatly depending on the etiology and extent of disease and can include neck pain radiating to the arm, numbness/paresthesias, pathologic gait, lower extremity weakness, and many others.
- Treatment can also vary based on severity and begins with nonoperative treatment. Operative management is indicated for neurological symptoms that are refractory to nonoperative management and for "red flag" symptoms such as bowel/bladder dysfunction and acutely progressive symptoms.

History

- History must rule out other, nonmechanical causes of symptoms including neoplasms, infection, metastases, or traumatic/pathologic fractures.

- Determine type of pain: axial neck pain, radiculopathy, or myelopathy.
  - Axial neck pain: exclusively in the cervical, occipital, and scapular areas. Axial neck pain is usually musculoskeletal in origin, resulting from muscle strain.
    - More immediate onset pain
    - Often persistent
  - Radiculopathy: Nerve root compression (see Fig. 108.1D) causing neck pain radiating into the arm. Can include weakness and numbness of the arm.
    - Insidious onset headache with radiating pain
    - Unilateral pain, numbness and tingling, with dermatomal distribution
  - Myelopathy: spinal cord compression with various causes including congenital stenosis. Symptoms include progressive gait imbalance and hand clumsiness.
    - Can present with neck stiffness or occipital headache
    - Instability with gait
    - Progressive clumsiness, fine motor difficulty

Physical Examination
(Figs. 108.2 and 108.3)

- Look for neck pain and stiffness of muscles. Determine if pain or spasms are present with palpation.
- Observe muscle tone and if any atrophy is present in neck, shoulders, arms, and hands.
- Observe gait and posture changes.
- Determine range of motion.
- Full neurological examination.
- Special tests include: Spurling test, shoulder abduction test, finger escape, and Hoffman sign among others
  - Radiculopathy: examination findings are dependent upon nerve root level.
    - C5—deltoid and biceps weakness
    - C6—wrist extension weakness, thumb paresthesias
    - C7—wrist flexion weakness, diminished triceps reflex, index and middle finger paresthesias
    - C8—weakness of distal phalanx flexion, little finger paresthesias
    - Spurling test—pain with neck extension and ipsilateral bending, relief from neck flexion with deviation opposite to symptomatic side
    - Shoulder abduction test—relief of pain/symptoms with abduction of shoulders
  - Myelopathy: motor and sensory signs along with gait instability and upper motor neuron signs
    - Weakness may be present, though difficult to ascertain

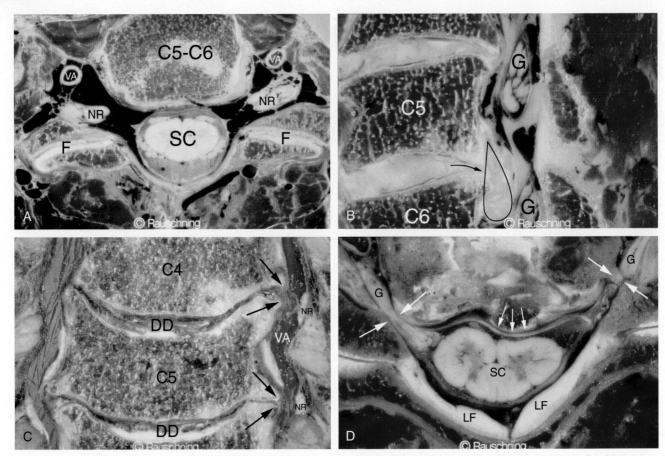

Fig 108.1 Normal **(A)** and degenerative **(B–D)** cervical spine anatomy. **(A)** Axial cross-section showing a normal C5-C6 level and the relationship of nerve roots *(NR)*, facets *(F)*, spinal cord *(SC)*, and vertebral artery *(VA)*. **(B)** Parasagittal section showing a teardrop-shaped disc extrusion (herniation), compressing the ganglion (G) of the C6 nerve root. **(C)** Coronal section showing severe disc degeneration (DD; cervical spondylosis), collapse, and uncinate process osteophytes *(arrows)*. **(D)** Axial section showing late-stage cervical disc disease, with osteophytes centrally *(small arrows)* and peripherally compressing the ganglia *(large arrows)*, as well as thickened ligamentum flava *(LF)*. (From Gallego J, Schnuerer AP, Manuel C. *Basic Anatomy and Pathology of the Spine.* Memphis: Medtronic Sofamor Danek, 2001; photographs by Wolfgang Rauschning, MD, PhD.)

- Test paresthesias and decreased pain sensation with pinprick
- Spasticity is noted on exam; clonus or Babinski may be present
- Hoffman sign—snap of distal phalanx of middle finger results in flexion of other fingers
- Finger escape may occur with fingers extended and adducted (small finger drifts away due to muscle weakness)
- Lhermitte sign—cervical flexion will result in shock-like pain shooting down spine and may radiate into extremities
- Grip and release test—patients have difficulty with making a fist and releasing in succession

Imaging
Radiography (Fig. 108.4A and B)
- Common findings on radiography include osteophytes, narrowed disc spaces, decreases in sagittal diameter, sagittal or coronal malalignment, and degenerative changes in anteroposterior and lateral views.

- Flexion/extension imaging may reveal angular (>11 degrees) or translational (>3.5 mm) instability and may also demonstrate compensatory subluxation.
- Oblique view findings include foraminal stenosis, usually not needed.
- With older age, radiographic findings of degeneration become common in asymptomatic individuals and may not correlate with the clinical presentation.

Computed Tomography
- Aids in evaluation of bony elements
- Can determine level of bony cord compression and foraminal stenosis and can also evaluate ossification of posterior longitudinal ligaments

Magnetic Resonance Imaging (see Fig. 108.4C)
- Indicated in patients with suspected disc disease or herniation.
- Can evaluate surrounding soft tissues, spinal cord lesions, tumors, infections, and other spinal cord changes/compression.
- Disc degeneration can be evaluated.

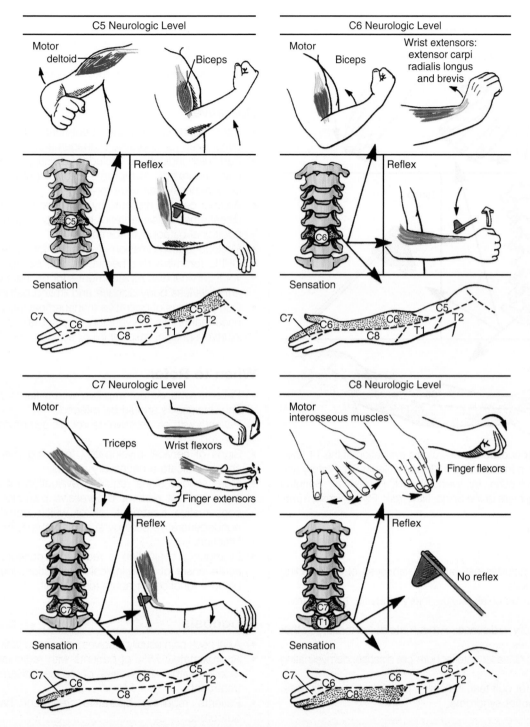

Fig 108.2 Upper extremity neurologic evaluation of C5-C8. (Modified with permission from Klein JD, Garfin SR. History and physical examination. In: Weinstein JN, Rydevik B, Sonntag VKG, eds. *Essentials of the Spine.* New York: Raven Press; 1995:71–95.)

- Magnetic resonance imaging (MRI) findings must correlate with the clinical presentation as abnormal findings on MRI are common in asymptomatic patients.

- Discography is rarely used in cervical spondylosis patients due to the risk of esophageal puncture and infection.

Additional Tests

- Computed tomography myelography with contrast aids in evaluation in patients where MRI is contraindicated.

Differential Diagnosis

- Neoplasm: includes metastases, primary bony tumors, superior sulcus tumor, cord tumors

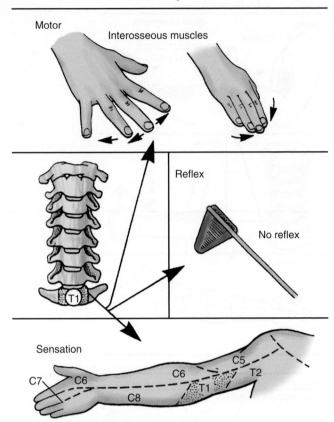

T1 Neurologic Level

Motor

Interosseous muscles

Reflex

No reflex

Sensation

C5
C6
C7
C6
C8
T1
T2

Fig 108.3 Upper extremity neurologic evaluation of the T1 level. (Modified with permission from Klein JD, Garfin SR. History and physical examination. In: Weinstein JN, Rydevik B, Sonntag VKG, eds. *Essentials of the Spine*. New York: Raven Press; 1995: 71–95.)

- Infection: includes osteomyelitis, abscess of surrounding tissue, diskitis
- Traumatic: brachial plexus injury, muscle sprain/strain, instability
- Inflammatory disease: rheumatoid arthritis, other arthropathies
- Neurologic disease: anterior horn cell disease, demyelinating diseases
- Misc: rotator cuff tear, instability, peripheral nerve disease, thoracic outlet syndrome

Treatment (Fig. 108.5)
Nonoperative Methods
- A majority of patients recover without operative intervention.
  - Most patients recover within 12 weeks of conservative treatment.
- Rest or decrease in activity, soft collar may be used
  - Some patients benefit from immobilization for short periods.
- Ice/heat with or without antiinflammatory medications for added pain relief, including nonsteroidal antiinflammatory drugs (NSAIDs) or steroids for more severe pain

- Medications also include gamma-aminobutyric acid (GABA) inhibitors, muscle relaxants, and narcotics.
- Stretching/physical therapy for patients who do show improvement with rest and analgesics.
- Corticosteroid injections may be used for nerve root pain relief.

Operative
- After failed conservative treatment, patients may be considered for operative management.
- Particular indications include persisting pain, disabling pain, neurologic symptoms (radiculopathy, myelopathy, or weakness), gait symptoms.
- Anterior cervical discectomy with fusion—for cervical disc disease/herniation, anterior pathology, radiculopathy, and additional osteophyte formation.
- Posterior decompression +/– fusion—for multilevel disease, OPLL, foraminal disc herniation, and pseudoarthrosis.
- Total cervical disc replacement—for patients with minimal arthrosis/less bony disease and limited pathology.
- Complications of operative management include infection, pseudoarthrosis, nerve injury, implant failure, esophageal injury/dysphagia, vascular injury, adjacent segment disease.

When to Refer
- Patients who do not improve with initial treatment, rest, and analgesics should be referred.
- Patients with progressive neurologic symptoms should be referred.
- Signs of cervical myelopathy, including pathologic gait, should indicate a necessary referral.
- More serious signs requiring evaluation include pain at night, pain at rest, or progressive pain not relieved by conservative treatment, all of which could indicate a nondegenerative etiology such as trauma, malignancy, or infection.
- Emergency evaluation is required if patients suffer from acute onset of neurological dysfunction, loss of bowel/bladder function, or acute loss of gait.

Prognosis
- Axial neck pain usually resolves with conservative treatment.
- Approximately 75% of patients with radicular symptoms recover within 12 weeks of conservative/nonoperative treatment.
- Patients requiring operative treatment have variable outcomes.
  - Anterior cervical discectomies are the gold standard treatment for radiculopathy and have favorable outcomes.
  - Posterior foraminotomies have favorable outcomes in a large majority of patients.
  - Recurrence is often not predictable.

Troubleshooting
- A proper and thorough history and physical should be conducted to rule out nondegenerative etiologies.
- Patients should have adequate follow-up visits after initial diagnosis.

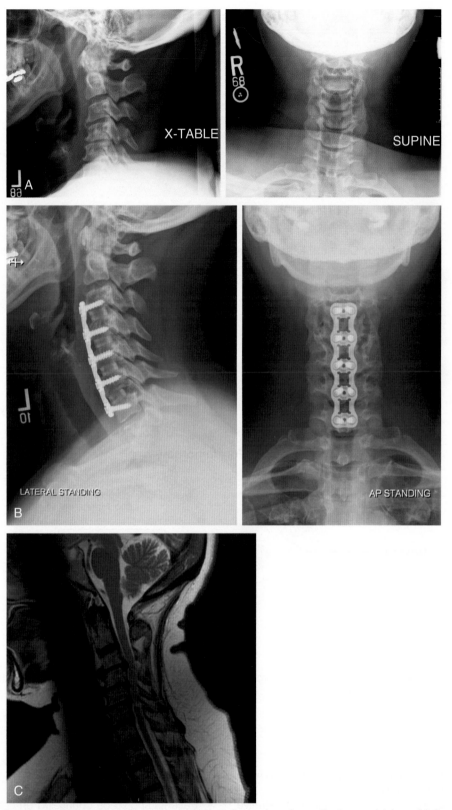

Fig 108.4 (A) Sagittal and anteroposterior (AP) cervical spine radiographs of a patient complaining of left upper extremity pain, numbness, and tingling with evidence of disc space narrowing and loss of lordosis. (B) Postoperative sagittal and AP cervical radiographs showing anterior cervical discectomies and fusion spanning C3-C7. (C) Cervical spine magnetic resonance imaging showing degenerative disc disease as well as central canal narrowing at C3-C4, C4-C5, C5-C6, and C6-C7.

A   **Epidural Steroid Injection**

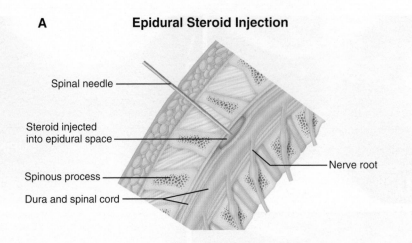

Spinal needle

Steroid injected into epidural space

Spinous process

Dura and spinal cord

Nerve root

B   **Anterior Cervical Discectomy with Fusion or Total Disc Replacement**

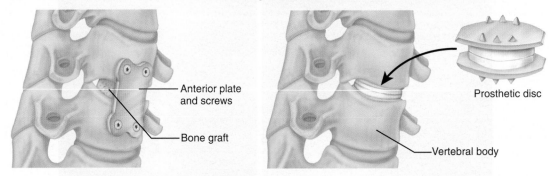

Anterior plate and screws

Bone graft

Prosthetic disc

Vertebral body

C   **Posterior Foraminotomy**

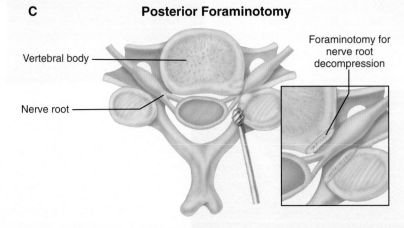

Vertebral body

Nerve root

Foraminotomy for nerve root decompression

Fig 108.5 Treatment modalities. **(A)** Epidural corticosteroid injection. **(B)** Anterior cervical discectomy with fusion or total disc replacement. **(C)** Posterior foraminotomy.

- Particularly patients with neurological symptoms to allow for assessment of progression
- Surgical complications can occur and postoperative management must include close in-hospital monitoring and follow-up office visits.
  - Dysphagia is particularly common and patients should be treated accordingly.
- Patients at risk for infection should be monitored more closely for postoperative infection.

Patient Instructions

- Patients should be counseled on conservative treatment and the benefits of rest and physical therapy.
- Patients should be given information regarding operative management in case conservative treatment fails.
- Preoperatively, patients should be counseled regarding surgical risks and postoperative expectations in terms of both functionality and pain.

- Whether undergoing operative or nonoperative treatment, patients should be given instructions to return for follow-up in the event that symptoms persist after treatment.

Considerations in Special Populations

- Patients with chronic pain/pain syndromes need to be counseled on expectations and should have close follow-up. If pain does not subside after surgery, referral to pain management may be necessary.
  - Additionally, chronic pain patients should undergo physical therapy and conditioning both before and after surgery.
  - Close attention should be paid to pain medications, particularly narcotics consumption.
- Patients with inflammatory arthritis should be evaluated more carefully for trauma and neurologic dysfunction.

Suggested Readings

Bohlman HH, Emory SE, Goodfellow DB, Jones PK. Robinson anterior cervical discectomy and arthrodesis for cervical radiculopathy. *J Bone Joint Surg*. 1993;75(9):1298–1307.

Burkett CJ, Greenberg MS, et al. Cervical and thoracic spine degenerative disease. In: Baaj AA, Mummaneni PV, Uribe JS, eds. New York: Thieme; 2011:146–150.

Nakashima H, Yukawa Y, Suda K, et al. Abnormal findings on magnetic resonance images of the cervical spines in 1211 asymptomatic subjects. *Spine*. 2015;40(6):392–398.

Toledano M, Bartleson JD. Cervical spondylotic myelopathy. *Neurol Clin*. 2013;31(1):287–305.

Woods BI, Hilibrand AS. Cervical radiculopathy: epidemiology, etiology, diagnosis, and treatment. *J Spinal Disord Tech*. 2015;28(5):E251–E259.

Chapter 109 Cervical Spinal Stenosis

Brett A. Freedman, Nathan Wanderman, S. Tim Yoon

ICD-10-CM CODES
M47.812 *Spondylosis without myelopathy or radiculopathy, cervical region*
M48.02 *Spinal stenosis, cervical region*
M50.00 *Cervical disc disorder with myelopathy, unspecified cervical region*

Key Concepts

- Cervical spondylotic myelopathy is the most common cause of spinal cord dysfunction (paresis/paralysis) in patients older than 55 years of age.
- Cervical spinal stenosis is a multifactorial phenomenon, with acquired and congenital etiologies, which results in a reduced anteroposterior (AP) canal diameter.
- Cervical spondylotic myelopathy likely represents a combination of compressive and ischemic insults. Long tract signs tend to occur first (biceps hyperreflexia), followed by hypertonia and pathologic reflexes
- Axial neck pain or radiculopathy do not correlate with the severity of stenosis or presence of myelopathy.
- Myelopathy is usually progressive. Surgical intervention to decompress the spinal cord should be considered when there are functional deficits. Surgery ceases progression of myelopathy and leads to neurologic improvement in as many as 75% of cases.
- The diagnosis of myelopathy is a clinical one, based on history and examination findings, with imaging studies providing corroborating evidence.

History

- Typical symptom onset at age 50 to 60 years; younger in congenital stenosis
- Natural history patterns: no progression, stepwise progression (most common; 75%), slow steady decline, and rapid progression (least common)
- Hand clumsiness; decreased dexterity with buttons, coins, and handwriting
- Altered gait: problems with balance, new need for walking aid
- Generalized weakness, increased fatigability, decreased walking tolerance
- Neck pain can be present but tends not to be a prominent component.
- Key elements of history of present illness (HPI): duration of symptoms, previous treatments and results, bowel/bladder/erectile function, medical history (previous neck trauma or surgery, history of cancer), smoking, and occupation

Physical Examination

- Observation
  - Previous scars, altered cervical spine alignment (loss of lordosis)
- Palpation
  - Identify masses, tender points, deformity, and paraspinal spasm
- Special tests
  - Complete motor, sensory, and reflex examination
  - Rectal examination: Record tone, sensation, wink (reflexive anal contraction when skin contacted), or bulbocavernosus reflex (pinch glans/clitoris or tug on Foley catheter to elicit reflexive anal sphincter contraction).
  - Wide-based, shuffling gait; inability to perform tandem gait
  - Stand on toes to check plantarflexion strength and balance
  - Myelopathy signs: Hoffmann, hyperreflexia (absent in 30%), abnormal reflexes (inverted radial reflex), clonus, Babinski, dysdiadochokinesia (alternating clapping, grip release test), Lhermitte (flexing/extending neck shoots electric pain down spine)
  - Postvoid residual: sterile catheter placed after patient attempts to fully void, should be less than 100 mL; also check urinalysis
  - Nurick score for myelopathy (as many as 75% of patients improve one grade with surgery)
    - 0: Signs/symptoms of radiculopathy, but no myelopathy
    - 1: Myelopathy signs, but no difficulty walking
    - 2: Myelopathy, slight difficulty walking, does not restrict employment
    - 3: Myelopathy, difficulty walking, no full-time job, still independent
    - 4: Myelopathy, assisted ambulation only
    - 5: Myelopathy, wheelchair only

Imaging

- Because spondylosis is present in more than 70% of normal elderly patients, imaging studies alone cannot diagnose cervical spondylotic myelopathy.
- Radiographs: AP, lateral, and flexion/extension lateral views
  - Spondylosis: disc height loss, osteophytes, retrolisthesis (typically C3-C4 or C4-C5), lost cervical lordosis, signs of fractures or other pathology
  - Spinal canal AP diameter: normal, more than 17 mm on lateral view; cord compression (from spinal stenosis) occurs with canal diameter of less than 13 mm

- Torg ratio (AP canal diameter/AP vertebral body length): describes the congenital component of cervical spinal stenosis (normal is > 1; cervical stenosis is suggested with values < 0.8.
- Flexion/extension views demonstrate dynamic stenosis and intervertebral instability. Listhesis of more than 2 to 3.5 mm decreases canal dimensions.
- Computed tomography
  - Best for defining bony anatomy and quality. Computed tomography myelography is useful for patients intolerant of magnetic resonance imaging or those with previous metallic implants.
  - The AP canal dimension is most useful for cervical stenosis. In addition, a cross-sectional area of less than 30 to 50 mm^2 has been correlated with poor outcomes.
  - Osteophytes, facet malalignment (trauma), facet hypertrophy, and extraosseous calcifications including chronic disc protrusions or ossification of the posterior longitudinal ligament may contribute to stenosis (Fig. 109.1).
- Magnetic resonance imaging
  - Best for visualizing soft-tissue structures compressing the spinal cord, detecting ligamentous injuries, and demonstrating cord signal changes—a relative prognosticator of poor outcome

- Myelomalacia (softening of the cord) results from repeated ischemic and hemorrhagic insults to the spinal cord, seen on T2-weighted images as a white grainy signal within the normally gray cord (Fig. 109.2).
- With progressive stenosis, the T2-weighted cerebrospinal fluid signal is reduced and the cord becomes deformed, usually in the AP direction (bean shaped).
- Myelopathic signs/symptoms are usually present when the AP diameter of the cord is reduced to 30% of its normal value.

Additional Tests

- Electromyography may distinguish peripheral neuropathy from radicular and myelopathic conditions.
- Advanced brain imaging studies may rule out a central cause of symptoms.

Differential Diagnosis

- Peripheral neuropathy (compressive, metabolic, or diabetes related)
- Cerebral vascular accident
- Progressive intrinsic neurologic or muscular disorders: multiple sclerosis, metabolic myopathy, Parkinson disease, amyotrophic lateral sclerosis (Lou Gehrig disease)
- Syringomyelia, Arnold-Chiari malformation, hydrocephalus
- Primary or metastatic intramedullary spinal cord tumor
- Infection: epidural abscess, vertebral osteomyelitis, spondylodiscitis

Treatment

- Nonoperative management
  - Typically progressive, so surgery is the preferred treatment in symptomatic patients.
  - Most patients have congenital narrowing of their canal that becomes critical with acquired changes with aging or acutely after trauma.
  - Watchful waiting can be tried in patients with mild symptoms or those with a high risk of severe surgical complications.
  - Collars or exercises can be used, but their efficacy is unproven.
  - Corticosteroids can be useful as a temporizing measure in patients with new cord compression and progressive myelopathy.
- Surgical management
  - Surgical options are based on the etiology and level of stenosis.
  - Posterior approaches: laminectomy with or without posterior spinal fusion or laminoplasty (Fig. 109.3); more commonly considered for multilevel (more than three levels) stenosis. Severe fixed kyphosis is a contraindication to a posterior-only approach.
  - Anterior approaches: anterior cervical discectomy and fusion or corpectomy and fusion (see Figs. 109.2 and 109.4); allows direct decompression of the spinal cord—useful in cases of >10 degrees of cervical kyphosis. Transient dysphagia is common, but typically resolves within 6 months
  - Combined approaches: reserved for complex cases

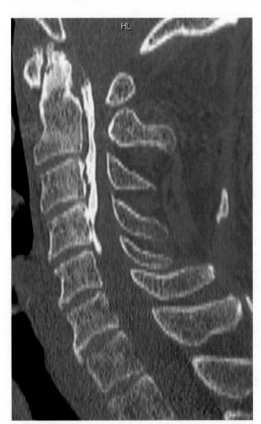

Fig 109.1 Midsagittal reconstructed image from a noncontrast computed tomography scan demonstrating advanced ossification of the posterior longitudinal ligament from C2 to C4 causing severe cervical stenosis.

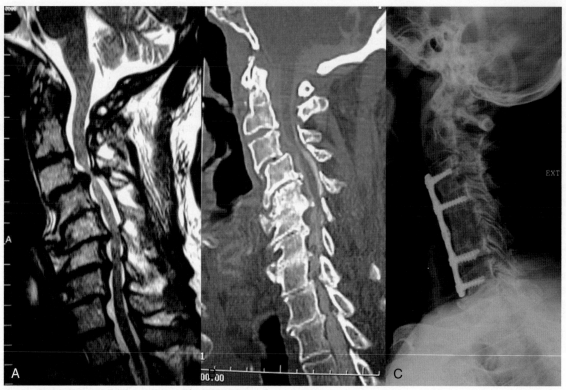

Fig 109.2 Severe multilevel cervical spondylotic myelopathy. Note the classic imaging findings of cervical myelopathy seen on T2-weighted sagittal magnetic resonance image (A) and sagittal reconstruction of the computed tomography myelogram (B). (C) This complex compressive pathology was treated with a hybrid anterior technique (C3-C4 and C6-C7 anterior cervical discectomy and fusion and C5 corpectomy with strut allograft).

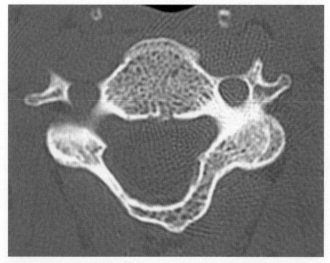

Fig 109.3 Axial computed tomography image 12 months after an open-door laminoplasty in which a cortical allograft was used to hold "the door" open. The hinge is healed on the left, and the bone graft on the right has incorporated and remodeled.

When to Refer

- Cervical stenosis without signs or symptoms of myelopathy is usually not a surgical disease.
- When myelopathy is present, prompt referral is warranted.
- If myelopathy is progressing, urgent referral is indicated.

Prognosis

- The natural history of cervical spondylotic myelopathy is progressive neurologic deterioration in the majority of patients.
- With surgical treatment, progression of myelopathy is prevented, and the majority of patients have some improvement in neurologic function.
- Cord signal changes on magnetic resonance imaging, an AP canal diameter less than 13 mm, and preoperative nonambulatory status (high Nurick grade) predict a poor outcome.

Troubleshooting

- Establish realistic expectations. The main goal of surgery in patients with myelopathy is to halt progression of the disease.
- Document the neurologic examination immediately preoperatively and postoperatively. Serial examination should be performed during the in-patient stay.

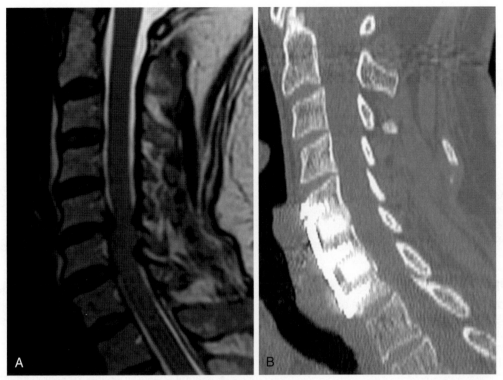

Fig 109.4 T2-weighted sagittal magnetic resonance images demonstrating cord compression at the C5-C6 and C6-C7 levels from disc herniations. **(A)** In addition, there is posterior compression from ligamentum flavum infolding. **(B)** Healed two-level anterior cervical discectomy and fusion with cortical allograft and anterior cervical plate fixation.

- Rule out other causes. 14% of patients with poor outcomes after surgery for cervical spondylotic myelopathy were later determined to have alternative or additional diagnoses such as myopathy, Parkinson disease, and cerebellar ataxia.
- Poor neurologic recovery or deterioration should prompt repeat imaging.

Patient Instructions

- If a nonoperative approach is tried, the surgeon must clearly instruct the patient to report any evidence of a progressive neurologic deficit. This warning should include the obvious (muscle weakness, sensory deficits), as well as the not so obvious (changes in bowel/bladder/erectile function, altered gait and balance, reduced hand dexterity).

Considerations in Special Populations

- Football players
  - Cervical cord neurapraxia is a condition associated with cervical canal stenosis.
  - Spear tackling (axial load and hyperflexion) may result in acute, transient (typically 10–15 minutes), burning sensations in the upper extremities, with or without motor deficits.
  - Cervical cord neurapraxia does not predict future permanent neurologic deficit; however, the recurrence rate is 56%.

- Return to play requires careful discussion. Return is contraindicated in patients with a Torg ratio of less than 0.8, loss of cervical lordosis, or evidence of cord damage on magnetic resonance imaging.
- Stenotic myelopathy secondary to ossification of the posterior longitudinal ligament is often a multilevel process, and progressive enlargement is expected. Thus it is important to establish the specific diagnosis (computed tomography) and plan surgery that addresses the global nature of the disorder (laminoplasty).
- Patients with Klippel-Feil syndrome frequently have congenitally narrowed spinal canals.

Suggested Readings

Bohlman HH, Emery SE. The pathophysiology of cervical spondylosis and myelopathy. *Spine*. 1988;13:843–846.

Clarke E, Robinson PK. Cervical myelopathy: A complication of cervical spondylosis. *Brain*. 1956;79:483–510.

Emery SE. Cervical spondylotic myelopathy: diagnosis and treatment. *J Am Acad Orthop Surg*. 2001;9:376–388.

Hilibrand AS, Carlson GD, Palumbo MA, et al. Radiculopathy and myelopathy at segments adjacent to the site of a previous anterior cervical arthrodesis. *J Bone Joint Surg Am*. 1999;81A:519–528.

Nurick S. The natural history and the results of surgical treatment of the spinal cord disorder associated with cervical spondylosis. *Brain*. 1972;95:101–108.

Torg JS, Naranja RJ Jr, Pavlov H, et al. The relationship of developmental narrowing of the cervical spinal canal to reversible and irreversible injury of the cervical spinal cord in football players. *J Bone Joint Surg Am*. 1996;78A:1308–1314.

Chapter 110 Spinal Cord Injury

Bradley M. Anderson, D. Greg Anderson

ICD-10-CM CODES
ES14.** *Cervical spinal cord injury*
S24.** *Thoracic spinal cord injury*
S34.** *Lumbar spinal cord injury*

Key Concepts

- Approximately 11,000 spinal cord injuries occur each year in North America, the majority in young, active individuals as a result of trauma.
  - Motor vehicle accidents are the most common cause, followed by diving, sporting events, falls, and acts of violence.
- No effective means of treatment exists to repair the neural injury and restore spinal cord function below the level of injury.
- After an acute traumatic spinal cord injury, two mechanisms of damage occur:
  - Primary injury: acute contusion of the cord, which occurs at the time of injury as a result of a spinal column fracture, dislocation, or acute cord compression
  - Secondary injury: begins over the hours and days after the acute injury and involves an inflammatory cascade and secondary pathologic changes that worsen the primary insult to the cord
  - Using a pharmacologic means of blocking a secondary injury (e.g., high-dose steroid protocol) is an area of research and debate.
- Stabilization of the injury and medical support are accepted means of treating a patient with an acute, traumatic spinal cord injury, and are best performed in a center with experience treating spinal cord injured patients.

History

- Mechanism of injury, including thorough history regarding traumatic event
- Associated injuries
  - Bowel injury in seatbelt mechanism
  - Facial injuries in cervical hyperextension mechanism
- Search for noncontiguous fractures (image the entire spinal axis).

Physical Examination

- Observation
  - Airway, breathing, and circulation
  - Paradoxical diaphragmatic breathing pattern
  - Neurogenic shock; results from loss of sympathetic tone with hemodynamic instability, including bradycardia and hypotension
- Palpation
  - Log roll patient to examine spine from occiput to sacrum during secondary examination
  - Tenderness, swelling, deformity
  - Reproducible, focal spinous process tenderness is a sensitive indication of spinal column injury.
  - Palpable gaps between spinous processes indicative of distraction injury
- Special tests
  - Complete neurologic examination
  - Sacral sparing (perianal sensation intact) represents an incomplete spinal cord lesion with a better prognosis.
  - Bulbocavernosus reflex: anal contraction on squeezing the glans penis or pulling on the Foley urinary catheter; return of the bulbocavernosus reflex (or a window of 48 hours) signals the end of spinal shock
  - American Spinal Injury Association Impairment Scale (Table 110.1): standard for assessing and classifying spinal cord injury; the level of neurologic function is defined as the most caudal level with at least grade III motor function

Imaging

- Radiographs: anteroposterior, lateral, and odontoid views of the cervical spine
  - Occiput to T1: if unable to visualize C7-T1, other techniques are employed (e.g., swimmer's view, oblique view, computed tomography)
  - Eighty-five percent of all traumatic injuries are visualized on the lateral radiograph.
  - Soft-tissue swelling in the retropharyngeal space (>7 mm at C2) may suggest spinal column injury.
  - If a cervical spinal fracture is found, the entire spine needs to be imaged because there is a 10% chance of noncontiguous spinal injuries.
- Computed tomography
  - Most sensitive imaging modality in diagnosing fractures of the cervical spine
- Magnetic resonance imaging
  - Not as sensitive in identifying cervical spine fractures as radiographs and computed tomography
  - Gold standard in soft-tissue assessment, including the spinal cord
  - Required before open or closed reduction if patient is not awake and alert

TABLE 110.1 American Spinal Injury Association Impairment Scale

A	Complete	No motor or sensory function preserved in the sacral segments S4-S5
B	Incomplete	Sensory, but no motor function preserved below the neurologic level; includes the sacral segments S4-S5
C	Incomplete	Motor function preserved below the neurologic level; more than half of the key muscles below the neurologic level have a muscle grade <3
D	Incomplete	Motor function preserved below the neurologic level; at least half of the key muscles below the neurologic level have a muscle grade ≥3
E	Normal	Sensory and motor functions are normal

Differential Diagnosis

- Complete spinal cord injury: no motor or sensory function below level of injury
- Incomplete spinal cord injury: Below the level of injury, the spinal cord acts as an upper motor neuron injury, whereas at the level of injury, the cord produces lower motor neuron findings.
  - Brown-Séquard syndrome (best prognosis): penetrating trauma or unilateral facet dislocation and/or fracture; results in ipsilateral muscle paralysis and loss of proprioception/vibratory sense with contralateral loss of pain and temperature sensation below the level of injury
  - Central cord syndrome (second best prognosis): hyperextension injury, typically in older individuals with spinal stenosis; upper extremities (especially hands) weaker than the lower extremities
  - Anterior cord syndrome (poorest prognosis): flexion-compression injury; results in minimal distal motor function; injury to the spinothalamic tracts leads to loss of sensitivity to pain and temperature
  - Posterior cord syndrome (very rare): isolated injury to the dorsal columns; results in loss of proprioception, vibration sense, and deep pressure

Treatment

- At diagnosis
  - The goal for cervical fractures and dislocations is to achieve an anatomic, pain-free, and mobile spine without neurologic deficit. Trauma protocols should be instituted at the initial presentation, including spine immobilization.
  - Neurogenic shock requires aggressive hemodynamic monitoring to maintain appropriate cardiac output and a mean blood pressure of 85 to 90 mm Hg.
    - The goal is to maintain cord perfusion to minimize secondary damage.
    - Best treated with vasopressors and atropine

- Medical therapies are directed at limiting the effect of secondary injuries that follow the initial insult to the spinal cord.
  - Methylprednisolone: 30 mg/kg intravenous (IV) bolus and 5.4 mg/kg/h for 23 hours for patients with spinal cord injury less than 8 hours to treatment
- Later
  - There is little question about the benefits of spinal cord decompression.
  - The surgical approach is typically dictated by the injury pattern.

When to Refer

- All patients with spinal cord injuries require referral to a center experienced in spinal cord injuries.

Prognosis

- Greater functional recovery occurs when there is more initial sparing of motor and sensory function distal to the level of injury. The root return phenomenon has been observed after decompression of the spinal cord in patients with complete cervical neurologic injuries.

Considerations in Special Populations

- In elderly patients with preexisting stenosis, hyperextension injuries may result in central cord syndrome.

Suggested Readings

Aebi M, Mohler J, Zach GA, et al. Indications, surgical technique, and results of 100 surgically treated fractures and fracture-dislocations of the cervical spine. *Clin Orthop Relat Res*. 1986;203:244–257.

Bracken MB. Treatment of acute spinal cord injury with methylprednisolone: results of a multicenter, randomized clinical trial. *J Neurotrauma*. 1991;8:S47–S50.

Bracken MB, Shepard MJ, Collins WF, et al. A randomized, controlled trial of methylprednisolone or naloxone in the treatment of acute spinal cord injury. *N Engl J Med*. 1990;322:1404–1411.

Bracken MB, Shepard MJ, Holford TR, et al. Administration of methylprednisolone for 24 or 48 hours or tirilazad mesylate for 48 hours in the treatment of acute spinal cord injury. Results of the third national acute spinal cord injury randomized controlled trial. *JAMA*. 1997;277:1597–1604.

Bracken MB, Shepard MJ, Holford TR, et al. Methylprednisolone or tirilazad mesylate administration after acute spinal cord injury: 1 year follow up. Results of the third national acute spinal cord injury randomized controlled trial. *J Neurosurg*. 1998;89:699–706.

Fehlings MG, Martin AR, Tetreault LA, et al. A clinical practice guideline for the management of patients with acute spinal cord injury: recommendations on the role of baseline magnetic resonance imaging in clinical decision making and outcome prediction. *Global Spine J*. 2017;3(suppl):221S–230S.

Fehlings MG, Tator CH. An evidence-based review of decompressive surgery in acute spinal cord injury: rationale, indications, and timing based on experimental and clinical studies. *J Neurosurg*. 1999;91:1–11.

Fehlings MG, Tetreault LA, Aarabi B, et al. A clinical practice guideline for the management of patients with acute spinal cord injury: recommendations on the type and timing of anticoagulant thromboprophylaxis. *Global Spine J*. 2017;3(suppl):212S–220S.

Fehlings MG, Tetreault LA, Wilson JR, et al. A clinical practice guideline for the management of patients with acute spinal cord injury and central cord syndrome: recommendations on the timing (≤24 hours versus >24 hours) of decompressive surgery. *Global Spine J.* 2017;3(suppl): 195S–202S.

Hurlbert RJ. Strategies of medical intervention in the management of acute spinal cord injury. *Spine.* 2006;31:S16–S21.

Levi L, Wolf A, Rigamonti D. Anterior decompression in cervical spine trauma: does the timing of surgery affect the outcome? *Neurosurgery.* 1991;29:216–222.

Tsutsumi S, Ueta T, Shiba K, et al. Effects of the second national acute spinal cord injury study of high-dose methylprednisolone therapy on acute cervical spinal cord injury—results in spinal injuries center. *Spine.* 2006;31(26):2992–2996.

Chapter 111 Burners/Stingers (Brachial Plexopathy)

Sanjitpal S. Gill, Andrew S. Donnan III

ICD-10-CM CODE
G54.2 *Injury to brachial plexus, cervical roots*

Key Concepts

- Burners and stingers are injuries to the brachial plexus resulting from traction, compression, or direct trauma.
- The brachial plexus is composed of cervical nerve roots C5 through T1 (Fig. 111.1A).
- C5-C6 most commonly affected (see also Fig. 111.1B)
  - Deltoid, biceps, rotator cuff (supraspinatus, infraspinatus) muscles
- Reversible, unilateral upper extremity pain, radiculopathy, and weakness
- One of the most common cervical spine injuries in athletes.
- Most underreported by the athlete.
- Most common in collision and contact sports; as many as 65% of college football players report stingers during their 4-year career
- 87% of athletes had previous burners or stingers.
- Symptoms typically resolve within minutes of the injury.
- Limited evidence-based guidelines make return to activity decisions difficult, especially after recurrent episodes.

History

- Posttraumatic syndrome
  - Traction: sudden shoulder depression with lateral head deviation, more common in the younger athlete
  - Compression: extension, ipsilateral compression, rotation to affected side
- Root injury in narrowed foramen; more common in mature athletes, may be related to congenital spinal stenosis.
  - Direct trauma: direct blow or compression from shoulder pad and superior medial scapula (Erb point); poorly fitted equipment can play a role.
- Unilateral burning or tingling sensation in the entire arm
- Transient inability to actively use the arm (dead arm syndrome)
- Neurologic symptoms rarely follow a strict dermatomal pattern.
- If symptoms are bilateral, the concern is for cervical spine injury or transient quadriparesis.

Physical Examination

- Observation
  - Splinting of the affected arm (Fig. 111.2)
  - Shoulder depression

- Palpation
  - Rule out tenderness over the spinous processes and clavicle
  - May have positive Tinel sign at Erb point
- Range of motion
  Always perform active motion first.
- Special tests
  - Spurling test: cervical extension, lateral flexion to the side of the injury, and gentle axial compression reproduce radicular symptoms (Fig. 111.3).
- Testing for compression through stenotic foramen
  - Thorough neurologic examination

Imaging

- Radiographs
  - Anteroposterior view: coronal alignment
  - Lateral view: may have loss of cervical lordosis from spasm
  - Oblique views: to evaluate cervical foramina
  - Flexion/extension views: instability, less useful in acute setting
  - Torg ratio: ratio of sagittal spinal canal width to sagittal vertebral body width; measures degree of congenital spinal stenosis
  - A ratio of less than 0.8 suggests an increased risk of recurrence
- Magnetic resonance imaging
  - To evaluate suspected spinal cord or nerve root injury, herniated cervical disc, foraminal stenosis, canal stenosis, spinal cord edema

Additional Tests

- Electromyography
- Not useful in the acute setting
  - Most useful 2 to 4 weeks after injury if persistent symptoms
  - After clinical return of normal strength, as many as 80% of patients show electromyographic abnormalities that may persist for more than 5 years.

Differential Diagnosis

- Cervical spine injury
- Cervical cord neurapraxia (transient quadriparesis)
- Clavicle fracture
- Herniated cervical disc
- Rotator cuff injury
- Stress fracture of first rib

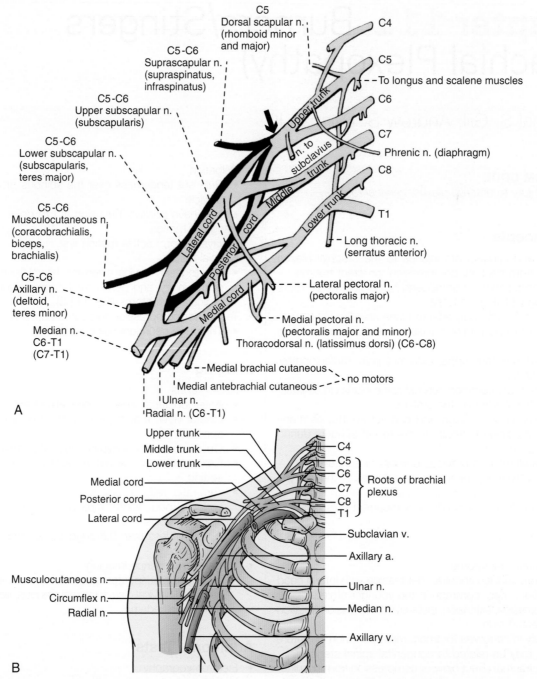

Fig 111.1 (A) Stingers and burners commonly affect the upper trunk of the brachial plexus creating weakness of the deltoid, biceps, and rotator cuff muscles. **(B)** The relationship of the brachial plexus to the surrounding anatomic structures including the chest wall. (A, modified from DeLee JC, Drez D Jr, Miller MD, (eds). *DeLee & Drez's Orthopaedic Sports Medicine.* Vol. 1, 2nd ed. Philadelphia: WB Saunders, 2003:797; B, modified from Warner CJ, Roddy SP, Darling RC. Upper extremity arterial disease. In Sidawy AN, Perler BA (eds). *Rutherford's Vascular Surgery and Endovascular Therapy*, 9th ed. Philadelphia, Elsevier, 2019.)

- Thoracic outlet syndrome
- Parsonage-Turner syndrome

Treatment

- At diagnosis
  - If applicable, remove from competition until complete resolution of symptoms and cervical spine injury excluded.

- Treatment is largely supportive; a sling may help rest the affected extremity until symptoms improve.
- Later
  - Rehabilitation program to restore strength and motion of cervical spine and upper extremity
  - Athletes should not be allowed to return to competition without a full, pain-free cervical range of motion, negative Spurling test, negative brachial plexus stretch test, and

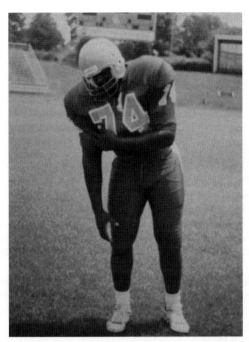

Fig 111.2 Common clinical presentation of an athlete with a stinger that has to support the weight of the arm while leaving the field due to pain or muscle weakness. (From Pritchard JC. Football and other contact sports injuries: diagnosis and treatment. In: Buschbacher RM, Braddom RL, eds.: *Sports Medicine and Rehabilitation: A Sport Specific Approach.* Philadelphia: Hanley and Belfus; 1994:172.)

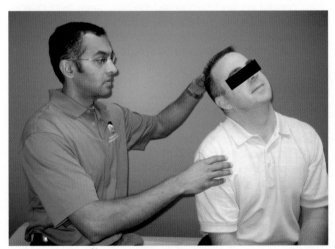

Fig 111.3 Spurling test is used to recreate foraminal stenosis by ipsilateral extension and rotation.

negative axial compression test. This is paramount in preventing more serious spinal cord injury.

- The use of neck rolls, a neck-shoulder-cervical orthosis (cowboy collar), and/or pads at the base of the neck in football players can help minimize recurrence.

When to Refer

- If cervical spine injury is suspected (axial neck pain), immobilization and full radiographic evaluation are warranted.
- Specialist referral if symptoms last longer than 1 week and there are positive findings suggestive of nerve root injury, bilateral symptoms, or recurrent symptoms.

Prognosis

- It varies depending on severity.
  - Grade 1: neurapraxia. All nerve structures remain intact (most common). Complete resolution of symptoms typically occurs in minutes, but may take as long as 6 weeks.
  - Grade 2: axonotmesis. There are axonal disruption and Wallerian degeneration distal to the injury site. Recovery is complete, but it may take months. An intact epineurium allows axonal regrowth at a rate of approximately 1 mm/day.
  - Grade 3: neurotmesis. Complete disruption of axons, endoneurium, perineurium, and epineurium. The prognosis varies, with complete loss common.

Troubleshooting

- Red flags include bilateral symptoms, lower extremity involvement, painful range of motion, axial tenderness, persistent burning, neurologic deficit, and altered consciousness.
- Immobilize and perform a complete clinical/radiographic evaluation.

Patient Instructions

- Patients should continue sling use until pain resolves. Monitor for elbow stiffness.
- Instruct athletes to report all instances of recurrence.
- Patients may resume activity when full, pain-free range of motion and the return of full upper extremity strength.

Suggested Readings

Chao S, Pacella MJ, Torg JS. The pathomechanics, pathophysiology and prevention of cervical spinal cord and brachial plexus injuries in athletics. *Sports Med.* 2010;40(1):59–75.

Concannon LG, Harrast MA, Herring SA. Radiating upper limb pain in the contact sports athlete: an update on transient quadriparesis and stingers. *Am Coll Sports Med.* 2012;11(1):28–34.

Feinberg JH. Burners and stingers. *Phys Med Rehabil Clin N Am.* 2000;11: 771–784.

Hoppenfeld S. Physical examination of the cervical spine. In: Hoppenfeld S, eds. *Physical Examination of the Spine and Extremities.* Norwalk, CT: Appleton-Century-Crofts; 1976:105–132.

Kasow DB, Curl WW. "Stingers" in adolescent athletes. *Instr Course Lect.* 2006;55:711–716.

Kelley JD. Brachial plexus injuries: evaluating and treating "burners.". *J Musculoskel Med.* 1997;14:70–80.

Olson DE, McBroom SA, Nelson BD, et al. Unilateral cervical nerve injuries: brachial plexopathies. *Curr Sports Med Rep.* 2007;6:43–49.

Safran MR. Nerve injury about the shoulder. Part 2: long thoracic nerve, spinal accessory nerve, burners/stingers, thoracic outlet syndrome. *Am J Sports Med.* 2004;32:1063–1076.

Weinberg J, Rokito S, Silber JS. Etiology, treatment, and prevention of athletic "stingers". *Clin Sports Med.* 2003;22:493–500.

Chapter 112 Thoracolumbar Strain

Eric Magrum, Michael McMurray

ICD-10-CM CODES
S39.012A *Strain of muscle, fascia, and tendon of lower back, initial encounter*
M54.5 *Low back pain*

Key Concepts

- Low back pain (LBP) affects more than 90% of the adult population at some point in their lifetime.
- Screening and risk stratification for patients with poor coping mechanisms and high fear avoidance behavior have a higher prevalence of progression of disability; this should be utilized to guide treatment decision making (Fig. 112.1B).
- Nonspecific LBP is a heterogeneous condition and includes a number of different clinical entities.
- Previous research suggested a wait-and-see approach for acute LBP.
- A treatment-based classification system has been proposed for acute LBP, based on response to specific treatment interventions (see Fig. 112.1A).
- Manipulation may be successful in alleviating pain in patients with recent onset of LBP and no lower extremity symptoms.
- Patients with impaired motor control and movement abnormalities benefit from core stabilization exercises.

History

- Localized LBP
- Utilization of prognostic tools (i.e., Start Back Screening Tool) to help clinicians identify modifiable risk factors (biomedical, psychological, and social) for back pain disability
- Stratification of low, medium, high risk with matched treatment
- A stratified management approach in which prognostic screening and treatment targeting were combined resulted in improved primary care efficiency, leading to higher health gains for patients with back pain than did existing nonstratified best care (see Fig. 112.1B).
- Those factors include: high pain intensity, symptoms below the knee, psychological distress or depression, fear of movement or reinjury, passive coping strategies.
- Red flags requiring special attention should be identified (Table 112.1).

Physical Examination

- Observation
  - Postural assessment: lateral shift may be present with disc pathology; flexed spine may be present with stenosis; hyperlordosis may be present with hypermobility.
- Palpation
  - Tenderness of paraspinal musculature, sacroiliac joints, and pubic symphysis
- Range of motion
  - Often decreased secondary to pain
  - Evaluate hip and knee range of motion.
  - Evaluate for aberrant motions (e.g., Gowers sign: using hands to walk up thighs to return from forward bending in standing).
  - Repeated motions: have patient perform active lumbar flexion and extension to assess for symptoms centralization or peripheralization (SP 94, +LR 6.7; SN 92, –LR 0.12).
- Special tests
  - Neurologic examination
  - Nerve tension tests: straight leg raise (sciatic nerve) (SN 92 –LR 0.29), prone knee bend (femoral nerve)
  - Crossed straight leg raise (straight leg raise in uninvolved leg reproduces symptoms in involved leg); useful in detecting disc herniation (SP 90 +LR 2.8)
  - Provocative tests for sacroiliac dysfunction: posterior shear/thigh thrust test (Fig. 112.2), iliac compression and gapping, Gaenslen test, and sacral thrust
  - Slump test: seated nerve tension test useful for chronic conditions and suspected central canal dysfunction, dural irritability (SN 83 –LR 0.32)
  - Quadrant test (extension-rotation): (Fig. 112.3) useful in determining facet mediated symptoms (SN 100; –LR 0.0)

Imaging

- Imaging modalities have frequent false positive and false negative results, limiting their utility in identification of active anatomic pain generators; routine ordering of imaging for LBP should be discouraged.
- The primary utility of imaging lies in interventional and/or surgical planning or in determining the presence of serious medical conditions. For these purposes, lumbar MRI represents the most useful tool in particular.
- Current recommendations are that imaging is only indicated for severe progressive neurological deficits or when red flags are suspected, and routine imaging does not result in clinical benefit and may lead to harm.

Differential Diagnosis

- Facet syndrome: pain aggravated by extension biased movements, that is, quadrant testing (see Fig. 112.3); relieved by recumbency, diagnostic block
- Spinal stenosis: pain relieved with flexion; advanced age; previous lumbar history; lower extremity (LE)/radicular symptoms

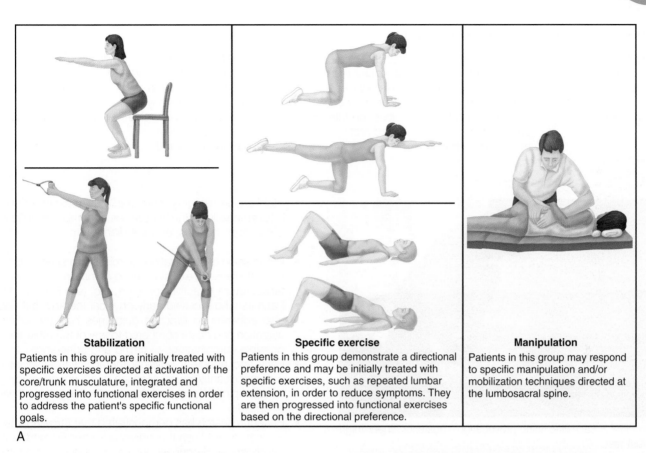

Stabilization

Patients in this group are initially treated with specific exercises directed at activation of the core/trunk musculature, integrated and progressed into functional exercises in order to address the patient's specific functional goals.

Specific exercise

Patients in this group demonstrate a directional preference and may be initially treated with specific exercises, such as repeated lumbar extension, in order to reduce symptoms. They are then progressed into functional exercises based on the directional preference.

Manipulation

Patients in this group may respond to specific manipulation and/or mobilization techniques directed at the lumbosacral spine.

A

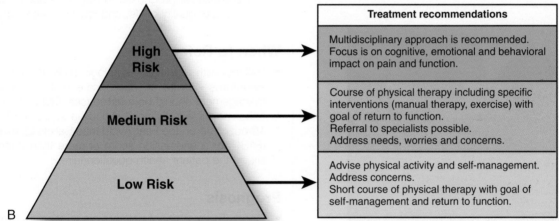

Treatment recommendations
Multidisciplinary approach is recommended. Focus is on cognitive, emotional and behavioral impact on pain and function.
Course of physical therapy including specific interventions (manual therapy, exercise) with goal of return to function. Referral to specialists possible. Address needs, worries and concerns.
Advise physical activity and self-management. Address concerns. Short course of physical therapy with goal of self-management and return to function.

High Risk

Medium Risk

Low Risk

B

Fig 112.1 (A) Treatment classifications for patients with low back pain. **(B)** Stratification for progression to chronicity of low back pain.

- Spondylolysis/listhesis: pain with or without instability with extension, radiographs
- Sacroiliac dysfunction: cluster of provocative tests

Treatment

- Symptomatic treatments should be instituted. Early referral for physical therapy may help to determine the appropriate classification and direct treatment (see Fig. 112.1A). Recent

onset and lack of pain below the knee indicate a high likelihood of a positive response to lumbosacral manipulation.
- Treatment-based classification system (Fig. 112.4)
  - Specific exercise category: initial treatment to include repeated movements that centralize symptoms (e.g., repeated extension causes leg symptoms to decrease or centralize into low back).
  - Manipulation category: initial treatment with lumbosacral manipulation or specific segmental manipulation

TABLE 112.1 Red Flags for Low Back Pain

Fractures	Cauda Equina Syndrome	Cancer	Ankylosing Spondylitis	Spinal Infection
Fracture due to major trauma; or minor trauma in elderly	Saddle numbness; bladder dysfunction of recent onset; severe or rapidly progressive neurologic deficit	Age older than 50 yr; history of cancer; unexplained weight loss; no relief with bed rest	Male; morning stiffness; age younger than 35 yr at onset; no relief with lying down; relief with exercise or movement; chest expansion restricted	Recent fever; recent bacterial infection; IV drug abuse; immunosuppression

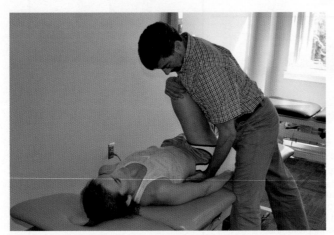

Fig 112.2 Sacroiliac joint provocation—posterior shear/thigh thrust test.

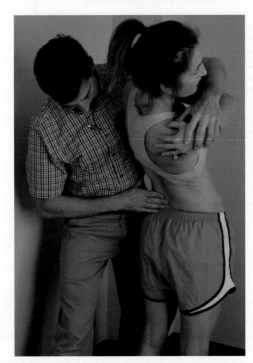

Fig 112.3 Combined movement/quadrant test.

- Stabilization category: core stabilization exercises with initial emphasis on the transversus abdominis, multifidus, pelvic floor muscles, and the diaphragm
- Later
  - Progression of stabilization exercises into specific functional therapeutic exercise based on patient goals, work tasks, return to activity or sport, etc. (see Fig. 112.1A)
  - Patients who received early physical therapy that was also adherent to practice guidelines had the lowest utilization and costs compared to any of the other three possible combinations of timing and adherence.
  - Early and adherent physical therapy was associated with significantly lower utilization of advanced imaging, lumbar spinal injections, lumbar spine surgery, and use of opioids.
  - Recent research has demonstrated that targeted interventions to address the individual's specific modifiable psychosocial prognostic indicators reduces disability, increases quality of life, and lowers health care costs.

When to Refer

- Patients with red flags, neurologic findings, or persistent symptoms despite an appropriate trial of conservative management should be referred (see Table 112.1).
- Other possible indications include a score of more than 19 out of 24 on the Fear Avoidance Beliefs Questionnaire (FABQ) or a depression score of more than three out of six on the patient health questionnaire.

Prognosis

- Good: The majority of patients are successfully managed with conservative treatments.
- A history of depression is prognostic for a slow recovery from back pain.

Troubleshooting

- Patients with pain lasting longer than 4 to 6 weeks need to be referred to a specialist and the biopsychosocial aspects of the patient's case considered.
- One percent to 2% of LBP is due to radiculopathy secondary to disc herniation.

Patient Instructions

- Patients should be encouraged to stay active and avoid bed rest.

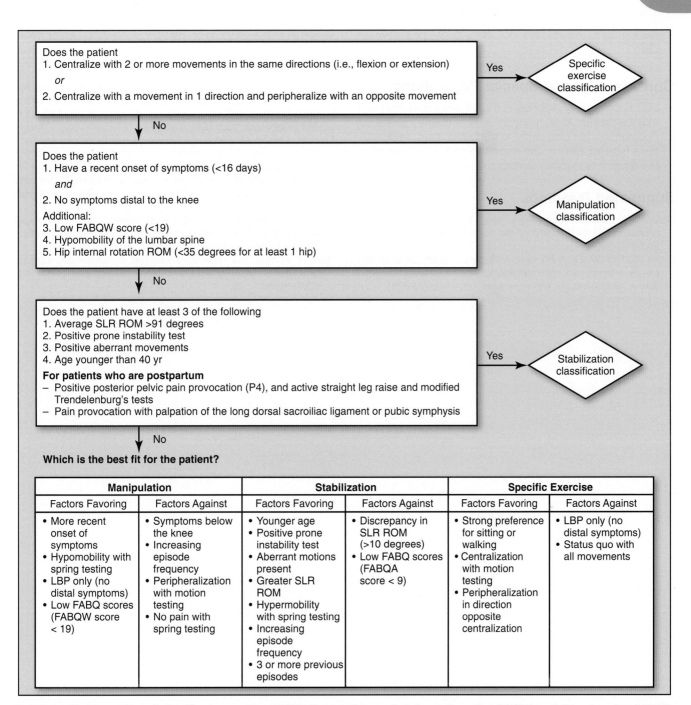

Does the patient
1. Centralize with 2 or more movements in the same directions (i.e., flexion or extension)
   or
2. Centralize with a movement in 1 direction and peripheralize with an opposite movement

→ Yes → Specific exercise classification

↓ No

Does the patient
1. Have a recent onset of symptoms (<16 days)
   and
2. No symptoms distal to the knee
Additional:
3. Low FABQW score (<19)
4. Hypomobility of the lumbar spine
5. Hip internal rotation ROM (<35 degrees for at least 1 hip)

→ Yes → Manipulation classification

↓ No

Does the patient have at least 3 of the following
1. Average SLR ROM >91 degrees
2. Positive prone instability test
3. Positive aberrant movements
4. Age younger than 40 yr
For patients who are postpartum
– Positive posterior pelvic pain provocation (P4), and active straight leg raise and modified Trendelenburg's tests
– Pain provocation with palpation of the long dorsal sacroiliac ligament or pubic symphysis

→ Yes → Stabilization classification

↓ No

Which is the best fit for the patient?

Manipulation		Stabilization		Specific Exercise	
Factors Favoring	Factors Against	Factors Favoring	Factors Against	Factors Favoring	Factors Against
• More recent onset of symptoms • Hypomobility with spring testing • LBP only (no distal symptoms) • Low FABQ scores (FABQW score < 19)	• Symptoms below the knee • Increasing episode frequency • Peripheralization with motion testing • No pain with spring testing	• Younger age • Positive prone instability test • Aberrant motions present • Greater SLR ROM • Hypermobility with spring testing • Increasing episode frequency • 3 or more previous episodes	• Discrepancy in SLR ROM (>10 degrees) • Low FABQ scores (FABQA score < 9)	• Strong preference for sitting or walking • Centralization with motion testing • Peripheralization in direction opposite centralization	• LBP only (no distal symptoms) • Status quo with all movements

Fig 112.4 Treatment-based classification system. *FABQ,* Fear-avoidance belief questionnaire; *FABQA,* activity subscale of FABQ; *FABQW,* work subscale of FABQ; *LBP,* low back pain; *ROM,* range of motion; *SLR,* straight leg raise. (Modified from Fritz JM, Cleland JA, Childs JD. Subgrouping patients with low back pain: evolution of a classification approach to physical therapy. *J Orthop Sports Phys Ther.* 2007;37:290–302.)

- Radiographic results are not necessarily predictive of LBP.

Considerations in Special Populations

- LBP is commonly reported in the athletic population and may be present in as many as 20% of sports injuries.
- Postpartum females with lumbopelvic pain frequently have hypermobility at the sacroiliac joint and respond to stabilization and motor control exercises.

Suggested Readings

Benedetti F, Lanotte M, Lopiano L, et al. When words are painful: unraveling the mechanisms of the nocebo effect. *Neuroscience*. 2007;147:260–271.

Childs JD, Fritz JM, Flynn TW, et al. A clinical prediction rule to identify patients with low back pain most likely to benefit from spinal manipulation: A validation study. *Ann Intern Med*. 2004;141:920–928.

Cleland JA, Fritz JM, Brennan GP. Predictive validity of initial fear avoidance beliefs in patients with low back pain receiving physical therapy: is the FABQ a useful screening tool for identifying patients at risk for a poor recovery? *Eur Spine J*. 2008;17:70–79.

Fritz JM, Childs JD, Flynn TW. Pragmatic application of a clinical prediction rule in primary care to identify patients with low back pain with a good prognosis following a brief spinal manipulation intervention. *BMC Fam Pract*. 2005;6:29.

Fritz JM, Cleland JA, Childs JD. Subgrouping patients with low back pain: evolution of a classification approach to physical therapy. *J Orthop Sports Phys Ther*. 2007;37:290–302.

Laslett M, Aprill CN, McDonald B, et al. Diagnosis of sacroiliac joint pain: validity of individual provocation tests and composites of tests. *Man Ther*. 2005;10:207–218.

Mens JM, Vleeming A, Snijders CJ, et al. Validity of the active straight leg raise test for measuring disease severity in patients with posterior pelvic pain after pregnancy. *Spine*. 2002;27:196–200.

Tsao H, Hodges PW. Immediate changes in feedforward postural adjustments following voluntary motor training. *Exp Brain Res*. 2007;181:537–546.

Chapter 113 Thoracolumbar Disc Disease

Tinnakorn Pluemvitayaporn, Frank M. Phillips, R. Todd Allen

ICD-10-CM CODES

M51.34	*Degeneration of thoracic disc(s)*
M51.36	*Degeneration of lumbar disc(s)*
M48.04	*Foraminal encroachment (compression) of nerve root, thoracic*
M99.53	*Foraminal encroachment (compression) of nerve root, lumbar*
M54.17	*Thoracic neuritis or radiculitis*
M51.17	*Lumbosacral neuritis or radiculitis*
M51.24	*Thoracic disc disorder without myelopathy*
M51.04	*Thoracic disc disorder with myelopathy*
M51.26	*Lumbar disc disorder without myelopathy*
M51.06	*Lumbar disc disorder with myelopathy*

Key Concepts
Intervertebral Disc

- Intervertebral disc, the layers of fibrocartilage and fibers, plays an important role in the functional spinal unit (one intervertebral disc and the adjacent vertebral bodies).
- This structure consists of an outer annulus fibrosus (AF) and an inner nucleus pulposus (NP) (Fig. 113.1), and is structurally made mostly of water, collagen, and proteoglycans (PGs).
- Function of the intervertebral disc is to cushion the vertebrae, provide spinal motion, and promote spinal stability.

Degenerative Disc Disease and Pathogenesis

- Disc degeneration is a natural process, and occurs with aging.
- Sequence of disc degenerative changes: small circumferential tear in AF → increase in size and form radial fissure → expand into NP → loss of PGs and water content → decrease disc height/disc collapse.
- In the 1970s, Kirkaldy-Willis first described the three phases of the "degenerative cascade," comprised of disc dysfunction, instability, and restabilization.
- Disc degeneration begins with decreased NP water and PG content, impairing its load-bearing ability. As degeneration progresses, type II collagen replaces type I and tears/fissures develop in the AF. Vertebral endplates calcify, impairing nutrient diffusion to the intervertebral disc (see Fig. 113.1).
- With degeneration, protrusions, herniation, or extrusion may occur; facet joints may become arthritic and hypertrophy; vertebral body osteophytes develop, and the ligamentum flavum thickens. The result is often spinal canal narrowing (stenosis), which can result in neural compression (central, lateral recess, or foraminal).

Prevalence and Incidence

- Thoracic disc herniation: most asymptomatic; usually occur third to sixth decades
  - Of all symptomatic herniations, less than 4% occur in the thoracic spine.
  - Thoracic spinal kyphosis increases susceptibility to injury from herniation.
- Lumbar herniated NP (HNP); most common at L4-L5, then L5-S1
  - Mean age at onset: less than 35 years, *unusual* at less than 20 or greater than 60 years
  - Rare in children; slippage of entire disc and endplate (apophyses) may mimic HNP
- Conus medullaris syndrome versus cauda equina syndrome (Table 113.1).

History
Clinical Feature

- In general, the most common symptom of degenerative disc disease (DDD) is deep aching low back or thoracic back pain.
- Lumbar back pain associated with DDD is often mechanical (increased with spinal loading) and exacerbated by lumbar flexion and sitting (increases intradiscal pressure).
- *"Band-like" radicular pain* along the course of the intercostal nerve is the most common symptom for thoracic radiculopathy.
- Red flag "warning" signs for patients with atypical low back pain include:
  - Age (>50 or <20); history of malignancy
  - History of recent infection or trauma; immune suppression
  - Unexplained weight loss; fever/chills; rest/night pain
  - Constant aching/throbbing pain (query infection); pain duration over 1 month
  - Cauda equina syndrome (surgical emergency)
- Thoracic DDD and herniated disc
  - Highly variable presentation; onset typically insidious; often axial thoracic pain.
  - Valsalva maneuver typically worsens pain.
  - Nerve root compression may result in radicular pain, or dermatomal sensory changes (paresthesias, dysesthesias), radiating around the chest wall in a dermatomal pattern.
  - Spinal cord compression may lead to thoracic myelopathy with lower extremity hyperreflexia, spasticity/clonus, unsteady gait, numbness, variable weakness, and/or more severe findings of bowel/bladder dysfunction.

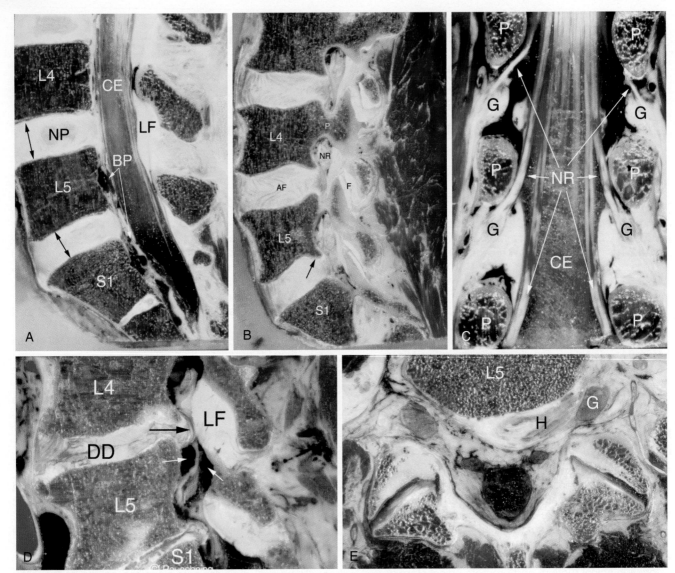

Fig 113.1 Normal and degenerative lumbar spine anatomy. Midsagittal **(A)**, parasagittal **(B)**, and coronal **(C)** views of a normal lumbar spine. Note maintained disc heights, nerve roots (NR) exiting below the pedicles and out the neural foramen. The coronal section shows the cauda equina *(CE)* and the location of nerve root ganglia (G) in relation to the pedicle. **(D)** Sagittal view of a degenerative lumbar segment. Note the narrowed degenerative disc *(DD)*, posterior disc bulge, ligamentum flavum *(LF)* hypertrophy, and narrowed intervertebral foramen for the exiting nerve root. **(E)** Axial view of a herniated disc. *AF,* Annulus fibrosus; *BP,* Batson plexus; *F,* facet joint; *G,* nerve root ganglia; *NP,* nucleus pulposus; *P,* pedicle. (From Gallego J, Schnuerer AP, Manuel C. *Basic Anatomy and Pathology of the Spine*. Memphis, TN: Medtronic Sofamor Danek, USA, Inc.; 2001; photographs by Wolfgang Rauschning, MD, PhD.)

- Lumbar DDD and herniated disc
  - Classically presents with sciatica or radiating leg pain (with or without paresthesia, dysesthesia) in a dermatomal distribution.
    - Usually worse with coughing or sneezing (increased intraspinal pressure), with sitting or lumbar flexion (nerve root stretch), and with raising a straight leg with toes upward
  - May lead to dermatomal sensory, motor, or reflex loss.
  - Posterolateral herniations impinge on the traversing nerve root (e.g., L5 root with L4-L5 posterolateral herniation), while far lateral or foraminal herniation impinges on exiting nerve root (e.g., L4 root with L4-L5 foraminal herniation).

- Central herniations: axial pain with or without unilateral (or even bilateral) radiculopathy; if large enough, watch for cauda equina syndrome.

Physical Examination

- Inspection
  - Sagittal plane alignment.
    - Normal thoracic kyphosis: 20 to 40 degrees
    - Normal lumbar lordosis: 40 to 60 degrees
  - Coronal plane alignment
    - Presence or absence of shoulder tilt, hemipelvis elevation, leg length discrepancy, etc.
  - Skin abnormality/lesion(s)

TABLE 113.1 Distinguishing Features of Conus Medullaris and Cauda Equina Syndromes

	Conus Medullaris Syndrome	Cauda Equina Syndrome
Affected levels	Sacral cord (conus) and lumbar nerve roots	Lumbosacral nerve roots
Clinical presentation	Usually bilateral	Unilateral or bilateral (depends on involved nerve roots)
	Combination of UMN and LMN symptoms	LMN symptoms
	More low back pain	More radicular pain
Sensory	Symmetrical	Asymmetrical
	More localized in perianal area	More localized in saddle area
	Sensory dissociation: yes	Sensory dissociation: no
Motor	Symmetrical	Usually asymmetrical
Reflex	Hyperreflexia	Hyporeflexia or areflexia

LMN, Lower motor neuron; *UMN*, upper motor neuron.

TABLE 113.2 Neurological Examination in Thoracic and Lumbar Spine

	Sensory/Dermatome	Motor/Myotome (Autonomous Zone)
T1	Ulnar antecubital fossa	Intrinsic muscles (interossei)
T4	Nipple	—
T6	Xyphoid	—
T10	Umbilicus	—
L2	Mid-anterior thigh	Hip flexors (iliopsoas)
L3	Medial femoral condyle	Knee flexors (quadriceps)
L4	Medial malleolus	Ankle dorsiflexors (tibialis anterior)
L5	Second dorsal web space of foot	Big toe extensors (extensor hallucis longus)
S1	Lateral heel	Ankle plantar flexors (gastrocnemius, soleus)

TABLE 113.3 Common Provocative Tests for Radiculopathy

Test	Outcome
SLR, sitting and supine	Reproduction/aggravation of radicular pain in exact dermatomal pattern of involved root with elevation of involved leg (sciatic nerve involvement should produce pain distal to knee)
Contralateral SLR	SLR of nonpainful limb causes tension of involved root but from opposite side, causing radiculopathy; may suggest sequestered or extruded large disc fragment
Bowstring sign	Pressure over popliteal fossa aggravates SLR radicular pain
Lasègue's sign	Ankle dorsiflexion aggravates SLR radiculopathy
Femoral nerve stretch test	While patient is prone, examiner extends hip/leg (with or without flexed knee) to stretch femoral nerve roots L2-L4; painful if irritated

SLR, Straight leg raise.

- Palpation
  - Paravertebral muscle spasm/tenderness, rotational changes
  - Spinous process tenderness/rotation or step off
  - Rib cages tenderness/mass
  - Sciatic notch tenderness (in radiculopathy)
  - Sacroiliac joint tenderness (e.g., inflammatory arthritis, infection, ankylosing spondylitis); can be associated with positive flexion-abduction-external rotation (FABER) test
- Gait disturbance: UMN lesion → spastic gait, broad-based gait, stomping gait
  - LMN lesion → steppage gait, waddling gait, antalgic gait
- Range of motion
  - Low back pain in extension suggests posterior element pathology (facet arthritis); low back pain with flexion (loads intervertebral disc) suggests discogenic pain; leg pain with lumbar flexion (increased nerve tension) suggests radiculopathy.
  - With a posterolateral HNP, ipsilateral lateral bending may exaggerate the radiculopathy as the root is stretched over the herniated disc.
  - In axillary herniated discs, lateral bending away from symptomatic side will stretch the root.
  - Neurological examination.
    - Sensory/motor (Table 113.2)
    - Deep tendon reflex: pathognomonic levels
      - C5-C6 → biceps reflex, brachioradialis reflex
      - C6-C7 → triceps reflex (mainly C7)
      - L3-L4 → knee jerk reflex (mainly L4)
      - S1 → ankle jerk reflex
  - Special tests (Table 113.3)
  - Complete motor/sensory/reflex examination (Fig. 113.2)
  - Waddell's nonorganic tests: assess for malingering or secondary gain
    - Nonanatomic superficial tenderness; stimulation tests (axial loading and rotation); flip test (straight leg raise positive while supine, but negative while sitting); nonanatomic weakness and sensory findings; overreaction

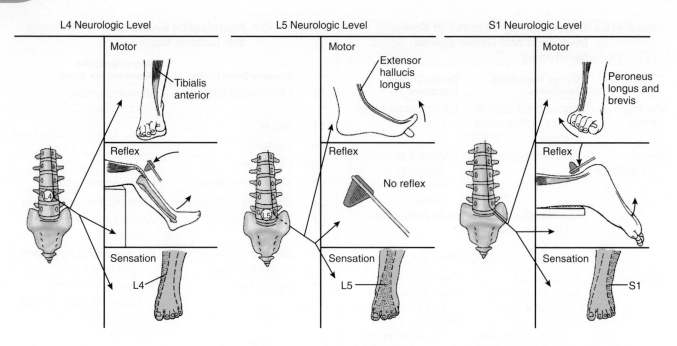

Fig 113.2 Neurologic evaluation of the lower extremity, L4-S1 levels. (Modified from Klein JD, Garfin SR. History and physical examination. In: Weinstein JN, Rydevik B, Sonntag VKG, eds. *Essentials of the Spine.* New York: Raven Press; 1995:71–95.)

Imaging

- 80% of individuals older than 55 years of age have radiographic degenerative changes; most are asymptomatic, making correlation with the history/examination most important.
- Radiographs: anteroposterior, lateral, and oblique views.
  - Degenerative findings: disc space narrowing, endplate sclerosis, osteophytes, facet arthrosis/hypertrophy.
  - Deformity/instability: coronal (anteroposterior) and sagittal (lateral) plane spinal alignment.
  - Assess for scoliosis, kyphosis, pelvic obliquity, and spondylolysis/spondylolisthesis.
  - May detect tumors (pedicle destruction, e.g., winking owl sign) or fractures (trauma).
- Magnetic resonance imaging (MRI) (Fig. 113.3)
  - Imaging study of choice, but high incidence of abnormalities in asymptomatic patients.
  - Gadolinium increases accuracy of complex pathology (tumor, infection).
  - According to a recent systematic review, the most reliable method to classify and grade herniated discs based on MRI is the Combined Task Force (CTF) classification, which defined lumbar discs as normal, focal protrusion, broad-based protrusion, or extrusion. More recently, they have excluded "disc bulges," which is a source of confusion and disagreement among many practitioners.
- Computed tomography myelography (CT myelogram).
  - More than 80% sensitivity for a herniated disc or stenosis but invasive (with myelography); radiation dose relatively high.
  - Useful if MRI contraindicated or in patients with complex problems.

Additional Tests

- Discography (controversial): reproduces concordant pain with intradiscal injection; may be useful in surgical workup of axial back pain (may promote degeneration long term).
- Electromyography (EMG) may help to rule out nonspinal etiologies of neural dysfunction.

Differential Diagnosis

- Trauma, neoplasms, and infections
- Inflammatory conditions: rheumatoid arthritis, seronegative spondyloarthropathies
- Neurologic conditions: demyelinating disease, anterior horn cell disease, intraspinal cyst
- Visceral conditions: abdominal/renal problems, inflammatory bowel disease
- Other: cardiac disorders, pulmonary disorders, herpes zoster, polymyalgia rheumatica, myofascial syndrome, psychogenic disorders, etc.

Treatment

- Nonoperative Options
  - Acute phase: nonsteroidal antiinflammatory drugs (NSAIDs), short-term analgesics, ice/heat, ± oral steroids, and activity modifications with gradual mobilization. Physical therapy with core strengthening, lumbar stabilization, and a cardiovascular program can be beneficial (prevents deconditioning).
  - Epidural steroid injections for acute/subacute radiculopathy (not axial back pain).

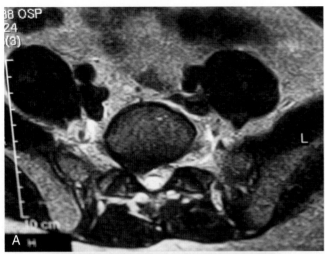

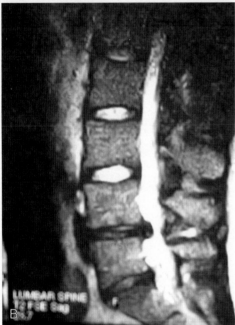

Fig 113.3 (A) Axial magnetic resonance image of a herniated disc at L4-L5. (B) Sagittal magnetic resonance image of L4-L5 and L5-S1 disc degeneration. Note the loss of disc height, decreased signal intensity, and disc herniation at L4-L5, causing pain and L5 radiculopathy in this patient.

- Prolonged bed rest (more than 24 hours) and long-term use of muscle relaxants or braces may lead to deconditioning, longer recovery, and delays in return to work and function.
- One 2-year follow-up study of nonoperative treatment for thoracic disc disease and herniation showed 78% of patients returned to their prior level of activity. Meanwhile, 20% had progressive pain and weakness requiring surgery.
- Operative Options
  - Surgical indications include severe radicular pain unresponsive to a comprehensive nonoperative program (at least 6 to 12 weeks), spinal cord dysfunction/myelopathy (thoracic HNP), and progressive or profound motor

deficit/cauda equina syndrome (lumbar HNP) that may require emergent surgical intervention.
- Surgical procedures
  - HNP with radiculopathy: discectomy; more than 90% success rate
  - Degenerative disc disease with axial low back pain: fusion, disc replacement may be an option in carefully selected patients
- Recent less invasive or "minimally invasive spine surgery" (MISS) options are available.

When to Refer

- Patients with progressive or profound neurologic symptoms, signs of myelopathy, or HNP and pain (without neurologic findings), and in those with persistent pain or weakness in whom a reasonable course of nonsurgical care fails.
- The presence of any red flags requires more aggressive evaluation, and in cases of acute neurologic change/cauda equina or conus syndrome, emergent referral is warranted.

Prognosis

- Asymptomatic or minimally symptomatic HNPs generally have a benign clinical course and can be managed nonoperatively.
- Recovery in a patient with symptomatic lumbar HNPs causing radiculopathy is approximately 50% in 1 month, with 75% recovery by 1 year.
- For low back pain, 50–60% of patients recover in 1 week and 95% recover in 3 months.
- Surgical success for HNP is enhanced if radicular pain is associated with positive tension signs and imaging studies correlate with the clinical picture.
- Surgery results in more rapid improvement of sciatica than nonsurgical care, but differences become less pronounced over time.

Troubleshooting

- Close, serial follow-up is essential.
- A comprehensive history and examination are critical to an accurate diagnosis.
- Consider referral if the diagnosis is uncertain.

Patient Instructions

- Counsel patients on expectations with nonoperative treatment, when to return if failing to improve or worsening, and risks/benefits/anticipated outcomes of surgery.
- Patients with low back pain should be instructed to stay in shape, improve core strength, quit smoking (risk factor for disc degeneration), maintain their ideal weight, and learn proper ergonomic techniques of sitting, standing, lifting, and pushing/pulling.

Suggested Readings

An HS, Singh K, eds. Synopsis of Spine Surgery. 2nd ed. New York: Thieme; 2007.

Andersson GB. Epidemiological features of chronic low-back pain. Lancet. 1999;354:581–585.

Baker HL Jr, Love G, Uihlein A. Roentgenologic features of protruded thoracic intervertebral disks. *Radiology*. 1965;84:1059–1065.

Brown CW, Deffer PA Jr, Akmakjian J, et al. The natural history of thoracic disc herniation. *Spine*. 1992;17(6 suppl):S97–S102.

Buttermann GR. Treatment of lumbar disc herniation: epidural steroid injection compared with discectomy: A prospective, randomized controlled study. *J Bone Joint Surg Am*. 2004;86A:670–679.

Dworkin RH, Johnson RW, Breuer J, et al. Recommendations for the management of herpes zoster. *Clin Infect Dis*. 2007;44(suppl 1): S1–S26.

Gardocki RJ, Park AL. Degenerative disorders of the thoracic and lumbar spine. In: Azar FM, Beaty JH, Canale ST, eds. *Campbell's Operative Orthopaedics*. 13th ed. Philadelphia: Elsevier; 2017:1644–1727.

Goergen S, Maher C, Leech M, Kuang R *Acute low back pain. Education modules for appropriate imaging referrals. Royal Australian and New Zealand College of Radiologists*. 2015. Available at https://www.ranzcr.com/our-work/quality-standards/education-modules. Accessed April 24, 2018.

Grauer JN, Beiner JM, Albert TJ. Lumbar disc disease. In: *VacARro Ar*. Orthopaedic Knowledge Update 8: Home Study Syllabus. Rosemont, IL: American Academy of Orthopaedic Surgeons; 2005:539–552.

Grauer JN, Beiner JM, Albert TJ. Thoracic disc disease. In: *VacARro Ar*. Orthopaedic Knowledge Update 8: Home Study Syllabus. Rosemont, IL: American Academy of Orthopaedic Surgeons; 2005:535–538.

Haak M. History and physical examination. In: Spivak J, Connolly P, eds. *Orthopaedic Knowledge Update Spine 3*. Rosemont, IL: American Academy of Orthopaedic Surgeons; 2006:43–56.

Haldeman SD, Kirkaldy-Willis WH, Bernard TN. Spinal degeneration. In: *The Encyclopedia of Visual Medicine Series: An Atlas of Back Pain*. New York: Parthenon; 2002:19–28.

Jordan J, Konstantinou K, O'Dowd J. Herniated lumbar disc. *BMJ Clin Evid*. 2009;1118:pii.

Leerar P, Boissonnault W, Domholdt E, Roddey T. Documentation of red flags by physical therapists for patients with low back pain. *J Man Manip Ther*. 2007;15(1):42–49.

Li Y, Fredrickson V, Resnick DK. How should we grade lumbar disc herniation and nerve root compression? A systematic review. *Clin Orthop Relat Res*. 2015;473(6):1896–1902.

Rao R, Bagaria V. Pathophysiology of degenerative disk disease and related symptoms. In: Spivak J, Connolly P, eds. *Orthopaedic Knowledge Update Spine 3*. Rosemont, IL: American Academy of Orthopaedic Surgeons; 2006:35–42.

Singh K, Phillips FM. The biomechanics and biology of the spinal degenerative cascade. *Sem Spine Surg*. 2005;17(3):128–136.

Vanichkachorn JS, Vaccaro AR. Thoracic disk disease: diagnosis and treatment. *J Am Acad Orthop Surg*. 2000;8:159–169.

Videman T, Battie MC, Gibbons LE, et al. Associations between back pain history and lumbar MRI findings. *Spine*. 2003;28:582–588.

Chapter 114 Cauda Equina Syndrome

Ali Nourbakhsh, Anuj Singla

ICD-10-CM CODE
G83.4 *Cauda equina syndrome*

Key Concepts

- The group of nerve roots that originate from the conus medullaris inside the thecal sac are termed the cauda equina (horse's tail).
- These nerves include L2-L5 and all the sacral and coccygeal nerves.
- Symptoms and signs of cauda equina compression include back pain, unilateral or bilateral sciatica with or without weakness, decreased sensation of the perineal area (saddle anesthesia), and loss of bowel or bladder function.
- Incomplete cauda equina syndrome (CES) presents with decreased urinary sensation, desire to urinate, and urinary stream. Unilateral or partial perineal sensation might also be present.
- Complete CES presents with painless urinary retention, overflow incontinence, and complete perineal sensation loss.
- Etiologies include large lumbar disc herniation, smaller disc herniation with preexisting lumbar spinal stenosis, epidural hematoma or abscess, fractures, spine tumors, primary and metastatic neoplasms, and spinal trauma.

History

- Patients usually present with variable combinations of:
  - Back pain
  - Radicular leg pain
  - Bladder/bowel incontinence/ retention (Fig. 114.1)
  - Sexual dysfunction

Physical Examination Signs

- Decreased perineal sensation and the tone of anal sphincter
- Saddle anesthesia
- Absent or diminished bulbocavernosus reflex
- Post-void residue scan: If the post-void residue was more than 100 to 200 mL, urinary retention is present.
- Straight leg raise: to evaluate radicular symptoms
- Leg weakness
- Decreased or absent deep tendon reflexes

Imaging

- Anteroposterior and lateral views of the lumbar and thoracolumbar spine should be obtained.
- Radiographs can aid in the evaluations for degenerative disc disease, fractures, tumors, and spondylolisthesis.
- Urgent magnetic resonance imaging (MRI) of the entire spine may show severe stenosis on the axial and sagittal views (Fig. 114.2).
- Computed tomography myelography (if MRI cannot be done)

Differential Diagnosis

- Amyotrophic lateral sclerosis: weakness, atrophy, fasciculations
- Diabetic neuropathy: numbness, impotence, dysesthesia, muscle weakness
- Human immunodeficiency virus myelopathy: urinary hesitancy, clumsiness
- Spinal cord infarction: sudden and severe back pain with possible sciatica, bilateral weakness, paresthesias, numbness, and inability to urinate or defecate within hours
- Syringomyelia: myelopathy and urinary incontinence

Treatment

- Surgical decompression is recommended to be performed as soon as possible. Decompression done between 24 and 48 hours from the onset of symptoms may provide better outcomes. Surgical decompression of cauda equina is the mainstay of treatment.
- Laminectomy is performed for spinal stenosis and herniated disc.
- For spine metastasis, posterior laminectomy with or without anterior corpectomy and reconstruction is performed in case of anterior compression of the cord.

Prognosis

- Incomplete CES has a better prognosis than the complete form.
- Almost 75% of patients with CES cases will gain acceptable urological function, with possible motor/sensory deficit of the lower extremities and chronic back pain.

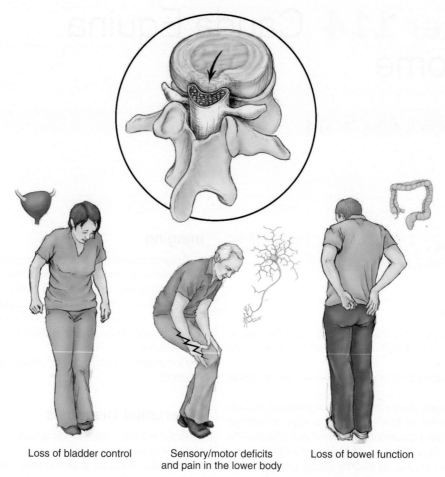

Loss of bladder control | Sensory/motor deficits and pain in the lower body | Loss of bowel function

Fig 114.1 Central disc herniation and resultant common cauda equine syndrome.

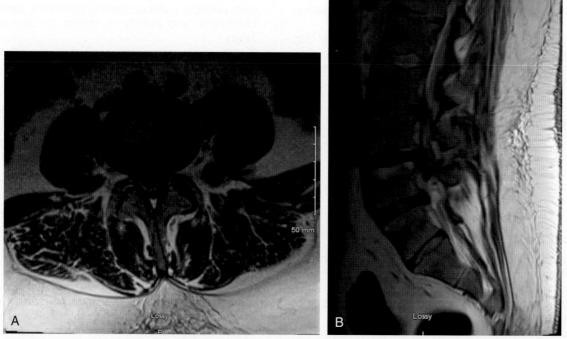

Fig 114.2 (A) Axial image showing severe central canal stenosis. (B) T2 W sagittal image showing large disc herniation at L3-L4 with significant stenosis.

- 20% of these patients will have sexual dysfunction, need for self-catheterization, colostomy, or urological and gynecological surgery.

Patient Instructions

- Patients who are at risk of developing cauda equina such as known metastasis to the spine or disc herniation should seek medical assistance if they are having any symptoms consistent with CES.

Suggested Readings

Ahn UM, Ahn NU, Buchowksi JM, et al. Cauda equina syndrome secondary to lumbar disc herniation: a meta-analysis of surgical outcomes. *Spine.* 2000;25:1515–1522.

Gardner A, Gardner E, Morley T. Cauda equina syndrome: a review of the current clinical and medico-legal position. *Eur Spine J.* 2011;20:690–697.

Gleave JR, Macfarlane R. Cauda equina syndrome: what is the relationship between timing of surgery and outcome? *Br J Neurosurg.* 2002;16:325–328.

Kohles SS, Kohles DA, Karp AP, et al. Time-dependent surgical outcomes following cauda equina syndrome diagnosis—comments on a meta-analysis. *Spine.* 2004;29:1281–1287.

Quraishi NA, Giannoulis KE, Manoharan SR, Edwards KL, Boszczyk BM. Surgical treatment of cauda equina compression as a result of metastatic tumours of the lumbo-sacral junction and sacrum. *Eur Spine J.* 2013;22(suppl 1):S33–S37.

Shapiro S. Cauda equina syndrome secondary to lumbar disc herniation. *Neurosurgery.* 1993;8:317–322.

Small SA, Perron AD, Brady WJ. Orthopedic pitfalls: cauda equina syndrome. *Am J Emerg Med.* 2005;23:159–163.

Chapter 115 Thoracolumbar Stenosis

Larry Lee, Kaku Barkoh, Jeffrey Wang

ICD-10-CM CODES

M48.06	*Stenosis lumbar region*
M99.53	*Intervertebral disc stenosis of neural canal of lumbar region*
M48.061	*Spinal stenosis without neurogenic claudication*
M99.63	*Osseous subluxation stenosis of intervertebral foramina in lumbar region*
M47.61	*Other spondylosis with myelopathy, lumbar region*
M99.73	*Connective tissue and disc stenosis of intervertebral foramina of lumbar region*
M48.05	*Spinal stenosis of the thoracolumbar region*
M48.04	*Stenosis thoracic region*
M99.42	*Connective tissue stenosis of the thoracic region*
M99.52	*Intervertebral disc stenosis of neural canal of thoracic region*
M99.62	*Osseous and subluxation stenosis of the thoracic spine*
M47.14	*Other spondylosis with myelopathy, thoracic region*

Thoracic Spine
Key Concepts

- Stenosis is defined as a narrowing of the spinal canal or the neural foramina (Fig. 115.1).
  - This can lead to compression of the spinal cord, the conus, individual nerve roots causing thoracic myelopathy, thoracic and lumbar radiculopathy, cauda equina syndrome depending on where the compression is located.
- Stiffer construct than both the cervical and lumbar spine.
  - Anterior connection to ribs contribute to rigidity.
- The cross-sectional area of the thoracic spinal canal is relatively constant from T2-10 averaging 198 mm^2, T1 and T11-12 did have higher averages at 280 mm^2.
  - The cross-sectional area of the thoracic spinal cord ranges from 40 to 50 mm^2.
- Thoracic stenosis incidence rates are significantly lower than cervical and lumbar stenosis rates
- Primary causes of thoracic stenosis:
  - Spinal disc degeneration
    - Osteophyte formation
    - Thoracic disc herniations
  - Facet hypertrophy

- Ligamentum flavum hypertrophy
  - Includes buckling of the ligamentum flavum into the spinal canal
  - Ossification of the ligamentum flavum (OLF)
    - Ligamentum flavum calcification
- Ossification of the posterior longitudinal ligament (OPLL)
  - More rare than cervical OPLL
  - Beaked versus flat OPLL
    - Beaked: Protrusion into the canal behind the disc space
- Tumors
  - Metastasis, most common spine tumors
    - Breast
    - Lung
    - Thyroid
    - Kidney
    - Prostate

History/Physical Examination

- Compression at the thoracic levels can lead to either radiculopathy or myelopathy or a combination of both
  - Thoracic radiculopathy
    - Can present as chest wall pain, in a band distribution
  - Thoracic myelopathy
    - Presents as upper motor neuron signs in the lower limbs
      - Brisk reflexes
      - Clonus
      - Upwards going Babinski
      - Gait disturbances, trouble walking in a tandem gait
      - Balance issues
      - Bowel and bladder disturbances

Imaging

- X-ray/radiograph
  - Helpful in the diagnosis of degenerative disc disease, spinal alignment, and OPLL.
  - Limited in use for diagnosis for thoracic stenosis.
- CT
  - Gives better imaging of the spinal canal.
  - Better assessment of protruding osteophytes, OPLL, OLF, facet hypertrophy, and other potential radiopaque structures that could be impinging in the spinal canal.
  - Does not provide an adequate image of the neural structures, that is, spinal cord, spinal nerves.
    - Not a reliable way to directly image compression.
  - CT myelogram
    - Contrast is injected into the intradural space.
    - Allows a better image of spinal cord impingement.

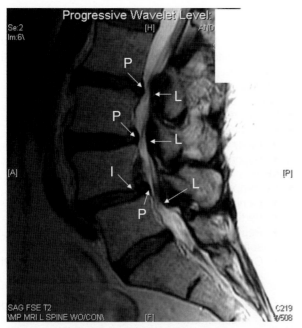

Fig 115.1 Axial T2-weighted magnetic resonance image of an elderly patient with three-level degenerative lumbar stenosis at L2–3, L3–4, and L4–5, as well as degenerative spondylolisthesis *(I)* at L4–5, at the level of L4–5. Significant compression of the thecal sac occurs secondary to disc protrusion *(P)*, hypertrophic deformity of the osteoarthritic facet joints *(F)*, and thickened ligamentum flavum infolding *(L)*.

- MRI
  - Gold standard in assessment of thoracic stenosis
    - Allows the best visualization of spinal cord impingement.
    - Visualization of herniated disc, hypertrophied ligaments, other soft tissue pints of compression.

Differential Diagnosis
- Cervical myelopathy
  - Compression at in the cervical spine can lead to myelopathic symptoms.
- Upper motor neuron disease
- Shingles

Treatment
- Conservative
  - Reserved for patients without symptoms of myelopathy.
  - Injections and nerve modulators for patients who develop radiculopathy.
- Operative
  - Laminectomy with or without fusion
    - Laminectomy without fusion
      - Motion preserving, less motion inherent to the thoracic system.
    - Depending on site of compression, allows direct versus indirect decompression of the spinal cord.
    - Removal of ligamentum flavum, and bony impingement
    - Could use transpedicular approach the anterior aspect of the canal.

- Depending on the amount of bone taken, stability may be an issue, necessitating a fusion.
- Anterior decompression
  - Access through the lateral window
  - Corpectomy/discectomy
    - Allows for better access to anterior impingement structures than posterior approaches.
    - Direct decompression versus indirect decompression.

Lumbar Stenosis
Key Concepts
- Narrowing of the spinal canal, nerve root canals, or intervertebral foramina.
- Can be subdivided into three main types of stenosis
  - Central stenosis—thecal sac compression
    - Area posterior to the posterior longitudinal ligament and medial to the superior articular facets.
    - Potential causes
      - Soft tissues, such as hypertrophied ligamentum flavum, bulging discs, and facet capsule.
      - Overgrown/hypertrophied facets
      - Lumbar segmental spondylolisthesis
      - Congenital stenosis, decreased area for the spinal canal.
        - Less margin for compression
    - Disease of age
      - As degenerative changes lead to hypertrophying of the spinal canal structures, risks increase.
    - Absolute stenosis
      - Less than 10 mm anterior to posterior distance of the spinal canal, or cross-sectional area of less than 100 mm^2.
  - Lateral recess stenosis—nerve compression, traversing nerve root.
    - Area between the posterolateral border of the vertebral body and the articular facets.
    - Potential causes
      - Medial overgrowth of the facet joint, the superior articular process.
    - More likely to affect the traversing nerve root.
      - Exiting nerve root has already exited the foramen.
  - Foraminal stenosis—nerve compression, exiting root.
    - Bordered by the pedicles above and below.
    - Foraminal height is usually 20 to 30 mm.

History/Physical Exam
- Neurogenic claudication
  - Pain in the lower extremities, posterior thigh/buttock cramping, altered sensation.
  - Patients can report that the pain is mitigated through flexion of their backs.
- Lumbar radiculopathy
  - Depending on the individual nerve being compressed, patients can present with pain that radiates to specific dermatomes in the lower extremities.
  - Further compression can lead to chronic nerve damage including weakness in the specific myotome groups.
  - Potential for decreased reflexes.

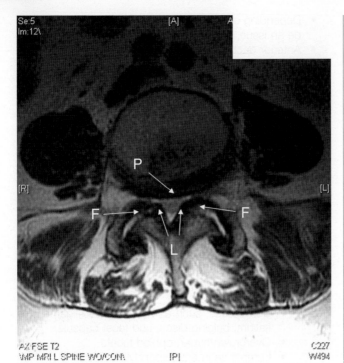

Se:5
Im:12\
[A]

[R]

P

F
F
L

[L]

AX FSE T2
MP MRI L SPINE WO/CON
[P]

C227
W494

Fig 115.2 Sagittal T2-weighted magnetic resonance image of the same patient. Disc protrusions *(P)* and thickened ligamentum flavum infolding *(L)* contribute to marked narrowing of the thecal sac.

Imaging

- X-rays
  - AP/lateral
    - Interspace narrowing due to disc degeneration.
    - Medially placed facets.
    - Flattening of the lordotic curve.
    - Subluxation and alignment.
  - Flexion/extension
    - Allows assessment of dynamic instability.
- CT
  - Osteophyte formation
  - Look for axial canal morphology.
- MRI
  - Allows for visualization of the thecal sac and surrounding structures (Fig. 115.2).
    - Hypertrophy of the ligamentum flavum.
    - Foraminal stenosis and nerve impingement.
    - Evaluation for malignancy.
  - If there is dynamic instability, the slip could reduce while the patient lies supine.
- Electromyography/nerve conduction study
  - Potentially effective to differentiate between radiculopathy versus peripheral neuropathy.
  - Can be user dependent

Treatment

- Conservative: No conservative treatment can change the inherent architecture of the stenosis, but could bring the patient relief.
  - Physical therapy
  - Nonsteroidal antiinflammatory drugs (NSAIDs)
  - Weight reduction
  - Epidural steroid injections
    - Likely a short-term treatment.
    - Secondary use for diagnostic purposes.
- Surgery
  - Decompression of the neural elements.
    - Laminectomy
    - Partial medial facetectomy
    - Removal of ligamentum flavum and other impinging soft tissues.
    - Care must be paid to not destabilize spine at the level of decompression.
      - Maintain 1 cm of pars
      - Care when performing the partial medial facetectomy.
    - Residual stenosis is a common reason for persistent symptoms.
- Fusion: Indicated in the following
  - Segmental instability on flex/ex x-rays.
    - Degenerative or isthmic spondylolisthesis
    - Degenerative scoliosis
  - Surgical instability
    - Pars fracture
    - Removing too much of the medial facet.
- Outcomes
  - SPORT Trial showed significant improvement versus nonoperative improvement at 4 years.
    - SF-36 Bodily Pain and Function
    - Oswestry Disability Index
  - Both operative and nonoperative groups showed improvement form baseline.

Suggested Readings

Arnoldi CC, Brodsky AE, Cauchoix J, et al. Lumbar spinal stenosis and nerve root entrapment syndromes. Definition and classification. *Clin Orthop Relat Res.* 1976;115:4–5.

Cheung JPY, Ng KKM, Cheung PWH, et al. Radiographic indices for lumbar developmental spinal stenosis. *Scoliosis Spinal Disord.* 2017;12:3.

Genevay S, Atlas SJ. Lumbar spinal stenosis. *Best Pract Res Clin Rheumatol.* 2010;24(2):253–265.

Hitchon PW, Abode-Iyamah K, Dahdaleh NS, et al. Risk factors and outcomes in thoracic stenosis with myelopathy: A single center experience. *Clin Neurol Neurosurg.* 2016;147:84–89.

Hoang S, et al. *Spinal Stenosis. StatPearls [Website].* Treasure Island, FL: StatPearls Publishing; 2017.

Machado GC, Ferreira PH, Yoo RI, et al. Surgical options for lumbar spinal stenosis. *Cochrane Database Syst Rev.* 2016;(11):CD012421.

Chapter 116 Spondylolysis and Spondylolisthesis

Michael T. Nolte, Christopher J. DeWald

ICD-10-CM CODES
M43.0 *Spondylolysis*
M43.1 *Spondylolisthesis*
Q76.2 *Congenital spondylolisthesis*

Key Concepts
Spondylolysis

- Defect or stress fracture in the pars interarticularis, or junction between the superior and inferior facets, of the lumbar spine (Fig. 116.1).
- Due to repetitive impact from the inferior facet of the cranial vertebral segment on the adjacent caudal vertebral segment through the pars interarticularis.
- Common cause of back pain, with a childhood prevalence of approximately 4%, and an adult prevalence of 6-12%.
- Particularly prevalent in adolescent athletes who experience repetitive hyperextension (e.g., gymnasts, divers, football linemen).

Spondylolisthesis

- Forward translation of one vertebral segment on another.
- Grading scale based on the percentage of displacement: I, less than 25%; II, 25-50%; III, 50-75%; IV, 75-100%; V, more than 100%.
- Lytic spondylolisthesis occurs most commonly in the lower lumbar spine (85% at L5-S1 and 10% at L4-L5).
- Historical classification of Wiltse (Box 116.1) and functional classification of Marchetti and Bartolozzi (Box 116.2).
- Higher grade slips and dysplastic slips are more likely to progress in severity.
- Adolescent to young adult population: continuum of spondylolysis to low-grade isthmic/lytic spondylolisthesis (L5-S1 most common) resulting in foraminal nerve root compression.
- Older adult population: degenerative spondylolisthesis resulting from disc degeneration without previous spondylolysis, leading to spinal stenosis with neurogenic claudication (L4-L5 most common) affecting the traversing nerve roots.

History

- Patients with either spondylolysis or spondylolisthesis may be asymptomatic or have mild to moderate low back pain.
- Spondylolysis typically occurs during youth and is the most common identifiable cause of back pain in children.
- Most common presenting symptom in lytic spondylolisthesis is the development of radicular pain at the level of the lysis or stenosis.

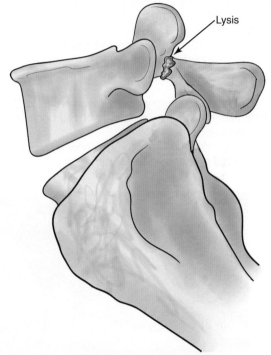

Fig 116.1 Diagram of vertebral body with lysis of the pars interarticularis.

- Degenerative spondylolisthesis may present as neurogenic claudication in older patients (i.e., pain or heaviness in legs with standing/walking, improved with bending/sitting).

Physical Examination

- General Inspection
  - Typically normal
  - Children with progressive high-grade spondylolisthesis and radicular pain may exhibit Phalen-Dickson gait and posture (Fig. 116.2).
  - High-grade spondylolisthesis is also characterized by accentuated lumbar lordosis.
- Palpation
  - Typically nontender
  - Prominence of the spinous process of the lytic vertebral segment's spinous process with step-off to the cephalad spinous process.
- Range of motion
  - Normal in most cases
  - Extension limited due to pain in adolescents with spondylolysis.

- Tight hamstring muscles in adolescents with spondylolisthesis.
- Extension substantially limited in adults with degenerative spondylolisthesis.
- Neurologic examination
  - Typically normal in most cases.
  - Achilles reflexes may be diminished with degenerative spondylolisthesis.

BOX 116.1 Wiltse Classification

1. Dysplastic: congenital defect of the upper sacrum or the arch of L5 allowing for vertebral segment translation
2. Isthmic: defect in the pars interarticularis
   a. Lytic: fatigue fracture of the pars
   b. Elongated but intact pars
   c. Acute fracture
3. Degenerative: long-standing intersegmental instability
4. Traumatic: fractures in areas of the bony hook other than the pars
5. Pathologic: destruction of the posterior elements from generalized or localized bone pathology

---

- Decreased motor strength can occur in degenerative spondylolisthesis with long-standing severe stenosis.

Imaging
Radiographs

- Supine anteroposterior, lateral, and oblique lumbosacral views.
  - To evaluate for the presence of spondylolysis (Fig. 116.3) and/or spondylolisthesis (Figs. 116.4 and 116.5).

BOX 116.2 Marchetti-Bartolozzi Classification

Developmental

High dysplastic with lysis or elongation
Low dysplastic with lysis or elongation

Acquired

Traumatic, due to acute or stress fracture
Postsurgical, caused by direct or indirect surgery
Pathologic, due to local or systemic pathology
Degenerative, found in primary or secondary degenerative conditions

---

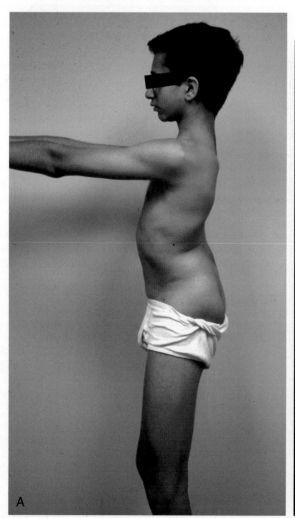

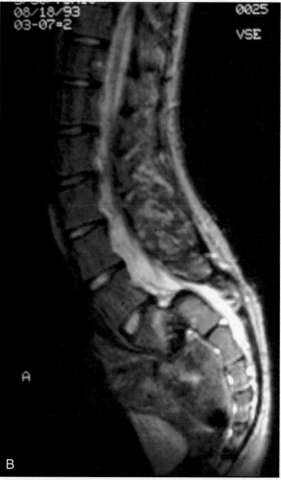

Fig 116.2 **(A)** Phalen-Dixon sign in an adolescent with high-grade spondylolisthesis. **(B)** Magnetic resonance image of developmental high-grade spondylolisthesis.

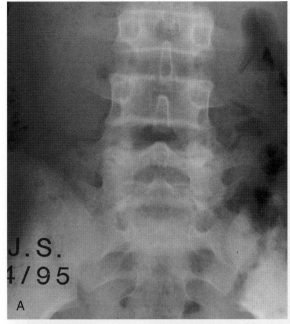

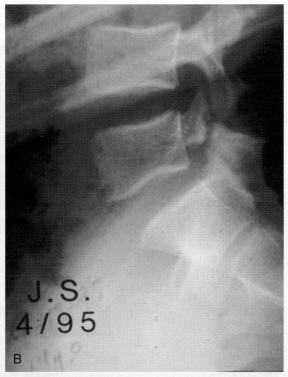

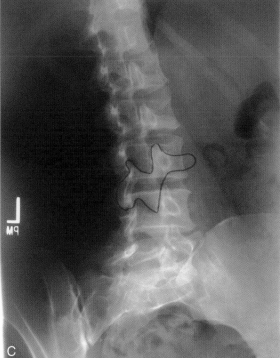

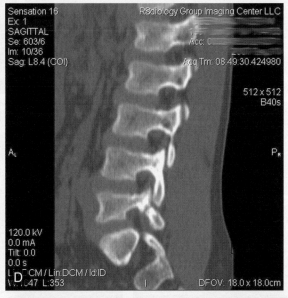

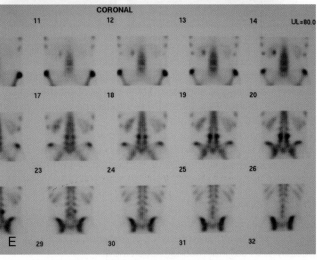

Fig 116.3 L5 spondylolysis. Anteroposterior (A), lateral (B), and oblique (C) radiographs. Note the lysis just inferior to the pedicle of L5 at the "neck of the Scotty dog." (D) Sagittal computed tomography clearly demonstrates the lysis. (E) Single-photon emission computed tomography images showing uptake at the pars interarticularis bilaterally at L5.

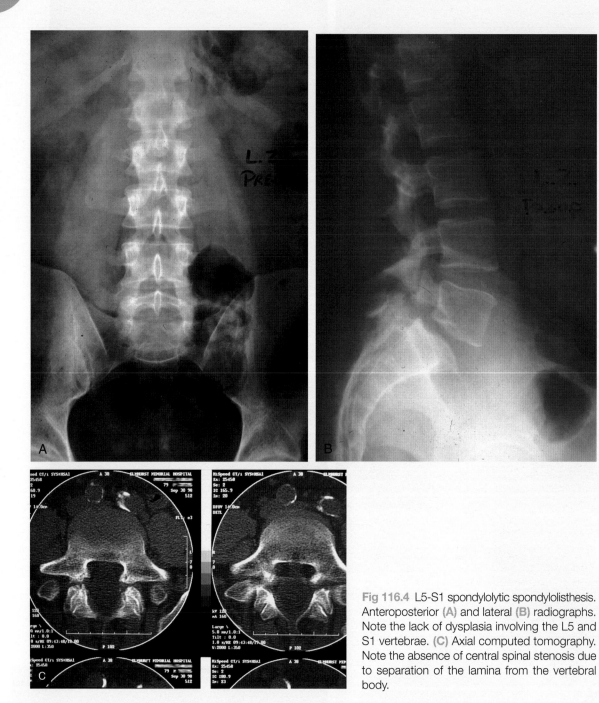

Fig 116.4 L5-S1 spondylolytic spondylolisthesis. Anteroposterior **(A)** and lateral **(B)** radiographs. Note the lack of dysplasia involving the L5 and S1 vertebrae. **(C)** Axial computed tomography. Note the absence of central spinal stenosis due to separation of the lamina from the vertebral body.

- To determine the degree of bony dysplasia (trapezoidal L5, rounded sacral endplate, spina bifida of posterior elements, sacral verticalization, elongated pars).
- Standing lateral lumbosacral view
  - Required to determine grade of spondylolisthesis.
  - Measures the true severity and instability (compared to the supine view) of anterior translation of vertebral segment.

Computed Tomography

- Best study to confirm presence of spondylolysis (see Fig. 116.3) and determine presence or absence of healing, especially with sagittal reconstruction view.

- Not necessary in most cases of spondylolisthesis, as slip is typically evident on plain radiographs.
- Assists in defining bony anatomy of dysplastic spondylolisthesis.

Bone Scan

- Solely used to determine acuity in adolescent spondylolysis; "hot" scan suggests acute fracture or stress reaction.
- Single-photon emission computed tomography (CT) images are required to determine the location of uptake at the pars (see Fig. 116.3).
- A "cold" scan does not rule out the presence of a spondylolysis.

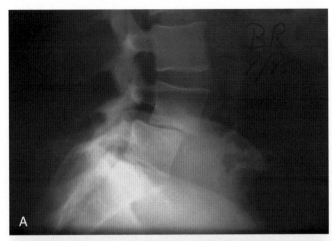

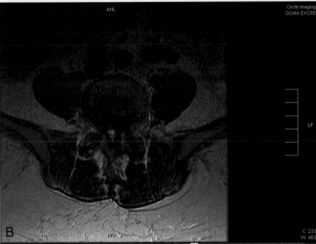

Fig 116.5 Degenerative spondylolisthesis. **(A)** Lateral radiograph depicting the severity of slippage. **(B)** Magnetic resonance imaging revealing the severity of the associated stenosis. Compare this with the lack of stenosis typically found in lytic spondylolisthesis as shown in Fig. 116.4. Note the facet hypertrophy and anterior subluxation of the inferior facets resulting in the spinal stenosis.

Magnetic Resonance Imaging

- Not necessary for the diagnosis or effective treatment of spondylolysis.
- Can determine edema associated with stress reaction or acute spondylolysis.
- Less radiation than CT scan
- Best method to assess for other etiologies of back pain in adolescents (e.g., herniated nucleus pulposus, soft tissue tumor, infection).
- Valuable study for patients with spondylolisthesis to assess for concurrent spinal stenosis (see Fig. 116.5).

Differential Diagnosis

- Herniated nucleus pulposus
- Osseous tumor (e.g., osteoid osteoma)
- Infection (e.g., discitis, osteomyelitis)

- Mechanical back pain
- Low back strain

Treatment
Spondylolysis

- At time of diagnosis
  - Treatment is based on symptoms.
  - Stop the contributing activity or sport, start nonsteroidal anti-inflammatory drugs, and consider physical therapy.
  - If the patient remains symptomatic or a bone scan reveals uptake (hot) at the pars, a hypolordotic lumbosacral orthosis is used for 6 to 12 weeks.
- Later in course
  - For patients with persistent pain, surgical options include L5-S1 posterior spinal fusion (younger patients) or a surgical repair of the pars defect (adolescents, midlumbar lysis).

When to Refer

- Significant back pain lasting more than 1 to 2 weeks should be referred for further evaluation.
- Referral is not necessary for patients with radiographic spondylolysis in the absence of spondylolisthesis who are asymptomatic.

Prognosis

- Good
  - The majority of patients respond well to conservative management, whether or not the spondylolysis heals.
  - The results of surgical intervention are also successful if patients do not improve with activity modification, bracing, and physical therapy.
  - Patients may return to sports once symptoms resolve.

Spondylolisthesis

- At time of diagnosis
  - Treatment is dependent on age and severity of the slip.
  - Nonoperative treatment includes nonsteroidal antiinflammatory drugs, physical therapy, and consideration of bracing in the adolescent patient.
- Later in course
  - In adult patients, selective nerve blocks or epidural injections can be used in those with spondylolytic or degenerative spondylolisthesis, respectively.
  - Surgical treatment includes posterior spinal fusion with instrumentation in adolescent and adult patients (Fig. 116.6) and without instrumentation in pediatric patients.
  - Due to high risk for progression, skeletally immature patients with developmental high-grade spondylolisthesis must be recognized by the treating physician as they often require surgical stabilization (fusion) even in the absence of symptoms.

When to Refer

- Refer patients younger than age 12 with spondylolisthesis, radiographic evidence of bony dysplasia, or high-grade slips (grade 2 or higher).
- Adult and adolescent patients not responding to nonoperative treatment should be referred for surgical discussion.

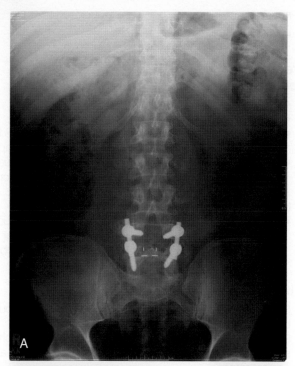

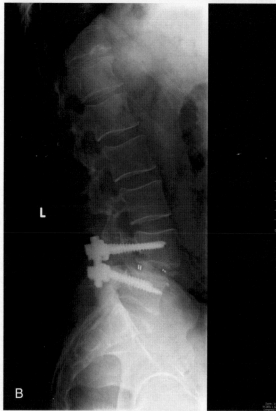

Fig 116.6 Posterior spinal fusion and instrumentation of an adult with spondylolytic spondylolisthesis at L4-5. Anteroposterior **(A)**, and lateral **(B)** radiographs.

Prognosis

- The prognosis of spondylolisthesis following surgical treatment for both adult and pediatric patients is generally good.
- Surgical management of degenerative spondylolisthesis typically consisting of decompression and single-level posterior spinal fusion is particularly successful.
- The need to reduce high-grade spondylolisthesis in adolescents is continually debated.

Points to Remember

- Back pain in adolescents is unusual. If pain is significant or persistent, further workup is warranted.
- A change in or cessation of a specific sport or activity will often be sufficient to decrease pain and avoid surgery.
- When patient experiences unrelenting low back or radicular pain, surgical intervention may be indicated.
- Surgical risks include blood loss, infection, nerve root injury, pseudarthrosis, revision surgery, instrumentation failure, and adjacent disc degeneration.

Patient Instructions

- Except for developmental highly dysplastic spondylolisthesis, patients with spondylolysis or spondylolisthesis can be treated based on symptoms. If the patient's pain is controlled with nonoperative measures, surgery can be avoided.

Suggested Readings

Beck NA, Miller R, Baldwin K, et al. Do oblique views add value in the diagnosis of spondylolysis in adolescents? *J Bone Joint Surg Am.* 2013;95(10):e65.

Beutler WJ, Fredrickson BE, Murtland A, et al. The natural history of spondylolysis and spondylolisthesis: 45-year follow-up evaluation. *Spine.* 2003;28:1027–1035.

Carragee EJ. Single-level posterolateral arthrodesis, with or without posterior decompression, for the treatment of isthmic spondylolisthesis in adults. A prospective, randomized study. *J Bone Joint Surg Am.* 1997;79A:1175–1180.

Deguchi M, Rapoff AJ, Zdeblick TA. Posterolateral fusion for isthmic spondylolisthesis in adults: analysis of fusion rate and clinical results. *J Spinal Disord.* 1998;11:459–464.

Endler P, Ekman P, Moller H, Gerdhem P. Outcomes of posterolateral fusion with and without instrumentation and of interbody fusion for isthmic spondylolisthesis: a prospective study. *J Bone Joint Surg Am.* 2017;99:743–752.

Fischgrund JS, Mackay M, Herkowitz HN, et al. Degenerative lumbar spondylolisthesis with spinal stenosis: A prospective randomized study comparing decompressive laminectomy and arthrodesis with and without spinal instrumentation. *Spine.* 1997;22:2807–2812.

Hammerberg KW. Spondylolysis and spondylolisthesis. In: DeWald RL, eds. *Spinal Deformities. The Comprehensive Text.* New York: Thieme; 2003:787–808.

Herkowitz HN, Kurz LT. Degenerative lumbar spondylolisthesis with spinal stenosis. A prospective study comparing decompression and intertransverse process arthrodesis. *J Bone Joint Surg Am.* 1991;73A:802–808.

Hsu WK, Jenkins TJ. Management of lumbar conditions in the elite athlete. *J Am Acad Orthop Surg.* 2017;25:489–498.

Hu SS, Tribus CB, Diab M, et al. Spondylolisthesis and spondylolysis: an instructional course lecture. American Academy of Orthopedic Surgeons. *J Bone Joint Surg Am*. 2008;90A:656–671.

Molinari RW, Bridwell KH, Lenke LG, et al. Complications in the surgical treatment of pediatric high-grade isthmic dysplastic spondylolisthesis. A comparison of three surgical techniques. *Spine*. 1999;24:1701–1711.

Moller H, Hedlund R. Instrumented and noninstrumented posterolateral fusion in adult spondylolisthesis. A prospective randomized study: part 2. *Spine*. 2000;25:1716–1721.

Sakai T, Tezuka F, Yamashita K, et al. Conservative treatment for bony healing in pediatric lumbar spondylolysis. *Spine*. 2017;42: 716–720.

6

SECTION

The Pelvis/Hip

Chapter 117 Hip and Pelvis Overview

Michelle E. Kew, F. Winston Gwathmey, Jr.

Key Concepts

- The hip and pelvis serve many roles including the attachment site for the appendicular and axial skeleton, protector of vital internal organs, and structural support for locomotion.
- The hip and pelvis are commonly injured sites and account for approximately 5% to 24% of activity-related injuries in adults and children, respectively.
- The hip and pelvic areas are also often involved in referred pain from the lumbar spine and knee.
- The hip joint is a major weight-bearing joint (up to 3 to 5 times body weight with activity) and subject to both acute traumatic as well as chronic degenerative injury from repetitive loading.
- A thorough history, physical examination, and a good working knowledge of the anatomy of this region are essential for proficient diagnosis.
- Further evaluation such as the use of plain film radiographs, magnetic resonance imaging, and bone scan can be helpful to confirm the diagnosis.

Bones and Landmarks

- Hip and pelvis are made up of many bones that are listed in Table 117.1.

TABLE 117.1 Bones and Landmarks

Bone	Components	Features
Sacrum	Sacral promontory	Convex anterior; forms posterior margin of pelvic inlet
	Anterior, posterior sacral foramina	4 paired foramen that allow transmission of branches of sacral plexus and lateral sacral arteries
Coccyx	3–5 fused vertebra attached to distal end of sacrum	Attached to distal end of sacrum
		Provides support to rectum, pelvic floor
Femur	Head	Articulates with acetabulum; lined with hyaline cartilage; 15 degrees anteversion relative to knee
	Greater trochanter	Lateral prominence; attachment site for many muscles
	Lesser trochanter	Superomedial prominence; psoas muscle insertion site
	Neck	At an angle of 120 degrees from shaft, at 15 degrees anteversion; is a common site for injury
	Fovea capitis	Depression in femoral head where ligament to head of femur attaches
Innominate		
Ilium	Anterior inferior iliac spine	Inferior to origin of sartorius; forms upper ring of acetabulum
	Anterior superior iliac spine	Anterior margin of iliac crest
	Greater sciatic notch	Inferior to posterior superior iliac spine; is site of passage for many important structures
	Lesser sciatic notch	Obturator internus muscle and nerve; pudendal vessels enter pelvis through this opening
	Iliac tuberosity	Posterior prominence of ilium; attachment for low back muscles, sacroiliac ligament
	Posterior inferior iliac spine	Superior boundary of greater sciatic notch
	Posterosuperior iliac spine	Posterior margin of iliac crest; attachment site for sacrotuberous and sacroiliac ligaments
Ischium		Consists of a body, 2 rami; forms the posteroinferior portion of the pelvis
	Ischial ramus	Inferior margin of obturator foramen
	Ischial spine	Site of attachment for sacrospinous ligament
	Ischial tuberosity	Strongest part of the hip bone
		Major weight-bearing structure during sitting
		Site of attachment of many muscles
Pubis	Superior and inferior pubic rami	Form part of pubic symphysis
		Common site of muscle insertion
	Pubic tubercle	Medial prominence of pubic bone
		Site of attachment for inguinal ligament

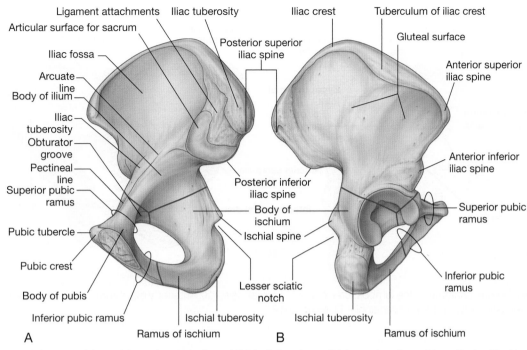

Fig 117.1 Bony landmarks of the pelvis and acetabulum. **(A)** Medial surface. **(B)** Lateral surface. (From Drake RL, Vogl AW, Mitchell A, eds. *Gray's Basic Anatomy*. 2nd ed. Philadelphia: Elsevier; 2018.)

- Pelvis is made up of innominate bones (ilium, ischium, pubis; Fig. 117.1).
- Hip joint is composed of the femur and acetabulum to create a ball-and-socket joint.

Joints and Ligaments

- Hip joint is the primary joint which allows multiaxial movement with inherent stability provided by ligamentous and muscle constraints.
- Sacroiliac joint is the articulation between the lateral sacral wings and the ilium; both surfaces are lined with articular cartilage; motion at the sacroiliac joint is limited in all planes due to the joint's extensive ligamentous attachments (Fig. 117.2).
- Sacrococcygeal symphysis: This articulation between the apex of the sacrum and base of the coccyx allows little movement and also contains a small fibrocartilage disc.
- Lumbosacral joint: Articulation between the fifth lumbar vertebra and disc and the first sacral vertebra (Fig. 117.3)
- Important joints and ligaments are listed in Table 117.2.

Muscles

- A number of muscles are located in the pelvis or exert their influence here.
- Pelvic muscles generally provide stability to the trunk or function in the transmission of load to the lower extremities.
- The muscles of the hip are divided into four compartments: anterior (hip flexion), posterior (hip extension), medial (hip adduction), and lateral (hip abduction).
- Table 117.3 lists the main muscles that exert action in the hip or pelvis.

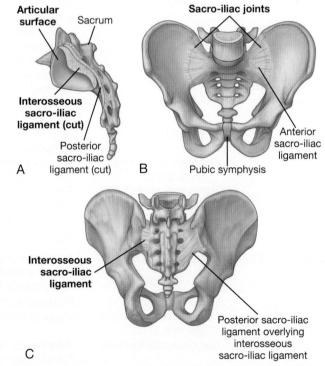

Fig 117.2 Ligamentous anatomy of the sacroiliac joint. **(A)** Lateral view. **(B)** Anterior view. **(C)** Posterior view. (From Drake RL, Vogl AW, Mitchell A, eds. *Gray's Basic Anatomy*. 2nd ed. Philadelphia: Elsevier; 2018.)

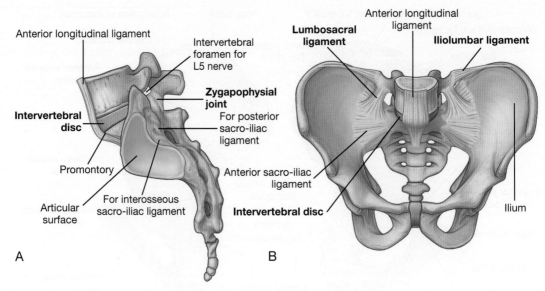

Fig 117.3 Ligamentous anatomy of the lumbosacral joint. **(A)** Lateral view. **(B)** Anterior view. (From Drake RL, Vogl AW, Mitchell A, eds. *Gray's Basic Anatomy*. 2nd ed. Philadelphia: Elsevier; 2018.)

TABLE 117.2 Joints and Ligaments

Bone	Components	Features
Hip joint	Acetabulum	Socket portion of the ball-and-socket hip joint
		Joint stability due to superior bony ridge, depth of acetabular cup, degree of acetabular anteversion, degree of femoral head coverage
	Femoral head	Joint mechanics are affected by the size, shape, and angle of femoral head
	Joint capsule	Capsule includes iliofemoral ligament; provides anterior support to joint capsule from inferior border of the ilium
		Ischiofemoral ligament: primary restraint in hip internal rotation
		Ligamentum orbicularis: surrounds hip capsule
		Pubofemoral ligament: primary restraint in hip abduction
	Acetabular labrum	Ring of fibrocartilage
		Deepens cavity to help distribute stress
	Ligament of the head of the femur	Attaches femoral head to acetabulum
		Carries some arterial supply to femoral head
	Transverse acetabular ligament	Provides inferior reinforcement of labrum, hip joint
		Connects ends of acetabular notch
Pelvis	Pubic symphysis	Cartilaginous joints between superior rami of pubic bones
		Stabilized by anterior, inferior, posterior, superior pubic ligaments
Sacroiliac joint	Sacroiliac ligament	Anterior and posterior components
		Attach anterolateral sacrum and posterior sacrum to ilium
		Responsible for rotational and vertical stability of the pelvis
		Posterior component is strongest
	Interosseous sacroiliac ligament	Deep to posterior sacroiliac ligament
	Sacrospinous ligament	Attaches to sacrum and ischial spine ventrally
		Contributes to rotational stability
		Boundary for greater and lesser sciatic notches
	Sacrotuberous ligament	Attaches sacrum to ischial tuberosity
		Major stabilizer: contributes to vertical stability
		Forms inferior border of lesser sciatic notch
	Iliolumbar ligament	Process of L5 with the ilium

TABLE 117.2 Joints and Ligamentsc—cont'd

Bone	Components	Features
Sacrococcygeal symphysis	Sacrococcygeal ligaments	Anterior, posterior, lateral components Provides stability to sacrococcygeal joint
Lumbosacral joint	Anterior longitudinal ligament	Stabilizes the spine from axis to sacrum Located on anterior vertebra
	Ligamentum flavum	Connects vertebral lamina from C1 to S1
	Posterior longitudinal ligament	Stabilizes the spine from axis to sacrum Located on posterior vertebra
	Supraspinous ligament	Connects spinous process from C7 through sacrum

TABLE 117.3 Major Muscles of the Hip and Pelvis

Muscle	Origin	Insertion	Action
Iliacus	Anterior iliac fossa	Lesser trochanter	Hip flexion
Psoas major	Vertebral body, transverse process, disc T12-L4	Lesser trochanter	A primary hip flexor
Tensor fascia latae	Iliac crest, anterosuperior iliac spine	Iliotibial band	Hip abduction, flexion, internal rotation
Gluteus medius	Posterior ilium	Greater trochanter (superior, lateral)	Primary hip abductor, internal rotator
Gluteus minimus	Posterior ilium	Greater trochanter (anterior, lateral)	Abduction, internal rotation
Gluteus maximus	Posterior ilium, sacrum	Femur, iliotibial band	Primary hip extensor, external rotation
Piriformis	Anterior sacrum	Greater trochanter	External rotation
Obturator externus	Ischiopubic rami, obturator membrane	Trochanteric fossa	External rotation
Obturator internus	Ischiopubic rami, obturator membrane	Greater trochanter	External rotation, abduction
Superior gemellus	Ischial spine	Greater trochanter	External rotation
Inferior gemellus	Ischial tuberosity	Greater trochanter	External rotation
Quadratus femoris	Ischial tuberosity	Intertrochanteric crest	External rotation
Sartorius	Anterosuperior iliac spine	Pes anserinus	Flexion, external rotation of hip
Rectus femoris	Anterosuperior iliac spine	Patella, tibial tuberosity	Flexion of hip, extension of knee
Vastus lateralis	Greater trochanter, femur	Patella, tibial tuberosity	Leg extension
Vastus intermedius	Femoral shaft	Patella, tibial tuberosity	Leg extension
Vastus medialis	Intertrochanteric line	Patella, tibial tuberosity	Leg extension
Adductor longus	Pubis	Femoral shaft	Adduction
Adductor brevis	Pubic body, inferior rami	Femoral shaft	Adduction
Adductor magnus	Ischiopubic ramus, ischial tuberosity	Femoral shaft, adductor tubercle	Adduction, flexion, extension
Gracilis	Pubic body, inferior rami	Pes anserinus	Adduction, flexion, internal rotation
Pectineus	Superior pubic ramus	Femoral shaft	Adduction, flexion
Semitendinosus	Ischial tuberosity	Pes anserinus	Hip extension, knee flexion
Semimembranosus	Ischial tuberosity	Tibia	Hip extension, knee flexion
Biceps femoris	Ischial tuberosity	Fibular head (long head), lateral tibia (short head)	Hip extension, knee flexion

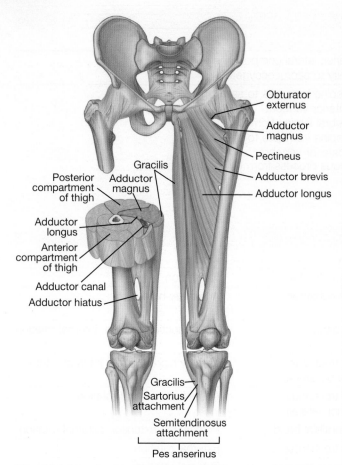

Fig 117.4 Muscle attachments of the pelvis and leg. (From Drake RL, Vogl AW, Mitchell A, eds. *Gray's Basic Anatomy*. 2nd ed. Philadelphia: Elsevier; 2018.)

- Origin, insertion, and main muscle activity with regard to function in the hip or pelvis are noted (Fig. 117.4).

Soft Tissues

- Femoral triangle: Formed by the adductor longus (medially), sartorius (laterally), and inguinal ligament (superiorly).
- The femoral artery and inguinal lymph nodes are palpable within the triangle.
- The femoral nerve lies lateral to and the femoral vein lies medial to the femoral artery.
- The organization of the structures can be remembered by the pneumonic NAVEL (lateral to medial for the structures): nerve, artery, vein, empty space, lymphatics.

Neurovascular Structures and Bursae

- Nerves related to the hip and pelvis are listed in Table 117.4.
- Lumbar plexus: Originate as roots from the anterior divisions of T12 nerve and lumbar nerves L1-L4. These further divide to form the upper and lower trunks in the case of L1 and L2 nerves or anterior and posterior branches in the case of L2-L4 nerves.

- Terminal branches of the anterior division supply flexor muscles, whereas the posterior division supplies extensor and abductor muscles.
- In addition, many of these terminal branches provide sensory innervation to the pelvis and lower extremities.
- Sacral plexus: Provides important sensory and motor innervation in the pelvis and upper thigh and is formed by the anterior division of sacral nerves S1-S3 as well as the anterior division of the lumbar trunk (lumbar nerves L4-L5).
- The anterior branches of the plexus supply the flexor muscles, and the posterior branches supply the extensor and abductor muscles of the limb.
- The sacral plexus continues on to supply the lower extremities as the sciatic nerve, the largest nerve in the body.
- Pudendal plexus: Formed from the anterior divisions of S2-S4 and the coccygeal nerve, provides sensory and motor supply to the deep pelvic muscles and perineum.

Bursae

- Bursae function as lubrication sacs to decrease friction between musculoskeletal structures. Because of excessive friction, poor biomechanics, or trauma, these sacs can fill with fluid and become painful (bursitis). Common areas of involvement in the hip and pelvis include the trochanteric, iliopectineal, and ischial bursae.

Hip and Pelvis Biomechanics

- Hip joint: range of motion
- Abduction: 35 to 50 degrees (examine supine)
- Adduction: 20 to 35 degrees (examine supine)
- Flexion: 110 to 130 degrees (examine supine)
- Extension: 30 degrees (examine prone)
- Internal rotation: 30 to 35 degrees (examine with hip both extended and flexed)
- External rotation: 45 to 50 degrees (examine with hip both extended and flexed)
- Biomechanical force generation by the hip and pelvis muscles is extremely complex. Muscle length, tension, and the degree of hip or knee flexion are but a few of the factors that determine force transmission.
- Pubic symphysis: Motion at the pubic symphysis has been demonstrated to be very limited. Rotation is limited to 2 to 3 degrees, whereas translations of only 1 to 2 mm are common.
- Sacroiliac joint: Motion at the sacroiliac joint does occur in all three planes, but is also extremely limited to approximately 2 to 4 degrees of rotation and 1 to 2 mm of translation. This may increase slightly during pregnancy.

History

- The examiner should attempt to discern the following before examining the hip and pelvis:
  - Symptom onset: acute or chronic, duration, quality of pain, character, location
  - Groin pain (most commonly affects the hip joint), buttock or posterior thigh (spine), lateral thigh (trochanteric bursitis), anterior thigh (femur)
  - Exacerbating or relieving factors; pain with standing, ambulation, movement

TABLE 117.4 Nerves

Nerve	Location	Function
Lumbar Plexus Anterior Division		
Iliohypogastric nerve	From lumbar trunk L1	Provides sensory innervation to pubic region via anterior cutaneous branch Provides sensory innervation to posterolateral buttocks via lateral cutaneous branch
Ilioinguinal	From lumbar trunk L1	Provides sensory innervation to inguinal region, scrotum, base of penis
Genitofemoral	From lumbar trunks L1-L2	Provides sensory innervation to anteromedial high via lumboinguinal branch Provides motor innervation for cremasteric function via external spermatic branch Provides sensory innervation to scrotum and pubic region
Obturator	From ventral portion of L2-L4	Provides sensory innervation to inferior medial thigh Provides motor function to external oblique, adductor longus/brevis/magnus, gracilis, pectineus, obturator externus
Lumbar Plexus Posterior Division		
Lateral femoral cutaneous	From dorsal division of lumbar trunks L2-L3	Provides sensory innervation to lateral thigh through anterior and posterior branches
Femoral	From ventral lumbar trunks, L2-L4	Provides sensory innervation to anteromedial thigh Provides motor innervation to iliacus, pectineus, psoas, vastus lateralis/intermedius/medialis, rectus femoris, sartorius
Sacral Plexus Anterior Division		
Nerve to quadratus femoris	From L4-L5, S1 trunks	Provides innervation to quadratus femoris, inferior gemelli
Neve to obturator internus	From L5, S1-S2 trunks	Provides motor innervation to obturator internus, superior gemelli
Sciatic	From L4-L5, S1-S3 trunks Branches into tibial and common peroneal nerves	Provides motor innervation to biceps femoris long and short head, semimembranosus, semitendinosus, and distal lower leg musculature
Sacral Plexus Posterior Division		
Superior gluteal	From L4-L5, S1-S2	Provides motor innervation to gluteus medius, gluteus minimus, tensor fascia latae
Inferior gluteal	From L5, S1-S2 trunks	Provides motor innervation to gluteus maximus
Posterior femoral cutaneous nerve	From anterior and posterior divisions of S1-S3 trunks	Provides sensory innervation to posterior thigh, perineum, gluteal areas
Nerve to piriformis	From S2 trunk	Provides motor innervation to piriformis
Pudendal Plexus		
Pudendal nerve	From S2-S4 trunks	Provides sensory innervation to perineum, penis, urethral sphincter, anal sphincter

- Paresthesia or weakness, muscle atrophy or fatigue, cool extremities
- Snapping, popping, slipping sensation, clicking, catching, grinding
- Trauma, falls, or overuse (premeditative loading) factors

Suggested Readings

Armstrong AD, Hubbard MC, eds. *Essentials of Musculoskeletal Care*. 5th ed. Rosemont, IL: American Academy of Orthopaedic Surgeons; 2016.

Braly B, Beall DP, Martin HD. Clinical examination of the athletic hip. *Clin Sports Med*. 2006;25:199–210.

Cohen SP. Sacroiliac joint pain: a comprehensive review of anatomy, diagnosis, and treatment. *Anesth Analg*. 2005;101:1440–1453.

Gray H. *Anatomy of the Human Body*. Philadelphia: Lea & Febiger; 1918.

Hoppenfeld S. *Physical Examination of the Spine and Extremities*. Norwalk, CT: Appleton-Century-Crofts; 1976.

Miller MD, Thompson SR, eds. *DeLee and Drez's Orthopaedic Sports Medicine: Principles and Practices*. 4th ed. Philadelphia: Elsevier; 2015.

Netter FH, Colacino S, eds. *Atlas of Human Anatomy*. Summit, NJ: CIBA-GEIGY; 1989.

Thompson JC. *Netter's Concise Orthopaedic Anatomy*. 2nd ed. Philadelphia: Elsevier; 2016. (Updated Edition).

Tory MR, Schenker ML, Martin HD, et al. Neuromuscular hip biomechanics and pathology in the athlete. *Clin Sports Med*. 2006;25: 179–197.

Walheim GG, Selvik G. Mobility of the pubic symphysis. In vivo measurements with an electromechanic method and a roentgen stereophotogrammetric method. *Clin Orthop Relat Res*. 1984;191:129–135.

Chapter 118 Physical Examination of the Hip and Pelvis

F. Winston Gwathmey, Jr., Benjamin A. Tran

ICD-10-CM CODES
M25.559 *Pain in unspecified hip*
M70.70 *Bursitis of unspecified hip*
M24.85 *Other specific joint derangements of hip, not elsewhere classified*
M25.859 *Femoroacteabular impingement*

It should be noted that lumbar spine, knee, and intra-abdominal pathology can manifest with hip symptoms. Thus, systematic physical examination of the hip should also include a clinical assessment of the lumbar spine and knee.

Inspection

- Begin by inspecting the patient in a standing position
  - Observe pelvic and spine alignment, noting any kyphosis, lordosis, or scoliosis.
  - Examine the patient's skin for scars from previous surgeries, effusion, discoloration, erythema, and muscle atrophy.
  - Assess stance for symmetry. In a standing position, flexion of the hip and ipsilateral knee is commonly observed in patients with an irritated hip

- Evaluate the patient's gait for symmetry, speed, Trendelenburg gait, antalgic gait, or other abnormalities
- Measure true leg length with the patient in a supine position (Table 118.1)

Palpation

- Palpate bony landmarks, including iliac crest, to assess for iliac crest apophysitis, anterosuperior iliac spine (site of origin of sartorius muscle), anteroinferior iliac spine (insertion site of rectus muscle), pubic symphysis to assess for stress fracture and osteitis pubis, ischium, greater trochanter, trochanteric bursa, and sacroiliac joint.
- Palpate soft tissues including muscles around the hip, femoral pulse, lymph nodes, and the sciatic nerve as it exits the sciatic notch.

Range of Motion (Video 118.1)

- Evaluate both active and passive range of motion with special note taken of any clicking, catching, popping, or snapping during examination (Figs. 118.1 and 118.2). Normal range of motion parameters are noted in Table 118.2.

TABLE 118.1 Special Physical Examination Tests of the Hip

Test	Physical Maneuver	Positive Test	Suggested Diagnosis
90–90 straight leg	With patient supine, flex hip and knee to 90 degrees, stabilize pelvis and have patient extend knee	Unable to extend knee to full extension	Hamstring muscle tightness
Ely test	With patient prone, passively flex knee	Ipsilateral hip flexion	Rectus femoris tightness
FABER (Patrick's) test (see Fig. 118.1C)	With the patient supine, passively flex, abduct, and externally rotate hip and place ipsilateral ankle over the contralateral knee. Apply downward traction on knee	1. Ipsilateral sacroiliac joint pain 2. Ipsilateral groin pain	1. Sacroiliac joint involvement 2. Anterior hip capsular irritation
Leg length	With the patient supine, measure from anterosuperior iliac spine to medial malleoli	>1 cm of side-to-side difference	Leg length discrepancy
Log roll	With patient supine and hip extended, passively rotate hip internally and externally	Loss of motion, pain	Hip joint irritability
Ober's test (see Fig. 118.1B and Video 118.2)	With patient lying on side and hip extended, flex knee 90 degrees and passively abduct hip	Leg stays in abduction when support is removed	Tight hip abductors (Iliotibial band)

Continued

TABLE 118.1 Special Physical Examination Tests of the Hip—cont'd

Test	Physical Maneuver	Positive Test	Suggested Diagnosis
Piriformis test	With patient on side, abduct and flex hip and apply downward traction on upper flexed knee while lower leg is fully extended	Pain in hip or pelvis, may resemble shooting pain down leg	Piriformis involvement, consider impingement on sciatic nerve by piriformis
Straight leg raise	With patient supine, passively flex hip and extend knee until tight or pain	Radiation of pain down leg (ipsilateral or contralateral)	Herniated disc with radiculopathy
Resisted hip flexion (Stinchfield test) (see Fig. 118.2A)	With patient supine and hip actively flexed 30 degrees and knee extended, apply downward traction proximal to knee	Groin pain	Iliopsoas tendonitis or intra-articular pathology
Thomas test	With patient supine, stabilize lumbar spine and passively flex knee to chest	Elevation of contralateral hip or flexion of contralateral knee	Hip flexion contracture
Trendelenburg's sign	With patient standing on involved hip, lift the contralateral leg	Pelvis on contralateral side drops	Hip abductor or gluteus weakness
Anterior impingement sign (FADDIR test) (see Fig. 118.1D)	With patient supine, passively hyperflex, adduct, and internally rotate hip	Reproduction of pain and symptoms along anterior groin	Femoroacetabular impingement or labral tear
Resisted sit-up (see Fig. 118.2B)	With patient supine, stabilize hips and have patient perform a sit-up	Pain in groin	Athletic pubalgia

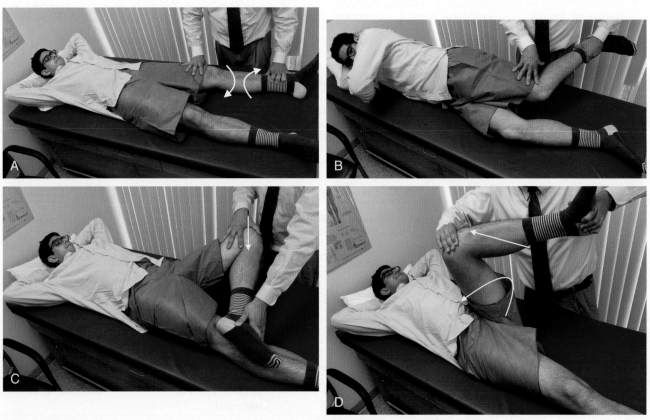

Fig 118.1 Passive special tests of hip. (A) Log roll. (B) Ober's test. (C) FABER (Patrick) test. (D) FADDIR test.

TABLE 118.2 Normal Hip Range of Motion

Motion	Flexion	Extension	Abduction	Adduction	Internal Rotation	External Rotation	Flexed External Rotation	Flexed Internal Rotation
Range in degrees	120	0–15	30–50	30	30	40–60	60	30

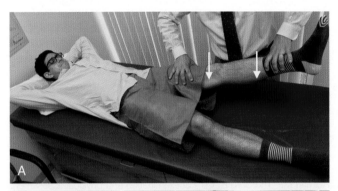

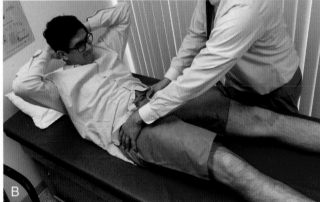

Fig 118.2 Active special tests of hip. **(A)** Resisted hip flexion (Stinchfield test). **(B)** Resisted sit-up.

- Extension may best be measured with the patient laying prone and passively lifting the patient's ankle upward off the table.
- The log roll maneuver (see Fig. 118.1A) provides a basic assessment of hip internal and external rotation. However, with the patient supine, flex the patient's hip and ipsilateral knee to 90 degrees and passively rotate the hip for consistent and accurate measurements of internal and external rotation.
  - In this maneuver, internal rotation of the hip occurs when the ankle is moved outward laterally and external rotation occurs when the ankle is passively moved inward (Fig. 118.3).

Strength Testing

- Test the patient's active range of motion against resistance to assess strength of the four functional muscle groups including anterior flexors, lateral abductors, medial adductors, and posterior extensors
- Grade the patient's bilateral hip strength on a scale of 0 to 5
- The physical maneuvers for strength testing are detailed in Table 118.3

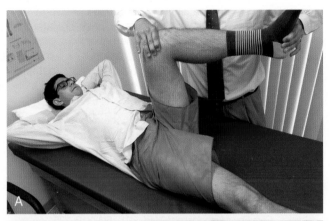

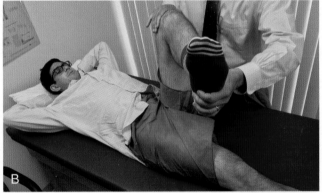

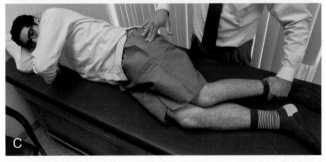

Fig 118.3 Assess range-of-motion internal rotation **(A)** and external rotation **(B)** in supine position. Palpation of greater trochanter **(C)**.

Neurovascular

- Complete neurovascular examination of bilateral lower extremities, including measuring peripheral pulses (posterior tibialis and dorsalis pedis pulses), and test sensation in dermatome distribution (L1-S2 sensory nerve distribution).

The previous physical examination serves as a basic screening of the hip. Special tests are used to further assess for hip pathology (see Table 118.1).

TABLE 118.3 Strength Testing of Hip Muscles

Muscle Groups	Flexors	Extensors	Abductors	Adductors	Internal Rotation	External Rotation
Physical Maneuver	With the patient in a seated position, ask the patient to lift their thigh against applied downward resistance	With the patient in a seated position and thigh flexed, ask the patient to extend hip against resistance	With the patient supine, apply resistance against lateral proximal knee while patient abducts hips	With the patient supine, apply resistance against medial proximal knee while patient adducts hips	With the patient supine, flex the hip and knee to 90 degrees, stabilize the knee and apply resistance to medial malleolus and have patient to internally rotate hip	With the patient supine, flex the hip and knee to 90 degrees, stabilize the knee and apply resistance to lateral malleolus and have patient to internally rotate hip

Suggested Readings

Byrd JWT. Evaluation of the hip: history and physical examination. *N Am J Sports Phys Ther*. 2007;2(4):231–240.

Martin HD, Palmer IJ. History and physical examination of the hip: the basics. *Curr Rev Musculoskelet Med*. 2013;6(3):219–225.

Poultsides LA, Bedi A, Kelly BT. An algorithmic approach to mechanical hip pain. *HSS J*. 2012;8(3):213–224.

Reiman MP, Thorborg K. Clinical examination and physical assessment of hip joint-related pain in athletes. *Int J Sports Phys Ther*. 2014;9(6): 737–755.

Chapter 119 Femoroacetabular Impingement

Kyle Hammond, Ryan Urchek

ICD-10-CM CODES
M25.851	*Femoroacetabular impingement, right*
M25.852	*Femoroacetabular impingement, left*
M21.951	*Hip deformity, right*
M21.952	*Hip deformity, left*
S73.191A	*Labral tear, right*
S73.192A	*Labral tear, left*
M24.051	*Loose body, right*
M24.052	*Loose body, left*

Key Concepts

- Femoroacetabular impingement (FAI) is abnormal contact between the proximal femur and acetabulum that leads to chondral and/or labral damage and symptoms
- "Pincer deformity" describes acetabular overcoverage, more common in middle-aged women and more likely to cause labral pathology (Fig. 119.1)
- "Cam deformity" describes a nonspherical femoral head with decreased head-neck offset, more common in young athletic males and more likely to cause articular damage (see Fig. 119.1)
- Most cases of FAI are a combined disorder
- More than 90% of labral tears occur in conjunction with FAI
- FAI may lead to early-onset osteoarthritis
- Appropriate treatment must match the appropriate patient

History

- Due to the overlap of symptoms, it is important to differentiate between potential back, hip, and pelvis etiologies
- Most patients with FAI complain of pain in the anterior groin or lateral hip with insidious onset and no specific injury
- A subset of patients (25%) may complain of lumbar spine, buttock, or referred pain to the knee
- Patients may display the classic "C" sign with their hand when describing the location of the pain
- Pain is often worse with activity and exacerbated by hip flexion

Physical Examination

- Observation
  - Antalgic gait
  - Positive Trendelenburg gait if abductor weakness is present
- Palpation
  - Assess for tenderness which may rule out other etiologies such as trochanteric bursitis
- Range of motion
  - Examine while supine at full extension and at 90 degrees of hip flexion, compare to contralateral limb
  - Hallmark feature is less than 10 to 20 degrees of painful internal rotation while the hip is at 90 degrees of flexion
- Special Tests
  - Anterior impingement test causes pain with flexion, adduction, and internal rotation (Fig. 119.2)
  - Log roll and Stinchfield tests are sensitive but not specific for intra-articular hip pathology
  - Apprehension with hip extension and external rotation may indicate hip dysplasia or instability, while pain with this maneuver may indicate posterior impingement

Imaging

- Radiographs: standing AP pelvis, false profile, Dunn view, frog-lateral views
  - A high-quality AP pelvis assesses for osteoarthritis, proximal femur deformity, acetabular depth and coverage. Findings can include coxa profunda, coxa protrusio, crossover sign, posterior wall sign, ischial spine sign, os acetabulum, and/or "pistol-grip" deformity (Fig. 119.3). Measurement of lateral center edge angle should be performed
  - False profile view may reveal excessive anterior overcoverage
  - Dunn and frog-lateral views are used for femoral cam morphology assessment with α angle values >50 degrees indicating significant cam deformity (Fig. 119.4)
    - 45-degree Dunn may be more sensitive than 90-degree Dunn view
- Computed tomography (CT)
  - 3D reconstruction is helpful for surgical planning of bony resection
- Magnetic resonance imaging (MRI) arthrogram
  - Helpful in diagnosing concomitant labral tears or chondral damage
  - Helpful for diagnosis if intra-articular anesthetic injection is performed at same time

Differential Diagnosis

- Osteoarthritis: chronic stiffness, aching, narrow joint space on radiographs

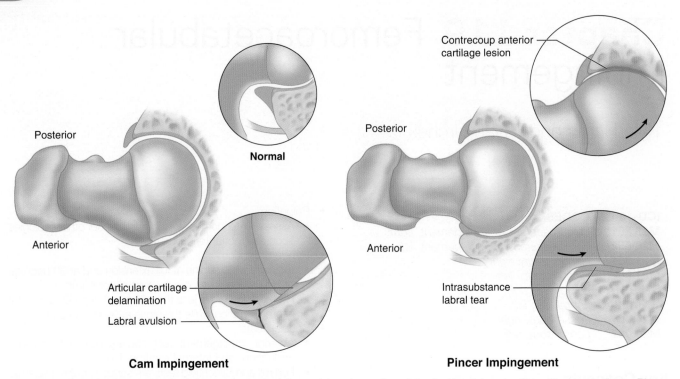

Fig 119.1 Cam impingement depicting nonspherical femoral head causing delamination injury to the articular cartilage. Pincer impingement depicting overcoverage of the femoral head by the acetabulum injuring the entrapped labrum. (From Thompson SR, Miller MD. Sports medicine. In: Miller MD, Thompson SR eds. *Miller's Review of Orthopaedics.* 7th ed. Philadelphia: Elsevier; 2016:364, Fig 4.23.)

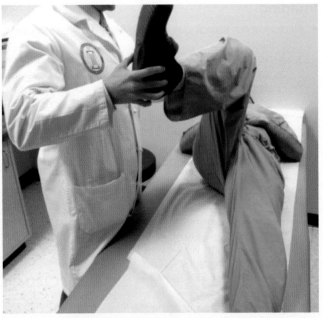

Fig 119.2 Anterior hip impingement test, aka FADIR test. The examiner flexes, adducts, and internally rotates the patient's hip, which with a positive test will recreate groin/hip articular symptoms.

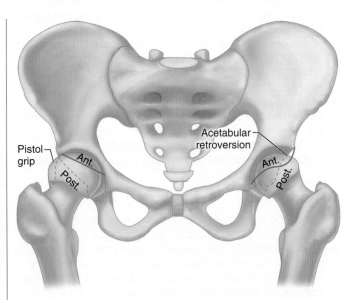

Fig 119.3 Right hip depicting pistol grip deformity commonly seen on x-ray with cam impingement. Left hip depicting the crossover sign seen on x-ray with acetabular retroversion. (From Thompson SR, Miller MD. Sports medicine. In: Miller MD, Thompson SR eds. *Miller's Review of Orthopaedics*. 7th ed. Philadelphia: Elsevier; 2016:365, Fig 4.24.)

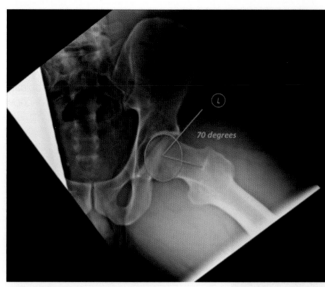

Fig 119.4 Dunn lateral radiograph of the left hip, which shows an outline of how one might calculate the alpha angle of the femoral CAM lesion, as the bone contour exits the circle around the femoral head.

70 degrees

- Lumbar spine pathology: back pain with radiating symptoms past the knee
- Loose bodies: mechanical symptoms with history of trauma
- Ruptured ligamentum teres: forceful twisting injury, catching, and popping
- Trochanteric bursitis: point tenderness of greater trochanter, negative radiographic signs of FAI
- Athletic pubalgia: pain with resisted sit-ups and negative radiographic signs of FAI
- Coxa Saltans: snapping hip on history/exam with negative radiographic signs of FAI

Treatment

- Nonsurgical management
  - Initial activity modification, antiinflammatory medications, and physical therapy
  - Although therapy may help symptoms, it is unlikely to affect natural history of FAI or alter progression of degenerative changes
- Surgical management
  - Indicated when above conservative treatment fails. Treatment can be performed via open surgical hip dislocation and/or arthroscopic techniques.
  - Arthroscopic options (Fig. 119.5) include acetabuloplasty, labral repair versus debridement, cam deformity resection (femoroplasty), ligamentum teres debridements, loose body removal, cartilage restoration techniques, capsular management, and benign neoplasm removal.
  - Periacetabular osteotomy may be indicated in patients with structural deformity of acetabulum with poor coverage of femoral head, resulting in dysplasia.

- Total hip arthroplasty is indicated if end-stage hip arthritis is present.

When to Refer

- In patients where appropriate workup has included ruling out lumbar spine, hip, and other pelvis etiology who have failed conservative treatment for FAI and/or labral tear
- Having appropriate XRs, CT, and/or MRI prior to referral may assist in diagnosis and expedient treatment for surgical candidates
- Younger patients with normal cartilage may benefit from hip-preserving procedures such as hip arthroscopy
- Older patients with advanced degenerative changes may benefit from hip joint arthroplasty procedures

Prognosis

- Proper patient selection is critical to successful surgical treatment of FAI
- Reduced pain and improved function is seen in the majority of patients after the appropriate surgical treatment is performed
- Presence of Outerbridge grade 3 or higher, or Tonnis grade 2 or higher, osteoarthritis is strongest predictor for poor outcomes following hip arthroscopy
- Residual impingement is leading cause of continued postoperative pain and revision surgery following arthroscopy

Troubleshooting

- The patient should be counseled on the benefits and risks of surgery
  - Risks specific to hip arthroscopy in this setting can include nerve injuries secondary to traction or aberrant portal placement, iatrogenic chondral or labral injuries, femoral neck fractures in the setting of excessive cam resection, heterotopic ossification, osteonecrosis, intraabdominal fluid extravasation, or failure to adequately resect requiring revision surgery

Patient Instructions

- Physical therapy focusing on core strength, hip muscular mobility, and strengthening
- Low-impact activities such as stationary bike or swimming should be encouraged
- Protected weight bearing with gradual increase in activity following hip arthroscopy depending on the procedure performed

Considerations in Special Populations

- It is important to match the proper surgical treatment to the individual patient
- Older patients, longer duration of symptoms, more severe preoperative pain, and poorer functional scores are associated with poorer outcomes following hip arthroscopy
- Patients with hip dysplasia and less than 20 degrees may be more appropriate for a periacetabular osteotomy instead of hip arthroscopy

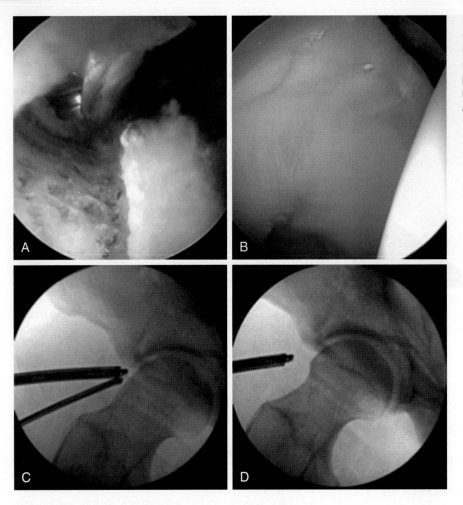

Fig 119.5 Intraoperative procedures. **(A)** Acetabuloplasty of the right hip; **(B)** Completed labral repair of the right hip; **(C)** Delineation of the femoral CAM lesion prior to femoroplasty on intraoperative fluoroscopy; and **(D)** Completed femoroplasty assessment on intraoperative fluoroscopy.

Suggested Readings

Bohunovic L, Nho SJ. Femoroacetabular impingement. In: *Orthopaedic Knowledge Update, Sports Medicine*. 5th ed. Rosemont, IL: American Academy of Orthopaedic Surgeons; 2016:127–140.

Byrd JWT. Femoroacetabular impingement in athletes. *Am J Sports Med*. 2013;42(3):737–751.

Byrd JWT, Jones KS. Arthroscopic management of femoroacetabular impingement in athletes. *Am J Sports Med*. 2011;39(suppl 1):7S–13S.

Kahn M, Habib A, Larson C, et al. Arthroscopy up to date: hip femoroacetabular impingement. *Arthroscopy*. 2016;32(1):177–189.

Miller MD, Thompson SR. Femoroacetabular impingement. In: *Miller's Review of Orthopaedics*. 7th ed. Philadelphia: Elsevier; 2016:364–365.

Nepple JJ, Byrd JWT, Siebenrock KA. Overview of treatment options, clinical results, and controversies in the management of femoroacetabular impingement. *J Am Acad Orthop Surg*. 2013;21(suppl 1):S53–S58.

Nepple JJ, Prather H, Trousdale RT, et al. Clinical diagnosis of femoroacetabular impingement. *J Am Acad Orthop Surg*. 2013;21(suppl 1):S16–S19.

Nepple JJ, Prather H, Trousdale RT, et al. Diagnostic imaging of femoroacetabular impingement. *J Am Acad Orthop Surg*. 2013;21(suppl 1):S20–S26.

Chapter 120 Hip Instability

Kyle Hammond, Andrew Schwartz

ICD-10-CM CODES
S73.005A *Unspecified dislocation of hip, left*
S73.005B *Unspecified dislocation of hip, right*
M25.559 *Pain: hip*
Q65.9 *Congenital deformity of hip, unspecified (dysplasia of hip)*

Key Concepts

- The hip joint is intrinsically stable and requires significant force to dislocate (Fig. 120.1).
- Ligaments of hip
  - Iliofemoral: anterior inferior iliac spine to intertrochanteric line
  - Pubofemoral: superior pubic ramus to femoral neck
  - Ischiofemoral: posterior acetabular/ischial rim to intertrochanteric crest
- The labrum is predominantly fibrocartilage and circumferentially covers the acetabulum (Fig. 120.2). The labrum deepens the acetabulum, enhancing stability and articular congruity, while contributing 10% of femoral head coverage.
- The vascular supply to the femoral head arises from the ring anastomosis of the medial (predominant) and lateral circumflex arteries. A minor contribution comes from the obturator artery via the ligamentum teres.
- The sciatic nerve runs posterior to the hip joint and may be stretched or compressed with posterior dislocations, or become incarcerated in associated acetabular fractures.
- The obturator nerve runs through the superolateral obturator foramen. The femoral nerve is anteromedial to the hip. Both are at risk with anterior dislocations.
- Mechanism of injury
  - The direction of the dislocation and associated injuries are dependent on the position of the hip and the direction of the force vector (Table 120.1).
  - Posterior dislocation (Figs. 120.1B and 120.3): axial load through the knee with a flexed and possibly adducted hip or knee driven into immovable object during hip flexion (i.e., knee driven into ground during football tackle)
    - Posterior dislocations comprise more than 80% of traumatic dislocations and approximately 90% of those occurring during athletic competitions.
  - Anterior dislocation (Figs. 120.1B and 120.4): flexed hip forced into extreme abduction and external rotation (i.e., performing splits during gymnastics)
  - Associated injuries: ipsilateral fractures of the proximal and diaphyseal femur, pelvis, patella, and acetabulum. Ipsilateral connective tissue injuries include knee ligaments, and neurovascular compromise (sciatic nerve, obturator nerve, femoral nerve/artery).

History

- Posterior dislocation: acute pain in buttock/groin after force to flexed hip and knee, with possible sensorimotor complaints in sciatic distribution
- Anterior dislocation: acute pain in thigh/groin after external rotation of abducted hip or direct blow to posterior hip, with possible sensorimotor complaints in femoral and/or obturator distributions

Physical Examination

- Posterior dislocation: leg flexed, adducted, and internally rotated. Leg length discrepancy with ipsilateral leg shortening, possible sciatic nerve palsy
  - Peroneal division (more commonly affected): foot eversion/dorsiflexion, lateral leg and dorsum of the foot sensation
  - Tibial division: foot plantarflexion, posterior leg and plantar foot sensation
- Anterior dislocation: leg flexed or extended, abducted, and externally rotated. Leg length discrepancy with ipsilateral leg shortening or lengthening, possible femoral/obturator nerve palsies
  - Femoral nerve: anteromedial thigh, hip and knee flexion
  - Obturator nerve: inferomedial thigh, thigh adduction
- Distal vascular exam: dorsalis pedis, posterior tibial arteries

Imaging

- Single anteroposterior (AP) view of the pelvis for diagnosis (see Figs. 120.1B, 120.3, and 120.4)
- Postreduction radiographs to identify associated injuries (femur, acetabular fractures, pelvic fractures) and to verify concentric reduction
  - Pelvis views: AP, Judet acetabular, pelvic inlet/outlet
  - Hip views: AP/lateral
- Computed tomography to better characterize associated injuries, identify intra-articular loose bodies
- Magnetic resonance imaging (MRI) to diagnose cartilaginous injuries, capsular injuries, and osseous issues, such as osteonecrosis (AVN)
  - MRI 2 to 6 weeks after hip dislocation to evaluate for femoral head ischemia to intervene prior to osteonecrosis (AVN); however MRI may need to be repeated at a later date as well because AVN can have a delayed presentation after a dislocation.

Differential Diagnosis

- Acetabulum fracture with noncongruent joint or intra-articular loose body

A Stable Hip Joint   B Diagnostic AP Pelvis X-ray   C Evaluation and Treatment

Anterior dislocation (superior)

Line of attachment
around head of femur
of synovial membrane
Iliofemoral ligament
Fibrous membrane
Zona orbicularis
(inner circular
fibers of fibrous
membrane)
Head of femur

Synovial membrane
reflects back to
attach to margin of
acetabulum
Zona orbicularis
(inner circular
fibers of fibrous
membrane)

Pubofemoral
ligament

Synovial
membrane

Posterior dislocation

- X-ray, femoral head is dislocated, femur is externally rotated
- Closed reduction Manager: Gentle hip flexion, adduction w: axial traction and slow internal rotation

- Early CT to evaluate for associated fractures
- Early range of motion as tolerated, delayed weightbearing for soft tissue healing
- Delayed MRI to evaluate for AVN

- X-ray, femoral head is dislocated, femur is internally rotated
- Closed reduction Manager: Flex hip Knee internally rotated hip w: axial traction

Fig 120.1 (A) The anatomy of a stable hip joint. **(B)** X-rays of anterior and posterior hip dislocations. **(C)** Management recommendations. *AVN,* Avascular necrosis; *CT,* computed tomography. (A, From Drake RL, Vogl AW, Mitchell AWM, et al, eds. *Gray's Atlas of Anatomy.* 2nd ed. Philadelphia, PA: Churchill Livingstone; 2015:299.)

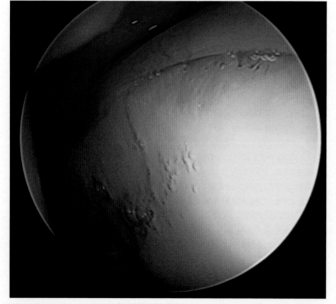

Fig 120.2 Arthroscopic imaging of a normal anatomic labrum around the periphery of the acetabulum in a left hip.

TABLE 120.1 Direction of the Dislocation Dependent on the Position of the Hip and Direction of the Force Vector

Hip Position, Force Vector	Type of Dislocation
Flexion, adduction, internal rotation	Posterior hip dislocation
Partial flexion, +/− adduction, internal rotation	Posterior fracture-dislocation
Flexion, abduction, external rotation	Anterior-inferior dislocation (obturator foramen)
Extension, abduction, external rotation	Anterior-superior dislocation (superior to superior pubic ramus)

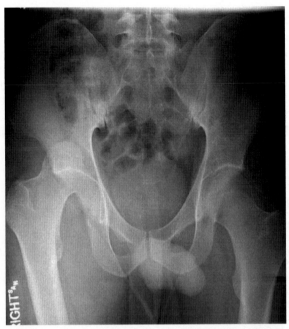

Fig 120.3 AP pelvis radiograph of a posterior hip dislocation.

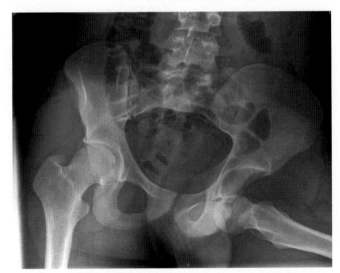

Fig 120.4 AP pelvis radiograph of an anterior hip dislocation.

- Femoral head or neck fracture
- Intertrochanteric/subtrochanteric femur fracture

Treatment (see Fig. 120.1C)

- At diagnosis
  - Urgent closed reduction under complete sedation in the supine position while an assistant stabilizes the hemipelvis
    - Posterior dislocation: hip and knee maximally flexed to relax the hamstring musculature. Steady axial traction

to overcome muscular spasm and elastic restraints is applied to the internally rotated and adducted extremity.
    - Anterior dislocation: steady axial traction to overcome muscular spasm and elastic restraints is continuously applied in line with the deformity with gentle hip flexion, adduction, and internal rotation to achieve reduction.
- Later
  - Active and passive hip range of motion should begin as soon as possible to avoid intra-articular adhesions and stiffness associated with immobilization.
  - Standard anterior or posterior hip precautions should be applied during the first 6 weeks after the injury to allow capsular and soft-tissue restraints adequate time to heal.
  - Toe-touch weight bearing progressing to weight bearing as tolerated by 6 weeks, during which time aggressive physical therapy is initiated to maintain range of motion and strengthen hip rotators.
  - Return to high-demand athletics should be delayed until the strength of the hip normalizes and the hip is pain free, as well as once all intra-articular processes have been treated to lessen recurrent injury or damage with sports.

When to Refer

- Patient reports mechanical symptoms (catching, locking) or sharp pain localized to the hip region.
- Patient reports continued symptoms of hip instability.
- Treatment considerations
  - Hip arthroscopy to address loose bodies and identify labral tears and cartilage lesions (femoral and acetabular), which may be amenable to repair, débridement, or chondroplasty, and to address impingement lesions that may predispose to recurrent instability and/or capsular procedures.

Prognosis

- The outcome ranges from a normal hip to a severely painful/degenerated hip joint.
- 48% to 95% of patients have a good or excellent outcome after pure posterior dislocations, with outcomes varying depending on associated injuries (fractures).
- Arthritis
  - Most common complication
  - Increased incidence after posterior dislocations and fracture-dislocations
  - Seen in approximately 50% of fracture-dislocations
- Avascular necrosis (AVN), also referred to as osteonecrosis
  - Rates vary in the literature from 1% to 40%.
  - Increased incidence after posterior dislocation, which correlates with the duration of the dislocation
  - The literature suggests that reduction of the hip joint within 6 hours of dislocation reduces the rate to 0% to 10%.
  - Symptoms and/or radiographic findings may likely present years after injury.

Troubleshooting

- Sciatic nerve dysfunction
  - Occurs in 5% to 30% of posterior hip dislocations
  - If sciatic nerve injury occurs after closed reduction, then entrapment of the nerve is possible and surgical exploration may be indicated; otherwise, nonsurgical management (physical therapy, ankle-foot orthosis) and observation are indicated for as long as 1 year.
- Indications for open reduction after hip dislocation
  - Irreducible/nonconcentric dislocation
  - Ipsilateral femoral neck fracture

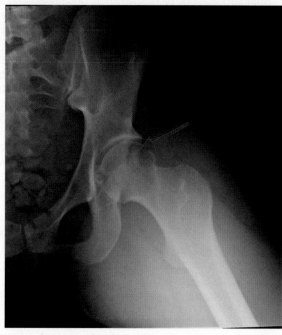

Fig 120.5 Lateral radiograph of the hip. *Arrow* shows a residual posterior acetabular wall fracture that has gone on to a nonunion, 1 year postinjury in a collegiate basketball player after a hip instability event.

Considerations in Special Populations

- Hip subluxation
  - Occurs when a patient falls on a flexed knee and hip or suddenly stops and pivots vigorously over the weight-bearing extremity causing the femoral head to shift out of the joint onto the acetabular rim and then spontaneously reduce
  - Radiographs and advanced imaging can define injury patterns in athletes.
    - Posterior acetabular lip fracture (Fig. 120.5)

Suggested Readings

Begly JP, Robins B, Youm T. Arthroscopic treatment of traumatic hip dislocation. *J Am Acad Orthop Surg*. 2016;24(5):309–317.

Dumont GD. Hip instability: current concepts and treatment options. *Clin Sports Med*. 2016;35:435–447.

Foulk DM, Mullis BH. Hip dislocation: evaluation and management. *J Am Acad Orthop Surg*. 2010;18(4):199–209.

Ilizaliturri VM Jr, Gonzalez-Gutierrez B, Gonzalez-Ugalde H, Camacho-Galindo J. Hip arthroscopy after traumatic hip dislocation. *Am J Sports Med*. 2011;39(suppl):50s–57s.

Mullis BH, Dahners LE. Hip arthroscopy to remove loose bodies after traumatic dislocation. *J Orthop Trauma*. 2006;20(1):22–26.

Pallia CS, Scott RE, Chao DJ. Traumatic hip dislocation in athletes. *Curr Sports Med Rep*. 2002;1(6):338–345.

Philippon MJ, Kuppersmith DA, Wolff AB, Briggs KK. Arthroscopic findings following traumatic hip dislocation in 14 professional athletes. *Arthroscopy*. 2009;25(2):169–174.

Poggi JJ, Callaghan JJ, Spritzer CE, et al. Changes on magnetic resonance images after traumatic hip dislocation. *Clin Orthop Relat Res*. 1995;319:249–259.

Sahin V, Karakas ES, Aksu S, et al. Traumatic dislocation and fracture-dislocation of the hip: a long-term follow-up study. *J Trauma*. 2003; 54(3):520–529.

Upadhyay SS, Moulton A, Srikrishnamurthy K. An analysis of the late effects of traumatic posterior dislocation of the hip without fractures. *J Bone Joint Surg Br*. 1983;65(2):150–152.

Yang RS, Tsuang YH, Hang YS, Liu TK. Traumatic dislocation of the hip. *Clin Orthop Relat Res*. 1991;265:218–227.

Chapter 121 Hip Osteoarthritis

Quanjun (Trey) Cui, Emanuel C. Haug

Key Concepts

- Osteoarthritis (OA) of the hip, also known as degenerative joint disease, is common in patients older than 40 years of age.
- OA can be classified into primary (or idiopathic) and secondary.
  - Risk factors for primary OA are shown in Box 121.1.
  - Risk factors for secondary OA are shown in Box 121.2.
- OA was once considered a normal process with aging, but is now recognized as a multifactorial process involving overuse, mechanical forces, joint integrity, local inflammation, and a possible genetic predisposition.
- Studies vary, but the incidence of symptomatic OA of the hip is estimated to be 88/100,000 per year.
- In 2010, the CDC reported 310,800 total hip replacements being done in patients above the age of 45 years.
- By 2030, the NIH estimates that 20% of Americans will be at risk of developing symptomatic OA, given the overall aging of the population.
- The pathogenesis of OA is poorly understood, but likely begins with injury to articular cartilage by the mechanical forces of macrotrauma or repeated microtrauma. There is growing evidence that this damage leads to inflammation and deranged chondrocyte metabolism. This in turn leads to thickening of the subchondral bone, abnormal bone structure (osteophytes), and synovial inflammation.
- Hip OA can be diagnosed by hip pain plus two of the following:
  - Erythrocyte sedimentation rate less than 20 mm/h
  - Radiographic evidence of femoral or acetabular osteophytes
  - Radiographic evidence of joint space narrowing (superior, axial, or medial)
  - This classification yields a sensitivity of 89% and specificity of 91%.
- Five percent of the population older than 65 years of age have radiographic evidence of hip OA. There is an inconsistent relationship between clinical symptoms and radiographic evidence, resulting in underestimation of the true prevalence.

- Nonoperative treatments include weight loss and low-impact aerobic exercises. Nonsteroidal antiinflammatory drugs (NSAIDs) and intra-articular steroid injections can be used to improve patient's pain and function.
- The most common surgical option, total hip arthroplasty (THA), is a highly successful procedure, having favorable long-term outcomes in terms of improvement of physical functioning, survivorship, and self-reported quality of life.

History

- Hip pain aggravated by activity and relieved with rest.
- Pain in the groin and buttock is most common in OA of the hip.
- Decreased range of motion of the hip joint due to pain and/or deformity.
- Morning stiffness of the hip joint that resolves in 30 to 60 minutes.
- As OA progresses, it may result in pain at rest or at night; this pain can radiate from the hip to the knee on the affected side.

Physical Examination

- Key findings on physical examination in advanced disease (note: the examination may be unremarkable in some patients)
  - Antalgic gait
  - Reduced internal rotation (<15 degrees)
  - Lack of full extension (>5 degrees flexion contracture)
  - Reduced hip flexion (<115 degrees)
  - Hip pain exacerbated by internal and external rotation with the knee in full extension

Imaging

- Obtain AP and lateral plain films of the hip and standing AP of pelvis.
- Key findings suggestive of OA, seen on weight-bearing anteroposterior pelvis plain radiographs (Fig. 121.1)
  - Joint space narrowing (normal is 4 to 5 mm)
  - Sclerosis along the joint space (subchondral sclerosis)
  - Osteophyte formation
  - Subchondral cyst formation
- Magnetic resonance imaging is typically not warranted for the diagnosis of OA but may be helpful when the diagnosis is in question.

Grading

- Kellgren and Lawrence described five radiographic stages of OA of the hip:

- Grade 0: normal
- Grade 1: possible narrowing of the joint space medially and possible osteophytes around femoral head
- Grade 2 (mild OA): definite narrowing of the joint space inferiorly, definite osteophytes, and slight sclerosis
- Grade 3 (moderate OA): marked narrowing of the joint space, slight osteophytes, some sclerosis and cyst formation, and deformity of the femoral head and acetabulum
- Grade 4 (severe OA): gross loss of joint space with sclerosis and cysts, marked deformity of the femoral head and acetabulum, and large osteophytes

---

BOX 121.1 **Risk Factors for Primary Osteoarthritis**

Older age
Female gender
Obesity (increased body mass index)
Muscle weakness
Proprioceptive deficits
Sports activities
Genetics
Occupations requiring heavy lifting or prolonged standing (farmers, construction workers)

BOX 121.2 **Risk Factors for Secondary Osteoarthritis**

Trauma (hip dislocation, intra-articular fractures)
Osteonecrosis
Rheumatoid arthritis
Gout
Developmental disorders (developmental dysplasia, slipped capital femoral epiphysis)
Septic arthritis
Calcium pyrophosphate crystal deposition disease
Paget disease
Legg-Calvé-Perthes disease
Diabetes mellitus
Hypothyroidism
Hyperparathyroidism
Acromegaly
Hemochromatosis
Hyperlaxity syndromes

- It is important to keep in mind that radiographic grading does not correlate to functional or pain impairment experienced by the patient.
- Tönnis classification is also commonly used to grade hip arthritis.

Differential Diagnosis

- Please see Box 121.3.

Treatment

- At diagnosis
  - Pain relief and function preservation are the primary treatment goals. At present, there are no disease-modifying agents.
  - The American Academy of Orthopaedic Surgeons (AAOS) updated their treatment recommendations in 2017.
  - Strong evidence supports that NSAIDs improve short-term pain, function, or both in patients with symptomatic OA of the hip. Drugs with clinical significance include naproxen, celecoxib, and diclofenac.
  - Literature does not support the use of glucosamine sulfate because it does not perform better than placebo for improving function, reducing stiffness, or decreasing pain for patients with symptomatic OA of the hip.
  - Modification of risk factors such as weight loss and avoidance of high-impact activities can slow the progress of the disease.

BOX 121.3 **Differential Diagnosis**

Trochanteric bursitis
Inflammatory arthritides
Septic joint
Osteonecrosis
Femoroacetabular impingement
Crystalline diseases
Lumbar radiculopathy
Lumbar spinal stenosis
Cancer (primary or metastatic)
Meralgia paresthetica
Iliotibial band syndrome
Vascular claudication

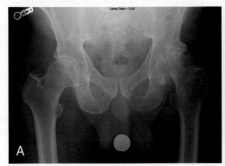 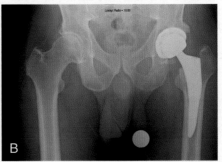

Fig 121.1 Weight-bearing anteroposterior plain pelvic radiograph of an 81-year-old male with chronic left hip pain. **(A)** shows the left hip with complete loss of joint space, subchondral sclerosis, cyst and osteophyte formation indicating Kellgren Grade 4 osteoarthritis, which was treated with total hip replacement **(B)**; while his right hip shows Grade 2 arthritis with joint space narrowing, slight sclerosis, and small osteophyte formation **(A and B)** that was managed conservatively.

- Strong evidence supports the use of physical therapy as a treatment to improve function and reduce pain for patients with OA of the hip and mild to moderate symptoms.
- May use assistive devices (e.g., cane, walker) as indicated.
- In only the most severe flare-ups, opioids can be prescribed for short-term use.
- Later
  - Steroid injections (under fluoroscopic guidance): Strong evidence supports the use of intra-articular corticosteroids to improve function and reduce pain in the short-term for patients with symptomatic OA of the hip.
  - Literature does not support the use of intra-articular hyaluronic acid because it does not perform better than placebo for function, stiffness, or pain in patients with symptomatic OA of the hip.

When to Refer

- When the patient experiences significant pain and/or disability despite conservative management, he or she may be a candidate for a total joint replacement.
- Severe deformity of the joint that may compromise successful surgery if delayed too long.

Prognosis

- Hip OA is a progressive disease.
- Total hip replacement is effective for reducing pain and disability.

Troubleshooting

- Counsel patients regarding the chronic nature of this condition.

- Counsel patients that they can slow the progression of this disease and delay (or avoid) the need for joint replacement if they modify their risk factors and restrict their exposure to high-impact activities.

Patient Instructions

- Follow physician and physical therapist instructions closely with respect to the type and quantity of activities that are acceptable: low-impact activities are recommended.
- Home- and community-based exercises are vital to the overall management of this disease process and should be performed diligently and regularly.
- Work to change those risk factors that are modifiable such as obesity.

Suggested Readings

American Academy of Orthopaedic Surgeons. *Management of osteoarthritis of the hip. OrthoGuidelines (website)*. Available at http://www.orthoguidelines.org/topic?id=1021. Accessed March 19, 2018.

Hochberg MC, Altman RD, April KT, et al. American College of Rheumatology 2012 recommendations for the use of nonpharmacologic and pharmacologic therapies in osteoarthritis of the hand, hip, and knee. *Arthritis Care Res (Hoboken)*. 2012;64(4):465–474.

Kellgren JH, Lawrence JS. Radiological assessment of osteo-arthrosis. *Ann Rheum Dis*. 1957;16(4):494–502.

Koenig L, Zhang Q, Austin MS, et al. Estimating the societal benefits of THA after accounting for work status and productivity: A Markov Model approach. *Clin Orthop Relat Res*. 2016;474(12):2645–2654.

Lane NE. Osteoarthritis of the hip. *N Engl J Med*. 2007;357:1413–1421.

National Institute on Aging. *Osteoarthritis (website)*. Available at https://www.nia.nih.gov/health/osteoarthritis. Accessed March 19, 2018.

Chapter 122 Osteonecrosis of the Hip

Quanjun (Trey) Cui

ICD-10-CM CODES

M87	*Osteonecrosis*
M87.0	*Idiopathic aseptic necrosis of bone*
M87.051	*Idiopathic aseptic necrosis of right femur*
M87.052	*Idiopathic aseptic necrosis of left femur*
M87.1	*Osteonecrosis due to drugs*
M87.151	*Osteonecrosis due to drugs, right femur*
M87.152	*Osteonecrosis due to drugs, left femur*
M87.2	*Osteonecrosis due to previous trauma*
M87.251	*Osteonecrosis due to previous trauma, right femur*
M87.252	*Osteonecrosis due to previous trauma, left femur*

Key Concepts

- Osteonecrosis (ON) of the femoral head is also known as avascular necrosis (AVN), aseptic necrosis, or ischemic necrosis of the femoral head. Association Research Circulation Osseous (ARCO) recommended using *osteonecrosis* to replace the old term *avascular necrosis*.
- ON generally occurs in younger patients; therefore early diagnosis and timely treatment is critical for preservation of the native hip joint.
- Pathogenesis of ON is poorly understood. Although many theories have been proposed, no one pathophysiologic mechanism has been identified as the etiology for the development of ON. Most authors believe that the mechanism involves impaired circulation to a specific area that ultimately becomes necrotic.
- Causes of ON fall under two major categories: traumatic and atraumatic. Traumatic causes mainly include femoral neck fracture and hip dislocation (with or without fracture). Atraumatic causes are many, but steroid use and alcoholism remain the most common risk factors (Box 122.1). The risk of ON associated with corticosteroids may not be clearly defined, but it has become a common cause of lawsuits.
- The prevalence of ON is unknown, but an estimated 10,000 to 20,000 cases are newly diagnosed each year in the United States.
- ON occurs more commonly in men with a male-to-female ratio 8:1 and in their most productive age with an average age of 38 (most common in their 30s, 40s, and 50s).
- The key to an early diagnosis is a high level of suspicion and clarification of known risk factors. Early diagnosis is best, but unfortunately most cases are diagnosed late in the disease process.

BOX 122.1 **Risk Factors Associated With Nontraumatic Osteonecrosis**

Systemic corticosteroid use
Heavy alcohol use
Systemic lupus erythematosus
Gaucher disease
Caisson disease (decompression sickness)
Sickle cell disease
Chronic renal failure
Organ transplantation
Pancreatitis
Hyperlipidemia
Radiation
Hypertension
Thrombosis
Cigarette smoking
Gout
Human immunodeficiency virus infection
Genetic predisposition (polymorphisms in VEGF, GR, 11β-HSD2, COL2A1, PAI1, *P*-glycoprotein)
Idiopathic

- X-rays are the first diagnostic test though are not sensitive for early stages of the disease. Therefore if suspicion is high, magnetic resonance imaging (MRI) should be performed.
- The size and location of the lesion and the stage of the disease will dictate prognosis and outcome of treatments. Core decompression with or without bone graft or stem cell therapy and total hip arthroplasty are the most common procedures for precollapse and postcollapse stages of the disease, respectively.
- Refer patients to an orthopaedic surgeon as soon as the ON diagnosis is confirmed so the joint preservation procedure can be performed in a timely manner.
- Variants of ON in children include Legg-Calvé-Perthes disease and that resulting from a slipped capital femoral epiphysis.

History

- Young adults with dull ache or throbbing pain in the groin or buttock area.
- With history significant for chronic use of glucocorticoid steroids and alcohol, or with associated risk factors such as organ transplant, chemotherapy, sickle cell disease, or lupus (see Box 122.1)

- Pain exacerbated with weight bearing and movement. Rest pain occurs in two thirds and night pain occurs in one third of the patients with ON.

Physical Examination

- Pain is usually deep in groin, no radiating pain.
- Gait and hip range of motion are generally normal until an advanced stage.
- Antalgic gait and limping when femoral head collapses and arthritis develops
- Once range limitations exist, severe pain can be produced with internal and external hip rotation.

Imaging

- Anteroposterior pelvis including both hips and cross table lateral, or frog leg lateral plain radiographs are the first line of study. Findings may include:

- Patchy areas of sclerosis and cyst formation of the femoral head (Fig. 122.1)
- The pathognomonic "crescent sign" (subchondral lucency) indicates collapse of the subchondral bone (see Fig. 122.1).
- Later findings include collapse of the femoral head and/or loss of its sphericity, joint-space narrowing, and degenerative changes of the joint (Fig. 122.2).
- If plain radiographs are normal and the index of suspicion remains high, MRI is sensitive and specific (both in the range of 97% to 100%) for this disease process (see Fig. 122.1). MRI is the study of choice for the early diagnosis of ON. The classic finding is the "double line sign" at the border between the necrotic and reparative zones. MRI of the bilateral hips and pelvis allows detection of additional lesions that may suggest a diagnosis other than ON.
- Scintigraphy may be useful if MRI is contraindicated or not available. Sensitivity of scintigraphy with single-photon emission computed tomography for detecting ON is approximately 88%. It is important to remember that

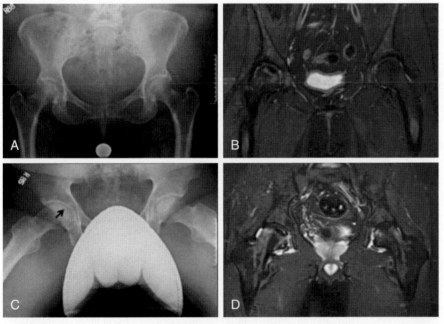

Fig 122.1 (A) Forty-year-old male patient with symptomatic osteonecrosis of the right hip. The plain AP radiograph looks unremarkable. But the T2 MRI **(B)** shows bone marrow edema indicating ARCO stage I osteonecrosis. **(C)** A crescent lucent subchondral line resulting from a subchondral fracture in a 35-year-old male patient *(black arrow)* indicating ARCO early-stage III osteonecrosis. **(D)** T2 MRI of the same patient shows subchondral edema around the fracture line.

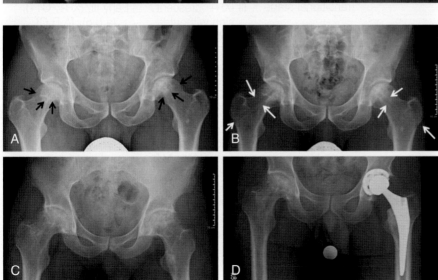

Fig 122.2 Sclerosis surrounding an osteopenic area in both hips (**A,** *black arrows*) but no collapse of the femoral head, indicating ARCO stage II disease, treated by core decompression *(white arrows)* and stem cell therapy (**B,** image obtained 5 years after surgery). **(C)** Collapsed femoral head in both hips with arthritic changes involving acetabulum. The current best treatment option available for this late stage disease is total hip arthroplasty **(D)**.

an abnormal bone scan can be the result of a number of other conditions affecting the hip joint.

Differential Diagnosis

- Osteoarthritis
- Femoroacetabular impingement (FAI)
- Septic joint
- Inflammatory arthritides
- Trochanteric bursitis
- Lumbar radiculopathy
- Lumbar spinal stenosis
- Meralgia paresthetica
- Iliotibial band syndrome

- Vascular claudication
- Crystalline diseases
- Cancer (primary or metastatic)

Classification

- Staging systems inform physicians about prognosis and treatment options.
- Association Research Circulation Osseous (ARCO) international system is commonly used with many features encompassing the older systems (Table 122.1).
- Other commonly used classification systems include Ficat and Arlet, Steinberg (The University of Pennsylvania), and the Japanese (see Table 122.1).

TABLE 122.1 Evolution and Comparison of Different Classification and Staging Systems for Osteonecrosis

	Marcus and Enneking (Florida)	Ficat and Arlet (French)	Modified Ficat and Arlet (French)	Steinberg (Philadelphia)	ARCO (International)
Year of introduction	1973	1977	1985	1984	1993
Pathology			0 (asymptomatic, XR–)		
Clinically at risk and symptomatic		I (symptomatic, XR–, biopsy+)	I (symptomatic, XR–, biopsy+)	0 (normal or nondiagnostic XR, bone scan, and MRI)	0 (all imaging studies negative)
Infarct/hyperemic marrow border	I (XR+/–)	II	II	I (XR–, bone scan+, MRI+), [A: mild <15%, B: moderate 15–30%, C: severe >30%]	I (XR–, CT–, scintigraph+, MRI+), {a: medial, b: central, c: lateral}, [area involvement: minimal A: <15%, moderate B: 15–30%, extensive C: >30%]
Granulation tissue repair, lucent, sclerosis, cysts, calcified marrow	II (XR+)			II (XR+), [A,B,C]	II (XR+, CT+, scintigraph+, MRI+), {a,b,c}, [A,B,C]
Subchondral fracture (crescent sign)	III		Transitional stage	III (XR+: crescent sign without collapse), [A,B,C]	Early III, (XR+, CT+), {a,b,c}, [A,B,C]
Collapse	IV	III	III	IV (XR+: flattening), [A,B,C]	Late III, (XR+, CT+), {a,b,c}, [A,B,C]
Early arthritis	V	IV	IV	V	IV (XR+)
Advanced arthritis	VI			VI	IV (XR+)
Contribution	Initial staging system	Acknowledged the need for a biopsy to confirm functional changes in bone	Acknowledged presence of ONFH with negative XR	Added MRI criteria and lesion size and category for subchondral fracture with no collapse	Added location of lesion

–, Negative; +, positive; (), general imaging tools; {}, location of the lesion; [], volume or size of the lesion; *ARCO*, Association Research Circulation Osseous; *ONFH*, osteonecrosis of the femoral head; *XR*, x-rays.

Modified from Cheng EY, from *Oxford Textbook of Orthopaedics and Trauma, Volume 2*, edited by Bulstrode, et al. (2002), by permission of Oxford University Press. In Choi HR, Steinberg ME, Cheng EY: Osteonecrosis of the femoral head: diagnosis and classification systems. *Curr Rev Musculoskelet Med.* 2015;8(3):210–220, Table 2.

Treatment

- The treatment of ON is controversial. The primary goal is to preserve the native joint for as long as possible.
- Although nonsurgical treatment options such as medications or using crutches can relieve pain and slow the progression of the disease, the most successful treatment options are surgical.
- Patients with very early stages of disease (prior to femoral head collapse) are good candidates for hip-preserving procedures such as core decompression and bone grafting/stem cell therapy (see Fig. 122.2).
- If ON has advanced to femoral head collapse or the acetabulum is involved, the most successful treatment is total hip replacement (see Fig. 122.2).

When to Refer

- At diagnosis

Prognosis

- Dependent on the lesion size and location, as well as the stage of the disease
- If diagnosed early (before femoral head collapse) and core decompression is performed (with or without bone grafting or stem cell therapy), the prognosis is better despite the various levels of reported success.
- If extensive (large lesion), lateral in location, prognosis is worse; total hip arthroplasty is the best treatment available.

Troubleshooting

- Counsel patients regarding the progressive and chronic nature of this condition.
- Counsel patients that the treatment of ON is controversial; eventually will need total hip replacement.

Patient Instructions

- See an orthopaedic surgeon as soon as the diagnosis is established.
- Follow physician and physical therapist instructions closely with respect to the type and quantity of activities that are acceptable; generally low-impact activities are recommended.
- Home- and community-based exercises are vital to the overall management of this disease process and should be performed diligently and regularly.
- Work to change those risk factors that are modifiable.

Considerations in Special Populations

- Legg-Calvé-Perthes disease (see Chapter 212)
- Slipped capital femoral epiphysis (see Chapter 213)

Suggested Readings

Kaushik AP, Das A, Cui Q. Stem cells in osteonecrosis: cons. In: Koo KH, Mont MA, Jones LC, eds. *Osteonecrosis*. New York: Springer; 2014:285–290.

Malizos KN, Karantanas AH, Varitimidis SE, et al. Osteonecrosis of the femoral head: etiology, imaging and treatment. *Eur J Radiol*. 2007;63:16–28.

Miller MD: *Osteonecrosis of the hip. OrthoInfo (website). American Academy of Orthopaedic Surgeons (AAOS)*, 2011. http://orthoinfo.aaos.org/topic.cfm?topic=a00216. Accessed April 24, 2018.

Mont MA, Cherian JJ, Sierra RJ, et al. Nontraumatic osteonecrosis of the femoral head: where do we stand today? A ten-year update. *J Bone Joint Surg Am*. 2015;97(19):1604–1627.

National Institutes of Health; *National Institute of Arthritis and Musculoskeletal and Skin Diseases: Osteonecrosis (website)*. 2015. https://www.niams.nih.gov/health-topics/osteonecrosis#tab-overview. Accessed April 24, 2018.

Weinstein RS. Glucocorticoid-induced osteonecrosis. *Endocrine*. 2012;41(2):183–190.

Chapter 123 Femoral Stress Fractures

Steven J. Magister, F. Winston Gwathmey, Jr.

ICD-10-CM CODE
M84.38   *Stress fracture, other site*

Key Concepts

- Femoral stress fractures have a variable incidence, constituting 7% to 20% of all stress fractures. Higher rates are seen in select populations where overuse mechanisms are more prominent, such as endurance athletes, and, classically, military recruits.
- Factors associated with an increased risk of femoral stress fractures are sudden increase in activity level, poor bone health, and femoral malalignment.
- Can be classified based on mechanism (overuse vs. insufficiency) or location (femoral neck vs. shaft)
  - Femoral neck stress fractures are further subdivided into tension type and compression type (Fig. 123.1).
- Overuse mechanisms are classically seen in runners, endurance athletes, and military recruits.
- Insufficiency mechanisms are secondary to poor bone quality and can be seen in osteoporosis, prolonged glucocorticoid or bisphosphonate use, and as a result of underlying medical conditions such as chronic kidney disease.
- Mainstay of treatment is conservative but can vary depending on fracture location (Fig. 123.2).

History

- Often insidious onset without history of a specific inciting event
- History of overuse or sudden increase in use is often present.
- Poorly localized pain is the most common presenting symptom.
  - Pain can be localized to the hip, inner groin, or thigh based on the location of the stress fracture.
- Pain is often worse with activity and relieved by rest.
- History can be overall unremarkable.

Physical Examination

- Often nonspecific pain that is reproducible by palpation and both active and passive range of motion
  - Hip range of motion exacerbates pain typically for femoral neck stress fractures as opposed to shaft fractures, but there may be some overlap.
- Fulcrum test is a specific but not sensitive test for femoral shaft stress fractures (Fig. 123.3).

Imaging

- Begin with plain radiographs
  - Often negative early in disease progression, but provides a baseline for follow-up imaging
- MRI is imaging modality of choice, especially in the setting of persistent pain with negative plain films (Fig. 123.4).
- MRI can show decreased cortical signal on T1-weighted images with corresponding increased cortical signal and marrow edema on T2 imaging.
- Bone scan has also been used historically but is widely being replaced by MRI.

Additional Tests

- Not needed. However, in the setting of an unclear etiology basic laboratory tests may be useful in evaluating for an underlying systemic cause.

Differential Diagnosis

- Differential is broad given nonspecific presentation and includes but not limited to:
  - Labral tear
  - Femoral acetabular impingement (FAI)
  - Muscular strain/tear
  - Ligamentous sprain/tear
  - Tendinous avulsion
  - Avascular necrosis
  - Osteoarthritis
  - Referred pain from abdominal or other musculoskeletal pathologies
  - Neoplasm

Treatment

- Mainstay of treatment is a trial of rest and reduced activity with possible period of non–weight bearing.
- Specific recommendations
  - Femoral neck
    - Conservative treatment employed for compression side fractures that span <50% of the femoral neck.
    - Operative treatment with closed reduction and percutaneous pinning (CRPP) or dynamic hip screw (DHS) placement for tension side fractures, compression fractures that span >50% of the femoral neck, or fractures that have failed nonoperative management (Fig. 123.5).

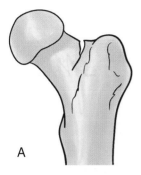
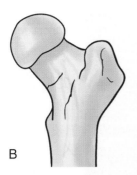
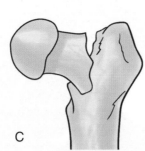

A B C

Fig 123.1 Fullerton and Snowdy classification of femoral neck stress fractures. **(A)** Tension type occurring along the superolateral portion of the femoral neck. **(B)** Compression type occurring along the inferomedial portion of the femoral neck. **(C)** Displaced type.

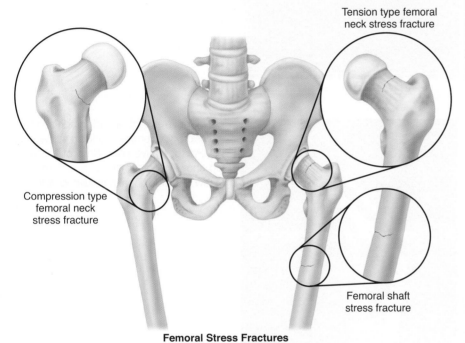

Tension type femoral neck stress fracture

Compression type femoral neck stress fracture

Femoral shaft stress fracture

Femoral Stress Fractures

Fig 123.2 Classification, presentation, and treatment strategies of femoral stress fractures.

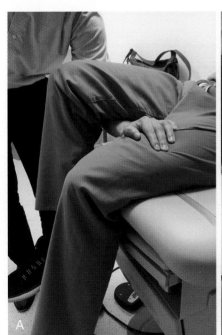
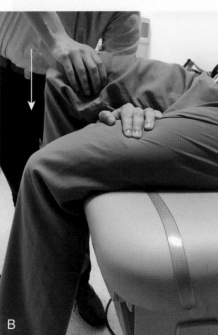

A B

Fig 123.3 Fulcrum test for femoral shaft stress fractures. **(A)** With the patient in a seated position and legs overhanging an exam table, the examiner places one arm under the affected leg around the mid-thigh and levers it on the contralateral leg as shown. **(B)** A downward force is then applied to the affected leg around the distal thigh. A positive test is increased pain on downward force.

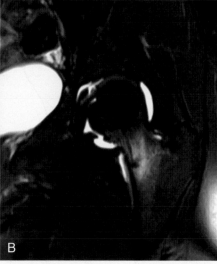

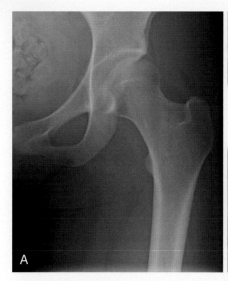

Fig 123.4 **(A)** Normal left hip radiograph without evidence of any pathologic fracture. **(B)** Corresponding T2-weighted coronal MRI showing marrow edema with an associated compression-type femoral-neck stress fracture.

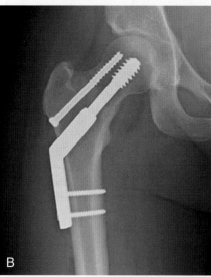

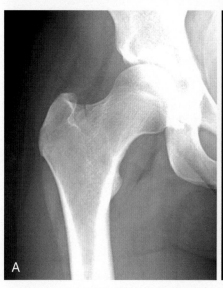

Fig 123.5 **(A)** Right hip radiograph showing a tension-type femoral-neck stress fracture. **(B)** Postoperative plain films of the right hip showing placement of a dynamic hip screw and additional cannulated screw.

- Femoral shaft
  - Often treated nonoperatively
  - Operative intramedullary (IM) nailing considered in older patients with low bone mass as a prophylactic measure to prevent complete femoral shaft fracture.

When to Refer

- Orthopaedic referral for a femoral stress fracture should take place when a period of activity modification fails to resolve symptoms, the fracture shows evidence of displacement or propagation, or there is evidence of a tension side femoral neck fracture.

Prognosis

- Nondisplaced femoral neck and shaft fractures often heal without significant sequelae after a period of reduced activity and weight-bearing restriction.

- Given tenuous blood supply of the femoral neck and head, avascular necrosis is a concern in displaced and tension-type femoral neck stress fractures.
- Nonunion, malunion, or refracture can be also be seen in those who fail to adequately rest the affected limb.

Troubleshooting

- Normal initial plain films should be met with apprehension in those suspected of a femoral stress fracture and advanced imaging should be employed when clinical suspicion is high.

Patient Instructions

- Patients should be advised that strict weight bearing adherence is critical to proper healing. This should be stressed in high-performance athletes who may find it difficult to endure a prolonged period of rest.

Considerations in Special Populations

- Female athletes
  - The female athlete triad is a well-known constellation of amenorrhea, disordered eating, and osteoporosis. Any female who presents with a stress fracture should be evaluated for these underlying conditions.

Suggested Readings

Biz C, Berizzi A, Crimi A, et al. Management and treatment of femoral neck stress fractures in recreational runners: a report of four cases and review of the literature. *Acta Biomed*. 2017;88(4–S):96–106.

Boden BP, Osbahr DC. High-risk stress fractures: evaluation and treatment. *J Am Acad Orthop Surg*. 2000;8(6):344–353.

Clough TM. Femoral neck stress fracture: the importance of clinical suspicion and early review. *Br J Sports Med*. 2002;36(4):308–309.

Fullerton LRJ, Snowdy HA. Femoral neck stress fractures. *Am J Sports Med*. 1988;16(4):365–377.

Johnson AW, Weiss CBJ, Wheeler DL. Stress fractures of the femoral shaft in athletes—more common than expected. A new clinical test. *Am J Sports Med*. 1994;22(2):248–256.

Katsougrakis I, Apostolopoulos AP, Tross SZ. Conservative management of a femoral neck stress fracture in a female athlete. A case report and review of the literature. *J Long Term Eff Med Implants*. 2016;26(1):7–12.

Wright AA, Taylor JB, Ford KR, et al. Risk factors associated with lower extremity stress fractures in runners: a systematic review with meta-analysis. *Br J Sports Med*. 2015;49(23):1517–1523.

Chapter 124 Traumatic Hip Fractures

Brandon S. Huggins, Michael S. Sridhar

ICD-10-CM CODES

S72.041A *Displaced fracture of base of neck of femur, closed, right*

S72.042A *Displaced fracture of base of neck of femur, closed, left*

S72.051A *Unspecified fracture of head of femur, closed, right*

S72.052A *Unspecified fracture of head of femur, closed, left*

S72.141A *Displaced intertrochanteric fracture of femur, closed, right*

S72.142A *Displaced intertrochanteric fracture of femur, closed, left*

Key Concepts

- Traumatic hip fractures occur in a bimodal age distribution as a result of high-energy trauma in the young and low-energy falls in the elderly.
- Femoral head fractures have a high association with posterior hip dislocations and rapid reduction is essential to prevent vascular compromise to the femoral head.
  - Elderly hip fractures are associated with 6% in-hospital mortality and 30% mortality within the first year after injury.
- Intertrochanteric femur fractures account for 50% of proximal femur fractures.
  - Timely management within 48 hours after injury is essential to decrease morbidity and mortality.
  - Risk factors in the elderly include osteoporosis, female gender, advanced age, and positive maternal history.
  - Treatment is directed at mobilizing the patient as soon as possible while optimizing bone health to achieve bony union and prevent future fractures.

History
Elderly Patients

- A history of a low-energy trauma, such as a fall from standing height, is involved.
- Determining medical co-morbidities and baseline level of function is imperative in the workup.
- Those with a history of frequent falls may have chronic hip injury findings on imaging studies. Magnetic resonance imaging (MRI) is helpful in these instances for determining acuity.

Younger Patients

- Most often associated with a history of high-energy trauma such as a motor vehicle collision or fall from height.
- Femoral head fractures most commonly seen in this population which have a high association with hip dislocation

(5% to 15%), concomitant acetabular and femoral neck fracture, and ipsilateral ligamentous knee injury.

Physical Examination

- A shortened, malrotated lower extremity with pain on passive log roll movement is the classic presentation for proximal femur fractures (Fig. 124.1A).
- A complete musculoskeletal examination should be performed to evaluate for concomitant injuries especially at the ipsilateral knee.
- Patients with nondisplaced intertrochanteric and valgus impacted femoral neck fractures may have minor pain with exam and be able to bear weight.
- Neurovascular exam is essential particularly with femoral head fracture–posterior dislocations as sciatic nerve neuropraxia occur in up to 10% of cases.
- In younger patients, higher-energy injury is usually involved, and thus a full trauma workup is warranted.

Imaging

- An anteroposterior view of the pelvis; anteroposterior, and lateral views (frog leg or cross-table) of the hip; anteroposterior view and lateral of entire ipsilateral femur should be obtained (see Fig. 124.1).
- If an occult femoral neck or intertrochanteric fracture is suspected based on history and exam but plain radiographs are negative, MRI of the hip is the imaging of choice (Fig. 124.2).
- If MRI is contraindicated (i.e., pacemaker), 2 mm thin-slice computed tomography (CT) can assist in diagnosis.

Classification
Femoral Head Fractures

- The Pipkin classification describes femoral head fractures associated with a posterior hip dislocation and provides a basis for treatment (Fig. 124.3).

Femoral Neck Fractures

- Garden classification is the most commonly used. In general, increased displacement results in a higher risk of avascular necrosis and influences the choice of surgical treatment (Fig. 124.4).
- More vertical fracture patterns have a higher risk of displacement and are more common in high-energy injuries.

Intertrochanteric Femur Fractures

- The AO/ASIF classification describes the fracture as stable versus unstable and helps guide treatment (Fig. 124.5).

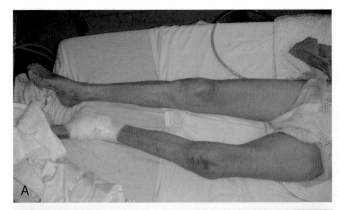

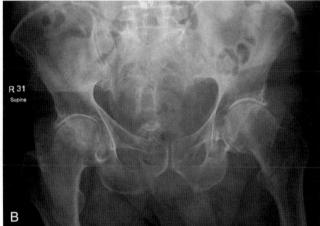

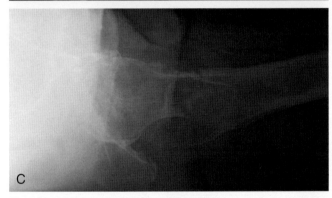

Fig 124.1 **(A)** A patient with a left intertrochanteric femur fracture lying in a typical position with a shortened and externally rotated lower extremity. **(B)** Preoperative anteroposterior radiograph demonstrating left intertrochanteric femur fracture. **(C)** Preoperative crosstable lateral radiograph.

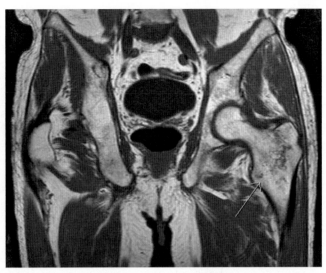

Fig 124.2 T1-weighted magnetic resonance imaging of the pelvis. The *arrow* demonstrates an occult left intertrochanteric femur fracture.

Additional Tests

- Outpatient dual-energy x-ray absorptiometry (DEXA) and osteoporosis laboratory workup is recommended in elderly individuals if they have not already been evaluated for osteoporosis.
- Elderly patients often require a workup for the etiology of their fall, which can include syncope, heart disease, stroke, metabolic abnormality, delirium/dementia, and other medical conditions.

Differential Diagnosis

- Hip dislocation
- Pelvic fracture
- Femoral shaft fracture
- Soft-tissue contusion
- Trochanteric bursitis

Treatment
Femoral Head Fractures

- Closed reduction of an associated hip dislocation should be promptly performed to lower risk of avascular necrosis (AVN), followed by post-reduction CT.
- Nonoperative management with protected weight bearing is acceptable if reduction is maintained and fracture is outside the weight-bearing portion of the femoral head.
- Operative management
  - Open reduction and internal fixation of a femoral head fracture and of associated femoral neck or acetabular fractures are required if reduction cannot be obtained or maintained by closed means (Fig. 124.6).
  - Hip arthroplasty is an operative consideration in the older patient population.

Femoral Neck Fractures

- Femoral neck fractures nearly always require surgical intervention in order to mobilize the patient quickly.
  - Surgical options depend upon the location of the fracture, amount of displacement, and the activity level of the patient.
- Nonoperative management may be acceptable in limited cases of nondisplaced, minimally symptomatic fractures, in cases of extreme comorbidity for surgery and family wishes, and in chronic cases (particularly valgus impacted femoral neck fractures).

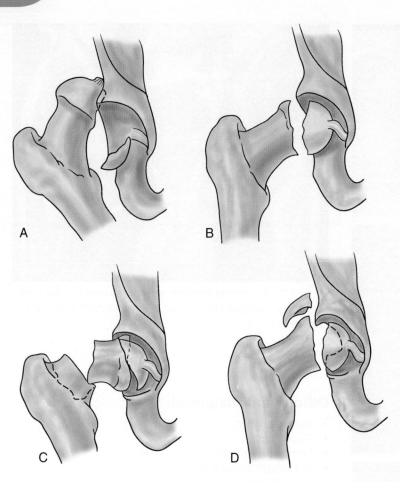

Fig 124.3 Pipkin classification of femoral head fractures. **(A)** Type I: below the fovea centralis. **(B)** Type II: above the fovea centralis. **(C)** Type III: either type I or II along with associated fracture of the femoral neck. **(D)** Type IV: either type I or II along with associated acetabular fracture. (Modified from Browner BD, Jupiter JB, Levine AM, Trafton PG, eds. *Skeletal Trauma: Fractures, Dislocations, Ligamentous Injuries*. Philadelphia, PA: WB Saunders; 1992:1339.)

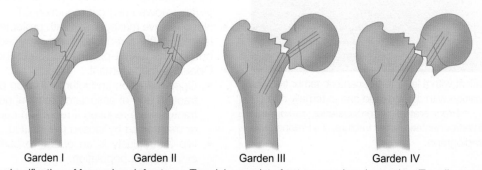

Garden I   Garden II   Garden III   Garden IV

Fig 124.4 Garden classification of femoral neck fractures. Type I: incomplete fracture or valgus impaction. Type II: complete, nondisplaced fracture. Type III: complete, partially (<50%) displaced fracture. Type IV: complete, fully displaced fracture. (From Sud A, Ranjan R: Pelvis and hip injuries. In: *Textbook of Orthopaedics*, New Delhi, India, Elsevier, 2018, pp 299-310.)

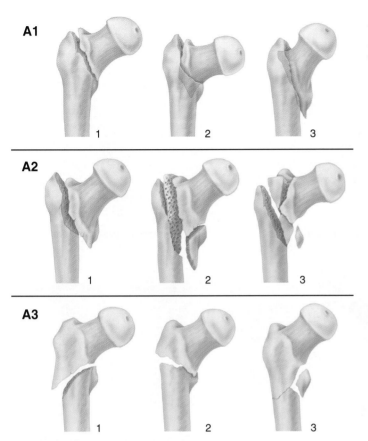

Fig 124.5 AO (Arbeitsgemeinschaft für Osteosynthesefragen)/ The Association of the Study of Internal Fixation (ASIF) classification of intertrochanteric femur fractures. A1: Simple two-part fracture pattern, lateral cortex remains intact. A2: Complex fracture pattern with loss of posteromedial buttress, lateral cortex remains intact. A3: Fracture extending into the lateral cortex including reverse oblique fracture pattern.

- Younger patients (typically defined as younger than 50) require timely open reduction and internal fixation within 24 hours is essential to try to preserve the viability of the femoral head.
- Elderly patients (typically defined as older than 50).
  - Nondisplaced fractures may be treated with percutaneous internal screw fixation or rarely a sliding hip screw (see Fig. 124.6).
  - Displaced fractures typically require hemiarthroplasty (replacement of the head) versus total hip arthroplasty (replacement of the head and socket) in the more active population (see Fig. 124.6).

Intertrochanteric Fractures

- Nonoperative management is infrequent and usually only considered in patients who have a very high surgical risk or who are nonambulatory.
- Operative management should proceed as soon as possible and usually involves closed more often than open reduction and internal fixation with a cephalomedullary nail with a screw(s) into the femoral head/neck using an indirect approach to the fracture site. Alternative surgical treatment is a plate/screw construct requiring a direct approach to the fracture site (see Fig. 124.6).

When to Refer

- Always

Prognosis

- Prognosis is generally related to the degree of injury and the timeliness of care as well as the age and medical status of the patient.
- Elderly patients have an extremely high rate of mortality within 1 year of a proximal femur fracture, up to 30%.
- Complications include avascular necrosis, nonunion, malunion, limb length and rotational discrepancy, peri-implant fracture, posttraumatic arthritis, cardiopulmonary demise, cerebrovascular accident, deep venous thrombosis, mortality, and other medical comorbidities.

Troubleshooting

- If radiographs are inconclusive, MRI is the preferred imaging modality. If patient has contraindications to MRI (i.e., incompatible pacemaker), CT is preferred.

Patient Instructions

- Weight-bearing and activity restrictions will vary by situation; however, the goal remains early weight bearing in the elderly.

Considerations in Special Populations

- Elderly patients warrant further investigation of the etiology of their fall as well as for other associated fractures sustained at the same time.

Surgical Management of Traumatic Hip Fractures

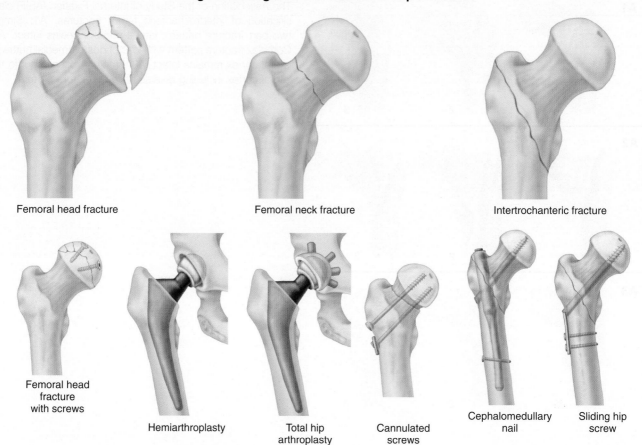

Fig 124.6 Surgical treatment options for fractures involving the femoral side of the hip joint. *Left to right*, Femoral head fracture: Femoral head screws. Femoral neck fracture: Hemiarthroplasty versus total hip arthroplasty versus cannulated screws. Intertrochanteric femur fractures: cephalomedually nail versus sliding hip screw.

Suggested Readings

Droll KP, Broekhuyse H, O'Brien P. Fracture of the femoral head. *J Am Acad Orthop Surg*. 2007;15:716–727.

Haidukewych GJ, Rothwell WS, Jacofsky DJ, et al. Operative treatment of femoral neck fractures in patients between the ages of fifteen and fifty years. *J Bone Joint Surg Am*. 2004;86A:1712–1716.

Iwata T, Nozawa S, Dohjima T, et al. The value of T1-weighted coronal MRI scans in diagnosing occult fracture of the hip. *J Bone Joint Surg Am*. 2012;94B:969–973.

Koval KJ, Zuckerman JD. Hip fractures: I. Overview and evaluation and treatment of femoral-neck fractures. *J Am Acad Orthop Surg*. 1994;2:141–149.

Koval KJ, Zuckerman JD. Hip fractures: II. Evaluation and treatment of intertrochanteric fractures. *J Am Acad Orthop Surg*. 1994;2:150–156.

Yu L, Wang Y, Chen J. Total hip arthroplasty versus hemiarthroplasty for displaced femoral neck fractures: meta-analysis of randomized trials. *Clin Orthop Relat Res*. 2012;470:2235–2243.

Chapter 125 Pelvic and Acetabular Fractures

Michael S. Sridhar, Brandon S. Huggins

ICD-10-CM CODES
S32.401A *Unspecified fracture of acetabulum, right*
S32.402A *Unspecified fracture of acetabulum, left*
S32.501A *Unspecified fracture of pubis, right*
S32.502A *Unspecified fracture of pubis, left*
S32.10 *Unspecified fracture of sacrum*
S32.2 *Fracture of coccyx*

Key Concepts

- Pelvic fractures, including acetabular fractures (intra-articular fractures involving hip socket), are usually associated with high-energy trauma in the young and low-energy falls in the elderly.
- Acetabular fractures, especially those involving the posterior wall, have a high association with hip dislocation requiring timely reduction to mitigate risk of femoral head avascular necrosis (AVN).
- Major vascular and neurologic structures pass through the pelvic ring and about the hip; there is great potential for serious complications or death with disruption.
- Large volumes of blood may be lost into the pelvis, with no external evidence of bleeding. Hemodynamic instability requires immediate attention and treatment involving an orthopaedist promptly.
- Pelvic fractures are often separated into two groups: stable and unstable. This distinction determines much of the management and prognosis of the injury.
  - Stable injuries are those that will not deform in the presence of normal physiologic forces.
  - Unstable injuries may display rotational instability, vertical instability, or both. These injuries often require surgical fixation and weight-bearing restrictions.
- Other "lesser" fractures of the pelvis, such as avulsion fractures, isolated iliac wing fractures, rami fractures, sacral buckle and coccygeal fractures, respond well to nonoperative treatment without weight-bearing restrictions.
- Pelvic anatomy distortion after fracture can cause obstetric issues for women of childbearing age, sometimes resulting in the need for a cesarean section.

Anatomy

- The pelvis is a ring structure composed of three bones: the sacrum and the left and right innominate bones (Fig. 125.1).
  - The innominate bone is composed of the ilium, ischium, and pubis.
- The center of fusion of these three bones forms the acetabulum.
- The pelvis, in the sagittal plane, may be considered to have two functional columns: anterior and posterior.
  - The anterior column is also known as the iliopectineal line and extends from the iliac crest to the pubic symphysis.
  - The posterior column, or ilioischial line, extends from the superior gluteal notch to the ischial tuberosity.
- The innominate bones join the sacrum posteriorly at the sacroiliac joint and join each other anteriorly at the symphysis pubis.
- The major sources of pelvic stability are the ligamentous structures posteriorly and anteriorly.
  - Posterior: the posterior, interosseous, and anterior sacroiliac ligaments, the sacrospinous and sacrotuberous ligaments; provide the main weight-bearing stability of the pelvis in a multiplanar fashion
  - Anterior: the symphysis pubis; provides rotational stability and control of flexion/extension

History

- The most severe cases typically involve high-energy trauma, including motor vehicle collisions, vehicle-pedestrian impacts, crush mechanisms, or falls from height.
- Some low-energy fractures can also occur and include patterns such as avulsions (often seen in pediatric and adult athletic injuries) (Fig. 125.2), osteoporotic rami fractures, sacral insufficiency fractures, iliac wing fractures, and coccygeal fractures.
- Understanding the mechanism of injury will often aid in identifying and fully characterizing the fracture pattern.

Physical Examination

- Patients with higher-energy mechanisms require a full-scale trauma evaluation with primary, secondary, and tertiary surveys.
- Early assessment of the neurovascular status is essential. Vascular injury, typically bridging veins, bleeding bone, or arterial injury can lead to major hemorrhage and hemodynamic instability. A rectal and vaginal exam is essential to evaluate for concomitant injury in high-energy mechanisms. With inspection, the patient with a pelvic fracture may have a visible deformity, including a limb length discrepancy or an internally or externally rotated lower extremity.
  - Ecchymosis may be present, especially anteriorly near the pubis or into the labia or scrotum and around the iliac crests.

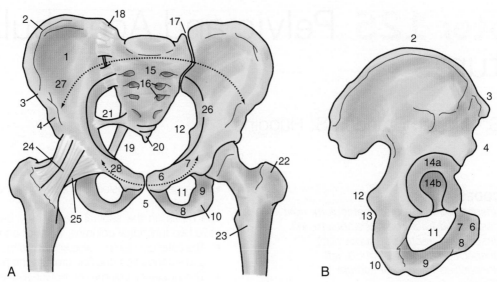

Fig 125.1 Pelvic anatomy. **(A)** Anterior view of the pelvis; **(B)** lateral view of the right innominate bone. *1*, Iliac fossa; *2*, iliac crest; *3*, anterior superior iliac spine; *4*, anterior inferior iliac spine; *5*, symphysis pubis; *6*, body of the pubis; *7*, superior ramus of the pubis; *8*, inferior ramus of the pubis; *9*, ramus of the ischium; *10*, ischial tuberosity; *11*, obturator foramen; *12*, ischial spine; *13*, lesser sciatic notch; *14*, acetabulum (14a, articular surface; 14b, fossa); *15*, sacrum; *16*, anterior sacral foramina; *17*, sacroiliac joint; *18*, anterior sacroiliac ligament; *19*, sacrotuberous ligament (sacrum to ischial tuberosity); *20*, coccyx; *21*, sacrospinous ligament; *22*, greater trochanter of the femur; *23*, lesser trochanter of the femur; *24*, iliofemoral ligament; *25*, pubofemoral ligament; *26*, arcuate line; *27*, posterior or femorosacral arch through which main weight-bearing forces are transmitted; *28*, anterior arch. (Modified from Cwinn AA. Pelvis. In: Marx JA, ed. *Rosen's Emergency Medicine: Concepts and Clinical Practice*. 6th ed. Philadelphia: Elsevier; 2006.)

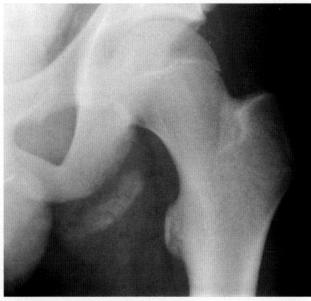

Fig 125.2 Ischial avulsion. (From Adam A, Dixon AK, eds. *Grainger & Allison's Diagnostic Radiology: A Textbook of Medical Imaging*. 5th ed. Philadelphia, PA: Churchill Livingstone; 2008.)

- There may be tenderness to palpation over the site of the injury, and there may also be crepitus.
- A unique consideration in pelvic fracture is genitourinary injury, which occurs in approximately 15% of pelvic trauma cases, with higher rates reported in males.
  - Signs include blood at the urethral meatus or, in males, a "floating" prostate on rectal examination. These findings preclude an immediate Foley catheter and require advanced imaging and urgent urology consultation.
- Lower-energy injuries will have more localized and less severe findings, including mild tenderness, local ecchymosis, and pain with certain resisted motions (such as challenged hip extension with hamstring avulsion fractures).

Imaging

- Radiographs: Anteroposterior, inlet/outlet, and Judet views (for acetabular fractures) of the pelvis should be obtained (Fig. 125.3).
- If pelvic stability is unclear, stress views may be useful, with the patient under anesthesia. More than 0.5 to 1 cm of motion at a fracture or dislocation of the symphysis or sacroiliac joint may be considered unstable.
- In cases of a suspected acetabular fracture, it is essential to get Judet views of the pelvis that include obturator and iliac oblique views (see Fig. 125.3).
- Computed tomography: Fine-slice computed tomography should also be performed. Recent studies have suggested

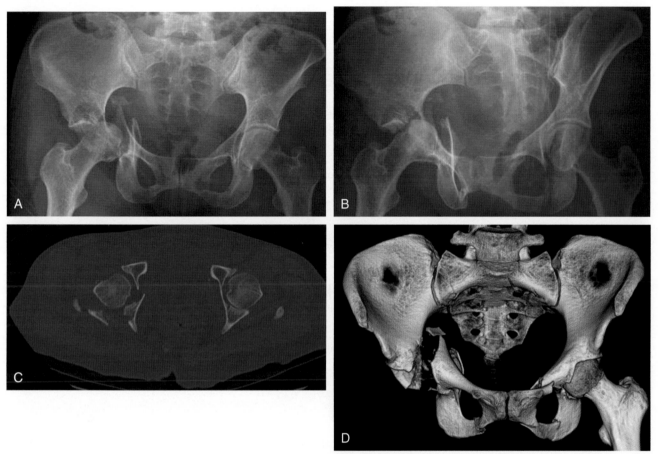

Fig 125.3 Separate images of a 40-year-old female involved in an motor vehicle collision (MVC) sustaining a right central hip dislocation with associated T-type acetabulum fracture and multiple pubic rami fractures. **(A)** Plain anteroposterior radiograph. **(B)** Plain radiograph taken in the Judet view (iliac oblique). **(C)** Axial computed topography image. **(D)** Three-dimensional reconstruction computed topography.

that computed tomography scanning should be considered the "gold standard" for evaluation of bony injury to the pelvis (including acetabulum) and for defining the true extent of a fracture, especially injury to the iliac wing, sacrum, or coccyx (see Fig. 125.3).

Classification

- The most common classification system for pelvic injury is the Young and Burgess system (Fig. 125.4), which is based on the mechanism of injury.
- Tile had previously defined a classification system based on stability.
  - It is divided into types A, B, and C. Type A injuries are stable; type B injuries are rotationally unstable but vertically stable; and type C injuries are both rotationally and vertically unstable.
- The Letournel and Judet classification scheme (Table 125.1) is used to describe fractures involving the acetabulum and has two subdivisions, simple/elementary (Fig. 125.5) and complex/associated (Fig. 125.6).

TABLE 125.1 Letournel and Judet Classification Scheme

Simple/Elementary	Complex/Associated
Posterior wall	Transverse and posterior wall
Posterior column	Posterior column and posterior wall
Anterior wall	T-shaped
Anterior column	Anterior column/posterior hemitransverse
Transverse	Both columns

Additional Tests

- Retrograde urethrography, voiding cystourethrography, or computed tomography cystography if a genitourinary injury is suspected.
- Angiography and possible intervention in the presence of uncontrolled hemorrhage from a pelvic fracture.

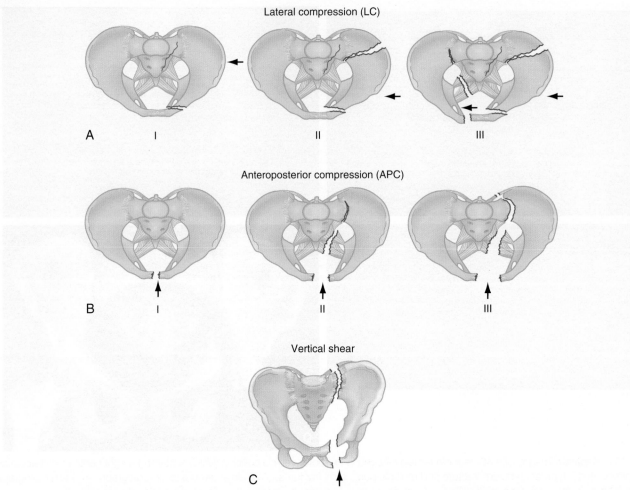

Fig 125.4 Young-Burgess classification. **(A)** Lateral compression. Type I: an internally directed force causing a sacral fracture and horizontal pubic ramus fractures. Type II: internally directed force causing horizontal pubic ramus fractures with fracture/dislocation of the ipsilateral sacroiliac joint ("crescent fracture"). Type III: an internally directed force that is continued, causing external rotation of the contralateral hemipelvis ("windswept pelvis"). **(B)** Anteroposterior compression. Type I: symphysis disrupted but with intact posterior ligamentous structures. Type II: continuation of type I fracture with anterior sacroiliac joint opening. Type III: continuation force disrupts the posterior sacroiliac ligaments in addition to anterior sacroiliac ligaments ("open-book pelvis"). **(C)** Vertical shear: vertical fractures in the rami and disruption of all posterior ligaments and sacroiliac joint. *Arrow* indicates the direction of force. (Modified from Young JWR, Burgess AR. *Radiologic Management of Pelvic Ring Fractures*. Baltimore, MD: Urban & Schwarzenberg; 1987.)

Differential Diagnosis

- Femoral head fracture
- Hip fracture
- Hip dislocation
- Femur fracture
- Hamstring strain
- Quadriceps strain
- Hip pointer (iliac wing contusion)

Treatment

- Treatment of a pelvic fracture will vary depending on the patient, the injury, and the institution. Multidisciplinary care is of the utmost importance with these injuries to expedite time to definitive treatment safely.

- The goals of treatment are to address/prevent life-threatening injuries, restore anatomy and function, and minimize long-term sequelae.
- The first decision to be made is determination of stability. Stable injuries can be managed nonoperatively.
  - In some circumstances, there is a lower threshold for surgical fixation in the polytrauma patients in an effort to mobilize them sooner.
  - Rehabilitation should focus on early mobilization despite any weight-bearing precautions. The patient should be followed with serial radiographs after mobilization.
- Most unstable pelvic fractures should be treated initially with a pelvic binder and with skeletal traction in the vertically unstable pelvis. External fixation may have a role as a temporizing measure in cases in which pelvic binder is

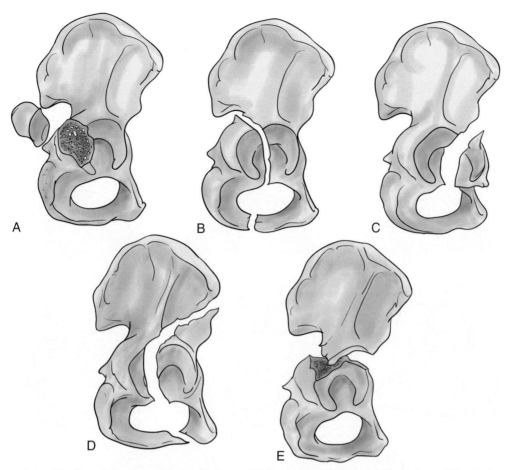

Fig 125.5 Letournel classification of simple acetabular fractures. **(A)** Posterior wall; **(B)** posterior column; **(C)** anterior wall; **(D)** anterior column; **(E)** transverse. (Modified from Browner BD, ed. *Skeletal Trauma: Basic Science, Management and Reconstruction*. 3rd ed. Philadelphia, PA: Elsevier; 2003.)

ineffective or is contraindicated (i.e., significant underlying soft tissue injury). Early open reduction and internal fixation is the ultimate goal (Fig. 125.7).
- Acetabular fractures must be treated with the goal of minimizing the risk for posttraumatic arthritis.
  - Initial management can include placement in skeletal traction if the hip is unstable after closed reduction or if surgical intervention will be delayed.
  - Operative treatment should be used in certain circumstances, including fractures with displacement greater than 2 to 3 mm, displaced/dislocated fractures that cannot be reduced by closed methods, and those in which a congruent joint cannot be maintained out of skeletal traction. In addition, loose intra-articular fragments need to be removed operatively (see Fig. 125.7).

When to Refer
- Higher-energy pelvic and acetabular fractures should all be referred to an orthopaedist early for inpatient care.
- Lower-energy pelvic fractures such as avulsion fractures, isolated iliac wing fractures, rami fractures, sacral buckle, and coccygeal fractures also require referral to an orthopaedist on an outpatient basis.

Prognosis
- Open pelvic fractures, hemorrhagic shock on admission, associated head and abdominal injuries, genitourinary injury, and nerve injury have a poorer prognosis. In unstable fractures, posterior disruption has a higher incidence of blood loss and mortality.
- Acetabular fracture: Injury to cartilage or bone of the acetabulum and femoral head have a higher incidence of posttraumatic arthritis and a worse long-term prognosis.

Troubleshooting
- In the setting of a pelvic fracture and hemodynamic instability, a sheet or pelvic binder should be emergently applied to assist in clot formation

Considerations in Special Populations
- Heterotopic ossification (HO) may occur in as many as 70% of patients requiring acetabulum fracture repair. The use of indomethacin and radiation therapy for HO prophylaxis has fallen out of favor due to risk of nonunion and wound issues. HO rarely needs to be surgically excised unless it is restricting motion and/or painful.

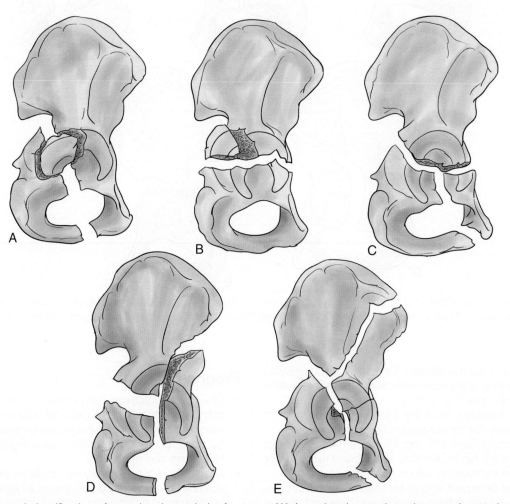

Fig 125.6 Letournel classification of associated acetabular fractures. **(A)** Associated posterior column and posterior wall fractures; **(B)** associated transverse and posterior wall fractures; **(C)** T-shaped fracture; **(D)** associated anterior and posterior hemitransverse fractures; **(E)** both-column fracture. (Modified from Browner BD, ed. *Skeletal Trauma: Basic Science, Management and Reconstruction*. 3rd ed. Philadelphia, PA: Elsevier; 2003.)

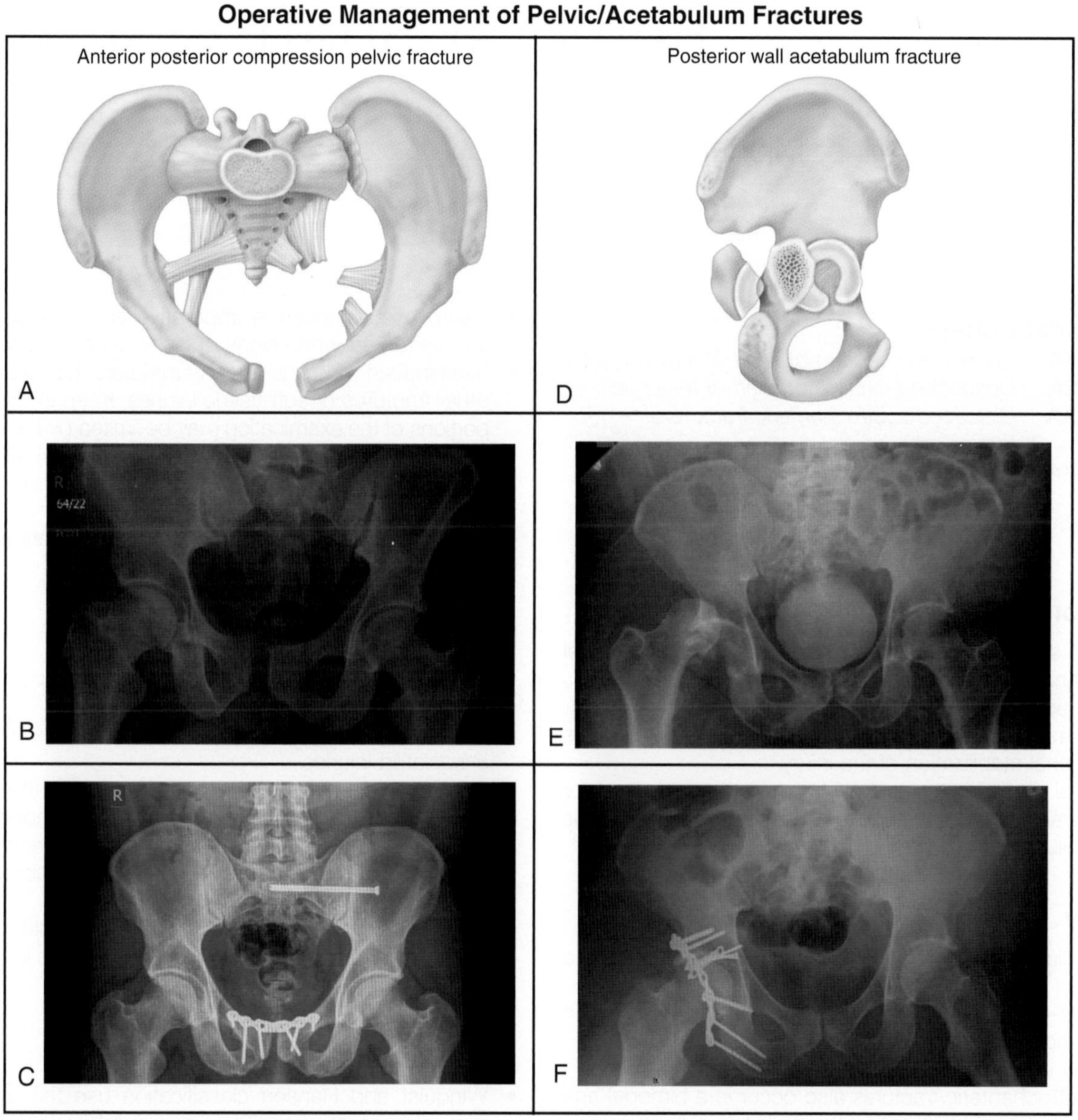

Operative Management of Pelvic/Acetabulum Fractures

Fig 125.7 Surgical treatment of pelvic and acetabulum fractures. **(A)** Young-Burgess anteroposterior (AP) compression-II pelvic fracture. **(B)** AP plain radiograph demonstrating APC II pelvic fracture. **(C)** Postoperative plain radiograph demonstration open reduction internal fixation of symphyseal disruption and percutaneous screw fixation of left sacroiliac joint. **(D)** Letournel posterior wall acetabulum fracture. **(E)** AP plain radiograph of right posterior hip dislocation with associated posterior wall fracture. **(F)** Postoperative AP plain radiograph demonstrating concentric reduction of right hip and open reduction internal fixation of posterior wall acetabulum fracture.

Suggested Readings

Hak DJ, Smith WR, Takashi S. Management of hemorrhage in life-threatening pelvic fracture. *J Am Acad Orthop Surg.* 2009;17:447–457.

Langford JR, Burgess AR, Liporace FA, Haidukewych GJ. Pelvic fractures: part 1. Evaluation, classification, resuscitation. *J Am Acad Orthop Surg.* 2013;21:448–457.

Langford JR, Burgess AR, Liporace FA, Haidukewych GJ. Pelvic fractures: part 2. Contemporary indications and techniques for definitive surgical management. *J Am Acad Orthop Surg.* 2013;21:458–468.

Mehta S, Auerbach JD, Born CT, Chin KR. Sacral fractures. *J Am Acad Orthop Surg.* 2006;14:656–665.

Schiller J, DeFroda S, Blood T. Lower extremity avulsion fractures in the pediatric and adolescent athlete. *J Am Acad Orthop Surg.* 2017; 25:251–259.

Tornetta P 3rd. Displaced acetabular fractures: indications for operative and nonoperative management. *J Am Acad Orthop Surg.* 2001;9:18–28.

Chapter 126 Femoral Shaft Fractures

Brandon S. Huggins, Michael S. Sridhar

ICD-10-CM CODES
S72.301A *Unspecified fracture of shaft of femur, right*
S72.302A *Unspecified fracture of shaft of femur, left*
S72.21XA *Displaced subtrochanteric fracture of femur, right*
S72.22XA *Displaced subtrochanteric fracture of femur, left*

Key Concepts

- Timely surgical treatment is usually required for femoral shaft and subtrochanteric fractures.
- Acute application of traction to the leg or a knee immobilizer may result in reduction of blood loss as it provides provisional stabilization of the injury.
- Femoral shaft fractures should always be evaluated for ipsilateral femoral neck fractures and ipsilateral ligamentous knee injury.

History

- Both diaphyseal and subtrochanteric fractures follow a bimodal distribution.
  - High-energy trauma such as motor vehicle collisions in young patients
  - Low-energy falls in elderly patients
  - Subtrochanteric fractures also occur in a bimodal age distribution. Elderly subtrochanteric femur fractures are associated with long-term bisphosphonate use and can be pathologic in nature.
- A complete history includes the injury mechanism, any known associated injuries (such as visceral injuries, other fractures, vascular compromise, neurologic injury, and head injury), the time elapsed from the injury, and other comorbidities that may alter the treatment decision (i.e., bisphosphonate use and history of malignancy).

Physical Examination

- Lower extremity rotational and angular deformity, swelling, thigh fullness, and often ecchymosis is typically observed.
- Skin should be checked circumferentially. Any breakage of the skin should be considered an open fracture until proven otherwise.
- Although rare, thigh compartment syndrome can occur with femoral shaft fractures. Etiology is blunt force trauma in 90% of cases. Please see Chapter 13 for compartment syndrome diagnostic criteria.

- Neurovascular exam is imperative and vascular studies are warranted when signs of ischemia are present.
- Examination must include the ipsilateral hip and knee for other fractures or soft-tissue injuries. Keep in mind, some portions of the examination may be limited by the injury due to pain (e.g., ligamentous knee examination). Remainder of examination can be performed in operating room after definitive treatment.
- Full primary, secondary, and tertiary surveys are warranted in the multitrauma setting.

Imaging

- Orthogonal view radiographs (usually anteroposterior and lateral views) of the entire femoral shaft
- Dedicated radiographs of the hip and knee to rule out associated injuries
- Contralateral femur films are a requirement in the setting of pathologic fracture, especially with bisphosphonate use to evaluate for a contralateral subtrochanteric stress reaction.
- Computed tomography helps to rule out associated femoral neck fractures.
- Magnetic resonance imaging of the knee should be considered if ligamentous knee examination is positive for instability.

Classification
Diaphyseal Fractures

- Winquist and Hansen classification use the amount of cortical contact of proximal and distal fragments to rate the fracture severity (Fig. 126.1).
  - Grade 0: no comminution at the fracture site
  - Grade I: minimal comminution at the fracture site, does not affect stability after intramedullary nailing and may be treated as though it were not comminuted
  - Grade II: cortical contact retained in more than 50% of shaft circumference at the fracture site, allowing control of length and rotation
  - Grade III: cortical contact retained is less than 50% of shaft circumference at the fracture site; shortening, rotation, and translation may occur
  - Grade IV: 0% of cortical contact retained; no intrinsic stability

Subtrochanteric Fractures

- Defined as fractures of the proximal femoral shaft within 5 cm below the lesser trochanter
- There are several classifications, mostly based on the location of the fracture line relative to the lesser trochanter and penetration through the piriformis fossa above.

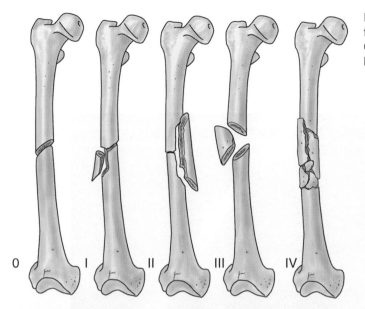

Fig 126.1 Winquist and Hansen classification of femoral shaft fractures. (Modified from Bucholz RW, Heckman JD, Court-Brown CM, eds. *Rockwood and Greene's Fractures in Adults*. 6th ed. Philadelphia: Lippincott Williams & Wilkins; 2006:1849.)

0   I   II   III   IV

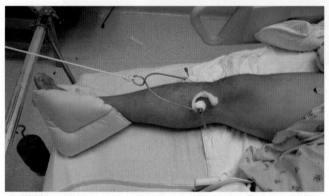

Fig 126.2 Patient with midshaft femur fracture in traction before operative fixation. (Photo courtesy of Tim Murphy, 2007.)

Differential Diagnosis

- Associated injuries, especially of the hip or knee, may contribute to the lower extremity deformity.
- Pathologic fracture from neoplastic disease, metabolic disease, or bisphosphonate use; the subtrochanteric region is the most common site for pathologic fractures of the femur and any lesion of the lesser trochanter is presumed malignant until proven otherwise.

Treatment

- Initial stabilization with a knee immobilizer followed by operative treatment within the first 24 hours reduces morbidity and mortality.
- Preoperative traction can be considered in cases in which significant delay to the operating room is anticipated (Fig. 126.2).
- Nonoperative treatment is reserved only for isolated cases with extenuating circumstances that contraindicate surgery.

Diaphyseal Fractures

- For adults, operative treatment is pursued in nearly all cases.
  - External fixation can be used as a temporizing method in damage control situations.
  - A reamed, locked intramedullary nail (Fig. 126.3) is the most common definitive treatment. The nail acts as a load-sharing device that allows the patient to begin early mobilization and weightbearing.
- Intramedullary nailing is usually performed with closed reduction to reduce blood loss and avoid soft-tissue devitalization. Open nailing is indicated when adequate reduction cannot be accomplished by closed means necessitating direct access.
- Plating of shaft fractures may also be performed in certain situations (such as previous malunion or deformity of femur), but it is much less commonly used than intramedullary nailing (Fig. 126.4).
- In skeletally immature patients younger than 5 years of age, closed treatment is often effective with immediate immobilization followed by closed reduction and spica casting until healing occurs (see Fig. 126.4).
  - In children younger than 6 months of age, Pavlik harness is an option as opposed to spica cast (see Fig. 126.4).
  - Internal fixation with a submuscular plate/screw construct may also be considered in this age range if fracture and/or patient are not amenable to spica cast (see Fig. 126.4).
- Internal fixation with flexible nailing is another viable option, especially in children between the ages of 6 and 10 and weighing less than 100 lbs (see Fig. 126.4). Beyond the age of 11 and/or weighing greater than 100 lbs, standard intramedullary nail should be considered (see Fig. 126.4).

Subtrochanteric Fractures

- Due to the mechanical forces placed on the fracture fragments by muscular attachments, the proximal piece is pulled into flexion, external rotation and abduction making these fractures notoriously difficult to treat.

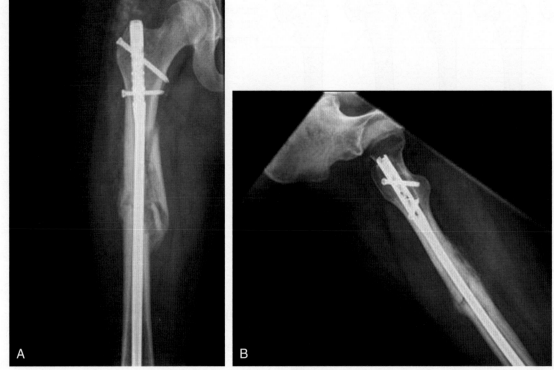

Fig 126.3 Anteroposterior **(A)** and lateral **(B)** radiographs of subtrochanteric femur fracture with diaphyseal extension treated with statically locked antegrade intramedullary nail.

- Operative treatment is almost always indicated unless the patient's comorbidities mandate nonoperative treatment.
  - Operative treatment involves internal fixation using an intramedullary nail, although a fixed angle plate is feasible depending on the configuration of the fracture and associated injuries (see Fig. 126.4).
  - With operative fixation, patients are typically able to weight bear as tolerated in the immediate postoperative period depending upon the quality of fixation.

Prognosis

- Diaphyseal fractures have a good prognosis, with healing rates of 95-99% with intramedullary nailing ("gold standard").
- Subtrochanteric fractures in the elderly have a worse prognosis, with a mortality rate reported as high as 30% in the first year after injury.
  - The fracture usually heals within 3 to 4 months.
  - Similar to hip fractures, subtrochanteric fractures often result in patients needing to use an assistive device (e.g., cane, walker) after treatment.

When to Refer

- Always

Troubleshooting

- Femur fractures are known for fat embolism and adult respiratory distress syndrome, especially when they occur

bilaterally. Close observation for respiratory changes is critical in the acute recovery period.
- It is common for patients to lose several units of blood into the thigh after femur fractures. This is often difficult to detect by clinical examination, and thus close monitoring of the hemodynamic status should be maintained in concert with compartment checks. Early immobilization or traction application can help to control blood loss.
- Neurovascular injury must be carefully evaluated and documented because compartment syndrome may develop.
- Late complications can include infection, deep venous thrombosis, and pulmonary embolus, malunion/nonunion, limb length discrepancy, and joint stiffness.

Patient Instructions

- Patients are typically allowed to weight bear as they can tolerate after surgical fixation using an intramedullary nail, although protected weightbearing may be used in certain cases.

Considerations in Special Populations

- Fractures in children are often complicated by overgrowth of the injured leg, which occurs through the physes at each end of the bone.
- Fractures in the elderly create a unique situation because there is often a combination of osteopenic bone and multiple medical comorbidities that make fixation and healing a challenge. However, immobility in this patient population leads to increased mortality.

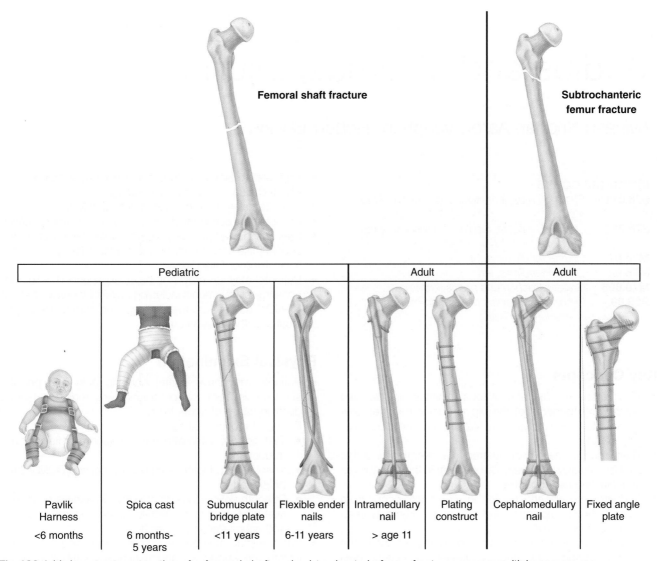

Femoral shaft fracture

Subtrochanteric femur fracture

Pediatric				Adult		Adult	
Pavlik Harness	Spica cast	Submuscular bridge plate	Flexible ender nails	Intramedullary nail	Plating construct	Cephalomedullary nail	Fixed angle plate
<6 months	6 months–5 years	<11 years	6-11 years	> age 11			

Fig 126.4 Various treatment options for femoral shaft and subtrochanteric femur fractures across multiple age groups.

Suggested Readings

Brumback RJ, Virkus WW. Intramedullary nailing of the femur: reamed versus nonreamed. *J Am Acad Orthop Surg.* 2000;8:83–90.

Flynn JM, Schwend RM. Management of pediatric femoral shaft fractures. *J Am Acad Orthop Surg.* 2004;12:347–359.

Lundy DW. Subtrochanteric femoral fractures. *J Am Acad Orthop Surg.* 2007;15:663–671.

Matullo KS, Gangavalli A, Nwachuku C. Review of lower extremity traction in current orthopaedic trauma. *J Am Acad Orthop Surg.* 2016;9:600–606.

Nork SE. Fractures of the shaft of the femur. In: Bucholz RW, Heckman JD, Court-Brown CM, eds. *Rockwood and Greene's Fractures in Adults.* 6th ed. Philadelphia: Lippincott Williams & Wilkins; 2006:1846–1913.

Pape HC, Tornetta P, et al. Timing of fracture fixation in multitrauma patients: the role of early total care and damage control surgery. *J Am Acad Orthop Surg.* 2009;9:541–549.

Peljovich AE, Patterson BM. Ipsilateral femoral neck and shaft fractures. *J Am Acad Orthop Surg.* 1998;2:106–113.

Chapter 127 Abductor (Gluteus Medius and Minimus) Injuries

Avinash Sridhar, Aaron Vaughan, Robert Boykin

ICD-10-CM CODES

S76.011	Strain of, muscle, fascia, and tendon of hip, right
S76.012	Strain of, muscle, fascia, and tendon of hip, left
M76.01	Gluteal tendinitis. right
M76.02	Gluteal tendinitis. left
M79.605	Greater trochanteric pain syndrome
R26.89	Other abnormalities of gait and mobility—Trendelenburg gait

Key Concepts

- The gluteus medius and gluteus minimus muscles are primary components of the hip abductor complex that plays a vital role in hip strength, stability, and gait mechanics (Fig. 127.1).
- These muscles have been referred to as the "rotator cuff of the hip," stabilizing the femoral head within the acetabulum and initiating hip abduction.
- Abductor muscle and tendon injuries rarely occur from acute traumatic episodes and are more commonly seen as a result of overuse.
- Gluteus medius and minimus tendinopathy are one of the three conditions that comprise greater trochanteric pain syndrome (GTPS) (the others being trochanteric bursitis and external coxa saltans or "snapping hip").
- The initial management for gluteal tendinopathy and GTPS is nonsurgical, including rest, activity modification, nonsteroidal antiinflammatory drugs (NSAIDs), and directed physical therapy.
- Although large isolated tears to the abductor tendon complex are a relatively infrequent cause of lateral hip pain, this should be considered in all patients who are unresponsive to nonsurgical management.
- Tendon tears in the hip range from interstitial to full-thickness tears, and management is based on the size of the tear, symptoms, duration, and quality of the remaining muscle.
  - Smaller tears may improve with nonoperative measures or biologic treatment options, whereas symptomatic full-thickness tears are considered for operative management.

History

- Patients typically present with chronic pain and tenderness over the proximal lateral aspect of the hip, usually directly on or anterior to the greater trochanter.
- Aggravating factors include side-bending, sleeping on the affected side, and prolonged sitting.
- Older females are more commonly affected.
- Patients may complain of a limp or other gait abnormalities.
- Previous hip arthroplasty via the anterolateral approach should raise concern for abductor insufficiency secondary to avulsion or failed repair.
- Patients may or may not have experienced relief with nonsurgical treatments including physical therapy, ice/heat, NSAIDs, use of assistive devices, and corticosteroid plus local anesthetic injections.

Physical Examination

- Patients may have peritrochanteric pain and possible ecchymosis from the peritrochanteric region extending distal in cases of acute injury.
- Range of motion testing:
  - Test flexion, internal/external rotation in flexion, and abduction.
  - In isolated abductor tendinopathy, passive ROM is often preserved.
  - Strength deficits include objective weakness on manual strength testing of resisted abduction in standing, supine, and lateral decubitus positions.
- When testing strength, ensure that the knee is flexed to isolate the abductors and minimize contribution of the iliotibial band (ITB).
- Clinical signs of a significant gluteus medius tear may include presence of a Trendelenburg gait.
  - A positive Trendelenburg test demonstrates the patient's torso leaning to the affected side while the contralateral side of the pelvis will sag (Fig. 127.2).
- Special tests:
  - Ober test: Perform with hip in extension, neutral, and flexion while assessing for contractures of the ITB, gluteus medius, and gluteus maximus, respectively (Fig. 127.3; see also Video 118.2 in Chapter 118).
  - Impingement testing, log roll, FABER (Flexion, ABduction, External Rotation) test, and straight leg raise are often normal.
- Carefully examine the hips for an intra-articular source of pain (labral tear, femoroacetabular impingement, loose body, etc.). These pathologies may coexist with peritrochanteric sources of pain and should be identified.

Imaging

- Plain radiography:
  - Hip x-ray/hip series: anteroposterior (AP) pelvis radiograph with lateral view of the hip (cross table, frog, or Dunn).

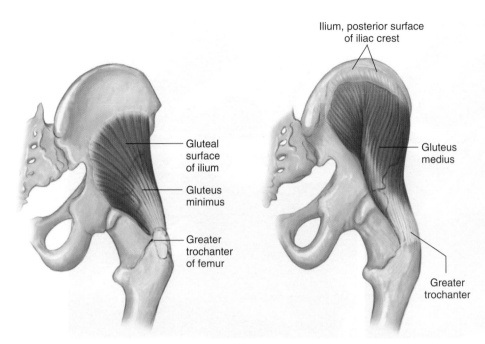

Fig 127.1 Gluteus medius, gluteus minimus, and surrounding bony architecture. (Modified from Patton KT, Thibodeau GA. Anatomy of the muscular system. In: Patton KT, Thibodeau GA, eds. *Anatomy and Physiology*. 7th ed. St. Louis, MO: Elsevier; 2010.)

Ilium, posterior surface of iliac crest

Gluteal surface of ilium

Gluteus minimus

Greater trochanter of femur

Gluteus medius

Greater trochanter

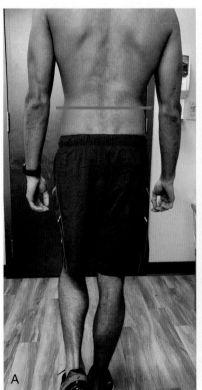
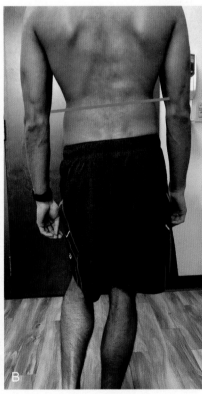

Fig 127.2 (A and B) Trendelenburg sign indicating abductor weakness of the right lower extremity.

- Plain radiographs are usually unremarkable but helpful in ruling out fracture, hip degenerative joint disease, femoroacetabular impingement, hip dysplasia, and calcification.
- Peritrochanteric calcifications:
  - May be present but are a nonspecific finding.
  - Sclerosis and irregular borders along the anterior edge of the greater trochanter, intrabursal calcification, calcific abductor tendinosis, and enthesophytes are frequently seen.
- Ultrasonography:
  - Diagnosis of abductor tendon pathology: Sensitivity 79–100%, positive predictive value 95–100%.
  - Gluteus medius pathology: The ultrasound probe can be used to palpate different areas of the tendon for pain and to perform diagnostic injection for pain resolution.

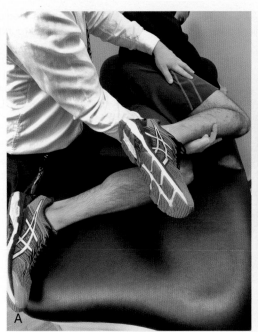
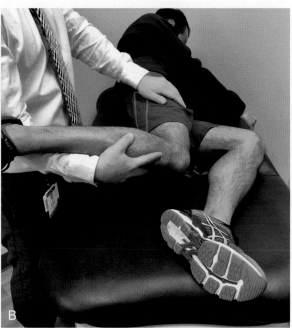
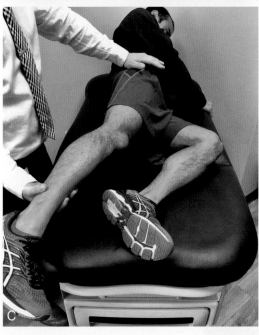

Fig 127.3 Ober test: flexion **(A)**, neutral **(B)**, and extension **(C)** positions.

- Dynamic evaluation is beneficial for confirming presence of external coxa saltans (snapping hip).
- Magnetic resonance imaging (MRI):
  - MRI is the primary means for evaluating GTPS and abductor pathology because it allows visualization of intra-articular and extra-articular structures.
  - Sensitivity of 73% and specificity of 95% when compared with definitive operative findings.
  - Arthrography is useful for labral tears and intra-articular pathology but not required for identifying peritrochanteric pathology.
  - T2-weighted sequences:
    - Trochanteric bursitis: Increased signal is seen in the trochanteric bursa.

- Tendinosis: Thickened tendon and increased signal intensity without focal discontinuity.
- Partial-thickness tears: Focal discontinuity of tendon fibers.
- Full-thickness/complete tears: Focal discontinuity of tendon fibers with retraction of tendon.
- T1 sequences are useful to evaluate fatty infiltration and/or atrophy of the muscle in large tears (similar to in the rotator cuff).

Differential Diagnosis

- GTPS:
  - Trochanteric bursitis.

- Swelling and tenderness at the greater trochanter.
- May observe a fluid collection or increased signal on ultrasound or MRI.
- Commonly with ITB/tensor fascia lata (TFL) tightness on Ober testing.
  - External coxa saltans (snapping hip)
    - Gait examination revealing short-leg limp.
    - To elicit a mechanical symptom, move affected leg from flexion, abduction, and external rotation to extension, adduction, and internal rotation.
- Occult fracture of the proximal femur:
  - Patient is unable to perform a resisted straight-leg raise while lying supine.
  - Deep-seated pain with weight bearing.
- Labral tears and femoroacetabular impingement:
  - Positive anterior impingement sign.
  - Increased side-to-side distance with FABER testing.
  - Predominately anterior with anterior groin pain.
- Extra-articular hip:
  - Piriformis/hip external rotator disorders
  - Hamstring complex disorders
  - Lumbar spondylosis and spinal stenosis:
    - Pattern of pain is radicular rather than localized to the greater trochanter, although patients may still present with a limp and hip abductor weakness.

Treatment

- Nonsurgical:
  - Initial period of relative rest and activity modification.
  - Antiinflammatory medications (NSAIDs).
  - Physical therapy focused on ITB/TFL stretching, gait training, and gluteal and core hip strengthening.
  - Corticosteroid injections:
    - Useful in reducing inflammation in trochanteric bursitis and abductor tendinopathy.
    - Less efficacious in larger abductor tears.
    - Accuracy may be improved with the use of ultrasound.
  - The use of biologic treatments such as platelet-rich plasma (PRP) may be effective based on limited supportive data in cases of gluteus medius and gluteus minimus tendinopathy and partial tears.
- Surgical:
  - Surgical management in cases of tendinopathy and partial tearing is typically reserved for patients with symptoms that have been present for a minimum of 6 to 12 months and in whom nonsurgical treatment has been unsuccessful.
    - This may include débridement, trochanteric bursectomy, and selective ITB fractional lengthening.
  - In symptomatic full-thickness or retracted abductor tears, surgical repair can be considered early to avoid further retraction and fatty infiltration/atrophy of the muscle.
  - Open and arthroscopic treatment options exist for management of abductor tendon injuries and peritrochanteric space pathology.
    - Arthroscopic management of abductor tears has shown significant progress with good clinical outcomes, improved pain and strength, and a low risk of complications.

- In patients with chronic, complete avulsions of the gluteus medius, mobilizing the tendon back to its trochanteric attachment for repair may not be possible.
- In these rare cases, there are limited data in small case series to support allograft augmentation or muscle transfer.

When to Refer

- Patients with lateral hip pain (with preserved strength and gait) refractory to nonsurgical treatment options for 6 to 12 months.
- Patients with lateral hip pain and weakness who have previously undergone total hip arthroplasty performed through an anterolateral approach.
- Patients presenting with objective weakness in abductor testing and/or Trendelenburg gait.
- Patients with imaging evidence of partial-thickness or full-thickness tears of the gluteus medius or minimus tendons.

Prognosis

- Most patients with lateral hip pain secondary to gluteus medius and medius tendinopathy and partial tearing improve with conservative therapy.
- For patients with abductor tendinopathy refractory to 6 to 12 months of conservative therapy, surgical management has shown promise in providing good pain relief as well as improved strength and function in limited series.
- In cases of full-thickness tears, the outcome is excellent if these are repaired early before progression to muscle wasting and atrophy.

Troubleshooting

- It is often difficult to distinguish hip abductor injuries from other causes of hip pain.
- Gluteus medius and gluteus minimus tendinopathy is often present with other conditions, particularly trochanteric bursitis and external coxa saltans (snapping hip), which make up the condition known as GTPS.
- Accurate diagnosis with focused history and physical examination, as well as appropriate imaging modalities, will help to ensure proper treatment that may include surgical intervention when appropriate.

Patient Instructions

- Continue stretching and strengthening exercises, as well as targeted physical therapy, to prevent recurrence of pain.
- If pain recurs, activity modification is necessary to prevent exacerbation and progression of injury.
- If surgery is required, a postoperative physical therapy protocol specific to the procedure is required for an optimal outcome.

Considerations in Special Populations

- Tearing of the hip abductor tendon complex is a relatively infrequent cause of lateral trochanteric hip pain but should be considered in all patients, particularly older females, with lateral hip pain and abductor weakness that are unresponsive to nonsurgical management.

- Patients who have had previous total hip arthroplasty performed through an anterolateral or transgluteal approach.

Suggested Readings

Bunker TD, Esler CN, Leach WJ. Rotator-cuff tear of the hip. *J Bone Joint Surg Br*. 1997;79(4):618–620.

Byrd JWT, Jones KS. Endoscopic repair of hip abductor tears: outcomes with two-year follow-up. *J Hip Preserv Surg*. 2017;4(1):80–84.

Chandrasekaran S, Lodhia P, Gui C, et al. Outcomes of open versus endoscopic repair of abductor muscle tears of the hip: a systematic review. *Arthroscopy*. 2015;31(10):2057–2067, e2.

Flack NA, Nicholson HD, Woodley SJ. The anatomy of the hip abductor muscles. *Clin Anat*. 2014;27(2):241–253.

Hendry J, Biant LC, Breusch SJ. Abductor mechanism tears in primary total hip arthroplasty. *Arch Orthop Trauma Surg*. 2012;132(11): 1619–1632.

Howell GE, Biggs RE, Bourne RB. Prevalence of abductor mechanism tears of the hips in patients with osteoarthritis. *J Arthroplasty*. 2001; 16(1):121–123.

Lachiewicz PF. Abductor tendon tears of the hip: evaluation and management. *J Am Acad Orthop Surg*. 2011;19(7):385–391.

Lindner D, Shohat N, Botser I, et al. Clinical presentation and imaging results of patients with symptomatic gluteus medius tears. *J Hip Preserv Surg*. 2015;2(3):310–315.

McCormick F, Alpaugh K, Nwachukwu BU, et al. Endoscopic repair of full-thickness abductor tendon tears: surgical technique and outcome at minimum of 1-year follow-up. *Arthroscopy*. 2013;29(12):1941–1947.

Patton T, Thibodeau GA. Anatomy of the muscular system. In: *Anatomy & Physiology*. 7th ed. St. Louis: Elsevier; 2010.

Redmond JM, Chen AW, Domb BG. Greater trochanteric pain syndrome. *J Am Acad Orthop Surg*. 2016;24(4):231–240.

Stanton MC, Maloney MD, Dehaven KE, Giordano BD. Acute traumatic tear of gluteus medius and minimus tendons in a patient without antecedant peritrochanteric hip pain. *Geriatr Orthop Surg Rehabil*. 2012; 3(2):84–88.

Strauss EJ, Nho SJ, Kelly BT. Greater trochanteric pain syndrome. *Sports Med Arthrosc*. 2010;18(2):113–119.

Williams BS, Cohen SP. Greater trochanteric pain syndrome: A review of anatomy, diagnosis and treatment. *Anesth Analg*. 2009;108(5): 1162–1670.

Chapter 128 Peritrochanteric Disorders and External Snapping Hip

Jeffrey Dart, Kevin deWeber

ICD-10-CM CODES
S76.01 *Gluteus medius/minimus tendinopathy*
M70.61 *Trochanteric bursitis*
M76.1 *Snapping hip syndrome*

Key Concepts

- Greater trochanteric pain syndrome (GTPS) is a common cause of lateral hip pain, and is a diagnosis that encompasses several conditions involving the lateral hip area:
  - Tendinopathy and partial tears of the hip abductors (gluteus medius and minimus) are the most common conditions.
  - Trochanteric bursitis (uncommon)
  - External snapping hip (external coxa saltans)
- The greater trochanter has several facets for the insertion of the gluteal tendons (Fig. 128.1):
  - The wide fan-shaped gluteus medius consolidates into two tendon bundles that insert on the superoposterior facet and cranial portion of the lateral facet. Most of the lateral facet comprises a "bald spot" with no tendinous attachment but over which the iliotibial band (ITB) passes.
  - Gluteus minimus inserts mainly on the anterior facet.
  - The superoposterior facet and its gluteus medius tendon insertion are the location for the preponderance of peritrochanteric pathology.
- The ITB consists of three fused layers (fibers from gluteus maximus, iliac crest, and tensor fascia lata); it passes over the greater trochanter and inserts distally on the lateral knee.
- The peritrochanteric space includes at least three bursae. Tendinopathy, trauma, or altered gait leading to friction can lead to bursitis, which is an uncommon finding in isolation.
  - The trochanteric bursa is located between the greater trochanter's "bald spot" of the lateral facet and the overlying ITB/gluteus maximus.
  - The subgluteus medius bursa lies posterior and superior to the greater trochanter.
  - The subgluteus minimus bursa lies anterior and superior to the greater trochanter.
- External snapping hip syndrome is the result of forward movement of the proximal ITB over the greater trochanter during hip flexion, often causing a popping sound with or without pain and leading to thickening of the trochanteric bursa and/or ITB.
- Patients often have 2 or more diagnoses in the GTPS group contributing to their pain.

History

- Lateral hip pain is the most common complaint, often worse with side-bending, prolonged sitting, or pressure on the affected side (e.g., lying on the side).
- Pain may radiate distally down the thigh or posteriorly into the gluteal region.
- Coxa saltans presents with painful snapping, catching, or popping with a specific movement demonstrated by the patient, typically flexion of the adducted and internally rotated hip.
- Patients with coxa saltans often have a history of repetitive physical activity/chronic overuse involving extremes of hip motion such as athletes, specifically dancers.

Physical Examination

- The patient may exhibit an antalgic gait or Trendelenburg gait, which indicates either hip joint disease or GTPS. A short-leg limp may indicate limb-length discrepancy or ITB pathology.
- Tenderness to palpation over the greater trochanter is a common finding:
  - Tenderness over the superoposterior facet correlates with gluteus medius pathology.
  - Tenderness only over the lateral facet may correlate with trochanteric bursitis or coxa saltans.
- A positive Trendelenburg test indicates abductor weakness or insufficiency (downward tilt of the contralateral hemipelvis during single-leg stance on the affected side).
- Pain with resisted hip abduction is common with gluteus medius/minimus pathology.
- The Patrick (flexion, extension, external rotation [FABER]) test can reproduce pain from hip joint or sacroiliac (SI) joint pathology, which can both radiate to the lateral hip.
- The Ober test can detect contractures of the ITB or gluteus medius/maximus.
- Test for external snapping hip by moving the affected extremity from flexion, abduction, and external rotation to extension, adduction, and internal rotation. Alternatively, having the patient demonstrate the motion causing pain can help localize pathology.
- Leg length discrepancy should be ruled out by clinical measurement from the anterior superior iliac spine (ASIS) to the distal medial malleolus.

Imaging

- Radiography is rarely needed when the diagnosis is clear but may be useful when the diagnosis is uncertain or when ruling out hip degenerative joint disease and other sources

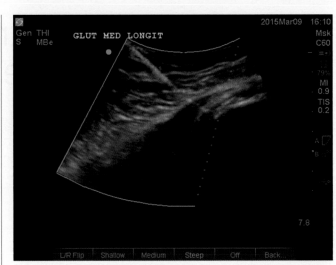

Fig 128.2 An injection of lidocaine under ultrasound guidance can provide more specific localization of the pathologic structure.

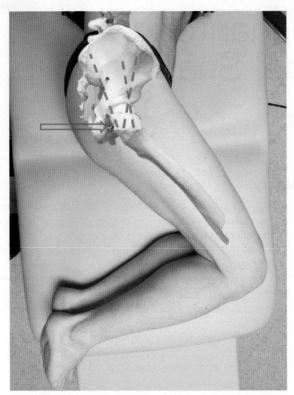

Fig 128.1 Th greater trochanter has three facets for insertion of the gluteal tendons. Gluteus medius tendon *(red dashed lines)*, gluteus minimus tendon *(green dashed line)*, and common point of maximal tenderness at superoposterior facet *(open arrow)*.

of referred pain. Nonspecific findings of GTPS include intrabursal calcification, calcific abductor tendinosis, and enthesophytes.
- Ultrasound can reveal abductor tendinosis or tears, thickened ITB, or bursitis. Accuracy diminishes with rising adiposity.
- Dynamic ultrasound can reveal snapping of the ITB against the trochanter to demonstrate external snapping hip.
- MRI is the most comprehensive modality for hip joint and extra-articular structures but is rarely needed, as in cases not responding to conservative measures or when the diagnosis is uncertain.

Differential Diagnosis

- Gluteus medius tendon rupture
- Tensor fascia lata strain
- Low back pathology radiating distally
- Osteoarthritis of the hip, and other intra-articular disorders
- Rectus femoris tendon origin injury
- Leg length discrepancy

Treatment

- Conservative therapies
  - Antiinflammatory medications, ice, and brief activity modification help control acute pain.
  - Rehabilitative exercise (hip abductor stretches and strength) is essential, initially at home or under supervision of physical therapy if needed.

- Corticosteroid injection at the point of maximal tenderness is very effective and lasts for weeks to months. Ultrasound guidance is useful in patients with large body habitus. Repeated injections (minimum 3-month intervals) should only be done in patients doing high-quality rehabilitative exercise to minimize tendon atrophy.
- Extracorporeal shock wave therapy can improve pain and function in GTPS patients.
- Needle tenotomy, prolotherapy, and platelet-rich plasma injection are unproven but may be considered in refractory cases. These are best done under ultrasound guidance (Fig. 128.2).
- Surgical therapies (open or endoscopic procedures) are rarely used in refractory cases.
  - Bursectomy, open and arthroscopic ITB lengthening, or release for bursitis and snapping hip.
  - Treatment of hip abductor tears.

When to Refer

- Patients failing to respond to nonoperative management, including quality rehabilitative exercise, for at least 12 months and if high-grade tears of the hip abductor tendons are seen on ultrasound or MRI.

Prognosis

- The majority of patients (75%) will see return to sport or work within 3 months during a course of conservative management and corticosteroid injection.
- Up to 25% of patients will have complete resolution of symptoms at 12 months, and two-thirds of patients will report some relief in that time.

Troubleshooting

- Failure of initial management, despite good adherence to recommendations, may indicate intra-articular hip or low back pathology, and the provider should maintain a low threshold for broadening the differential.

TABLE 128.1 Components of Trochanteric Bursa Injection

Syringe	Needle	Anesthetic Agent	Corticosteroid
10 mL	22- or 25-gauge, 1.5 inch or longer	3–5 mL total volume of 1% lidocaine	40 mg triamcinolone or 6 mg betamethasone

- Injecting local anesthetic to the point of maximal tenderness can be both temporarily therapeutic as well as diagnostic for localizing the source of pain (Table 128.1).

Patient Instructions

- Activity modification is necessary for snapping hip.
- Stretching/strengthening exercises should be continued after resolution of symptoms to prevent recurrence.
- Notify physician if patient is unable to tolerate physical therapy; corticosteroid injection of tendinopathy to reduce pain may facilitate quality rehab exercise.

Considerations for Special Populations

- For elderly patients, low back or intra-articular hip pathology must always be considered in the differential for GTPS.

Suggested Readings

Barratt PA, Brookes N, Newson A. Conservative treatments for greater trochanteric pain syndrome: a systematic review. *Br J Sports Med.* 2017;51:97–104.

Flato R, Passanante GJ, Skalski MR, et al. The iliotibial tract: imaging, anatomy, injuries, and other pathology. *Skeletal Radiol.* 2017;46:605–622.

Grimaldi A, Mellor R, Hodges P, et al. Gluteal tendinopathy: a review of mechanisms, assessment and management. *Sports Med.* 2015;45(8):1107–1119.

Ho GW, Howard TM. Greater trochanteric pain syndrome: more than bursitis and iliotibial tract friction. *Curr Sports Med Rep.* 2012;11(5):232–238.

Jacobson JA, Yablon CM, Henning PT, et al. Greater trochanteric pain syndrome: percutaneous tendon fenestration versus platelet-rich plasma injection for treatment of gluteal tendinosis. *J Ultrasound Med.* 2016;35:2413–2420.

Redmond JM, Chen AW, Domb BG. Greater trochanteric pain syndrome. *J Am Acad Orthop Surg.* 2016;24:231–240.

Reid D. The management of greater trochanteric pain syndrome: a systematic literature review. *J Orthop.* 2016;16:15–28.

Shrestha A, Wu P, Ge H, Cheng B. Clinical outcomes of arthroscopic surgery for external snapping hip. *J Orthop Surg Res.* 2017;12(1):81.

Chapter 129 Iliopsoas Disorders and Internal Snapping Hip

Patrick King, Patricia Feeney, Aaron Vaughan, Robert Boykin

ICD-10-CM CODES
M25.551 *Hip pain, right*
M25.552 *Hip pain, left*
S76.001 *Unspecified injury of muscle, fascia, and tendon of hip,*
S76.002 *Unspecified injury of muscle, fascia, and tendon of hip, left*
M24.851 *Other specific joint derangements of hip, not elsewhere classified, right*
M24.852 *Other specific joint derangements of hip, not elsewhere classified, left*
M76.11 *Psoas tendinitis, right*
M76.12 *Psoas tendinitis, left*

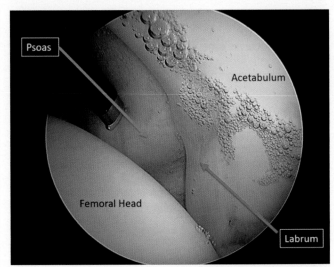

Fig 129.1 Left hip arthroscopic image. A tight psoas tendon is seen indenting the capsule and labrum in the anterior region of the acetabulum.

Key Concepts

- Coxa saltans or snapping hip syndrome
- Most common in young, active women 15 to 40 years of age
- More common in sports that require repetitive hip flexion, extension, and abduction
  - Dancers, distance runners, rowers, and cyclists
  - 50–90% of ballet dancers
- Iliopsoas disorders
  - Pathologic involvement of iliopsoas muscle or surrounding structures; strain, tendinitis/tendinopathy, bursitis, abscess, hematoma
  - "Psoas Impingement": a tight iliopsoas may create impingement on the far anterior labrum and lead to labral tearing (Fig. 129.1)
- Internal snapping hip
  - Occurs when a portion of the iliopsoas tendon slides over a bony prominence, usually the iliopectineal eminence, acetabular rim, or femoral head, creating tension and a resulting "snap"; can cause resultant iliopsoas bursitis (Fig. 129.2)
- Refer to Table 129.1 for differentiation of the types of snapping hip.

TABLE 129.1 Differentiation of the Types of Snapping Hip

Type	Anatomic Structure Implicated	Cause
External	Greater trochanter	Iliotibial band or gluteus maximus muscle snapping over greater trochanter
Internal	Iliopsoas tendon	Iliopsoas tendon snapping over iliopectineal eminence or femoral head
Intra-articular	Hip joint	Loose bodies, osteochondral fractures, labral tears, synovial chondromatosis

History

- Asymptomatic snapping may be common, does not require treatment
- Iliopsoas disorders
  - Pain localized to groin, possibly lower back or lower abdomen
  - Repeated forceful hip flexion (i.e., hurdlers, jumpers)
  - May be associated with trauma (i.e., bursitis, hematoma), overuse (i.e., tendinopathy, bursitis), recent hip or lumbar

spine surgery (i.e., abscess, hematoma), or arthritis (i.e., osteoarthritis, rheumatoid arthritis, septic arthritis)
- May have similar symptoms to labral tear, or other intrinsic disorders of hip
  - Psoas disorders may occur concomitantly with labral pathology as seen in psoas impingement of the labrum
- Consider abscess in setting of systemic symptoms; fever present in up to 75% of cases of psoas abscess

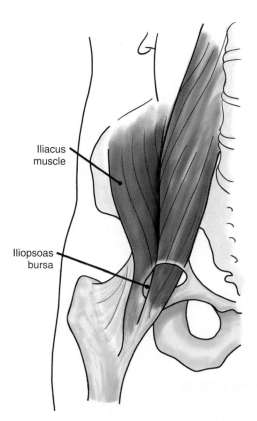

Fig 129.2 Iliopsoas bursa between the distal portion of the iliacus muscle and the psoas muscle. (Modified from Morelli V, Weaver V. Groin injuries and groin pain in athletes: part 1. *Prim Care.* 2005;32(1):163–183, Fig. 3.)

- Also can be seen after a total hip arthroplasty procedure, especially if there is anterior prominence to the acetabular component causing irritation of the psoas
- Internal snapping hip
  - Patient reports audible and/or typically anterior painful snapping, popping, or clicking sound/sensation with hip flexion to extension
  - Symptoms are most common during exercise but may be present afterward
  - May progress from painless snapping to debilitating pain
  - Consider as a potential cause of pain in patients after a total hip arthroplasty

Physical Examination

- Gait observation
  - Rule out muscular imbalance or neurologic impairment (i.e., Trendelenburg gait)
- Iliopsoas disorders
  - Painful hip extension or resisted hip flexion; may improve with hip flexion and lumbar lordosis which decreases tensile strain
  - Tight, painful hip flexors
  - Painful or painless mass below inguinal ligament (i.e., psoas abscess, hematoma)
- Internal snapping hip
  - Patients often voluntarily demonstrate snapping
  - Bringing the hip from the flexion, abduction, external rotation position to the extension, adduction, and internal rotation position reproduces symptoms as the iliopsoas tendon moves and snaps over the bony prominence (Fig. 129.3)

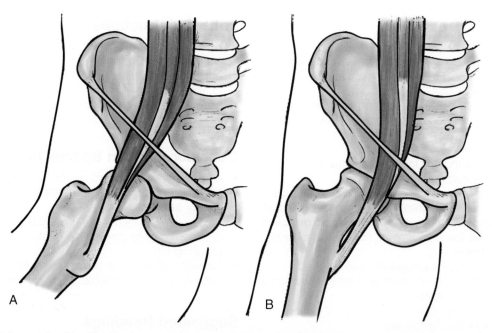

A   B

Fig 129.3 Internal snapping hip. The iliopsoas tendon snaps back and forth over the iliopectineal eminence. **(A)** The hip shown in the FABER (flexion, abduction, external rotation) position. The iliopsoas tendon lies lateral to the center of the femoral head. **(B)** The hip is brought into the EADIR (extension, adduction, internal rotation) position. The iliopsoas tendon snaps in the medial position. (Modified from Byrd JWT. Snapping hip. *Oper Tech Sports Med.* 2005;13(1):46–54, Fig. 1.)

Imaging

- Plain radiographs typically normal; however, helpful to rule out bony pathology
  - Assess for anterior overhang of the acetabular component in total hip arthroplasty
- Dynamic ultrasonography may be able to visualize snapping and/or demonstrate tendinopathy and bursitis
- Computed tomography can be useful to define bony deformity in femoroacetabular impingement (large pincer lesion, cam deformity)
- Magnetic resonance imaging improves definition of soft tissues and adjacent structures and is useful for evaluation of an abscess, hematoma, and musculotendinous pathology, although not essential to diagnosing iliopsoas disorders or internal snapping hip
  - With arthrography if labral tear suspected
  - Consider psoas impingement if far anterior labral tear (3 o'clock position)

Differential Diagnosis

- External snapping hip
  - Iliotibial band or gluteus maximus
- Intra-articular snapping hip
  - Osteoarthritis, loose bodies, osteochondral fractures, labral tears, synovial chondromatosis, hip instability
- Femoral neck stress fracture
- Avascular necrosis
- Septic arthritis
- Retrocecal appendicitis
- Pediatric
  - Legg-Calvé-Perthes disease, slipped capital femoral epiphysis, inflammatory/infectious synovitis, avulsion fracture

Treatment

- Initial treatment based on working differential diagnoses
  - Primary goal is pain relief and correction of modifiable biomechanical factors
  - Graded return to activity as symptoms allow
  - Nonsteroidal antiinflammatory drugs (NSAIDs), other analgesics
  - Activity modification/relative rest
  - Formal physical therapy for iliopsoas stretching
  - Consider osteopathic therapy
  - Injection (corticosteroid and/or lidocaine) of iliopsoas bursa and/or tendinous sheath, which may be diagnostic and therapeutic. Ultrasound or fluoroscopic guidance should be used due to proximity to neurovascular bundle.
- Continued treatment
  - Reevaluation to see if symptoms have resolved
  - Consider prolotherapy: i.e., dextrose, platelet rich plasma (PRP), stem cells—limited data
  - Consider hydrodissection
  - Consider tendinous fenestration
- Hematoma: correct coagulopathy, drainage based on size, close monitoring
- Abscess: antibiotics and consult for surgical versus interventional radiology drainage

When to Refer

- Patients with symptoms after 3 to 6 months of conservative therapy
- Consider if concomitant intra-articular pathology discovered and recalcitrant to conservative measures
- Surgical treatment options for iliopsoas tendinopathy: endoscopic versus open debridement, or fractional lengthening
- Surgical treatment considerations for internal snapping hip: endoscopic versus open release (fractional lengthening). Can be accomplished endoscopically/arthroscopically at the level of the labrum through the joint, in the peripheral compartment, or at the level of the lesser trochanter. The tendinous portion is transected, leaving the muscular fibers intact. Caution in dysplastic patients as this may cause increased symptoms of hip instability.

Prognosis

- Excellent prognosis with few patients requiring surgical intervention
- Full return to activity likely after 6 to 8 weeks of appropriate conservative measures

Troubleshooting

- Internal and intra-articular snapping hips are difficult to distinguish clinically
  - Use imaging and diagnostic injections to differentiate
- Correction of biomechanical factors may hasten recovery time
- If unresponsive to conservative modalities, make sure to reevaluate differential and consider referral to orthopaedic surgeon

Patient Instructions

- Work on focused iliopsoas stretching, avoid strengthening until psoas is nonpainful
- Attempt to modify activity to avoid positions that predispose to hip snapping
- If pain worsens with stretching and physical therapy, notify the physician immediately

Considerations in Special Populations

- An external snapping hip can be seen in geriatric patients after hip arthroplasty due to lateral displacement of the greater trochanter
- With pediatric patients, the presence of hip dysplasia and/or instability may predispose to internal or intra-articular snapping hip
- Consider adhesions or prominent implants in postoperative patients, possible abscess (although rare)

Suggested Readings

Anderson CN. Iliopsoas: pathology, diagnosis, and treatment. *Clin Sports Med*. 2016;35(3):419–433.

Anderson K, Strickland SM, Warren R. Hip and groin injuries in athletes. *Am J Sports Med*. 2001;29:521–533.

Byrd JWT. Snapping hip. *Oper Tech Sports Med*. 2005;13:46–54.

Chalmers BP, Sculco PK, Sierra RJ, et al. Iliopsoas impingement after primary total hip arthroplasty: operative and nonoperative treatment outcomes. *J Bone Joint Surg Am*. 2017;99(7):557–564.

de Sa D, Alradwan H, Cargnelli S, et al. Extra-articular hip impingement: a systematic review examining operative treatment of psoas, subspine, ischiofemoral, and greater trochanteric/pelvic impingement. *Arthroscopy*. 2014;30(8):1026–1041.

Dobbs MB, Gordon E, Luhmann SJ, et al. Surgical correction of the snapping iliopsoas tendon in adolescents. *J Bone Joint Surg Am*. 2002;84A:420–424.

Domb BG, Shindle MK, McArthur B, et al. Iliopsoas impingement: a newly identified cause of labral pathology in the hip. *HSS J*. 2011;7(2):145–150.

James SL, Ali K, Pocock C, et al. Ultrasound guided dry needling and autologous blood injection for patellar tendinosis. *Br J Sports Med*. 2007;41:518–521.

Kelly BT, Williams RJ, Philippon MJ. Hip arthroscopy: current indications, treatment options, and management issues. *Am J Sports Med*. 2003;31:1020–1037.

Lee YT, Lee CM, Su SC, et al. Psoas abscess: a 10 year review. *J Microbiol Immunol Infect*. 1999;32(1):40–46.

Morelli V, Smith V. Groin injuries in athletes. *Am Fam Physician*. 2001;64:1405–1414.

Perets I, Hartigan DE, Chaharbakhshi EO, et al. Clinical outcomes and return to sport in competitive athletes undergoing arthroscopic iliopsoas fractional lengthening compared with a matched control group without iliopsoas fractional lengthening. *Arthroscopy*. 2018;34(2):456–463.

Wahl CJ, Warren RF, Adler RS, et al. Internal coxa saltans (snapping hip) as a result of overtraining: a report of 3 cases in professional athletes with a review of causes and the role of ultrasound in early diagnosis and management. *Am J Sports Med*. 2004;32:1302–1309.

Winston P, Awan R, Cassidy JD, Bleakney RK. Clinical examination and ultrasound of self-reported snapping hip syndrome in elite ballet dancers. *Am J Sports Med*. 2007;35:118–126.

Yelland MJ, Sweeting KR, Lyftogt JA, et al. Prolotherapy injections and eccentric loading exercises for painful achilles tendinosis: a randomized trial. *Br J Sports Med*. 2011;45:421–428.

Chapter 130 Hip Flexor and Groin Strain

Alexander Knobloch, Cole Taylor

ICD-10-CM CODES
S76.01 *Strain of muscle, fascia and tendon of hip*
S76.11 *Strain of quadriceps muscle, fascia and tendon*
S76.21 *Strain of adductor muscle, fascia and tendon of thigh*

Key Concepts

- Hip flexor and groin (adductor) strains are common injuries in athletes, especially those in sports that involve kicking, cutting, and sprinting, such as soccer, football, and ice hockey.
- Among soccer players, groin injuries account for 8–18% of all injuries.
- A number of muscles are involved in flexion of the hip, including the iliopsoas, rectus femoris, sartorius, tensor fasciae latae, pectineus, and the adductor muscles. The iliopsoas and rectus femoris muscles, which are innervated by the femoral nerve (L2-L4), are the major hip flexors that are most commonly involved in injuries (Fig. 130.1).
- The adductor muscle group is made up of the adductor longus, magnus, and brevis, along with the gracilis, obturator externus, and pectineus (see Fig. 130.1). All the adductor muscles are innervated by the obturator nerve (L2-L4) except the pectineus (femoral nerve, L2-L4) and the adductor magnus (both obturator and tibial nerve [L2-S3]).
- Prior adductor or hip flexor strain, decreased strength in these muscle groups, and higher level of play have been associated with an increased risk of adductor and hip flexor injuries.
- Returning athletes to play before they can perform pain-free, sport-specific activities can lead to prolonged recovery or chronic injury.

History

- Pain localized to the proximal anterior, middle anterior, or medial thigh
- May be an insidious onset with progressive pain or a sudden, painful event, especially after a sudden change in direction or sudden increase in acceleration, kicking, or other forceful eccentric contraction of the hip flexor or adductor muscles. Pain after hyperextension of the hip may also be reported in hip flexor injuries.
- In an acute injury, the patient commonly reports "ripping" or "stabbing" pain in the groin or the medial thigh that

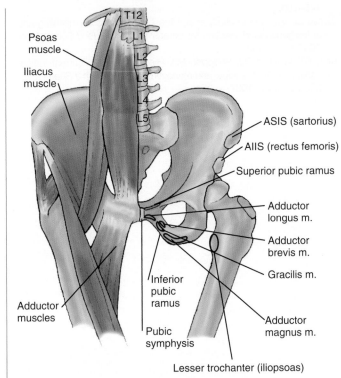

Fig 130.1 Applied anatomy of the groin with muscle insertions and origins. *AIIS,* Anteroinferior iliac spine; *ASIS,* anterosuperior iliac spine; *m,* muscle.

is intensified with passive abduction (adductor strain) or passive hip extension (hip flexor strain). This pain is replaced by an intense dull ache.
- In a chronic injury, the pain is often described as a diffuse dull ache that may be felt deep in the groin (iliopsoas strain), radiate distally along the anterior aspect of the thigh (rectus femoris strain), or radiate distally along the medial aspect of the thigh (adductor strain).
- In patients with pain unrelated to a specific injury or repetitive exercise, genitourinary, gynecologic, and gastrointestinal symptoms that suggest a nonmusculoskeletal etiology should also be explored.

Physical Examination

- A detailed and thorough examination, along with an understanding of the anatomy, will help to distinguish hip flexor and groin (adductor) strains from other causes of groin pain (Table 130.1).

TABLE 130.1 Differential Diagnosis of Groin Pain

Condition	Differentiating Features	Chapter Reference
Groin (adductor) strain	Painful resisted hip adduction and tenderness along the adductor muscle group.	
Hip flexor (iliopsoas or rectus femoris) strain	Painful resisted hip flexion and pain on hip flexor stretching. May have tenderness near the insertion of the iliopsoas on the femur or along the length of the rectus femoris.	
Osteitis pubis	Palpable tenderness at the pubic symphysis; may also see loss of rotation of one or both hips, positive pubic spring test, positive lateral compression test. Radiographs, magnetic resonance imaging, and/or bone scan can help to determine the diagnosis.	137
Athletic pubalgia	Previously referred to as sports hernia, groin disruption. Suspected to occur due to disruption of the rectus abdominus insertion at the pubic bone and a weakened posterior inguinal wall. Pain located in the region of the inguinal canal, pubic tubercle, or at or near the rectus insertion. No palpable inguinal hernia. Pain increases with resistance testing of the abdominal muscles and Valsalva.	136
Obturator neuropathy/ nerve entrapment	Deep ache near the adductor origin on the pubic rami that worsens with exercise and may radiate down medial thigh toward the knee. Spasm, weakness, and paresthesias of the adductors can also occur. Pain with hip abduction and external rotation and with resisted hip internal rotation (all causing nerve stretch). Electromyography or obturator nerve block can support the diagnosis. Also consider ilioinguinal, genitofemoral, and iliohypogastric nerve entrapments.	18
Pelvic avulsion fracture/ apophysitis	Pain and tenderness at the anterosuperior iliac spine, anteroinferior iliac spine, pubic rami, or lesser trochanter after an acute injury. More likely in pediatric and adolescent patients. Plain radiographs can confirm fracture.	225
Stress fracture	Medial thigh or groin pain that worsens with exercise, relieved with rest. Associated with repetitive overuse, endurance athletes. Most commonly occurs at the femoral neck or pubic ramus, leading to vague pain localization. Inability to complete single-leg hop due to pain. MRI or bone scan can confirm diagnosis.	123
Intra-articular hip sources of groin pain	Wide differential that includes femoroacetabular impingement, acetabular labral injury, hip osteoarthritis, hip avascular necrosis, slipped capital femoral epiphysis, Legg-Calvé-Perthes disease. Will often see painful or limited hip internal rotation, particularly with FADIR test (flexion, adduction, internal rotation). Plain radiographs and magnetic resonance imaging can be useful for clarifying diagnosis.	119–122, 212–213
Nonmusculoskeletal sources of groin pain	If history and exam do not suggest one of the above etiologies, consider evaluating the patient for the presence of gastrointestinal, genitourinary, or gynecologic conditions.	

- Ecchymosis or swelling can be observed at the proximal medial or anterior thigh or along the course of the adductor muscles.
- Adductor strains
  - Palpable tenderness along the adductor muscles or near their origin along the pubic bone
  - Pain and tightness with passive stretching of the adductor muscles with hip abduction
  - Pain with resisted hip adduction
- Hip flexor strains
  - Involving the iliopsoas
    - Palpable tenderness just medial to the anterosuperior iliac spine (ASIS) in the femoral triangle or along the psoas muscle above the inguinal ligament
  - Involving the rectus femoris

- Palpable tenderness can be found anywhere from its origin at the anteroinferior iliac spine (AIIS) to more distally along the anterior thigh
- Pain with resisted hip flexion
- Pain and tightness with passive stretching of the iliopsoas and rectus femoris with hip extension or a modified Thomas test (which involves maximally flexing the contralateral hip while stretching the affected hip flexor)

Imaging

- Imaging is generally unnecessary if history and exam suggest a hip flexor or groin (adductor) strain.
- If bony tenderness is present at the origin of the adductor muscles (pubic rami), the origin of the rectus femoris (AIIS),

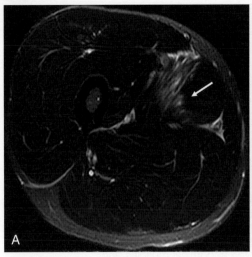
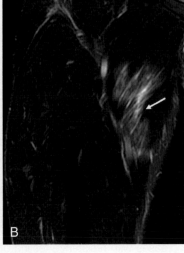

Fig 130.2 Axial **(A)** and coronal **(B)** fat-saturation fast spin-echo T2-weighted magnetic resonance imaging showing an adductor longus muscle strain *(arrows)*, with approximately 50–60% circumferential involvement of the muscle. (From McSweeney SE, Naraghi A, Salonen D, et al. Hip and groin pain in the professional athlete. *Can Assoc Radiol J.* 2012;63:87–99.)

or the insertion of the iliopsoas (lesser trochanter) after an acute onset of pain, plain radiographs can be useful in ruling out an avulsion fracture.

- In cases of diagnostic uncertainty or for injuries unresponsive to therapy, ultrasound and magnetic resonance imaging (MRI) are the modalities of choice to confirm injury to these muscle groups (Fig. 130.2).
- Ultrasound has a sensitivity of up to 84% when compared to the gold standard of MRI for the detection of muscle strains.
  - Advantageous in the ability to use sonopalpation to dynamically reproduce a patient's pain with palpation of a sonographically abnormal finding
- MRI can yield prognostic information about muscle strains and tears. Although there are no studies to date involving specific prognosis for adductor or iliopsoas strains seen on MRI, tears involving larger cross-sectional areas and tears located at specific locations (such as the central tendon of the rectus femoris) are generally associated with prolonged recovery.

Additional Tests

- None are required for hip flexor or adductor strains.
- If the history or physical examination suggests a nonmusculoskeletal source of the patient's groin pain, additional studies may be indicated.

Differential Diagnosis

- Please see Table 130.1.

Treatment

- Treatment principles are similar for both hip flexor and adductor strains (Fig. 130.3). Rehabilitation should follow a stepwise progression through the following phases:
- Phase 1: Range of motion and isometric exercises
  - Range of motion exercises can be performed multiple times per day. Avoid exercises that cause moderate to severe pain (>5/10).
  - Isometric exercises should be performed daily, with increasing resistance and increasing duration as tolerated.

- This phase should also include PRICE (Protection, Relative Rest [avoid painful activities, consider using crutches for a few days in acute strains], Ice, Compression, Elevation).
- Short courses of nonsteroidal antiinflammatory drugs can also be given.
- Modalities such as electrical stimulation and massage can help to alleviate muscle spasm.
- Once the patient is able to engage in normal activities of daily living without pain and has no pain with range of motion and isometric exercises, they can progress to the next phase.
- Phase 2: Progressive strengthening
  - Eccentric and concentric exercises with gradually increasing load while varying repetitions to achieve increased strength and neuromuscular coordination. Exercises should occur three times a week with at least one rest day in between each session.
  - Aerobic exercises can be introduced but should avoid cutting or aggressive changes in speed.
  - Once the patient can straight-line run and advance through the strengthening program without pain, they can progress to the next phase.
  - Other biomechanical abnormalities should be sought and corrected if found.
- Phase 3: Proprioception, dynamic sport-specific exercises, and return to play/activity
  - Return to play/activity goals
    - Patient has restored the vast majority of his or her strength compared with the contralateral side.
    - Patient has pain-free full range of motion.
    - Patient can perform sport-specific exercises without pain or alteration of mechanics.

When to Refer

- Although the vast majority of adductor and hip flexor injuries can be successfully managed conservatively, refer patients with chronic hip flexor or adductor strains that fail to respond after at least 6 months of conservative treatment.
  - Experienced orthopaedists or sports medicine physicians may have experience in treating these conditions with

Hip Flexor and Groin Strains

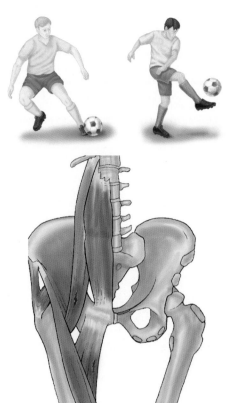

- **MOI:** Kicking, cutting, and sprinting

- **PE:** Tenderness along the affected muscle; pain with resisted hip flexion/passive hip extension or resisted adduction/passive abduction

- **Tx:** Progressive rehabilitation
  - Phase 1: PRICE, ROM, and isometrics
  - Phase 2: Progressive strengthening
  - Phase 3: Proprioception, dynamic sport-specific exercises, return to play

- **Return to Play:**
  - Return of strength compared to contralateral side
  - Pain-free ROM
  - Pain-free with sports-specific exercises

Fig 130.3 Summary of hip flexor and groin (adductor) muscle strain diagnosis and management. *MOI*, Mechanism of injury; *PE*, physical exam; *PRICE*, protection, rest, ice, compression, elevation; *Tx*, treatment; *ROM*, range of motion.

advanced injections (prolotherapy, platelet-rich plasma [PRP], etc.), dry needling, or acupuncture.
- Rare indications for surgical referral include chronic tendinopathy refractory to the aforementioned interventions, where a tenotomy may be considered, and a large bony avulsion at the tendon origin or insertion.

Prognosis

- Many athletes with minor injuries advance rapidly through their rehabilitation program and are able to return to sports in less than 1 week. More significant injuries may take 4 to 8 weeks for recovery and require careful advancement through their rehabilitation program.
- In chronic injuries, rehabilitation may take anywhere from 2 to 6 months before return to sports.

Troubleshooting

- The patient must be pain free with sports-specific activities to return to sports to avoid risk of reinjury or chronic injury.
- The use of corticosteroid injections in hip flexor and adductor strains is controversial. Although corticosteroids are likely to improve pain and inflammation in the short term, there is concern that steroids could weaken the tendon and predispose to chronic or recurrent injury.

Patient Instructions

- Counsel patients that these injuries respond well to conservative therapies and will benefit from long-term maintenance of hip flexor and adductor strength.
- Follow physician, physical therapist, and/or athletic trainer instructions closely with respect to the type, quantity, and timing of exercises and activities that are appropriate for the stage of injury.
- Counsel patients regarding symptoms that may suggest an alternative diagnosis or require immediate evaluation (see Table 130.1).

Considerations in Special Populations

- Those caring for athletes (particularly in sports involving kicking, cutting, and sprinting) will commonly encounter this condition.
- Treatment for athletes with hip flexor and adductor injuries requires a team approach and an understanding of the athlete's practice and competition schedule.
- Hip flexor and groin strains are recurrent in up to 50% of athletes, with highest rates of recurrence in ice hockey.
- Studies have shown mixed results regarding the efficacy of preseason and in-season exercise programs designed to prevent groin pain in competitive athletes.

Suggested Readings

Bayer ML, Magnusson SP, Kjaer M. Early versus delayed rehabilitation after acute muscle injury. *N Engl J Med*. 2017;377:1300–1301.

Eckard TG, Padua DA, Dompier TP, et al. Epidemiology of hip flexor and hip adductor strains in national collegiate athletic association athletes, 2009/2010-2014/2015. *Am J Sports Med*. 2017;45:2713–2722.

Hölmich P, Hölmich LR, Bjerg AM. Clinical examination of athletes with groin pain: an intraobserver and interobserver reliability study. *Br J Sports Med*. 2004;38:446–451.

Lee SC, Endo Y, Potter HG. Imaging of groin pain: magnetic resonance and ultrasound imaging features. *Sports Health*. 2017;9:428–435.

Morelli V, Weaver V. Groin injuries and groin pain in athletes: part 1. *Prim Care*. 2005;32:163–183.

Morelli V, Weaver V. Groin injuries and groin pain in athletes: part 2. *Prim Care*. 2005;32:185–200.

Serner A, Tol JL, Jomaah N, et al. Diagnosis of acute groin injuries: a prospective study of 110 athletes. *Am J Sports Med*. 2015;43:1857–1864.

Tyler TF, Silvers HJ, Gerhardt MB, Nicholas SJ. Groin injuries in sports medicine. *Sports Health*. 2010;2:252–261.

Weir A, Brukner P, Delahunt E, et al. Doha agreement meeting on terminology and definitions in groin pain in athletes. *Br J Sports Med*. 2015;49:768–774.

Chapter 131 Quadriceps Contusions

Tracy R. Ray, Ryan L. Freedman

ICD-10-CM CODES

S76.1 *Injury of quadriceps muscle, fascia and tendon*
M61.059 *Myositis ossificans traumatica of thigh*

Key Concepts

- A crush injury to the quadriceps musculature due to a direct blow causing either an intramuscular or intermuscular hematoma secondary to capillary damage.
- Very common occurrence in contact sports (e.g., football, rugby, martial arts).
- Many contusions go unreported and untreated.
- An intramuscular hematoma takes longer to resolve and may be associated with the major complications of the injury (e.g., myositis ossificans, and acute compartment syndrome).
- Most often involves the anterior (quadriceps femoris and sartorius muscles) and lateral (vastus lateralis) compartments.
- Damaged tissue is replaced by a fibrous connective tissue scar that usually resolves, leaving no sign of injury after 3 to 4 weeks.
- Complications
  - Myositis ossificans (MO): heterotopic bone formation within muscular tissue
    - Pathogenesis still poorly understood, related to increased bone turnover.
    - Likelihood of occurrence increases with increasing grade of injury and with reinjury during recovery.
    - May reabsorb over time.
    - May be promoted by early surgery.
  - Acute compartment syndrome: increased pressure within anterior compartment secondary injury
    - Pain out of proportion to injury
    - Paresthesia distal to injury (later sign)
    - Severe pain with passive range of motion
- Please see Table 131.1 and Fig. 131.1.

History

- Presentation
  - History of blow to thigh in contact sport (e.g., football, rugby, soccer, judo/karate), could not return to play, or worsened 24 to 48 hours after initial injury
- Symptoms
  - Painful to bear weight
  - Difficulty with knee flexion due to pain
  - Tightness of affected thigh

TABLE 131.1 Quadriceps Contusion Grading

Grade	Range of Motion	Symptoms/Presentation
1	>90-degree flexion	Minimal effect on ambulation No/minimal discomfort with resisted extension Feeling of "tightness" in the thigh Little, if any, swelling
2	45–90-degree flexion	Antalgic gait Pain reproducible with palpation Pain with resisted extension Likely, swelling
3	<45-degree flexion	Significant limp; crutches often required Immediate and significant swelling Quadriceps contraction with leg in extension is painful Unable to oppose resisted extension due to pain

Physical Examination

- Inspection
  - Observe gait.
  - Note any ecchymosis.
  - Measurement of thigh girth (as much as a 4-cm difference can be normal)
- Palpation
  - Consider deferring to last piece of examination secondary to discomfort.
  - Note warmth and amount of tension in the thigh.
  - There may be a palpable hematoma.
  - Examine for a muscular of quadriceps/patellar tendon defect.
  - Perform patellar range of motion.
  - Assess neurovascular status.
  - Most reliable findings for assessing severity of injury include degree of firmness, circumference, range of motion (ROM), or assessment for joint effusion.
- Motion
  - Measure the flexion and extension of the knee.
  - Note the degree of passive flexion at which pain commences.
  - Measure degree of active flexion at which pain commences.
  - Perform straight leg raise (may be painful, but possible unless damage to extensor mechanism).

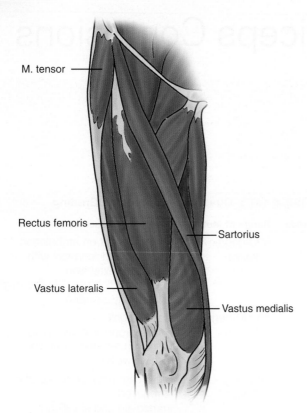

M. tensor

Rectus femoris

Sartorius

Vastus lateralis

Vastus medialis

Fig 131.1 Thigh anatomy. *M,* Musculus.

- Stability
  - Test ligamentous stability about the knee if swelling or effusion is present.

Imaging

- Radiographs
  - They should be obtained initially if there is any suspicion of bony injury; obtain additional radiographs if recovery is not progressing as expected (e.g., loss of flexion or worsening pain).
  - Radiographs may reveal MO as early as 2 weeks postinjury (Fig. 131.2).
- Magnetic resonance imaging (MRI)
  - There is no definite indication for MRI unless considering a surgical procedure or for localization of unresolved or complicating hematoma or swelling.
  - Abnormalities on MRI may last longer than symptoms and functional impairment.
- Ultrasound
  - Can be used for distinguishing between contusions and strains
  - May be used to evaluate for presence or the size of a hematoma; however, this is not likely to change necessary treatment
  - Current literature supports Jackson and Feagin classification for injury prognosis rather than ultrasound due to lack of comparison trials.

Differential Diagnosis

- Please see Table 131.2.

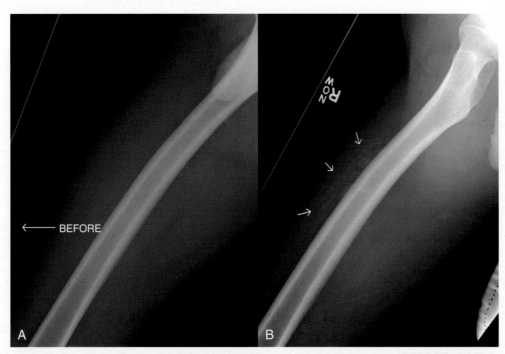

BEFORE

A   B

Fig 131.2 Radiograph of myositis ossificans. **(A)** Radiograph performed shortly after trauma *(BEFORE).* **(B)** Follow-up radiograph two weeks later shows the formation of myositis ossificans *(arrows).*

TABLE 131.2 Differential Diagnosis

Diagnosis	Features	Chapter Reference
Quadriceps contusion	Swelling, ecchymosis, history of traumatic blow	131
Myositis ossificans	Palpable mass, radiographic findings, decreased range of motion after period of improvement	14
Compartment syndrome	Pain out of proportion, neurologic symptoms	13
Quadriceps strain	No traumatic blow	

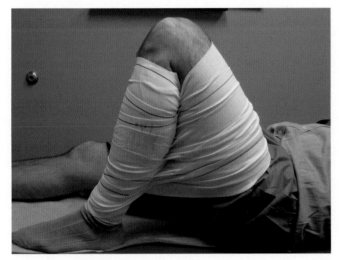

Fig 131.3 Example of patient immobilized in flexion using elastic wrap. Note that a postoperative or other locking knee brace can be used as well.

Treatment

- At time of diagnosis
  - Rest
  - Ice
  - Compression
  - Nonsteroidal antiinflammatory medications should be avoided in moderate to severe cases for 48 to 72 hours due to bleeding risk.
  - Treatment with intramuscular corticosteroid currently is not recommended due to delayed healing.
  - Immobilization of the knee in maximum painless flexion soon after injury may decrease the time to return to play; this should be maintained for 24 to 48 hours postinjury (Fig. 131.3).
- Early recovery
  - Active and passive painless ROM stressing flexion multiple times daily as soon as immobilization is discontinued
  - Perform painless isometric strengthening exercises as soon as possible.
  - Nonsteroidal antiinflammatory medication

- Late recovery
  - Noncontact functional rehabilitation
  - Return to sport with full ROM, no strength deficits, and successful completion of noncontact rehabilitation
- MO
  - Seen in 9–20% of military academy members following quadriceps contusion
  - Conservative treatment usually successful
  - Overly aggressive early therapy may stimulate growth of the ossification; avoid aggressive massage and forced motion and use pain as a guide.
  - Maintain range of motion.
  - In adults with stable MO (i.e., mature), excision of the mass may be considered if the ROM is significantly limited or pain is severe, but this can potentially result in recurrence and more extensive ossification.
  - One case report has shown successful treatment of MO with intravenous pamidronate, but no prospective trials have been completed.
- Acute compartment syndrome
  - Surgical emergency requiring a high level of clinical suspicion
  - Fasciotomy is sometimes performed, but a conservative approach involving rest, ice, compression, and elevation has shown promise.
  - If treating conservatively, monitor closely for muscular necrosis and renal compromise.

When to Refer

- Considered emergently if any signs or symptoms of acute compartment syndrome arise
- Considered if development of MO is accompanied by continuing symptoms that are affecting desired activities and/or significantly limiting ROM
- Considered if hematoma fails to resolve

Prognosis

- Length of recovery has been shown to be correlated with degree of severity in Jackson and Feagin classification.
- Risk factors that may prolong recovery in one study included:
  - Knee flexion ROM <120 degrees
  - Injury secondary to football
  - Previous quadriceps injury
  - Symptomatic knee effusion
  - Delayed treatment >3 days
- Generally, recovery is favorable because most patients are able to return to their previous level of activity without significant sequelae.
- Surgery is usually unnecessary and recovery is usually complete.
- Return to play should be allowed when motion, strength, and skill have returned.
- Unrecognized compartment syndrome can lead to muscular death, scarring, limb contractures, and nerve damage.

Troubleshooting

- Early, aggressive massage and forced motion may worsen muscle damage and increase the chances of MO.

- Counsel patients that surgery carries the risk of recurrence, infection, and extensor mechanism damage.
- Heat is not encouraged in early treatment.

Patient Instructions

- Maintaining the ROM is imperative.
- Avoiding reinjury in the recovery/rehabilitation phase is of significant importance.
- Home therapy and patient initiative are required to allow the quickest return to activity.
- Close follow-up and communication between patient, physician, and therapist/trainer are needed.
- Take care not to return to activity too early; always discuss return to play with the physician.
- Inform the physician of worsening symptoms including neurologic symptoms.

Suggested Readings

Aronen JG, Garrick JG, Chronister RD, McDevitt ER. Quadriceps contusions: clinical results of immediate immobilization in 120 degrees of knee flexion. *Clin J Sport Med*. 2006;16:383–387.

Beiner JM, Jokl P. Muscle contusion injuries: current treatment options. *J Am Acad Orthop Surg*. 2001;9:227–237.

DeLee JC, Drez D Jr, Miller MD, eds. *DeLee & Drez's Orthopaedic Sports Medicine: Principles and Practice*. Vol. 1. Philadelphia: WB Saunders; 2003:12 and Vol. 2, 1858–1860.

Diaz JA, Fischer DA, Rettig AC, et al. Severe quadriceps muscle contusions in athletes. *Am J Sports Med*. 2003;31:289–293.

Lamplot JD, Matava MJ. Thigh injuries in American football. *Am J Orthop*. 2016;45(6):E308–E318.

Mani-Babu S, Wolman R, Keen R. Quadriceps traumatic myositis ossificans in a football player: management with intravenous pamidronate. *Clin J Sport Med*. 2014;24(5):e56–e58.

Newton M, Walker J. Acute quadriceps injury: a case report. *Emerg Nurse*. 2004;12:24–29.

Chapter 132 Hamstring Strains and Tears

Tracy R. Ray, Donella Herman

ICD-10-CM CODES

S76.311A,D,S	Strain of muscle/fascia/tendon of the posterior muscle group at thigh level, right thigh
S76.312A,D,S	Strain of muscle/fascia/tendon of the posterior muscle group at thigh level, left thigh
S76.319A,D,S	Strain of muscle/fascia/tendon of the posterior muscle group at thigh level, unspecified thigh
S76.811A,D,S	Strain of other specified muscles/fascia/tendon at thigh level, right thigh
S76.812A,D,S	Strain of other specified muscles/fascia/tendon at thigh level, left thigh
S76.819A,D,S	Strain of other specified muscles/fascia/tendon at thigh level, unspecified thigh
S76.911A,D,S	Strain unspecified muscle/fascia/tendon at thigh level, right thigh
S76.912A,D,S	Strain unspecified muscle/fascia/tendon at thigh level, left thigh
S76.919A,D,S	Strain unspecified muscle/fascia/tendon at thigh level, unspecified thigh
M62.151	Other rupture of muscle (nontraumatic), right thigh
M62.152	Other rupture of muscle (nontraumatic), left thigh
M62.159	Other rupture of muscle (nontraumatic), unspecified thigh
M66.851	Spontaneous rupture of other tendons, right thigh
M66.852	Spontaneous rupture of other tendons, left thigh
M66.859	Spontaneous rupture of other tendons, unspecified thigh

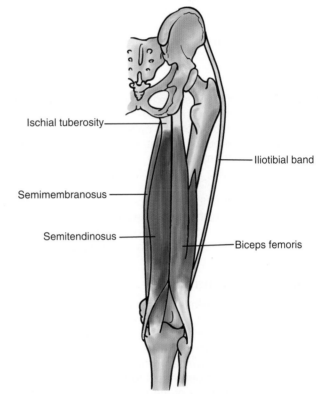

Fig 132.1 The muscles of the hamstring group.

Key Concepts

- Three muscles make up the hamstring group, from medial to lateral (Fig. 132.1):
  - Semimembranosus
  - Semitendinosus
  - Biceps femoris
- Hamstring injuries are the most common muscular injury in athletes.
- Rate of reinjury of hamstring is up to 34%.

- Three common locations of injury
  - Proximal/origin
    - Avulsion
    - Partial tears
    - Apophyseal injuries in pediatric population
  - Central/musculotendinous junction
    - Proximal or distal
    - Most common site of injury
  - Distal/insertion
- Grading of injury severity
  - Grade 1: Minor
  - Grade 2: More significant, partial tear
  - Grade 3: Complete tear, severe
- Biomechanics
  - Injury most often occurs as result of eccentric force during swing phase of gait, as the muscle develops tension in lengthening
  - Can occur with concentric force in the stance phase

- Avulsion injuries occur with hip flexed and knee in extension
- Risk factors
  - Most common risk factor for hamstring injury is previous hamstring injury.
  - Muscular imbalances
    - Hamstring strength imbalance ≥10% between right and left hamstring
    - Flexor to extensor strength ratio <0.5 to 0.6
    - Changes in activation timing and sequence in the posterior chain during prone hip extension have been shown to be a predictor for hamstring injury
  - Inadequate warmup
  - Lack of flexibility
  - Fatigue
  - Poor running mechanics

History

- Patient will complain of sudden onset of pain in the posterior thigh during strenuous exercise
- Description of injury from the patient:
  - Tightness or pulling sensation in the posterior thigh, generally with milder, grade 1 injuries
  - Feeling of being kicked or stabbed in the thigh while running
  - Frequently describe audible pop
- Grasping of the thigh is often diagnostic
- May or may not fall or be able to bear weight
- Pain generally limits continuation of high-level activity

Physical Examination

- Observe gait as patient ambulates to room or during your examination if patient can tolerate
- Place patient in prone position with knee flexed to 90 degrees to reduce tension (Figs. 132.2 and 132.3)
  - Observe for ecchymosis, which may be at the site of injury or in areas dependent to the injury
  - Palpate the entirety of the muscle, from origin at the ischial tuberosity to the insertions at the knee
    - Feel for defect, comparing bilaterally

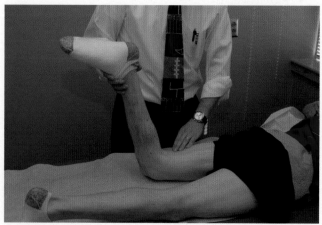

Fig 132.2 Examination of a hamstring injury.

- Mild activation of the muscle may make the defect more obvious to palpation, revealing a "Popeye" appearance similar to a biceps brachii rupture in the upper arm
- Evaluate and document range of motion of both the knee and the hip
- Evaluate for sensory changes in the lower extremity
- Evaluate vascular status in the lower extremity

Imaging

- Plain Radiographs (Fig. 132.4)
  - Rarely of value unless an avulsion fracture has occurred
  - Should be obtained in pediatric patients as they are at higher risk for avulsion fractures
  - Anteroposterior (AP) pelvis is the radiograph of choice if avulsion fractures are suspected

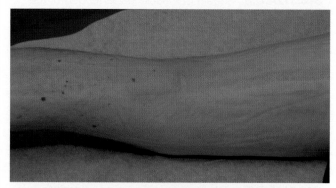

Fig 132.3 Ecchymosis after hamstring strain.

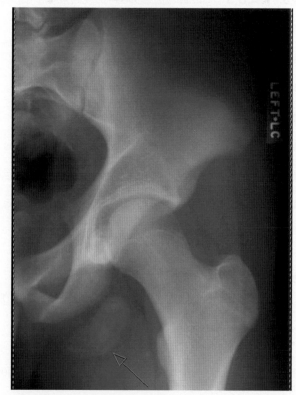

Fig 132.4 Ischial tuberosity avulsion fracture.

- MRI (Fig. 132.5)
  - Often unnecessary in mild injuries
  - Can help differentiate between partial and complete disruption of the muscle fibers in more severe injuries
- Ultrasound (Fig. 132.6)
  - Increasingly used to identify muscular injury
  - Muscles should be visualized in both the long and short axis in their entirety over the area of concern with comparison to the contralateral side
  - Doppler should be used to identify active blood flow and prior to performing any injections
- Bone Scan
  - May be helpful to differentiate femoral stress fractures from hamstring injury

Differential Diagnosis

- See Table 132.1

Treatment

- Rest, ice, compression, and elevation are early mainstays of treatment.
  - Initiate mobilization after brief period of rest to improve range of motion
  - Early mobilization in 1 to 3 days may reduce development of hematoma
- Oral nonsteroidal antiinflammatory medications may be of benefit.
- Formal Therapy
  - Acute period should focus on reduction of edema and hematoma
  - Advance to restoration of strength and range of motion
  - Restoring flexibility in the quadriceps and hamstring
  - Core strengthening for proper pelvic mechanics when return to sport

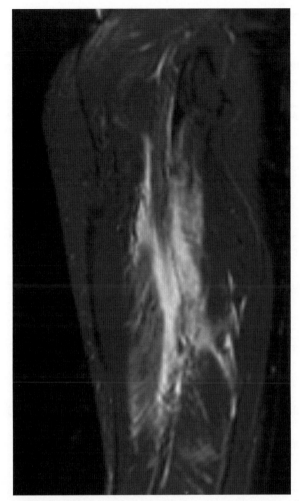

Fig 132.5 Magnetic resonance imaging of grade II hamstring strain. (Courtesy D. Dean Thornton, MD.)

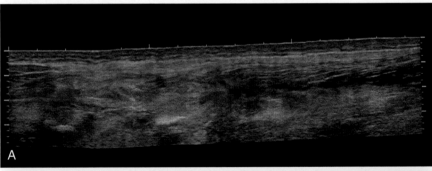

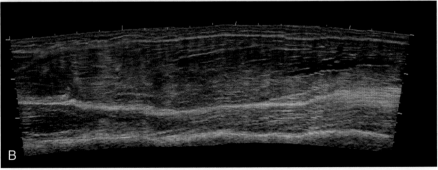

Fig 132.6 Hamstring injury, injured and uninjured. (A) Disorganization of muscle fibers in long axis in a traumatic hamstring injury. (B) Normal linear fibers of the contralateral hamstring in the same patient. (Images courtesy Dr. Blake Boggess, DO.)

TABLE 132.1 Differential Diagnosis in Hamstring Injury

Differential Diagnosis	Differentiating Factors	Chapter Reference
Adductor strain	More medial injury Pain with adduction	
Baker cyst	Pain is distal and medial May have pain with knee flexion and ankle plantarflexion, relieved by placing knee at 45 degrees Ultrasound is helpful in identifying	152
Gastrocnemius strain	Distal pain Pain with resisted plantarflexion	161
Gluteal strain	More proximal injury Pain with hip extension rather than knee flexion	117
Ischial bursitis	Chronic pain, insidious onset Pain localized at ischial bursa	117
Iliotibial band friction syndrome	Gradual onset Lateral pain	155
Popliteus strain	Pain at lateral knee with resisted knee internal rotation.	
Posterior thigh compartment syndrome—chronic exertional compartment syndrome	Diffuse aching pain at a predictable time of exertion Resolution with cessation of activity	160
Sciatica	Neurological symptoms Pain radiating from the back	113
Stress fracture	Overuse injury Seen on magnetic resonance imaging Can involve femoral neck, shaft, or pelvis	123

- Late therapy should focus on functional activities.
- Patient can return to sport when strength is restored and they are able to perform functional activities without pain.
- There have been some reports of using corticosteroid or platelet-rich plasma injections early after injury to reduce secondary injury and shorten return to play, but there is no definitive research to support these treatments at this time.

When to Refer

- Complete rupture of proximal or distal tendon
  - Early surgical intervention is preferred to later intervention, although both result in significant improvements in function
- Bony avulsion injuries are generally recommended for surgical intervention if displacement is greater than 20 mm

Prognosis

- Prognosis varies considerably based on patient activity level, degree of disruption of fibers, and management
- Healing can take from days to months
- Reinjury rate can be as high as 35%

Complications

- Sciatic nerve impingement
- Myositis ossificans
- Reinjury

Troubleshooting

- Hamstring muscle injuries can be difficult to treat, and the recovery time varies considerably on a case-by-case basis.
- Keep in mind the nature and level of activity the patient will be returning to.
- They must be pain free with activity prior to return to sport.
- If surgical intervention is necessary, counsel the patient on the risk of neurologic injury.

Patient Instructions

- Patients should be aware of the slow healing process and potential for recurrence
- Adequate warmup followed by thorough stretching regimen should be implemented prior to any activity
- Patients should not return to explosive activity until they are pain free with activity and have addressed flexibility and strength balance through a progressive rehabilitation program

Considerations in Special Populations

- Hamstring injuries are very common in the athletic population
- Athletes should be encouraged to stretch before exercise and develop well-balanced muscle groups
- Muscle strains are less likely to occur in the pediatric population, but they are at high risk for apophyseal injuries
- Pediatric patients with proximal posterior thigh pain should undergo radiography to assess for apophyseal avulsion injury

Suggested Readings

Clanton T, Coupe K. Hamstring strains in athletes: diagnosis and treatment. *J Am Acad Orthop Surg*. 1998;6:237–248.

Cohen S, Bradley J. Acute proximal hamstring rupture. *J Am Acad Orthop Surg*. 2007;15:350–355.

Drezner J. Practical management: hamstring muscle injuries. *Clin J Sport Med*. 2003;13:48–52.

Lempainen L, Sarima J, Mattila K, et al. Distal tears of the hamstring muscles: review of the literature and our results of surgical management. *Br J Sports Med*. 2007;41:80–83.

Levine WN, Bergfelt JA, Tessendorf W, et al. Intramuscular corticosteroid injection for hamstring injuries: a 13-year experience in the national football league. *Am J Sports Med*. 2000;28:297–300.

Mann G, Shabat S, Friedman A, et al. Hamstring injuries. *Orthopedics*. 2007;30:536–540.

Mason DL, Dickens V, Vail A. Rehabilitation for hamstring injuries. *Cochrane Database Syst Rev*. 2007;(1):CD004575.

Scheurmans J, Van Tiggelen D, Witvrouw E. Prone hip extension muscle recruitment is associated with hamstring injury risk in amateur soccer. *Int J Sports Med*. 2017;38(9):696–706.

Chapter 133 Piriformis Syndrome

Thomas M. Howard

ICD-10-CM CODE
G57.00 *Piriformis syndrome*

Key Concepts

- Definition: Sciatic nerve irritation caused by mechanical compression or chemical irritation of the sciatic nerve or its branches as it passes beneath or through the piriformis muscle.
- Often manifest as buttock pain that may radiate down the leg to the level of the knee.
- There has been significant historical controversy as to whether piriformis syndrome exists as a distinct entity. Recent literature and medical opinion support the existence of piriformis syndrome.
- Functional anatomy of the piriformis muscle.
  - Origin
    - Anterior of the S2-S4 vertebrae
    - Sacrotuberous ligament
    - Upper margin of the greater sciatic foramen
  - Insertion
    - Traverses greater sciatic notch to insert on the superior surface of greater trochanter of femur

- Function
  - Hip extended: primary external rotator of the femur
  - Hip flexed: abductor of the hip
- Relationship to sciatic nerve
  - Six possible anatomic relationships as originally described by Beaton (Fig. 133.1)
- Epidemiology
  - Low back pain has an estimated lifetime incidence of more than 90% in the general population.
  - Piriformis syndrome has an estimated prevalence of 6 cases per 100 cases of sciatica.
  - 6:1 female-to-male ratio

History

- Chronic pain in the buttock
  - Pain may radiate to leg and worsens with squatting and walking.
  - Pain is worse with active external rotation or abduction of the femur.
  - Pain is often prominent as the patient gets out of bed when lying on asymptomatic side. This maneuver requires active abduction and external rotation of the affected extremity, selectively activating the piriformis muscle.

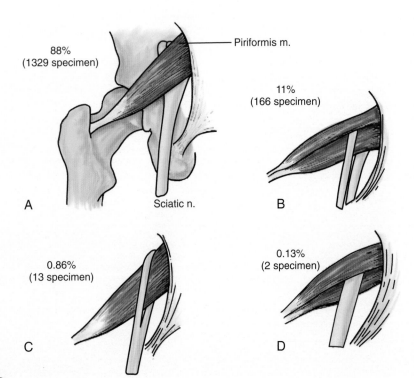

Fig 133.1 Beaton classification of anatomic variation in the piriformis muscle and sciatic nerve. Relationship of the sciatic nerve to the piriformis muscle in 1510 extremities studies. **(A)** Single-bodied piriformis muscle overlies sciatic nerve. **(B)** One branch of underlying sciatic nerve penetrates bifurcated piriformis muscle. **(C)** Single-bodied piriformis muscle penetrates sciatic nerve. **(D)** Sciatic nerve penetrates bifurcated piriformis muscle.

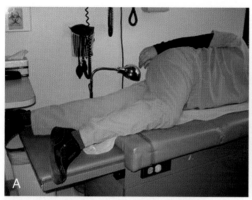
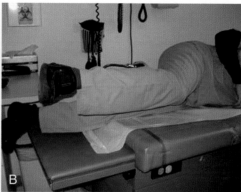

Fig 133.2 Beatty maneuver. Symptomatic leg resting **(A)** and actively lifted several inches **(B)**.

- History of trauma to the gluteal region in less than 50% of cases
  - Trauma is often subacute and may precede symptoms by months.
- Pain is often exacerbated by sitting.
- May be manifest as painful bowel movements in both sexes and dyspareunia in women

Physical Examination

- Tenderness on palpation of the piriformis muscle or its origin on the sacrum
- Palpable gluteal mass, sometimes described as sausagelike
- Tenderness on palpation of lateral wall during rectal or pelvic examination
- Lack of lower extremity motor weakness or deep tendon reflex change
- Special attention should be paid to Morton foot, pes planus, and hyperpronation, which may lead to an overuse syndrome due to compensatory contraction of the piriformis muscle.
- Gluteus maximus hypertrophy may be present in advanced or severe cases.
- Beatty maneuver (Fig. 133.2)
  - Selectively contracts the piriformis muscle
  - The patient is placed in a side-lying position on the unaffected side.
  - The knee of the affected side is rested on the examination table.
  - The patient lifts the affected leg several inches off the table and holds this position, resulting in active abduction and external rotation of the lower extremity.
  - The test is positive when the maneuver is painful.
- Pace test
  - The patient is placed in a seated position.
  - A positive test is marked by pain with resisted leg abduction.
- Freiberg test (Fig. 133.3)
  - The patient is placed in the supine position.
  - Pain upon passive internal rotation of the femur with hip neutral

Imaging

- Magnetic resonance imaging

- Useful to rule out tumor, herniated disc, and spinal stenosis
- May demonstrate hypertrophy of the piriformis muscle on T1-weighted images; usually no signal change on T2-weighted images
- Computed tomography
  - Useful to characterize the degree of underlying arthritis, assess for spinal stenosis
  - May identify mass anterior to the piriformis muscle
- Ultrasonography
  - May demonstrate painful hypertrophy of the piriformis muscle

Additional Tests

- Electromyography
  - Usually negative in piriformis syndrome.
  - May demonstrate the specific pattern of gluteus maximus and piriformis abnormalities in piriformis syndrome.
  - Positive tests usually indicate other diagnoses such as a herniated disc.
- H-reflex
  - The Hoffman reflex, or H-reflex, elicits the Achilles reflex through stimulation of the sciatic nerve at the popliteal fossa.
  - An abnormal H-reflex in the anatomic position is usually indicative of disc herniation.
- FAIR (flexion, adduction, internal rotation of the hip) test
  - The FAIR test compares the H-reflex in the anatomic position and in flexion, adduction, and internal rotation, stretching the piriformis muscle.
  - Prolongation of the H-reflex by 1.86 ms indicates pathologic compression of the sciatic nerve and is considered diagnostic of piriformis syndrome.
- Diagnostic injection
  - Diagnostic lidocaine injection of the piriformis muscle may be performed transcutaneously, transvaginally, or transrectally.
  - Ultrasound-guided transcutaneous injection is believed to be the best approach to injection of the piriformis.
  - Relief of pain on provocative testing is suggestive of piriformis syndrome.

Differential Diagnosis

Please see Table 133.1.

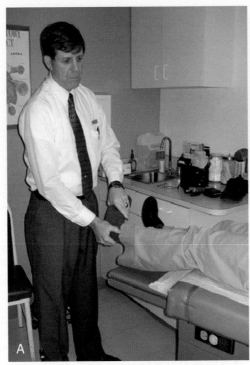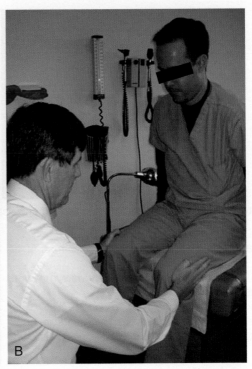

Fig 133.3 Freiberg **(A)** and Pace **(B)** tests.

TABLE 133.1 Differential Diagnosis of Low Back and Buttock Pain

Diagnosis	Differentiating Features	Chapter Reference
Piriformis syndrome	Positive Beatty maneuver, positive FAIR test, rule out other hip and spine pathology	N/A
Herniated lumbosacral disc	Motor weakness, altered deep tendon reflexes, radiology	113
Spinal stenosis	Neurogenic claudication, pain with back extension, radiology	115
Lumbosacral discogenic pain syndrome	Pain with Valsalva maneuver	113
Spondylolysis or spondylolisthesis	Pain with back extension, radiology	116
Sacroiliac joint pain	Positive FABER (flexion, abduction, external rotation) test; positive Gaenslen test; positive SI compression	138
Lumbosacral muscle or ligament sprain/strain	Pain with back flexion	112
Proximal Hamstring injury	Pain with resisted leg extension	132
Facet pain	Pain with back extension, radiology	106
Pelvic or cord mass, tumor, or endometriosis	History, radiology	N/A
Gluteal abscess	Constitutional symptoms, radiology	N/A
Aneurysm of inferior or superior gluteal artery	Radiology	N/A
Bursitis: trochanteric, ischial, or obturator	Palpation, diagnostic injection	128
Strain or tendinitis of the gluteal muscles, obturator muscle, etc.	Provocative muscle testing	117

FAIR, Flexion, adduction, internal rotation; *N/A,* not applicable; *SI,* sacroiliac.

Treatment

- At diagnosis
  - Avoid prolonged sitting and other exacerbating activities.
  - Home stretches, heat, ice, massage
- Physical therapy
  - Stretching, often preceded by moist heat or ultrasound
  - Soft-tissue massage
  - Myofascial release by therapist
  - Cold packs or electrical stimulation after physical therapy
  - Hip and core stability and flexibility exercises

- Later
  - Consider diagnostic or therapeutic injection with ultrasound guidance.
    - Local anesthetic agents, steroids, and botulinum toxin have demonstrated efficacy.
  - Consider advanced imaging studies (e.g., electromyography) not already performed.

When to Refer

- Physical therapy
  - Consider immediate referral.
- Neurologist
  - Consider referral for electromyography when diagnosis is unclear or the patient is not improving.
- Gynecologist
  - Consider referral for unclear diagnosis if pelvic pain is present.
- Surgery
  - Avoid surgical intervention with less than 6 months of conservative therapy.
  - Surgery has been demonstrated to be effective after failure of conservative therapy in select cases.
  - Has shown greatest efficacy in posttraumatic piriformis syndrome

Prognosis

- As with most causes of low back pain, the majority of patients respond to conservative therapy.
- Symptoms often resolve with 6 weeks of conservative therapy.
- Less than 10% of patients require surgical evaluation.

Patient Instructions

- Counsel patients that this is rarely a disabling condition and typically responds well to conservative therapies.
- Provide instruction on active rest to include
  - Activity modification
  - Heat, ice, massage
  - Specific stretches for the piriformis muscle
  - Use of analgesics or nonsteroidal antiinflammatory drugs

- Counsel patients regarding symptoms that may suggest an alternative diagnosis or require immediate evaluation.
  - Progressive weakness
  - Urinary retention
  - Constitutional symptoms

Considerations in Special Populations

- Sports medicine considerations
  - Look for abnormalities in the kinetic chain that may predispose to injury.
  - Consider dynamic gait examination.
  - Consider training habits that predispose to overuse injury with attention to frequency, intensity, duration, hill running, and so on.
  - Consider appropriate footwear.

Acknowledgment

The author acknowledges Dr. Edward J. Lewis for his contributions to the previous edition of this chapter.

Suggested Readings

Beatty R. The piriformis syndrome: a simple diagnostic maneuver. *Neurosurgery*. 1994;34:512–514.

Benzon HT, Katz J. Piriformis syndrome: anatomic considerations, a new injection technique, and a review of the literature. *Anesthesiology*. 2003;98:1442–1448.

Finnoff JT, Hurdle MF, Smith J. Accuracy of ultrasound-guided versus fluoroscopically guided contrast-controlled piriformis injections: a cadaveric study. *J Ultrasound Med*. 2008;20(8):1157–1163.

Fishman LM, Dombi GW, Michaelson C, et al. Piriformis syndrome: diagnosis, treatment, and outcome—a 10-year study. *Arch Phys Med Rehabil*. 2002;83(3):295–301.

Fishman LM, Konnoth C, Rozner B. Botulinum neurotoxin type B and physical therapy in the treatment of piriformis syndrome: a dose-finding study. *Am J Phys Med Rehabil*. 2004;83:42–50.

Foster M. Piriformis syndrome. *Orthopedics*. 2002;25:821–825.

Koes B, van Tulder M, Peul W. Diagnosis and treatment of sciatica. *Br Med J*. 2007;334:1313–1317.

Shah S, Wang TW: *Piriformis syndrome*. Available at www.emedicine.com/sports/topic102.htm. Accessed March 19, 2018.

Chapter 134 Meralgia Paresthetica

Mark Rogers

ICD-10-CM CODES
G57.1   *Meralgia paresthetica*
G57.10 *Unspecified lower limb*
G57.11 *Right lower limb*
G57.12 *Left lower limb*
G57.13 *Bilateral lower limbs*

Key Concepts

- Also known as lateral femoral cutaneous nerve compression syndrome or entrapment; Bernhardt-Roth disease, syndrome, or paresthesia; and British officer's cavalry disease.
- Mononeuropathy of the lateral femoral cutaneous nerve (from the primary ventral rami of L2 and L3 roots).
- Purely sensory nerve that innervates anterolateral thigh (Fig. 134.1).
- Diagnosis is made primarily on history and physical examination; additional studies may help to confirm the diagnosis.
- Most common cause of damage is from entrapment at the level of the inguinal ligament.
- Incidence rates reported at 3 to 4 cases per 10,000 primary care patients.
  - Most common in males in the 5th or 6th decade and a body mass index at or above 30.
  - Eighty percent of cases are unilateral.
- Generally self-limiting over weeks to months.

History

- Commonly presents with burning, numbness, and pain in the anterolateral thigh.
- Although not absolute, standing and hip extension often aggravate symptoms, whereas sitting and hip flexion may relieve symptoms.
- Mechanical causes:
  - Direct trauma (e.g., seatbelts, gun or hammer holsters, tight trousers, postsurgical)
  - Leg length discrepancy
  - Pregnancy
  - Obesity or rapid weight changes
  - Intra-abdominal or bone tumors
  - Anatomic variants (Fig. 134.2)
- Metabolic causes:
  - Diabetes, through one of two mechanisms: (1) abnormalities in metabolism of pyruvate, sorbitol, and lipids resulting in slowed nerve conduction; or (2) swelling of the nerve due to decreased axoplasmic transport, making it more vulnerable to compression
  - Thyroid disease

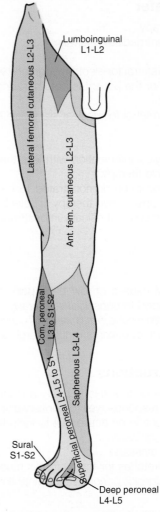

Fig 134.1 Diagram of the segmental distribution of the cutaneous nerves of the right lower extremity. Front view.

- Alcoholism
- Inflammatory diseases (e.g., systemic lupus erythematosus)

Physical Examination

- The patient will not typically demonstrate gross motor deficits or reflex changes.
- Palpation over a point 1 cm inferior and 1 cm medial to the anterosuperior iliac spine (ASIS) may reproduce symptoms or pain.
- Positive pelvic compression test (Fig. 134.3).
- Appropriate physical examination to rule out lumbar disc disease (see appropriate section).

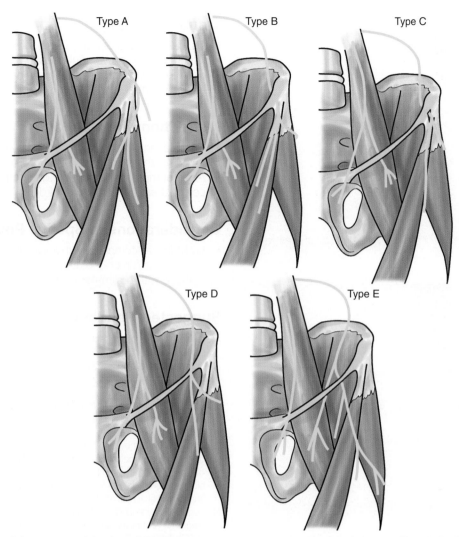

Fig 134.2 Variation of the course of the lateral femoral cutaneous nerve as it exits the abdomen. Type A (4%) courses across the iliac crest. In type B, it may be ensheathed by the inguinal ligament (27%). In type C (23%), it is ensheathed in the tendinous origin of the sartorius muscle. In type D (26%), it is deep to inguinal ligament and medial to sartorius muscle. In type E (20%), it is medial to iliopsoas muscle, contributing the femoral branch to the genitofemoral nerve. (Modified with permission from Aszmann OC, Dellon ES, Dellon AL. Anatomical course of the lateral femoral cutaneous nerve and its susceptibility to compression and injury. *Plast Reconstr Surg*. 1997;100:600–604.)

Imaging

- X-rays are often obtained to assess the lumbopelvic architecture and to rule out bony tumors.
- Ultrasonography may be useful to evaluate entrapment and morphology of the nerve.
- Magnetic resonance imaging may be useful to further evaluate and rule out other etiologies.
- Additional tests:
  - Complete blood count (CBC) and complete metabolic panel (CMP).
  - Erythrocyte sedimentation rate (ESR) and C-reactive protein (CRP).
  - Electromyography (EMG); nerve conduction studies (NCS) with somatosensory evoked potentials may help to rule out lumbar plexopathies.

Differential Diagnosis

- Lumbar radiculopathy or neuropathy
- Increased retroperitoneal pressure from a tumor

Treatment

- Conservative treatment relieves symptoms in more than 90% of patients.
  - Avoid compressive agents.
  - Nonsteroidal antiinflammatory drugs (NSAIDs).
  - Topical creams (e.g., diclofenac 1% or 2%, capsaicin, compounded creams with anesthetics and/or NSAIDs) or 5% lidocaine patch.
  - Local anesthetic injection with or without steroids, or hydrodissection of the nerve.

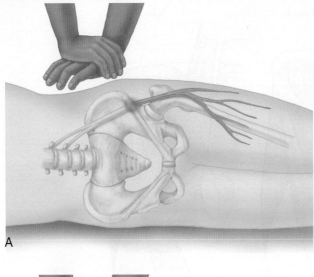

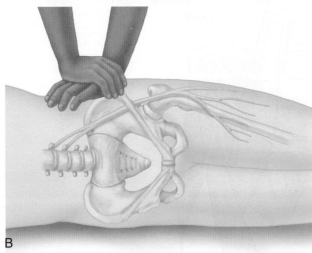

Fig 134.3 Pelvic compression test. **(A)** The patient is positioned in the lateral recumbent position. **(B)** Downward pressure is applied and maintained for approximately 45 seconds. A positive test result is when the patient's symptoms improve. (Redrawn from Nouraei SAR, Anand B, Spink G, O'Neill KS. A novel approach to the diagnosis and management of meralgia paresthetica. *Neurosurgery*. 2007;60:696–700.)

- • Osteopathic manipulation to correct functional leg length discrepancy and pelvis asymmetries.
- • Acupuncture or other trigger point treatments.
- Surgical management.
  - • Referral maybe an option if symptoms are intractable despite conservative measures for at least 6 months.

Troubleshooting

- Typically this is a benign, self-resolving disease; however, if there is no improvement despite conservative measures or if the history and physical examination suggest another etiology, further workup should be considered.

Instructions for the Patient

- Educate the patient about the typically benign, self-resolving nature of the diagnosis.
- Avoid compressive agents (e.g., hammer or gun holsters, cell phones, tight trousers, girdles).

Considerations in Special Populations

- In children as compared with adults, the course of symptoms may be more chronic, bilateral, and more frequent, especially in those with a slimmer body habitus.

Suggested Readings

Alexander RE. Clinical effectiveness of electroacupuncture in meralgia paresthetica: A case series. *Acupunct Med*. 2013;31(4):435–439.

Aszmann OC, Dellon ES, Dellon AL. Anatomical course of the lateral femoral cutaneous nerve and its susceptibility to compression and injury. *Plast Reconstr Surg*. 1997;100:600–604.

Ducic I, Dellon AL, Taylor NS. Decompression of the lateral femoral cutaneous nerve in the treatment of meralgia paresthetica. *J Reconstr Microsurg*. 2006;22:113–117.

Grossman MG, Ducey SA, Nadler SS, Levy AS. Meralgia paresthetica: diagnosis and treatment. *J Am Acad Orthop Surg*. 2001;9:336–344.

Hurdle MF, Weingarten TN, Crisostomo RA, et al. Ultrasound-guided blockade of the lateral femoral cutaneous nerve: technical description and review of 10 cases. *Arch Phys Med Rehabil*. 2007;88:1362–1364.

Nouraei SAR, Anand B, Spink G, O'Neill KS. A novel approach to the diagnosis and management of meralgia paresthetica. *Neurosurgery*. 2007;60:696–700.

Onat SS, Ata AM, Ozcakaar L. Ultrasound-guided diagnosis and treatment of meralgia paresthetica. *Pain Phys*. 2016;19:E667–E669.

Richer LP, Shevell MI, Stewart J, Poulin C. Pediatric meralgia paresthetica. *Pediatr Neurol*. 2002;26:321–323.

Zhu J, Zhao Y, Lui F, et al. Ultrasound of the lateral femoral cutaneous nerve in asymptomatic adults. *BMC Musculoskeletal Disord*. 2012;13:227–231.

Chapter 135 Iliac Crest Contusion/ Hip Pointer

Myro A. Lu, Chad D. Hulsopple

ICD-10-CM CODES
S70.02XA *Contusion of left hip, initial encounter*
S70.02XD *Contusion of right hip, initial encounter*

Key Concepts

- A hip pointer is a traumatic subperiosteal hematoma of the iliac crest (Fig. 135.1).
- It is a common injury in players of contact sports such as football, ice hockey, soccer, and rugby.
- The mechanism of injury is blunt trauma to the iliac crest.
- If not identified early, this injury can lead to significant pain and a prolonged recovery.
- Other conditions must be ruled out, such as hip injuries with similar presentations (muscle strains, apophyseal injuries, and fractures) as well as concomitant injuries in neighboring anatomy (abdomen/pelvis).

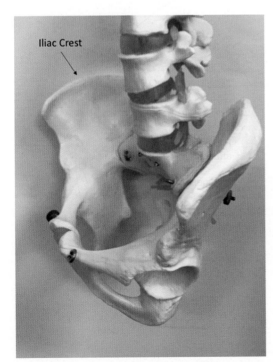

Fig 135.1 The iliac crest is the most common site for a hip pointer.

Iliac Crest

History

- Direct blow to the iliac crest
- Localized pain and tenderness over the iliac crest
- Antalgic gait
- Localized swelling and fluctuance present with a hematoma
- Contusion (immediate or delayed 24 to 48 hours)
- Pain with active flexion and abduction of the hip

Physical Examination

- Observe for antalgic gait or for the inability to bear weight.
- Evaluate for swelling, ecchymosis, and deformities.
- Evaluate for localized tenderness to palpation over the iliac crest.
  - Pain is usually localized over the anterior third of the iliac crest.
- Evaluate active and passive range of motion (ROM) of the hip.
- Evaluate strength and exacerbation of pain with resisted motion of the hip and abdominal oblique muscles.
- Perform complete abdominal exam to rule out concomitant injuries.

Imaging

- Radiographs are unnecessary unless there is a concern for a physeal injury or fracture.
- A radiographic evaluation should include pelvic anteroposterior, cross-table lateral, iliac oblique, and frog-leg lateral views.
  - Contralateral radiographs should be considered in skeletally immature individuals to identify physeal injuries.
- If the diagnosis remains in question,
  - MRI is the most sensitive and specific imaging modality.
  - A skilled sonographer can also help to better elucidate a hip pointer.

Differential Diagnosis

- Muscle or soft-tissue contusion.
- Avulsion fractures (Fig. 135.2).
  - Common injuries that can mimic hip pointers include avulsion fractures of the iliac crest, anterosuperior iliac spine (ASIS), and anteroinferior iliac spine (AIIS).
- Muscle strain (see Fig. 135.2)
  - Most common in sprinters, jumpers, soccer players, and football players.

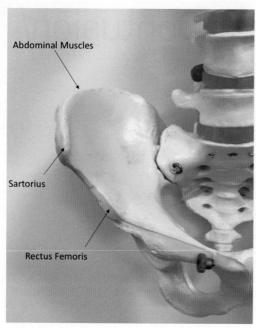

Fig 135.2 Myotendinous sites are common in the case of muscle strains, avulsion fractures, and apophyseal injuries.

Labels on Fig 135.2:
- Abdominal Muscles
- Sartorius
- Rectus Femoris

- Common muscle strain sites that can mimic hip pointers
  - Sartorius attachment to ASIS
  - Direct head of rectus femoris attachment to the AIIS
  - External oblique, internal oblique, and transversus abdominis muscles attachment to iliac crest
- Apophyseal avulsion injuries (see Fig. 135.2)
  - Most common age range is 13 to 25 years.
  - Common locations that can mimic hip pointers are the ASIS, AIIS, and iliac crest.
  - May not be obvious on plain radiographs if ossification has not yet occurred; with increased suspicion, further ultrasonography or MRI studies may be warranted.

Treatment (Fig. 135.3)

- Pain and inflammation control
  - Pain control (local anesthetics can provide temporary pain relief)
  - Protection, relative rest, ice, compression, elevation
  - Consider crutches or assistive devices
- Restore ROM
  - Start treatment with active assisted ROM exercises, progress to active ROM exercises, with a final phase of resisted ROM exercises.
  - Consider adding proprioceptive neuromuscular facilitation stretching in this phase to improve ROM.
  - Advance as tolerated based on the patient's injury and pain control.

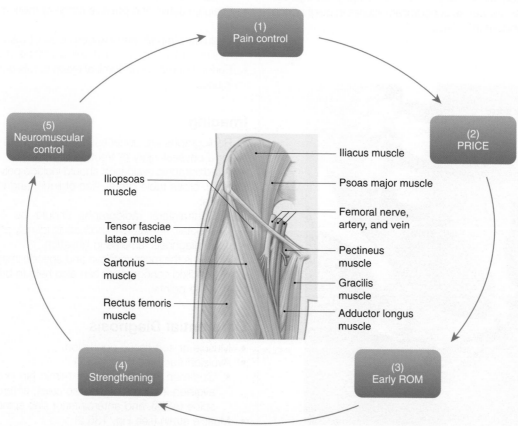

Labels on Fig 135.3:
- (1) Pain control
- (2) PRICE
- (3) Early ROM
- (4) Strengthening
- (5) Neuromuscular control
- Iliacus muscle
- Psoas major muscle
- Femoral nerve, artery, and vein
- Pectineus muscle
- Gracilis muscle
- Adductor longus muscle
- Iliopsoas muscle
- Tensor fasciae latae muscle
- Sartorius muscle
- Rectus femoris muscle

Fig 135.3 Stepwise treatment approach for hip pointers. *ROM,* Range of motion. (Center illustration modified from Moses KP, Banks JC, Nava PB, Petersen DK. *Atlas of Clinical Gross Anatomy*. 2nd ed. Philadelphia: Elsevier; 2013:498.)

- Strengthening
  - Begin with isometric exercises to strengthen ROM arc of the extremity.
  - Functional strength rehabilitation with eccentric and concentric exercises including progressive overloading with increased resistance.
  - Rehabilitation program including sport-specific exercises with the goal of restoring full strength and function.
- Neuromuscular control
  - Assess for deficits in balance, movement patterns, and sport-specific goals.
  - Build movement patterns for specific sport through active ROM, foam rollers, balance boards, and progress to plyometric training.
- Return to play
  - Full pain-free ROM.
  - Strength equal to that of the opposite leg.
  - Able to perform sport-specific exercises with the equipment required for the sport.
  - Evaluate protective padding for correct fit and location.
  - May initially benefit from extra padding until bony tenderness resolves.
  - Premature return to play often leads to reinjury.

When to Refer

- Prolonged pain with inability to return to sport.
- Consider consultation with an orthopaedic provider for fractures or apophyseal injuries.

Prognosis

- The patient returns to sport within 1 to 2 weeks, but bony tenderness may persist for months.
- Rare long-term disability.

Troubleshooting

- Avoid a premature return to play by testing for full pain-free ROM and strength as well as the ability to perform in full sports-related equipment before returning play.

- Counsel the patient that bony tenderness may persist for months.

Instructions for the Patient

- Initial treatment consists of protection, rest, ice, elevation, compressive dressing, and pain medication.
- Early activity modification, progressive ROM, strengthening, correction of movement pattern deficits, and return to play.
- Physical therapy or home exercises to speed return of strength and motion.
- Additional padding for comfort may be required upon return to sport.

Considerations in Special Populations

- In young athletes, one must consider injury or avulsion of an apophysis. These are most common between ages 13 and 25 years.
- Avulsion injuries require protected weight bearing with an extended period of rest until pain-free ROM has returned, then progressive rehabilitation is started.

Suggested Readings

Arkader A, Skaggs DL. Physeal injuries. In: *Green's Skeletal Trauma in Children*. 5th ed. Philadelphia: Elsevier; 2015:16–35.

Blankenbaker DG. The role of ultrasound in the evaluation of sports injuries of the lower extremities. *Clin Sports Med*. 2006;25:867–897.

Hall M, Anderson J. Hip pointers. *Clin Sports Med*. 2013;32(2):325–330.

LaBella CR. Common acute sports-related lower extremity injuries in children and adolescents. *Clin Pediatr Emerg Med*. 2007;8(1):31–42.

McMillan S, Busconi B, Montano M. Hip and thigh contusions and strains. In: DeLee JC, Drez D Jr, Miller MD, eds. *DeLee and Drez's Orthopaedic Sports Medicine*. 4th ed. Philadelphia: Elsevier; 2015:1006–1014.

Stracciolini A, Yen Y, d'Hemecourt P, et al. Sex and growth effect on pediatric hip injuries presenting to sports medicine clinic. *J Pediatr Orthop B*. 2016;25(4):315–321.

6

Chapter 136 Athletic Pubalgia and Core Muscle Injury (Sports Hernia)

David Hryvniak, Nicholas Anastasio

ICD-10-CM CODE
S39.81XA *Other specified injuries of abdomen, initial encounter*

Key Concepts

- Athletic pubalgia in characterized by lower abdominal or groin pain worsened by physical exertion and relieved with rest.
- There is no consensus on etiology. Traditionally athletic pubalgia is due to an occult hernia in the posterior inguinal wall.
- Other proposed etiologies include strain/tear of the conjoined tendon, inguinal ligament, transversalis fascia, rectus abdominis aponeurosis, and external/internal obliques (Fig. 136.1).
- The unifying terms *pubic inguinal pain syndrome* (PIPS) and *core muscle dysfunction* have been proposed because of the overlap with other syndromes.
- Athletic pubalgia is most common in sports that require sudden changes in direction or twisting (e.g., soccer, ice hockey, wrestling, football).
- Clinical diagnosis is one of exclusion with no specific assessment tool.
- Athletic pubalgia may occur concurrently with other groin pathology (e.g., osteitis pubis, adductor strain).
- It typically affects men more than women.
- In one study it was found in 50% of athletes with groin pain of more than 8 weeks' duration.

History

- Unilateral pain in the groin area. Typically of insidious onset.
- In some cases, can progress to bilateral pain over time.
- Often described as a "deep" pain in the lower abdomen or groin.
- Pain occurs with kicking, sprinting, cutting, coughing, sneezing, or performing situps.
- Often disabling, preventing many athletes from achieving a satisfactory level of play.
- Pain is typically relieved with rest and returns with the of onset of activity.
- Pain may radiate to the testis, suprapubic region, or origin of the adductor longus.

Physical Examination

- Tenderness to palpation in the groin or above the pubis, especially over the anterior pubic tubercle, conjoined tendon, and mid-inguinal region.
- The external inguinal ring is often dilated and/or tender.
- No obvious detectable or visible hernia bulge.
- Pain with lower abdominal and hip flexion (performing a situp).
- Pain with resisted hip adduction.
  - Adductor squeeze test: patient lies supine with hips abducted and flexed at 80 degrees. Positive if pain occurs with resisted adduction.

Risk Factors

- Reduced hip range of motion.
- Pelvic muscle imbalance, typically with strong adductors and relatively weak lower abdominal muscles.
- Limb length discrepancy.

Imaging

- Most imaging studies are normal, but they are useful to rule out alternative diagnoses.
- X-ray: Erect pelvic and flamingo stress-views of the pubic symphysis. Greater than 2 mm of motion across the symphysis pubis in the flamingo view identifies instability. However, functional instability can occur at less than 2 mm.
- MRI: Low specificity. Many athletes have no pathologic findings on MRI, but it is useful to rule out stress fractures and osteonecrosis of the femoral head. There is often concurrent osteitis pubis and adductor strain (see Fig. 136.1).
- Bone scan: Lacks specificity. Associated risks are well known. Helpful to rule out osteitis pubis, symphyseal instability, osteoarthritis, and tumor.
- Herniography: Popular in Europe but rarely used in the United States. Controversial due to potential risks and high false-positive rate. It involves injecting a radioopaque dye into the peritoneal cavity.
- Ultrasound: Results are of limited use owing to interoperator variability. Allows visualization during dynamic maneuvers (e.g., a situp) that can be used to bring out a convex anterior bulge and ballooning of the inguinal canal. However, there is a high prevalence of abnormal findings in asymptomatic athletes.

Athletic Pubalgia—"Sports Hernia"

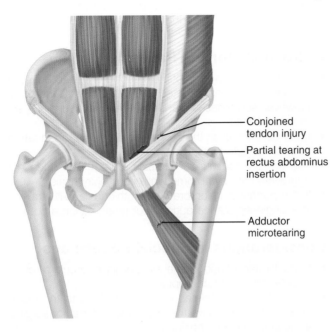

Conjoined tendon injury

Partial tearing at rectus abdominus insertion

Adductor microtearing

Imaging:
- XR and MRI useful to rule out other diagnoses
- US may be useful to display occult hernia

Tx:
- NSAIDs, oral corticosteroids, local corticosteroid injection
- PT
- Surgical repair (open vs. laparoscopic)

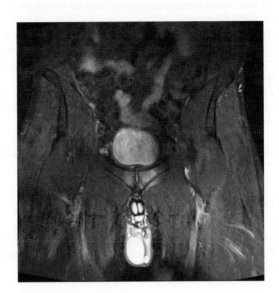

MOI:
- Repetitive twisting and kicking motions
- Pelvic muscle imbalance (adductors > low abdominals)

Pathophysiology:
- Occult hernia in the posterior inguinal wall
- Strain/tear of conjoined tendon, inguinal ligament, transversalis fascia, rectus abdominis aponeurosis and/or obliques

Fig 136.1 Athletic pubalgia. Magnetic resonance image of the pelvis displaying concurrent adductor longus strain (hyperintense signal at adductor origin) with osteitis pubis. This image depicts the anatomy of adductor strain, partial tearing of the rectus abdominis insertion, and conjoint tendon injury. *MOI,* Method of injury; *Tx,* treatment.

Additional Tests

- If the patient does not have a history of activity that might lead to a sports hernia or has developed a fever or subjective chills, one should consider ruling out of osteomyelitis of the pubic symphysis or genitourinary pathology. A complete blood count (CBC) with erythrocyte sedimentation rate (ESR) as well as urinalysis should be obtained. Blood cultures may be considered based on clinical presentation.

Differential Diagnosis

- Adductor strain—typically adductor longus
- Iliopsoas strain, bursitis, or tendonitis
- Rectus abdominis strain
- Osteitis pubis
- Stress fracture—proximal femur, femoral neck, superior pubic ramus
- Apophyseal avulsion fracture in a skeletally immature athlete
- Ilioinguinal nerve entrapment neuropathy
- Intra-articular hip pathology
- Inguinal hernia
- Lumbar disc disease
- Slipped capital femoral epiphysis
- Snapping hip syndrome
- Seronegative spondyloarthropathies

- Osteomyelitis
- Genitourinary pathology—urinary tract infection, prostatitis, urolithiasis, endometriosis, ovarian torsion, ovarian cysts
- Abdominal disorders
- Other groin pathology: Gilmore groin, gracilis syndrome, hockey groin syndrome

Treatment

- Fundamentals include rest, antiinflammatory medication, physical therapy, and possible surgical repair.
- First 7 to 10 days: avoidance of activities that produce pain, with relative rest encouraged.
- A course of nonsteroidal antiinflammatory drug therapy should be attempted.
- For severe pain: consideration for a short course of oral corticosteroids or local corticosteroid injection. Recently some providers have attempted prolotherapy or injections of platelet-rich plasma (PRP) prior to surgical referral.
- After 2 weeks: initiate physical therapy with a focus on improving strength and flexibility in the abdominal and inner thigh muscles via graduated stretching and strengthening.
  - Focus on adductor muscles, abdominal wall muscles, iliopsoas, quadriceps, and hamstrings. Important to focus on motor control and strength in single-leg stance.

- Should progress from strengthening to functional activity to sport-specific exercise.
- Rehabilitation can include manual therapy, joint manipulation, acupuncture, therapeutic modalities, taping techniques, sport-specific rehabilitation, and plyometrics.
- Two rehabilitation protocols well described in the literature include a four-phase rehabilitation program by Larson and Lohnes and a divided regimen of manual therapy and exercise rehab by Kachingwe and Grech.
- Conservative therapy should be tried for 4 to 6 weeks prior to surgical repair.
- There is no consensus to support any one surgical repair over another. However, some data suggests a faster return to play with laparoscopic (2–6 weeks) versus open (1–6 months) repair.
- Fundamentals of surgical repair involve reinforcement of the posterior abdominal wall with mesh followed by postoperative rehabilitation.
  - Concomitant repair of the conjoint tendon, transverse adductor tenotomy, and obturator nerve release may be attempted.

When to Refer

- Failed conservative therapy after 4 to 6 weeks
- Athlete recalls an acute tearing or ripping sensation
- Professional athletes for whom a long trial of conservative rehabilitation is not possible

Prognosis

- Many cases may resolve with 4 to 6 weeks of physical therapy, although some studies suggest that conservative therapy often fails to provide relief.
- For athletes requiring surgery, most are able to return to sports 6 to 12 weeks after surgery.
- Return to activity following surgical repair (across all surgical approaches) ranges from 62% to 100%. However, many surgical approaches report greater than 90% success rates.
- Maintaining rotational control and stability of the pelvis is the most important factor in preventing injury and reinjury.

Troubleshooting

- Asymptomatic direct inguinal hernias are common in the general population. Patients must have pain during exercise or provocative maneuvers and an appropriate examination and/or imaging findings for proper diagnosis.
- Return to sport can occur when the following are displayed: pain-free and strong adductor squeeze test, minimal adductor guarding, pain-free pubic symphysis shear test into

extension, pain-free brisk walking before running. There should be no pain with sport-specific drills and movements prior to full return to sport.

Instructions for the Patient

- This condition may sometimes resolve with 6 to 8 weeks of rehabilitation as directed by your physical therapist. However, some cases that do not resolve require surgery to achieve relief.
- Most patients, even those who require surgery, can return to sport or activity within 3 months.
- You should continue a fitness program that does not aggravate your symptoms while your injury heals.
- It is important to incorporate strength and flexibility training in a single-leg stance during your rehabilitation process.

Considerations in Special Populations

- Consideration of apophyseal avulsion injury should be given in skeletally immature populations.
- For professional athletes who are unwilling to try a long course of conservative therapy, earlier referral for surgical evaluation may be considered.

Suggested Readings

American Academy of Orthopedic Surgeons and the American Orthopedic Society for Sports Medicine. *Sports Hernia (Athletic Pubalgia)*. OrthoInfo: 2010.

Campanelli G. Pubic inguinal pain syndrome: the so-called sports hernia. *Hernia*. 2010;14(1):1–4.

Cohn M. Understanding sports hernias: University of Maryland doctor says condition can be tough to diagnose. *Baltimore Sun*. 2012;http://articles.baltimoresun.com/2012-10-03/health/bs-hs-ask-the-expert-hernia-20121003_1_sports-hernia-common-sports-groin-pain. Accessed December 15, 2014.

Farber AJ, Wilckens JH. Sports hernia: diagnosis and therapeutic approach. *J Am Acad Orthop Surg*. 2007;15(8):507–514.

Garvey JF, Read JW, Turner A. Sportsman hernia: what can we do? *Hernia*. 2010;14(1):17–25.

Hölmich P, Uhrskou P, Ulnits L, et al. Effectiveness of active physical training as treatment for long-standing adductor-related groin pain in athletes: randomized trial. *Lancet*. 1999;353(9151):439–443.

Kachingwe AF, Grech S. Proposed algorithm for the mangement of athletes with athletic pubalgia (sports hernia): a case series. *J Orthop Sports Phys Ther*. 2008;38(12):768–781.

Kemp S, Batt ME. The 'sports hernia': a common cause of groin pain. *Phys Sportsmed*. 1998;25(1):36–44.

LeBlanc KE, LeBlanc KA. Groin pain in athletes. *Hernia*. 2003;7(2):68–71.

Moeller JL. Sportsman's hernia. *Curr Sports Med Rep*. 2007;6(2):111–114.

Morelli V, Smith V. Groin injuries in athletes. *Am Fam Physician*. 2001;64(8):1405–1414.

Chapter 137 Osteitis Pubis and Pubic Symphysis Disorders

Christopher J. Pexton, Kevin deWeber

ICD-10-CM CODES
M85.30 *Osteitis pubis*
026.719 *Pubic symphysis diastasis*
N94.9 *Pain of female symphysis pubis*

Key Concepts

- The pubic symphysis is composed of a nonsynovial amphi-arthrodial joint articulating the hyaline cartilage surfaces of pubic bones through a fibrocartilaginous disc.
- Four ligaments protect it from shear and tensile stresses: inferior (arcuate), superior, anterior, and posterior (Figs. 137.1 and 137.2).
- The gap between cortical surfaces of the articulating cartilage is 4 to 5 mm in women and it increases during pregnancy, increasing risk of diastasis.
- Men have a smaller gap, increasing overuse, and friction pathology, such as osteitis pubis.

Osteitis Pubis (Fig. 137.3)

- A self-limited, inflammatory overuse disorder of the pubic symphysis and surrounding attachments
- Hypothesized that shearing forces from repetitive hip adduction or flexion cause inflammation of the joint and the surrounding periosteum. Contributing biomechanical factors may include:
  - Sacroiliac joint instability leading to a secondary stress reaction at the pubic symphysis
  - Muscle counterforce disequilibrium due to injury of hip adductors or recti abdominis
  - Leg length discrepancy causing unequal shear forces across the symphysis
- Most likely to occur during the third or fourth decade of life, and is more common in men
- Occurs mostly in sports that require rapid acceleration and deceleration, running, kicking, or change of direction (i.e., running, hockey, soccer); prevalence from 0.5% to 6.2% of athletes

Pubic Symphysis Diastasis (Fig. 137.4)

- Separation of the pubic symphysis without concomitant fracture
- Most common in women, due to wider pubic symphysis gap
- Highest incidence during pregnancy, but also occurs in high-impact trauma, particularly horseback riding

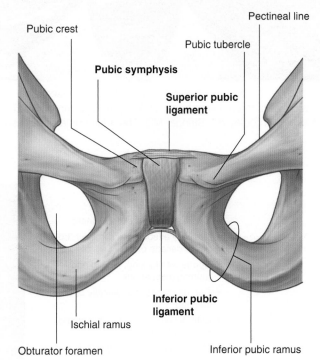

Fig 137.1 Bony and ligamentous anatomy of the pubic symphysis. (From Drake RL, Vogl AW, Mitchell AWM, eds. *Gray's Anatomy for Students*. 3rd ed. Philadelphia, PA; Elsevier; 2015:448.)

- Relaxin hormone, released during pregnancy, breaks down collagen in pelvic joints, creating greater ligament laxity
- Prevalence from 0.1% to 0.3% of all pregnancies; occurs any time throughout pregnancy, most commonly during labor

History
Osteitis Pubis

- Gradual onset of progressively worsening anterior or medial groin pain
- Pain often starts unilaterally; may progress to bilateral with radiation to the lower abdomen, hip, thigh, testicle, or perineum
- Classically described as sharp, stabbing, or burning; less often as dull or achy
- Pain typically relieved by rest
- Exacerbated by running, pivoting, kicking, hip adduction, or flexion and rectus abdominis muscle activation; sit-ups may cause pain; may have difficulty lying supine

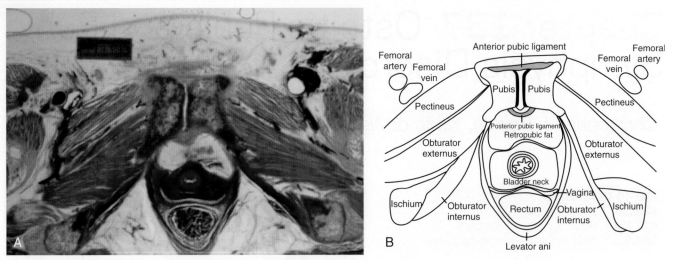

Fig 137.2 (A) and **(B)** Transverse cadaveric cross-sectional anatomy of the pubic symphyseal region. ([A], Courtesy W.D. Trotter Anatomy Museum, Department of Anatomy and Structural Biology, University of Otago, Dunedin, New Zealand. [A] and [B], From Becker I, Woodley SJ, Stringer MD. The adult human pubic symphysis: a systematic review. *J Anat*. 2010;217[5]:475–487.)

- Overuse injury, insidious onset
- Typically affects males in their 3rd or 4th decade of life
- Sports with kicking, cutting and running most at risk
- Can be diagnosed clinically or on imaging
- Lateral compression, pubic spring test may be positive
- Most cases will resolve in 2–6 months with physical therapy

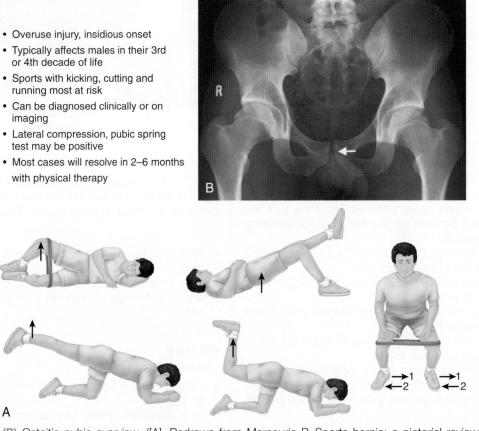

Fig 137.3 (A) and **(B)** Osteitis pubis overview. ([A], Redrawn from Mercouris P. Sports hernia: a pictorial review. *S Afr J Radiol*. 2014;18(2):1–4. [B], From Selkowitz DM, Beneck GJ, Powers CM. Which exercises target the gluteal muscles while minimizing activation of the tensor fascia lata? Electromyographic assessment using fine-wire electrodes. *J Orthop Sports Phys Ther*. 2013;43[2]:54–64.)

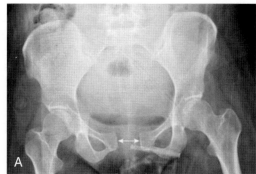

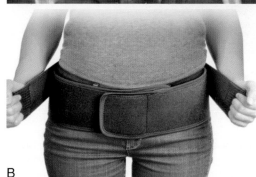

Fig 137.4 (A) and (B) Pubic symphysis diastasis overview. ([A] From Khorashadi L, Petscavage JM, Richardson ML. Postpartum symphysis pubis diastasis. *Radiol Case Rep*. 2011;6[3]:542.)

- Acute injury, focal swelling and antalgic gain
- Most common in pregnancy due to physiologic joint widening
- Also with OA or trauma, particularly horseback riding
- >10 mm gap on XR diagnostic
- >25 mm may need surgery
- Pelvic binder and early physical therapy results in fastest healing

- If instability is present, palpable clicking sensation at the pubic symphysis with certain activities (e.g., arising from a seated position, turning in bed, walking on uneven surfaces)

Pubic Symphysis Diastasis

- Pubic symphysis diastasis should be considered if there is history of pregnancy (especially with complicated or multiple vaginal deliveries), pelvic trauma, pelvic osteoarthritis, multiple pubic symphysis steroid injections, and a significant amount of horseback riding

Physical Examination

- Tenderness to palpation over the pubic symphysis suggests osteitis pubis, diastasis, or infection
- Tenderness in adjacent areas such as the superior and inferior pubic rami suggests tendinopathy, secondary muscle spasm (hip flexors or abdominal muscles), or stress fracture (Fig. 137.5)
- Decreased internal rotation of the hip suggests groin or pubic symphysis pathology

Osteitis Pubis

- Groin pain elicited with passive hip abduction and resisted hip adduction suggests osteitis pubis
- Pubic spring test may be positive: Place your fingers over the left and right pubic rami, a few cm lateral to the pubic symphysis. Apply downward pressure, one side at a time. Pain at the pubic symphysis is a positive test
- Lateral compression test may be positive: Pain in the pubic symphysis area with lateral compression over the iliac wing with the patient in the lateral decubitus position

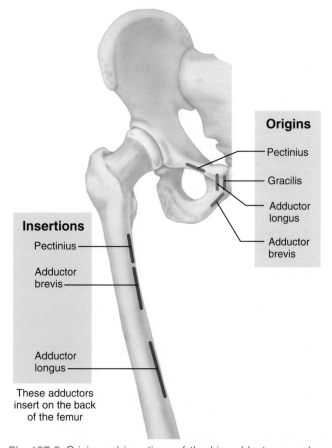

Fig 137.5 Origin and insertions of the hip adductor muscles. (From Keil D. The adductors: what are the adductor muscles? *Yoga Anat*. 2017. Used with permission of Lotus Publishing.)

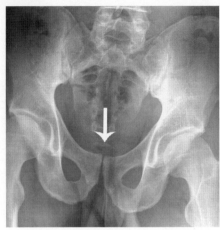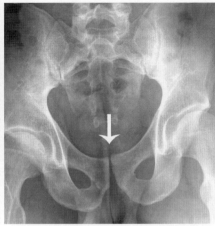

Fig 137.6 "Flamingo" view showing vertical symphyseal instability. (From Palisch A, Zoga AC, Meyers WC: Imaging of athletic pubalgia and core muscle injuries. *Clin Sports Med.* 2013;32(3):427-447.)

Pubic Symphysis Diastasis

- Noticeable edema over the pubic symphysis suggests diastasis with moderate to severe pain
- The patient may have antalgic or wide-based gait and difficulty with transfers

Imaging

- Plain radiographs—anteroposterior (AP), lateral, and "flamingo" views (AP with left foot raised, AP with right foot raised)
  - Radiographic abnormalities can lag behind clinical symptoms by 4 to 6 weeks in osteitis pubis
  - Typical findings for osteitis pubis include symphysis widening, sclerosis, cystic changes, or erosions in the subchondral bone (see Fig. 137.3A)
  - Greater than 10 mm between pubic symphysis edges is diagnostic for diastasis
  - Greater than 20 mm suggest concurrent SI joint instability (see Fig. 137.4A)
  - On "flamingo" views, greater than 2 mm of vertical shift between superior rami or widening of 7 mm of more is diagnostic for instability (Fig. 137.6)
- Magnetic resonance imaging (MRI)
  - Usually not needed, but preferred advanced imaging modality; consider MRI if diagnosis uncertain or symptoms are present for more than 6 weeks and not improving
  - May detect early osteitis pubis, stress fracture, or adductor muscle strain
  - Secondary cleft sign represents inferior extension of symphysis fibrocartilage due to microtear of the adductor enthesis
  - Bone marrow edema, fluid in the pubic symphysis joint, and periarticular edema are present in earlier stage of osteitis pubis (>6 months)
  - Subchondral sclerosis or resorption, bony margin irregularities, and osteophytes are present with chronic osteitis pubis (>6 months)
- Computed tomography
  - Less sensitive than MRI for early osteitis pubis
  - Marginal "stamp erosions" of the symphysis are seen with osteitis pubis

- Ultrasound
  - Helpful to rule out hernia and visualize widening of the pubic symphysis
  - May also detect adductor muscle or tendon pathology

Additional Tests

- Sudden onset of nontraumatic pubic symphysis pain with signs of systemic illness (fever, chills, or diaphoresis) should prompt workup for osteomyelitis of the pubic symphysis. Consider complete blood count with differential, c-reactive protein, blood culture, and urine culture in initial laboratory workup.

Differential Diagnosis

- Adductor strain (usually adductor longus muscle) or tendinopathy (see Fig. 137.5)
- Iliopsoas strain/bursitis
- Sports hernia (athletic pubalgia)
- Apophyseal avulsion fractures (skeletally immature athletes)
- Pubic rami stress fractures
- Entrapment neuropathy (ilioinguinal nerve)
- Snapping hip syndrome
- Intra-articular hip pathology
- Inguinal hernia
- Lumbar disc disease
- Seronegative spondyloarthropathies (reactive arthritis, ankylosing spondylitis)
- Osteomyelitis
- Urinary tract infection
- Prostatitis
- Urolithiasis
- Abdominal disorders

Treatment
Osteitis Pubis

- Pain-producing activity should be avoided; encourage relative rest to maintain state of general fitness.
- Course of oral nonsteroidal antiinflammatory drugs

- Consider a short course of oral corticosteroids for severe pain.
- Physical rehabilitation is the cornerstone of therapy. Begin a graduated, stepwise approach to therapy (restore range of motion, strength exercises, sport-specific exercise) that emphasizes stretching and strengthening of the hip joint muscles (specifically hip adductors, flexors, and rotators).
- Maintain a physical therapy program focusing on the muscles of the pelvis, back, and abdomen; include a core strengthening program.
- Intra-articular steroid injection therapy is controversial. Small, nonrandomized studies have yielded variable results. Injections early in disease course allowed more rapid return to play, but with high recurrence rates within 6 months.
- Dextrose injections have shown promise in refractory cases that have not improved with conservative therapy in small studies. Multiple injection sites have been utilized in trials, including the pubic symphysis and multiple muscle attachments into the pubic rami.

Pubic Symphysis Diastasis

- Consider abdominal/pelvic binder or pelvic stabilizing belt.
- Early physical therapy (within the first 2 weeks) is associated with quicker recovery time (3 months vs. 6 months with bed rest and supportive care).

When to Refer

- Chronic cases of osteitis pubis (>6 months' duration) that are unresponsive to conservative therapy and/or demonstrate vertical instability of the pubic symphysis may warrant operative treatment. Surgical therapies for osteitis pubis include curettage, wedge resection, wide resection, and arthrodesis (fusion of pubic symphysis with or without bone grafting).
- Pubic symphysis diastasis greater than 25 mm warrants surgical consideration.

Prognosis

- Osteitis pubis has an average healing time of 2 to 6 months with proper treatment.
- Healing time relates to severity, which is classified into four stages:
  - Stage I—Pain localized to the kicking leg, unilaterally, aggravated after exercise
  - Stage II—Pain extending bilaterally into inguinal regions, aggravated only after exercise
  - Stage III—Bilateral inguinal regions and lower abdominal muscle pain is noted. Exacerbation of pain during kicking, fast running, change in direction, and changes in stance
  - Stage IV—Inguinal, lower abdominal and lower back regions are painful, with pain reported when defecating, sneezing, or even walking
- Successful symptom resolution occurs in 90% to 95% of cases with structured conservative rehabilitation program; the recurrence rate is 25%.
- Return to play when the patient is pain free with activity, has full range of motion of the hip, and strength greater than 90% of the contralateral hip/leg.

- Pubis symphysis diastasis appropriate for conservative treatment alone may take 6 to 12 weeks depending on severity and physical therapy guidance.

Troubleshooting

- Utilize specialized exam tests to differentiate hip capsule, hip flexor, and abdominal pathology from pubis symphysis diagnoses.
- Sacroiliac joint pathology is often present with pubic symphysis pathology.

Patient Instructions

- Osteitis pubis is a self-limited condition that typically resolves in 2 to 6 months with rest.
  - Continue a fitness program that does not aggravate symptoms but provides cardiovascular fitness benefit.
  - Flexibility training is a key component of therapy and should become a part of the athlete's daily routine.
- Pubic symphysis diastasis often resolves without surgery in 6 to 12 weeks.
  - Recovery is fastest with early initiation of physical therapy (within the first 2 weeks) and with pelvis girdle support initially.

Considerations in Special Populations

- In skeletally immature populations, consider apophyseal avulsion injuries.
- Patients with hyperparathyroidism may have subchondral resorption within the pubic symphysis.
- The pubic symphysis is a common site for CPP (calcium pyrophosphate) crystal deposition disease, which can have a similar presentation.

Suggested Readings

Andrews SK, Carek PJ. Osteitis pubis: a diagnosis for the family physician. *J Am Board Fam Pract*. 1998;11:291–295.

Angoules Antonios G. Osteitis pubis in elite athletes: diagnostic and therapeutic approach. *World J Orthop*. 2015;6(9):672–677.

Goitz HT. Osteitis pubis. *Medscape (website)*. 2018. Available at: http://emedicine.medscape.com/article/87420-overview. Accessed July 12, 2018.

Hiti CJ, Stevens KJ, Jamati MK, et al. Athletic osteitis pubis. *Sports Med*. 2011;41(5):361–376.

Johnson R. Osteitis pubis. *Curr Sports Med Rep*. 2003;2(2):98–102.

Khorashadi L, Petscavage JM, Richardson ML. Postpartum symphysis pubis diastasis. *Radiol Case Rep*. 2011;6(3):542–545.

Moorman CT, et al. *Sports Medicine for the Orthopedic Resident*. World Scientific; 2016:233–237, and 291–294.

Morrison P. Musculoskeletal conditions related to pelvic floor muscle overactivity. In: Padoa A, Rosenbaum TY, eds. *The Overactive Pelvic Floor*. New York: Springer; 2016:91–112.

Read J. Pubic instability. *Sports Medicine Imaging (website)*. 2013. Available at: http://sportsmedicineimaging.com/topics/pubic-instabilty/. Accessed July 12, 2018.

Seidenberg PH, Bowen JD, King DJ, eds. *The Hip and Pelvis in Sports Medicine and Primary Care*. 2nd ed. New York: Springer; 2017: 117–120.

Chapter 138 Sacroiliac Joint Disorders

Per Gunnar Brolinson, David Leslie

ICD-10-CM CODES
M53.3 *Sacrococcygeal disorders, not otherwise specified*
M53.88 *Sacroiliac joint dysfunction*

Key Concepts

- The sacroiliac (SI) joint is a common source of low back pain in both the general (as many as 20%) and the athletic (as many as 50%) patient populations.
  - The diagnosis and treatment of SI joint problems are controversial due to its complex anatomy and biomechanics (Fig. 138.1).
  - There is no specific historical issue or single clinical examination technique that is both sensitive and specific for the diagnosis of SI dysfunction.
- The SI joint has been described as both a diarthrodial and synovial joint and has a well-defined, L-shaped articulation with an upper long vertical pole and a shorter lower horizontal pole.
  - The sacropelvic region serves as a force transfer link between the spine and the lower extremities.
- There have been conflicting studies regarding the mobility of the SI joints. Clinicians now believe that motion occurs throughout life.
- Integral to the biomechanics of SI joint stability is the concept of a self-locking mechanism. The SI joint is the only joint in the body that has a flat joint surface that lies almost parallel to the plane of maximal load (Fig. 138.2).

History

- Elements of the history should include the following factors:
  - The age of the patient. Many conditions occur within certain age ranges (e.g., in ankylosing spondylitis, the onset of symptoms is usually between the ages of 20 to 40 vs. osteoarthritis, which will become gradually more symptomatic after the age of 50 but can occur earlier in life if a joint is predisposed to an injury or surgery).
  - The type of sport or activity in which the patient is routinely involved.
  - The acuity or chronicity of the pain: it is important to differentiate between an acute, traumatic injury and a chronic, repetitive injury.
  - The mechanism of injury and identification of provocative and palliative measures.
  - The duration and frequency of the pain and the quality and intensity of the pain.
    - The presence of radiation or referred pain (usually unilateral, dull, and deep with radiation to buttock, posterior thigh, or groin).
  - Notation of previous low back injuries, with treatments and outcomes.
  - For active, pregnant women, remember that pregnancy causes laxity of the SI joint and predisposes women to pain or injury.
- The presence of red flags signaling more serious pathology include, but are not limited to, weight loss, night pain, and night sweats (cancer); fevers and chills (infection); dysuria and hematuria (nephrolithiasis); epigastric pain with nausea, vomiting, and/or heartburn (peptic ulcer disease or pancreatitis); left-sided abdominal pain with melena, hematochezia, diarrhea, and/or constipation (diverticular disease); pulsating abdominal pain with radiation to groin (abdominal aortic aneurysm); and numbness, tingling, weakness, and/or incontinence (radiculopathy or cauda equina syndrome).

Physical Examination

- Evaluate the patient in the standing, supine, and prone positions and assess the symmetry of the heights of the iliac crests, anterosuperior iliac spine, posterosuperior iliac spine, ischial tuberosities, gluteal folds, and greater trochanters. In addition, assess the symmetry of the sacral sulci, inferior lateral angles, and pubic tubercles.
- Determine whether there is any leg length discrepancy. This could be acquired or congenital, and management of such is dependent on proper diagnosis.
- Dynamic observation assesses for any asymmetry during both gait and specific motions characteristic of the patient's sport or usual activities.
- Always perform a thorough examination of the lumbar spine, hips, and knees because pathology in these areas can refer pain to the SI joint.
- A neurologic examination for radiculopathy should also be conducted, in addition to evaluating abdominal/core strength and overall flexibility.
- There have been numerous functional (motion) and provocative (pain-producing) tests reported in the literature; however, none have consistently been shown to reliably diagnose SI joint dysfunction. A detailed discussion of the numerous tests described for diagnosing the SI joint is beyond the scope of this review.

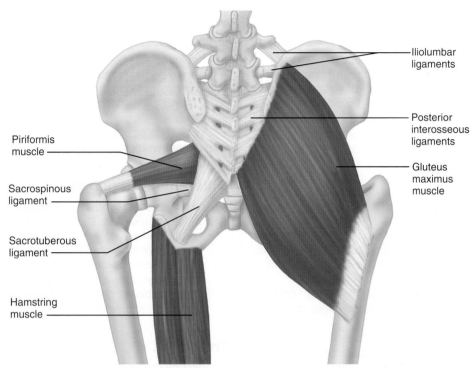

Fig 138.1 Surrounding structures, specifically the ligamentous and muscular structures, that contribute to the stability of the sacroiliac (SI) joint. On the left, the deep structures are depicted. On the right, the more superficial structures are identified. The multitude of these attached and surrounding structures contributes to the complexity of SI pathology, as many different factors may play a role and can certainly prevent improvement if not addressed in treatment.

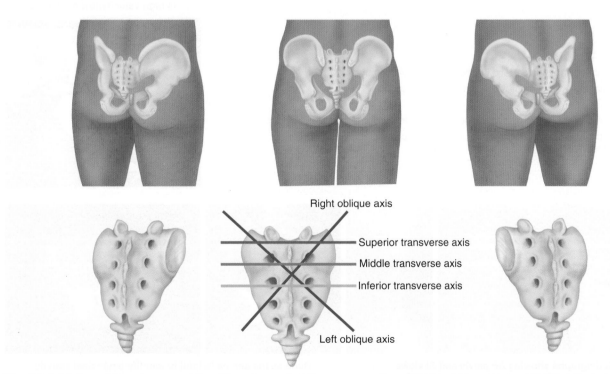

Fig 138.2 Motion of the sacrum and the different axes that it possesses. Sacral motion is complex and involves flexion, extension, and rotational components on multiple axes. During ambulation, two oblique axes are engaged. There are also three transverse axes of the sacrum, which are individually engaged with respiration and craniosacral motion *(superior transverse)*, posture *(middle transverse)*, and innominate *(hip)* motion about the sacrum *(inferior transverse)*.

- Common tests include standing forward flexion, sitting forward flexion, stork (Gillet), Gaenslen, supine-to-sit, Patrick (FABER [Flexion, ABduction, External Rotation]) test, side-lying approximation, and supine gapping.
- Accurate diagnosis must be based on a combination of historic clues, along with findings from static palpatory examination, segmental and regional motion testing, overall functional biomechanical examination, and appropriate diagnostic testing.

Imaging

- There is no specific gold standard imaging test to diagnose the SI joint, largely because of the location of the joint and visualization difficulties due to overlying structures. However, standard radiographs taken at 25 to 30 degrees from the anteroposterior axis coupled with lateral views may show degenerative changes, ankylosis, demineralization, or fracture (Fig. 138.3).
- Note that in adolescents, the SI joints may normally show widening and irregularity and therefore can make radiographic diagnosis more difficult.
- Bone scans identify osteoblastic activity and may signal infection, tumor, fracture, or a metabolic process.
- Computed tomography will identify fractures, osteoid osteomas, and degenerative changes.

- Magnetic resonance imaging helps to identify fractures, tumor, soft-tissue pathology, and lumbar disc disease and is most sensitive for identifying inflammatory sacroiliitis.
- Ultrasound can be also be considered to identify the anatomy and surrounding periarticular structures. In addition, it can be utilized to test SI motion dynamically in an office visit, and can also provide needle guidance for SI joint injections.
- Doppler ultrasound imaging can capture SI motion in pregnant women with SI pain.

Differential Diagnosis

- The differential diagnosis is extensive and should include, but not be limited to, the following:
  - Arthritis including ankylosing spondylitis, SI joint dysfunction (microinstability), lumbar radiculopathy, tumor, sacral stress fracture, lumbar facet syndrome, lumbar degenerative disc disease, abdominal aortic aneurysm, nephrolithiasis, diverticular disease, referred pain from pelvic organs, herpes zoster, and joint sepsis.

Treatment

- Accurate diagnosis is the key to successful treatment, and pain relief is an important early goal.

OMT directed at the SI joint. The technique being positioned is high velocity/low amplitude

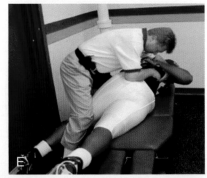

- Diagnosis
- Physical exam findings, history, and functional testing all contribute
- Consider imaging—radiographs, bone scan, MRI, ultrasound
- Treatment
  - Conservative—osteopathic manipulation, physical therapy are good starting points
  - Other options—SI joint injections (can be diagnostic and therapeutic), surgery if conservative options fail

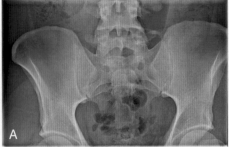
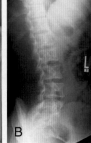
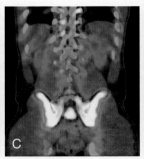
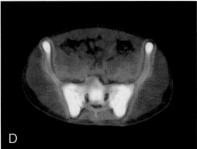

Radiographs showing AP pelvis and SI views Assess for SI asymmetry and irregularities   **Bone scans can be helpful to identify osteoblast activity**

Fig 138.3 Diagnostic and treatment options for sacroiliac *(SI)* joint dysfunction. Radiographs, both anteroposterior *(AP)* and SI views **(A)** and **(B)**, are shown as well as bone scan images **(C)** and **(D)** that focus on the SI joint. These can aid in diagnosis. In addition, osteopathic manipulation is a treatment option, and a technique is demonstrated in **(E)**.

- The use of nonsteroidal antiinflammatory drugs and non-narcotic analgesics, as well as physical therapy modalities, can be beneficial.
- Gross SI joint instability is rare, but microinstability is a relatively common component seen in patients with recurrent SI joint pain.
  - This microinstability often leads to chronic pain syndromes and must be identified and treated.
  - Instability often occurs as a result of the loss of the functional integrity of any of the systems of the lumbosacral and pelvic region that provide stability.
  - The myofascial, osteoarticular, ligamentous, and neural control components may be affected and should be a focus of intervention.
- Formal physical therapy can be helpful in both acute and chronic SI joint pain syndromes.
  - Rehabilitation must focus on the entire abdominolumbosacropelvic-hip complex addressing articular, muscular, neural, and fascial restrictions, inhibitions, and deficiencies.
  - A principle-centered, functional approach to evaluation and rehabilitation must be undertaken.
  - The transversus abdominis muscle has been shown to be the key muscle to functional core retraining due to its observed patterns of firing before and independent of the other abdominal muscles.
  - Exercise techniques that promote independent contraction of the transversus abdominis muscle have been shown to lower recurrence rates after an acute low back pain episode and lower pain and disability in chronic low back pain.
- Several joint mobilization or osteopathic manipulative techniques can be used in the treatment of SI joint pain syndromes, including soft-tissue technique, muscle energy, myofascial release, functional technique, strain/counterstrain, craniosacral technique, and high velocity/low amplitude. Fig. 138.3 shows the positioning for a treatment technique.
- Explanations of these techniques and their specific applications to the SI joint can be found in several excellent sources (see Suggested Readings).
- More recently, surgical intervention has become more popular as a treatment option for chronic SI joint pain in patients who have failed conservative treatment. Surgical techniques include minimally invasive surgery that involves fusion of the SI joint through an implant device or system, among others. Minimally invasive surgical intervention has demonstrated positive results in clinical trials; however, suboptimal outcomes from this type of intervention have been noted in these studies as well. Strict patient selection for surgical intervention may help to decrease the incidence of negative outcomes.

Prognosis

- A comprehensive functional approach based on historic clues and appropriate diagnostic testing will lead to the best clinical result.
- Clinical experience is that a multimodal approach works best. This includes aggressive pain control, functional therapeutic exercise, and potentially SI joint mobilization or manipulation.

- Identification and correction of functional or anatomic leg length discrepancy and optimization of posture are important, but often overlooked, clinical entities.

Troubleshooting

- Gravitational stress is a constant and greatly underestimated systemic stressor leading to postural imbalance, which is a systemic neuromuscular dysfunction.
- For patients with SI pain and dysfunction not responding to standard management, optimization of posture can be very beneficial. This can be achieved through the use of one or more of the following modes of treatment:
  - Contoured orthotics worn in the shoes to optimize foot and lower extremity biomechanics.
  - A flat orthotic of sufficient thickness to correct anatomic leg length discrepancy and level the sacral base.
  - Manipulation and/or mobilization directed to restore resilience to soft tissues and improve motion of restricted joint segments.
  - Daily practice of therapeutic postural exercise for 20 minutes to counter the bias of soft tissues reflective of the initial posture.
  - Use of pelvic belts (sacral belts) for sacropelvic support during postural retraining
- SI joint injections (local anesthetic with or without cortisone) have not been consistently shown to be effective, although they may at least help diagnose the SI joint as the source of pain.
- Periarticular injections, including prolotherapy and platelet-rich plasma (PRP), show promising results and can be clinically useful in the appropriately selected patient. In longitudinal, follow-up studies, the use of prolotherapy and PRP have been shown to be efficacious and are becoming more and more popular for both short-term and long-term management. The increasing availability and popularity of performing these procedures under ultrasound has the potential to increase the efficacy of treatment, as direct visualization of the needle can ensure that the solution or blood product is delivered to specific, pathologic anatomic areas.

Patient Instructions

- Follow physician and physical therapist instructions closely with respect to the type and quantity of exercise and acceptable job-related activities.
- Home-based exercises including postural retraining are vital to overall management and should be performed regularly.
- Consistently and diligently manage pain using physical therapy modalities. Also consider oral medications as appropriate.

Considerations in Special Populations

- Those caring for active patients will encounter this condition commonly and should be vigilant for its potential presence in any patient presenting with low back pain.
- One must be aware of this condition in the active pregnant female. Osteopathic manipulation has been shown to be an effective option for this patient population.

- For elderly patients, be particularly aware of issues potentially related to osteoporosis, and be sure to screen for underlying occult malignancy.
- For adolescent patients, watch carefully for sacral and pelvic stress fractures as well as lumbar spondylolysis.

Suggested Readings

Bandinelli F, Melchiorre D, Scazzariello F, et al. Clinical and radiological evaluation of sacroiliac joints compared with ultrasound examination in early spondyloarthritis. *Rheumatology*. 2013;52: 1293–1297.

Brolinson PG, Gray G. Principle-centered rehabilitation. In: Garrett WE, Kirkendall DT, Squire DH, eds. *Principles and Practice of Primary Care Sports Medicine*. Philadelphia: Lippincott Williams & Wilkins; 2001:645–652.

Brolinson PG, Kozar AJ, Cibor G. Sacroiliac dysfunction in athletes. *Curr Sports Med Rep*. 2003;2:47–56.

Dreyfuss P, Dreyer S, Griffin J, et al. Positive sacroiliac screening tests in asymptomatic adults. *Spine*. 1994;19:1138–1143.

Greenman PE. *Principles of Manual Medicine*. 5th ed. Philadelphia: Lippincott Williams & Wilkins; 2017.

Hancock MJ, Maher CG, Latimer J, et al. Systemic review of tests to identify the disc, SIJ or facet joint as the source of low back pain. *Eur Spine J*. 2007;16:1539–1550.

Kancherla VK, McGowan SM, Audley BN, et al. Patient reported outcomes from sacroiliac joint fusion. *Asian Spine J*. 2017;11:120–126.

Kim WM, Lee HG, Jeong CW, et al. A randomized controlled trial of intra-articular prolotherapy versus steroid injection for sacroiliac joint pain. *J Altern Complement Med*. 2010;16:1285–1290.

Lasslett M, April CN, McDonald B, et al. Diagnosis of sacroiliac joint pain: validity of individual provocation tests and composites of tests. *Man Ther*. 2005;10:207–218.

Peebles R, Jonas CE. Sacroiliac joint dysfunction in the athlete: diagnosis and management. *Curr Sports Med Rep*. 2017;16:336–342.

Polly DW, Cher DJ, Wine KD, et al. Randomized controlled trial of minimally invasive sacroiliac joint fusion using triangular titanium implants vs nonsurgical management for sacroiliac joint dysfunction: 12-month outcomes. *Neurosurgery*. 2015;77:674–691.

Richardson CA, Snijders CJ, Hides JA, et al. The relation between the transversus abdominis muscles, sacroiliac joint mechanics, and low back pain. *Spine*. 2002;27:399–405.

Slipman CW, Sterenfeld EB, Chou LH, et al. The predictive value of provocative sacroiliac joint stress maneuvers in the diagnosis of sacroiliac joint syndrome. *Arch Phys Med Rehabil*. 1998;79:288–292.

Van der Wurff P, Hagmeijer RHM, Meyne W. Clinical tests of the sacroiliac joint: A systematic methodological review. Part I: reliability. *Man Ther*. 2000a;5:30–36.

Van der Wurff P, Hagmeijer RHM, Meyne W. Clinical tests of the sacroiliac joint: A systematic methodological review. Part II: validity. *Man Ther*. 2000b;5:89–96.

Willard FH, et al. The muscular, ligamentous and neural structure of the low back and its relation to back pain. In: Vleeming A, Mooney V, Dorman T, eds. *Movement, Stability, and Low Back Pain: The Essential Role of the Pelvis*. New York: Churchill Livingstone; 1997.

Chapter 139 Trochanteric Bursa Injection

Stephen Shaheen, Tracy R. Ray

CPT CODE
20610 *Arthrocentesis, aspiration and/or injection; major joint or bursa (e.g., shoulder, hip, knee joint, subacromial bursa)*

ICD-10-CM CODES
70.61 *Trochanteric bursitis, right hip*
70.62 *Trochanteric bursitis, left hip*

Equipment

- Sterile skin prep solution (e.g., povidone-iodine, chlorhexidine)
- 10-mL syringe
- Needle:
  - long enough to make contact with bone
  - 20- or 22-gauge, 1.5-inch needle
  - consider a spinal needle for patients with increased subcutaneous tissue
- Ethyl chloride spray
- Gloves
- Medication:
  - Anesthetic (3 to 5 mL):
    - 1% lidocaine (Xylocaine) and/or
    - 0.5% bupivacaine (Marcaine)
  - Corticosteroid:
    - Intermediate acting: methylprednisolone (Depo-Medrol) or triamcinolone acetonide (Kenalog) and/or
    - Long acting: dexamethasone (Decadron) or beta-methasone sodium phosphate (Celestone)
- Sterile 4 × 4 adhesive bandage

Contraindications

- Sensitivity to selected medications
- Skin disease (e.g., cellulitis, rash) overlying injection site
- Poorly controlled diabetes mellitus (i.e., considerable HA1C, consistent FSBG >300 mg/dL)
- Underlying coagulopathy or poorly controlled anticoagulant therapy
- Lack of response to multiple prior injections

Considerations in Special Populations

- Diabetic: postinjection transient hyperglycemia
- Coagulopathic/anticoagulated: consider last international normalized ratio (INR) or recent medication dose changes prior to procedure

Instructions/Technique

- Obtain informed consent
  - Associated risks
    - Skin atrophy, depigmentation, or hyperpigmentation
    - Localized infection
    - Localized bleeding
    - Allergic or anaphylactic reaction
    - Systemic effects
      - Transient hyperglycemia (especially in diabetic patients)
      - Transient decrease in cortisol production
- Confirm the patient's allergies and previous adverse reactions
- Steps (Figs. 139.1 to 139.5)

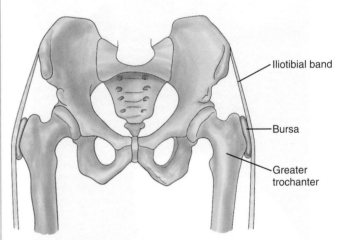

Iliotibial band

Bursa

Greater trochanter

Fig 139.1 Relevant anatomy.

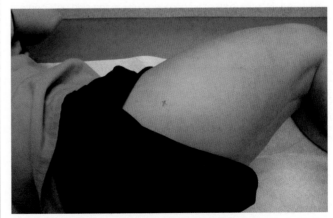

Fig 139.2 Patient in lateral decubitus position with affected side up. Area of maximal tenderness marked.

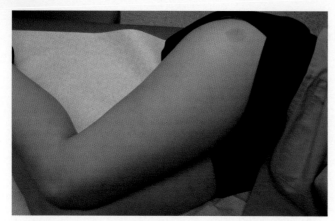

Fig 139.3 Injection site is cleaned with skin prep solution.

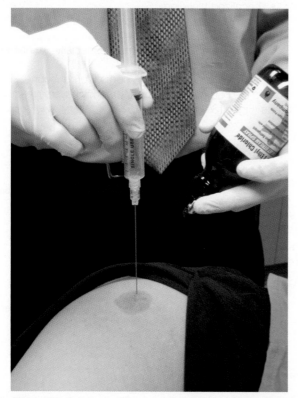

Fig 139.4 Needle is inserted perpendicular to the skin until contact with bone is made.

- Place the patient in the lateral decubitus position, affected side up.
- Locate the greater trochanter by palpating proximally from the diaphysis of the femur until an area of bony protrusion, lateral to the hip, is felt.
- Identify the point of maximal tenderness and mark before skin preparation.
- Clean the area of injection with sterile skin prep solution.
- Prepare provider and field to appropriate level of sterility.
- Apply topical anesthetic agent (e.g., ethyl chloride) as desired.
- Insert the needle perpendicular to the skin until contact with the greater trochanter is made.

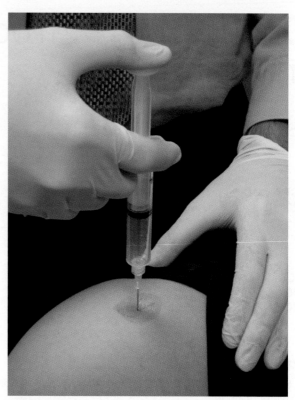

Fig 139.5 Aspirate to confirm that the needle is not in a vascular structure and then inject.

- Withdraw the needle approximately 1 to 2 mm—the bevel is now located in the bursa—and aspirate to make sure the needle is not in a vascular structure.
- Inject the mixture in 1- to 2-mL boluses, beginning at the site of maximal discomfort then fanning out to cover the surrounding area—the "wagon-wheel" technique.
- Apply an adhesive dressing.

Ultrasound (Fig. 139.6)

- Evaluated with a linear or curvilinear probe
- Bursa identification:
  - located next to the posterior facet of the greater trochanter, lateral and superficial to the insertion of the gluteus medius and deep to the gluteus maximus
  - hypoechoic, semilunar structure
- Gluteal tendinopathy can mimic bursitis—evaluate the tendon for acute (i.e., thinning, anechoic defects) or chronic (i.e., muscle wasting) injury.
- Injection:
  - Posterolateral approach: trochanteric bursa
  - Anterolateral approach: subgluteus medius and minimus bursa

Troubleshooting

- Resistance to injection? Consider withdrawing the needle slightly.
- Tight iliotibial band? Try placing a pillow between the patient's legs.

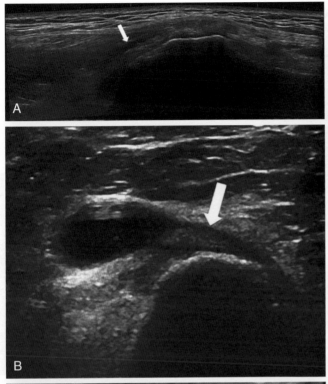

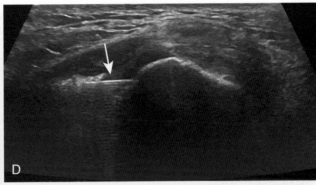

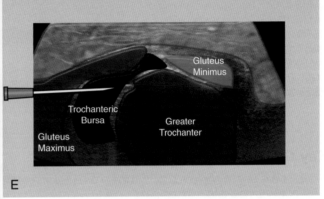

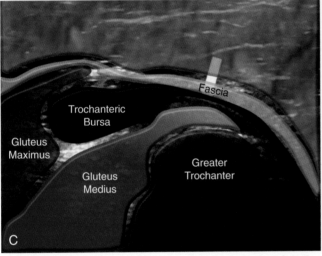

Fig 139.6 (A to E) Ultrasound evaluation and injection guidance. (From McNally E. Disorders of the groin and hip: lateral and posterior. In: *Practical Musculoskeletal Ultrasound*. 2nd ed. Philadelphia: Churchill Livingstone; 2014:210.)

Patient Instructions

- It is common to be sore immediately after the procedure, a result of local tissue swelling in response to the injection.
- Approximately 3% of patients will have a self-limited increase in their symptoms, a postinjection flare. This is well controlled with ice, acetaminophen, and antiinflammatory medications; the patient should consult the medical team if pain or swelling continues or worsens.
- Although the anesthetic provides some immediate relief, it is possible that symptoms may return. The steroid effect begins in 24 to 48 hours and continues building for several days, depending on the medication used.
- Limit activity to that necessary for daily living with a gradual return to baseline over the next 2 to 3 days.

Suggested Readings

Adkins SB, Figler RA. Hip pain in athletes. *Am Fam Physician*. 2000;61: 2109–2118.

Cardone DA, Tallia AF. Joint and soft tissue injection. *Am Fam Physician*. 2002;66:283–290.

Cardone DA, Tallia AF. Diagnostic and therapeutic injection of the hip and knee. *Am Fam Physician*. 2003;67:2147–2152.

Griffin LY, ed. Trochanteric bursitis injection. In: *Essentials of Musculoskeletal Care*. 3rd ed. Rosemont, IL: American Academy of Orthopaedic Surgeons; 2005:464–465.

McNally EG. Disorders of the groin and hip: lateral and posterior. In: *Practical Musculoskeletal Ultrasound*. 2nd ed. Philadelphia: Churchill Livingstone; 2014:201–210.

Chapter 140 Musculoskeletal Ultrasound of the Hip and Pelvis

Jennifer Pierce

Key Concepts

- Hip pain is cryptic and complex with many potential sources of both intrinsic and referred pain.
- Ultrasound (US) is a flexible imaging modality that can more easily and cost-effectively examine the area of interest, examine the contralateral side for comparison, and cover a larger anatomic area than magnetic resonance imaging (MRI).
- Dynamic US imaging using patient motion allows US to be a direct extension of the physical exam.
- US is technically more difficult in the hip because of the complex anatomy. Many of the hip anatomic structures are not superficial, and the depth of tissue in question may make US evaluation challenging.
- US is a less-desirable imaging modality for the evaluation of intra-articular processes.
- Using the correct US transducer is important to visualize structures and obtain better images. Lower-frequency transducers provide improved imaging for deeper anatomic structures; linear (9 MHz) or curvilinear (6 MHz) transducers are recommended.

Intra-Articular

- MRI and computed tomography (CT) are the better imaging modalities for tears of the cartilage and labrum, bone disease, fractures, and bone infarcts involving the hip joint.
- US can be used for the detection of a hip joint effusion (Fig. 140.1).
- US is an excellent modality for image-guided joint aspirations and injections.

Iliopsoas Tendon/Bursa

- Iliopsoas muscle is composed of the psoas and iliacus (Fig. 140.2). It functions as a hip flexor and to straighten the upper body. The iliopsoas tendon inserts onto the

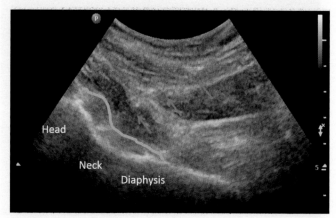

Fig 140.1 Longitudinal ultrasound image of the hip demonstrates a joint effusion with elevation of the anterior joint capsule *(orange line)*. A needle *(arrows)* is placed along the anterior hip, with the needle tip at the femoral head-neck junction.

lesser trochanter of the femur. Iliopsoas bursa surrounds the tendon where it passes over the ilium and distally.
- Iliopsoas (internal) snapping syndrome is a painful audible or palpable snapping due to abnormal motion of the tendon complex. Dynamic US is the "gold standard" for diagnosis. Commonly seen in ballet dancers.
- Iliopsoas bursitis is caused by repetitive motion, acute trauma, and rheumatoid arthritis.
- US-guided injection is both a useful diagnostic test and treatment for iliopsoas issues. It is also a good predictor of favorable surgical iliopsoas release outcome.

Adductor Aponeurosis/Core Muscle Injury

- Occurs most commonly in athletes and can be the primary cause of hip/groin pain in 40–50% of cases in the athlete.
- Tears occur due to the imbalance of forces (in athletes, leg muscles overpower the abdominal musculature) along the rectus abdominis–adductor aponeurosis/plate (Fig. 140.3).
- MRI is the most comprehensive imaging modality for this diagnosis; however, tears in the adductor aponeurosis and muscles can be detected with US (see Fig. 140.3).
- US-guided steroid injection can be performed as a diagnostic test to assist in localization of the pain and confirm the diagnosis. Efficacy needs more investigation.

Meralgia Paresthetica

- Entrapment of the lateral femoral cutaneous nerve as it courses near the proximal sartorius and inguinal ligament.

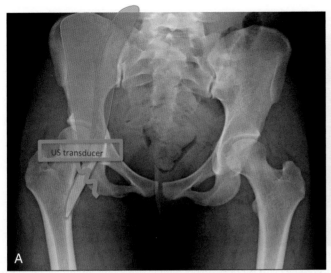

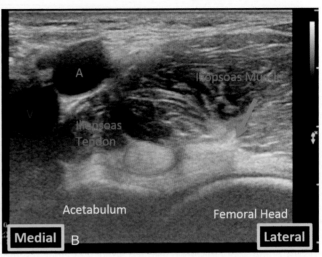

Fig 140.2 **(A)** Pelvic radiograph with the iliopsoas muscle *(red)*, tendon *(yellow),* and surrounding bursa *(blue)* drawn. The transducer is placed along the superior hip joint anteriorly in the transverse orientation. **(B)** Transverse ultrasound image of the superior hip joint where the medial acetabulum and superior aspect of the femoral head is visualized. The iliopsoas tendon and muscle are located directly anterior to the hip joint. The iliopsoas tendon is outlined and shaded with an accessory iliopsoas tendon *(arrow)*. *A,* Femoral artery; *V,* Femoral vein.

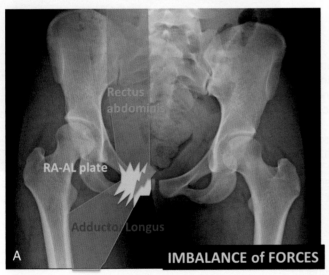

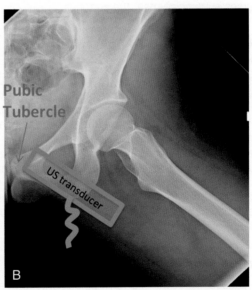

Fig 140.3 **(A)** Pelvic radiograph with the rectus abdominis and adductor longus muscle with the rectus abdominis adductor longus *(RA-AL)* aponeurosis or plate drawn. The imbalance of forces causes the RA-AL plate and the muscles to tear. **(B)** Radiograph of the left hip in frog leg position. To visualize the RA-AL plate, the transducer is placed just lateral to the pubic symphysis and oriented parallel to the femur. *Continued*

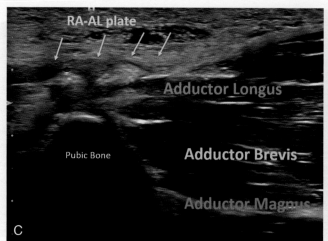
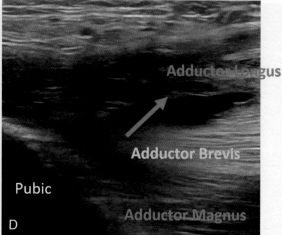

Fig 140.3, cont'd **(C)** Longitudinal ultrasound image of the RA-AL plate *(arrows)* also shows the pubic bone and the three stratified muscles of the adductor group with the adductor longus the most superficial. **(D)** Longitudinal plane ultrasound image of the pubic bone and adductor group muscles demonstrates a tear and hematoma of the adductor longus with retracted tendon *(arrow)*.

This causes sensory deficits and pain in the anterolateral thigh.
- US-guided injection of the nerve is diagnostic and can be therapeutic. The injection is performed along the nerve as it courses superficially near the sartorius.

Gluteal Tendons and Their Respective Subjacent Bursae

- Gluteus minimus (subgluteus minimus bursa), gluteus medius (subgluteus medius bursa), and gluteus maximus (trochanter bursa) all may account for pain and tenderness over the greater trochanter. Pain can be due to tendinosis, tears, calcific tendinosis, and bursitis.
- US-guided needle lavage is an effective treatment for calcific tendinosis by removing the calcifications and eliminating pain.
- US-guided bursal steroid injections targeting the trochanter and subgluteus medius bursae can be performed for the treatment of painful bursitis and trochanteric pain.

Piriformis Syndrome

- Pain caused by sciatic nerve impingement from either abnormal piriformis muscle morphology or aberrant course of the sciatic nerve; 6–8% of low back pain/radiculopathy symptoms can be attributed to piriformis syndrome.
- Once the diagnosis is confirmed by physical exam and/or MRI, US-guided localization of the piriformis muscle and steroid injection can be performed (Fig. 140.4).

Hamstring Tendon Complex/Ischial Bursa

- Hamstring tendon complex consists of the semimembranosus, semitendinosus, and biceps femoris.
- Pain is located at the ischial tuberosity or gluteal fold region and aggravated with sitting, walking uphill, or active knee flexion against resistance. Older patients typically have

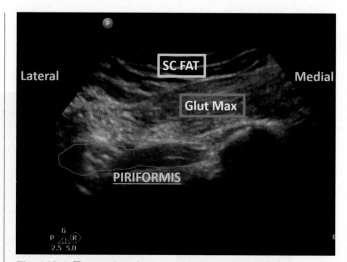

Fig 140.4 The patient is prone and the transducer is placed obliquely inferior to the sacroiliac joint. Transverse ultrasound image of the piriformis shaded in red subjacent to the gluteus maximus.

degenerative tendinosis/tears. Younger patients typically have suffered acute sports trauma.
- US evaluation
  - Detect tears and disruption of the tendon fibers (Fig. 140.5).
  - Localize the torn, retracted tendon for the surgeon.
  - Visualize associated hematomas and muscle tears.
  - With tendinosis, see intact fibers but the tendon is thickened and hypoechoic (darker than normal tendon) (see Fig. 140.5).
- US-guided injection can be performed targeting the ischial bursa which surrounds the hamstring origin.

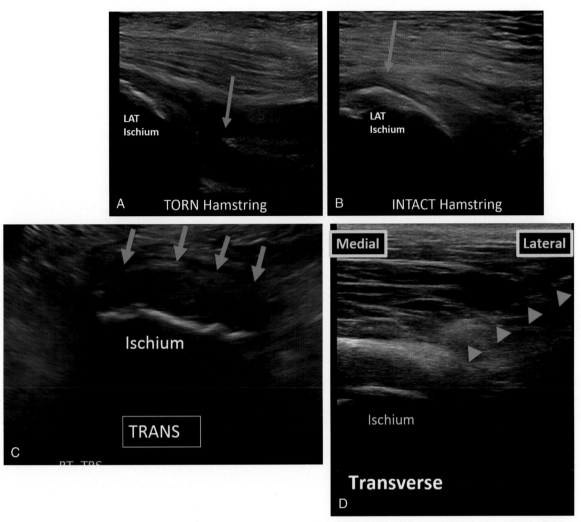

Fig 140.5 Longitudinal ultrasound image at the lateral ischium. **(A)** The hamstring tendon is intact with normal linear echogenic fibrillary architecture. **(B)** The hamstring tendon is torn at the ischium and mildly retracted *(arrow)*. There is surrounding dark, anechoic fluid representing hemorrhage and blood. **(C)** Transverse ultrasound image of the hamstring tendon at the ischium shows a thickened hypoechoic tendon compatible with tendinosis. **(D)** Ultrasound-guided hamstring injection. Transverse ultrasound image of the hamstring tendon at the ischium shows a needle *(arrow heads)* outlining a needle placed superficial to the tendon along the ischial bursa.

Suggested Readings

Finnoff JT, Hurdle FB, Smith J. Accuracy of ultrasound-guided versus fluoroscopically guided contrast-controlled piriformis injections a cadaveric study. *J Ultrasound Med*. 2008;27:1157–1163.

Jacobson JA. *Fundamentals of Musculoskeletal Ultrasound*. 2nd ed. Philadelphia: Elsevier; 2013.

Jose J, Buller LT, Fokin A Jr, et al. Ultrasound-guided corticosteroid injection for the treatment of athletic pubalgia: a series of 12 cases. *J Med Ultrasound*. 2015;23(2):71–75.

McEvoy JR, Lee KS, Blankenbaker DG, et al. Ultrasound-guided corticosteroid injections for treatment of greater trochanter pain syndrome: greater trochanteric bursa versus subgluteus medius bursa. *Am J Roentgen*. 2012;201:313–317.

Rowbotham EL, Grainger AJ. Ultrasound-guided intervention around the hip. *Am J Roentgen*. 2011;197(1):122–127.

Tagliafico A, Ferafini G, Lacelli F, et al. Ultrasound-guided treatment of meralgia paraesthetica (lateral femoral cutaneous neuropathy): technical description and results of treatment in 20 consecutive patients. *J Ultrasound Med*. 2011;30(10):1341–1346.

Zissen MH, Wallace G, Stevens KJ, et al. High hamstring tendinopathy: MRI and ultrasound imaging and therapeutic efficacy of percutaneous corticosteroid injection. *Am J Roentgen*. 2010;195:993–998.

7

SECTION

The Knee and Lower Leg

Chapter 141 Overview of the Knee and Lower Leg

Mark D. Miller, Ian J. Dempsey

Anatomy
Bones and Joint

- The knee joint is made up of the articulation of the distal femur and the proximal tibia and fibula (Fig. 141.1).
- This articulation allows flexion and extension of the joint, as well as a rolling (screw home) motion, during terminal extension.
- The patella, which is the largest sesamoid bone in the body, also articulates with the femur.

Femur

- The articular surface of the distal femur is composed of two condyles.
  - The medial condyle has a larger surface area, but the lateral condyle is longer.
- The intercondylar area serves as an attachment for the cruciate ligaments: the anterior cruciate ligament laterally and the posterior cruciate ligament medially.
- The medial epicondyle serves as the attachment for the medial collateral ligament.
- The lateral epicondyle serves as the attachment for the lateral collateral ligament.
- A groove distal to the epicondyle is where the popliteus tendon lies; it inserts distal and anterior to the lateral collateral ligament.

Tibia

- The tibia also has medial and lateral condyles.
  - The medial condyle is broad and concave.
  - The lateral condyle is smaller, more circular, and convex.
- The tibial eminences (spines) serve as the border of the anterior cruciate ligament.
- The posterior cruciate ligament lies between two bony prominences posteriorly, distal to the joint line.
- The patellar tendon inserts onto the tibial tuberosity.
- Gerdy tubercle is the attachment site for the iliotibial band.

Fibula

- The fibula articulates with the tibia and serves as the attachment for the lateral collateral ligament.

Patella

- The patella has the thickest articular cartilage in the body.
- It has two facets: a larger lateral facet and a smaller medial facet, separated by a vertical ridge.
- The medial patellofemoral ligament originates near the medial epicondyle and inserts on the upper border of the medial patella; it is the primary restraint to lateral displacement of the patella.
- The knee is the largest joint in the body and includes the following structures:
  - Ligaments
    - Anterior cruciate ligament: resists anterior translation
    - Posterior cruciate ligament: resists posterior translation
    - Medial collateral ligament: resists valgus displacement
    - Lateral collateral ligament: resists varus displacement
    - Posteromedial and posterolateral corner structures: resist rotation
  - Menisci
    - Medial: semicircular and broader posteriorly
    - Lateral: more circular and covers a larger portion of the articular surface

Muscles

- A variety of muscles cross the knee and cover the leg (Fig. 141.2). These are perhaps best considered in groups or compartments.
  - Anterior thigh
    - Quadriceps muscle (extends the leg)
    - Vastus lateralis, intermedius, medialis, and rectus femoris muscles
  - Posterior thigh
    - Hamstrings (flex the leg)
    - Lateral: biceps femoris muscle
    - Medial: semimembranosus, semitendinosus, sartorius, and gracilis muscles
  - Medial thigh
    - Adductors (adduct the leg)
    - Adductor magnus, longus, and brevis muscles
  - Anterior leg (extend/invert the foot/ankle)
    - Tibialis anterior, extensor hallucis longus, extensor digitorum longus muscles
  - Posterior leg (flex the foot/ankle)
    - Gastrocnemius, soleus, flexor hallucis longus, flexor digitorum longus, tibialis posterior muscles
  - Lateral leg (evert the foot/ankle)
    - Peroneus brevis, longus, and tertius muscles

Nerves

- The nerves that cross the knee and continue on into the leg are extensions of nerves from the lumbosacral plexus (Fig. 141.3).
- The femoral nerve (L2-L4 roots) innervates the quadriceps muscles.

- The obturator nerve (L2-L4 roots) innervates the adductors.
- The sciatic nerve (primarily S2-S4 nerve roots) innervates the hamstrings and divides in the midthigh into tibial and peroneal divisions.
- The tibial nerve continues distally to innervate the posterior compartments of the lower leg.
- The common peroneal nerve divides into superficial and deep branches after coursing around the fibular head.
- The superficial peroneal nerve innervates the lateral compartment of the leg and the deep peroneal nerve innervates the anterior compartment.

Vascularity

- The femoral artery divides in the thigh into deep (or profundus) and superficial branches.
- The artery passes posteriorly, becoming the popliteal artery as it passes between the origins of the gastrocnemius muscle and then bifurcates into the anterior and posterior tibial arteries.
- The peroneal artery is the first branch of the posterior tibial artery (Fig. 141.4).

Cross-Sectional Anatomy

- It is often very helpful to have a good understanding of the cross-sectional anatomy of the thigh and especially the leg (Fig. 141.5).
- Three compartments are commonly recognized in the thigh and four in the leg:
  - Thigh
    - Anterior compartment
      - Vastus medialis, vastus intermedius, vastus lateralis, rectus femoris, sartorius muscles
      - Superficial femoral artery and vein
      - Femoral nerve branches

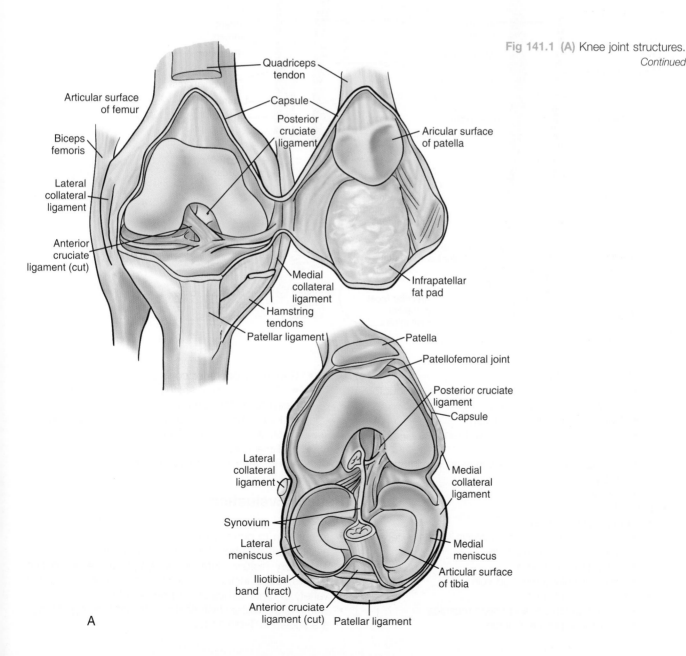

Fig 141.1 (A) Knee joint structures.
Continued

A

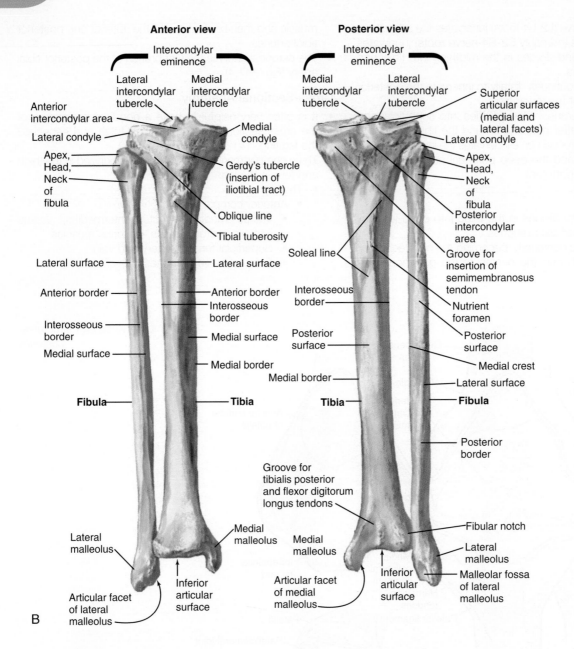

Anterior view

Intercondylar eminence

Lateral intercondylar tubercle

Medial intercondylar tubercle

Anterior intercondylar area

Lateral condyle

Medial condyle

Apex,
Head,
Neck of fibula

Gerdy's tubercle (insertion of iliotibial tract)

Oblique line

Tibial tuberosity

Lateral surface — Lateral surface

Anterior border — Anterior border
Interosseous border

Interosseous border — Medial surface

Medial surface — Medial border

Fibula — **Tibia**

Lateral malleolus

Medial malleolus

Articular facet of lateral malleolus

Inferior articular surface

Posterior view

Intercondylar eminence

Medial intercondylar tubercle

Lateral intercondylar tubercle

Superior articular surfaces (medial and lateral facets)

Lateral condyle

Apex,
Head,
Neck of fibula

Posterior intercondylar area

Soleal line

Groove for insertion of semimembranosus tendon

Interosseous border

Nutrient foramen

Posterior surface

Posterior surface

Medial crest

Medial border

Lateral surface

Tibia — **Fibula**

Posterior border

Groove for tibialis posterior and flexor digitorum longus tendons

Fibular notch

Medial malleolus

Medial malleolus

Lateral malleolus

Articular facet of medial malleolus

Inferior articular surface

Malleolar fossa of lateral malleolus

B

Fig 141.1, cont'd
(B) The tibia and fibula are the bones in the leg. (Modified from Miller MD, Chhabra AB, Browne JA, Park J, Shen F, Weiss, D. *Orthopaedic Surgical Approaches.* 2nd ed. Philadelphia: Elsevier; 2015:341.)

- Medial compartment
  - Adductor longus, adductor brevis, adductor magnus, gracilis muscles
  - Deep femoral artery and vein
  - Femoral and obturator nerve branches
- Posterior compartment
  - Biceps femoris, semitendinosus, semimembranosus muscles
  - Sciatic nerve
- Lower leg
  - Anterior compartment
    - Tibialis anterior, extensor hallucis longus, extensor digitorum longus muscles
    - Deep peroneal nerve
    - Anterior tibial artery and vein
  - Lateral compartment
    - Peroneus longus and brevis muscles
    - Superficial peroneal nerve

- Superficial posterior compartment
  - Gastrocnemius, soleus, plantaris muscles
- Deep posterior compartment
  - Flexor hallucis longus, flexor digitorum longus, tibialis posterior muscles
  - Tibial nerve
  - Posterior tibial artery and vein

Patient Evaluation
History

- In addition to demographic information, it is important to ask the patient about his or her symptoms.
- The injury history, duration of symptoms, exacerbating factors, pain, instability, mechanical symptoms, and a variety of other issues should be included.
- Some of the classic historical events and their significance are shown in Table 141.1.

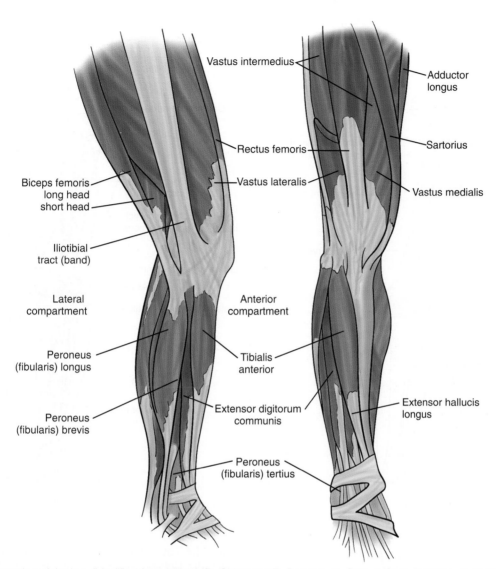

Fig 141.2 The muscles of the leg. (Modified from Miller MD, Chhabra AB, Browne JA. Park J, Shen F, Weiss, D. *Orthopaedic Surgical Approaches*. 2nd ed. Philadelphia: Elsevier; 2015:344.)

TABLE 141.1 Key Knee Historical Points

Historical Point	Significance
Noncontact pivoting injury with effusion	Anterior cruciate ligament tear
Blow to anterior tibia (dashboard injury)	Posterior cruciate ligament tear
Fall on leg with plantarflexed foot	Posterior cruciate ligament tear
Blow to the outside (lateral side) of the knee	Medial collateral ligament injury
Blow to the inside (medial side) of the knee	Posterolateral corner and or lateral collateral ligament injury
Fall directly onto patella with dorsiflexed foot	Patellar injury
Mechanical locking/catching after a twisting injury	Meniscal tear
Pain with prolonged sitting/stair climbing	Patellofemoral syndrome

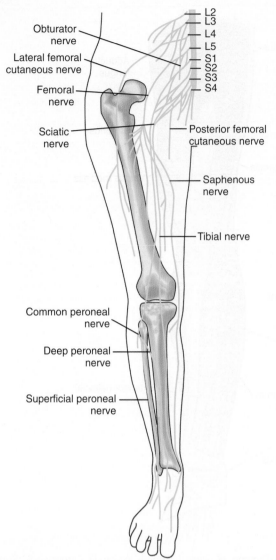

Fig 141.3 The nerves of the lower extremity. (Modified from Miller MD, Chhabra AB, Browne JA, Park J, Shen F, Weiss, D. *Orthopaedic Surgical Approaches*. 2nd ed. Philadelphia: Elsevier; 2015:347.)

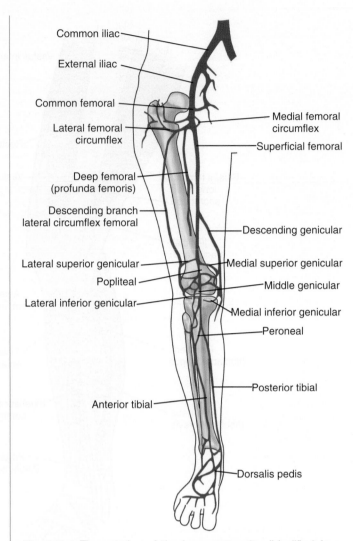

Fig 141.4 The arteries of the lower extremity. (Modified from Miller MD, Chhabra AB, Browne JA, Park J, Shen F, Weiss, D. *Orthopaedic Surgical Approaches*. 2nd ed. Philadelphia: Elsevier; 2015:347.)

- Ask patients about prior knee injuries or prior knee surgery.
  - If prior knee surgery present, obtaining prior operative report is key as patient reports are often incomplete or inaccurate

Physical Examination (Video 141.1)

- It is important to observe the patient.
  - Look for asymmetry, skin lesions, effusions, and other findings.
  - Look grossly at the patient's mechanical alignment.
  - Observe the patient's gait. Some classic gaits and their descriptions can be found in Table 141.2.
  - Check for an antalgic (painful) gait, a lateral or medial thrust, or other abnormalities.

- Next, evaluate the patient's passive and active range of motion (typically full extension or as much as 10 degrees of hyperextension and 130 to 140 degrees of flexion).
- Palpate the knee for an effusion (patellar ballottement or wave test) and locate the point of maximal tenderness (especially important in patients with meniscal tears).
- Attempt to displace the patella laterally and note whether the patient has apprehension (associated with patellar instability).
- Flex and rotate the knee and note whether the patient has popping (McMurray test) or increased joint line tenderness.
- Next, individual knee ligaments can be tested with specific examinations. The key maneuvers are shown in Table 141.3.

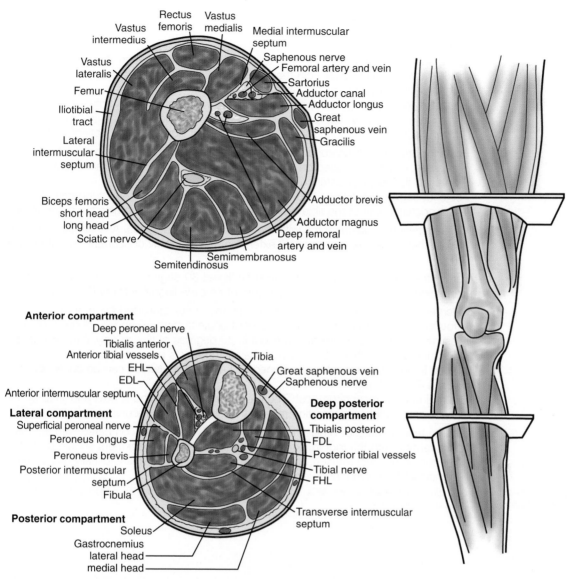

Fig 141.5 Cross-sectional anatomy of the thigh and leg. *EDL,* Extensor digitorum longus; *EHL,* extensor hallucis longus; *FDL,* flexor digitorum longus; *FHL,* flexor hallicus longus. (Modified from Miller MD, Chhabra AB, Browne JA, Park J, Shen F, Weiss, D. *Orthopaedic Surgical Approaches.* 2nd ed. Philadelphia: Elsevier; 2015:348.)

TABLE 141.2 Classic Injury Gait Patterns

Gait Pattern	Explanation
Antalgic gait	Patient may walk with limp on affected side, manifested as decreased stance phase of injured extremity
Trendelenburg gait	Patient leans to the side with weak hip abductors to compensate for this weakness causing a periodic lean during ambulation
Quadriceps avoidance gait	Patient leans forward when ambulating to lock the knee attempting to avoid the use of the quadriceps on the affected side
Varus recurvatum gait	Patient's affected knee hyperextends with relative varus during the stance phase of the affected limb

TABLE 141.3 Key Knee Examination Findings

Ligament/Structure	Examination
ACL	Lachman test: anterior force applied to proximal tibia with knee in 30 degrees of flexion. A pillow under the knee will help the patient to relax. Lachman test is more specific than the anterior drawer test (Fig. 141.6). Pivot shift test: valgus force applied to the knee with foot internally rotated. As you flex the knee from full extension to approximately 30 degrees of flexion, it will "jump" or pivot as it reduces from a subluxed position. This examination is best done with the patient under anesthesia.
PCL	Posterior drawer test: posterior force applied to the proximal tibia with the knee flexed to 90 degrees. Grading is based on displacement in relation to the medial femoral condyle (I, anterior; II, flush; III, posterior) (Fig. 141.7). Posterior sag sign: the knee and hip are flexed to 90 degrees while supporting the ankle. There is a posterior shift of the tibia best noted by observing the prominence of the tibial tubercle.
MCL	Valgus stress test: valgus force with the knee flexed 30 degrees. Assess the medial opening. Note that if the knee opens in full extension, there is likely concurrent cruciate ligament injury (Fig. 141.8).
LCL	Varus stress test: varus force with the knee flexed 30 degrees. Assess lateral opening. Again, opening in full extension implies concurrent cruciate ligament injury (Fig. 141.9).
PLC	External rotation asymmetry or Dial test: with the knees stabilized by an assistant, externally rotate the feet and compare the thigh-foot angle in both 30 and 90 degrees of knee flexion. If asymmetry (of ≥15 degrees) is present in 30 degrees of flexion only, it represents an isolated PLC injury (or an ACL-PLC injury). If the asymmetry is present at both 30 and 90 degrees of knee flexion, it represents a combined PCL-PLC injury (which can be confirmed with other tests) (Fig. 141.10). External rotation recurvatum test: The great toe of the affected is held and lifted off the examination table. Observation reveals the leg falling into recurvatum and varus (Fig. 141.11).
PMC	Slocum test: an anterior drawer test with the foot in neutral is compared with an anterior drawer test with the foot in external rotation. Anterior displacement should be reduced with the foot in external rotation, unless there is a PMC injury. This is usually associated with a significant MCL injury and valgus laxity (Fig. 141.12).

ACL, Anterior cruciate ligament; *LCL,* lateral collateral ligament; *MCL,* medial collateral ligament; *PCL,* posterior cruciate ligament; *PLC,* posterolateral corner; *PMC,* posteromedial corner.

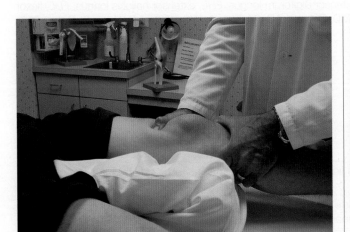

Fig 141.6 The Lachman examination. Note that the hand closest to the head of the patient grasps the thigh and the opposite hand performs the examination with the thumb close to the joint line. A pillow can be placed under the knee to help the patient relax.

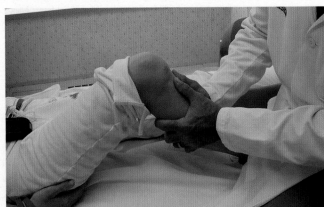

Fig 141.7 The posterior drawer examination. Note that the starting point is evaluated by palpating the medial tibial plateau in relation to the medial femoral condyle before applying a posteriorly directed force.

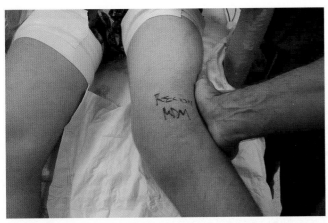

Fig 141.8 Valgus stress testing. A valgus stress is applied across the knee. This examination is done in both 30 degrees of knee flexion and full extension. Opening in full extension implies concurrent injury to the cruciate ligament(s).

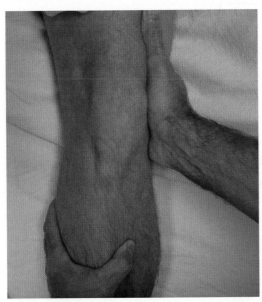

Fig 141.9 Varus stress testing. A varus stress is applied across the knee. This examination is done in both 30 degrees of knee flexion and full extension. Opening in full extension implies concurrent injury to the cruciate ligament(s).

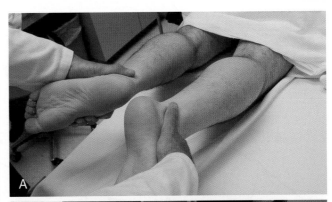

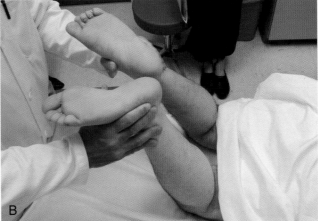

Fig 141.10 External rotation asymmetry. With the knees stabilized, both feet are passively externally rotated and the thigh-foot angle is measured. Asymmetry of 15 degrees or more implies injury to the posterolateral corner structures. The test is performed in both 30 degrees **(A)** and 90 degrees **(B)** of knee flexion. Asymmetry in both 30 and 90 degrees implies injury to both the posterolateral corner and the posterior cruciate ligament.

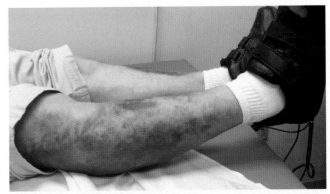

Fig 141.11 External rotation recurvatum test. The great toe of the affected is held and lifted off the examine table. Observation reveals the leg falling into recurvatum and varus.

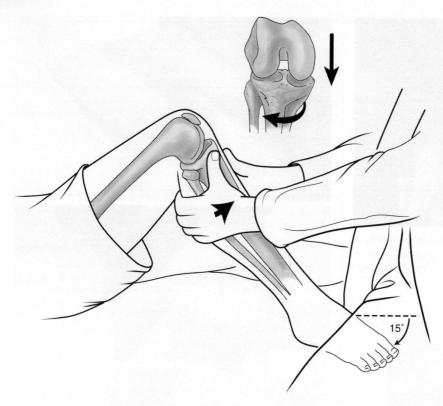

Fig 141.12 Slocum test. An anterior drawer is done in external rotation, and the anterior translation is compared with the same test done with the foot in neutral. The displacement should decrease with the knee in external rotation; if it does not, then a posteromedial corner injury should be suspected. (Modified from Tria AJ, Klein K. *An Illustrated Guide to the Knee*. New York: Churchill Livingstone; 1992.)

Imaging

- Plain radiographs
  - Standard radiographs include orthogonal (anteroposterior and lateral) views and a patellar (sunrise or Merchant) view.
  - Radiographic findings may include those listed in Table 141.4 and are shown in Fig. 141.13.
  - In older patients, it is very helpful to obtain a 45-degree posteroanterior flexion weight-bearing (Rosenberg) view (Fig. 141.14).
- Stress radiographs
  - Varus and valgus stress radiographs can be helpful in patients with open physes to determine whether there is a ligamentous or physeal injury.
  - They can also be helpful in multiple ligament–injured knees when the collateral ligament status is unknown.
  - Stress radiographs have also become the standard for reporting posterior cruciate ligament injuries and treatment.
    - A 15-kDa force is applied to the proximal tibia with the knee flexed 90 degrees and a lateral radiograph is obtained (Fig. 141.15).
    - Measurements are done posteriorly, and side-to-side comparisons are made.
    - Displacement of 10 mm implies an isolated posterior cruciate ligament injury. Displacement of 20 mm or more implies a combined posterior cruciate ligament–posterolateral corner injury.
- Magnetic resonance imaging
  - Unfortunately, most sports fans believe that the diagnosis of any sports injury must await the results of magnetic

TABLE 141.4 Key Knee Radiographic Findings

Finding	Significance
Segond fracture (lateral capsular sign)	Highly associated with ACL tear (although it is not common)
Calcification of the proximal MCL (Pellegrini-Stieda)	Chronic MCL injury
Patella alta	Patellar instability
Patella baja	Arthrofibrosis (chronic stiff knee)
Squaring, ridging, narrowing (Fairbanks changes)	Postmedial meniscectomy DJD
Lucency lateral aspect MFC	Osteochondritis dissecans
Widened/cupping laterally	Discoid meniscus

ACL, Anterior cruciate ligament; *DJD*, degenerative joint disease; *MCL*, medial collateral ligament; *MFC*, medial femoral condyle.

resonance imaging. In reality, magnetic resonance imaging should be a confirmatory examination.
  - It is very accurate for ligament injuries, meniscal tears, and other problems (Fig. 141.16).
  - Historically, it has not been as helpful for articular cartilage injuries, although techniques are improving.
- Computed tomography
  - Computed tomography can be useful for the evaluation of bony pathology (e.g., fractures, tumors, revision surgery with bone defects).

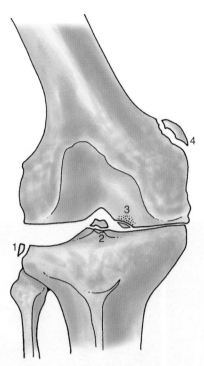

Fig 141.13 Illustration showing multiple radiographic findings. (1) Segond fracture (lateral capsular sign); (2) tibial eminence fracture; (3) osteochondritis dissecans; (4) Pelligrini-Stieda lesion. (Modified from Miller MD. Sports medicine. In: Miller MD, Thompson SR, eds. *Review of Orthopaedics*. 7th ed. Philadelphia: Elsevier; 2016:343.)

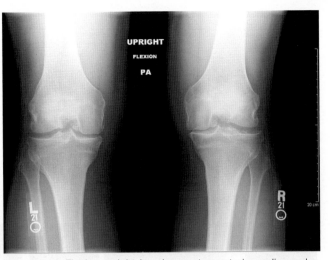

Fig 141.14 Flexion weight-bearing posteroanterior radiographs. This test is done in 45 degrees of flexion and demonstrates postmeniscectomy medial compartment arthrosis (right greater than left).

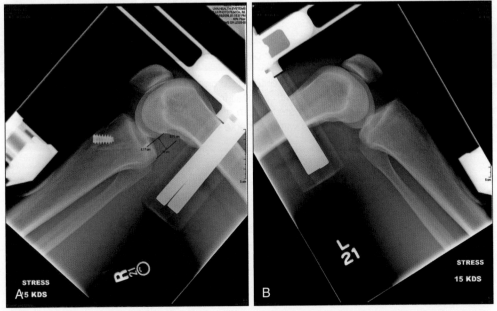

Fig 141.15 Telos stress radiograph with 15 kDa of force in a patient with a failed previous posterior cruciate ligament reconstruction (A). Note that the posterior displacement is measured and compared with the opposite normal knee (B).

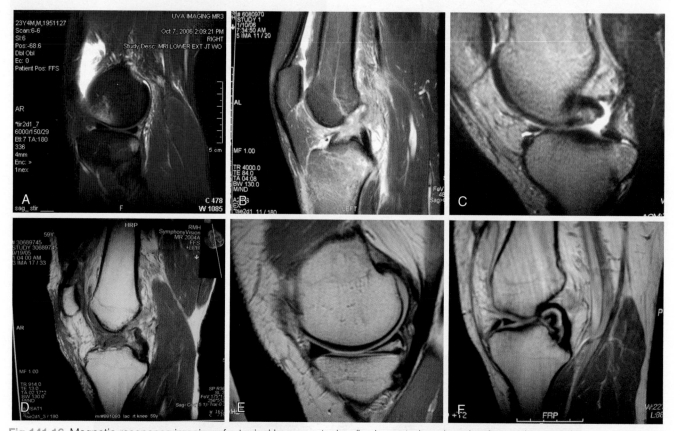

Fig 141.16 Magnetic resonance imaging of a typical bone contusion (bruise or trabecular microfracture) associated with an anterior cruciate ligament (ACL)-injured knee **(A)**; an ACL injury with a linear fracture **(B)**; a posterior cruciate ligament (PCL) injury **(C)**; a combined ACL and PCL-injured knee **(D)**; a complex posterior horn medial meniscal tear with a "picture frame" meniscus **(E)**; and a displaced bucket-handle tear of the medial meniscus with a "double PCL sign" **(F)**.

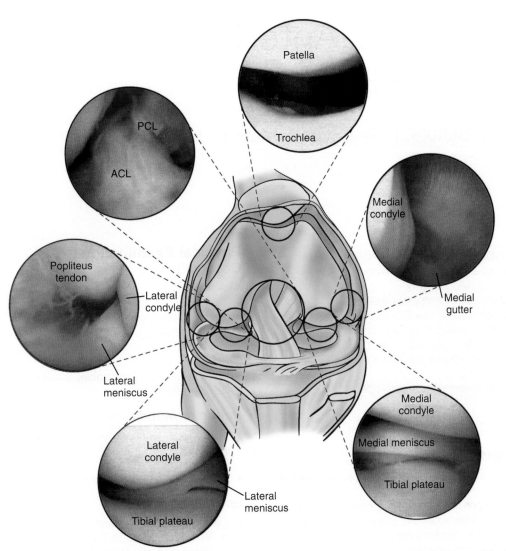

Fig 141.17 Diagnostic knee arthroscopy. *ACL*, Anterior cruciate ligament; *PCL*, posterior cruciate ligament. (Modified from Miller MD, Chhabra AB, Browne JA, Park J, Shen F, Weiss, D. *Orthopaedic Surgical Approaches*. 2nd ed. Philadelphia: Elsevier; 2015:388.)

- Arthroscopy
  - Arthroscopy is typically done with the patient in the supine position with a leg holder or post.
  - The inferolateral portal is typically used for visualization and the inferomedial portal for instrumentation.
  - Additional portals are made as necessary.
  - A thorough and complete examination of the knee is performed and pathology addressed (Fig. 141.17).

Suggested Readings

Ellis H. The applied anatomy of examination of the knee. *Br J Hosp Med*. 2007;68:M60–M61.

Hoppenfeld S. *Physical Examination of the Spine and Extremities*. Norwalk, CT: Appleton & Lange; 1976.

Hughston JC, Andrews JR, Cross MJ, Moschi A. Classification of knee ligament instabilities. Part I. The medial compartment and cruciate ligaments. *J Bone Joint Surg Am*. 1976;58(2):159–172.

Lubowitz JH, Bernardini BJ, Reid JB III. Current concepts review: comprehensive physical examination for instability of the knee. *Am J Sports Med*. 2008;36:577–594.

Malanga GA, Andrus S, Nadler SF, McLean J. Physical examination of the knee: a review of the original test description and scientific validity of common orthopedic tests. *Arch Phys Med Rehabil*. 2003;84(4):592–603.

Miller MD, Howard RF, Plancher KD. *Surgical Atlas of Sports Medicine*. Philadelphia: WB Saunders; 2003.

Miller MD, Sekiya JK. *Sports Medicine: Core Knowledge in Orthopaedics*. Philadelphia: Elsevier; 2006.

Post WR. Anterior knee pain: diagnosis and treatment. *J Am Acad Orthop Surg*. 2005;13:534–543.

Slocum DB, Larson RL. Rotatory instability of the knee: its pathogenesis and a clinical test to demonstrate its presence. *J Bone Joint Surg Am*. 1968;50A:211–225.

Tria AJ Jr. *An Illustrated Guide to the Knee*. New York: Churchill Livingstone; 1992.

Wojtys EM, Chan DB. Meniscus structure and function. *Instr Course Lect*. 2005;54:323–330.

Chapter 142 Anterior Cruciate Ligament Injury

Siobhan M. Statuta, Kelly E. Grob, Mark D. Miller

ICD-10-CM CODES
S83.519	*Acute anterior cruciate ligament injury— unspecified laterality*
S83.511	*Acute anterior cruciate ligament injury—right*
S83.512	*Acute anterior cruciate ligament injury—left*
M23.50	*Chronic anterior cruciate ligament injury— unspecified laterality*
M23.51	*Chronic anterior cruciate ligament injury—right*
M23.52	*Chronic anterior cruciate ligament injury—left*

Key Concepts

- The anterior cruciate ligament (ACL) is one of four major knee ligaments.
- The ACL is the primary restraint to anterior translation of the tibia and provides rotational stability to the knee.
- It originates on the medial lateral femoral condyle, runs obliquely, and inserts anterior to the center of the tibial intercondylar area region (Fig. 142.1).
- Injury to the ACL results in abnormal translation and rotation of the knee, leading to increased forces on other knee structures (e.g., menisci, articular cartilage), risking additional acute or chronic injury.
- Approximately half of acute ACL injuries are associated with meniscal tears.
- A triad of injuries commonly occurs in conjunction: ACL, medial collateral ligament (MCL), and lateral meniscus.
- Rarely, ACL injuries are involved with multiple knee ligament injury that may require emergent knee reduction and confirmation of neurovascular status.

History
Acute Injury

- Noncontact, pivoting injury to the knee
- Associated with a "pop" sensation and results in immediate swelling
- Unable to continue in activity

Chronic Injury

- Recurrent swelling with activity
- Instability with pivoting maneuvers

Physical Examination
Observation

- Abrasions
- Deformity
- Effusion (intra-articular swelling)
- Difficulty bearing weight

Palpation

- Patellar effusion (ballottable)
- Tenderness

Range of Motion

- Rule out a "locked knee" (lacking full extension) from an ACL tear in conjunction with a displaced bucket handle tear of the meniscus
- Loss of flexion can occur from an effusion

Special Tests

- Lachman test (gold standard) (Fig. 142.2 and Video 142.1)
  - With knee in 20 to 30 degrees of flexion, stabilize the femur and pull forward on the tibia along the plane of the joint line
  - A positive test is excessive forward tibial translation compared to the unaffected knee
- Anterior drawer sign
  - Place knee in 70 to 90 degrees of flexion, apply an anterior force, and assess the endpoint (not as sensitive as the Lachman test)
  - Positive test is endpoint laxity in anterior direction
- Pivot shift test (Video 142.2)
  - A valgus force is applied while knee is being flexed
  - Positive test is the appreciation of a rotational jerk or "clunk" in movement

Other Helpful Tests

- McMurray test (to assess for an associated meniscal tear)
  - Flexion and rotation of the knee with varus and valgus forces applied
  - Positive test is pain or a "click" as the meniscus displaces
- Posterior drawer sign (to evaluate for a posterior cruciate ligament [PCL] tear)
  - Knee in 70 to 90 degrees of flexion, apply a posterior force to assess the endpoint
  - Positive test is endpoint laxity in posterior direction

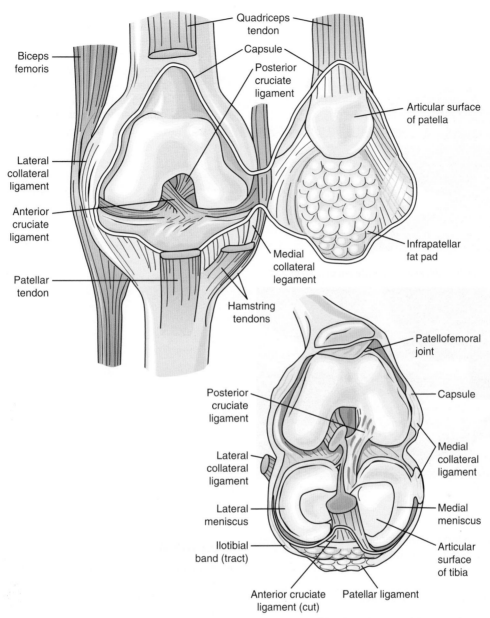

Fig 142.1 Front *(top)* and cut-away *(bottom)* views of the knee joint demonstrating the location of the anterior cruciate ligament.

- Dial test (associated posterolateral corner or PCL injury)
  - With patient prone and knees flexed 30 and 90 degrees, externally rotate bilateral feet
  - Asymmetrical rotation in both 30 and 90 degrees of flexion suggests a combined posterolateral corner and PCL injury
  - Asymmetrical rotation only in 30 degrees of flexion suggests an isolated posterolateral corner injury or with an associated ACL injury
- Patellar apprehension test (to determine patellar dislocation or instability)
  - With knee in extension, attempt to displace the patella laterally or medially
  - Positive test is the provocation of patient apprehension

Imaging
Radiographs

- Posteroanterior flexion weight-bearing view
  - Determine presence of arthritis (especially in older patients)
  - Assess for a lateral tibial avulsion (Segond fracture), which is highly associated with an ACL tear
- Lateral view
  - Determine patellar height
  - A high-riding patella (alta) may be associated with patellar instability or a patellar tendon rupture
  - A low-riding patella (baja) is associated with a stiff knee (arthrofibrosis)

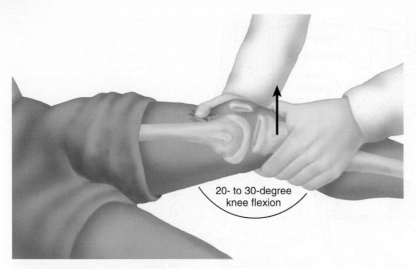

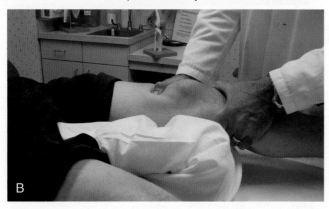

20- to 30-degree
knee flexion

A Tibia pulled anteriorly while femur is stabilized

B

Fig 142.2 (A) Lachman test is the gold standard for evaluating an anterior cruciate ligament–injured knee. It is helpful to place a pillow under the knee to relax the hamstring muscle and gain the patient's confidence. **(B)** Note that the examiner faces the injured knee and uses the hand that is closer to the patient's head to stabilize the thigh and the other hand to displace the tibia anteriorly.

- Assess for posterior tibial slope (slopes >12 degrees are hypothesized to correlate with greater risks of ACL injury)
- Sunrise view
  - Evaluate for patellar subluxation/tilt

Magnetic Resonance Imaging (Fig. 142.3)

- Not required for diagnosis
- Evaluate for ligament disruption in sagittal view and classic bone bruise pattern.

Additional Tests

- KT1000/KT2000 knee arthrometers
  - Instruments that provide objective measurement of anterior tibial translation
  - Often used after ACL reconstruction
  - Methods to test rotation are under development

Differential Diagnosis

- Patellar instability
- Patellar or quadriceps tendon rupture
- PCL rupture
- Meniscal tear

Treatment

- At diagnosis of ACL tear, treatment focuses on:
  - Decreasing the effusion (consider aspiration, ice, compression)
  - Physical therapy with focus of closed-chain quadriceps rehabilitation. Important to maximize range of motion, quadriceps tone, and pain control (Fig. 142.4)
- Later
  - ACL reconstruction unless otherwise contraindicated

When to Refer

- All but sedentary, inactive patients should consult with an orthopedic surgeon.
- The presence of a locked knee requires immediate referral with a goal to salvage as much of the associated healthy meniscus as possible.
- Isolated ACL injuries may be referred at any time (reconstruction after improvement in effusion, range of motion is regained, and quadriceps tone restored).
- ACL reconstruction involves first removing the torn ACL (the disrupted ends cannot be repaired, as they are immediately coated with a myofibrinous cap). A "new ACL" is created using a tendon (Autograft: typically a folded portion of

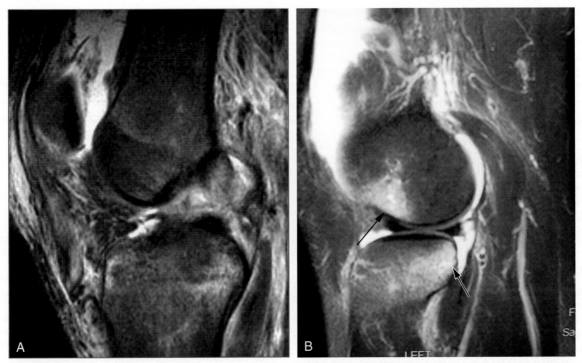

Fig 142.3 Sagittal magnetic resonance imaging demonstrating anterior cruciate ligament disruption **(A)** and classic bone bruise **(B)** (see *arrows*).

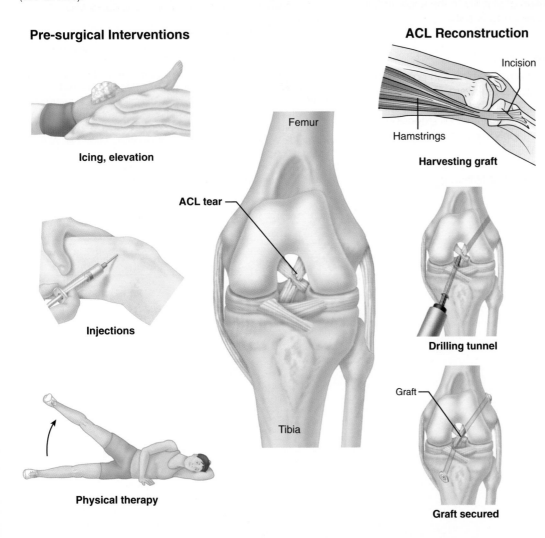

Pre-surgical Interventions

Icing, elevation

Injections

Physical therapy

Femur

ACL tear

Tibia

ACL Reconstruction

Incision

Hamstrings

Harvesting graft

Drilling tunnel

Graft

Graft secured

Fig 142.4 Anterior cruciate ligament *(ACL)* reconstruction overview. In the acute period, treatment should focus on controlling the knee effusion and maintaining both strength and range of motion. To reconstruct, an autograft must be harvested, prepared, new tunnels surgically placed prior to fixation of the graft.

Section 7 The Knee and Lower Leg

the semitendinosus and gracilis hamstring tendons, or the central one-third of the patellar tendon. Alternatively, an allograft from a cadaver.). This tendon is then passed through surgically created tunnels in the tibia and femur and secured with screws or other fixation devices (see Fig. 142.4).

Prognosis

- ACL reconstruction—Good, given improvement of stability and recovery of function. Patients with uncomplicated ACL reconstructions should return to sports in approximately 6 months.
- Nonoperative treatment—Fair. Recurrent instability may occur, often resulting in additional injuries (meniscal and/or articular cartilage).

Surgical Risks and Benefits

- Risks include bleeding, infection, nerve injury (numbness is not uncommon after patellar tendon or hamstring harvesting from incision or retraction of the infrapatellar branches of the saphenous nerve), loss of motion, and recurrence. When patellar tendon autografts are used, there is also a slight risk of a patellar fracture and late anterior knee pain typically with kneeling.
- Benefits include restoration of stability to the knee and, in most cases, successful return to activity.

Patient Instructions

- It is important to achieve full range of motion prior to ACL reconstruction and immediately afterward. Patients should be encouraged to use a pillow or bolster under their heel rather than under the knee to maintain full extension.
- Control swelling with ice (apply for periods of 15 to 20 minutes several times daily).
- Quadriceps strengthening (stationary cycle, elliptical trainer, etc.) is a crucial part of the rehabilitation process.

- Patients should avoid running and activities involving sudden changes in direction both preoperatively and for at least 3 months after surgery.

Considerations in Special Populations

- Inactive and sedentary patients should be treated nonoperatively. Arthroscopic management of an associated meniscal tear (and not for ACL reconstruction) may be considered.
- Obesity can make surgery challenging, but should be performed nonetheless for any knee instability.

Suggested Readings

Ardern CL, Webster KE, Taylor NF, et al. Return to sport following anterior cruciate ligament reconstruction surgery: a systematic review and meta-analysis of the state of play. *Br J Sports Med*. 2011;45(7):596–606.

Benjaminse A, Gokeler A, van der Schans CP. Clinical diagnosis of an anterior cruciate ligament rupture: a meta-analysis. *J Orthop Sports Phys Ther*. 2006;36:267–288.

Chhabra A, Starman JS, Ferretti M, et al. Anatomic, radiographic, biomechanical, and kinematic evaluation of the anterior cruciate ligament and its two functional bundles. *J Bone Joint Surg Am*. 2006;33(4):2–10.

Fithian DC, Paxton EW, Stone ML, et al. Prospective trial of a treatment algorithm for the management of the anterior cruciate ligament-injured knee. *Am J Sports Med*. 2005;33:333–334.

Iobst CA, Stanitski CL. Acute knee injuries. *Clin Sports Med*. 2000;19:621–635.

Sanders TG, Miller MD. A systematic approach to magnetic resonance imaging interpretation of sports medicine injuries of the knee. *Am J Sports Med*. 2005;33:131–148.

Schub D. Saluan p: anterior cruciate ligament injuries in the young athlete: evaluation and treatment. *Sports Med Arthrosc*. 2011;19(1):34–43.

Solomon DH, Simel DL, Bates DW, et al. The rational clinical examination. Does this patient have a torn meniscus or ligament of the knee? Value of the physical examination. *JAMA*. 2001;286:1610–1620.

Spindler KP, Wright RW. Anterior cruciate ligament (ACL) tear. *N Engl J Med*. 2008;2135-2142.

Utukuri MM, Somayaji HS, Khanduja V, et al. Update on pediatric ACL injuries. *Knee*. 2006;13:345–352.

Chapter 143 Posterior Cruciate Ligament Injury

Robert G. Marx

ICD-10-CM CODES

S83529A	*Sprain of the posterior cruciate ligament unspecified knee initial encounter*
S83521A	*Sprain of the posterior cruciate ligament right knee initial encounter*
S835122A	*Sprain of the posterior cruciate ligament left knee initial encounter*
M23622	*Other spontaneous disruption of the posterior cruciate ligament of the left knee*
M23621	*Other spontaneous disruption of the posterior cruciate ligament of the right knee*

Key Concepts

- The posterior cruciate ligament (PCL) is the primary restraint to posterior translation of the tibia.
- The PCL injury accounts for 3-20% of all knee ligament injuries.
- The PCL resists 85-100% of a posteriorly directed knee force at 30 and 90 degrees.
- The PCL runs obliquely, originating from the lateral border of the medial femoral condyle and inserting 1 to 1.5 cm inferior to the posterior rim of the tibia in a depression called the PCL facet (Fig. 143.1A).
- There are two main bundles of the PCL, the anterolateral (stronger, larger) and the posteromedial, a concept that is important for reconstruction (see Fig. 143.1B).
- The mechanism of injury for isolated PCL tear is usually related to trauma ("dashboard injury") or sports (fall on flexed knee with plantarflexed foot or isolated hyperflexion).
- Frequently injured in combination with other ligaments (posterolateral corner, anterior cruciate, collaterals); isolated injuries less than 50%
- Partial tears may heal due to their extrasynovial position and good blood supply.
- After PCL rupture, contact forces increase in the medial and patellofemoral compartments and may lead to arthritis.
- Results after reconstruction are encouraging, but acute surgery is generally not indicated in the setting of an isolated PCL injury.

History

- Acute injury
  - Minimal to large effusion.
  - Patient may complain of instability.
- In the setting of trauma, rule out associated injuries including occult knee dislocation.
- Determine time from injury.
- Chronic injury
  - Anterior and/or medial knee pain
  - Feeling of instability, especially with twisting, impact activities, and stairs
  - Mild effusion, worsened with activities

Physical Examination

- Inspection for effusion
- Bruising or anterior abrasions
- Deformity (rule out dislocation)
- Special tests
  - Lachman test: rule out associated anterior PCL injury. Patient may have increased translation with good end point if PCL is injured with an intact anterior cruciate ligament (ACL).
  - Posterior drawer test (Video 143.1): imparts a posterior force on the proximal tibia. Posterior translation is greatest at 70 to 90 degrees of knee flexion. The tibia must be reduced to its normal anatomic position before testing (Fig. 143.2).
    - Grade I (0 to 5 mm): tibial condyles anterior to femoral condyles
    - Grade II (5 to 10 mm): tibial condyles flush with femoral condyles, usually partial injury
    - Grade III (10 to 15 mm): tibial condyles posterior to femoral condyles, complete tear, may indicate concomitant posterolateral corner injury
  - Posterior sag: hip and knee flexed to 90 degrees; gravity applies posterior force to tibia; look for "sag" of tibia on the injured side compared with the normal side (Fig. 143.3).
  - Posterolateral spin test: check lateral tibial plateau step-off compared with lateral condyle with an external rotation force applied to the tibia and look for side-to-side difference.
  - Passive external rotation (dial test): Test at 30 and 90 degrees, prone or supine, and compare with the other side. More than a 10-degree difference is positive.
    - External rotation increased at 30 degrees only: isolated posterolateral corner injury
    - External rotation increased at 90 degrees only: isolated PCL
    - External rotation increased at both 30 and 90 degrees: PCL plus posterolateral corner injury

Posterior cruciate ligament injuries

PCL injury treatment

- **Isolated PCL**
  - No bony fragment
    - Non-operative
    - Rehabilitation
    - Brace
  - Large bony fragment
    - Surgical fixation
    - Open reduction
- **Chronic PCL**
  - Surgery after failed rehabilitation
- **Combined injury**
  - Reconstruction
    - Single or double bundle

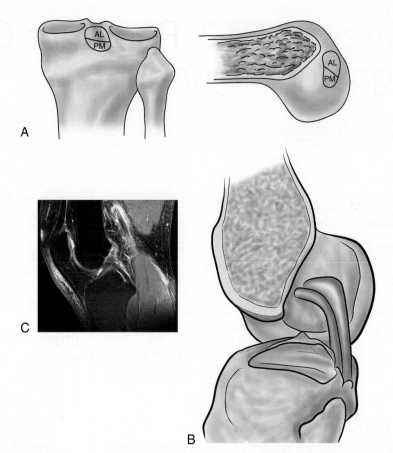

Fig 143.1 **(A)** Insertion sites of the posterior cruciate ligament. **(B)** Anterolateral and posteromedial bundles of the posterior cruciate ligament. **(C)** Magnetic resonance image of an intact posterior cruciate ligament. *AL,* anterolateral; *PM,* posteromedial.

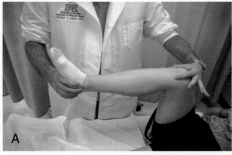
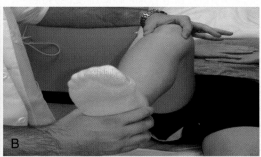

Fig 143.2 **(A)** Hand position for the posterior drawer/sag test. **(B)** The anterior joint line is palpated to determine the relationship of the proximal tibia to the femoral condyles.

Imaging

- Radiographs: weight-bearing anteroposterior, lateral, and merchant views
  - Look for PCL avulsion fragment from posterior tibia in acute injuries (Fig. 143.4).
  - Evaluate for degenerative joint disease and osteochondral injury.
- Stress radiographs: taken with a posterior force applied to proximal tibia at 90-degree knee flexion
  - A Telos device may be used to reliably reproduce this force.
  - Useful in suspected chronic injuries.

- Magnetic resonance imaging (see Fig. 143.1C)
  - Useful to evaluate complete and partial PCL injuries.
  - Identifies other associated ligament, meniscal, and chondral injuries.
  - Magnetic resonance imaging should be interpreted with caution in the chronic setting; PCL may appear healed in patients with laxity due to postinjury lengthening of the ligament.

Differential Diagnosis

- Anterior cruciate ligament rupture.
- Occult knee dislocation (multiligamentous knee injury).

- Isolated posterolateral corner injury.
- Tibial plateau fracture.
- May be missed in polytrauma patient, ipsilateral long bone fractures or ipsilateral floating knee.

Treatment
Isolated Posterior Cruciate Ligament Injuries

- At diagnosis (acute injuries)
  - Treatment is dependent on grade of injury and the presence or absence of avulsion fragments.
    - Grade I and II: no/small bony fragment
      - Nonoperative with aggressive rehabilitation program concentrating on quadriceps strengthening and range of motion.

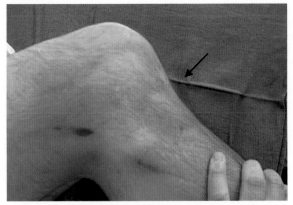

Fig 143.3 Positive posterior sag test. Note the position of the tibia *(arrow)*.

- Return to play in approximately 1 month when quadriceps strength nearly normal (time to play can vary).
  - Children may require repair.
- Grade I and II: large bony fragment
  - Refer for surgical fixation of fragment.
- Grade III
  - Refer for operative consultation: Double- versus single-bundle reconstructions and arthroscopically assisted versus all-arthroscopic options exist.
- Later (chronic injuries)
  - Alignment and degree of joint degeneration must be taken into account.
  - Patients may require high tibial or sagittal plane osteotomy.

When to Refer

- Indications for referral include acute PCL injuries with large bony fragments amenable to fixation, grade III PCL injuries (usually not isolated injuries), and all multiligamentous knee injuries (see Chapter 145).

Prognosis

- The PCL has a greater capacity to heal than the anterior cruciate ligament.
- A good therapy program focusing on quadriceps strengthening is successful in most cases of isolated PCL injury.

Troubleshooting

- Large bony avulsions that are amenable to open reduction and internal fixation should be fixed.

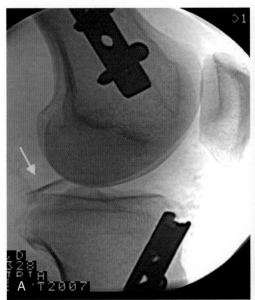
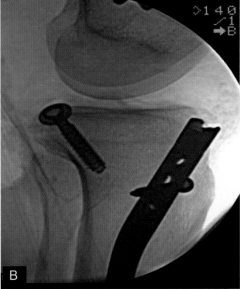

Fig 143.4 Radiographs depicting avulsion of the posterior cruciate ligament. **(A)** *Arrow* denotes fragment of large bony avulsion (also note the associated fractures). **(B)** Same fragment after open reduction and internal fixation.

- Chronic injuries should be considered for surgery if nonoperative management has failed and the patient has persistent instability.
- Careful examination is critical to rule out associated knee pathology and occult knee dislocation.

Instructions for the Patient

- Patients should be counseled that not all injuries require surgery.
- The prognosis is favorable in most cases of isolated PCL injury with a good quadriceps strengthening program.
- The PCL-deficient knee may be at risk of developing a more rapid rate of medial compartment and patellofemoral arthrosis.
- Multiligament injuries generally require surgery.

Suggested Readings

Arnoczky SP, Grewe SR, Paulos LE, et al. Instability of the anterior and posterior cruciate ligaments. *Instr Course Lect*. 1991;40:199–270.

Campbell RB, Jordan SS, Sekiya JK. Arthroscopic tibial inlay for posterior cruciate ligament reconstruction. *Arthroscopy*. 2007;23:1356e1–1356e4.

Campbell RB, Torrie A, Hecker A, et al. Comparison of tibial graft fixation between simulated arthroscopic and open inlay techniques for posterior cruciate ligament reconstruction. *Am J Sports Med*. 2007;35:1731–1738.

Marx RG, Shindle MK, Warren RF. Management of posterior cruciate ligament injuries. *Operat Tech Sports Med*. 2009;17(3):162–166.

Miller MD, Bergfeld JA, Fowler PJ, et al. The posterior cruciate ligament injured knee: principles of evaluation and treatment. *Instr Course Lect*. 1999;48:199–207.

Parolie JM, Bergfeld JA. Long-term results of nonoperative treatment of isolated posterior cruciate ligament injuries in the athlete. *Am J Sports Med*. 1986;14:35–38.

Sekiya JK, West RV, Ong BC, et al. Clinical outcomes after isolated arthroscopic single-bundle posterior cruciate ligament reconstruction. *Arthroscopy*. 2005;21:1042–1050.

Sekiya JK, Whiddon DR, Zehms CT, Miller MD. A clinically relevant assessment of PCL and posterolateral corner injuries. Part I: evaluation of isolated and combined deficiency. *J Bone Joint Surg Am*. 2008;90(8):1621–1627.

Shelbourne KD, Davis TJ, Patel DV. The natural history of acute, isolated, nonoperatively treated posterior cruciate ligament injuries: a prospective study. *Am J Sports Med*. 1999;27:276–283.

Veltri DM, Warren RF. Isolated and combined posterior cruciate ligament injuries. *J Am Acad Orthop Surg*. 1993;1:67–75.

Whiddon DR, Zehms CT, Miller MD, et al. Double compared with single-bundle open inlay posterior cruciate ligament reconstruction in a cadaver model. *J Bone Joint Surg Am*. 2008;90(9):1820–1829.

Chapter 144 Medial Collateral Ligament Injury

Matthew H. Blake, Darren L. Johnson

ICD-10-CM CODES
S83.41 *Medial collateral ligament sprain*
M23.50 *Chronic medial collateral ligament tear*

Key Concepts

- The medial collateral ligament (MCL) is the primary stabilizer to valgus stress on the knee (Fig. 144.1).
- The MCL is a secondary stabilizer to anterior drawer and external rotation.
- The MCL is the most commonly injured knee ligament.
- Injuries to the MCL can occur concomitantly with other ligaments injuries, with anterior cruciate ligament (ACL) tears occurring most frequently.
- Of the four major knee ligaments, the MCL has the greatest capacity to heal.
- Tears of the MCL can be classified as acute or chronic and are often described by location of injury (i.e., femoral, midsubstance, tibial, or a bony avulsion).
- MCL tears are graded as sprains: I, II, or III.
- Isolated grade III MCL tears are uncommon.
- Most MCL injuries are treated nonoperatively in a hinged brace.
- MCL with posterior oblique ligament (POL) injuries have valgus and rotational instability, resulting in worse patient outcomes if treated nonoperatively.

History

- Incidence is 0.24 per 1000 person-years.
- These injuries frequently occur in isolation.
- Acute
  - Valgus force: contact or noncontact.
  - Medial-side knee pain with or without feeling a "pop."
  - Patient may be able to walk.
  - Knee may feel unstable.
- Chronic
  - Medial knee pain
  - Feeling of instability
  - With or without effusion, depending on concomitant injuries

Physical Examination

- Inspection
  - Medial knee swelling, ecchymosis, and/or deformity
  - Abrasions/contusions on lateral knee
  - With or without antalgic gait/valgus thrust

- Palpation
  - Medial: Femur versus tibial
  - Effusion: None unless there is concomitant ligament/meniscal injury
- Range of Motion
  - Flexion/extension: Usually near full. Swelling may limit extremes of motion.
  - Locked knee: Superficial medial collateral ligament (sMCL) incarcerated in the joint, concomitant bucket-handle meniscal tear or loose body.
- Special Tests
  - Valgus stress at 30 degrees of flexion (Fig. 144.2 and Video 144.1).
  - Grade I: 1–4 mm laxity with end point.
  - Grade II: 5–9 mm laxity with end point.
  - Grade III: >10 mm laxity without end point.
  - Opening to valgus stress at full extension is a grade III MCL injury, and the physician must rule out concomitant ligament injury
  - A stable knee with anterior draw in external rotation rules out POL injury.
  - A subluxating meniscus while valgus testing indicates a meniscotibial ligament injury.
  - Full ligamentous knee exam.

Imaging

- Radiographs
  - Standing posteroanterior, Rosenburg, lateral, Merchant, and full-length standing.
  - Most often normal.
  - Pellegrini-Stieda lesions significant for a chronic MCL injury (Fig. 144.3).
  - Valgus stress at 20 degrees of flexion.
  - Normal is <2 mm of widening in comparison to contralateral side.
  - Opening >3.2 mm more than the contralateral knee is a grade III sMCL injury.
  - >9.8-mm widening in comparison to the contralateral knee indicates a complete medial side injury.
- Magnetic resonance imaging
  - Not required unless additional pathology is suspected.
  - Evaluation of the MCL is best seen on coronal views.
  - Femur, midsubstance, tibial injury, or bony avulsions.
  - Stener-like lesions: Tibia-based avulsion where the sMCL lies on top of the pes anserine tendons.
  - May have sMCL entrapment in the medial joint space (Fig. 144.4).

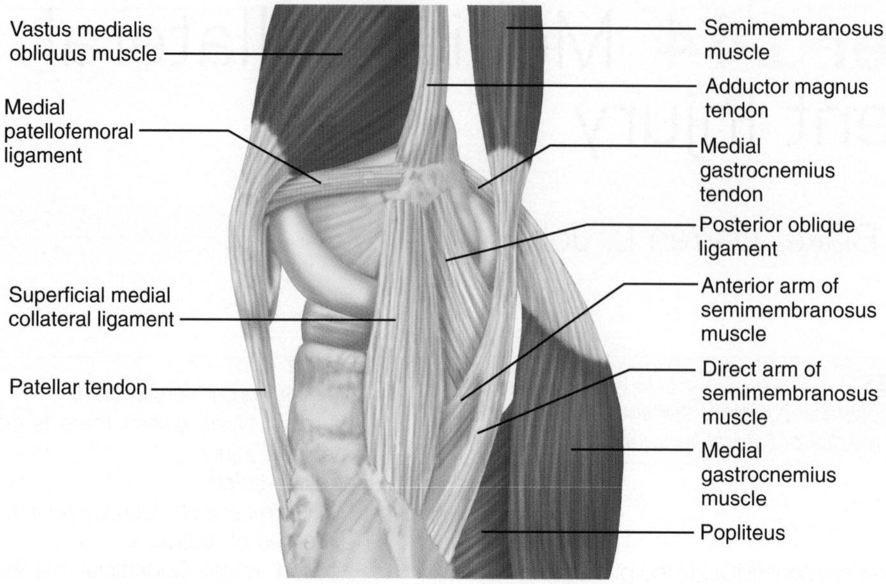
Vastus medialis obliquus muscle
Medial patellofemoral ligament
Superficial medial collateral ligament
Patellar tendon
Semimembranosus muscle
Adductor magnus tendon
Medial gastrocnemius tendon
Posterior oblique ligament
Anterior arm of semimembranosus muscle
Direct arm of semimembranosus muscle
Medial gastrocnemius muscle
Popliteus

Fig 144.1 Anatomy of the medial side of the knee. (Redrawn from LaPrade RF, Engebretsen AH, Ly TV, et al. The anatomy of the medial part of the knee. *J Bone Joint Surg Am*. 2007;89:2000–2010.)

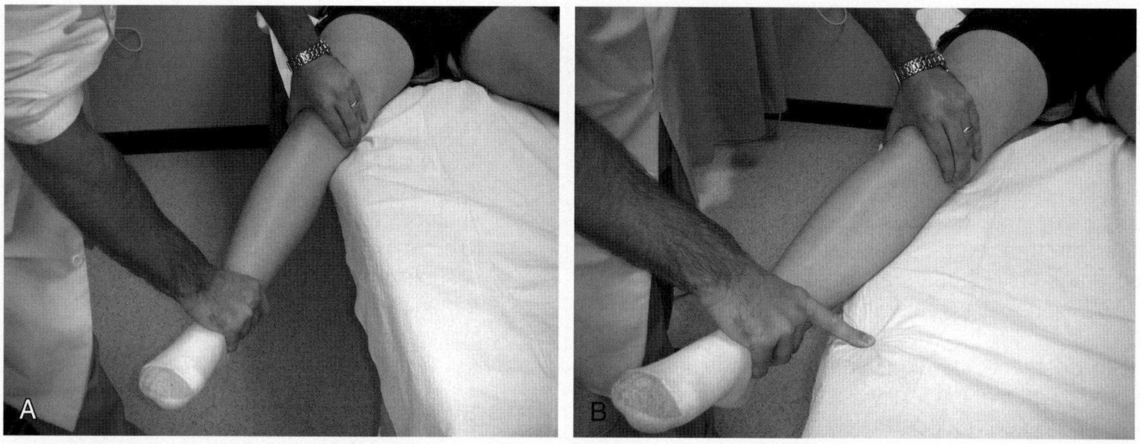
A
B

Fig 144.2 Valgus stress performed at 30 degrees of flexion (A) and full extension (B). The examiner pulls the lower leg away from midline while stabilizing the femur. By palpating the joint line, the examiner can determine the amount of laxity and ensure assessment of true laxity rather than rotation.

- Bony edema of the lateral femoral condyle and lateral tibial plateau (Fig. 144.5).
- Evaluate for concomitant ligament injury, medial meniscus tear, or meniscal root tear.

Differential Diagnosis

- Distal hamstring strain
- Medial meniscus tear
- ACL tear
- Patellar subluxation/dislocation

Treatment

- Acute
  - Ice, elevation, compressive dressing, with knee immobilization in slight flexion.
  - Weight bearing as tolerated in hinged knee brace when pain allows.
  - Begin motion and strengthening when pain subsides.
  - Return to play based on severity.
  - Grade I injuries usually require 10 days.
  - Grade II injuries usually require 20 days.
  - Grade III injuries usually require at least 4 weeks.
- Chronic
  - Bracing
  - Reconstruction
  - May need osteotomy for malalignment

When to Refer/Surgical Intervention

- Stener-like lesions.
- Incarceration of the sMCL in the joint.
- MCL with POL injury.

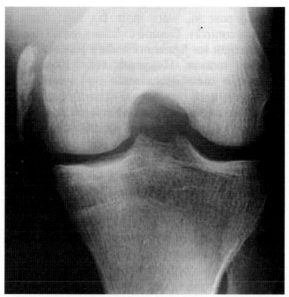

Fig 144.3 Pellegrini-Stieda lesion. Calcification of the medial collateral ligament due to traumatic injury.

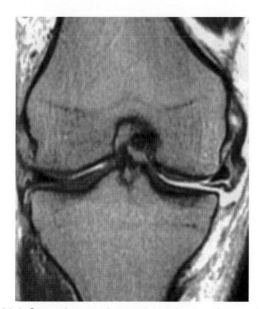

Fig 144.4 Coronal magnetic resonance image of an avulsion of the distal medial collateral ligament with entrapment in the medial joint space.

- Bony avulsions.
- Valgus knee alignment.
- Symptomatic valgus patholaxity. These usually occur from tibia-based avulsions.
- Multiligament knee injury.

Prognosis

- MCL injuries (including some grade III injuries) heal well with nonoperative treatment.
  - May have residual laxity
- Combined injuries require specialized treatment.

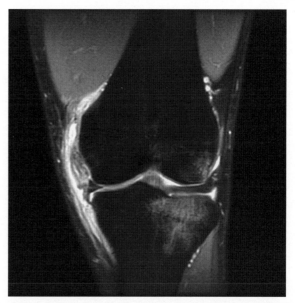

Fig 144.5 Coronal magnetic resonance image showing a tear of the medial collateral ligament with bone edema in the lateral femoral condyle and lateral tibial plateau due to a valgus impact.

Troubleshooting

- Avoid prolonged immobilization to prevent stiffness.
  - Start range-of-motion exercise in 1 week.
- An effusion indicates intra-articular pathology. Should obtain MRI.
- Multiligament injuries usually require surgery.
- Degenerative changes or valgus malalignment may complicate recovery.

Instructions for the Patient

- Wear a hinged knee brace during weight-bearing activities until physical examination reveals pain-free motion and ambulation.
- Avoid heat in the acute phase of injury.
- Use NSAIDs judicially.

Considerations in Special Populations

- Obtain stress radiographs in skeletally immature patients to rule out physeal injuries.
- Contact sport athletes may need a brace to return to sport.
- Arthritic knees will have a higher risk of stiffness.

Suggested Readings

Elliott M, Johnson DL. Management of medial-sided knee injuries. *Orthopedics.* 2015;38(3):180–184.

Geeslin AG, LaPrade RF. Outcomes of treatment of acute grade-III isolated and combined posterolateral knee injuries: a prospective case series and surgical technique. *J Bone Joint Surg Am.* 2011;93(18):1672–1683.

Laprade RF, Bernhardson AS, Griffith CJ, et al. Correlation of valgus stress radiographs with medial knee ligament injuries: an in vitro biomechanical study. *Am J Sports Med.* 2010;38(2):330–338.

LaPrade RF, Engebretsen AH, Ly TV, et al. The anatomy of the medial part of the knee. *J Bone Joint Surg Am*. 2007;89(9):2000–2010.

Marchant MH Jr, Tibor LM, Sekiya JK, et al. Management of medial-sided knee injuries, part 1: medial collateral ligament. *Am J Sports Med*. 2011;39(5):1102–1113.

Smyth MP, Koh JL. A review of surgical and nonsurgical outcomes of medial knee injuries. *Sports Med Arthrosc*. 2015;23(2):e15–e22.

Stephenson DR, Rueff D, Johnson DL. MRI and arthroscopic analysis of collateral knee ligament injuries in combined knee ligament injuries. *Orthopedics*. 2010;33(3):187–189.

Tibor LM, Marchant MH Jr, Taylor DC, et al. Management of medial-sided knee injuries, part 2: posteromedial corner. *Am J Sports Med*. 2011;39(6):1332–1340.

Chapter 145 Lateral Collateral Ligament and Posterolateral Corner Injury

Matthew D. LaPrade, Samantha L. Kallenbach, Robert F. LaPrade

ICD-10-CM CODES
S83.42 *Sprain of lateral collateral ligament of the knee*
M23.50 *Chronic lateral collateral ligament tear*

Key Concepts

- The lateral collateral ligament (LCL), or fibular collateral ligament (FCL), is the primary stabilizer against varus stress on the knee.
- The LCL originates on the lateral epicondyle of the femur and inserts on the fibular head.
- The posterolateral corner is composed of several ligaments on the outside of the knee, including the LCL, popliteofibular ligament (PFL), and popliteus tendon (Fig. 145.1); combined, these ligaments resist varus stress and external rotation of the knee.
- The posterolateral corner is a static and dynamic stabilizer of the knee and provides secondary restraint for anterior cruciate ligament (ACL) and posterior cruciate ligament (PCL) injuries.
- Isolated LCL injuries are rare; therefore it is important to look for additional injuries to other ligaments.

History

- Acute
  - Varus force, hyperextension (contact or noncontact related)
  - Patient feeling of side-to-side instability
- Chronic
  - Lateral or medial knee pain
  - Instability on near extension, cutting exercises, or stair climbing
  - Swelling following physical activity

Physical Examination

- Presentation
  - Swelling or abrasions following a medial force on the knee.
  - Lateral knee pain.
  - Deformity.
  - Varus thrust gait may be present.
- Palpation
  - Tenderness over the lateral knee or fibular head.
  - Swelling over lateral knee.

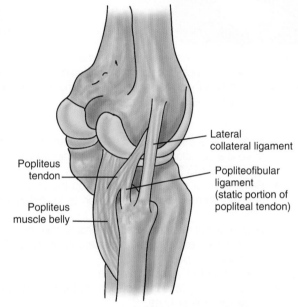

Fig 145.1 Anatomy of the posterolateral aspect of the knee. (Modified from Larson RV, Tingstad E: Lateral and posterolateral instability of the knee in adults. In: DeLee JC, Drez Jr D, Miller M, [eds]. *DeLee and Drez's Orthopaedic Sports Medicine.* 2nd ed. Philadelphia: WB Saunders; 2002:1968–1994.)

- Range of Motion
  - Swelling may limit extremes of flexion and extension.
  - Locked knee (cannot fully extend) may indicate bucket-handle meniscal tear.
- Special Tests
  - Neurovascular Examination
    - Evaluate for common peroneal nerve injury
    - Foot drop or weak dorsiflexion
    - Sensory changes on dorsal foot
    - Tinel sign at fibular neck
    - Evaluate distal pulses
  - Knee Examination (see Video 144.1)
    - LCL: Varus stress testing at 30 degrees of flexion (Fig. 145.2); if there is laxity in full extension, there is a grade III LCL injury with or without concomitant cruciate injury.
    - Popliteus tendon/popliteofibular ligament: Dial test with increased external rotation at 30 degrees of

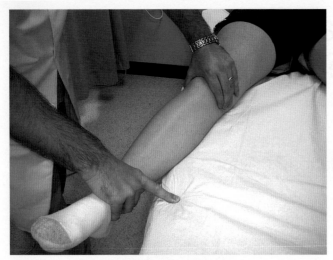

Fig 145.2 The varus stress test is performed at 30 degrees and 0 degrees of flexion. Apply force on the leg toward midline while stabilizing the femur with the other hand. By keeping one's fingers along the joint line, one can estimate laxity.

flexion; if it is also increased at 90 degrees of flexion, there is a combined posterolateral corner (PLC)/PCL injury (Fig. 145.3).
- Reverse pivot shift: Valgus stress on the knee as it is taken from 90 degrees of flexion to full extension with the foot externally rotated; this may indicate posterolateral rotatory instability. This is often positive in normal knees with genu recurvatum, so check the contralateral knee.
- Assessment of varus thrust gait.
- ACL/PCL: Increased translation on Lachman's and posterior drawer tests.

Imaging

- Radiographs: Highly Recommended
  - Anteroposterior and lateral views: Check for avulsion fracture of fibular head.
  - Posteroanterior flexion weight-bearing view: Degenerative changes, especially in the medial compartment.
  - Look for degenerative changes on patellofemoral views.
  - Bilateral varus stress views: >2.7 mm of increased gapping is seen with LCL tear, >4.0 mm of gapping is seen with a complete PLC tear (Fig. 145.4).
- Magnetic Resonance Imaging (MRI): Highly Recommended
  - Look for disruption of LCL on coronal views (Fig. 145.5).
  - Popliteus tendon/PFL is more difficult to image but is also typically seen on coronal views.
  - Look for bone bruising in the medial femoral condyle and medial tibial plateau.
  - Evaluate for concomitant injuries (ACL, PCL, meniscal tears).

Differential Diagnosis

- Lateral meniscus tear
- Multiligamentous knee injury
- Bone bruise

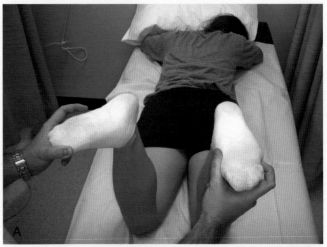

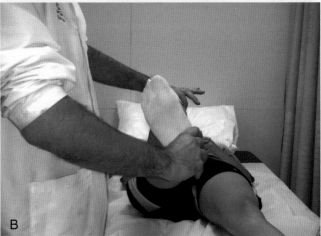

Fig 145.3 The dial test may be performed prone **(A)** or supine **(B)**. Posterolateral corner injury is indicated by increased external rotation of the affected side at 30 degrees of flexion. Combined posterolateral corner and posterior cruciate ligament injury is indicated by increased external rotation at 90 degrees of flexion.

- Knee dislocation/multiligament damage
- Medial compartment arthritis with medial compartment pseudolaxity

Treatment

- Acute
  - RICE: rest, ice, compression, elevation
  - Knee immobilization in extension or slight flexion
  - Toe touch or partial weight bearing for 2 to 4 weeks followed by progressive rehabilitation for grade I and grade II injuries
  - Surgical intervention for grade III injuries
  - Surgical reconstruction should be performed within 3 weeks of injury
- Chronic
  - Surgical reconstruction is necessary.
  - Bracing can be beneficial (medial compartment unloaders).
  - Osteotomies are necessary when varus alignment is present.

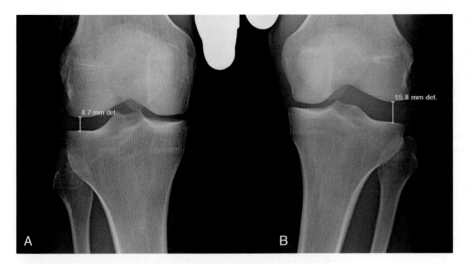

Fig 145.4 Bilateral varus stress radiographs demonstrating 7.1 mm of increased lateral compartment gapping in the left knee **(B)** compared with the right knee **(A)**, indicating a complete posterolateral corner injury.

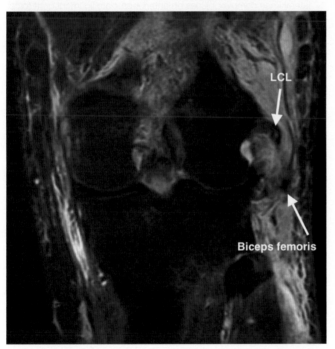

Fig 145.5 Proton density coronal knee magnetic resonance imaging in a left knee demonstrating a tear of the biceps femoris off the fibular head *(lower arrow)* and a tear of the lateral collateral ligament *(LCL) (upper arrow)* and popliteus tendon.

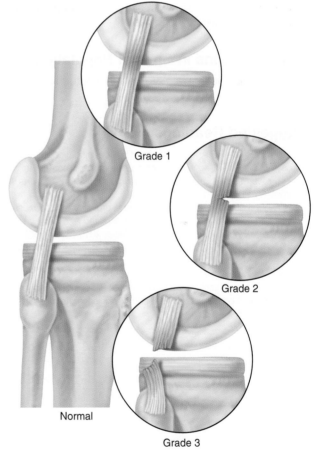

Fig 145.6 The prognoses/treatments for various lateral collateral ligament strains/tears.

When to Refer

- Grade III injuries should be referred immediately because optimal outcomes are obtained for surgery within 3 weeks. In more chronic cases, reconstructive procedures are necessary.
- Vascular injury is an emergent condition.
- Common peroneal (fibular) nerve involvement.
- Combined ligamentous injuries.
- Chronically unstable knee.
- Patients with varus alignment and chronic injuries.
- Avulsion fractures may be amenable to reduction and fixation and should be referred as soon as possible.

Prognosis

- Isolated grade I/II: often heal without surgical intervention (Fig. 145.6).
- Grade III: often require surgical reconstruction; lack of reconstruction can lead to chronic knee instability.
- Complete LCL ruptures or combined ligamentous injuries require surgical intervention; if untreated, these injuries can lead to chronic instability.

- The increase in risk of osteoarthritis after these injuries is unknown.

Troubleshooting

- The presence of degenerative changes or malalignment may complicate recovery.
- Physeal injuries in the skeletally immature patient may present similarly to ligamentous injuries.
- These injuries can become chronically disabling if not addressed appropriately.

Instructions for the Patient

- Avoid heat in the acute phase.
- Wear brace during weight-bearing activities for 2 to 4 weeks for partial tears.
- Report any giving way or instability
- Seek medical attention with signs of deep venous thrombosis or vascular compromise.

Considerations in Special Populations

- High-level athletes warrant referral to determine return to sport activities.

Suggested Readings

Arthur A, LaPrade RF, Agel J. Proximal tibial opening wedge osteotomy as the initial treatment for chronic posterolateral corner deficiency in the varus knee: a prospective clinical study. *Am J Sports Med*. 2007;35(11):1844–1850.

Geeslin AG, LaPrade RF. Location of bone bruises and other osseous injuries associated with acute grade III isolated and combined posterolateral knee injuries. *Am J Sports Med*. 2010;38(12):2502–2508.

Geeslin AG, Moulton SG, LaPrade RF. A systematic review of the outcomes of posterolateral corner knee injuries, part 1: surgical treatment of acute injuries. *Am J Sports Med*. 2016;44(5):1336–1342.

LaPrade RF. Arthroscopic evaluation of the lateral compartment of knees with grade 3 posterolateral knee complex injuries. *Am J Sports Med*. 1997;25(5):596–602.

LaPrade RF, Gilbert TJ, Bollom TS, et al. The magnetic resonance imaging appearance of individual structures of the posterolateral knee. A prospective study of normal knees and knees with surgically verified grade III injuries. *Am J Sports Med*. 2000;28(2):191–199.

LaPrade RF, Heikes C, Bakker AJ, Jakobsen RB. The reproducibility and repeatability of varus stress radiographs in the assessment of isolated FCL and grade-III posterolateral knee injuries. An in vitro biomechanical study. *J Bone Joint Surg Am*. 2008;90(10):2069–2076.

LaPrade RF, Johansen S, Agel J, et al. Outcomes of an anatomic posterolateral knee reconstruction. *J Bone Joint Surg Am*. 2010;92(1):16–22.

LaPrade RF, Johansen S, Wentorf FA, et al. An analysis of an anatomical posterolateral knee reconstruction: an in vitro biomechanical study and development of a surgical technique. *Am J Sports Med*. 2004;32(6):1405–1414.

LaPrade RF, Muench C, Wentorf F, Lewis JL. The effect of injury to the posterolateral structures of the knee on force in a posterior cruciate ligament graft: a biomechanical study. *Am J Sports Med*. 2002;30(2):233–238.

LaPrade RF, Resig S, Wentorf F, Lewis JL. The effects of grade III posterolateral knee complex injuries on anterior cruciate ligament graft force. A biomechanical analysis. *Am J Sports Med*. 1999;27(4):469–475.

LaPrade RF, Spiridonov SI, Coobs BR, et al. Fibular collateral ligament anatomical reconstructions: a prospective outcomes study. *Am J Sports Med*. 2010;38(10):2005–2011.

LaPrade RF, Terry GC. Injuries to the posterolateral aspect of the knee: association of anatomic injury patterns with clinical instability. *Am J Sports Med*. 1997;25:433–438.

LaPrade RF, Wentorf F. Acute knee injuries: on-the-field and sideline evaluation. *Phys Sportsmed*. 1999;27(10):55–61.

LaPrade RF, Wentorf F. Diagnosis and treatment of posterolateral knee injuries. *Clin Orthop Relat Res*. 2002;402:110–121.

Long JL, Miller BS. Lateral collateral ligament and posterolateral corner injury. In: Miller MD, Hart JA, MacKnight JM, eds. *Essential Orthopaedics*, 1st ed. Philadelphia: Elsevier; 2009:624–627.

Moulton SG, Geeslin AG, LaPrade RF. A systematic review of the outcomes of posterolateral corner knee injuries, part 2: surgical treatment of chronic injuries. *Am J Sports Med*. 2016;44(6):1616–1623.

Moulton SG, Matheny LM, James EW, LaPrade RF. Outcomes following anatomic fibular (lateral) collateral ligament reconstruction. *Knee Surg Sports Traumatol Arthrosc*. 2015;23(10):2960–2966.

Terry GC, LaPrade RF. The posterolateral aspect of the knee. Anatomy and surgical approach. *Am J Sports Med*. 1996;24(6):732–739.

Chapter 146 Knee Dislocation

Gregory C. Fanelli, Matthew G. Fanelli, David G. Fanelli

ICD-10-CM CODE
S83.106A *Knee dislocation*

Key Concepts

- Multisystem injury complex
  - Ligaments
  - Vessels (arteries, veins)
  - Skin
  - Nerves (peroneal nerve, tibial nerve)
  - Bones (fractures: tibia, femur, patella, pelvis, spine)
  - Head injury (heterotopic ossification, spasticity)
  - Other organ system trauma
- Vascular injury
  - Knee dislocation—same incidence as bicruciate knee ligament injury.
  - Hyperextension mechanism results in popliteal artery rupture.
  - Flexed knee posterior tibial displacement ("dashboard knee") results in popliteal artery intimal tear.
- Classification
  - Direction of displacement of the tibia relative to the femur (anterior, posterior, medial, lateral)
  - Number of ligaments involved
  - Energy level of the injury mechanism
    - High (motor vehicle accident)
    - Low (sports)
    - Ultra low (stepping off a curb)
      - Morbidly obese
      - High incidence of neurovascular injury
- Extensor mechanism may be involved
  - Patellar tendon or quadriceps tendon disruption

History

- Mechanism
  - Energy level (high, low, ultra low)
- Visible dislocation
- Spontaneous reduction
- Time from injury
  - Acute
  - Chronic
- Loss of sensation
  - Muscle function

Physical Examination

- Observation
  - Deformity
  - Skin condition (bruising, abrasions, dimple sign)
  - Effusion
  - Tense compartments

- Vascular evaluation
  - Symmetric pulses.
  - Ankle-brachial index (ABI).
  - Asymmetric pulses and/or ABI less than 0.9 indicate the need for arteriogram, magnetic resonance (MR) angiography, or computed tomography (CT) angiography.
  - Beware popliteal artery intimal tear.
  - Deep venous thrombosis (DVT).
    - Acute: posttraumatic
    - Chronic
    - May or may not have calf pain
    - High index of suspicion
      - Screening venous Doppler examination
- Nerve injury
  - Peroneal nerve injury more common than tibial nerve injury.
  - Sensation.
  - Motor function.
  - Test both peroneal nerve and tibial nerve.
- Instability pattern
  - Intra-articular fractures
  - Extra-articular fractures
  - Anterior, posterior, axial rotation
  - Anterior translation of the tibia relative to the femur
    - Anterior cruciate ligament (ACL)
      - Lachman test
      - Anterior drawer test
      - Pivot shift test
  - Posterior translation of the tibia relative to the femur
    - Posterior cruciate ligament (PCL)
      - Posterior drawer
  - Medial side
    - Valgus laxity (medial collateral ligament [MCL])
    - Valgus laxity plus axial rotation (MCL and postero-medial corner [PMC])
    - External rotation asymmetry test
      - Medial tibial plateau rotates either anterior, posterior, or both
  - Lateral side
    - Varus laxity (lateral collateral ligament [LCL])
    - Varus laxity plus axial rotation (LCL plus posterolateral corner-PLC)
    - External rotation asymmetry test
      - Lateral tibial plateau rotates anteriorly, posteriorly, or both.

Imaging

- Radiographs
  - Prereduction: anteroposterior and lateral (Fig. 146.1)
  - Postreduction: anteroposterior, lateral, 30-degree anteroposterior patellar axial, intercondylar notch view

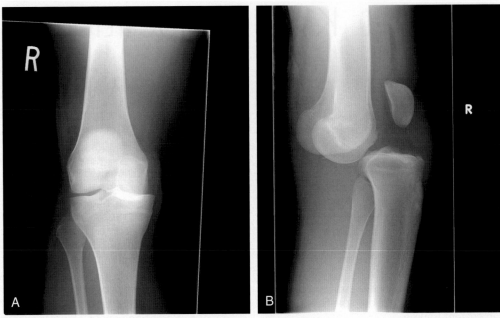

Fig 146.1 Anteroposterior **(A)** and lateral **(B)** view of a tibiofemoral knee dislocation.

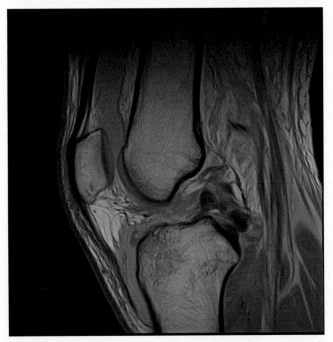

Fig 146.2 Magnetic resonance image combined posterior collateral ligament and anterior collateral ligament tears in a knee dislocation.

- Look for:
  - Proximal tibia and distal femur fractures
  - Avulsion fractures (cruciates, capsule)
  - Fibular head fractures
  - Osteochondral fractures
- Magnetic resonance imaging (MRI)
  - Preoperative planning
    - Arterial repair/reconstruction location
      - May need magnetic resonance arteriogram (MRA)
  - Identification of injury pattern (Figs. 146.2 to 146.4)

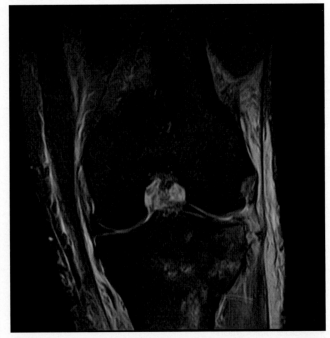

Fig 146.3 Magnetic resonance image of a lateral posterolateral corner injury in a knee dislocation.

- Ligaments
- Extensor mechanism
- Articular surface

Differential Diagnosis

- Isolated ACL injury
- Isolated PCL injury
- Isolated collateral ligament injury
- Distal femur or proximal tibia fracture

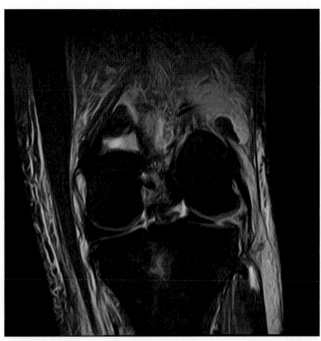

Fig 146.4 Magnetic resonance image of a medial posteromedial corner injury in a knee dislocation.

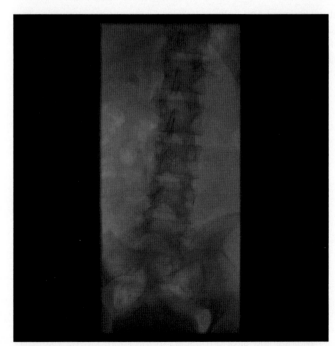

Fig 146.5 Placement of an inferior vena cava filter for post-traumatic deep venous thrombosis after a knee dislocation.

- Patellar dislocation
- "Minor knee sprain"

Treatment

- Acute knee dislocations (multiple ligament knee injuries)
  - Immediate reduction
  - Vascular and neurologic examination (Fig. 146.5)
  - Stabilization in splint or immobilizer

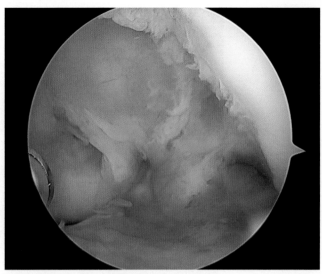

Fig 146.6 Arthroscopic intercondylar notch view showing combined posterior collateral ligament and anterior collateral ligament tears in a knee dislocation.

- Transfer to emergency department setting
- X-rays to assess reduction
- Vascular examination
  - Abnormal (asymmetric to the uninvolved extremity) or ABI less than 0.9 indicates the need for an arteriogram, computed tomography (CT) or MR angiography to evaluate for popliteal artery disruption or popliteal artery intimal flap tear.
- Current surgical treatment techniques can provide excellent functional outcomes.
- Surgical timing is dependent on injury severity and other associated injuries (blood vessels, skin, nerves, fractures, head injury, other organ system trauma).
- External fixation is utilized when it is not possible to maintain reduction with bracing, to protect an arterial repair, to observe compartment pressures, and to treat skin wounds.
- Chronic knee dislocations (multiple ligament knee injuries)
  - Patients present with functional instability during activity.
  - Critically important to make the correct diagnosis
    - Anteroposterior translation (PCL, ACL)
    - Varus-valgus laxity (LCL, MCL)
    - Axial rotation laxity (PMC, PLC)
  - Lower extremity alignment
    - Malunion of fractures
    - Abnormal gait pattern
  - Treatment plan
    - Correct malalignment if necessary.
      - High tibial osteotomy
      - Distal femoral osteotomy
    - Surgical ligament reconstruction
      - Address all planes of instability (Figs. 146.6 and 146.7).

When to Refer

- All patients with acute knee dislocations or bicruciate knee injuries should be sent to an emergency department for vascular evaluation and an orthopaedic surgeon notified.

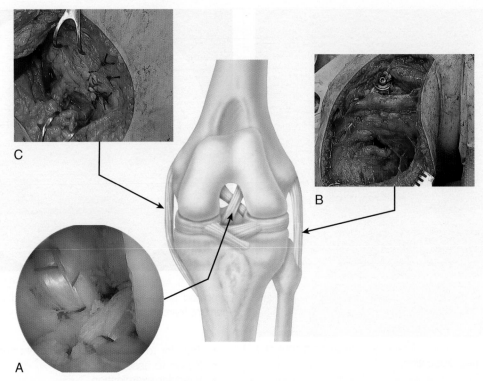

Fig 146.7 (A) Arthroscopic view showing combined posterior collateral ligament and anterior collateral ligament reconstruction in a knee dislocation. **(B)** Posterolateral reconstruction in a knee dislocation using the fibular head–based figure-of-eight surgical technique with semitendinosus allograft combined with a posterolateral shift. Peroneal nerve decompression is routinely performed to protect the nerve during the surgical procedure. **(C)** Posteromedial reconstruction using the posteromedial capsular shift procedure in a knee dislocation.

- Arterial injuries require emergent vascular surgery.
- Patients with vascular intact and stabilized acute and chronic multiple ligamentous knee injuries should be referred to an orthopaedic surgeon for surgical treatment as indicated.
- Nerve injuries may be treated by nerve repair, nerve grafting, nerve transfer, or tendon transfer.

Prognosis

- Knee dislocations are serious knee injuries.
- Surgical treatment can restore functional stability and return to preinjury Tegner level of function in 60% of cases, and 93% at the same or one Tegner grade lower level of activity in certain series; however, these will not be normal knees even with the restoration of functional stability.
- Posttraumatic degenerative arthrosis has been reported in 23-30% of cases.
- Good functional results have been reported in patients 18 years of age and younger with treatment of multiple-ligament-injured (dislocated) knees.

Troubleshooting

- Knee dislocations are potentially limb-threatening injuries.
- Bicruciate knee ligament injuries have the same risk of arterial injury as frank tibiofemoral knee dislocations.

- A knee injury with three or more knee ligaments injured should raise suspicion for a knee dislocation with possible arterial and venous injury.

Instructions for the Patient

- Surgical treatment will most likely improve knee stability but will not return the knee to normal.
- Posttraumatic arthrosis may occur.
- Residual ligament laxity may occur.
- Nerve injuries may leave residual deficits.
- Compliance with preoperative and postoperative rehabilitation instructions will improve the chances of a successful outcome.
- Maintaining strong muscles in the injured lower extremity will improve the chances of better function.

Considerations in Special Populations

- Head injury patients may develop heterotopic ossification.
- Lower extremity spasticity in head injury patients may cause redislocation.
  - Indication for external fixation
- Results are less predictable in obese patients.
- Surgical treatment of knee dislocations and multiple-ligament knee injuries in patients with open growth plates must respect the physis to avoid growth disturbances.

Suggested Readings

Edson CJ, Fanelli GC, Beck JD. Rehabilitation after multiple ligament reconstruction of the knee. *Sports Med Arthrosc Rev*. 2011;19(2):162–166.

Fanelli GC, ed. *The Multiple Ligament Injured Knee. A Practical Guide to Management*. 2nd ed. New York: Springer-Verlag; 2013.

Fanelli GC, ed. *Posterior Cruciate Ligament Injuries: A Practical Guide to Management*. 2nd ed. New York: Springer; 2015.

Fanelli GC, Beck JD, Edson CJ. How I treat the multiple-ligament injured knee. *Oper Tech Sports Med*. 2010;18(4):198–210.

Fanelli GC, Beck JD, Edson CJ. Combined PCL ACL lateral and medial side injuries: treatment and results. *Sports Med Arthrosc Rev*. 2011;19(2):120–130.

Fanelli GC, Edson CJ. Surgical treatment of combined PCL, ACL, medial, and lateral side injuries (global laxity): surgical technique and 2 to 18 year results. *J Knee Surg*. 2012;25(4):307–316.

Fanelli GC, Edson CJ, Orcutt DR, et al. Treatment of combined ACL-PCL-MCL-PLC injuries of the knee. *J Knee Surg*. 2005;18(3):240–248.

Fanelli GC, Edson CJ, Reinheimer KN. Evaluation and treatment of the multiple ligament injured knee. *Instr Course Lect*. 2009;58:389–395.

Fanelli GC, Fanelli DG. Knee dislocations in patients 18 years of age and younger. Surgical technique and outcomes. *J Knee Surg*. 2016;29(4):269–277.

Fanelli GC, Levy B, Whalen D, et al. Mangement of complex knee ligament injuries. *Instr Course Lect*. 2011;60:523–535.

Fanelli GC, Orcutt DR, Edson CJ. Current concepts: the multiple ligament injured knee. *Arthroscopy*. 2005;21(4):471–486.

Fanelli GC, Sousa P, Edson CJ. Long term follow-up of surgically treated knee dislocations: stability restored, but arthritis is common. *Clin Orthop Relat Res*. 2014;472(9):2712–2717.

Fanelli GC, Stannard JP, Stuart MJ, et al. Management of complex knee ligament injuries. *J Bone Joint Surg*. 2010;92-A(12):2235–2246.

Levy B, Dajani KA, Whalen DB, et al. Decision making in the multiple ligament injured knee: an evidence based systematic review. *Arthroscopy*. 2009;25(4):430–438.

Levy B, Fanelli GC, Whalen D, et al. Modern perspectives for the treatment of knee dislocations and multiligament reconstruction. *J Am Acad Orthop Surg*. 2009;17(4):197–206.

Malone JW, Verde F, Weiss D, Fanelli GC. MR imaging of knee instability. *Magn Reson Imaging Clin N Am*. 2009;17(4):697–724.

Peskun CJ, Levy BA, Fanelli GC, et al. Diagnosis and management of knee dislocations. *Phys Sportsmed*. 2010;38(4):101–111.

Chapter 147 Synovitis

Lisa A. Sienkiewicz, Eric J. Gardner, Geoffrey S. Baer

ICD-10-CM CODES
SYNOVITIS
M65.9   *Synovitis and tenosynovitis, unspecified*
M65.861   *Other synovitis and tenosynovitis, right lower leg*
M65.862   *Other synovitis and tenosynovitis, left lower leg*
PROLIFERATIVE (PIGMENTED) VILLONODULAR SYNOVITIS
M12.261   *Villonodular synovitis (pigmented), right knee*
M12.262   *Villonodular synovitis (pigmented), left knee*
M12.269   *Villonodular synovitis (pigmented), unspecified knee*
PLICA
M67.51   *Plica syndrome, right knee*
M67.52   *Plica syndrome, left knee*

CPT CODES
29875   *Arthroscopy, knee, surgical; synovectomy, limited (e.g., plica or shelf resection)*
29876   *Arthroscopy, knee, surgical: synovectomy, major, two or more compartments*

Key Concepts

- Synovitis is inflammation of the synovial membrane or synovium.
- Nonspecific proliferative lesion
- Synovium lines the cavities of all synovial joints.
  - Composed of fibrous and vascular connective tissue
  - Produces synovial fluid that is a combination of fluid produced by the synovium and an ultrafiltrate of blood plasma
- Synovial fluid lubricates the joint and provides nutrients for the articular cartilage.
- Contains hyaluronic acid, proteinase, lubricin (glycoprotein and key lubricating component), prostaglandins, and collagenases
- Void of red blood cells, hemoglobin, and clotting factors

History

- Isolated to a single joint or involving multiple joints
- Acute injury
  - Jarring or twisting of joint
  - Pain and swelling
  - Knee ligaments stable
- Chronic injury (degenerative changes)
- Knee pain with or without swelling; worse with activity and at night

Physical Examination

- Observation
  - Effusion (intra-articular swelling)
  - Erythema (increased blood flow)
  - Quadriceps atrophy
  - Antalgic gait
- Palpation
  - Effusion/patellar ballottement (intra-articular swelling)
  - Nonspecific soft-tissue tenderness
  - Warmth (increased blood flow)
- Range of motion
  - Often decreased
    - Painful due to inflamed synovium, distended joint
    - Effusion may prevent full range of motion.
    - Chronic underlying articular involvement may restrict range of motion due to degenerative changes (i.e., rheumatoid arthritis, osteoarthritis).
- Special tests
  - Crepitus with range of motion: degenerative changes
  - Joint line tenderness: meniscal tears or degenerative changes
  - McMurray test: meniscal tears
  - Lachman test, anterior/posterior drawer test, pivot shift test, reverse pivot shift test, dial test, varus/valgus stress test: ligamentous instability; may be associated with the synovitic process

Imaging

- Radiographs: bilateral weight bearing posteroanterior, 45 degrees of flexion posteroanterior (Rosenberg view), lateral, and 20 degrees of flexion patellofemoral view (Laurin view).
  - Typically normal but may show soft-tissue swelling and effusion
- Magnetic resonance imaging
  - If clinical and laboratory studies are inconclusive for septic arthritis, magnetic resonance imaging can be used as a confirmatory test.
  - Pigmented villonodular synovitis can often be diagnosed based on the magnetic resonance imaging appearance (Fig. 147.1).
  - Allows better characterization of soft tissues and/or evaluation of soft-tissue mass (Fig. 147.2)
- Bone scan
  - May identify other areas of involvement

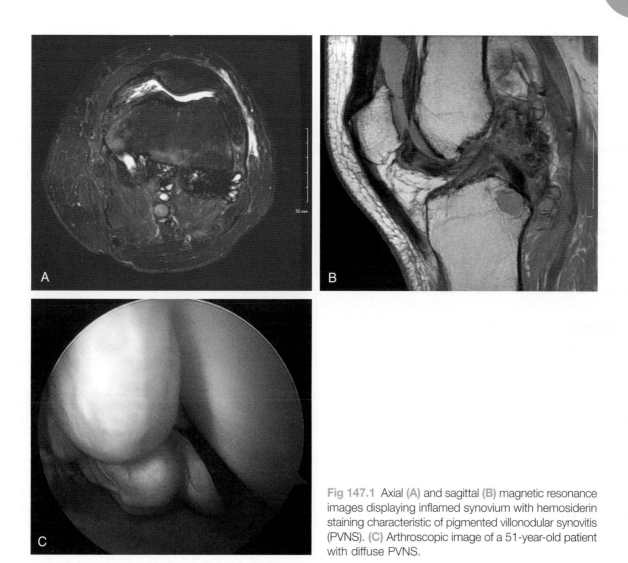

Fig 147.1 Axial **(A)** and sagittal **(B)** magnetic resonance images displaying inflamed synovium with hemosiderin staining characteristic of pigmented villonodular synovitis (PVNS). **(C)** Arthroscopic image of a 51-year-old patient with diffuse PVNS.

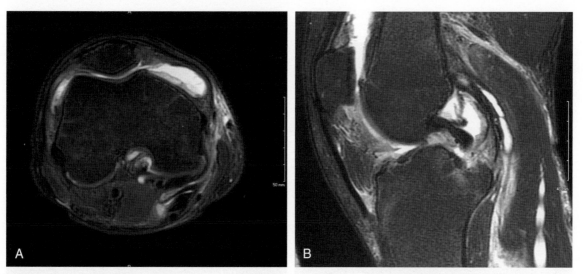

Fig 147.2 Axial **(A)** and sagittal **(B)** magnetic resonance images showing synovitis associated with gout in a 46-year-old patient.

Additional Tests

- Blood tests: complete blood count, erythrocyte sedimentation rate, C-reactive protein, serologic tests (i.e., rheumatoid factor)
- Aspiration: cell count, crystals, culture, and sensitivities

Differential Diagnosis

- Inflammatory arthritides: rheumatoid arthritis, juvenile rheumatoid arthritis, systemic lupus erythematosus, psoriatic arthritis, gout, pseudogout
- Infectious arthritides: septic arthritis, tuberculous arthritis, fungal arthritis, Lyme disease
- Noninflammatory arthritides: osteoarthritis, neuropathic joint
- Hemorrhagic arthritides: hemophilic arthropathy, sickle cell joint destruction, pigmented villonodular synovitis
- Others: toxic/transient synovitis, traumatic synovitis

Treatment

- At diagnosis
  - Rest, ice, compression, and elevation help to decrease swelling and pain; acetaminophen and nonsteroidal antiinflammatory drugs for pain control
- Later
  - Depending on the underlying cause of the synovitis, intra-articular corticosteroid, hyaluronic injections, or synovectomy may help to treat symptoms. Most inflammatory and noninflammatory arthritides can be treated conservatively.

When to Refer

- Soft-tissue infections can be diagnosed and treated without surgical consultation. When intra-articular infection is determined to be present, urgent surgical evaluation is required. Some causes of synovitis, such as gout and hemophilic arthropathy, are amenable to synovectomy after exhaustion of conservative means (Figs. 147.3 and 147.4).
- Recurrence of synovitis after synovectomy is common.
- Patients with degenerative joint changes predisposing them to joint pain that interferes with quality of life can be sent for evaluation for total knee arthroplasty.
- Patients with pigmented villonodular synovitis should be seen for potential open versus arthroscopic synovectomy.
- Otherwise, most other patients can be treated effectively with conservative measures by primary care physicians, rheumatologists, or infectious disease doctors.

Prognosis

- The prognosis depends on the underlying etiology. Most causes of synovitis have excellent prognoses when the underlying cause is treated. The prognosis of joint infections depends on timely surgical evaluation, irrigation and débridement, and appropriate antibiotic therapy.

Troubleshooting

- Aspiration should be performed in patients when there is concern for a septic joint.
  - The presence of purulent fluid, a positive Gram stain or cultures, or an elevated cell count suggestive of a septic joint are orthopaedic emergencies and demand immediate referral.

Patient Instructions

- The patient should be counseled on the risks and benefits of surgery to treat the underlying cause of synovitis.
  - Benefits: Treating the underlying cause of synovitis will lead to return of a nonswollen, painless knee.
  - Risks: Surgical management with arthroscopy or total knee arthroplasty risks bleeding, infection, nerve damage, and, of course, incomplete resolution of symptoms. Total

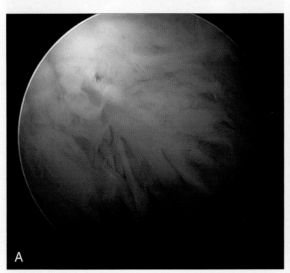 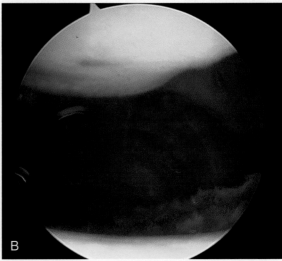

Fig 147.3 Arthroscopic images before **(A)** and after **(B)** resection of synovitis associated with gout that did not respond to conservative management.

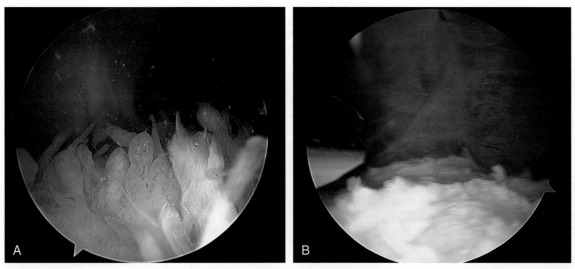

Fig 147.4 Arthroscopic images before **(A)** and after **(B)** resection of synovitis associated with advanced degenerative joint disease in a patient not interested in pursuing joint replacement.

knee arthroplasty adds the risks of prosthetic failure, deep venous thrombosis, pulmonary embolus, risks of anesthesia, and even death.

Considerations in Special Populations

- Young, highly active patients are not good candidates for total knee arthroplasty due to increased prosthetic wear and consequently early prosthetic failure.

Suggested Readings

Carl HD, Klug S, Seitz J, et al. Site-specific intraoperative efficacy of arthroscopic knee joint synovectomy in rheumatoid arthritis. *Arthroscopy*. 2005;21:1209–1218.

Comin JA, Rodriguez-Merchan EC. Arthroscopic synovectomy in the management of painful localized post-traumatic synovitis of the knee joint. *Arthroscopy*. 1997;13:606–608.

De Ponti A, Sansone V. Malchere m: results of arthroscopic treatment of pigmented villonodular synovitis of the knee. *Arthroscopy*. 2003;19:602–607.

Dines JS, DeBerardino TM, Wells JS, et al. Long-term follow-up of surgically treated localized pigmented villonodular synovitis of the knee. *Arthroscopy*. 2007;23:930–937.

Fiacco U, Cozzi L, Rigon C, et al. Arthroscopic synovectomy in rheumatoid and psoriatic knee joint synovitis: Long-term outcome. *Br J Rheumatol*. 1996;35:463–470.

Frick MA, Wenger DE, Adkins M. MR imaging of synovial disorders of the knee: an update. *Radiol Clin North Am*. 2007;45:1017–1031.

Gilbert MS, Radomisli TE. Therapeutic options in the management of hemophilic synovitis. *Clin Orthop Relat Res*. 1997;343:88–92.

Klug S, Wittmann G, Weseloh G. Arthroscopic synovectomy of the knee joint in early cases of rheumatoid arthritis: Follow-up results of a multicenter study. *Arthroscopy*. 2000;16:262–267.

Li TJ, Lue KH, Lin ZI, et al. Arthroscopic treatment for gouty tophi mimicking an intra-articular synovial tumor of the knee. *Arthroscopy*. 2006;22:910, e1–e3.

Wiedel JD. Arthroscopic synovectomy of the knee in hemophilia: 10 to 15 year follow-up. *Clin Orthop Relat Res*. 1996;328:46–53.

Chapter 148 Meniscus Tears

S. Evan Carstensen, Mark D. Miller

ICD-10-CM CODES

S83.2	Tear of meniscus, current injury
S83.21	Bucket-handle tear of medial meniscus
S83.22	Peripheral tear of medial meniscus
S83.23	Complex tear of medial meniscus
S83.24	Other tear of medial meniscus
S83.25	Bucket-handle tear of lateral meniscus
S83.26	Peripheral tear of lateral meniscus
S83.27	Complex tear of lateral meniscus
S83.28	Other tear of lateral meniscus

Key Concepts

- Medial meniscus (C-shaped) and lateral meniscus (circular) consist mainly of fibrocartilage, attached to the joint capsule at the periphery; the anterior and posterior horns of each meniscus have ligamentous anchors to the tibial plateau
- Limited vascular supply and healing potential: outer third (red-red zone) is vascular, inner third (white-white zone) is avascular, middle third (red-white zone) is intermediate
- Critical for normal knee function: load sharing, shock absorption, stability, and proprioception
  - Transmit 50-70% of load with knee extension and 85-90% with knee flexion.
  - The medial meniscus is a secondary stabilizer to anterior tibial translation, making it critical for stability in an anterior cruciate ligament (ACL)-deficient knee.
  - Lateral meniscus provides less stabilization but has twice the excursion compared with the medial meniscus.
- Removing the entire meniscus causes the overall knee contact area to decrease, resulting in increased contact stress, degenerative joint disease, and pain.
  - Lateral meniscectomy leads to joint degeneration much more rapidly than medial meniscectomy given the convex-convex design of the lateral femoral condyle and lateral tibial plateau
- Meniscus tears can occur as an acute injury or as a result of degenerative joint disease.
- The most common location for a meniscal tear with an acute ACL tear is the lateral meniscus, whereas knees with chronic ACL deficiency often result in medial meniscus injury.
  - Menisci assume role of primary stabilization in setting of ACL tears.
- Medial and lateral menisci supplied by the medial interior and lateral inferior geniculate arteries, respectively

History
Acute Injury

- Twisting or hyperflexion mechanism
- Acute pain with or without swelling
- Pain recurs with deep knee bending or twisting.
- Locking or catching (mechanical symptoms) may be present.
- Associated injuries include ACL tears and collateral ligament sprains.
- Audible pop may be heard at the time of injury

Chronic (Degenerative) Injury

- Older patients, associated with degenerative osteoarthritis
- Atraumatic mechanism, like walking on uneven ground or bending at the knees
- Chronic mild joint swelling, stiffness, joint line pain
- Mechanical symptoms may be present.
- Insidious onset of knee pain often noted

Physical Examination
Observation

- Effusion (intra-articular swelling)
- Quadriceps atrophy in subacute or chronic tears
- Antalgic gait

Palpation

- Medial and lateral joint line tenderness: most sensitive examination finding (74%)
  - Assess with knee flexed to 90 degrees.
  - Assess medial and lateral, anterior and posterior.
- Patellar ballottement (effusion); may see increased patellar excursion medially and laterally due to effusion presence

Range of Motion

- Displaced bucket-handle tears may cause a block to full extension, a locked knee (Fig. 148.1).
- Effusions may cause loss of flexion.

Special Tests

- McMurray test: flex and internally and externally rotate the knee; positive if there is a palpable "clunk" at the joint line as the torn meniscus displaces (Video 148.1)
  - Most specific (rule in) for meniscal tear (98%) but only 15% sensitive
  - Pain with McMurray test without palpable clunk is more sensitive and more likely to be elicited but less specific.
- Squat test: posterior knee pain with squatting or inability to squat (anterior knee pain may reflect patellofemoral joint pathology including a chondral defect of the patella trochlea)

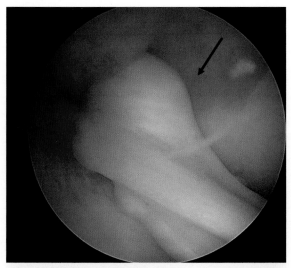

Fig 148.1 Displaced bucket handle tear *(arrow)* of the medial meniscus causing a mechanical block to full extension (locked knee).

- Patellar apprehension test to rule out patellar instability
- Lachman, anterior/posterior drawer, pivot shift, and varus/valgus stress tests to rule out associated ligamentous injuries

Imaging
Radiography

- Bilateral weight-bearing anteroposterior, lateral, 45 degrees of flexion posteroanterior (PA; Rosenberg view), and 20 degrees of flexion in patellofemoral view (Laurin view)
  - To rule out osteoarthritis, osteochondral fracture, osseous loose bodies, osteonecrosis of the femoral condyle, osteochondritis dissecans, plateau fracture, tibial eminence fracture, Segond fracture (ACL tear)
  - PA flexion weight-bearing view especially useful to look for osteoarthritis
    - Will reveal joint space narrowing
  - Laurin (Sunrise) view to look for patellofemoral arthritis

Magnetic Resonance Imaging

- Sensitive and specific, accuracy approximately 95%
- Meniscal tear pattern and displacement can often be determined by magnetic resonance imaging (MRI) (Figs. 148.2–148.4).
  - Vertical tears or displaced bucket handle tears require special attention because these often can be repaired (Fig. 148.5).
- Multiple types of tears may be appreciated on MRI (Fig. 148.6).

Differential Diagnosis

- Osteoarthritis: chronic stiffness, aching, joint space narrowed on radiographs
- Loose body: catching, mobile pain, osseous fragments on radiographs, cartilaginous fragments on MRI
- Patellar subluxation or dislocation: patellar apprehension test, pain at medial patella, patellar instability with freely mobile patella

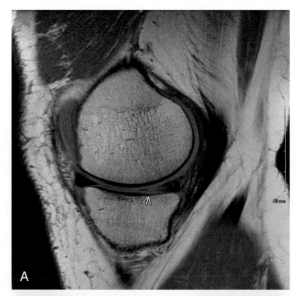

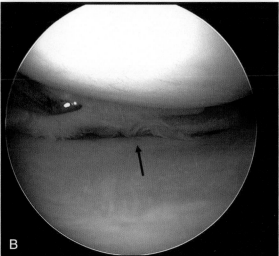

Fig 148.2 Complex tear of the medial meniscus *(arrows)*. **(A)** Sagittal magnetic resonance imaging. **(B)** Arthroscopic view.

- Osteochondritis dissecans: younger patient (often <18 years old), pain to palpation of condyle, seen on radiographs or MRI
- Articular cartilage lesions: often associated with meniscal or cruciate injuries, seen on MRI
- Tibial plateau fracture: higher-energy injury directly associated with trauma, seen on radiographs or computed tomography scans
- ACL tear: positive Lachman and anterior drawer tests, acute (within 8 hours) hemarthrosis, seen on MRI
- Collateral ligament sprain or tear: pain or instability to varus stress (lateral collateral ligament) or valgus stress (medial collateral ligament), medial or lateral joint space widening
- Pes anserine bursitis: pain on medial tibia distal to the joint line
- Fat pad impingement syndrome: positive Hoffa test (with knee in flexion, place pressure with thumbs along each side of patellar tendon; pain with knee extension indicates inflammation of the fat pad)

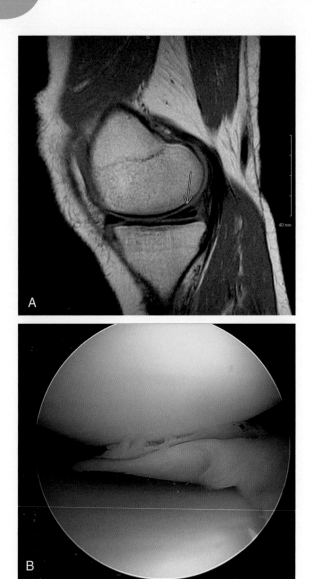

Fig 148.3 Oblique tear of the medial meniscus *(arrow)*. **(A)** Sagittal magnetic resonance imaging. **(B)** Arthroscopic view of displaced fragment.

- Symptomatic plica: painful snapping band across medial femoral condyle

Treatment
At Diagnosis
- Determining the type of tear is important as a myriad of tear types may be present (see Fig. 148.6).
- Young patients with acute meniscal tears and all patients with a locked knee should be referred to an orthopaedic surgeon. Otherwise, initial treatment is symptomatic.
- Rest, ice, compression, and elevation are helpful to decrease swelling and pain.
- Acetaminophen and/or nonsteroidal antiinflammatory drugs (NSAIDs) are useful for pain control.
- Physical therapy focused on restoring range of motion and reducing pain, while maintaining or improving muscle strength around the knee, is beneficial.

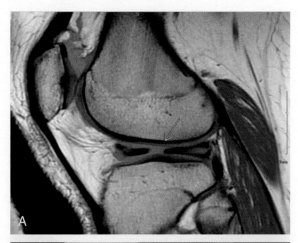

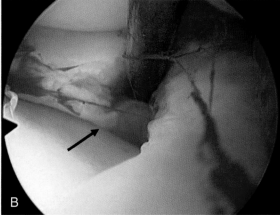

Fig 148.4 Radial tear of the lateral meniscus *(arrows)*. **(A)** Sagittal magnetic resonance imaging. **(B)** Arthroscopic view

Later
- Patients with degenerative meniscal tears may require arthroscopic surgery for débridement (partial meniscectomy) if symptoms are not responsive to conservative treatment.

When to Refer
- It is appropriate to refer patients with clinical and MRI evidence of a meniscus tear, particularly those who have pain, swelling, and feelings of apprehension that significantly limit their lives after a diligent trial of conservative treatment.
- The threshold for referral should be lower for acute tears, younger patients, and those with more active lifestyles as they may benefit from surgical intervention.
- Patients with vertical tears in the vascular zone of the meniscus should be referred early for meniscal repair (see Fig. 148.5C and D). Note that many asymptomatic tears are picked up on MRI, especially in older individuals with arthritis. MRI findings should be correlated with the history and examination before referral.

Prognosis
- The prognosis of partial meniscectomy is excellent when no concomitant cartilage damage is present.

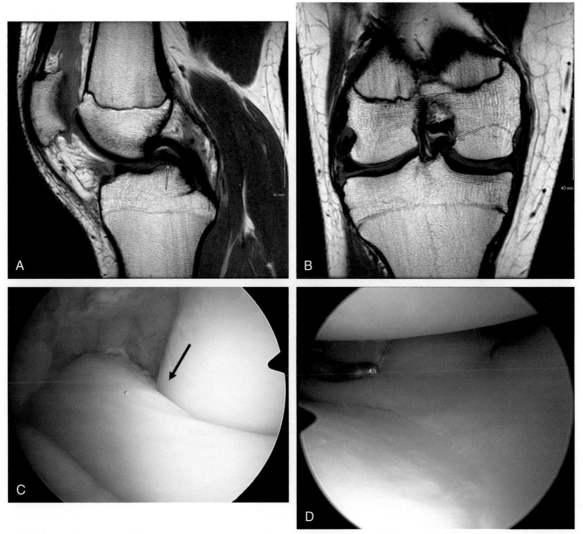

Fig 148.5 Displaced bucket handle tear of the medial meniscus. **(A)** Sagittal magnetic resonance imaging (MRI). Note double posterior cruciate ligament sign *(arrow)*. **(B)** Coronal MRI. Note meniscus displaced into the notch *(arrow)*. **(C)** Arthroscopic view of displaced meniscus draped over medial femoral condyle *(arrow)*. **(D)** Arthroscopic view of meniscus after reduction and inside-out meniscal repair.

- The results remain good if associated cartilage lesions are addressed appropriately.
- The prognosis of meniscal repair is also very good, depending on the location and vascularity of the tear.
- Meniscal repair should be performed concomitantly with ACL reconstruction because isolated meniscal repair in the setting of ACL-deficient knee has been proven to fail.

Troubleshooting

- Patients with degenerative meniscal tears and arthritic change may benefit from corticosteroid or hyaluronic acid injections. These patients may also continue to have arthritis-related pain after knee arthroscopy.
- Using NSAIDs to help minimize the inflammation may also be of benefit.

Patient Instructions

- The patient should be counseled on the benefits and risks of surgery.
  - The benefits include restoration of a smooth range of motion, decrease in pain, and return to sports, exercise, and activities of daily living.
  - The risks are minimal with arthroscopic surgery but include bleeding, infection, and nerve injury (particularly with inside-out meniscal repairs requiring a separate incision).

Considerations in Special Populations

- Sedentary patients should be given a trial of nonoperative management. However, if symptoms are adversely affecting

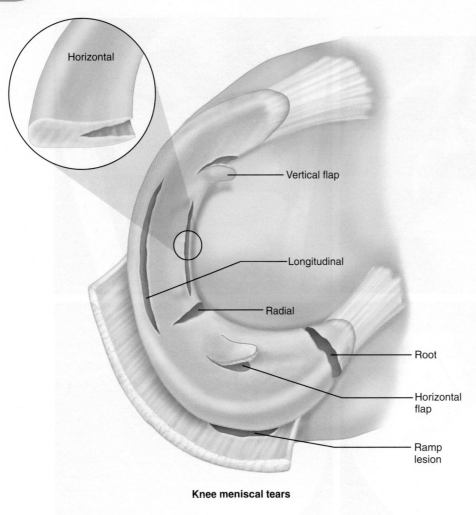

Fig 148.6 Various pathologic tears of the meniscus.

Horizontal

Vertical flap

Longitudinal

Radial

Root

Horizontal flap

Ramp lesion

Knee meniscal tears

daily activities, it is reasonable to perform arthroscopy with possible partial meniscectomy.

- Patient who have previously undergone partial meniscectomy should be counseled about the increased risk of joint degeneration with repeat meniscectomy.

Suggested Readings

Andersson-Molina H, Karlsson H, Rockborn P. Arthroscopic partial and total meniscectomy: A long-term follow-up study with matched controls. *Arthroscopy*. 2002;18:183–189.

Burks RT, Metcalf MH, Metcalf RW. Fifteen-year follow-up of arthroscopic partial meniscectomy. *Arthroscopy*. 1997;13:673–679.

Ericsson YB, Roos EM, Dahlberg L. Muscle strength, functional performance, and self-reported outcomes four years after arthroscopic partial meniscectomy in middle-aged patients. *Arthritis Rheum*. 2006;15:946–952.

Fox MG. MR imaging of the meniscus: review, current trends, and clinical implications. *Radiol Clin North Am*. 2007;45:1033–1053.

Hegedus EJ, Cook C, Hasselblad V, et al. Physical examination tests for assessing a torn meniscus in the knee: a systematic review with meta-analysis. *J Orthop Sports Phys Ther*. 2007;37:541–550.

Higuchi H, Kimura M, Shirakura K, et al. Factors affecting long-term results after arthroscopic partial meniscectomy. *Clin Orthop Relat Res*. 2000;377:161–168.

Katz JN, Brophy RH, Chaisson CE, et al. Surgery versus physical therapy for a meniscal tear and osteoarthritis. *N Engl J Med*. 2013;368(18):1675–1684.

Lee SJ, Aadalen KJ, Malaviya P, et al. Tibiofemoral contact mechanics after serial medial meniscectomies in the human cadaveric knee. *Am J Sports Med*. 2006;34:1334–1344.

Matsusue Y, Thomson NL. Arthroscopic partial medial meniscectomy in patients over 40 years old: A 5- to 11-year follow-up study. *Arthroscopy*. 1996;12:39–44.

Ryzewicz M, Peterson B, Siparsky PN, et al. The diagnosis of meniscus tears: the role of MRI and clinical examination. *Clin Orthop Relat Res*. 2007;455:123–133.

Sihvonen R, Paavola M, Malmivaara A, et al. Arthroscopic partial meniscectomy versus sham surgery for a degenerative meniscal tear. *N Engl J Med*. 2013;369(26):2515–2524.

Wheatley WB, Krome J, Martin DF. Rehabilitation programs following arthroscopic meniscectomy in athletes. *Sports Med*. 1996;21:447–456.

Chapter 149 Articular Cartilage Disorder

S. Evan Carstensen, Mark D. Miller

ICD-10-CM CODES
M23.8X1   *Chondral defect femoral condyle, right*
M23.8X2   *Chondral defect femoral condyle, left*
M23.91   *Articular cartilage disorder of the knee, right*
M23.92   *Articular cartilage disorder of the knee, left*
M93.261   *Osteochondritis dissecans (OCD), right*
M93.262   *Osteochondritis dissecans (OCD), left*

Key Concepts

- Cartilage (chondral) lesions can involve only articular cartilage or articular cartilage and subchondral bone defects (osteochondral lesions).
- Articular (hyaline) cartilage is uniquely suited for joint functions, such as axial loading and shear forces.
- Articular cartilage, composed mainly of type II collagen, is avascular with very limited regenerative potential.
- When a chondral defect is created, that gap does not simply heal and fill in.
- Osteochondral lesions violate the subchondral bone and create a bleeding healing response, causing the lesion to be partially filled with fibrocartilage (mainly type I collagen; poor mechanical properties compared with those of hyaline cartilage).
- Cartilage damage predisposes the joint to more rapid degeneration.
- Cartilage defects (chondral lesions) may be asymptomatic and symptoms/signs of chondral lesions overlap with those of other knee conditions (meniscal tears, arthritis, loose bodies).
- Treatment is a spectrum from symptomatic control through cartilage transplantation or regeneration.

History

- Acute injury
  - Athletic injury: Often associated with anterior cruciate ligament (ACL), meniscus, or collateral ligament injury
  - Patellar dislocation: Chondral injury to lateral femoral condyle and patellar facets.
  - Dashboard injury or other high-energy trauma: The patella is forced into the trochlea or an external object directly traumatizes the femoral condyles.
  - Lipohemarthrosis possible if the subchondral bone is fractured.

- Pain recurs with weight bearing or flexion-extension.
  - Locking or catching (mechanical symptoms) may be present, indicating an unstable cartilage flap or a loose body.
  - Symptomatic loose bodies often accompany acute chondral lesions; articular cartilage fragments may be displaced into the joint.
- Chronic (degenerative) lesion
  - Older patients with no traumatic mechanism; associated with degenerative osteoarthritis.
  - Chronic mild joint swelling, stiffness, joint line pain.
  - Mechanical symptoms may be present, especially if there are loose bodies or unstable flaps of articular cartilage.

Physical Examination

- Observation
  - Effusion (intra-articular swelling): Large hemarthrosis if subchondral fracture present.
  - Skin abrasions or ecchymosis in direct trauma to the knee.
  - Quadriceps atrophy for subacute or chronic symptomatic lesions.
  - Antalgic gait.
- Palpation
  - Assess joint-line tenderness with knee flexed to 90 degrees (possible meniscus tear).
  - Assess entire knee medial and lateral, anterior and posterior.
  - Tenderness over the femoral condyles or behind the patella.
  - Assess for crepitus while performing range of motion (ROM).
- Range of motion
  - Loose body, released from site of articular lesion, may cause block or catching during ROM.
  - Effusions may cause loss of flexion due to capsular stretch.
  - Crepitus with motion may indicate a large area of chondral damage.
  - A "clunk" with motion may indicate a displaced fragment.
- Special tests to identify other pathology or narrow the differential:
  - McMurray test, squat test, and joint-line tenderness for meniscal pathology.
  - Patellar facet tenderness and apprehension.
  - Ligament testing for cruciate or collateral ligament injury.

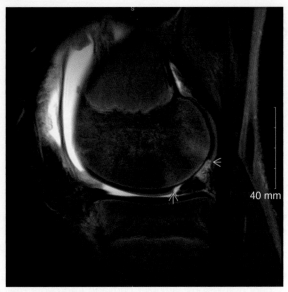

40 mm

Fig 149.1 Sagittal magnetic resonance imaging of a full-thickness osteochondral lesion of the medial femoral condyle (*arrows* indicate anterior and posterior extent of full thickness defect).

Imaging

- Radiographs: weight-bearing anteroposterior (AP), lateral, 45 degrees of flexion posteroanterior (Rosenberg view), 20 degrees of flexion patellofemoral (Laurin), and tunnel posteroanterior views
  - Rule out osteochondral fracture, osseous loose body, osteoarthritis, osteonecrosis of the femoral condyle, osteochondritis dissecans, plateau fracture, tibial eminence fracture, and Segond fracture (ACL tear).
  - Posteroanterior flexion weight-bearing view is especially useful to look for osteoarthritis.
  - Laurin view to look for patellofemoral arthritis.
  - Tunnel view is helpful to look for osteochondritis dissecans lesions.
- Computed tomography (CT)
  - Sensitive for identifying fractures as well as accurately sizing bone fragments.
  - Reconstructions give accurate depiction of injury and bony involvement.
- Magnetic resonance imaging (MRI)
  - Sensitive for cartilage injury and bony edema but underestimates damage (Fig. 149.1).
  - Bone edema may indicate local subchondral overloading in an area with chondral defect.
  - Identifies associated pathology of the meniscus, cruciate ligaments, collateral ligaments, and patellar retinaculum.

Differential Diagnosis

- Osteoarthritis: chronic stiffness, aching, narrow joint space on radiographs.
- Loose body without significant chondral defect: catching, mobile pain, osseous fragments on radiographs, cartilaginous fragments on MRI.
- Patellar subluxation or dislocation: patellar apprehension, pain at the medial patella.

- Osteochondritis dissecans: pain to palpation of the condyle, seen on radiographs, MRI, or computed tomography (CT).
- Tibial plateau fracture: high-energy injury, seen on radiographs or CT.
- ACL tear: positive Lachman/anterior drawer tests, acute (2 to 4 hours) hemarthrosis, seen on MRI.
- Collateral ligament sprain or tear: pain or instability to varus stress (lateral collateral ligament) or valgus stress (medial collateral ligament).
- Pes anserine bursitis: pain on medial side, 3 to 5 cm distal to the joint line.
- Fat pad impingement syndrome.
- Meniscal tear: medial/lateral joint line tenderness, effusion accumulating over 12 hours.
- Symptomatic plica: painful snapping band across medial femoral condyle (MFC).

Treatment

- At diagnosis
  - Traumatic injuries in which there is significant concern for fracture, unstable knee joint, or open knee require the consultation of an orthopaedic surgeon.
  - Acute chondral injuries from athletics or other activities, including those associated with tears of the cruciate or collateral ligaments, also warrant referral to an orthopaedic surgeon.
  - Young patients with potentially unstable chondral lesions should be referred to an orthopaedic surgeon for close evaluation and early intervention should the lesion become unstable or displace (Fig. 149.2).
- Otherwise, for chondral lesions found by radiologic evaluation for knee pain, initial treatment is symptomatic.
  - Rest, ice, compression, and elevation (RICE) are helpful to decrease swelling and pain.
  - Acetaminophen and/or nonsteroidal antiinflammatory drugs are useful for pain control and inflammation.
  - Physical therapy focused on restoring ROM and reducing pain while maintaining or improving muscle strength around the knee is beneficial to help support the knee.
  - If there is varus/valgus malalignment and overloading of the medial or lateral compartment, an unloader brace or heel wedge may be helpful to restore a more neutral mechanical axis.
- Failure of conservative treatment
  - If symptoms are not responsive to conservative treatment or if mechanical symptoms persist, the patient may be a surgical candidate with multiple treatment options available (Fig. 149.3).
  - Arthroscopic options include chondroplasty (débridement) and loose body removal, microfracture, cartilage transfer (osteochondral autograft or allograft transfer), or autogenous chondrocyte implantation (ACI) (Figs. 149.4 to 149.7).

When to Refer

- Acute injuries with a concern for fracture or articular cartilage injury should be referred immediately for orthopaedic evaluation.

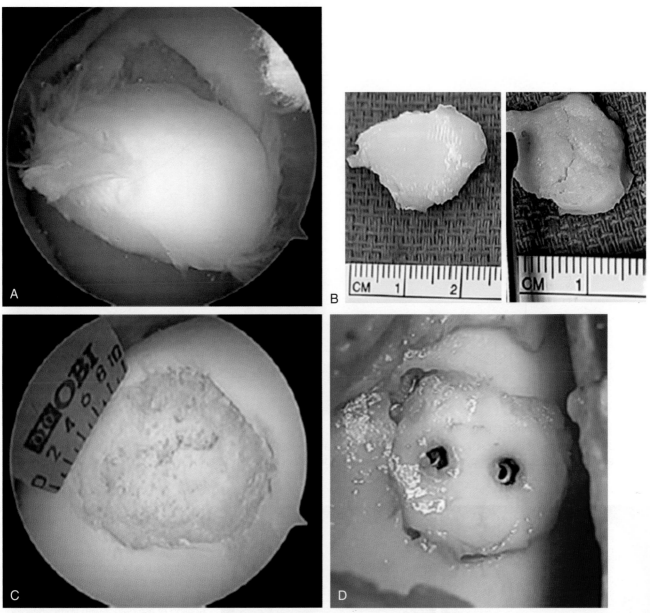

Fig 149.2 Acute osteochondritis dissecans (OCD) lesion of the medial femoral condyle (MFC). **(A)** The lesion is detached from base. **(B)** Articular surface seen with bone attached deep to cartilage. **(C)** Measurement of MFC defect. **(D)** Primary repair of the displaced OCD fragment with headless screw fixation.

- Knee pain without acute injury should be initially managed nonoperatively with the modalities previously mentioned.
  - Making sure that patients have attempted sufficient nonoperative measures prior to referring is paramount.
- Having appropriate x-rays, CT, and/or MRI prior to referral may assist in diagnosis and expedient treatment for surgical candidates.
  - X-ray: AP, lateral, and sunrise views are appropriate to obtain at initial imaging.
- Older patients with continued mechanical symptoms in whom conservative management has failed should also be referred.

Prognosis

- Many patients with symptomatic chondral lesions will improve with conservative therapy only.
- Patients with mechanical symptoms often respond well to arthroscopy for loose body removal and chondroplasty of loose cartilage flaps.
- Marrow stimulation techniques (microfracture) for cartilage defects have shown positive results, especially in the short term, but do not restore native hyaline cartilage.
- Osteochondral autograft transplantation has shown a high percentage of good to excellent results and, in limited

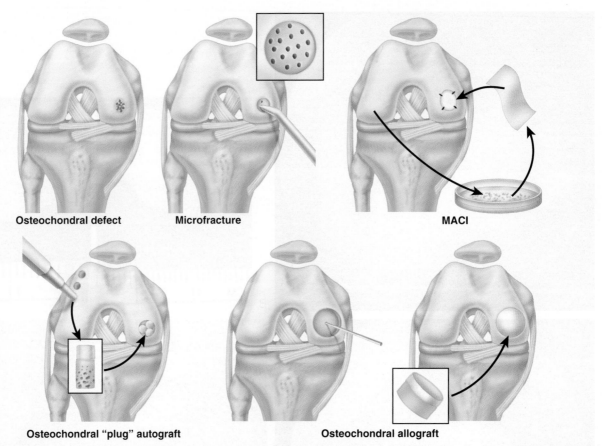

Osteochondral defect   **Microfracture**   **MACI**

Osteochondral "plug" autograft   **Osteochondral allograft**

Fig 149.3 Composite illustration demonstrating osteochondral treatment options. *Left to right,* Microfracture, osteochondral autograft "plug" transfer, autologous chondrocyte implantation, osteochondral allograft transplantation.

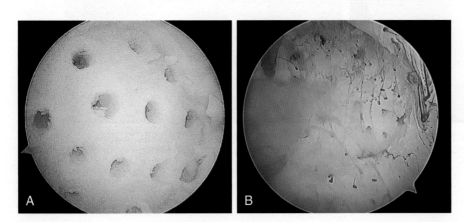

Fig 149.4 Full-thickness chondral lesion treated with microfracture. **(A)** Following removal of the calcified cartilage layer with a curette, a microfracture awl is used to penetrate the subchondral bone in 2 to 3 mm intervals. **(B)** Bleeding subchrondral bone is demonstrated, which facilitates healing of the defect with fibrocartilaginous tissue.

studies, was found to produce better results than microfracture for larger lesions.

- Results of autogenous chondrocyte implantation are mixed but generally positive.
- Overall it is imperative that patients attempt conservative management prior to proceeding with surgery.

Troubleshooting

- The patient should be counseled on the benefits and risks of surgery.

- Benefits include restoration of smooth ROM and decrease in pain with return to sports, exercise, and activities of daily living; however, this varies from patient to patient and depends on the treatment modality. Restoration of a more anatomic joint surface and joint mechanics will likely decrease the rate of progression to posttraumatic arthritis.
- Risks are minimal with arthroscopic débridement and loose body removal, but symptomatic relief cannot be guaranteed and may be only temporary.
- Microfracture, osteochondral autograft or allograft transfer, and autogenous chondrocyte implantation

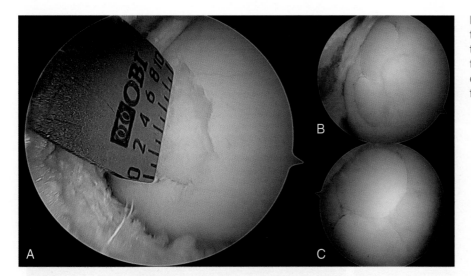

Fig 149.5 Full-thickness chondral defect treated with osteochondral autograft transfer. (A) Arthroscopic measurement of the cartilage defect. (B and C) Chondral defect is filled with two 8 mm plugs transferred into the lesion.

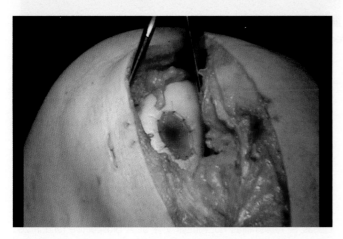

Fig 149.6 Autologous chondrocyte implantation. Sutured and sealed borders after cell implantation.

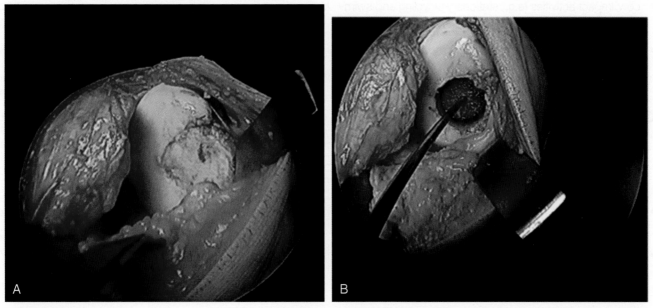

Fig 149.7 Allograft cartilage transfer. (A) Articular surface defect of lateral femoral condyle. (B) Trephine reamer with adequate osteochondral resection.

Continued

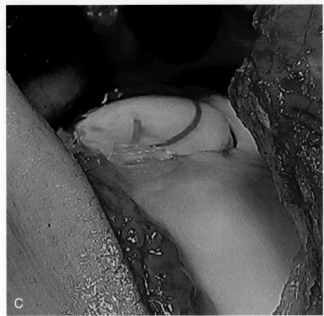

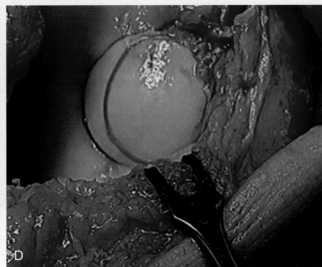

Fig 149.7, cont'd (C and D) Allograft chondrocyte plug transferred to defect.

require an extended period of non–weight bearing for 6 to 8 weeks, with results that are variable. Return to full activities often requires 6 to 12 months of rehabilitation.
- Effusions and swelling about the operative extremity may be present for months to years after surgery when compared with the contralateral limb.
- High-impact activities should be discouraged in patients who have had significant chondral injuries.

Instructions for the Patient

- Physical therapy focused on strengthening and ROM can help facilitate the return to activities.
- Low-impact activities (e.g., stationary bicycling and swimming) should be encouraged in patients with chondral injuries.
- Young patients with osteochondritis dissecans (OCD) lesions should be aware that a sudden loss in motion may indicate a displaced fragment that may require surgery.

Considerations in Special Populations

- Sedentary patients should be given a trial of nonoperative management. However, if symptoms are adversely affecting daily activities, it is reasonable to perform arthroscopy for chondroplasty, loose body removal, and potentially marrow stimulation techniques or grafting.
- It is important to match the individual patient and his or her physical demands with the treatment for the chondral lesion.
- Weight loss prior to the aforementioned procedures may prove helpful in reducing knee pain as well.

Suggested Readings

Alford JW, Cole BJ. Cartilage restoration, part 1: basic science, historical perspective, patient evaluation, and treatment options. *Am J Sports Med*. 2005a;33:295–306.

Alford JW, Cole BJ. Cartilage restoration, part 2: techniques, outcomes, and future directions. *Am J Sports Med*. 2005b;33:443–460.

Gracitelli GC, Moraes VY, Franciozi CE, et al. Surgical interventions (microfracture, drilling, mosaicplasty, and allograft transplantation) for treating isolated cartilage defects of the knee in adults. *Cochrane Database Syst Rev*. 2016;(9):CD010675.

Gudas S, Kalesinskas RJ, Kimtys V, et al. A prospective randomized clinical trial of mosaic osteochondral autologous transplantation versus microfracture for the treatment of osteochondral defects of the knee in young athletes. *Arthroscopy*. 2005;21:1066–1075.

Hangody L, Fules P. Autologous osteochondral mosaicplasty for the treatment of full-thickness defects of weight-bearing joints: ten years of experimental and clinical experience. *J Bone Joint Surg Am*. 2003;85A:25–32.

Mandelbaum BR, Browne JE, Fu F, et al. Articular cartilage lesions of the knee. *Am J Sports Med*. 1998;26:853–861.

Marcacci M, Kon E, Zaffagnini S, et al. Multiple osteochondral arthroscopic grafting (mosaicplasty) for cartilage defects of the knee: prospective study results at 2-year follow-up. *Arthroscopy*. 2005;21:462–470.

Messner K, Maletius W. The long-term prognosis for severe damage to weight-bearing cartilage in the knee. *Acta Orthop Scand*. 1996;67:165–168.

Peterson L, Minas T, Brittberg M, et al. Two- to 9-year outcome after autologous chondrocyte transplantation of the knee. *Clin Orthop Relat Res*. 2000;374:212–234.

Sharpe JR, Ahmed SU, Fleetcroft JP, et al. The treatment of osteochondral lesions using a combination of autologous chondrocyte implantation and autograft: Three-year follow-up. *J Bone Joint Surg Br*. 2005;87B:730–735.

Steadman JR, Briggs KK, Rodrigo JJ, et al. Outcomes of microfracture for traumatic chondral defects of the knee: average 11-year follow-up. *Arthroscopy*. 2003;19:477–484.

Chapter 150 Spontaneous Osteonecrosis of the Knee and Avascular Necrosis

Jeffrey Ruland, Harrison Mahon, David Diduch

ICD-10-CM CODES

M84.451A	*Insufficiency fracture of medial femoral condyle, right*
M84.452A	*Insufficiency fracture of medial femoral condyle, left*
M84.461A	*Insufficiency fracture of tibia, right*
M84.462A	*Insufficiency fracture of tibia, left*
M87.851	*Osteonecrosis of femur, right*
M87.852	*Osteonecrosis of femur, left*
M87.861	*Osteonecrosis of tibia, right*
M87.862	*Osteonecrosis of tibia, left*

Key Concepts

- Osteonecrosis (ON) refers to bone death.

Etiology

- Spontaneous osteonecrosis of the knee (SONK) and avascular necrosis (AVN) are of different etiologies.

Spontaneous Osteonecrosis of the Knee

- Spontaneous osteonecrosis is a misnomer, as it is caused by insufficiency fracture rather than interference of blood supply.
- Sudden increases in mechanical load across the knee joint—as with meniscal root tear or meniscectomy, with subsequent meniscal extrusion—leads to increased forces across bone. Over time, the bone remodels to handle the increased stress. But if the force is too great or bone health is not optimal, stress fracture will result (Figs. 150.1 and 150.2).
- Typically women older than 60 years of age (female-to-male ratio 3:1), especially those with osteoporosis, are affected.
- Osteonecrosis should always be considered in an elderly patient with a painful knee that appears normal radiographically.

Avascular Necrosis

- Interference of microcirculation to bone leads to edema and increased compartmental pressure, resulting in bone ischemia. If blood supply is restored before subchondral collapse, the lesion may heal and symptoms resolve.

- As blood supply to bone is lost, necrosis leads to segmental collapse of subchondral bone.
- Primary AVN is idiopathic; secondary AVN is due to trauma, long-term steroid therapy, alcoholism, renal transplantation, systemic lupus erythematosus, sickle cell anemia, or Gaucher disease.
- Most often patients are below 55 years of age.
- Osteoarthritis is typically the end stage of ON, whether resulting from SONK or AVN.

History

Spontaneous Osteonecrosis of the Knee

- Sudden onset of pain.
- Can be precipitated by minor trauma or meniscectomy.
- Pain from increased stress with edema of subchondral bone. This can progress to subchondral fracture and even collapse of the osteochondral surface. Often pain can be much improved even in the face of collapse once the fracture has had time to heal.
- Typically involves the medial femoral condyle or tibia and is unilateral in more than 99% of cases. Any pressure whatsoever to the medial side of the knee can be very uncomfortable.
- Pain worse at night in the acute phase (6 to 8 weeks)
- Pain may resolve or become chronic depending on the size and stage of the lesion.

Avascular Necrosis

- Insidious onset of pain
- AVN can involve the femoral condyles or tibial plateau; it is bilateral in the vast majority of cases and frequently involves both femoral condyles. Pain can thus be diffuse, lateral, or medial.
- It can be challenging to distinguish from SONK using history alone. History should be correlated with demographic factors.

Physical Examination

Spontaneous Osteonecrosis of the Knee

- Observation
  - Antalgic gait
  - Knee typically not red
  - Slight swelling possible (intra-articular effusion)

Progression of SONK

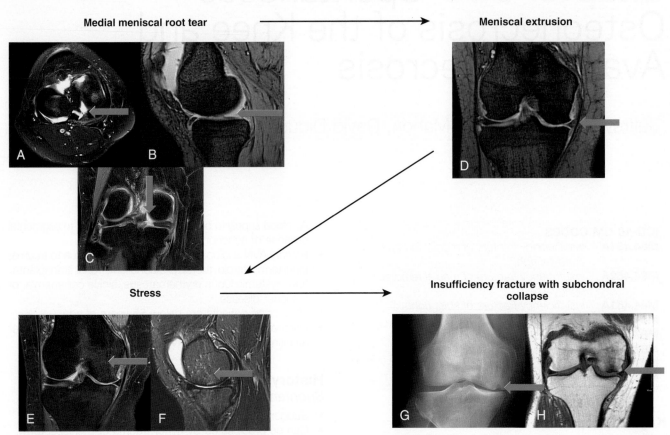

Fig 150.1 Progression of spontaneous osteonecrosis of the knee. **(A to C)** T2-weighted axial, sagittal, and coronal magnetic resonance imaging sections showing medial meniscal root tear. Note characteristic "ghost sign" in sagittal section **(B)**. **(D)** T2-weighted coronal MRI section demonstrating meniscal extrusion secondary to root tear. **(E and F)** T2-weighted coronal and sagittal MRI sections showing edema in the medial femoral condyle, indicative of increased stress across the joint. **(G and H)** Radiograph and T1-weighted coronal MRI section indicating insufficiency fracture with collapse of subchondral bone. *SONK,* Spontaneous osteonecrosis of the knee.

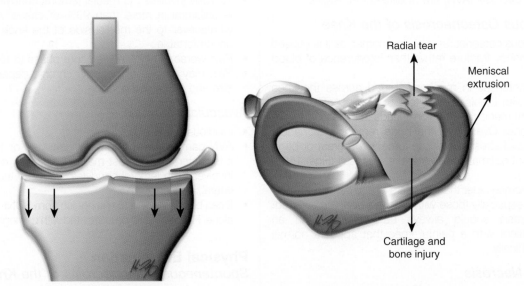

Fig 150.2 This illustration demonstrates how root tear leads to subsequent meniscal extrusion and increased pressure on the medial femoral condyle and tibia. The pressure across the joint can ultimately lead to spontaneous osteonecrosis of the knee. (From Tafur M, Bencardino JT. Imaging of the meniscus. In: Scott WN, ed. *Insall & Scott Surgery of the Knee.* 6th ed. Philadelphia: Elsevier; 2018:133–160.)

- Palpation
  - Patellar ballottement (effusion)
  - Exquisite tenderness to palpation over affected area (medial femoral condyle or tibia) or joint line (secondary degenerative changes)
  - Crepitus: degenerative changes and inflammation
- Range of motion
  - Acute phase: decreased due to pain, effusion, or synovitis
  - Chronic phase: decreased due to degenerative changes

Avascular Necrosis

- Similar physical exam findings
- Often with more diffuse tenderness over the affected joint

Imaging
Spontaneous Osteonecrosis of the Knee

- Findings are typically limited to subchondral bone and epiphysis
- Magnetic resonance imaging (MRI; recommended as first option)
  - Confirmatory test to delineate extent of pathology: lesions often more extensive than appreciated on radiographs.
  - Edema on MRI indicative of stress. May see halo of insufficiency fracture with collapse of trabeculae.
- Radiographs: bilateral weight-bearing posteroanterior, lateral, 45 degrees of flexion posteroanterior (Rosenberg), and 45 degrees of flexion patellofemoral (Merchant) views
  - Useful to track disease progression
  - Radiographic staging of ON/spontaneous osteonecrosis of the knee
  - Stage I: radiograph normal (positive bone scan)
  - Stage II: subtle flattening of articular surface
  - Stage III: typical lesion with radiolucent area in subchondral bone and a sclerotic halo
  - Stage IV: collapse of subchondral bone
  - Stage V: collapse with secondary degenerative changes
  - Joint space narrowing without osteophytes or subchondral sclerosis suggests SONK over osteoarthritis

Avascular Necrosis

- Similar findings with more extensive involvement through knee and potentially with other joint involvement including hips and shoulders.
- Typically involves a larger area of bone with extension into the epiphysis and potentially the metaphysis or the diaphysis (Fig. 150.3).
- Consider MRI of contralateral knee, bilateral hips, or other symptomatic joints, given the propensity for multiple joint involvement.

Differential Diagnosis

- Meniscal tear: joint line tenderness, swelling, mechanical symptoms, evident on MRI.
- Osteoarthritis: chronic stiffness, aching, often tricompartmental involvement on radiographs.
- Osteochondritis dissecans: discrete lesions involving separate fragment of bone detaching from vascular bony bed, most commonly in lateral aspect of medial femoral

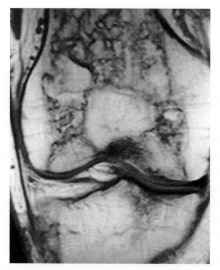

Fig 150.3 T1-weighted magnetic resonance imaging section showing avascular necrosis. Note extensive involvement of the joint with both femoral condyles and tibial plateau affected and extension into the metaphysis. (From Mont MA, Ragland PS. Osteonecrosis of the knee. In: Scott WN, ed. *Insall & Scott Surgery of the Knee*. 4th ed. Philadelphia: Churchill Livingstone; 2006: 460–480.)

condyle; peak incidence between 10 and 15 years of age, more common in males.
- Pes anserine bursitis: location of tenderness below the medial joint line.
- Iliotibial band tendinitis: lateral pain with positive Ober test.

Conservative Treatment
Spontaneous Osteonecrosis of the Knee

- Prior to subchondral collapse
  - Conservative treatment with analgesics, nonsteroidal antiinflammatory drugs (NSAIDs), protected weight bearing, and unloader bracing until the lesion has been defined (may take as long as 6 months).
  - Treatment of the insufficiency fracture is much like that of any other fracture. It needs time and reduced load to heal.
  - Bone health is critical. Look for vitamin D deficiency or other correctable causes of osteopenia/osteoporosis to increase healing potential.
  - Corticosteroid or hyaluronic acid injections may be considered in patients who do not respond, but injection will not affect bone pain.
- With subchondral collapse
  - Conservative treatment is recommended to allow the fracture to heal before considering operative procedures.
- Patients **with or without** collapse remaining painful after bone has healed or those who have had time for bone to heal from any stress fracture with correction of any bone health issues but remain symptomatic should be referred for joint replacement.

Avascular Necrosis

- Observation is recommended for asymptomatic lesions.
- Nonoperative management (NSAIDs, other analgesics, and protected weight bearing) of symptomatic lesions is associated with high rates of clinical failure and progression to more advanced lesions that may require arthroplasty.

Surgical Options

Spontaneous Osteonecrosis of the Knee

- High tibial osteotomy if patient is young.
- Unicompartmental knee arthroplasty (UKA) is an option for SONK, but not until the lesion is fully healed. Restoration of bone health is indicated by a normal pattern of subchondral sclerosis on radiography.
- If an associated meniscal root tear is present, partial meniscectomy can worsen the condition.
- Total knee arthroplasty (TKA) is reserved for lesions with subchondral collapse (stage IV).

Avascular Necrosis

- Drilling or core decompression (with or without grafting) are options for the treatment of AVN but not SONK. Patients who undergo these procedures do quite well. These may help prevent progression to more advanced lesions with need for more invasive procedures.
- UKA is not recommended because of frequent involvement of multiple condyles.
- Total knee arthroplasty (TKA) reserved for lesions with subchondral collapse (stage IV).

Prognosis

- Small lesions do well, but mild degenerative changes may develop.
- Ultimately the prognosis depends on the size of the initial lesion.
- Lesions that involve more than 50% of the condyle have a poor prognosis; these tend to deteriorate progressively to osteoarthritis.

Troubleshooting

- The patient should be counseled on the benefits and risks of surgery.
- Benefits of surgical intervention (e.g., drilling, grafting, high tibial osteotomy) include pain relief, restoration of quality of life, and slowing of degenerative changes. UKA and TKA remove degenerative joint surfaces to more closely approximate normal anatomy and function.

- The risks of UKA include early prosthetic failure and the possibility of revision surgery. The stress fracture in patients with SONK must be completely healed prior to UKA to support the prosthesis.
- Repair of meniscal root tears should be considered in young patients or those with relatively acute conditions with root tear and extruded meniscus.

Instructions for the Patient

- Patients should be counseled on the findings of ON. The size of the lesion and expectations for outcome should be discussed.
- Vitamin D supplementation should be encouraged to support bone health.
- Weight loss should be encouraged in obese patients in an effort to protect the knee and increase the likelihood of success with future surgical intervention.
- Physical therapy programs should be recommended to help improve strength and function.

Suggested Readings

Akgun I, Kesmezacar H, Oqut T, et al. Arthroscopic microfracture treatment for osteonecrosis of the knee. *Arthroscopy.* 2005;21:834–843.

Burrus MT, Diduch DR. Osteochondritis dissecans and avascular necrosis. In: Wiesel SW, eds. *Operative Techniques in Orthopaedic Surgery.* Philadelphia: Lippincott Williams & Wilkins; 2011:366–380.

Kim JY, Finger DR. Spontaneous osteonecrosis of the knee. *J Rheumatol.* 2006;33:1416.

Marulanda G, Seyler TM, Sheikh NH, et al. Percutaneous drilling for the treatment of secondary osteonecrosis of the knee. *J Bone Joint Surg Br.* 2006;88B:740–746.

Mont MA, Baumgarten KM, Rifai A, et al. Atraumatic osteonecrosis of the knee. *J Bone Joint Surg Am.* 2000;82A:1279.

Mont MA, Marker DR, Zywiel MG, et al. Osteonecrosis of the knee and related conditions. *J Am Acad Orthop Surg.* 2011;19:482–494.

Myers TG, Cui Q, Kuskowski M, et al. Outcomes of total and unicompartmental knee arthroplasty for secondary and spontaneous osteonecrosis of the knee. *J Bone Joint Surg Am.* 2006;88A:76–82.

Pape D, Seil R, Kohn D, et al. Imaging of early stages of osteonecrosis of the knee. *Orthop Clin North Am.* 2004;35:293–303.

Patel DV, Breazeale NM, Behr CT, et al. Osteonecrosis of the knee: current clinical concepts. *Knee Surg Sports Traumatol Arthrosc.* 1998;6:2–11.

Soucacos PM, Johnson EO, Soultanis K, et al. Diagnosis and management of the osteonecrotic triad of the knee. *Orthop Clin North Am.* 2004;35:371–381.

Valenti Nin JR, Leyes M, Schweitzer D. Spontaneous osteonecrosis of the knee: treatment and evolution. *Knee Surg Sports Traumatol Arthrosc.* 1998;6:12–15.

Yates PJ, Calder JD, Stranks GJ, et al. Early MRI diagnosis and nonsurgical management of spontaneous osteonecrosis of the knee. *Knee.* 2007;14:112–116.

Chapter 151 Osteoarthritis of the Knee

Nicholas E. Gerken, James A. Browne

ICD-10-CM CODES
OSTEOARTHRITIS OF KNEE
M17.10 *Unilateral primary osteoarthritis, unspecified knee*
M17.11 *Unilateral primary osteoarthritis, right knee*
M17.12 *Unilateral primary osteoarthritis, left knee*
M17.30 *Unilateral post-traumatic osteoarthritis, unspecified knee*
M17.31 *Unilateral post-traumatic osteoarthritis, right knee*
M17.32 *Unilateral post-traumatic osteoarthritis, left knee*
ADDITIONAL RELEVANT CODES
M06.861 *Other specific rheumatoid arthritis, right knee*
M06.862 *Other specific rheumatoid arthritis, left knee*
M08.961 *Unspecified juvenile RA, right knee,*
M08.962 *Unspecified juvenile RA, left knee*
M00.061 *Staph arthritis, right knee*
M00.062 *Staph arthritis, left knee*
M00261 *Strep arthritis, right knee*
M00262 *Strep arthritis, left knee*
M00.861 *Arthritis, right knee due to other bacteria*
M00.862 *Arthritis, left knee due to other bacteria*

Key Concepts

- Primary osteoarthritis (OA) is the most common cause of knee pain and disability in adult US population; approximately 85% of people older than 65 years of age have radiographically detectable OA.
- Age-related articular cartilage degeneration, often called "wear-and-tear arthritis," includes low-grade synovitis coupled with alterations in periarticular and subchondral bone.
- Obesity and jobs/lifestyles that require intense or repetitive loading of the knees may accelerate the disease and exacerbate symptoms.
- Articular (hyaline) cartilage is uniquely suited for joint functions (axial loading and shear forces) and has very limited regenerative potential (avascular).
- Secondary OA may occur at any age and is secondary to damage of the protective anatomy of the joint or the cartilage itself, which predisposes to further degradation. Examples of preceding events include intra-articular fracture, osteochondral defect, ligament instability, meniscus tear/meniscectomy, gout, pseudogout, or septic joint.

- An estimated 54.4 million adults (22.7%) annually have been diagnosed by their physician with some form of arthritis. By 2040 this number is estimated to rise to 78 million (26%) US adults ages 18 and older. Two-thirds of those will be women.
- Arthritis is the leading cause of work disability among U.S. adults.
- Estimated total medical costs and earnings losses due to arthritis is approximately 304 billion dollars; 164 billion dollars in lost wages is attributed to arthritis.
- Arthritis is much more common among those who have other chronic conditions: 49% of adults with heart disease have arthritis; 47% of adults with diabetes have arthritis; 31% of adults who are obese have arthritis.

History
Primary Osteoarthritis

- Older patients, often obese
- Typically unidentified trauma/injury or mild incident that exacerbates preexisting knee pain
- Chronic mild joint swelling, stiffness, joint line pain with periodic flares
- Pain with weight bearing, aggravated by stairs, hills, uneven ground, sit-to-stand motion. Relief with rest and nonsteroidal antiinflammatory drugs.
- More severe disease will cause pain even at night or at rest; patient may note instability or knee "giving way"/knee subluxation events.
- The medial compartment is the most commonly affected secondary to increased mechanical load, but tricompartmental disease in the older adult with OA is very common (Fig. 151.1).
- Mechanical symptoms (catching, locking), unstable articular cartilage flaps, or acute-on-chronic degenerative meniscal tears especially to posterior medial aspect of knee
- Fullness to back of the knee may represent a Baker cyst (a synovial fluid-filled cyst in the popliteal space).
- Important to assess impact of knee pain on activities of daily living (ADLs)/quality of life
- Key concept: Differentiate acute meniscal pathology clinically from OA via mechanical symptoms.

Secondary Osteoarthritis

- Often younger patients
- Posttraumatic (Fig. 151.2): Previous knee injury (cruciate/collateral ligament injury, meniscal tear requiring subtotal meniscectomy, intra-articular fracture, osteochondral lesion) or previous injury that is remote from the knee but causes

mechanical malalignment (slipped capital femoral epiphysis, hip fracture, femur fracture, tibia fracture, physeal injury with subsequent growth disturbance)

- Degenerative joint disease of the knee can also be secondary to a history of gout, pseudogout (calcium pyrophosphate dihydrate deposition syndrome), or a septic knee joint.

Physical Examination
Observation

- Varus malalignment with medial compartment OA (bow legged; Fig. 151.3); valgus malalignment with lateral compartment OA (knock knee)
- Quadriceps atrophy in chronic symptomatic knees
- Gait:
  - Antalgic gait
  - Varus thrust gait
  - In-toeing: excessive femoral anteversion
  - Out-toeing: relative femoral retroversion
- Previous surgical scars (arthroscopic portals)

Palpation

- Effusion, osteophytes, crepitus
- Tenderness secondary to reactive synovitis
- Joint line tenderness (may have associated meniscal pathology)
- Loose bodies (may cause decreased range of motion)
- Evaluate for tenderness at Gerdy tubercle and pes anserine
- Popliteal cyst (Baker cyst)

Range of Motion

- Decreased compared with contralateral knee
- Lack of full extension is common presentation.
- Competency of collateral ligaments in terminal extension and 90 degrees flexion:
  - Varus: lateral collateral ligament (LCL) laxity
  - Valgus: medial collateral ligament (MCL) laxity
- Note if coronal deformity is correctable with manual counter-manipulation.
- Patella tracking, lateral subluxation or grinding (typically more prominent in valgus knee secondary increased Q-ankle)

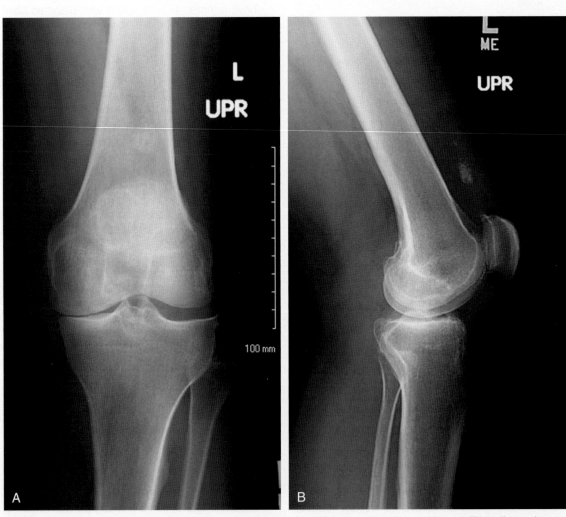

Fig 151.1 A 55-year-old man with isolated medial compartment pain. Anteroposterior **(A)** and lateral **(B)** radiographs reveal medial compartment degenerative joint disease.

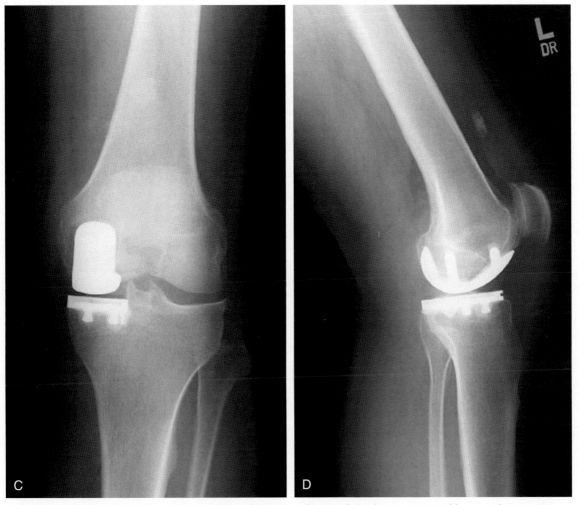

Fig 151.1, cont'd Anteroposterior **(C)** and lateral **(D)** radiographs after medial unicompartmental knee replacement.

- Always evaluate the hip and spine. Referred pain from obturator nerve versus lumbar spinal stenosis and radiculopathy.

Imaging
Radiographs

- Numerous classification systems available that attempt to grade severity of arthritis based on radiographic findings: Kellgren and Lawrence, Ahlback. Common themes include evaluation of the degree of joint space narrowing, subchondral sclerosis, reactive osteophyte formation, and, in more advanced disease, boney defect/loss.
- Always get weight-bearing films, typically four views (Fig. 151.4): Bilateral weight-bearing posteroanterior, lateral, 45 degrees of flexion posteroanterior (Rosenberg), and 20 degrees of flexion patellofemoral (Laurin) views.
- Posteroanterior flexion weight-bearing view is especially useful to look for OA.
  - May be more advanced on posterior condyles early in the disease
- Long cassette posteroanterior weight-bearing views can be helpful to assess limb mechanical and anatomic alignment: more useful in patients with advance disease and in

patients with congenital or acquired femoral deformities (see Fig. 151.3).

Magnetic Resonance Imaging
- Grossly overused in the arthritic patient population
- If weight-bearing radiographs demonstrate obvious joint space narrowing, then magnetic resonance imaging (MRI) is not indicated.
- When to use: only after obtaining weight-bearing knee radiographs and in:
  - Younger patient population (i.e., >50 without obvious joint space narrowing, typically for evaluation of osteonecrosis or acute traumatic knee injury)
  - Older population with osteopenia or osteoporosis to evaluate for insufficiency fracture (when symptoms appear out of proportion to degree of arthritis)

Differential Diagnosis
- Not all knee pain is OA, but after the age of 65, most of it is.
- Rheumatoid arthritis: Look for other signs of rheumatoid arthritis or autoimmune disease–centralized cupping deformity on tibia.

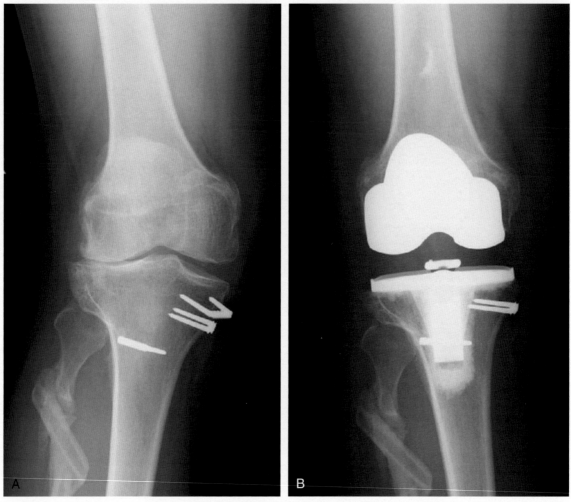

Fig 151.2 A 60-year-old man with posttraumatic degenerative change after traumatic knee dislocation. **(A)** Preoperative radiograph with tricompartmental degenerative change. **(B)** Postoperative radiograph after total knee arthroplasty.

- Septic arthritis: Fever; elevated white blood cell count, erythrocyte sedimentation rate, C-reactive protein; hot knee; intense pain with range of motion
- Meniscal tear: Mechanical symptoms; locking, often associated with OA
- Tibial plateau or femoral condyle fracture: History of fall or other trauma
- Osteonecrosis of the femur or tibia: Steroid use, alcoholism, female, blood dyscrasia
- L3-L4 radiculopathy: Worse with straining/coughing, positive femoral stretch test
- Pigmented villonodular synovitis: Recurrent hemarthroses
- Patellar tendinitis (jumper's knee)
- Prepatellar bursitis: Palpable fluid collection superficial to patella
- Iliotibial band syndrome: Lateral pain, worse with repetitive activity like cycling
- Pes anserine bursitis: Pain distal to the medial joint line
- Hip OA: Pain with internal rotation and flexion of the hip, often groin pain but may be referred to the knee

- Gout, pseudogout—radiographs may show significant chondrocalcinosis
- Hemophilia, sickle cell, thalassemias

Treatment

- Current treatment guidelines based on updated American Academy of Orthopaedic Surgeons (AAOS) second edition clinical practice guidelines for treatment of symptomatic OA of the knee in coordination with the American College of Rheumatology, American Academy of Family Practice, and American Physical Therapy Association
- Divided into four basic treatment categories: (1) conservative; (2) pharmacologic; (3) procedural; and (4) surgical
- Conservative
  - Strong recommendation for patients to participate in self-management programs (home exercise programs) aimed at low-impact aerobic exercise, neuromuscular education, strengthening
  - Moderate recommendation for weight loss for body mass index (BMI) greater than 25

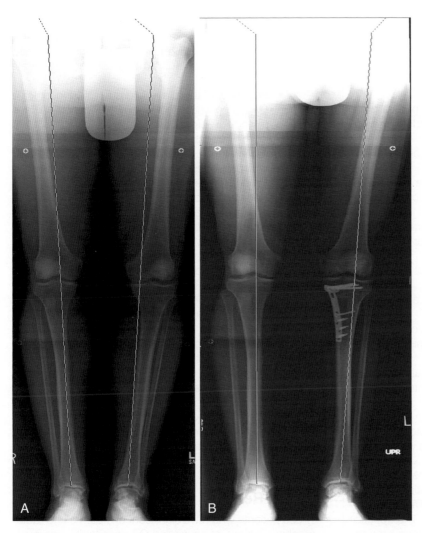

Fig 151.3 A 39-year-old man with left knee isolated medial compartment arthritis and varus malalignment. (A) Long cassette alignment radiograph depicting varus malalignment (mechanical axis shown). (B) Long cassette alignment after medial opening wedge high tibial osteotomy with correction of mechanical axis into the lateral compartment (mechanical axis shown).

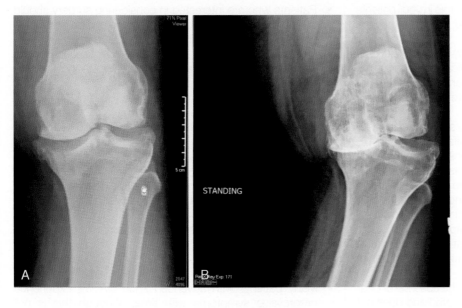

Fig 151.4 (A) Nonstanding anteroposterior radiograph demonstrating some arthritis but no significant malalignment. (B) Standing posteroanterior radiograph demonstrating advanced arthritis and gross malalignment.

- Inconclusive findings: manual therapy, physical agents (electrotherapeutic modalities), medial offloader braces, heel wedges
- Recommend against (strong) acupuncture, glucosamine, and chondroitin
  - Pharmacologic
    - Strong recommendation for oral or topical nonsteroidal antiinflammatory drugs (NSAIDs) or tramadol (Ultram)
    - Inconclusive evidence for acetaminophen
    - Recommend against opioids or pain patches
  - Procedural
    - Moderate recommendation against needle lavage
    - Strong recommendation against hyaluronic acid intra-articular injections
    - Inconclusive recommendation for corticosteroids, growth factor, or platelet-rich plasma intra-articular injections
  - Surgical
    - Limited recommendation for proximal tibial osteotomy in medial compartment disease
    - Strong recommendation against the use of arthroscopic lavage or débridement
    - Inconclusive evidence for or against arthroscopic partial meniscectomy in persons with a torn meniscus
  - Additional considerations
    - Clinical practice guidelines are recommendations based on best available evidence and not to be interpreted as dogma.
    - Conservative treatment
      - Tylenol is an appropriate option for symptomatic relief in conjunction with NSAIDs or in patients who cannot tolerate NSAIDs.
      - Corticosteroid intra-articular knee injections are a good option for both diagnostic and therapeutic treatment in conjunction with conservative treatment and in those patients with reactive synovitis. Therapeutic response in duration and efficacy is often related to severity of disease. Limited to three or four injections/years.
      - Offloader braces do have a limited role in your patients with single compartment disease; however, they are typically poorly tolerated.
      - Formal outpatient physical therapy can be useful on a limited basis in patients with significant deconditioning, lack of neuromuscular control, and in patients who are poor surgical candidates to optimize current functional status.
      - "Prehab" physical therapy prior to surgery has unclear benefits and may not be cost effective.
    - Surgical treatment: Surgical options are available for patients in whom conservative measures fail.
      - Arthroscopy does play a role in younger patients with limited radiographic evidence of arthritis and advanced imaging with identified unstable meniscal tears causing mechanical symptoms.
      - Patients should be counseled that symptomatic relief cannot be guaranteed and will likely be temporary if it occurs.
      - Routine arthroscopy for arthritis in the absence of clear mechanical symptoms is not indicated and does not appear to be superior to nonoperative management.
      - High tibial osteotomy (HTO)

- Young, active patients (laborers, higher-demand patients) with isolated medial or lateral compartment degenerative joint disease, mild deformity, with functional cruciate and collateral ligaments (see Fig. 151.3)
- Popularity of this procedure is decreasing for knee OA but continues to have a role alongside cartilage restoration procedures.
  - Unicompartmental knee arthroplasty (partial knee replacement)
    - Indications less defined and have expanded to younger patients
    - Potential candidates for a unicompartmental knee arthroplasty are similar to those considered for HTO. Isolated medial (most common) or lateral compartment degenerative joint disease with mild correctable deformity, intact cruciate and collateral ligaments, and possible restriction based on patient weight (see Fig. 151.1).
    - Generally considered to have more favorable functional outcomes when compared with HTO.
  - Potential limitations to HTOs and unicompartmental knee arthroplasties are their longevity. Compared with total knee replacement, rates of revision are significantly higher for unicompartmental arthroplasty.
  - Number one reason for revision for HTO and unicompartmental knee arthroplasty is advancement of disease in adjacent compartment.
  - Total knee arthroplasty: "gold standard" for knee arthritis (see Fig. 151.2)

When to Refer

- Those patients who have significant symptoms and radiographic evidence of advancing OA despite the previously listed therapies should be presented with surgical options and referred to an orthopaedic surgeon.
- Patients who are interested in considering surgery should be in the best possible physical condition and be committed to their health and rehabilitation after surgery.
- Medical conditions that may require optimization prior to proceeding with orthopaedic surgery for OA include:
  - Morbid obesity (BMI > 40)
  - Uncontrolled DM (hemoglobin A1c [Hb1Ac] >7.0 to 8.0)
  - Alcoholism
  - Poor nutritional status as noted by nutritional markers
  - Severe arthrofibrosis
  - Active infections or nonhealing wounds
  - Severe cardiopulmonary, renal, or liver disease, which makes the patient unfit to tolerate surgery
  - High doses of opioid pain medications
  - Smoking
  - Patients with unrealistic expectations

Prognosis

- Many patients with advanced knee OA will experience progressive symptoms with time, although this is not inevitable and the speed of disease progression cannot be predicted.

- The overall success rate of total knee arthroplasty is generally excellent in the appropriately selected, educated patient.
- Benefits include pain relief, improved quality of life and activities of daily living, regaining productivity with the workforce, and potentially returning to limited-impact activities and exercise.
- The cumulative life expectancy of a total knee replacement at 20 years approaches 90%.
- Younger (<55 age) male patients are at the highest risk for early failure.
- It is imperative to educate patient and set realistic expectations of the risks, benefits, limitations, and duration of recovery after a total knee replacement. Most patients experience improvements in pain and function but may still have some symptoms and limitations. Full recovery can take a year or more after surgery.
- Joint replacement, especially in the older population, carries a risk of intraoperative and postoperative medical complications such as deep venous thrombosis, pulmonary embolism, myocardial infarction, stroke, and even death. Arthroplasty also carries the risk of both early and late postoperative complications to include, but not limited to, infection, loosening of components, fracture, wear, debonding, instability, soft-tissue irritation, reactive synovitis, and potentially revision surgery.
- Changes in implant design and advancements in the load-bearing inserts known as polyethylene tibial inserts with more favorable wear characteristic may improve survivorship and longevity of total knee replacement.

Patient Instructions

- OA treatment is tailored to the individual patient and is based upon severity of pain and functional limitations, impact on quality of life and daily activities, and patient preferences.
- Overweight patients should be instructed on need for weight control to help relieve pain, as well as make them better candidates for joint replacement surgery.
- Morbidly obese patients may benefit from weight loss (including through bariatric surgery) prior to joint replacement surgery.
- Avoiding high-impact activities (running, jumping) and participating in low-impact exercise (cycling, swimming, elliptical training) can be helpful in decreasing stiffness and improving pain control.
- Surgical management is reserved for patients with severe OA who have failed nonoperative management and have appropriate and realistic expectations for the outcome of joint replacement.

- Younger patients should fully exhaust conservative measures and consider delaying unicompartmental or total knee arthroplasty because the life span for joint replacement is limited.

Future Considerations/Concerns

- Joint preservation: both conservative and surgical treatment
- Disease-modifying osteoarthritis drugs (DMOADs)
- Genetic component of OA
- Increasing demand for total knee arthroplasty both in the Baby Boomer population and younger patients
- Ever-expanding aging population with increasing life expectancy

Suggested Readings

American Academy of Orthopedic Surgeons: *Arthritis of the knee. OrthoInfo (website)*. Available at https://orthoinfo.aaos.org/en/diseases–conditions/arthritis-of-the-knee/. Accessed April 17, 2018.

American Academy of Orthopedic Surgeons: *Guidelines. Treatment of Osteoarthritis of the Knee. Evidence-Based Guideline*. 2nd Edition. Available at http://www.aaos.org/research/guidelines/guidelineoaknee.asp. Accessed April 17, 2018.

American Joint Replacement Registry (AJRR): #4. *2017 Annual Report*. IL, AJRR: Rosemont; 2017.

Fehring TK, Fehring K, Odum SM, Halsey D. Physical therapy mandates by medicare administrative contractors: effective or wasteful? *J Arthroplasty*. 2013;28(9):1459–1462.

Glassman AH, Lachiewicz PF, Tanzer M, eds. *Orthopaedic Knowledge Update: Hip and Knee Reconstruction*. 4th ed. American Academy of Orthopaedic Surgeons; 2011.

Leahy M. *Changing the Paradigm for Diagnosing and Treating Arthritis*. American Academy of Orthopaedic Surgeons; 2012. Available at: https://www.aaos.org/AAOSNow/2012/Nov/clinical/clinical6/. Accessed April 17, 2018.

Li CS, Karlsson J, Winemaker M, et al. Orthopedic surgeons feel that there is a treatment gap in management of early OA: international survey. *Knee Surg Sports Traumatol Arthros*. 2014;22(2):363–378.

Messier SP, Gutekunst DJ, Davis C, Devita P. Weight loss reduces knee-joint loads in overweight and obese older adults with knee osteoarthritis. *Arthritis Rheum*. 2005;52(7):2026–2032.

Morrey BF, Berry DJ, An K-N, et al, eds. *Joint Replacement Arthroplasty: Basic Science, Hip, Knee and Ankle, Fourth Centennial Edition*. Philadelphia: Lippincott Williams & Wilkins; 2011.

National Joint Registry: *14th Annual Report. Surgical Data to 31 December 2016*. Available at http://www.njrreports.org.uk/Portals/0/PDFdownloads/NJR%2014th%20Annual%20Report%202017.pdf. Accessed April 17, 2018.

Sridhar MS, Jarrett CD, Xerogeanes JW, Labib SA. Obesity and symptomatic osteoarthritis of the knee. *J Bone Joint Surg Br*. 2012;94(4):433–440.

Chapter 152 Baker Cyst (Popliteal Cyst)

Michael Rosen, Julie Dodds

ICD-10-CM CODES
M71.21 *Synovial cyst of popliteal space, right*
M71.22 *Synovial cyst of popliteal space, left*

Key Concepts

- Popliteal cysts, often also referred to as Baker cysts, are a common occurrence in the adult knee
- Classic cyst location is in posteromedial knee between the medial head of the gastrocnemius (MHG) muscle and the semimembranosus muscle
- Medial meniscal tears have been noted to be the most common pathology associated with popliteal cysts
- Asymptomatic cysts can be managed conservatively, whereas surgery is recommended for persistent cases
- There is a reproducible and straightforward arthroscopic treatment for this pathology, and open treatment is rarely indicated

History

- Posteromedial knee mass and aching are the most common presenting symptoms
- Sensation of fullness with intermittent posteromedial pain with cyst distension
- May see tibial nerve compression leading to pain, gastrocnemius weakness and atrophy, or paresthesias
- Popliteal cyst rupture has been known to cause acute compartment syndrome, necessitating fasciotomy
- May be incidental magnetic resonance imaging (MRI) finding or severe enough to cause nerve and/or vascular complications

Physical Exam

- Patient should begin supine with knee in full extension; posterior palpation will often reveal a firm, tender mass.
  - This should be repeated in various degrees of flexion for change in size or tenderness, known as "Foucher sign"
- A mass can usually be palpated at or just below the joint line slightly medial to the midline in the popliteal fossa.
- Medial position is due to the position of the cyst between the MHG muscle and the semimembranosus muscle (Fig. 152.1).

- Popliteal cysts can occasionally extend proximally, leading to fullness above the joint line in a more central location along the course of the semimembranosus tendon.
- Ruptured cysts can cause acute compartment syndrome findings, such as pain with passive dorsiflexion of the foot.
- Venous compression can cause swelling and lymphedema.
- Tibial nerve compression can cause gastrocnemius atrophy and weakness, or paresthesias.
- Cysts exceeding 5 cm are more likely symptomatic.
- Pain from popliteal cysts is often difficult to differentiate from other pathology such as posterior horn of medial meniscal tears.

Imaging
Magnetic Resonance Imaging

- Have been identified on 5% of all knee MRIs
- Essential for preoperative planning prior to arthroscopic treatment of the cyst
  - Although rare, popliteal artery aneurysms, synovial cell sarcomas, and hemangiomas can be mistaken for popliteal cysts on initial presentation
- MRI also is needed to define any underlying pathology that may predispose the patient to cyst, such as meniscal tears and chondral injury.
- The valvular communication between the cyst and the joint is almost always present between the MHG and the semimembranosus tendon.
- This is best identified on the axial sections.
- Locating the most superficial portion of the cyst on MRI is important if cyst excision or loose body excision is to be performed.
  - This can be best identified on both the sagittal and coronal sections (Fig. 152.2).

Ultrasound (US)

- Can also be used to diagnose and define a popliteal cyst
- Must have an excellent understanding of the images and have the ability to identify surrounding structures.
- It is essential to have knowledge of the actual shape and position of the cyst.

Differential Diagnosis

- Posterior horn of medial meniscal tear: joint line tenderness, mechanical symptoms such as locking, clicking, catching
- Degenerative joint disease: aching, stiffness

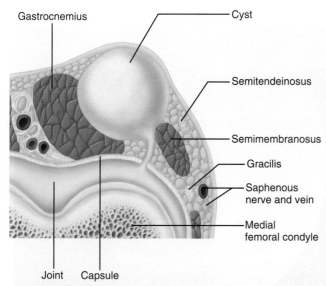

Fig 152.1 Axial view of knee demonstrating typical position of popliteal cyst medial to the medial head of the gastrocnemius muscle and lateral to the semimembranosus muscle.

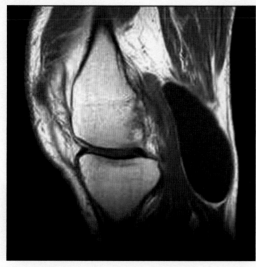

Fig 152.2 Sagittal magnetic resonance imaging of popliteal cysts with extension superior and inferior joint line extension.

- Deep venous thrombosis: calf edema, tenderness
- Although rare, must differentiate popliteal cyst from popliteal artery aneurysm, synovial cell sarcoma, or hemangioma

Treatment

- Nonsurgical treatment has consisted of nonsteroidal anti-inflammatory drugs (NSAIDs), intra-articular corticosteroid injection, compressive sleeves, and direct cyst aspiration with steroid injection
- If intra-articular pathology exists, complete nonsurgical treatment may be less effective
- Addressing the intra-articular pathology, such as performing meniscectomy, may be adequate to allow the joint effusion to dissipate and the cyst may resolve on its own

- However, in patients with intra-articular pathology that cannot be corrected by arthroscopic means, such as high-grade chondral lesions (grade 3 and 4), the cyst often remains following arthroscopy, leading to poor patient satisfaction
- Symptomatic popliteal cysts in these patients are amenable to arthroscopic decompression of the cyst
- Arthroscopic decompression (Fig. 152.3)
  - Spinal needle is used for localization under direct arthroscopic visualization
  - Transillumination may be used to identify and overlying vascular structures.
  - Valvular flap known as the posterior transverse synovial infold (PoTSI) has been consistently seen as cause of one-way valve effect and should be addressed to minimize risk of popliteal cyst recurrence.
  - "Puff" of cyst fluid frequently noted after decompression. This fluid is usually more viscous and more yellowish than the synovial fluid and can be easily identified.
  - Remove any intra-articular loose bodies that may be within popliteal cyst.
  - Complete cyst resection is generally unnecessary, as decompression alone often leads to resolution.

When to Refer

- Popliteal cysts without acute worsening can be initially managed nonsurgically as described previously, especially in the pediatric patient
- Appropriate diagnostic imaging may expedite treatment for symptomatic surgical candidates
- Large, symptomatic cysts, especially those >5 cm in size, should be evaluated for surgical management
- Patients presenting with signs concerning for neurovascular compression should be referred
- Acute cyst rupture leading to signs concerning for compartment syndrome, namely pain out of proportion, excessive pain on passive dorsiflexion of the foot, and firm compartments, necessitates emergent orthopaedic evaluation

Prognosis

- In adults, asymptomatic cysts may be monitored and managed conservatively
- High recurrence rate for nonsurgical measures that fail to address any underlying intra-articular pathology
- Symptomatic patients may be treated surgically after failure of nonoperative interventions
- Initial recommendations for arthroscopic surgery, with open excision rarely indicated

Troubleshooting

- Benefits and risks should be detailed for all surgical patients
  - Benefits include popliteal cyst resolution and decreased posterior knee fullness. Pain improvement may be noted posteriorly after the mass effect has been relieved.
  - Risks are minimal with arthroscopic decompression and namely involve incomplete decompression and recurrence.

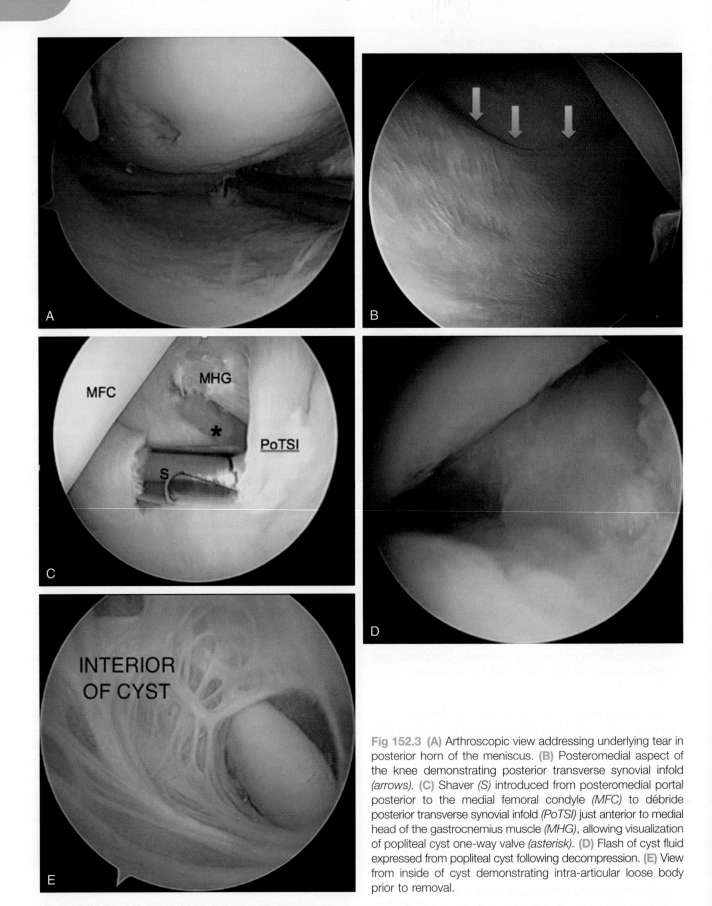

Fig 152.3 (A) Arthroscopic view addressing underlying tear in posterior horn of the meniscus. (B) Posteromedial aspect of the knee demonstrating posterior transverse synovial infold *(arrows)*. (C) Shaver *(S)* introduced from posteromedial portal posterior to the medial femoral condyle *(MFC)* to débride posterior transverse synovial infold *(PoTSI)* just anterior to medial head of the gastrocnemius muscle *(MHG)*, allowing visualization of popliteal cyst one-way valve *(asterisk)*. (D) Flash of cyst fluid expressed from popliteal cyst following decompression. (E) View from inside of cyst demonstrating intra-articular loose body prior to removal.

- Intra-articular loose bodies may be seen on preoperative MRI imaging and should be removed.
- Knee effusions and swelling are common after any arthroscopic procedure, and patients should be aware it may take several weeks or months to resolve.
- Popliteal cyst excision requires the creation of a postero-medial portal.
  - Only blunt trocars should be used to introduce the posteromedial cannula.
  - Care must be taken not to "plunge" into the compartment. The popliteal artery, vein, and nerve can lie directly in the path of the cannula if placed too deep.

Patient Instructions

- Compressive dressing is placed over the posteromedial knee, with care not to compromise the popliteal fossa.
- If cyst excision is performed, the patient is placed in intermittent pneumatic compression socks for 2 weeks to add additional compression.
- Full range of motion is allowed postoperatively.
- Leg elevation is essential to avoid knee and lower leg swelling.
- The patient is encouraged to bear weight as tolerated; discontinuing crutches as able and the performance of ankle pumps is advised to minimize risk of venous thrombosis.

- Gradual return to activities of daily living and sports activities, if applicable, is allowed.
- Patients usually return to all activities by 4 to 6 weeks postoperatively.

Considerations in Special Populations

- In children, cysts are generally self-limited and rarely associated with intra-articular pathology and should therefore be treated with observation

Suggested Readings

Baker WM. On the formation of synovial cysts in the leg in connection with disease of the knee-joint: 1877. *Clin Orthop Relat Res*. 1994;299:2–10.

Canoso JJ, Goldsmith MR, Gerzof SG, et al. Foucher's sign of the Baker's cyst. *Ann Rheum Dis*. 1987;46:228–232.

Johnson LL, van Dyk GE, Johnson CA, et al. The popliteal bursa (Baker's cyst): an arthroscopic perspective and the epidemiology. *Arthroscopy*. 1997;13:66–72.

Rauschning W. Anatomy and function of the communication between knee joint and popliteal bursae. *Ann Rheum Dis*. 1980;39:354–358.

Seil R, Rupp S, Jochum P, et al. Prevalence of popliteal cysts in children: a sonographic study and review of the literature. *Arch Orthop Trauma Surg*. 1999;119:73–75.

Stone KR, Stoller D, De Carli A, et al. The frequency of Baker's cysts associated with meniscal tears. *Am J Sports Med*. 1996;24:670–671.

Chapter 153 Patellofemoral Pain Syndrome

Scott Linger, Marc Tompkins

ICD-10-CM CODES
M22.2x1 *Patellofemoral disorders, right knee*
M22.2x2 *Patellofemoral disorders, left knee*
M22.2x9 *Patellofemoral disorders, unspecified knee*

Key Concepts

- Patellofemoral pain syndrome, or anterior knee pain, is defined as retropatellar or peripatellar pain resulting from physical and biomechanical changes in the patellofemoral joint.
- Spectrum of pathology from soft-tissue inflammation to severe arthritic changes.
- History and physical examination typically provide diagnosis.
- Treatment with activity modification, rest, and physical therapy is usually successful.

History

- Pain is localized to the anterior knee or "under" the patella.
- Pain interferes with work/sports.
- Daily living activities such as stair climbing, prolonged sitting, and rising from a seated position may exacerbate symptoms.
- May report symptoms consistent with depression or anxiety.

Physical Examination
Observation

- Gait
- Lower extremity alignment (knee valgus, femoral anteversion, tibial torsion, foot pronation)
- Weakness or poor neuromuscular control during single leg squat

Palpation

- Tenderness medial or lateral patellar facet
- Assess patellar mobility: with or without tight lateral retinaculum (Fig. 153.1)

Range of Motion

- Patellofemoral crepitus

Specific Tests

- +/− effusion
- Quadriceps weakness against resistance
- Patellar tests: tilt, grind, glide, and J sign

Imaging

- Radiographs: anteroposterior, lateral, and patellofemoral (20 degrees of flexion) views of the knee
  - May show patella tilting or patellofemoral joint space narrowing (Fig. 153.2)
  - Trochlear dysplasia or patella alta
- Magnetic resonance imaging
  - Typically not necessary; consider in cases of refractory symptoms
  - Effusion and patellofemoral chondral changes
  - Anatomic factors such as trochlear dysplasia, patella alta, or extensor mechanism malalignment
- Computed tomography
  - In cases of suspected tibial torsion or femoral anteversion

Differential Diagnosis

- Patellofemoral arthritis
- Hip arthritis, medial/lateral knee arthritis
- Patellar instability
- Stress fracture patella
- Chondral lesion/osteochondritis dissecans patella or trochlea
- Iliotibial syndrome
- Patellar or quadriceps tendinitis

Treatment
At Diagnosis

- Physical therapy including stretching and strengthening exercises (specifically vastus medialis oblique [VMO], core, and hip strengthening), ice, ultrasound, and electrical stimulation is beneficial (Fig. 153.3)
- McConnell or kinesio tape (KT) taping as adjunct to traditional exercise therapy
- Rest and activity modification
- Obesity should be addressed in cases in which it is a contributing factor
- Appropriate screening and treatment for depression and anxiety

Later

- Surgical intervention is considered only after failure of extensive conservative management including a formal physical therapy program
- Surgical procedures generally focused on decreasing the stress between patella and trochlea; may include lateral retinacular lengthening, tibial tubercle osteotomy, or derotational osteotomies

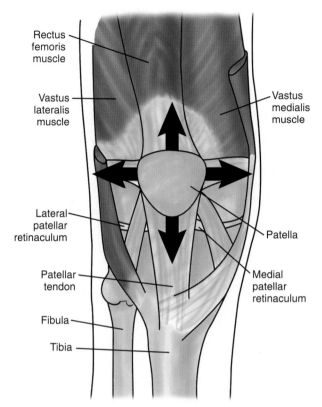

Fig 153.1 The patella is stabilized by dynamic (muscles) and static (retinaculum and tendon) restraints. In patellofemoral pain syndrome, the lateral retinaculum can become tight.

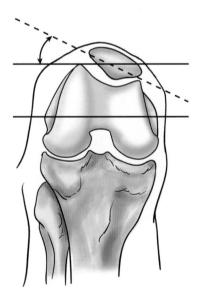

Fig 153.2 Patellar tilt is a function of the tightness in the lateral retinaculum.

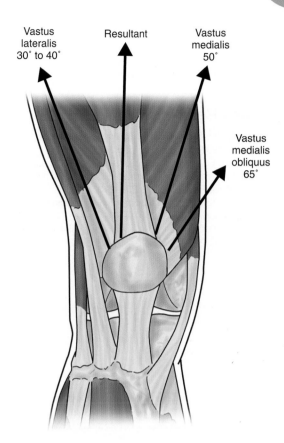

Fig 153.3 The quadriceps muscle influences the patella. Weakness in the quadriceps, or the core musculature, can have a significant influence on the forces experienced in the patellofemoral joint, which in turn has a role in patellofemoral pain.

When to Refer

- Failure of 3 to 6 months of appropriate conservative treatments, including rest, ice, activity modifications, and physical therapy warrants referral.

Prognosis

- Good
- Typically a self-limiting condition
- The majority of patients obtain symptom resolution with conservative management

Troubleshooting

- Consider multifactorial etiology: may include muscular (weak core/quadriceps muscles) (see Fig. 153.3), biomechanical (knee valgus, femoral anteversion, tibial torsion, foot pronation), and overuse issues.
- Psychiatric comorbidities such as anxiety and depression may be exacerbating factor.

Patient Instructions

- Diligence and patience with rehabilitation are critical.
- Notify your physician if symptoms of instability, loose body sensations, or mechanical symptoms such as locking and catching develop.

Acknowledgment

The authors wish to thank Dr. Richard Parker for his contributions to this chapter in the previous edition.

Suggested Readings

Cutbill JW, Ladly KO, Bray RC, et al. Anterior knee pain: A review. *Clin J Sport Med*. 1997;7:40–45.

Finestone A, Radin EL, Lev B, et al. Treatment of overuse patellofemoral pain. Prospective randomized controlled clinical trial in a military setting. *Clin Orthop Relat Res*. 1993;293:208–210.

Fulkerson JP. A practical guide to understanding and treating patellofemoral pain. *Am J Orthop*. 2017;46(2):101–103.

Koh TJ, Grabiner MD, De Swart RJ. In vivo tracking of the human patella. *J Biomech*. 1992;25:637–643.

Lester JD, Watson JN, Hutchinson MR. Physical examination of the patellofemoral joint. *Clin Sports Med*. 2014;33(3):403–412.

Logan CA, Bhashyam AR, Tisosky AJ, et al. Systematic review of the effect of taping techniques on patellofemoral pain syndrome. *Sports Health*. 2017;9(5):456–461.

Maclachlan LR, Collins NJ, Matthews MLG, et al. The psychological features of patellofemoral pain: a systematic review. *Br J Sports Med*. 2017;51(9):732–742.

Rothermich MA, Glaviano NR, Li J, Hart JM. Patellofemoral pain: epidemiology, pathophysiology, and treatment options. *Clin Sports Med*. 2015;34(2):313–327.

Thomee R, Renstrom P, Karlsson J, et al. Patellofemoral pain syndrome in young women. I. A clinical analysis of alignment, pain parameters, common symptoms and functional activity level. *Scand J Med Sci Sports*. 1995;5:237–244.

Tria AJ Jr, Palumbo RC, Alicea JA. Conservative care for patellofemoral pain. *Orthop Clin North Am*. 1992;23:545–554.

Chapter 154 Patellar Instability

Christopher E. Urband, Marc Tompkins

ICD-10-CM CODE
S83.0 *Subluxation and dislocation of patella*

Key Concepts

- The chief complaint is instability, not pain
- Can occur secondary to severe trauma or with minimal trauma
- Treatment varies depending on all components of the history, physical examination, imaging, and previous treatment
- Consider all potential factors contributing to instability and address as many as possible both nonsurgically and surgically

History

- Patient feels patella move out of place
- Patient reports pain; may note swelling
- Injury occurred
  - May be contact or noncontact
  - May be high or low energy
- Patient often presents with the fear that the patella will dislocate again
- The patient often can describe the injury(ies) and whether the patella subluxed, dislocated and spontaneously reduced, or had to be manually reduced
  - Important for understanding severity of injury and potential for chondral damage
- Can present as acute, subacute, or chronic patellar instability
- Inquire about loose body symptoms, duration of pain and swelling associated with instability episodes, number of instability events, if frequency of instability events is changing, activities associated with instability, and the degree of trauma required for the instability event
  - Important in surgical decision making

Physical Examination

- Observation
  - Gait
  - Neuromuscular coordination and movement patterns (i.e., anterior knee loading, valgus)
  - Lower extremity alignment
    - Q angle in both extension and flexion (tubercle sulcus angle)
    - Rotational malalignment
  - Effusion
    - Hemarthrosis is common, but with large effusion/hemarthrosis, must rule out anterior cruciate ligament (ACL) or meniscal tear.

- Palpation
  - Degree of lateral translation of patella by quadrant
  - Presence of end point during lateral translation
  - Tenderness, especially medial patella or lateral femoral condyle
  - Evaluate lateral retinaculum and if possible to tip patella to neutral
  - If loose body present, may palpate loose body
- Range of motion
  - Apprehension with forced lateral translation during range of motion
  - J sign
  - Crepitus
- Assess for generalized ligamentous laxity
- General knee exam including ligamentous exam

Imaging (Fig. 154.1)

- Radiographs: anteroposterior, true lateral, and patellofemoral (20 degree) views of the knee
  - May demonstrate trochlear dysplasia, patella alta, patella tilt, patellar degenerative change, or loose body
- Full-length standing radiographs—if excessive valgus suspected
- Magnetic resonance imaging
  - Evaluate for effusion, medial patellofemoral ligament disruption, loose body, chondral injury (medial patellar facet most common), subchondral edema of the lateral femoral condyle and/or medial patella (typical bone bruise pattern), trochlear dysplasia, patella alta, patella tilt, Q angle (tibial tubercle-trochlear groove distance or tibial tubercle-posterior cruciate ligament [PCL] distance)
- Computed tomography (CT) scan—if rotational malalignment suspected
  - Hip, knee, ankle to evaluate femoral version or tibial torsion

Differential Diagnosis

- Anterior cruciate ligament rupture
- Chondral injury with or without loose body
- Meniscus tear
- Patellofemoral pain syndrome

Treatment

- Nonoperative management
  - Ensure that the patella is reduced
  - Aspiration may be indicated if severe effusion exists and is affecting rehabilitation

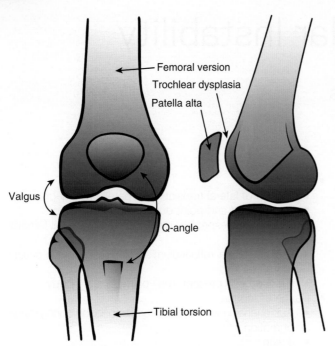

Fig 154.1 Potential sites of anatomic abnormalities.

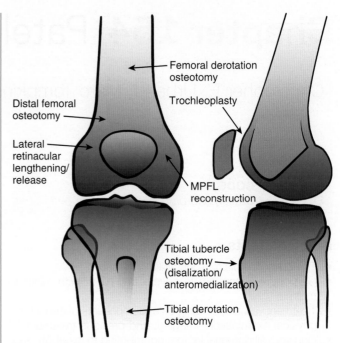

Fig 154.2 Types of potential surgical intervention. *MPFL,* Medial patellofemoral ligament.

- Initial immobilization is controversial but may be helpful in patients with severe swelling or pain; limit to a short duration only
- Bracing and taping (especially McConnell taping) may be helpful
- Physical therapy
  - Critical in nonoperative and postoperative rehabilitation
  - Must address poor neuromuscular coordination and at-risk movement patterns using various modalities
  - Strengthening includes vastus medialis obliquus/quadriceps muscles, as well as hip and core musculature
- Operative management (Fig. 154.2)
  - Surgery following primary dislocation generally reserved for a loose body or osteochondral fracture (at this time, standard of care for a first time dislocator is nonoperative management)
  - Patients with recurrent dislocations may be candidates for surgical intervention.
  - Arthroscopy is helpful to treat loose bodies and chondral pathology; however, open surgery is generally required to stabilize the patella
  - Proximal realignment
    - Medial patellofemoral ligament (MPFL) reconstruction (MPFL repair generally reserved for surgery that is necessary following primary dislocation but not recurrent dislocations)
    - Lateral retinacular lengthening or lateral release
  - Distal realignment
    - Tibial tubercle osteotomy with distalization, medialization, anteriorization, or a combination of the three
  - Trochleoplasty
    - Removal of supratrochlear spur
    - Trochlear groove deepening
  - Coronal plane
    - Distal femoral osteotomy

- Axial plane
  - Femoral or tibial derotational osteotomies
- Surgical approach depends on areas of anatomic abnormality—often a combination of the aforementioned procedures

When to Refer
- Recurrent dislocations
- Primary dislocations with osteochondral injury
- Failure of nonoperative management
- Athletes should be referred after a first-time dislocation

Prognosis
- Generally good but depends on thoughtful, step-wise approach
- Instability often can be improved, but alleviation of pain is less predictable
- Patients with recurrent dislocations and with bony anatomic abnormalities have higher risk of recurrence after treatment
- Risk of contralateral injury is present

Troubleshooting
- Important to consider and address underlying anatomic abnormalities
- Emphasize the importance of physical therapy, both nonoperative and postoperative
- Refer to expert if necessary

Patient Instructions
- Patients should be instructed to complete the nonoperative rehabilitation protocol because this is effective in preventing

recurrence in many patients and also helps with postoperative rehabilitation in patients that ultimately require surgery
- Patients should be instructed to report any recurrent episodes of instability or recurrent sensations of apprehension

Suggested Readings

Arendt EA, Moeller A, Agel J. Clinical outcomes of medial patellofemoral ligament repair in recurrent (chronic) lateral patella dislocations. *Knee Surg Sports Traumatol Arthrosc*. 2011;19(11):1909–1914.

Buckens CFM, Saris DBF. Reconstruction of the medial patellofemoral ligament for treatment of patellofemoral instability: A systematic review. *Am J Sports Med*. 2010;38(1):181–188.

Carstensen SE, Menzer HM, Diduch DR. Patellar instability: when is trochleoplasty necessary? *Sports Med Arthrosc*. 2017;25(2):92–99.

Charles MD, Haloman S, Chen L, et al. Magnetic resonance imaging-based topographical differences between control and recurrent patellofemoral instability patients. *Am J Sports Med*. 2013;41(2):374–384.

Drexler M, Dwyer T, Dolkart O, et al. Tibial rotational osteotomy and distal tuberosity transfer for patella subluxation secondary to excessive external tibial torsion: surgical technique and clinical outcome. *Knee Surg Sports Traumatol Arthrosc*. 2014;22(11):2682–2689.

Duerr RA, Chauhan A, Frank DA, et al. An algorithm for diagnosing and treating primary and recurrent patellar instability. *JBJS Rev*. 2016;4(9).

Liu JN, Steinhaus ME, Kalbian IL, et al. Patellar instability management: A survey of the international patellofemoral study group. *Am J Sports Med*. 2017;[E-pub ahead of print].

Magnussen RA, De Simone V, Lustig S, et al. Treatment of patella alta in patients with episodic patellar dislocation: A systematic review. *Knee Surg Sports Traumatol Arthrosc*. 2014;22(10):2545–2550.

Nelitz M, Dreyhaupt J, Williams SRM, et al. Combined supracondylar femoral derotation osteotomy and patellofemoral ligament reconstruction for recurrent patellar dislocation and severe femoral anteversion syndrome: surgical technique and clinical outcome. *Int Orthop*. 2015;39(12):2355–2362.

Ntagiopoulos PG, Byn P, Dejour D. Midterm results of comprehensive surgical reconstruction including sulcus-deepening trochleoplasty in recurrent patellar dislocations with high-grade trochlear dysplasia. *Am J Sports Med*. 2013;41(5):998–1004.

Pagenstert G, Wolf N, Bachmann M, et al. Open lateral patellar retinacular lengthening versus open retinacular release in lateral patellar hypercompression syndrome: A prospective double-blinded comparative study on complications and outcome. *Arthroscopy*. 2012;28(6):788–797.

Schneider DK, Grawe B, Magnussen RA, et al. Outcomes after isolated medial patellofemoral ligament reconstruction for the treatment of recurrent lateral patellar dislocations: A systematic review and meta-analysis. *Am J Sports Med*. 2016;44(11):2993–3005.

Sherman SL, Erickson BJ, Cvetanovich GL, et al. Tibial tuberosity osteotomy: indications, techniques, and outcomes. *Am J Sports Med*. 2014;42(8):2006–2017.

Steensen RN, Bentley JC, Trinh TQ, et al. The prevalence and combined prevalences of anatomic factors associated with recurrent patellar dislocation: A magnetic resonance imaging study. *Am J Sports Med*. 2015;43(4):921–927.

Swarup I, Elattar O, Rozbruch SR. Patellar instability treated with distal femoral osteotomy. *Knee*. 2017;24(3):608–614.

Weber AE, Nathani A, Dines JS, et al. An algorithmic approach to the management of recurrent lateral patellar dislocation. *J Bone Joint Surg Am*. 2016;98(5):417–427.

Chapter 155 Iliotibial Band Syndrome

Dennis Q. Chen, Brian C. Werner

ICD-10-CM CODES
M76.30   *Iliotibial band syndrome, unspecified leg*
M76.31   *Iliotibial band syndrome, right leg*
M76.32   *Iliotibial band syndrome, left leg*

Key Concepts

- Involves the distal iliotibial band (ITB) and lateral femoral epicondyle (LFE) (Fig. 155.1).
- Primarily an overuse injury seen in long-distance runners, cyclists, cross-country skiers, and military recruits following repetitive knee flexion and extension.
- Proposed etiologies include: friction of the ITB against the LFE, compression of soft tissues deep to the ITB, and chronic inflammation of the ITB bursa.
- Differential diagnosis includes lateral meniscus tear, lateral collateral ligament injury, arthritis, patellofemoral pain, patellofemoral instability, and osteochondroma of the lateral femoral condyle.
- Medical management consists of rest, ice, nonsteroidal antiinflammatory drugs, activity modification, stretching, and cortisone injection.
- Surgery may be considered in refractory cases after all conservative measures have been exhausted.
- Slow return to sport.

History

- Insidious onset, worsens with activity, and responds initially to rest
- Patient can point to exact area of involvement over the LFE

Physical Examination
Observation

- Swelling over area of tenderness with soft-tissue thickening

Palpation

- Minimal to no knee effusion
- Tender to palpation at the LFE but no lateral joint line tenderness

Range of Motion

- Tight ITB

Special Tests

- Noble test: With patient supine, the affected knee is flexed to 90 degrees. The knee is then extended with direct pressure

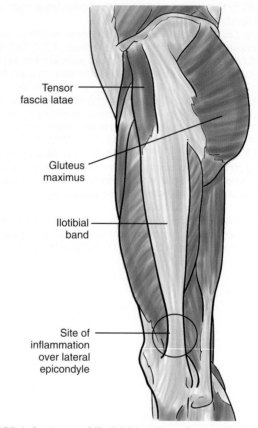

Tensor fascia latae

Gluteus maximus

Ilotibial band

Site of inflammation over lateral epicondyle

Fig 155.1 Anatomy of iliotibial band syndrome. Note the area of involvement over the lateral femoral epicondyle.

over the LFE. Reproducible pain near 30 degrees of knee flexion indicates a positive test.
- Ober test: With patient on his or her side (unaffected knee down and flexed to 90 degrees), the affected knee is flexed to 90 degrees with the hip in an extended and abducted position. The hip is then passively adducted by the examiner. Inability to adduct the leg to horizontal indicates a positive test.
- Thomas test: With the patient supine at the edge of the bed, the patient holds the unaffected leg to the chest while the affected leg is extended and lowered. Inability to completely extend and lower the affected leg to horizontal indicates a positive test.
- Negative McMurray test
- Stable knee ligament examination
- Benign patella examination

Imaging

- Radiographs of the knee are typically normal.
- Magnetic resonance imaging (MRI) shows increased fluid signal in the area between the LFE and ITB, often with associated reactive edema of the LFE and thickening of the ITB.
- Ultrasound (US) demonstrates edematous swelling of the soft tissues between the ITB and the LFE.

Additional Tests

- ITB injection may be diagnostic and therapeutic
  - Lidocaine (1%) injection test: Injecting 5 mL at the level of the LFE provides pain relief in the physician's office.
  - Bupivacaine (0.25%) injection test: Have the patient perform the aggravating activity (running) after the injection to determine whether symptoms are relieved.

Differential Diagnosis

- Lateral meniscus tear
- Lateral collateral ligament pathology
- Biceps femoris tendinopathy
- Knee arthritis
- Lateral femoral condyle osteochondroma
- Patellofemoral pain
- Patellofemoral instability
- Hip disease
- Stress fracture

Treatment
At Diagnosis

- Conservative measures are the mainstay of treatment and include rest, ice, physical therapy for stretching and strengthening, orthotics, and cross-training (Fig. 155.2).
- Cortisone injections to the area of maximal tenderness may also provide significant relief.

Later

- If all conservative measures have failed and the patient is unwilling to change sports/activities, surgical intervention may be considered.
- Surgery typically involves knee arthroscopy to rule out intra-articular knee pathology, followed by open exploration of the

Iliotibial band syndrome

- Overuse injury commonly seen in runners and cyclists (repetitive knee flexion and extension)

- Localized lateral tenderness worse with knee flexion to 30°

- Usually resolves with conservative treatment: rest, stretching, physical therapy, steroid injection, slow return to sport

- Elliptical excision or fenestration of the ITB and debridement of underlying tissue may be required in refractory cases

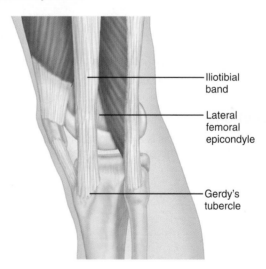

Iliotibial band

Lateral femoral epicondyle

Gerdy's tubercle

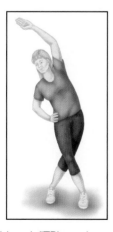
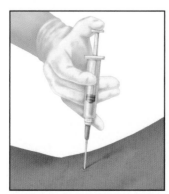
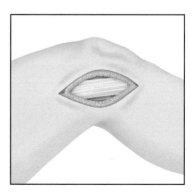

Fig 155.2 Iliotibial band *(ITB)* syndrome. Mainstay of treatment is conservative therapy with activity modification, rest, stretching, and cortisone injection. Surgery is reserved for refractory cases.

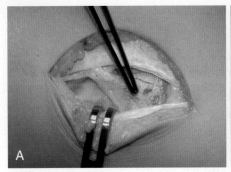 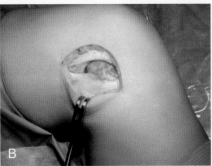

Fig 155.3 (A) Bursitis at the lateral femoral condyle. **(B)** After removal of bursitis, shaving of the lateral femoral epicondyle and excision of a portion of the iliotibial band is performed.

area with débridement of the synovium or bursa, shaving of any bony prominences, and excision or fenestration (piecrusting) of the ITB over the lateral femoral condyle (Fig. 155.3).
- Postsurgical rehabilitation is focused on slow strengthening, core strengthening, ITB stretching, orthotics, and slow return to sport.

When to Refer

- Patients who fail a minimum of 6 weeks of conservative treatment, including formal physical therapy, are appropriate for referral.

Prognosis

- Approximately 44% return to sport at 8 weeks and 91.7% return to sport at 6 months with conservative therapy alone.

Patient Instructions

- Patients should be aware that this is a diagnosis of exclusion, and recovery (after nonoperative or operative treatment) is slow.

Suggested Readings

Baker RL, Fredericson M. Iliotibial band syndrome in runners: biomechanical implications and exercise interventions. *Phys Med Rehabil Clin N Am.* 2016;27(1):53–77.

Beals C, Flanigan D. A review of treatments for iliotibial band syndrome in the athletic population. *J Sports Med.* 2013;2013:367169.

DeLee JC, Drez D Jr, Miller M, eds. *DeLee and Drez's Orthopaedic Sports Medicine: Principles and Practice.* 2nd ed. Philadelphia: WB Saunders; 1994.

Drogset JO, Rossvoll I, Grontvedt T. Surgical treatment of iliotibial band friction syndrome. A retrospective study of 45 patients. *Scand J Med Sci Sports.* 1999;9:296–298.

Fairclough J, Hayashi K, Toumi H, et al. The functional anatomy of the iliotibial band during flexion and extension of the knee: implications for understanding iliotibial band syndrome. *J Anat.* 2006;208(3):309–316.

Flato R, Passanante GJ, Skalski MR, et al. The iliotibial tract: imaging, anatomy, injuries, and other pathology. *Skeletal Radiol.* 2017;46(5):605–622.

Fredericson M, Cookingham CL, Chaudhari AM, et al. Hip abductor weakness in distance runners with iliotibial band syndrome. *Clin J Sport Med.* 2000;10:169–175.

Strauss EJ, Kim S, Calcei JG, Park D. Iliotibial band syndrome: evaluation and management. *J Am Acad Orthop Surg.* 2011;19(12):728–736.

Chapter 156 Quadriceps and Patellar Tendinitis

Michelle E. Kew, Brian C. Werner

ICD-10-CM CODES
M76.50   *Patellar tendinitis*
M76.51   *Patellar tendinitis*
M76.52   *Patellar tendinitis*
M70.50   *Quadriceps tendinitis*
M70.51   *Quadriceps tendinitis*
M70.52   *Quadriceps tendinitis*

Key Concepts

- Quadriceps and patellar tendinitis are usually secondary to overuse.
- Physical examination often reveals tight musculature and tenderness at the site.
- Magnetic resonance imaging can be helpful to isolate the area of discomfort; however, it is usually a clinical diagnosis.
- Treatment includes modification of activities, focus on eccentric exercises.

History

- Usually associated with overuse; associated with jumping sports, sudden increase in activity
- Gradual onset with pain in distal pole of the patella
- Symptoms improve with short periods of rest, but recur and can affect sports performance

Physical Examination

- Observation
  - Focal swelling, knee alignment
- Palpation
  - Identify areas of tenderness, especially at proximal patellar tendon or distal pole of the patella with leg fully extended
  - Minimal to no effusion
- Range of motion
  - Look for loss of flexibility in hamstring, quadriceps, and Achilles tendons
- Special tests
  - Evaluate core strength; may have quadriceps weakness
  - Decline squat test: Produces substantial load on patellar tendon, causing pain
  - Evaluate knee ligament exam and quadriceps/patellar tendon for evidence of rupture

Imaging

- Radiographs: Anteroposterior, lateral, and patellofemoral views of the knee
- Rule out fracture, evaluate for malalignment or patella alta, patella baja
- Magnetic resonance imaging
  - Shows increased signal in posterior proximal patellar tendon; may see tendon thickening (Fig. 156.1)
  - Can be used to rule out other intra-articular pathologies

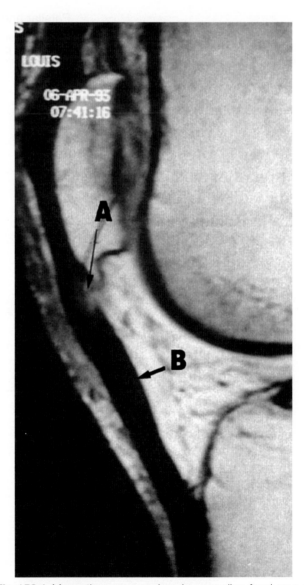

Fig 156.1 Magnetic resonance imaging revealing focal area of patellar tendinosis (A) compared with normal tendon signal (B). Note the area of tendinosis is located at the bone-tendon junction.

- Ultrasonography
  - Used to locate intratendinous lesions; will appear as areas of low echogenicity in posterior patellar tendon

Differential Diagnosis

- Quadriceps or patellar tendon rupture
- Partial tendon tear
- Patellofemoral pain syndrome
- Prepatellar bursitis

Treatment

- Nonoperative treatment
  - Patients should be encouraged to rest with activity modifications.
  - Eccentric exercises are used as the initial treatment for both athletes and nonathletes.

- Local modalities such as ultrasound, ice, and electrical stimulation are appropriate.
- Steroid injections not recommended; studies have failed to show long-term improvement.
- Extracorporeal shock wave therapy, platelet-rich plasma, hyaluronic acid have all been evaluated as potential therapies; however, further validation studies are required.
- Surgical treatment
  - Reserved for patients who fail nonoperative therapies, usually less than 10% of patients
  - Both open and arthroscopic techniques exist for patellar and quadriceps tendon debridement.
  - Goals of surgery are to excise abnormal tissue, induce repair process with patellar drilling, marginal resection.
  - Rehabilitation includes free range of motion, pain management, eccentric squats, strengthening (Fig. 156.2).

Patellar and Quadriceps Tendinitis

- Usually due to overuse, with exam revealing tenderness at proximal or distal pole of patella.
- Clinical exam is most important part of diagnosis.
- Mainstay of treatment is eccentric exercises, rest, may require operative debridement.

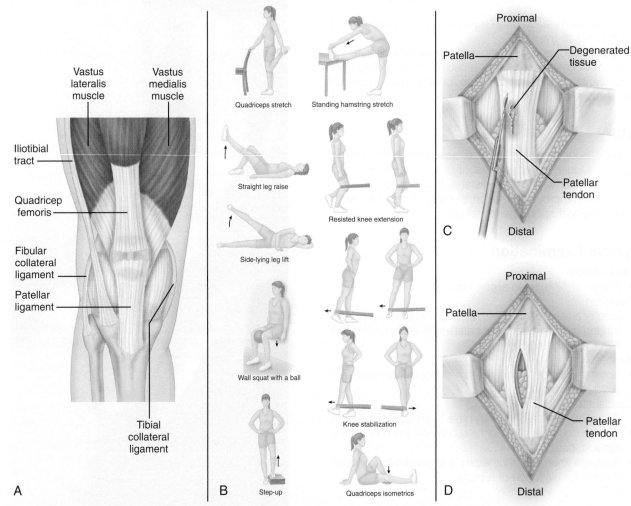

Fig 156.2 Patellar and quadriceps tendinitis. **(A)** Anatomy of patellar and quadriceps tendons showing anatomic location and local muscular and ligamentous structures. **(B)** Eccentric exercises are first step in treatment and encompass a wide variety of exercises as shown. **(C and D)** Schematic of operative debridement showing degenerative tissue **(C)** with excision **(D)**; this step in treatment is reserved for patients who fail lengthy nonoperative management.

When to Refer

- Referral is indicated after failure of appropriate conservative treatment for a minimum of 3 months.

Prognosis

- Good when recognized early and completely treated

Troubleshooting

- Beware of associated metabolic diseases.
- Do not underestimate the value of rest and core strengthening.

Patient Instructions

- Patients should be encouraged to adhere to the treatment regimen, specifically activity modification.
- Stretching and correction of training errors are imperative.

Suggested Readings

Basso O, Johnson DP, Amis AA. The anatomy of the patellar tendon. *Knee Surg Sports Traumatol Arthrosc*. 2001;9:2–5.

Figuero D, Figueroa F, Calvo R. Patellar tendinopathy: diagnosis and treatment. *J Am Acad Orthop Surg*. 2016;24:184–192.

Griesser MJ, Hussain WM, McCoy BW, Parker RD. Extensor mechanism injuries of the knee. In: Miller MD, Thompson SR, eds. *DeLee and Drez's Orthopaedic Sports Medicine: Principles and Practice*. 4th ed. Philadelphia: Elsevier; 2015:1272–1288.

Nordin M, Frankel VH. Biomechanics of the knee. In: *Basic Biomechanics of the Musculoskeletal System*. 4th ed. Philadelphia: Wolters Kluwer; 2012.

Chapter 157 Prepatellar Bursitis and Pes Anserine Bursitis

Christopher DeFalco, Marc Tompkins

ICD-10-CM CODES
M70.4   *Prepatellar bursitis*
M76.8   *Pes anserine tendinitis or bursitis*

Key Concepts
Pes Anserine Bursitis

- Pes anserine bursitis (tendinitis) involves inflammation of the bursa at the insertion of the pes anserine tendons on the medial proximal tibia (Fig. 157.1).
- The pes anserine is composed of the sartorius, gracilis, and semitendinosus tendons.
- Symptoms include swelling, pain to touch, warmth, and pain with hamstring activation.
- The cause is usually overuse.
- Common treatment involves modification of activities, icing, and physical therapy.
- Nonsurgical treatment usually resolves pes anserine bursitis.

Prepatellar Bursitis

- Prepatellar bursitis involves inflammation of the anterior knee bursa and not the knee joint itself (Fig. 157.2).
- May be the result of direct trauma to the anterior knee (fall) or repetitive, overuse injury (excessive kneeling)
- Results in swelling, and in chronic cases, the bursa may be thickened (Fig. 157.3)
- Septic bursitis involves an infection (typically *Staphylococcus aureus*) of the inflamed bursa, usually from a break in the skin, and may require surgical management.
- May be mistaken for septic/pyogenic arthritis of knee joint itself
- Nonsurgical treatment usually resolves prepatellar bursitis.

History
Pes Anserine Bursitis

- Often the result of repetitive friction in sports such as cycling, swimming, and running
- Increased incidence also seen with obesity, pes planovalgus, and genu valgum
- Abrupt onset with pain at night
- Pain and localized swelling over the anteromedial proximal tibia
- Often symptomatic with stairs and when rising from a seated position; typically deny pain with walking on level surfaces

- May have coexistent medial collateral ligament pathology (tenderness superior and posterior to the pes bursa)
- Bilateral symptoms in one-third of patients

Prepatellar Bursitis

- Anterior knee pain, particularly with activity
- Difficulty with ambulation and inability to kneel on the affected side
- History of repetitive, overuse injury, or occupation requiring excessive kneeling
- Direct blow to the front of the knee or fall onto the anterior knee (with presentation of symptoms up to 10 days after the incident)
- Septic bursitis is more common in children
- Inquire about history of gout, pseudogout, hemophilia, warfarin use, and inflammatory conditions

Physical Examination
Pes Anserine Bursitis

- Localized swelling and/or tenderness proximal anteromedial tibia; however, bursa usually not palpable unless effusion and thickening present
- Crepitus over the bursa occasionally present
- Absence of joint line pain
- Exostosis of the tibia may contribute to chronic symptoms in athletes.
- May have pain with resisted knee flexion or valgus stress

Prepatellar Bursitis

- Swelling and tenderness to palpation over anterior patella
- Crepitus over anterior patella
- Decreased flexion secondary to pain due to swelling
- Erythema may indicate septic bursitis.

Imaging
Pes Anserine Bursitis

- Radiographs: anteroposterior, lateral, and patellofemoral views of the knee
  - Can obtain if concerned for insufficiency fracture
  - Often negative, except for possible degenerative changes or presence of exostosis
- Magnetic resonance imaging
  - Axial view may demonstrate fluid around the pes anserine insertion.
  - Can rule out meniscus tears and medial collateral ligament pathology

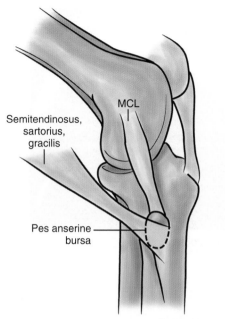

Fig 157.1 Location of the pes anserine bursa on the medial side of the knee. *MCL,* Medial collateral ligament.

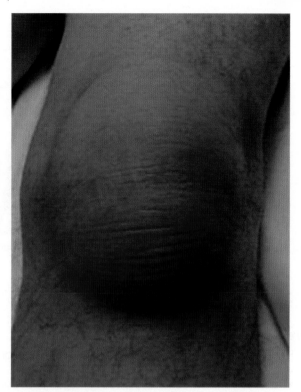

Fig 157.3 Patient with swollen prepatellar bursa.

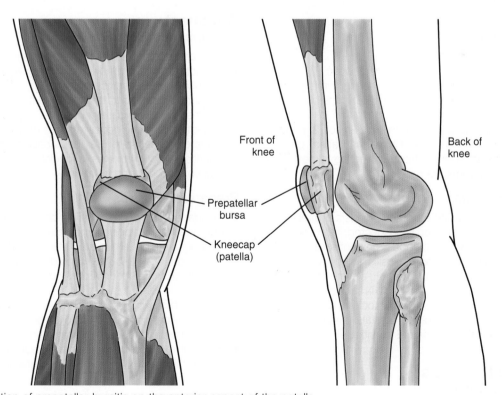

Fig 157.2 Location of prepatellar bursitis on the anterior aspect of the patella.

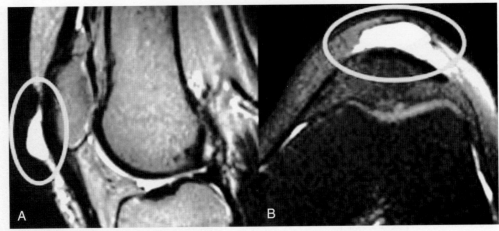

Fig 157.4 Sagittal **(A)** and axial **(B)** magnetic resonance images showing prepatellar bursitis.

Prepatellar Bursitis

- Radiographs: anteroposterior, lateral, and patellofemoral views of the knee
  - Can see anterior soft-tissue swelling, negative for bony pathology
- Magnetic resonance imaging
  - Axial view may demonstrate fluid in the prepatellar bursa (Fig. 157.4)

Additional Tests
Pes Anserine Bursitis

- Injections may be diagnostic and therapeutic
  - Lidocaine (1%) injection test: Injecting 2 mL into the pes anserine bursa provides pain relief in the physician's office.
  - Bupivacaine (0.25%) injection test: Inject 2 mL into the pes anserine bursa and have the patient perform the aggravating activity after the injection to determine whether symptoms are relieved.

Prepatellar Bursitis

- Aspiration is not indicated for the diagnosis of prepatellar bursitis; however, if infection is suspected, then aspiration is recommended, and fluid should be sent for analysis.
- Findings consistent with septic bursitis include a fluid white blood cell count greater than 5000/μL, elevated protein and lactate, decreased glucose, and bacteria seen on Gram stain.
- Crystal analysis may reveal monosodium urate crystals (gout), calcium pyrophosphate crystals (pseudogout), or cholesterol crystals (rheumatoid bursitis).

Differential Diagnosis
Pes Anserine Bursitis

- Medial meniscus tear
- Medial compartment osteoarthritis
- Medial tibial stress (insufficiency) fracture
- Superficial medial collateral ligament sprain at tibial insertion

- Patellar tendinitis
- Patellofemoral pain

Prepatellar Bursitis

- Patella fracture
- Patellar tendinitis
- Patellofemoral pain syndrome
- Septic knee

Treatment
Pes Anserine Bursitis

- Rest and nonsteroidal antiinflammatory drugs
- Physical therapy including stretching and strengthening, ice, ultrasound, electrical stimulation, and gait evaluation
- Small cushion placed between the thighs for sleeping
- Address obesity in cases in which it is a contributing factor
- Resection is rarely necessary but may be appropriate in refractory cases, such as those causing 6 to 8 weeks of limitation among athletes, especially if mature exostosis is present and causing irritation.

Prepatellar Bursitis

- Avoidance of the precipitating cause, use of knee pads, compression wrapping, and time
- Oral nonsteroidal antiinflammatory medication
- Aspiration of the bursa should be discouraged if not concerned for infection as this can cause a superimposed infection.
- If infection is excluded and conservative management fails, may consider corticosteroid injection into the bursa (again should be cautious, as this can lead to infection).
- Surgical excision of the bursa is reserved for infections and recalcitrant, symptomatic prepatellar bursitis.

When to Refer
Pes Anserine Bursitis

- Referral is indicated after failure of conservative treatment including rest, ice, and activity modification.

- Corticosteroid injections should be given 6 weeks to assess their effectiveness before referral.

Prepatellar Bursitis

- Referral is indicated in cases of septic bursitis and in patients in whom a course of conservative treatment including rest, ice, compression, and activity modification has failed.

Prognosis

- Excellent for both prepatellar and pes anserine bursitis
- Most patients will fully recover and return to pre-bursitis levels of activity with rare long-term sequelae.
- Even in cases of septic prepatellar bursitis, prognosis is excellent if recognized and treated early.

Troubleshooting
Pes Anserine Bursitis

- If symptoms persist, magnetic resonance imaging is helpful to rule out differential diagnoses.

Prepatellar Bursitis

- Remember infection and beware of methicillin-resistant *S. aureus*.
- Beware of aspiration and injections unless absolutely necessary, as these can seed an aseptic bursa and create septic bursitis.

Patient Instructions
Pes Anserine Bursitis

- Full resolution can take time, but conservative management is generally successful, especially if able to temporarily modify activities.

Prepatellar Bursitis

- Full resolution can take time, but conservative management is generally successful, especially if able to temporarily modify activities.

- If swelling becomes red and warm, contact your physician.
- Complete the treatment course of antibiotics (if infected) regardless of symptoms and appearance.

Acknowledgment

The authors thank Dr. Richard Parker for his contributions to this chapter in the previous edition.

Suggested Readings

Baumbach SF, Lobo CM, Badyine I, et al. Prepatellar and olecranon bursitis: literature review and development of a treatment algorithm. *Arch Orthop Trauma Surg*. 2014;134(3):359–370.

Dawn B, Williams JK, Walker SE. Prepatellar bursitis: a unique presentation of tophaceous gout in a normouricemic patient. *J Rheumatol*. 1997;24:976–978.

Donahue F, Turkel D, Mnaymneh W, Ghandur-Mnaymneh L. Hemorrhagic prepatellar bursitis. *Skeletal Radiol*. 1996;25:298–301.

Forbes JR, Helms CA, Janzen DL. Acute pes anserine bursitis: MR imaging. *Radiology*. 1995;194:525–527.

Handy JR. Anserine bursitis: a brief review. *South Med J*. 1997;90:376–377.

Khodaee M. Common superficial bursitis. *Am Fam Physician*. 2017;95(4): 224–231.

Muchnick J, Sundaram M. Radiologic case study. Pes anserine bursitis. *Orthopedics*. 1997;20:1092–1094.

Rennie WJ, Saifuddin A. Pes anserine bursitis: incidence in symptomatic knees and clinical presentation. *Skeletal Radiol*. 2005;34:395–398.

Sarifakioglu B, Afsar SI, Yalbuzdag SA, et al. Comparison of the efficacy of physical therapy and corticosteroid injection in the treatment of pes anserine tendino-bursitis. *J Phys Ther Sci*. 2016;28(7):1993–1997.

Wilson-MacDonald J. Management and outcome of infective prepatellar bursitis. *Postgrad Med J*. 1987;63:851–853.

Wood LR, Peat G, Thomas E, Duncan R. The contribution of selected non-articular conditions to knee pain severity and associated disability in older adults. *Osteoarthritis Cartilage*. 2008;16(6):647–653.

Chapter 158 Extensor Tendon Rupture

Jarred Holt, Marc Tompkins

ICD-10-CM CODE
S76.1 *Rupture of tendon, patellar or auadriceps tendon*

Key Concepts

- Patellar tendon rupture is usually due to a sports injury in patients younger than 40 years old.
- Quadriceps tendon rupture is more typical in patients older than 40 years of age.
- A force multiple times that of body weight is necessary to produce traumatic patellar rupture.
- Bilateral rupture of either tendon is uncommon and usually results from systemic disease (inflammatory disease, diabetes, chronic renal failure) and previous degenerative changes.
- Local and systemic steroid (corticosteroids or anabolic steroids) use has also been implicated in pathogenesis of low-energy injury.
- A palpable defect at the site of injury along with inability to actively extend the knee is often found.
- Although physical examination is often sufficient to make an accurate diagnosis, imaging (including plain radiographs and magnetic resonance imaging [MRI]) may be obtained if there is a question about the pathology.
- Surgical repair is usually indicated.

History

- Acute traumatic injury: stumble, fall, or a giving way of the knee
- Severe pain, immediate disability, and swelling
- Cannot lift leg and cannot support themselves with the injured leg
- With or without history of knee pain/tendinosis
- Inquire about history of medical steroid or anabolic steroid use

Physical Examination

- Observation
  - Diffuse, tender swelling and ecchymosis of anterior knee
- Palpation
  - Effusion and tenderness
  - Palpable defect at level of rupture (Fig. 158.1); this typically occurs at either the proximal or distal pole of the patella as majority of injuries are tendinous avulsions from the patella
- Range of motion
  - Active extension may be completely lost and the patient is unable to maintain the knee passively extended against gravity.
  - On rare occasion active knee extension may be maintained due to intact medial and lateral retinacular structures; weakness will be noted in this case.
  - Quadriceps rupture: The patella does not move with quadriceps contraction.
  - Patella tendon rupture: The patella moves with quadriceps contraction.
- Special tests
  - Knee ligament examination should be performed to rule out concomitant injury

Imaging

- Radiographs: anteroposterior, lateral, and patellofemoral views of the knee
  - Rule out fracture and assess patella position: alta/baja (Figs. 158.2 and 158.3)
- MRI
  - Recommended for documentation, localization of the tear, and identification of additional injuries (Fig. 158.4)
- Ultrasonography
  - May also document and localize tear

Differential Diagnosis

- Quadriceps or patellar tendinitis
- Patellar fracture
- Partial tendon tear
- Metabolic disease

Treatment

- At diagnosis
  - Surgical repair is indicated in all but the most medically unstable patients for optimal return of function.
  - Patients should be immobilized in extension, instructed in crutch use with weight bearing as tolerated in extension, and referred for surgical intervention.
- Later
  - Surgery is best performed as soon as possible and ideally within 2 weeks.
  - Repair of the patella or quadriceps tendon is performed with bone tunnels or suture anchors in the patella.

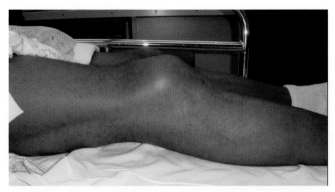

Fig 158.1 Clinical photograph of superior patellar swelling associated with quadriceps rupture.

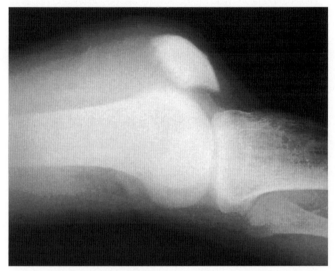

Fig 158.2 Lateral radiograph revealing soft-tissue swelling superior to the patella and patella baja consistent with quadriceps rupture. (Copyright 2006 by Elsevier, Inc.)

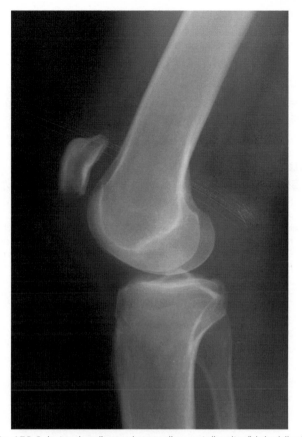

Fig 158.3 Lateral radiograph revealing patella alta (high riding), consistent with patellar tendon rupture.

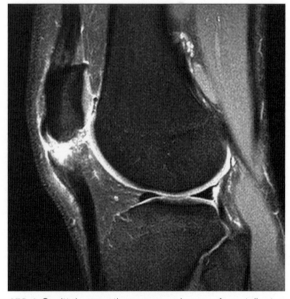

Fig 158.4 Sagittal magnetic resonance image of a patellar tendon rupture at the inferior pole of the patella.

When to Refer
- All patients with quadriceps or patellar tendon rupture should be referred on presentation and diagnosis of the rupture.

Prognosis
- Good for function, but often have residual quadriceps atrophy; may have slight extensor lag, and occasional loss of flexion.
- Majority of patients are able to return to preinjury level of function following appropriate repair.

Troubleshooting
- Beware of associated metabolic diseases.
- Beware of steroid use.

Patient Instructions
- Avoid smoking during the postoperative period (3 months).
- Avoid use of steroids when possible.

- Commit to postoperative rehabilitation.
- Adhere to postoperative deep venous thrombosis prevention exercises (ankle pumps).

Acknowledgment

The authors thank Dr. Richard Parker for his contributions to this chapter in the previous edition.

Suggested Readings

Clark SC, Jones MW, Choudhury RR, Smith E. Bilateral patellar tendon rupture secondary to repeated local steroid injections. *Emerg Med J.* 1995;12(4):300–301.

Greisser MJ, Hussein WM, McCoy BW, Parker RD. Extensor mechanism injuries of the knee. In: Miller M, Thompson S, eds. *Delee and Drez's Orthopaedic Sports Medicine: Principles and Practice.* 4th ed. Philadelphia: Elsevier; 2015:1272–1288.

Ilan DI, Tejwani N, Keschner M, Leibman M. Quadriceps tendon rupture. *J Am Acad Orthop Surg.* 2003;11(3):192–200.

Kannus P, Józsa L. Histopathological changes preceding spontaneous rupture of a tendon. *J Bone Joint Surg Am.* 1991;73:1507–1525.

Maffulli N, Papalia R, Torre G, Denaro V. Surgical treatment for failure of repair of patellar and quadriceps tendon rupture with ipsilateral hamstring tendon graft. *Sports Med Arthrosc Rev.* 2017;25(1):51–55.

Matava MJ. Patellar tendon ruptures. *J Am Acad Orthop Surg.* 1996;4(6): 287–296.

Meyer Z, Ricci WM. Knee extensor mechanism repairs: standard suture repair and novel augmentation technique. *J Orthop Trauma.* 2016; 30(suppl 2):S30–S31.

Serino J, Mohamadi A, Orman S, et al. Comparison of adverse events and postoperative mobilization following knee extensor mechanism rupture repair: A systematic review and network meta-analysis. *Injury.* 2017;48(12):2793–2799.

Woo SL, Maynard J, Butler D. Ligament, tendon, and joint capsule insertions to bone. In: Woo SL, Buckwalter JA, eds. *Injury and Repair of the Musculoskeletal Soft Tissues.* Park Ridge, IL: American Academy of Orthopaedic Surgeons; 1988:133–166.

Chapter 159 Medial Tibial Stress Syndrome (Shin Splints)

Andrew Kubinski, Annunziato Amendola

ICD-10-CM CODES
S86.891A *Medial tibial stress syndrome, right leg,*
initial encounter
S86.892A *Medial tibial stress syndrome, left leg, initial*
encounter

Key Concepts

- Medial tibial stress syndrome (MTSS) is an overuse or repetitive stress injury characterized by pain and tenderness over the posteromedial middle and/or distal third of the tibia.
- "Shin splints" is a broad, nonspecific term that has been used to describe exertional leg pain over the anterior or medial tibia, anterior compartment, or lateral compartment.
- MTSS is one of the most common causes of exertional leg pain, with an incidence of 13–17% of running injuries and 4–35% of military recruits in basic training.
- The etiology of MTSS is not well understood. Theories include inflammation/periostitis, traction injury, and bone stress reaction. The medial soleus muscle, flexor digitorum longus muscle, and crural fascia originate from the medial tibia in the area of symptoms.
- A benign stress fracture of the distal third of the tibia may be a continuum in severe recalcitrant cases of MTSS as a result of the bone stress reaction (enthesopathy → periostitis → periosteal remodeling → stress reaction).
- It is most common in repetitive running and jumping activities such as running, volleyball, basketball, football, dancing, and soccer.
- Risk factors for MTSS include overpronation of the foot during gait, training errors such as a rapid increase in training intensity (e.g., hill running) or duration, running on hard or uneven surfaces, running greater than 20 miles per week, improper shoes, muscle imbalance between dorsiflexors and plantar flexors with decreased dorsiflexion, and a history of previous lower extremity injury. The risk in women is twice that in men.

History

- Gradual onset, dull, vague, and diffuse pain over the middle and/or distal third of the posteromedial tibia. With increasing severity, the tenderness extends proximally over the soleal bridge.
- Early in MTSS, pain is worst at the beginning of exercise but subsides with activity and resolves with cessation of activity.
- Later stages of MTSS have an early onset of pain with less activity; this pain is more pronounced and persists throughout exercise.
- Pain may be present with ambulation and at rest, not completely resolving after exercise, which is in contrast to exertional compartment syndrome, which usually subsides with rest.
- Comprehensive exercise history includes exercise routine, running mileage, intensity, pace, terrain, and footwear.
- Pertinent negatives on reactive oxygen species (ROS) include change in foot color, paresthesia, weakness, swelling, or trauma.

Physical Examination

- Observation
  - Examine shoe wear patterns and gait.
  - Evaluate for pes planus, hindfoot valgus, and foot pronation during stance.
  - Look for leg-length discrepancy, femoral anteversion, tibial torsion, and excessive knee varus or valgus structure.
- Palpation
  - Diffuse tenderness over the middle and/or distal third of the posteromedial tibia.
  - With increasing severity, tenderness may extend proximally.
- Range of motion
  - Pain with stretching of the soleus muscle during passive ankle dorsiflexion or contraction of the soleus muscle during resisted ankle plantarflexion, standing toe raises, or jumping.

Imaging

- Imaging can help to differentiate stress fracture, stress reaction, and MTSS.
- Radiographs
  - Usually normal but indicated to exclude a stress fracture diagnosis.
  - Rarely, cortical hypertrophy or scalloping in the area of pain can be long-term findings.
- Triple-phase bone scan
  - Although bone scan has been the traditional method, MRI has generally become the imaging investigation of choice.

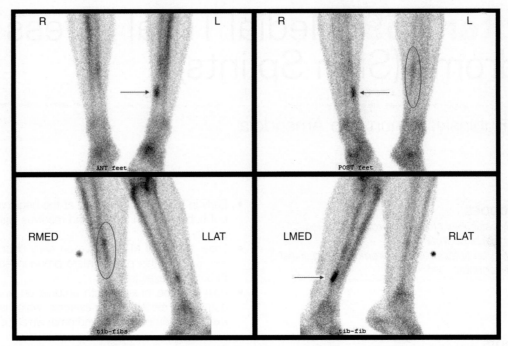

Fig 159.1 Delayed phase of triple-phase bone scan showing the difference between medial tibial stress syndrome *(right)* and stress fracture *(left)*. The right posteromedial middle third of the tibia has diffuse linear uptake *(red circle)*. The left distal posteromedial tibia has focal uptake *(arrows)*. *ANT*, Anterior view; *fib*, fibula; *L*, left; *LLAT*, left lateral view; *LMED*, left medial view; *POST*, posterior view; *R*, right; *RLAT*, right lateral view; *RMED*, right medial view; *tib*, tibia.

TABLE 159.1 Differential Diagnosis for Exercise-Related Leg Pain

	MTSS	Stress Fracture	Exertional Compartment Syndrome	Popliteal Artery Entrapment
Pain	Exercise ± rest	Exercise, rest, night	Exercise, gone 20 min after	Exercise: claudication
Palpation	Diffuse	Focal	± with exercise	± with exercise
Percussion	Negative	Positive	Negative	Negative
Range-of-motion pain	Positive or negative	Positive or negative	Negative, ± with exercise	Negative
Neurovascular	Normal	Normal	± with exercise	± with exercise
Bone scan	Diffuse	Focal	Negative	Negative
Magnetic resonance imaging	Bone diffuse	Bone focal	± in muscle compartment after exercise	Magnetic resonance arthrography or angiography

MTSS, Medial tibial stress syndrome.

- Diffuse, longitudinal linear uptake can be seen along the posteromedial tibia in the delayed phase (Fig. 159.1).
- Magnetic resonance imaging
  - Periosteal edema, periosteal reaction, bone marrow edema, fascial or muscle inflammation may be present (Figs. 159.2 and 159.3).

Differential Diagnosis (Table 159.1)

- Exertional compartment syndrome (acute or chronic)
- Tibial stress fracture
- Tendinopathy
- Lumbar radiculopathy
- Popliteal artery entrapment
- Fascial hernia
- Nerve entrapment syndrome
- Malignancy
- Osteomyelitis
- Deep venous thrombosis/venous stasis
- Peripheral vascular disease

Treatment

- Evidence is lacking regarding specific treatments and their effectiveness. Most treatments are based on expert opinion and clinical experience.

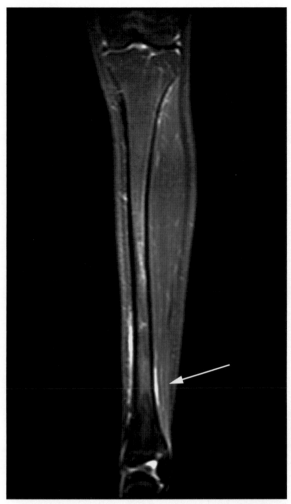

Fig 159.2 Magnetic resonance imaging coronal T1 short tau inversion recovery image of medial tibial stress syndrome. Note the periosteal and bone marrow edema *(arrow)* in the posteromedial middle and distal thirds of the tibia on the left side of the image.

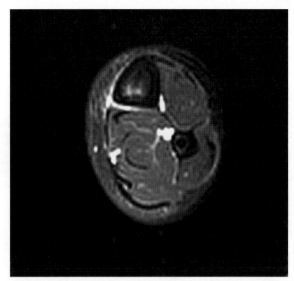

Fig 159.3 Magnetic resonance imaging axial T2-weighted fat-saturated image of medial tendon stress syndrome with periosteal edema at the posteromedial corner of the tibia, posterior bone marrow edema, and soft-tissue edema medial to the tibia.

- At diagnosis
  - Conservative treatment is effective in most cases.
  - Modification of activity, with relative rest by low-impact cross-training and decreasing running volume (distance, frequency, and intensity), is the mainstay of therapy (Fig. 159.4).
  - If pain continues to inhibit training, cease activity (absolute rest) until pain has disappeared, which may take 3 days to 3 weeks.
  - Correct training errors by decreasing mileage and modifying the training surface to avoid harder surfaces.
  - Modalities to decrease inflammation include ice, non-steroidal antiinflammatory drugs, local transcutaneous antiinflammatory modalities, leg wraps, and ultrasound.
  - Correct foot pronation and excessive hind foot motion with orthotics, supportive shoe wear, or taping.
  - Stretching and global strengthening of the gastrocnemius/soleus muscle, ankle dorsiflexors and plantar flexors, and foot inverters and evertors

- Later
  - Gradually increase mileage or activity with no more than 10% increase per week as long as there are no symptoms.

When to Refer

If conservative treatment fails after 6 to 12 months, consider referral. Operative therapy with fasciotomy of the medial deep posterior compartment and periosteal stripping can be beneficial for cases where conservative management has failed.

Prognosis

- Good with a graduated rehabilitation program.
- The majority will be able to return to their previous level of activity.
- Pain improves in more than 70% of those undergoing surgery.

Troubleshooting

- Avoid rapid conditioning, especially on hard surfaces.
- Pain may improve with taking a week off, and then gradually increase activity.
- Imaging may be used when the diagnosis is in question and to distinguish MTSS from other entities.

Instructions for the Patient

- Discuss proper shoe wear, training modifications, and training errors. Regular stretching and strengthening, soft-surface running, and avoiding hills. Recommendation for changing running shoes is every 250 to 350 miles.

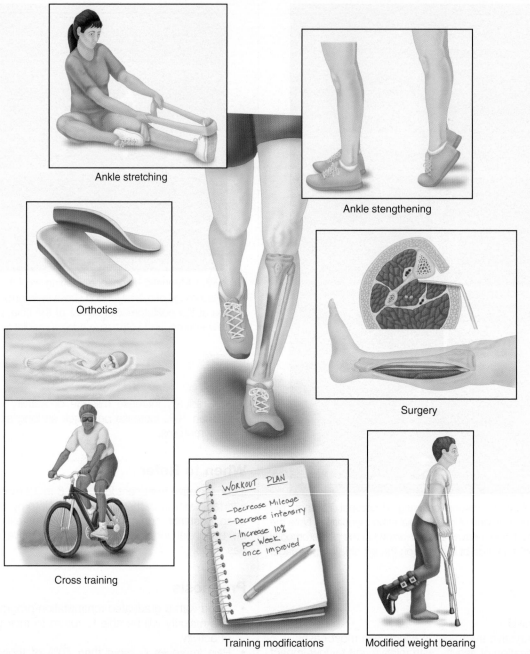

Ankle stretching

Ankle stengthening

Orthotics

Surgery

Cross training

Training modifications

Modified weight bearing

Fig 159.4 Location of pain in medial tibial stress syndrome is along the posteromedial aspect of the middle and distal thirds of the tibia *(shown by highlighted area)*. Various treatments can be used to treat medial tibial stress syndrome, including stretching, strengthening, orthotics, cross-training, training modifications, modified weight bearing, or surgery.

- Cross-training can maintain cardiovascular fitness. However, if pain continues, absolute rest is indicated, followed by gradual progression of activity.
- Pain may recur in the future, especially after a period of inactivity (e.g., off-season followed by initiation of training at the beginning of the next season).

Considerations in Special Populations

- MTSS may be more common in obese individuals.
- MTSS is prevalent in new military recruits.

- MTSS may be an early finding with the female athlete triad.

Suggested Readings

Batt ME, Ugalde V, Anderson MW, et al. A prospective controlled study of diagnostic imaging for acute shin splints. *Med Sci Sports Exerc*. 1998;30:1564–1571.

Beck BR, Osternig LR. Medial tibial stress syndrome: the location of muscles in the leg in relation to symptoms. *J Bone Joint Surg Am*. 1994;76A:1057–1061.

Galbraith RM, Lavallee ME. Medial tibial stress syndrome: conservative treatment options. *Curr Rev Musculoskelet Med*. 2009;3:127–133.

Plisky MS. Medial tibial stress syndrome in high school cross-country runners: incidence and risk factors. *J Orthop Sports Phys Ther*. 2007;37: 40–47.

Reshef N, Guelich DR. Medial tibial stress syndrome. *Clin Sports Med*. 2012;31(2):273–290.

Thacker SB, Gilchrist J, Stroup DF, et al. The prevention of shin splints in sports: a systematic review of literature. *Med Sci Sports Exerc*. 2002;34(1):32–40.

Winters M, Eskes M, Weir A, et al. Treatment of medial tibial stress syndrome: a systematic review. *Sports Med*. 2013;43(12):1315–1333.

Yates B, Allen MJ, Barnes MR. Outcome of surgical treatment of medial tibial stress syndrome. *J Bone Joint Surg Am*. 2003;85A:1974–1980.

Yates B, White S. The incidence and risk factors in the development of medial tibial stress syndrome among naval recruits. *Am J Sports Med*. 2004;32:772–780.

Chapter 160 Exertional Compartment Syndrome

David Hryvniak, Robert P. Wilder

ICD-10-CM CODES
M79.A21 *Nontraumatic compartment syndrome of right lower extremity*
M79.A22 *Nontraumatic compartment syndrome of left lower extremity*

Key Concepts

- Chronic exertional compartment syndrome is defined as reversible ischemia secondary to a noncompliant osseo-fascial compartment that is unresponsive to the expansion of muscle volume that occurs with exercise.
- Most commonly seen in the lower leg, exertional compartment syndrome in athletes has also been described in the thigh and medial compartment of the foot.
- Several factors contribute to increased compartment pressures during exercise.
  - Enclosure of compartment contents in an inelastic fascial sheath.
  - Increased volume of skeletal muscle due to blood flow and edema.
  - Muscle hypertrophy.
  - Myofiber damage from eccentric exercise causes release of protein-bound ions and subsequent increase in osmotic pressure.
- Increased compartment pressures have been identified in athletes taking creatine.
- There are four major compartments in the leg: the anterior compartment is most frequently involved, followed by the deep posterior, lateral, and superficial posterior compartments.
- Chronic compartment syndrome left untreated can develop into an acute syndrome.
- Resting intracompartmental pressure greater than 30 mm Hg is associated with diminished blood flow and resultant muscle and nerve ischemia.
- Women may be more susceptible to chronic lower leg compartment syndrome.

History

- Tight, cramp-like, squeezing pain localized over a specific compartment.
- Symptoms typically occur at a well-defined and reproducible point of exercise (distance, time, or intensity) and increase if training persists. Relief of symptoms occurs with cessation of activity.
- Neurologic symptoms (paresthesias, weakness) may or may not occur.

- In some cases the classic exertional component is not as evident, and patients report pain at rest or with daily activities.

Physical Examination

- Observation
  - Swelling
- Palpation
  - Tightness and tenderness over involved compartments.
  - Fascial hernia may be present.
- Special tests
  - Neurologic findings may be present.
- Anterior compartment: weakness of ankle dorsiflexion or toe extension (may include transient or persistent foot drop), sensory changes over dorsum of the foot (numbness in first web space).
- Deep posterior compartment: weakness of toe flexion and foot inversion, sensory changes on the plantar foot.
- Lateral compartment: weakness of ankle eversion, sensory changes in the anterolateral leg.
- Superficial posterior compartment: weakness of foot plantarflexion and sensory changes in dorsolateral foot.

Imaging

- Radiographs, bone scan, or magnetic resonance imaging (MRI) may identify stress fractures that can coexist with compartment syndrome. MR angiography may identify possible vascular causes, including popliteal entrapment syndrome.

Additional Tests

- Diagnosis based solely on clinical presentation can lead to misdiagnosis and therefore should be confirmed with exercise challenge and documentation of pressure elevation.
- Intracompartment pressure measurements are obtained at rest and after an exercise challenge (see Chapter 170). Generally accepted pressure criteria suggesting compartment syndrome: before exercise, ≥15 mm Hg; 1 minute after exercise, ≥30 mm Hg; 5 minutes after exercise, ≥20 mm Hg.

Differential Diagnosis

- Shin splints
- Stress fracture
- Entrapment neuropathy
- Lumbar radiculopathy
- Spinal stenosis
- Popliteal artery entrapment syndrome

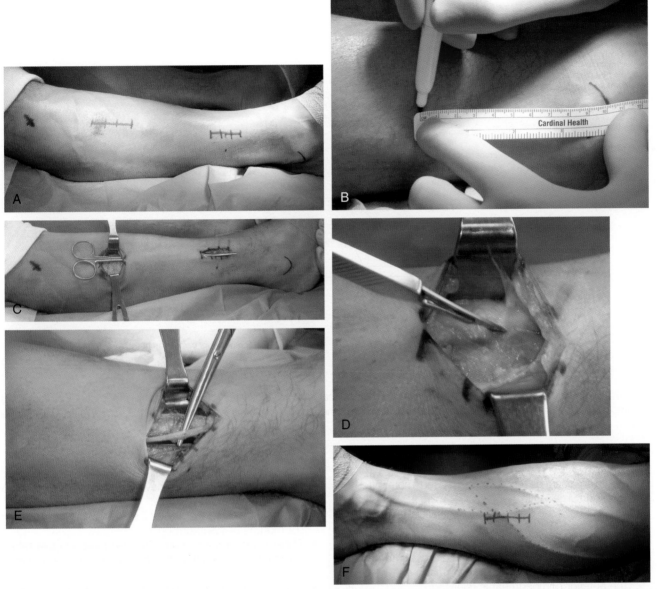

Fig 160.1 Surgical fasciotomy. **(A)** Dual lateral incisions for release of the anterior and lateral compartments. **(B)** The distal lateral incision is centered 10 to 12 cm proximal to the tip of the distal fibula, at the site where the superficial peroneal nerve penetrates the fascia. **(C)** Blunt dissection produces subcutaneous connection of the incisions to allow adequate release of the compartments throughout their lengths. **(D)** Anterior compartment fascial incision. The fascial incision is then extended proximally and distally under direct visualization. **(E)** Superficial peroneal nerve after release of the anterior and lateral compartments. It is important to freely mobilize the nerve. **(F)** Medial incision for release of the superficial and deep posterior compartments.

- Arterial insufficiency
- Deep venous thrombosis

Treatment

- At diagnosis
  - Conservative measures include relative rest (limiting activity to the level that avoids significant symptoms), nonsteroidal antiinflammatory drugs, stretching and strengthening of the involved muscles (especially the gastrocnemius-soleus complex), and orthotics (particularly in cases of excessive pronation).

- Gait retraining has been shown to decrease compartment pressures and to improve pain and function.
- Some athletes may simply choose to refrain from the causative activity, which is a viable option provided that they remain neurovascularly intact.
- Botox chemodenervation and ultrasound-guided fascial fenestration are more invasive procedures that may be considered for recalcitrant cases.
- Later
  - Surgical fasciotomy may alleviate persistent symptoms (Fig. 160.1). Single-incision, double-incision, and endoscopic techniques have been described. Fasciectomy

Exertional compartment syndrome

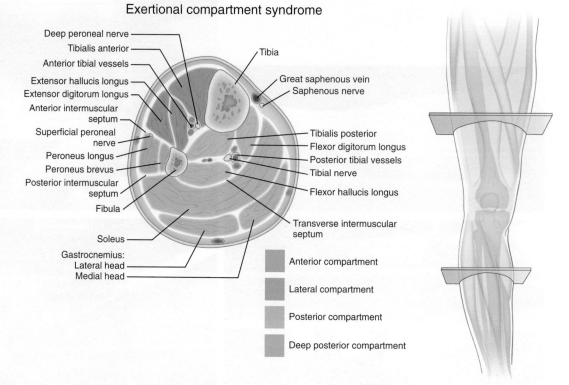

- Sx-Tight, cramping, squeezing pain, worse with activity, relieved by cessation, with possible neurological symptoms
- PE-Swelling, tightness/tenderness in muscles, sensory/motor changes
- Tests-MRI, compartment pressure testing
- Tx-PT, gait changes, Botox, fasciotomy

Deep peroneal nerve
Tibialis anterior
Anterior tibial vessels
Extensor hallucis longus
Extensor digitorum longus
Anterior intermuscular septum
Superficial peroneal nerve
Peroneus longus
Peroneus brevis
Posterior intermuscular septum
Fibula
Soleus
Gastrocnemius:
Lateral head
Medial head

Tibia
Great saphenous vein
Saphenous nerve
Tibialis posterior
Flexor digitorum longus
Posterior tibial vessels
Tibial nerve
Flexor hallucis longus
Transverse intermuscular septum

Anterior compartment
Lateral compartment
Posterior compartment
Deep posterior compartment

Fig 160.2 Exertional compartment syndrome: symptoms, physical examination, tests, and treatments. The image is of four lower leg compartments in cross section. (Illustration from Miller MD, Thompson SR, eds. *Miller's Review of Orthopaedics.* 7th ed. Philadelphia: Elsevier; 2016, Figure 2.54.)

has also been described and is used more often in revision surgery (Fig. 160.2).
- Regardless of the technique chosen, fascial hernias must be included in the fascial incision and the superficial peroneal nerve must be released.
- Owing to the high rate of coexistence, some authors advocate release of the lateral compartment whenever the anterior compartment is released.
- In performing deep posterior compartment release, attention must be given to adequate decompression of the tibialis posterior muscle.

When to Refer

- Referral for pressure measurements should be made when symptoms are present with daily activities, when symptoms fail to abate with rest from athletic activity and conservative care, or in the presence of neurologic symptoms.
- Surgical remediation should be considered if symptoms persist despite 6 to 12 weeks of conservative care and in cases of extreme pressure elevation (resting pressures > 30 mm Hg) or focal motor weakness.

Prognosis

- Early diagnosis and management are critical to minimize the risk for muscle necrosis or permanent neurologic deficit.

- Good to excellent results have been reported in 60–96% of patients after fasciotomy.
- The best results are obtained if surgery is performed within 12 months of symptom onset.
- Patients undergoing anterior release have a higher rate of satisfactory results than those undergoing deep posterior release.
- For unclear reasons, women may respond less favorably to fasciotomy than men.

Troubleshooting

- All potentially involved compartments must be tested; failure to identify all involved compartments is a cause for failure of surgical remediation.
- Potential complications may include bleeding, damage to neurologic structures, and recurrent symptoms.
- Patients with recurrent symptoms may require fasciectomy in addition to fasciotomy.

Instructions for the Patient

- Activity should be limited to the level at which symptoms are considered mild and abate within minutes of activity cessation.
- Activity should not produce weakness or limping.
- Cross-training may be substituted for running when necessary.

Suggested Readings

Barkdull T, Glorioso J, Wilckens J. Exertional leg pain. In: O'Connor F, Wilder R, Magrum E, eds. *The Textbook of Running Medicine*. 2nd ed. Monterey: Healthy Learning; 2014:332–352.

Glorioso J, Wilckens J. Compartment syndrome testing. In: O'Connor F, Wilder R, Magrum E, eds. *The Textbook of Running Medicine*. 2nd ed. Monterey: Healthy Learning; 2014:213–220.

Pedowitz RA, Hargens AR, Mubarak SJ, et al. Modified criteria for the objective diagnosis of chronic compartment syndrome of the leg. *Am J Sports Med*. 1990;18:35–40.

Rajasekaran S, Hall MM. Nonoperative management of chronic exertional compartment syndrome: a systematic review. *Curr Sports Med Rep*. 2016;15(3):191–198.

Wilder R, Sethi S. Overuse injuries: tendinopathies, stress fractures, compartment syndrome, and shin splints. *Clin Sports Med*. 2004;23:55–81.

Chapter 161 Medial Gastrocnemius Rupture (Tennis Leg)

Annunziato Amendola, Benjamin Boswell

ICD-10-CM CODES

S86.819A	*Rupture of medial head of gastrocnemius*
S86.811A	*Rupture of medial head of gastrocnemius, right, initial encounter*
S86.811S	*Rupture of medial head of gastrocnemius, right, sequela*
S86.811D	*Rupture of medial head of gastrocnemius, right, subsequent encounter*
S86.812A	*Rupture of medial head of gastrocnemius, left, initial encounter*
S86.812S	*Rupture of medial head of gastrocnemius, left, sequela*
S86.812D	*Rupture of medial head of gastrocnemius, left, subsequent encounter*

Key Concepts

- Medial gastrocnemius rupture or strain is often referred to as "tennis leg."
- Traumatic injury that involves tearing to the medial head of the gastrocnemius muscle, typically occurring at the musculotendinous junction.
- Can range from partial tear to complete rupture.
- Typically occurs in running or jumping in conjunction with sudden stopping or cutting.
- Mechanism of injury is a combination of ankle dorsiflexion with concomitant knee hyperextension (Fig. 161.1).
- More commonly occurs in middle-aged individuals or deconditioned athletes.
- Evaluate for compartment syndrome if clinical concern, as the posterior superficial compartment contains the gastrocnemius muscle.

History

- Occurs with knee extension and ankle dorsiflexion during active eccentric loading of gastrocnemius muscle, causing a tear at the musculotendinous junction.
- Typically a tennis injury, but can occur in any activity involving sudden contraction of the calf muscles.
- Patients sometimes give history of sudden audible "pop," but this may not always be the case.
- Patients often describe feeling of being kicked in the leg or being struck by an object.
- Patients will typically complain of painful ambulation after injury.

Physical Examination

- Swelling and ecchymosis will develop over the medial aspect of the calf within 24 to 48 hours.
- Palpable defect at the musculotendinous junction.
- Observation will likely reveal an antalgic gait.
- Patient may hold ankle in plantarflexion due to painful dorsiflexion.
- Tenderness to palpation along medial calf.
- Active and passive dorsiflexion will elicit pain.
- Ankle dorsiflexion and single toe raise will be weaker on affected leg.

Imaging

- This is typically a clinical diagnosis, but imaging can be performed when the diagnosis is in question or to evaluate for progression.
- Magnetic resonance imaging (MRI)
  - Will likely show high T2-signal fluid deep to medial gastrocnemius as well as a focal area of disruption of muscle continuity along the medial head of gastrocnemius, with associated edema.
  - May be used for diagnosis but also beneficial to rule out additional injury.
- Ultrasound (US).
- Demonstrates fluid deep to the medial gastrocnemius and superficial to the soleus muscle.
- Can evaluate for progression of healing.
- Duplex venous US can be used to rule out deep venous thrombosis (DVT).

Differential Diagnosis

- Plantaris tendon rupture
- Achilles tendon rupture
- DVT
- Muscle contusion/hematoma
- Thrombophlebitis
- Posterior superficial compartment syndrome

Treatment

- Initial management:
  - Conservative management similar to that for any muscle strain.
  - Protection, rest, ice, compression, elevation (PRICE) for 24 to 72 hours postinjury.

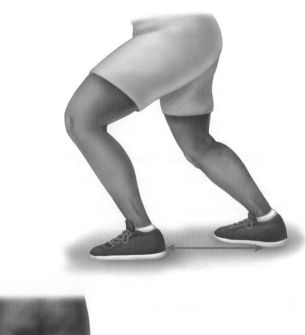

Fig 161.1 Center, Mechanism leading to medial gastrocnemius muscle rupture, such as the combination of ankle dorsiflexion with concomitant knee hyperextension and eccentric loading. Bottom Left: Compression device to reduce fluid accumulation between gastrocnemius and soleus muscles. Bottom Right: Band strengthening exercises.

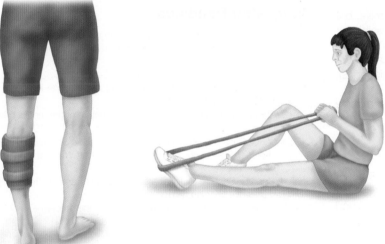

- Compression wrapping or device has been proven by US to decrease fluid accumulation between the gastrocnemius and soleus muscles (Fig. 161.1).
- Make patient non–weight bearing initially with use of crutches but for as short a time as possible until weight bearing is tolerated.
- Use of a heel lift (2 to 3 cm) is recommended to place patient in plantarflexion; this is well tolerated and minimizes pain with weight bearing.
- Decrease heel lift and begin ambulation as tolerated as soon as possible to increase healing.
- When patient is able to perform full active range of motion (AROM) without pain, progress to passive and then active stretching.
- Antiinflammatory medications; however, nonselective nonsteroidal antiinflammatory medications should be avoided in the first 48 hours due to increased risk of bleeding in the injured area.

- Late management
  - When the patient is able to tolerate pain-free active stretching, begin plantarflexion and dorsiflexion strengthening exercises (see Fig. 161.1).
  - May begin stationary cycling, resistance-band plantarflexion exercises, electrical stimulation, and cross-frictional massage.
  - As strength and range of motion exercises return to normal, return to sport participation may begin with close observation.
  - Full return to sport when strength and function of affected leg is similar to that of the unaffected leg.

When to Refer

- If there is any clinical suspicion for compartment syndrome, consider compartment measurements and referral emergently to surgery for possible fasciotomy, specifically of the superficial posterior compartment.

- If pain continues beyond the expected recovery time or there is recurrent injury, consider referral.

Prognosis

- After medial gastrocnemius injury and a staged rehabilitation program, the prognosis for recovery and return to participation is good, with a low recurrence rate.
- Partial tears take approximately 4 to 8 weeks for recovery, whereas severe tears to complete ruptures take approximately 8 to 12 weeks for recovery, depending on severity.

Troubleshooting

- Avoid using nonselective nonsteroidal antiinflammatory medications in the first 48 hours of injury to reduce risk of bleeding into injured area and improve healing.
- Healing is quicker when PRICE management is begun within 48 hours of injury.
- A heel lift is used in early stages of injury for pain relief, but it should be tapered and removed as early as possible for quicker return to ambulation.
- With inadequate rehabilitation, scar tissue formation will occur (which is weaker than muscle), causing a higher risk for injury recurrence.
  - Treat with cross-frictional massage, eccentric muscle strengthening, and stretching.

Instructions for the Patient

- Expect worsening ecchymosis and swelling for 48 hours postinjury.
- Expect 2 to 4 weeks of rehabilitation for minor strains and up to 12 weeks for severe injuries.

- Discuss and give patient information on what to expect during rehabilitation and discuss risk of reinjury if an attempt to return to sport is made prior to full recovery.
- The patient should continue strengthening and stretching exercises for several months after the injury to avoid reinjury.
- Even with adequate rehabilitation, reinjuries can occur, although this is rare.
- Strengthening exercises should be performed on the opposite leg as well, as contralateral injury is possible.

Considerations for Special Populations

- Injury is uncommon in athletes younger than 19 years of age.
- Risk of injury is higher for the deconditioned athlete attempting to return too soon from unrelated injury.
- Geriatric patients are at higher risk of injury to medial gastrocnemius muscle from lower-stress activities such as stepping out of a car or arising from bed.

Suggested Readings

Delgado GJ, Chung CB, Lektrakul N, et al. Tennis leg: clinical US study of 141 patients and anatomic investigation of 4 cadavers with MR imaging and us. *Radiology*. 2002;224:112–119.

Fromison AI. Tennis leg. *JAMA*. 1969;209:415–416.

Miller AP. Strains of the posterior calf musculature ("tennis leg"). *Am J Sports Med*. 1979;7:172–174.

Miller WA. Rupture of the musculotendinous juncture of the medial head of gastrocnemius muscle. *Am J Sports Med*. 1977;5(5):1913.

O'Connor FG, Casa DJ, Davis BA, et al, eds. *ACSM's Sports Medicine: A Comprehensive Review*. Philadelphia: Lippincott Williams & Wilkins; 2013:435–436.

Shah J, Shah B, Shah A. Pictorial essay: ultrasonography in 'tennis leg. *Indian J Radiol Imaging*. 2010;20(4):269–273.

Shields CL, Redix L, Brewster CE. Acute tears of the medial head of the gastrocnemius. *Foot Ankle*. 1985;5:186–189.

Chapter 162 Stress Fractures of the Tibia and Fibula

Robert H. Lutz, Annunziato Amendola

ICD-10-CM CODE
M84.369A *Stress fracture, unspecified tibia and fibula, initial encounter for fracture*

Key Concepts

- The tibia is the most common site of stress fracture (25–46%), followed by the fibula (5–12%).
- High-risk stress fractures for nonunion in the leg (under tension) include the anterior tibia and medial malleolus (Fig. 162.1).
- Low-risk stress fractures for nonunion in the leg (under compression) include the posteromedial tibia and fibula (see Fig. 162.1).
- Most tibia stress fractures occur in the proximal third (volleyball, basketball), followed by the distal and middle thirds (runners).
- The "dreaded black line" is a midshaft anterior tibia stress fracture seen on the lateral radiograph. It is notorious for delayed healing, with a high nonunion rate, and represents the majority of operatively treated stress fractures (Fig. 162.2).
- Most stress fractures of the fibula occur in the distal third.
- The pathophysiology of stress fractures involves accumulated stress to the bone without adequate time for repair, causing failure of bone remodeling.
- A stress reaction is a precursor to stress fracture with periosteal and bone marrow edema but no fracture line.
- Risk factors include younger age, white race, female gender, exercise-induced amenorrhea, recent increase in intensity/duration of exercise, previous inactivity, foot pronation, training on hard or uneven surfaces, previous stress fracture, and narrow intramedullary canal.

History

- Exertional pain of insidious onset after a change in activity level
- Exercise makes the pain worse, but the pain does not go away with rest
- Night pain possible
- Pain localized over a discrete area of bone
- Important to ask about a history of stress fractures

Physical Examination
Observation

- Antalgic gait with walking or running
- Focal swelling over the fracture site

Palpation

- Localized point tenderness, often transverse rather than longitudinal along the bone
- Periosteal edema or palpable bump

Special Tests

- Hop test: Hopping on one leg causes pain at the site of stress fracture.
- Tuning fork test: Vibration causes pain over the fracture site.
- Percussion test: Percussion of the bone at a site distant from the injury causes pain.
- Neurovascular examination is normal.

Imaging
Radiographs

Recommended first imaging study, consider repeat in 10 to 14 days if negative

- Only 20-30% positive at presentation; 50% later in the course
- Focal sclerosis, periosteal reaction, and cortical thickening (Fig. 162.3)
- Dreaded black line: linear transverse lucency in the anterior tibial cortex on the lateral view (see Fig. 162.2)
- If negative, consider repeating in 2 to 4 weeks or obtain additional studies.

Magnetic Resonance Imaging

- Recommended next imaging study if radiographs negative
- Periosteal edema, bone marrow edema, and fracture line (Figs. 162.4–162.7)
- Distinguishes between soft-tissue and bone injury

Computed Tomography

- May be used to define fracture lines or distinguish a fracture from other diagnoses
- May show evidence of healing with resolution of the lucency or bone sclerosis

High risk

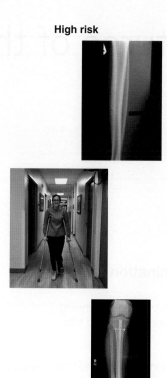

Low risk

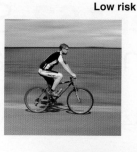

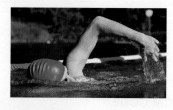

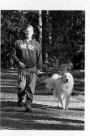

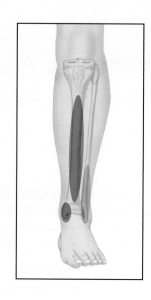

Fig 162.1 High-risk fractures (anterior tibia and medial malleolus) are identified by radiographs, treated in a non–weight-bearing cast or boot, and may require surgical fixation. Low-risk fractures (fibula and posterior tibia) are treated with relative rest and activity modification, replacing high-impact exercise with biking, swimming, or walking.

Bone Scan

- Focal area of uptake (versus diffuse linear uptake in medial tibial stress syndrome)
- Traditional "gold standard" for diagnosis: highly sensitive, less specific
- More radiation exposure and more time consuming than magnetic resonance imaging

Differential Diagnosis

- Medial tibial stress syndrome
- Exertional compartment syndrome
- Fascial hernia
- Neoplasm
- Nerve entrapment

Treatment
At Diagnosis

- Treatment varies depending on the fracture site.
- High-risk stress fractures may result in progression to complete fracture, nonunion, or recurrence if not treated aggressively.
- Low-risk stress fractures tend to heal with activity modification and nonaggressive treatment.
- Nonsteroidal antiinflammatory drugs and physical therapy modalities help to control pain.
  - Anterior tibia (high risk): strict avoidance of weight bearing; use crutches, casting, or bracing for 3 to 12 weeks

- More than 70% may require operative intervention.
- In competitive athletes, surgery may be considered initially.
- If there is a clear fracture line or 3 to 6 months of failed nonoperative treatment, operative treatment is indicated with intramedullary nailing or plating.
- Other surgical techniques include drilling or excising the fracture site with or without bone grafting and tension-band plating.
- Posteromedial tibia or fibula (low risk): Treatment depends on the athlete's goals, functional limitations, and timing of the season.
  - If no limitations and pain not progressive, activity level may be continued to complete the season
  - If functional limitation due to pain, activity modification with relative rest (cross-training)
  - If limitations in walking due to pain, bracing or crutches may be used with cross-training to remain pain free

Later

- Anterior tibia stress fractures should be healed and have painless activity before return to sport (average 7 months, range 3 to 10 months).
- After surgical management, the patient may weight bear as tolerated.
- Crutches and bracing are discontinued as soon as symptoms allow, followed by a gradual progression of activity based on symptoms.
- For low-risk stress fractures, gradually advance activity as tolerated to remain pain free.

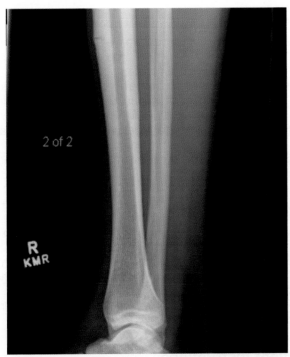

Fig 162.2 Radiograph showing the "dreaded black line" of an anterior tibia stress fracture with a thickened anterior cortex and a lucent line.

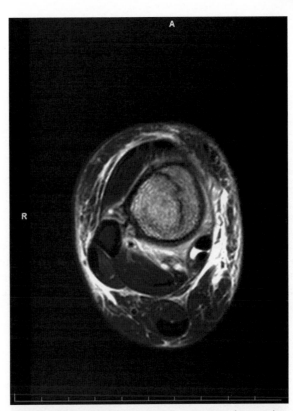

Fig 162.4 Axial T2-weighted magnetic resonance image showing a tibia stress fracture with the fracture line and severe periosteal and bone marrow edema.

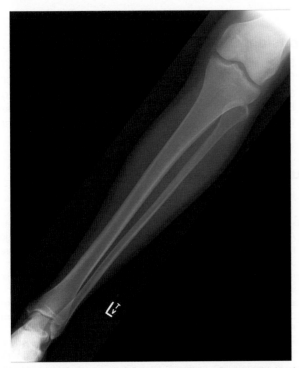

Fig 162.3 Radiograph showing scalloping, periosteal thickening, and cortical thickening at the medial distal tibia consistent with a stress fracture.

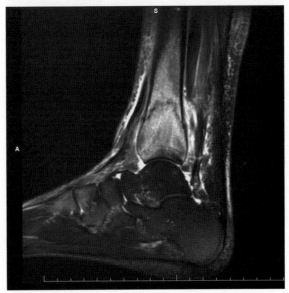

Fig 162.5 Sagittal T2-weighted magnetic resonance image showing a tibia stress fracture with the fracture line and severe periosteal and bone marrow edema.

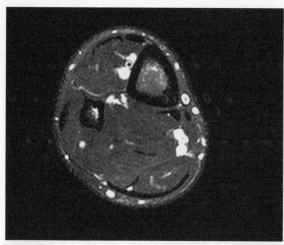

Fig 162.6 Axial T2-weighted, fat-saturated magnetic resonance image showing bone marrow edema with adjacent cortical thickening of the lateral fibula consistent with stress reaction.

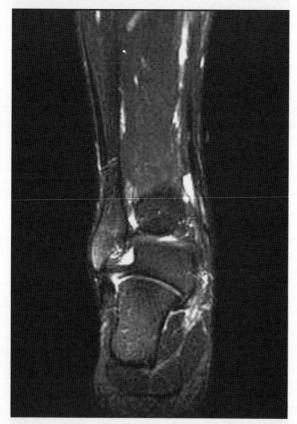

Fig 162.7 Coronal T2-weighted, fat-saturated magnetic resonance image showing bone marrow edema with cortical thickening of the lateral fibula consistent with stress reaction.

- If fracture does not heal with activity modification, implement complete rest, immobilization, or surgical treatment.

When to Refer

- Patients with high-risk stress fractures, low-risk stress fractures with progressive pain despite conservative treatment, and recurrent stress fractures should be referred.

Prognosis

- An anterior tibia stress fracture may take 6 to 12 months to heal, even with surgery can be a career-ending injury for a high-performance athlete.
  - Complications of intramedullary nailing include anterior knee pain, recurrent fracture, progression to complete fracture, nonunion, and infection.
- Fibula and posteromedial tibia stress fractures may take 1 to 3 months to heal with appropriate-level rest.
- Stress reactions (no definite fracture line) usually heal more quickly in 3 to 6 weeks.

Troubleshooting

- Worsening pain at a previously comfortable level should prompt investigation for progression of the fracture.
- Search for training errors that may be changed to avoid future injury because training errors are the most common cause of stress injuries.
- Pneumatic leg braces may be effective in speeding healing, decreasing pain, and returning to activity earlier.

Patient Instructions

- For an anterior tibia stress fracture, counsel the patient about the risk of progression to complete fracture and the prolonged recovery period so that activity is not advanced too early.

Considerations in Special Populations

- Stress fractures in female athletes require assessment for female athletic triad including menstrual history, nutritional assessment, and consideration of bone density testing.
- For recurrent stress fractures, consider a laboratory workup for metabolic bone disease, bone density testing, and nutritional assessment.

Suggested Readings

Brukner P, Bradshaw C, Khan KM, et al. Stress fractures: a review of 180 cases. *Clin J Sport Med*. 1996;6:85–89.

Expert Panel on Musculoskeletal Imaging, Bencardino JT, Stone TJ, et al. American College of Radiology appropriateness criteria: stress (fatigue/insufficiency) fracture, including sacrum, excluding other vertebrae. *J Am Coll Radiol*. 2017;14(5S):S293–S306.

Iwamoto J, Takeda T. Stress fractures in athletes: review of 196 cases. *J Orthop Sci*. 2003;8:273–278.

Jones BH, Thacker SB, Gilchrist J, et al. Prevention of lower extremity stress fractures in athletes and soldiers: a systematic review. *Epidemiol Rev*. 2002;24:228–247.

Robertson GAJ, Wood AM. Return to sport after stress fractures of the tibial diaphysis: a systematic review. *Br Med Bull*. 2015;114:95–111.

Rome K, Handoll HHG, Ashford R. Interventions for preventing and treating stress fractures and stress reactions of bone of the lower limbs in young adults. *Cochrane Database Syst Rev*. 2005;(2):CD000450.

Varner KE, Younas SA, Lintner DM, et al. Chronic anterior midtibial stress fractures in athletes treated with reamed intramedullary nailing. *Am J Sports Med*. 2005;33:1071–1076.

Chapter 163 Distal Femur and Proximal Tibia Fractures

Jonathan R. Helms, Michelle E. Kew, Seth R. Yarboro

ICD-10-CM CODES
S72.45*A *Supracondylar fracture of the femur, closed*
S72.45*B *Supracondylar fracture of the femur, open*
S72.46*A *Intercondylar fracture of the femur, closed*
S72.46*B *Intercondylar fracture of the femur, open*
S82.143A *Tibial plateau fracture, closed*
S82.143B *Tibial plateau fracture, open*

Key Concepts

- Supracondylar femur fractures involve the distal femoral metaphysis with or without intercondylar (intra-articular) extension.
- Radiographs and computed tomography (CT) are essential to characterize intra-articular extension (Fig. 163.1).
- Supracondylar femur fractures occurring proximal to total knee arthroplasty components are classified as periprosthetic fractures (Fig. 163.2).
- Open and high-energy distal femur fractures are frequently associated with a femoral condyle coronal plane (Hoffa) fracture (Fig. 163.3).
- Tibial plateau fractures are intra-articular fractures of the proximal tibia.
- Tibial plateau fractures are commonly classified using the Schatzker classification (Figs. 163.4 and 163.5).
- High-energy tibial plateau fractures can be associated with neurovascular injuries or compartment syndrome; both are indications for immediate surgical referral.
- Knee ligament and meniscal injuries are common.
- All periarticular knee fractures require orthopaedic surgery evaluation.

History

- High-energy mechanism (e.g., motor vehicle collision, polytrauma) in younger patients
- Low-energy mechanisms are common in older patients (see Fig. 163.2).
- Pain, swelling, and inability to bear weight
- Possible neurovascular symptoms

Physical Examination

- Observation
  - Deformity
  - Circumferential skin assessment: Evaluate any bleeding, lacerations, fracture blisters, or prior incisions and for the possibility of an open fracture.
- Palpation
  - Tenderness and crepitus.
  - Knee ligament examination is important after the fracture is stabilized.
  - Posterior tibial and dorsalis pedis pulses: use Doppler if nonpalpable.
    - The ankle-brachial index measures systolic pressure at the ankle compared with the upper extremity. Values less than 0.9 indicate a high probability of arterial injury, possibly requiring arteriography and/or vascular surgery consultation (Fig. 163.6).
  - Compartment syndrome evaluation: Primary sign is pain out of proportion (pallor, pulselessness, poikilothermia, paresthesias are late findings or associated with vascular injury); immediate surgical evaluation for consideration of fasciotomies.

Imaging

- Radiographs: anteroposterior, lateral, and 45-degree oblique views of the knee
  - Traction (manual or external fixator) may aid in fracture visualization (Fig. 163.7).
  - Evaluate fracture displacement and intra-articular extension.
  - Obtain radiographs of the joint above and below for associated injuries.
  - Periprosthetic fractures require full-length femur and/or tibia radiographs. Assess implant stability.
- Computed tomography with axial, coronal, and sagittal reconstructions, +/–3D
  - Mandatory to characterize intra-articular extension and articular depression (see Figs. 163.1 and 163.3).
- Magnetic resonance imaging may detect associated ligamentous and meniscal injuries.

Differential Diagnosis

- Distal femoral or proximal tibial shaft fracture
- Knee dislocation
- Pathologic fracture
- Compartment syndrome without fracture
- Proximal tibiofibular joint disruption

Treatment

- Initial management
  - Reduce and stabilize fracture to limit further soft-tissue injury with a padded, well-molded, three-sided long leg splint.

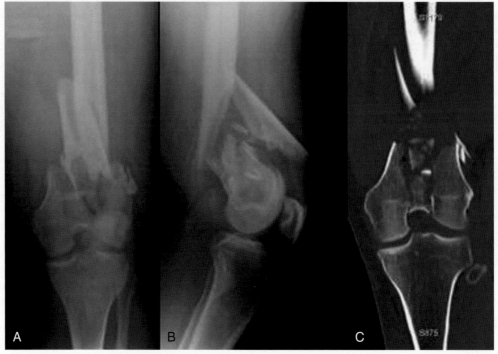

Fig 163.1 Open comminuted supracondylar femur fracture with intercondylar extension. Anteroposterior **(A)** and lateral **(B)** radiographs. **(C)** Computed tomography demonstrating the intra-articular extension.

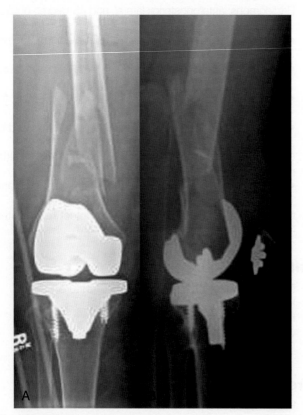

Fig 163.2 Periprosthetic distal femur fracture. Anteroposterior **(A)** and lateral **(B)** radiographs demonstrating fracture above a well-fixed total knee arthroplasty.

- Open fractures first require a sterile saline dressing in addition to appropriate antibiotic and tetanus prophylaxis (see Tables 165.2 and 165.3). Do not irrigate or probe the wound, remove bone fragments, apply tourniquets or clamps for vascular injury (address with direct pressure), or perform wound closure. After splint application, repeat physical examination and obtain radiographs. Patients with high-energy fractures should be admitted and monitored for compartment syndrome.
- Definitive management
  - Definitive treatment is determined by consulting an orthopaedic surgeon.
  - Nonoperative treatment is rarely indicated for isolated, nondisplaced, extra-articular distal femur fractures and more frequently for isolated lateral tibial plateau fractures with less than 3 mm of articular step-off and less than 10 degrees of varus/valgus instability with the knee extended.
    - A locked hinged knee brace and no weight bearing for 6 to 12 weeks are required.
    - Knee range of motion (ROM) is initiated at 2 to 4 weeks.
    - Occasionally, nonoperative treatment is also selected for nonambulatory patients with advanced medical conditions (severe dementia, paraplegia).
    - Physical therapy is essential, as are serial radiographs, to ensure maintenance of mechanical alignment.
    - Consider deep venous thrombosis prophylaxis with injectable low-molecular-weight heparin or aspirin.

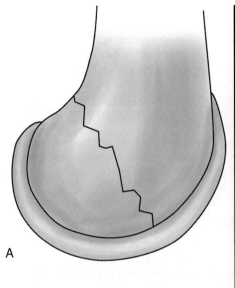

A

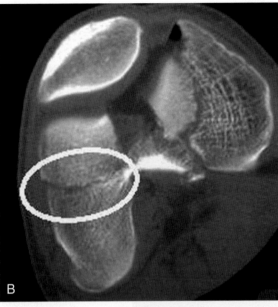

B

Fig 163.3 Hoffa fracture. Coronal shear injury of the femoral condyle, common in open fractures. **(A)** Lateral diagram of fracture orientation. **(B)** Computed tomography image of an open supracondylar femur fracture showing the coronal fracture fragment *(circle)*.

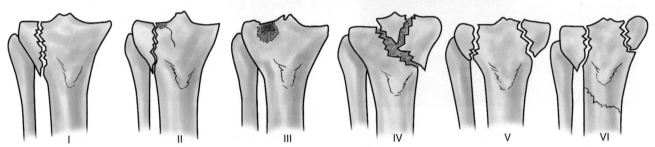

I   II   III   IV   V   VI

Fig 163.4 Schatzker classification of tibial plateau fractures. **I,** Lateral split; **II,** lateral split depression; **III,** lateral isolated depression; **IV,** medial; **V,** bicondylar; **VI,** bicondylar with metadiaphyseal dissociation.

Distal Femoral and Proximal Tibial Fractures

Fig 163.5 Overview of distal femur and proximal tibia fractures. *ROM,* Range of motion.

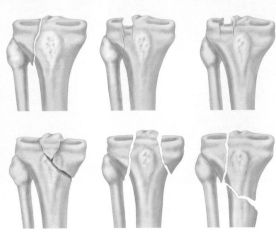

- Most distal femur fractures require surgery to restore stability and allow early ROM.

- Proximal tibial fractures require surgery if associated with 10 degrees of coronal plane stability.

- If stable and less than 3 mm displacement, closed traetment likely appropriate.

- If the fracture is shortened and not length-stable, temporizing external fixator may be required.

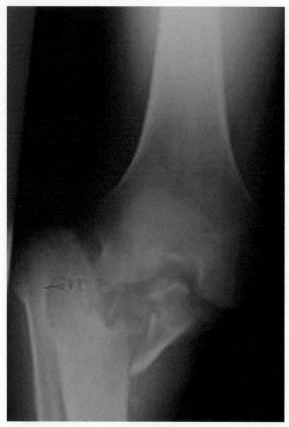

Fig 163.6 Anteroposterior radiograph of comminuted, high-energy, medial tibial plateau fracture (Schatzker grade IV). The patient had a vascular injury at the level of the popliteal fossa that was detected after reduction and ankle-brachial index determination (ankle-brachial index <0.9). This patient required hospital admission and urgent orthopaedic referral.

- Operative treatment is required for all other distal femur and tibial plateau fractures.
  - Temporizing external fixation is performed on all fractures with residual knee subluxation after traction and splinting or soft-tissue injuries that require close monitoring.
  - The duration of temporizing fixation ranges from 1 to 6 weeks and is generally dictated by the soft tissues (i.e., fracture blisters).
  - When the soft tissues improve, the treating surgeon will decide between definitive open reduction and internal fixation or definitive treatment in an external fixator.

When to Refer

- All patients with distal femur or tibial plateau fractures require referral to an orthopaedic surgeon.
- Delayed referral can be considered in patients with low-energy injuries, adequate reduction, soft compartments, and intact neurovascular status after appropriate immobilization.
- Emergent orthopaedic surgical consultation is required for open fractures, neurovascular injury, severe fracture displacement (e.g., Schatzker grade IV, V, VI), or knee subluxation requiring external fixation (see Figs. 163.6 and 163.7), and/or impending or established compartment syndrome.

Prognosis

- Varies from simple fracture patterns with minimal soft-tissue damage to severe limb-threatening injuries associated with neurologic, vascular, muscle, and skin damage.
- The prognosis also varies depending on patient comorbidities and social factors.

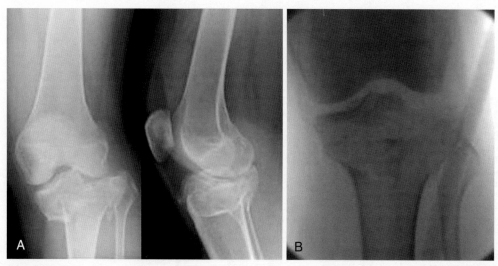

Fig 163.7 Bicondylar tibia plateau fracture (Schatzker grade V). **(A)** Anteroposterior and lateral radiographs demonstrating subluxation of the knee. **(B)** Radiograph obtained after application of temporizing external fixation (traction). This image assists with preoperative planning. Computed tomography should also be performed with the knee in a reduced position.

- Restoration of mechanical alignment and early postoperative knee motion are essential for good outcomes.
- Timely antibiotic administration in open fractures improves the prognosis.

Troubleshooting

- Delayed unions should be evaluated for the presence of infection (complete blood count with differential, erythrocyte sedimentation rate, and C-reactive protein) and are often associated with high-energy injuries and poor host factors (i.e., nicotine use, diabetes, thyroid conditions, vitamin D deficiency).
- Complications include malunion, nonunion, posttraumatic arthritis, nerve injury, vascular injury, deep venous thrombosis, pulmonary embolism, fat embolism, pain, weakness, knee stiffness, infection, hardware failure, and wound-healing issues.

Patient Instructions

- Patients should be counseled on weight-bearing restrictions, splint care, extremity elevation, and deep venous thrombosis prophylaxis.
- Patients should return or call if increased pain, swelling, or neurovascular changes.

Considerations in Special Populations

- Individuals who are at high risk for complication from anesthesia may benefit from nonoperative management.

- Nonoperative treatment may be considered in patients with low functional demands (i.e., nonambulatory patients).

Suggested Readings

Barei DP, Nork SE, Mills WJ, et al. Functional outcomes of severe bicondylar tibial plateau fractures treated with dual incisions and medial and lateral plates. *J Bone Joint Surg Am*. 2006;88A:1713–1721.

Bennett WF, Browner B. Tibial plateau fractures: a study of associated soft tissue injuries. *J Orthop Trauma*. 1994;8:183–188.

Borrelli J. Management of soft tissue injuries associated with tibial plateau fractures. *J Knee Surg*. 2014;27(1):5–10.

Ehlinger M, Ducrot G, Adam P, Bonnomet F. Distal femur fractures. Surgical techniques and a review of the literature. *Orthop Traumatol Surg Res*. 2013;99:353–360.

Gwathmey WF, Jones-Quaidoo SM, et al. Distal femoral fractures: current concepts. *J Am Acad Orthop Surg*. 2010;18:597–607.

Jeelani A, Arastu MH. Tibial plateau fractures—review of current concepts in management. *J Orthop Trauma*. 2017;31:102–115.

Miller M, Thompson SR, eds. *Review of Orthopaedics*. 7th ed. Philadelphia: Elsevier; 2016.

Mthethwa J, Chikate A. A review of the management of tibial plateau fractures. *Musculoskelet Surg*. 2017;[Epub ahead of print].

Nauth A, Ristevski B, Béqué T, Schemitsch EH. Periprosthetic distal femur fractures: current concepts. *J Orthop Trauma*. 2011;25(suppl 2):S82–S85.

Nork SE, Segina DN, Aflatoon K, et al. The association between supracondylar-intercondylar distal femoral fractures and coronal plane fractures. *J Bone Joint Surg Am*. 2005;87A:564–569.

Ruffolo MR, Gettys FK, Montijo HE, et al. Complications of high-energy bicondylar tibial plateau fractures treated with dual plating through 2 incisions. *J Orthop Trauma*. 2015;29:85–90.

Weigel DP, Marsh JL. High-energy fractures of the tibial plateau: knee function after longer follow-up. *J Bone Joint Surg Am*. 2002;84A:1541–1551.

Chapter 164 Patella Fractures

Seth R. Yarboro, Michelle E. Kew

Key Concepts

- Patella fractures are uncommon, comprising approximately 1% of all fractures.
- Patella fractures are twice as common in males.
- The diagnosis is made with physical examination and confirmed with radiographs. Advanced imaging is rarely required.
- Fractures are classified by the orientation of the fracture line(s) on radiographs (Fig. 164.1), the degree of displacement, and whether the fracture is open or closed.
- Displaced fractures have more than 2-mm articular step-off and/or 3-mm separation between fragments (gap).
- Patella fractures are rarely bilateral; bilateral radiographic findings may represent a bipartite patella.
- Displaced patella fractures disrupt the extensor mechanism and may result in an inability to actively extend the knee (Fig. 164.2).
- In fractures with an intact medial/lateral retinacula, active knee extension may be possible (Fig. 164.3). If there is minimal extension lag, nonoperative treatment is usually indicated.

History

- Usually a combination of direct trauma with (e.g., knee striking dashboard) with indirect force of quadriceps contraction.
- Patients report pain and swelling, difficulty with knee extension and ambulation (may report knee buckling with weight bearing).

Physical Examination

- Observation, palpation, range of motion (ROM), effusion may be noted (hemarthrosis).
- Circumferential skin assessment: Laceration or surrounding skin trauma must raise concern for possible traumatic knee arthrotomy or open fracture. A saline load test can further evaluate.
  - Saline load test: sterile arthrocentesis followed by intra-articular injection of at least 60 mL of sterile saline, with extravasation indicating traumatic arthrotomy

- Palpable defect may be noted with severely displaced fractures.
- Document active knee extension as either absent, intact, or with extension lag.
- Avoid routine aspiration of hematomas or instillation of intra-articular lidocaine to minimize the risk of iatrogenic septic arthritis. Patients with equivocal exam may be able to demonstrate extensor mechanism function if knee hemarthrosis is aspirated.

Imaging

- Radiographs: Anteroposterior and lateral radiographs are required. Sunrise view can be considered but painful for patient and of limited clinical value for most fractures.
- Evaluate fracture orientation (transverse, stellate [comminuted], or vertical), displacement, presence of effusion, presence of foreign materials or free air, and patella alta or baja (indicating patellar tendon or quadriceps tendon injury, respectively).
- Magnetic resonance imaging (MRI), computed tomography (CT) rarely indicated for isolated patellar fractures.

Differential Diagnosis

- Patella fracture
- Bipartite patella: round, smooth bony fragment at the superolateral corner of the patella with sclerotic borders (see Fig. 164.1)
- Femoral condyle fracture or chondral injury (Fig. 164.4)
- Quadriceps tendon or patella ligament injury
- Patella sleeve fracture (see Fig. 164.1)

Treatment

- Initial management: Stabilize fracture with a padded knee brace to limit further soft-tissue injury.
- Nonoperative management reserved for patellar fractures with intact extensor mechanism or patients with significant comorbidities.
  - Patients may weight bear as tolerated in hinged knee brace locked in extension.
- Operative treatment used for displaced or open fractures with the goal to reconstruct the extensor mechanism and patellar joint surface.
- Open fracture management: First apply sterile saline gauze and administer appropriate antibiotic and tetanus prophylaxis (see Tables 165.2 and 165.3). Do not irrigate or probe the wound, remove bone fragments, or perform wound closure.

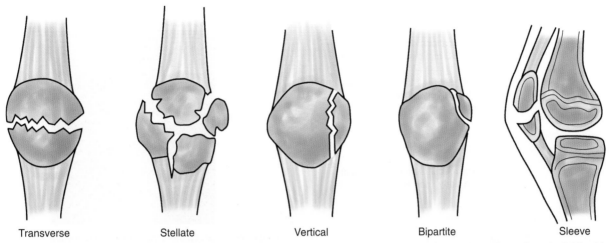

Fig 164.1 Patella fracture classification. Adult fracture patterns include transverse, stellate (comminuted), and vertical. The bipartite patella is frequently confused with a patella fracture. Patellar sleeve fractures are the most common patella fracture in the pediatric population.

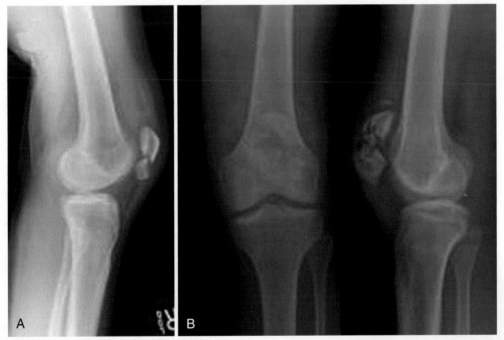

Fig 164.2 Radiographs of displaced patella fractures. **(A)** Lateral view of transverse patella fracture associated with loss of active knee extension. Note knee effusion and fracture displacement. The superior fragment is pulled by the quadriceps muscle while the inferior pole of the patella is pulled by the patellar ligament. **(B)** Anteroposterior and lateral views of stellate (comminuted) open patella fracture in a patient with loss of active knee extension.

- Operative options include open reduction and internal fixation (see Fig. 164.3), partial patellectomy, and total patellectomy (only indicated if patella nonreconstructible).

When to Refer

- All patients with patella fractures generally require referral to an orthopaedic surgeon.
- Closed, nondisplaced, or minimally displaced fractures with an intact extensor mechanism may be referred within 1 to 2 weeks. Patients should be placed in a knee immobilizer or ROM knee brace locked in extension.

Patients are allowed to bear weight in extension, but may benefit from crutches or walker in the early recovery period.
- Displaced fractures are likely operative and should be referred more acutely.
- Emergent orthopaedic surgical consultation is required in patients with open fractures or traumatic arthrotomy.

Prognosis

- Varies based on fracture type, associated injuries, and patient comorbidities

Patellar Fractures

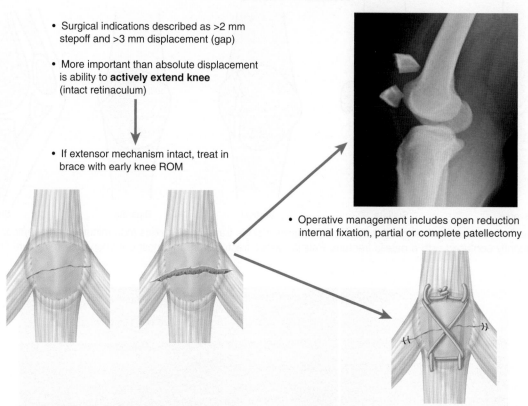

- Surgical indications described as >2 mm stepoff and >3 mm displacement (gap)

- More important than absolute displacement is ability to **actively extend knee** (intact retinaculum)

- If extensor mechanism intact, treat in brace with early knee ROM

- Operative management includes open reduction internal fixation, partial or complete patellectomy

Fig 164.3 Overview of patella fractures. *ROM,* Range of motion.

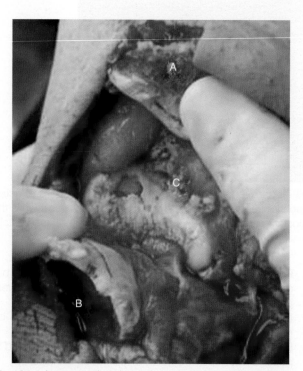

Fig 164.4 Intraoperative photograph of transverse patella fracture. This patient had direct patella trauma striking the dashboard during a motor vehicle collision. Superior patella fracture fragment (A). Inferior patella fracture fragment (B). Femoral condyle impaction fracture with articular cartilage damage and loss (C).

- Timely antibiotic administration in open fractures is considered to improve the prognosis.
- In general, fracture healing can be seen on radiographs 8 to 12 weeks after injury.
- Postoperatively, patients may have quadriceps weakness, knee stiffness, and surgical implant prominence.

Troubleshooting

- Patients should be informed of possible complications including loss of reduction or fixation requiring repeat surgery, nonunion or malunion, knee stiffness, persistent extensor lag, and prominent implants.

Patient Instructions

- Patients should be instructed on the importance of strict adherence to ROM restrictions and bracing. Surgeons may follow a postoperative protocol to regain motion gradually as healing occurs.
- Physical therapy is often employed and will be dictated by the treating orthopaedist.

Considerations in Special Populations

- After anterior cruciate ligament reconstruction with a patellar tendon autograft, patients may be at risk of a patella fracture.

- Patellar sleeve (osteochondral) fractures are the most common patella fracture in pediatric patients and require prompt reduction; internal fixation is usually necessary.

Suggested Readings

Bostrom A. Fracture of the patella: a clinical study of 422 patellar fractures. *Acta Orthop Scand*. 1921;143:1–80.

Browner B, Jupiter J, Krettek C, Anderson PA, eds. *Skeletal Trauma: Basic Science, Management, and Reconstruction*. 5th ed. Philadelphia: Elsevier; 2015.

Carpenter JE, Kasman R, Matthews LS. Fractures of the patella. *J Bone Joint Surg Am*. 1993;75A:1550–1561.

Catalano JB, Iannacone WM, Marczyk S, et al. Open fractures of the patella: long-term functional outcome. *J Trauma*. 1995;39:439–444.

Hunt DM, Somashekar N. A review of sleeve fractures of the patella in children. *Knee*. 2005;12:3–7.

Melvin JS, Mehta S. Patellar fractures in adults. *J Am Acad Orthop Surg*. 2011;19(4):198–207.

Miller M, Thompson SR, eds. *Review of Orthopaedics*. 7th ed. Philadelphia: Elsevier; 2016.

Okike K, Bhattacharyya T. Trends in the management of open fractures. A critical analysis. *J Bone Joint Surg Am*. 2006;88A:2739–2748.

Chapter 165 Tibial and Fibular Shaft Fractures

Thomas Schaller, Michael Hunter

ICD-10-CM CODES

S82.7	*Multiple fractures of lower leg*
S82.70	*Multiple fractures of lower leg, closed*
S82.71	*Multiple fractures of lower leg, open*
S82.40	*Fibula alone, closed*
S82.41	*Fibula alone, open*
S82.10	*Upper end, closed*
S82.11	*Upper end, open*
S82.20	*Shaft, closed*
S82.21	*Shaft, open*
823.4	*Torus fracture*
S82.90	*Unspecified part, closed*
S82.91	*Unspecified part, open*

Key Concepts

- The tibia is the major weight-bearing bone of the lower leg. Although the fibula is less significant in weight-bearing (6–17%), it does serve an important role in ankle stability.
- Tibial shaft fractures are the most common long bone diaphyseal fracture and frequently require surgical intervention.
- Fractures of the tibial shaft are frequently open fractures (24%). Timely tetanus and antibiotic prophylaxis is critical, along with immediate surgical referral.
- Tibia fractures are most frequently associated with fibula fractures (80%); they may also be associated with ligamentous injuries of the knee and ankle.
- High-energy tibia fractures may result in neurovascular injuries or compartment syndrome (1.2–9%)—most commonly in young males; both are indications for immediate surgical referral. Open fractures do not exclude the possibility of developing compartment syndrome.

History

- Acute injury
- Direct blow or indirect trauma (typically twisting injury)
- Low-energy (fall) or high-energy (motor vehicle collision) trauma (Fig. 165.1)
- Low- versus high-velocity penetrating injuries (gunshot wounds)
- Pain and inability to bear weight are common complaints
- Chronic injury
- Soldiers, dancers, and runners are susceptible to fatigue fractures. Must have high index of suspicion. This clinical scenario refers to failure of healthy bone under abnormally high amounts of stress

- Pathologic fractures may result from a tumor or metabolic condition causing mechanical weakening in the bony architecture. This clinical scenario occurs in the presence of weakened bone structure under normal amounts of stress

Physical Examination

- Inspection
- Deformity
- Be sure to assess entire extremity and patient for associated injuries
- Circumferential skin assessment: Any blood, lacerations, or surrounding skin trauma must raise concern for possible open fracture
- A compromised soft-tissue envelope (i.e., fracture blisters, abrasions) can alter the surgical plan
- Palpation
- Tenderness, crepitus
- Manual compression of leg compartments (see later in the chapter)
- Range of motion
- Assess for injuries to the knee and ankle. This can be challenging in the acute setting while the fracture is mobile and the patient is guarding due to pain
- Special tests
- Advanced Trauma Life Support protocol when indicated in a trauma setting, including secondary survey to assess for additional skeletal trauma and complete neurovascular examination
  - Posterior tibial and dorsalis pedis pulses; Doppler probe for signals if nonpalpable.
  - The ankle-brachial index measures systolic pressure at the ankle compared with that of the ipsilateral upper extremity. Values less than 0.9 indicate a high probability of arterial injury and warrant vascular consultation and possible arteriography.
  - Neurologic examination (Table 165.1) may be compromised in obtunded patients. Proximal fibula fractures (bumper injuries), in particular, may be associated with injury to the common peroneal nerve as it courses around the fibular neck.
- Compartment syndrome evaluation
  - This is a clinical diagnosis based on symptoms and physical exam findings; however, in the obtunded patient it can be exceptionally difficult and therefore requires objective compartment pressure measurement.
  - Elevated compartment pressures are common after significant leg trauma, but the elevated pressure does

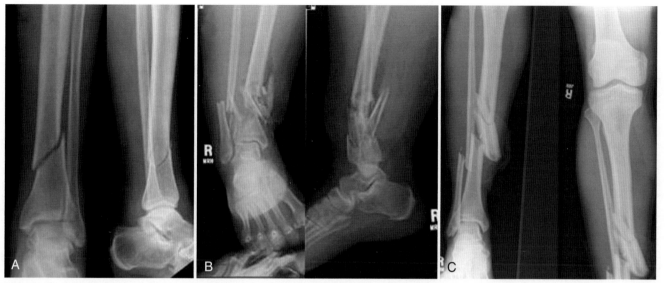

Fig 165.1 Anteroposterior and lateral radiographs. **(A)** Low-energy, distal, spiral tibial shaft fracture without associated fibula fracture. **(B)** High-energy, distal, comminuted, open tibial shaft fracture with associated fibula fracture. **(C)** High-energy, midshaft, segmental, comminuted, open tibial shaft fracture with associated fibula fracture.

TABLE 165.1 Examination of a Tibial Shaft Fracture

Nerve	Motor Function	Sensory Distribution
Sural	Foot plantarflexion	Lateral heel
Saphenous	None	Medial leg and ankle
Superficial peroneal	Foot eversion	Dorsum of foot including great toe
Deep peroneal	Great toe dorsiflexion	First web space of the foot
Tibial	Toe plantarflexion	Sole of foot

not necessarily lead to the development of the clinical syndrome.
- Maintain a high index of suspicion. Firmness to manual compression is a cause for concern.
- Pain out of proportion to the injury and pain that does not respond to appropriate medication are associated with the syndrome.
- Pain with passive stretch of the toes is a sensitive test but can be difficult to assess due to the presence of fracture-related pain.
- Patients often appear anxious, diaphoretic, or even writhing due to the intractable nature of the pain.
- When assessing the pressure directly, measurements should be obtained at the level of the fracture. ΔP (diastolic blood pressure – compartment pressure) of less than 30 mm Hg warrants emergent fasciotomy of all four leg compartments.

Imaging

- Radiographs: anteroposterior and lateral views of the tibia and fibula
- Optimal radiographs are obtained after gross realignment and prior to splinting to better characterize the fracture pattern (see Fig. 165.1B).
- Obtain radiographs of the joint above and below.
- Evaluate the radiographs for fracture location, comminution, malalignment, skin tenting, and the presence of foreign materials or free air.
- Bone scan or magnetic resonance imaging (MRI)
- May be useful in diagnosing fatigue or pathologic fractures
- Computed tomography (CT) scan may be used to define any intra-articular extension of the fracture

Differential Diagnosis

- Intra-articular fracture of the knee (plateau fracture) or ankle (pilon fracture)
- Compartment syndrome without fracture
- Pathologic, osteopenic, or stress fracture

Treatment
Tibial Shaft Fractures

- Initial management.
- Reduce and stabilize the fracture to limit further soft-tissue injury with a padded, well-molded, long leg splint.
- For open fractures, remove superficial loose gross contamination with sterile gloves, irrigate the wound with sterile saline, and apply a sterile saline dressing. Administer appropriate tetanus and antibiotic prophylaxis (Tables 165.2 and 165.3).

TABLE 165.2 Current Centers for Disease Control and Prevention Recommendations Regarding Tetanus Prophylaxis

Previous Doses of Absorbed TT	CLEAN MINOR WOUNDS <6 H OLD		ALL OTHER WOUNDS	
	Tdap or Td	TIG	Tdap or Td	TIG
Unknown or <3	Yes	No	Yes	Yes
≥3	No[a]	No	No[b]	No

[a]Yes, if ≥10 years since last TT-containing vaccine dose.
[b]Yes, if ≥5 years since last TT-containing vaccine dose.
The preferred vaccine preparation depends on the age of the child or adolescent:
<7 yr: DTaP
7–11 yr: Td
11–64 yr: Tdap for those who have never received Tdap.
Td is preferred to TT for those who received Tdap previously, when Tdap is not available, or for persons >64 years.
DTap, Diphtheria-tetanus-acellular pertussis; *Td*, adult tetanus; *Tdap*, booster tetanus toxoid-reduced diphtheria toxoid-acellular pertussis; *TIG*, human tetanus immune globulin; *TT*, tetanus toxoid.
Data from Centers for Disease Control and Prevention.

- Do not probe the wound, remove bone fragments, or perform wound closure.
- Use direct pressure to control hemorrhage in almost all circumstances; in rare cases a tourniquet may be needed for rapid hemorrhage not responding to firm pressure.
- Patients with high-energy or open injuries should be admitted and monitored for compartment syndrome with serial examinations for 24 hours.
- Definitive management.
- Definitive treatment determined by consulting an orthopaedic surgeon.
- Nonoperative treatment indicated for closed, low-energy fractures with acceptable alignment including angulation less than 5 degrees, shortening less than 12 mm, and translation less than 50% (Fig. 165.2).
  - Splint immobilization is converted to a long leg cast in 1 to 2 weeks as swelling improves.
  - Protected boot/brace or cast weight-bearing is initiated at 6 weeks.
- Operative treatment is indicated for many tibial shaft fractures.

TABLE 165.3 Recommended Antibiotic Prophylaxis for Open Fractures

Open Fracture Type (Gustilo)	Definition	Antibiotic
Grade I	<1 cm skin opening	First-generation cephalosporin
Grade II	Between 1- and 10-cm skin opening	First-generation cephalosporin
Grade III	A = 10 cm B = 10 cm requiring soft-tissue coverage C = vascular injury requiring repair	First-generation cephalosporin + gentamicin

Special Circumstances

High-velocity gunshot, shotgun close range, segmental fracture, open wound >8 h	Defined as a grade III	First-generation cephalosporin + gentamicin
Farm injury or grossly contaminated	Defined as a grade III	Cefazolin, gentamicin + penicillin G (12 million U/day q4h)
Freshwater-, saltwater-, or brackish water–related open fracture	Define using Gustilo Anderson classification	Consider the addition of fluoroquinolone

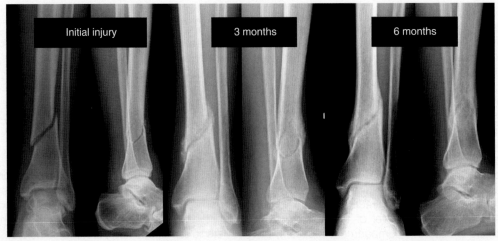

Fig 165.2 Nonoperative management: anteroposterior and lateral radiographs. Callus formation is noted in the 3-month radiograph, with healed fracture and acceptable alignment demonstrated 6 months after injury.

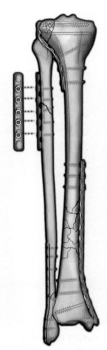

Fig 165.3 Operative management of fibular and tibial shaft fracture with plate fixation. (From Miller MD, Thompson SR, eds. *Miller's Review of Orthopaedics*. 7th ed. Philadelphia: Elsevier; 2016.)

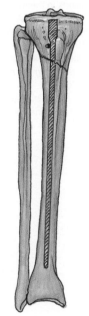

Fig 165.4 Operative management of tibial shaft fracture with intramedullary implant. (Reprinted with permission from Hiesterman TG, Shafiq BX, Cole PA. Intramedullary nailing of extra-articular proximal tibia fractures. *J Am Acad Orthop Surg*. 2011;19:690–700. © 2011 American Academy of Orthopaedic Surgeons.)

- Surgical intervention varies based on fracture type and condition of the soft-tissue envelope.
- Options include plate fixation (Fig. 165.3), intramedullary implant fixation (Fig. 165.4), or external fixation (temporary stabilization or definitive management).

- Amputation can be the best acute treatment for severe nonviable extremity injuries.

Isolated Fibular Shaft Fractures

- In isolated fibular shaft fractures from a direct blow, the fracture is generally stable and the patient can bear weight as tolerated in a functional brace or boot.
- Isolated proximal third spiral or oblique fibula fractures that result from a twisting injury to the leg can be associated with instability of the knee or the ankle and occasionally require plate fixation (see Fig. 165.3).

When to Refer

- All patients with a tibial or fibular shaft fracture require referral.
- Emergent orthopaedic surgical consultation is required in open fractures, neurovascular injury, and any with impending or established compartment syndrome.

Prognosis

- Varies from simple fracture patterns with minimal soft-tissue damage to severe limb-threatening injuries with associated neurovascular, muscular, and/or skin damage (see Fig. 165.1).
- Timely antibiotic administration in open fractures is shown to improve prognosis.
- In general, early fracture healing can be seen radiographically (callus) 4 to 12 weeks after injury (see Figs. 165.2 and 165.5).
- Normal tensile strength of bone is not restored until 8 to 12 months after fracture healing.

Troubleshooting

- Delayed unions should be evaluated for the presence of infection (complete blood count with differential, erythrocyte sedimentation rate, and C-reactive protein) and are often associated with high-energy injuries, open fractures, and poor host factors (i.e., nicotine use, diabetes, endocrine disorders).
- Fracture complications include malunion, nonunion (10%), neurovascular injury, deep venous thrombosis, pulmonary embolism, fat embolism, pain, weakness, and knee/ankle.
- Stiffness.
- Cast-related complications include skin irritation, skin breakdown, and cast saw burns.
- Specific surgery-related complications include infection, hardware failure, and wound healing issues.

Patient Instructions

- Patients should be instructed on the importance of weight-bearing restrictions, splint or cast care, extremity elevation, and deep venous thrombosis prophylaxis.
- Patients should call the physician if any increased pain, swelling, or neurovascular changes are noted.
- Frequently, due to changes in swelling or patient noncompliance issues (i.e., wet cast), adjustment or reapplication of the splint or cast is required.

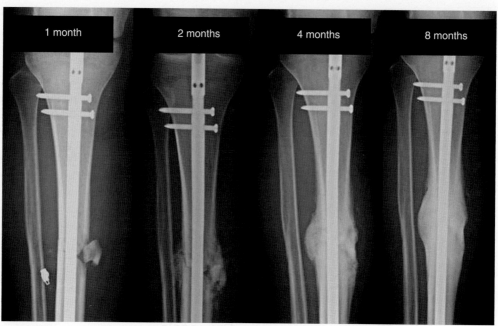

Fig 165.5 Operative management with intramedullary fixation: anteroposterior radiographs. Callus formation is noted in the 2-month postoperative radiograph. Note that surgery does not change the overall time required for fracture healing.

Suggested Readings

Bhandari M, Guyatt GH, Swiontkowski MF, et al. Treatment of open fractures of the shaft of the tibia. *J Bone Joint Surg Br*. 2001;83B:62–68.

Browner B, Jupiter J, Levine A, Trafton P. *Skeletal Trauma: Basic Science, Management, and Reconstruction*. 3rd ed. Philadelphia: Elsevier; 2003.

Court-Brown CM, McBirnie J. The epidemiology of tibial fractures. *J Bone Joint Surg Br*. 1995;77B:417–421.

Fletcher N, Sofianos D, Berkes M, et al. Prevention of perioperative infection. *J Bone Joint Surg Am*. 2007;89A:1605–1618.

Gustilo RB, Anderson JT. Prevention of infection in the treatment of one thousand and twenty-five open fractures of long bones: retrospective and prospective analyses. *J Bone Joint Surg Am*. 1976;58A:453–458.

Melvin SJ, Dombroski DG, et al. Open tibial shaft fractures: I. Evaluation and initial wound management. *J Am Acad Orthop Surg*. 2010;18(2):108–117.

Miller MD, Thompson SR. *Miller's Review of Orthopaedics*. 7th ed. Philadelphia: Elsevier; 2016.

Okike K, Bhattacharyya T. Trends in the management of open fractures. A critical analysis. *J Bone Joint Surg Am*. 2006;88A:2739–2748.

Patzakis MJ, Wilkins J. Factors influencing infection rate in open wounds. *Clin Orthop Relat Res*. 1989;243:36–40.

Shuler FD, Obremskey WT. Tibial shaft fractures. In: Stannard JP, Schmidt AH, Kregor PJ, eds. *Surgical Treatment of Orthopaedic Trauma*. New York: Thieme; 2007:742–766.

White TO, Howell GE, Will EM, et al. Elevated intramuscular compartment pressures do not influence outcome after tibial fracture. *J Trauma*. 2003;55:1133–1138.

Chapter 166 Knee Aspiration and/or Injection Technique

Mark D. Miller

CPT CODE
20610 *Aspiration and/or injection, large joint*

Procedure Name
- Knee aspiration (arthrocentesis) and injection

Equipment
- 25-gauge needle if local anesthesia planned
- Injection needle (21 gauge)
- Large-bore aspiration needle (16- to 18-gauge)
- Stopcock, optional for combined aspiration and injection
- Injection syringe (5 to 10 mL)
- Aspiration syringe (30 mL)
- Local anesthetic
- Sterile cup and/or appropriate laboratory tubes for aspiration
- Sterile tray
- Sterile gloves
- Sterile prep solution (e.g., povidone-iodine)
- Ethyl chloride, optional
- Injectable agent (steroid, hyaluronic acid)
- Sterile gauze and bandage

Indications
Aspiration
- Suspected joint infection
- Gouty arthritis
- Large painful effusion
- Loss of motion secondary to effusion

Injection
- Osteoarthritis
- Rheumatoid arthritis
- Pseudogout
- Patellar chondromalacia

Contraindications
- Aspiration
- Generalized sepsis without evidence of infected joint
- Injection
- Active or recent joint infection
- Overlying skin disease
- Impending surgical procedure

Technique (Video 166.1)
- Verbal patient consent is obtained and the correct knee is identified.
- The medication is prepared on a sterile tray with a stopcock and extra syringe available if aspiration is indicated.
- Ethyl chloride, if used, should be administered topically before sterile skin preparation (Fig. 166.1).
- With sterile gloves in place, the skin is prepared with a sterile prep solution (Fig. 166.2).
- If an effusion is present, a small needle is used to infiltrate the skin with local anesthetic before inserting the larger needle for aspiration (Fig. 166.3).
- A large-bore aspiration needle is passed into the supero-lateral pouch at a site just proximal and lateral to the superolateral border of the patella (Fig. 166.4).
- After feeling the needle pass into the joint capsule, apply gentle pressure to the plunger of the syringe to aspirate the fluid (Fig. 166.5).
- Using a stopcock will allow the same needle to be used for the injection after the aspiration is complete.
- After ensuring that the needle tip is unobstructed and in place inside the joint capsule, turn the stopcock and inject the steroid or hyaluronic acid preparation. Alternatively, the injection can be done without the use of a stopcock by using a second needle and syringe (Fig. 166.6).
- Apply dressing as per routine.

Considerations in Special Populations
- Multiple approaches have been described, but the supero-lateral approach (described here) and the direct lateral approach have been found to be the most accurate.
- Injections of morbidly obese patients may be made easier by using an inferomedial or inferolateral approach with the knee flexed to 90 degrees. This is also useful for patients who are unable to lie fully prone secondary to conditions such as back pain or orthopnea.
- If joint infection is suspected, synovial fluid obtained during aspiration should be sent for cell count, crystal analysis, Gram stain, and aerobic/anaerobic cultures.

Troubleshooting
- "Bumping" bone: Gently redirect the needle superiorly to enter the suprapatellar pouch above the femur.
- No fluid on aspiration: Make sure that the needle is in the synovial capsule and push the plunger back in to clear any obstructions in the needle tip.

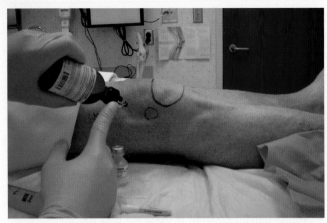

Fig 166.1 Optional use of ethyl chloride for anesthetizing the skin.

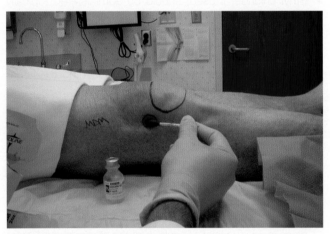

Fig 166.2 Skin preparation begins.

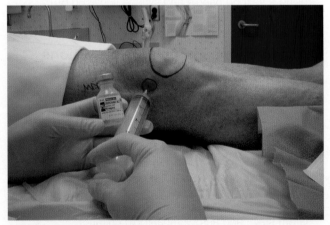

Fig 166.3 Local anesthetic is injected in the superolateral space.

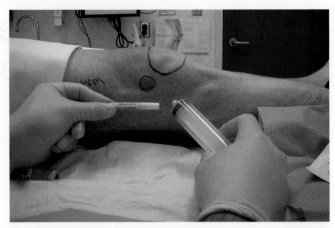

Fig 166.4 A large-bore needle and large syringe are prepared for arthrocentesis.

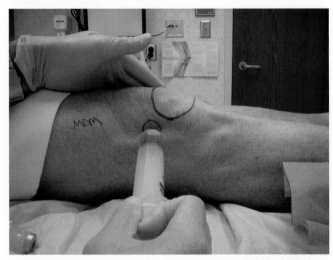

Fig 166.5 The plunger of the syringe is pulled back with gentle pressure for aspiration.

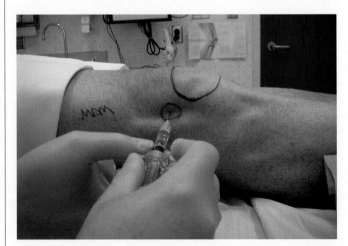

Fig 166.6 Injection of hyaluronic acid.

- Not all fluid removed: Gently "milk" the knee with your other hand, directing the fluid medially to laterally.

Instructions

may remove the dressing the following day.
t any local soreness at the injection site.

- Call the physician's office immediately if any redness, warmth, increased swelling, severe increase in pain, fever, or chills develop.
- Diabetic patients may notice slight transient elevations in the blood glucose level.

Chapter 167 Prepatellar Bursa Aspiration and/or Injection Technique

Mark D. Miller

CPT CODE

20610 *Arthrocentesis, aspiration, or injection of major joint or bursa*

Procedure Name

- Prepatellar bursa aspiration and injection

Equipment

- 25-gauge needle if local anesthesia planned
- Injection needle (21 gauge)
- Injection syringe (5 to 10 mL)
- Large-bore aspiration needle (16 to 18 gauge)
- Aspiration syringe (30 mL)
- Local anesthetic agent
- Sterile tray
- Sterile gloves
- Sterile prep solution (e.g., povidone-iodine)
- Ethyl chloride, optional
- Injectable agent (steroid, anesthetic)
- Sterile gauze and bandage

Indications

- Acute or chronic prepatellar bursitis refractory to conservative management

Contraindications

- Overlying cellulitis or skin disease

Technique (Video 167.1 ▶)

- Verbal patient consent is obtained, and the correct knee is identified.
- The medication is prepared on a sterile tray with an extra syringe available if aspiration is planned.
- The patient is placed in the supine position with the knee resting in a comfortable position. A small pillow may be placed under the knee for comfort and support (Fig. 167.1).
- The area over the patella is palpated for fluctuance (Fig. 167.2).
- Prepare the skin site by anesthetizing with ethyl chloride (Fig. 167.3) and sterilizing with povidone-iodine solution (Fig. 167.4).

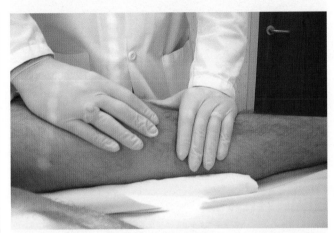

Fig 167.1 The patient is placed supine with a small support under the knee for comfort.

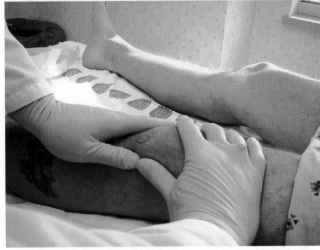

Fig 167.2 The prepatellar bursa is palpated and the injection site determined.

- If aspiration is planned, a small needle is used to infiltrate the skin with local anesthetic before inserting the larger aspiration needle.
- Aspiration and injection are performed by placing the needle directly into the fluid-filled bursa from the lateral side. Fluid should be aspirated from the bursa with a large-bore needle (Fig. 167.5) followed by injection with a corticosteroid (Fig. 167.6). If injecting, a hemostat is used to hold the needle in

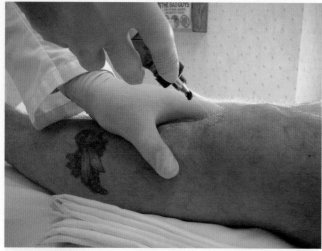

Fig 167.3 Optional use of ethyl chloride for anesthetizing the skin.

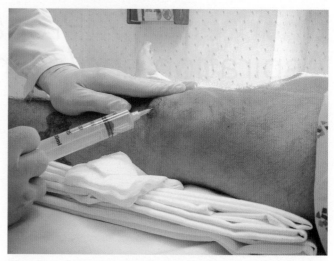

Fig 167.5 Aspiration of the bursa with large-bore needle.

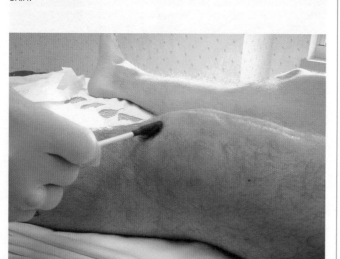

Fig 167.4 Sterile skin preparation.

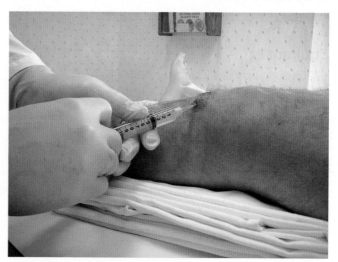

Fig 167.6 Injection of corticosteroid.

place while changing the syringe. Alternatively, a separate needle and syringe may be used for injection.
- Apply dressing per routine.

Considerations in Special Populations

- In the evaluation of a patient with prepatellar bursitis, the physician should be aware of possible underlying infection, fracture of the patella, or an associated intra-articular injury of the knee.
- Bursitis-related prepatellar swelling must be differentiated from an intra-articular effusion.

- If infection is suspected, bursal fluid obtained during aspiration should be sent for a cell count, a Gram stain, and aerobic/anaerobic cultures.

Patient Instructions

- The dressing may be removed the following day.
- Use ice to treat any local soreness at the injection site.
- Call the physician's office if any redness, warmth, increased swelling, fever, or chills develop.

Chapter 168 Pes Anserine Bursa Injection Technique

Mark D. Miller

CPT CODE
20610 *Aspiration or injection of major joint or bursa*

Procedure Name

- Pes anserine bursa injection

Equipment

- 25-gauge needle if local anesthesia planned
- Injection needle (21-gauge)
- Injection syringe (5 to 10 mL)
- Local anesthetic agent
- Sterile tray
- Sterile gloves
- Sterile prep solution (e.g., povidone-iodine)
- Ethyl chloride, optional
- Injectable agent (steroid, anesthetic)
- Sterile gauze and bandage

Indications

- Pes anserine bursitis

Contraindications

- Overlying cellulitis or skin disease

Technique (Video 168.1)

- Verbal patient consent is obtained, and the correct extremity is identified.
- The medication is prepared on a sterile tray.
- The patient is placed in the supine position with the knee slightly flexed.
- Identify the tendinous border of the medial hamstring muscle and follow it distal to the joint line to its insertion at the pes anserine. The pes anserine bursa is located at this site, along the medial aspect of the knee approximately 2 cm below the joint line.
- Prepare the skin site by anesthetizing with ethyl chloride and sterilizing with povidone-iodine solution (Fig. 168.1).
- The needle is inserted perpendicular to the tibia into the point of maximal tenderness. The needle is gently advanced to bone and then withdrawn 2 to 3 mm to perform the injection (Fig. 168.2).
- Apply a dressing per routine.

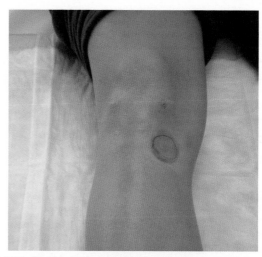

Fig 168.1 Sterile skin preparation.

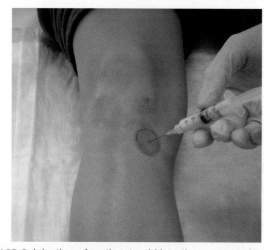

Fig 168.2 Injection of corticosteroid into the pes anserine bursa distal to the medial joint line.

Considerations in Special Populations

- Injection in this condition is often performed early in the course of treatment rather than after an extended trial of other modalities.

Patient Instructions

- The dressing may be removed the following day.
- Use ice to treat any local soreness at the injection site.
- Call the physician's office if any redness, warmth, increased swelling, fever, or chills develop.

Chapter 169 Iliotibial Band Injection Technique

Mark D. Miller

CPT CODE
20610 *Aspiration or injection of major joint or bursa*

Procedure Name
- Iliotibial band injection technique

Equipment
- 25-gauge needle if local anesthesia planned
- Injection needle (21-gauge)
- Injection syringe (5 to 10 mL)
- Local anesthetic agent
- Sterile tray
- Sterile gloves
- Sterile prep solution (e.g., povidone-iodine)
- Ethyl chloride, optional
- Injectable agent (steroid, anesthetic)
- Sterile gauze and bandage

Indications
- Iliotibial band syndrome

Contraindications
- Overlying cellulitis or skin disease

Technique
- Verbal patient consent is obtained and the correct extremity is identified.
- The medication is prepared on a sterile tray.
- The patient is placed in the lateral decubitus position with the knee flexed 20 to 30 degrees (Fig. 169.1).
- Palpate the course of the iliotibial band along the lateral thigh to its insertion at the Gerdy tubercle on the proximal tibia. Determine the site of maximal tenderness (Fig. 169.2).
- Prepare the skin site by anesthetizing with ethyl chloride (Fig. 169.3) and sterilizing with povidone-iodine solution (Fig. 169.4).
- The needle is inserted at the point of maximal tenderness in the region of the lateral femoral condyle, and the corticosteroid is injected (Fig. 169.5).
- Apply a dressing per routine.

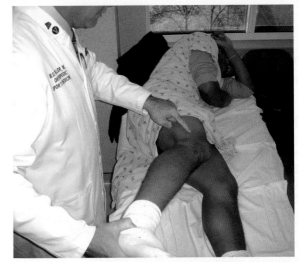
Fig 169.1 The patient is placed in the lateral decubitus position with the knee slightly flexed.

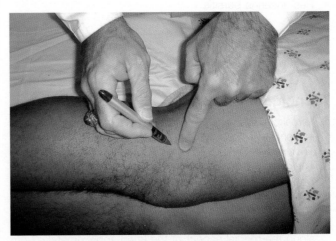
Fig 169.2 The site of maximal tenderness is identified.

Considerations in Special Populations
- Injection is typically reserved for patients in whom a program of iliotibial band stretching, hip abductor strengthening, and activity modification has failed.

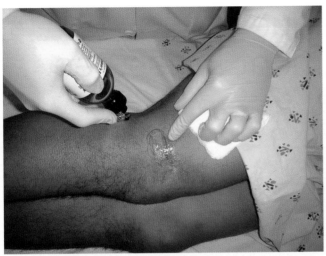

Fig 169.3 Optional use of ethyl chloride for anesthetizing the skin.

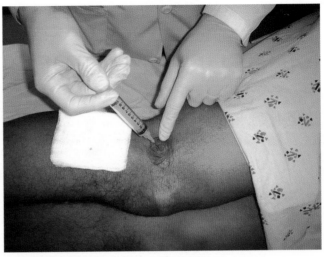

Fig 169.5 Injection of the corticosteroid.

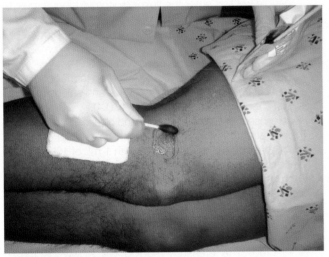

Fig 169.4 Sterile skin preparation.

Patient Instructions

- The dressing may be removed the following day.
- Use ice to treat any local soreness at the injection site.
- Call the physician's office if any redness, warmth, increased swelling, fever, or chills develop.

Chapter 170 Technique for Measuring Compartment Pressures

Mark D. Miller

CPT CODE

20950 *Monitoring of interstitial fluid pressure, muscle compartment syndrome*

Procedure Name

- Intramuscular compartment pressure monitoring

Equipment

- Sterile prep solution (e.g., alcohol, iodine)
- Local anesthetic agent
- Aspiration needle for local and injection needle (25-gauge) for local
- Ethyl chloride
- Sterile gloves
- Sterile gauze
- Adhesive bandages
- Stryker handheld pressure monitor (Fig. 170.1)
- Quick pressure monitor set (see Fig. 170.1)
  - 3-mL sodium chloride fluid-filled syringe
  - Sterile monitor pack (large-bore needle and monitor hub)

Indications

- Suspected compartment syndrome

Contraindications

- Local infection or overlying skin disease
- Anticoagulation (relative contraindication)

Technique

- Informed consent is obtained and the correct extremity identified.
- The needle, hub, and syringe of the quick pressure monitor set are attached to each other, maintaining sterility of the needle and hub. The hub is then placed into the port on the manometer. Saline is gently pushed through the apparatus until a drop is visualized at the tip of the needle.
- To avoid damage to neurovascular structures, each compartment should be approached with an understanding of anatomic contents (Table 170.1).
  - Anterior: Needle insertion is made into the muscle belly of the tibialis anterior muscle just lateral to the anterior tibial border at the level of the middle third of the tibia (Fig. 170.2).
  - Lateral: Needle insertion is into the bellies of the peroneus longus and brevis muscles midway between the fibular head and lateral malleolus (see Fig. 170.2).
  - Deep posterior: Needle insertion is posterior to the posteromedial tibia in its middle aspect, closely approximating the posterior aspect of the bone. The needle will first enter the flexor digitorum longus muscle and, when guided deeper, will enter the posterior tibial muscle. As long as the needle is not driven too deeply, this method will keep the needle anterior and medial to the neurovascular structures (Fig. 170.3).
  - Superficial posterior: Needle insertion is made into the muscle bellies of the gastrocnemius and soleus muscles just medial to the midline (Fig. 170.4).
- Needle insertion sites are marked and cleansed with alcohol. Topical anesthesia is achieved with ethyl chloride spray. Local anesthesia is then achieved with 1 mL of 1% lidocaine injected subcutaneously at each site.
- Each of the test insertion sites is then thoroughly prepped with alcohol and iodine.
- Before insertion, the needle is placed perpendicular to the insertion site and the monitor zeroed. The needle is inserted into the muscle compartment and 0.3 mL of saline is injected. The pressure reading will slowly decrease. Measurement is recorded as the value at which the pressure stops decreasing or after the pressure vacillates up and down a few times. After the resting test, the areas are cleansed with alcohol and adhesive bandages are placed.
- In suspected exertional compartment syndrome, the athlete then exercises until symptoms are reproduced. Athletes should perform the specific exercise that typically causes their symptoms, to the point at which they would normally have to stop or to a level of 8 out of 10.
- After exercise, each of the areas is again cleansed with alcohol, and testing is repeated for each of the compartments, entering the same insertion sites as used pre-exercise. The sites are then again thoroughly cleansed with alcohol, antibiotic ointment is applied (as long as it is not contraindicated), and adhesive bandages are placed.

Considerations in Special Populations

- Static (most common) and dynamic testing can be performed. Dynamic testing requires continuous monitoring with an indwelling catheter, which limits testing to a single compartment, requires the athlete to remain in one setting,

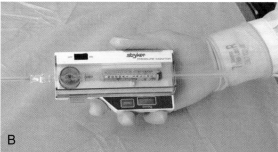

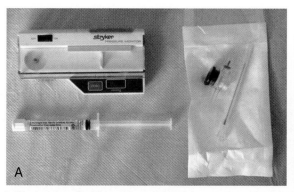

Fig 170.1 Stryker handheld monitor and quick pressure monitor set. **(A)** Preassembly. **(B)** Postassembly.

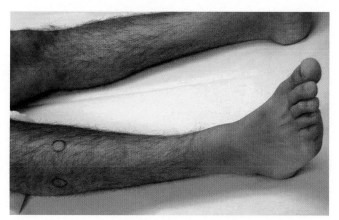

Fig 170.2 Insertion sites for anterior and lateral compartments.

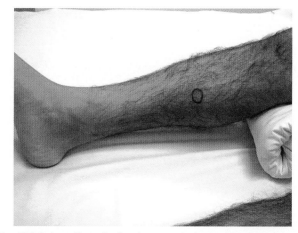

Fig 170.3 Insertion site for deep posterior compartment.

TABLE 170.1 Neurovascular Contents of Lower Leg Compartments

Compartment	Neurovascular Structures
Anterior	Deep peroneal nerve, tibial artery
Lateral	Superficial peroneal nerve
Deep posterior	Peroneal artery/vein, tibial nerve/artery
Superficial posterior	Sural nerve, saphenous vein

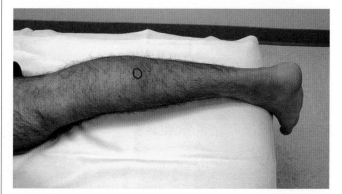

Fig 170.4 Insertion site for superficial posterior compartment.

and may result in the catheter failing to remain in place during the procedure.

- It is advised that anticoagulated patients be removed from anticoagulants before pressure measurements whenever possible.

Troubleshooting

- Several factors will ensure accurate pressure measurements.
  - Leg positioning, particularly of the knee and ankle, must be identical before and after exercise.
  - Exercise using the same activity that normally causes symptoms
  - No contact should be made with the limb tested other than with the pressure monitor.

- Patients are instructed to relax to prevent additional muscle contraction (which can result in an artificially high reading).
- All potentially involved compartments must be tested. Failure to identify all involved compartments is a cause of surgical remediation failure.

Patient Instructions

- Ice for 10 minutes three times daily for 3 days.
- Perform local wound care daily (alcohol wipe, antibiotic ointment if not contraindicated, and adhesive bandages) for 3 days.

- Call the physician's office if you experience swelling, severe pain, neurologic sequelae, or symptoms suggestive of infection.

Suggested Readings

Glorioso J, Wilckens J. Compartment syndrome testing. In: O'Connor F, Wilder R, eds. *The Textbook of Running Medicine*. New York: McGraw-Hill; 2001a:95–100.

Glorioso J, Wilckens J. Exertional leg pain. In: O'Connor F, Wilder R, eds. *The Textbook of Running Medicine*. New York: McGraw-Hill; 2001b:181–198.

Pedowitz RA, Hargens AR, Mubarak SJ, et al. Modified criteria for the objective diagnosis of chronic compartment syndrome of the leg. *Am J Sports Med*. 1990;18:35–40.

Wilder R, Sethi S. Overuse injuries: tendinopathies, stress fractures, compartment syndrome, and shin splints. *Clin Sports Med*. 2004;23:55–81.

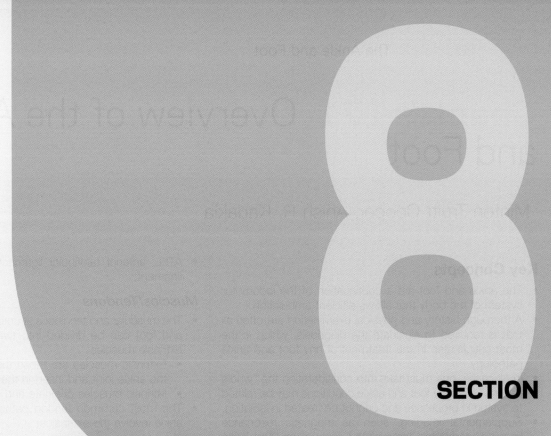

SECTION

The Ankle and Foot

Chapter 171 Overview of the Ankle and Foot

Minton Truitt Cooper, Anish R. Kadakia

Key Concepts

- The ankle and foot are a continuation of the locomotor system of the body that allows efficient ambulation.
- A thorough history and physical examination are often all that is required to elucidate the diagnosis, which is the most critical step in the treatment of any foot and ankle pathology.
- In all cases, one must take into consideration the "whole patient," as many foot and ankle conditions may be related to systemic processes and cannot be treated in isolation.
- Supplemental imaging, such as magnetic resonance imaging, computed tomography, technetium-99m bone scan, and ultrasonography, is often not required, and deferral to the specialist is appropriate for ordering these examinations in the vast majority of cases.
- The treatment of many ankle and foot conditions can be initiated in the office, minimizing the delay inherent in referral to a specialist.

Anatomy
Bones and Joints

- The primary articulation between the foot and the appendicular skeleton is the ankle joint.
- The joint is composed of the distal tibia, fibula, and talus, with articulations between all three (primarily the tibiotalar joint and the syndesmosis).
- The foot itself consists of 28 bones: talus, calcaneus, navicular, cuboid, cuneiforms (3), metatarsals (5), proximal phalanges (5), middle phalanges of the lesser toes (4), distal phalanges (5), and sesamoids of the great toe (2) (Figs. 171.1 to 171.5).
- The multiple joints in the foot can be divided into three distinct divisions: hindfoot, midfoot, and forefoot.
  - Hindfoot: talocalcaneal (subtalar), talonavicular, and calcaneocuboid joints
  - Midfoot: Naviculocuneiform and metatarsocuneiform (tarsometatarsal or Lisfranc) joints
  - Forefoot: Metatarsophalangeal, proximal interphalangeal, and distal interphalangeal joints

Ligaments

- Multiple ligaments in the ankle and foot impart the stability required for weight bearing.
- Those most commonly injured include the anterior talofibular ligament, calcaneofibular ligament, deltoid ligament, Lisfranc ligament, and spring ligament (Table 171.1). The anterior inferior tibiofibular and posterior tibiofibular ligaments may also be injured (high ankle sprain).

- ATFL, anterior talofibular ligament; CFL, calcaneofibular ligament.

Muscles/Tendons

- The muscular and tendinous structures that cross the ankle and foot can be divided into two groups: intrinsic and extrinsic muscles.
  - Extrinsic muscles are those that originate superior to the ankle joint and insert in the foot.
  - Intrinsic muscles originate and insert in the foot.
- The most common tendon pathologies of the foot and ankle involve the extrinsics.

Extrinsic

- Anterior: tibialis anterior, extensor hallucis longus, extensor digitorum longus, peroneus tertius
- Posterior: Achilles tendon
- Posterolateral: peroneus brevis and peroneus longus
- Posteromedial: tibialis posterior, flexor digitorum longus, flexor hallucis longus

Intrinsic

- Dorsum of foot: extensor digitorum brevis, extensor hallucis brevis
  - The extensor hallucis brevis is the medial portion of the extensor digitorum brevis, which originates from the anterior calcaneus. Innervation is by the deep peroneal nerve.
- Plantar foot: There are four layers of intrinsic muscles plantarly that are innervated by the medial and lateral plantar nerves (terminal branches of the tibial nerve)
  - Layer 1 (superficial): abductor hallucis, flexor digitorum brevis, abductor digiti minimi
  - Layer 2: quadratus plantae, lumbricals (four)
  - Layer 3: adductor hallucis, flexor hallucis brevis, flexor digiti minimi brevis
  - Layer 4 (deep): dorsal interossei (four), plantar interossei (three)

Nerves

- The sensation to the foot is provided by six terminal extensions of the lumbosacral plexus (Table 171.2).

Patient Evaluation
History

- The critical step in the diagnosis and treatment of foot and ankle disorders is obtaining a thorough history.
  - Injury history, duration of symptoms, exacerbating factors, pain, instability, mechanical symptoms, and a variety of other issues should be included.

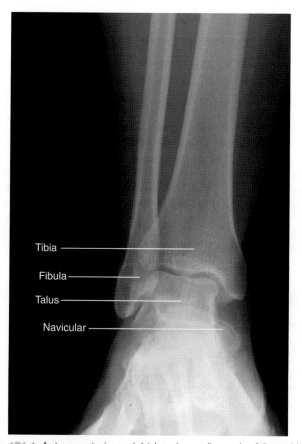

Fig 171.1 Anteroposterior weight-bearing radiograph of the ankle.

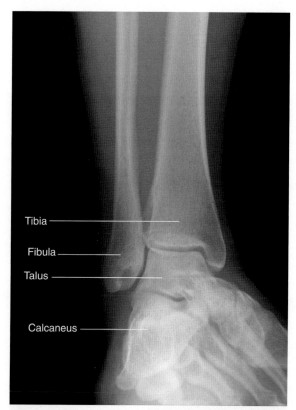

Fig 171.2 Mortise weight-bearing radiograph of the ankle.

TABLE 171.1 Ligaments of the Foot and Ankle

Ligament	Origin	Insertion
ATFL	Tip of the fibula	Talus
CFL	Tip of the fibula	Calcaneus
AITFL	Distal anterolateral tibia	Distal posterior fibula
PITFL	Distal posterior tibia	Distal posterior fibula
Deltoid	Tip of the medial malleolus	Talus and calcaneus
Lisfranc	Medial cuneiform	Base of the second metatarsal
Spring	Sustentaculum tali of calcaneus	Navicular

AFTL, Anterior talofibular ligament; *AITFL*, anterior inferior tibiofibular; *CFL*, calcaneofibular ligament; *PITFL*, posterior tibiofibular ligaments.

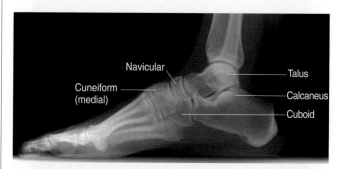

Fig 171.3 Lateral weight-bearing radiograph of the ankle and foot.

- Pain is a primary presenting symptom and can provide a wealth of information when analyzed critically. The common types of pain and their significance are presented in Table 171.3.
  - Instruct the patient to localize the source of the pain with one finger; this will allow a focused examination of the anatomic structures within the area, facilitating diagnosis.
- Instability or "giving out" can be associated with recurrent ankle sprains and incompetence of the lateral collateral

TABLE 171.2 Superficial Nerve Distribution of the Ankle and Foot

Nerve	Sensory Distribution
Superficial peroneal	Dorsum of ankle and foot
Deep peroneal	First web space
Saphenous	Medial ankle
Sural	Lateral aspect of heel and foot
Medial plantar	Plantar foot (medial toes)
Lateral plantar	Plantar foot (lateral toes)

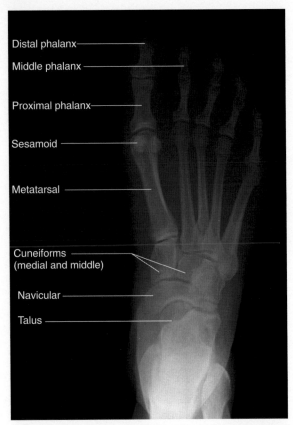

Distal phalanx
Middle phalanx
Proximal phalanx
Sesamoid
Metatarsal
Cuneiforms
(medial and middle)
Navicular
Talus

Fig 171.4 Anteroposterior weight-bearing radiograph of the foot.

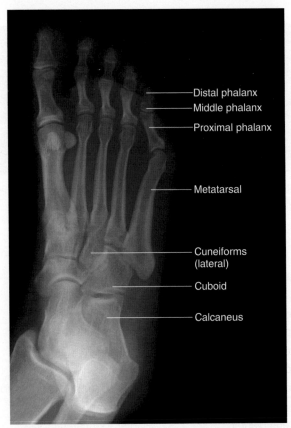

Distal phalanx
Middle phalanx
Proximal phalanx
Metatarsal
Cuneiforms
(lateral)
Cuboid
Calcaneus

Fig 171.5 Internal oblique view radiograph of the foot.

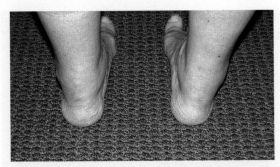

Fig 171.6 Posterior view of the heel demonstrating heel varus on the right side. Note how the heel turns toward the midline. Associated with stress fractures of the fifth metatarsal, instability, or hereditary sensory motor neuropathy. (From Miller MD, Thompson SR, eds. *Miller's Review of Orthopaedics*. 7th ed. Philadelphia: Elsevier; 2016.)

TABLE 171.3 **Pain Type and Clinical Correlation**

Type of Pain	Significance
Startup pain (at the initiation of activity)	Arthritis, fasciitis, tendinitis
Night pain (at the end of the day after activity)	Arthritis, impingement
Activity-related pain	Tendinitis, osteochondral lesions, impingement, stress fractures, trauma
Burning or tingling pain	Morton neuroma, tarsal tunnel, neuropathy
Shoe wear–related pain	Hallux valgus, hallux rigidus, claw or hammer toes, midfoot arthritis (osteophytes and deformity), accessory navicular, nail disorder

ligaments (anterior talofibular ligament and calcaneofibular ligament) or osteochondral lesions (paroxysmal instability in which the patient may feel that the joint is out of place and will not support them).

- In addition to the focused musculoskeletal history, evaluation for peripheral vascular disease, diabetes, inflammatory arthropathy, and neuropathy may aid in diagnosis and affect the course of treatment.
- Many foot and ankle conditions will present with a positive family history, which should be explored as well.

Physical Examination (Video 171.1 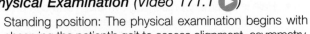)

- Standing position: The physical examination begins with observing the patient's gait to assess alignment, asymmetry, limp, knee thrust (varus, valgus, recurvatum), and foot position at heel strike. Evaluate for uneven shoe wear and assess the shape of the shoe compared with the shape of the foot. Examination with the patient in a standing position allows a true assessment of the longitudinal arch, heel alignment (varus or valgus), and position of the toes (Figs. 171.6 and 171.7). During a single limb heel rise (Fig. 171.8), failure of

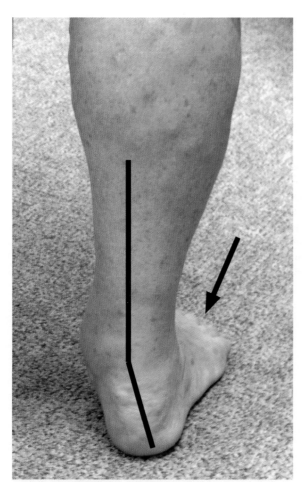

Fig 171.7 Posterior view of the heel demonstrating heel valgus. Note how the heel turns outward, away from the midline. "Too many toes" sign *(arrow)*. Less than 5 degrees is physiologic; if more, it can be associated with pes planovalgus (flatfoot), midfoot arthritis, or posterior tibial tendinitis.

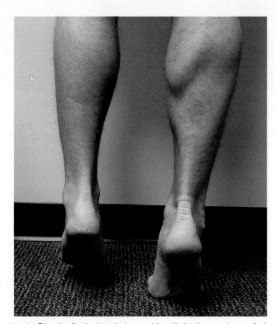

Fig 171.8 Single limb heel rise with slight inversion of the heel and normal longitudinal arch.

TABLE 171.4 Pain Location and Clinical Correlation

Location	Significance
Anterior ankle	Ankle arthritis, osteochondral lesion of the talus, anterior ankle impingement
Posteromedial ankle	Posterior tibial tendon dysfunction
Posterolateral ankle	Peroneal tendinitis
Posterior ankle: superficial	Achilles tendinitis or rupture (acute)
Posterior ankle: deep	Os trigonum or flexor hallucis longus tendinitis
Dorsal midfoot	Midfoot arthritis or Lisfranc injury, stress fracture
Inferior to the fibula	Ankle sprain
Between the tibia and fibula	High ankle sprain (syndesmotic injury)
Heel tenderness	Calcaneal stress fracture, fat pad atrophy, insertional Achilles tendinitis or rupture
Plantar foot	Plantar fasciitis
Great toe	Hallux rigidus or hallux valgus
Lesser toes	Synovitis or neuroma (burning/ tingling)

heel inversion, lack of a rise of the longitudinal arch, and external rotation of the leg are indicative of a pathologic process such as posterior tibial tendon dysfunction or an Achilles tendon disorder. However, it is important to note that this exam is not specific, as many patients are unable to perform this maneuver due to other factors (obesity, deconditioning, poor balance, other joint dysfunction).

- Sitting position: A systematic examination begins with the skin, evaluating for edema, callosities, ecchymosis, erythema, ulcers, or previous incisions. The two palpable pulses are the dorsalis pedis (dorsum of foot) and the tibialis posterior (posterior to medial malleolus).
  - The inability to palpate the pulses or loss of hair can indicate peripheral vascular disease.
  - The most sensitive test for the presence of neuropathy is the failure to sense a Semmes-Weinstein 5.07 monofilament. These are commercially available and should be a routine part in the examination of diabetic patients, as well as other patients with concern for sensory neuropathy.
  - Systematic palpation is very effective at localizing the source of the pain, given the superficial location of the bony, ligamentous, and tendinous structures of the foot and ankle (Fig. 171.9).
  - Some of the classic anatomic locations and their significance are shown in Table 171.4.
  - Range of motion is extremely helpful in understanding the pathologic process.
  - Asymmetry between extremities or pain at the extremes of motion is more relevant than the absolute value.

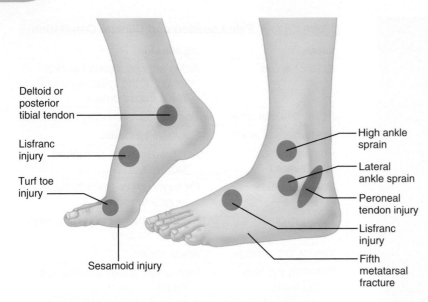

Deltoid or posterior tibial tendon

Lisfranc injury

Turf toe injury

Sesamoid injury

High ankle sprain

Lateral ankle sprain

Peroneal tendon injury

Lisfranc injury

Fifth metatarsal fracture

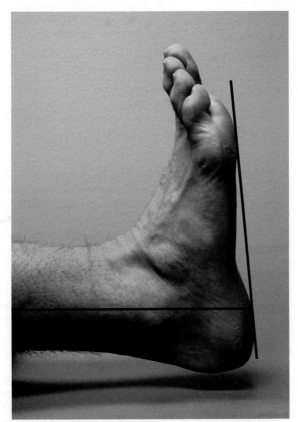

Fig 171.10 Dorsiflexion range of motion of the ankle.

- Maximal range of motion of the ankle is 10 to 23 degrees of dorsiflexion and 23 to 48 degrees of plantarflexion (Figs. 171.10 and 171.11). It is important to test ankle dorsiflexion differentially with the knee extended and flexed to test for isolated gastrocnemius contracture (Silfverskiöld test—positive if dorsiflexion improves greater than 10 degrees with knee flexion).
  - Maximal range of subtalar inversion is 5 to 50 degrees and eversion is 5 to 26 degrees (Figs. 171.12 and 171.13).

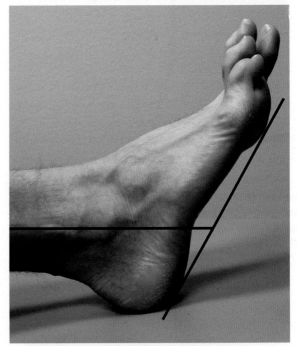

Fig 171.11 Plantarflexion range of motion of the ankle.

- Maximal range of motion for the first metatarso-phalangeal joint (great toe) is 45 to 90 degrees of dorsiflexion and 10 to 40 degrees of plantarflexion (Figs. 171.14 and 171.15).
- Motor strength should be tested with the patient actively firing the muscle group to be tested (Table 171.5).
  - The examiner then attempts to move the foot against the patient's resistance.
  - At full strength, the examiner should not be able to overcome the patient.
- The gastrocnemius/soleus complex is best tested with single limb heel rise (see Fig. 171.8). T5e gastrocnemius is more active when the knee is extended. The posterior tibial tendo5 can be isolated from the anterior tibial tendon using Fig. 4 position (Fig. 171.16).

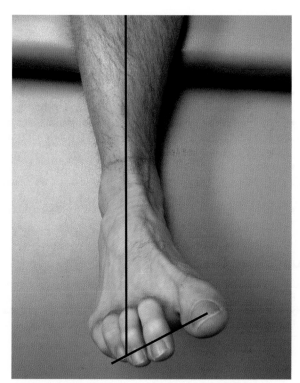

Fig 171.12 Inversion range of motion of the hindfoot.

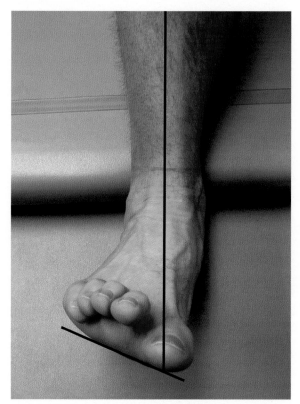

Fig 171.13 Eversion range of motion of the hindfoot.

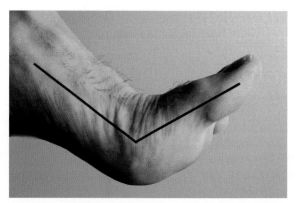

Fig 171.14 Dorsiflexion of the first metatarsophalangeal joint.

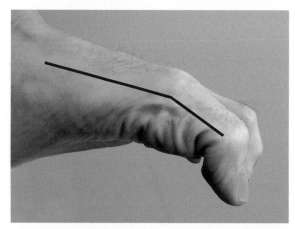

Fig 171.15 Plantarflexion of the first metatarsophalangeal joint.

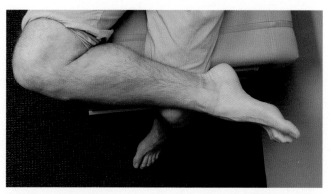

Fig 171.16 The figure 4 position to assess the strength of the posterior tibial tendon. Test-resisted inversion with the patient's foot in the plantarflexed position.

TABLE 171.5 **Motor Examination of the Ankle**

Muscle Group	Motion
Anterior tibialis	Dorsiflexion
Gastrocnemius/soleus (Achilles)	Plantarflexion
Posterior tibial tendon	Inversion
Peroneal tendons	Eversion

TABLE 171.6 Clinical Relevance of Common Radiographic Findings

Finding	Significance
Lucency in the talus	Osteochondral lesion of the talus
Small bone medial to the navicular	Accessory navicular (associated with posterior tibial tendon dysfunction)
Calcaneal spur (posterior)	Insertional Achilles tendinitis
Calcaneal spur (inferior)	Fasciitis (spur does not require removal)
Dorsal spur on first metatarsophalangeal	Hallux rigidus
Fleck at the base of the second metatarsal	Lisfranc injury

Imaging

- Plain radiographs are critical in the evaluation of foot and ankle pathology.
- All views should be weight bearing when possible.
- The ability to detect subtle alignment and arthritic conditions is improved with weight-bearing views.
- Standard views of the ankle include anteroposterior (see Fig. 171.1), mortise (15 degrees of internal rotation; see Fig. 171.2), and lateral (see Fig. 171.3).
- Standard views of the foot include anteroposterior (see Fig. 171.4), internal oblique (see Fig. 171.5), and lateral (see Fig. 171.3).
- Radiographic findings may include those shown in Table 171.6.

Suggested Readings

Chou LB, ed. *Orthopaedic Knowledge Update: Foot and Ankle 5.* Rosemont, IL: AAOS; 2014.

Coughlin MJ, Saltzman CL, Anderson RB, eds. *Mann's Surgery of the Foot and Ankle.* 9th ed. Philadelphia: Elsevier; 2014.

Chapter 172 Arthritis of the Ankle

Anish R. Kadakia, Milap S. Patel

ICD-10-CM CODES
M19.071	*Primary osteoarthritis, right ankle and foot*
M19.072	*Primary osteoarthritis, left ankle and foot*
M19.079	*Primary osteoarthritis, unspecified ankle and foot*
M19.171	*Posttraumatic osteoarthritis, right ankle and foot*
M19.172	*Posttraumatic osteoarthritis, left ankle and foot*
M19.179	*Posttraumatic osteoarthritis, unspecified ankle and foot*
M19.271	*Secondary osteoarthritis, right ankle and foot*
M19.272	*Secondary osteoarthritis, left ankle and foot*
M19.279	*Secondary osteoarthritis, unspecified ankle and foot*

Key Concepts

- Primary arthritis of the ankle is rare—6-9% (Fig. 172.1).
- Trauma is the most common cause of ankle arthritis— approximately 80% (malleolar ankle fracture, 39%; distal tibia pilon fracture, 16%; ligamentous injuries, 14%). Avascular necrosis of talus, hemophilia, gout, infection, and malalignment from paralytic deformity are some other causes.
- Many patients with ankle arthritis can be effectively managed without surgery.
- Historically, ankle arthrodesis has been the current gold standard for surgical treatment of ankle arthritis in which conservative measures have failed (Fig. 172.2).
- Ankle replacement is an alternative surgical treatment option for end-stage arthritis in carefully selected patients, although long-term results are less predictable (Fig. 172.3).

History

- Ankle stiffness, swelling, and pain
- Most often unilateral
- Difficulty with inclines and stairs secondary to impingement
- Often report history of trauma or instability (recurrent ankle sprains)
- Less commonly, history of inflammatory arthropathy, infection, or bleeding
- History of swelling, erythema, or warmth without significant pain in a patient with neuropathy may suggest Charcot (neuropathic) arthropathy, which is most frequently related to diabetes.

Physical Examination

- Observation
  - Effusion/swelling
  - Surgical scars
  - Deformity, limb/hindfoot malalignment
  - Gait
- Palpation
  - Tenderness at anterior ankle joint line
  - Lateral hindfoot pain indicates subtalar involvement.
- Range of motion
  - Ankle (dorsiflexion/plantarflexion); compare with contralateral side
  - Hindfoot motion (inversion/eversion); assess for concomitant hindfoot (subtalar) arthritis
- Special tests
  - Diagnostic injection: Injection of local anesthetic into the ankle or subtalar joint can help differentiate ankle from subtalar joint pain.
  - Use of contrast and fluoroscopy can ensure appropriate placement of the injection.
  - Addition of steroid can provide short-term relief.

Imaging

- Radiographs
  - Anteroposterior and mortise (15-degree oblique) views of the ankle (Fig. 172.4)
    - Assess for loss of joint space, syndesmosis, widening, angular deformity, subchondral sclerosis, evidence of previous trauma.
  - Lateral view of the ankle (Fig. 172.5)
    - Anterior or posterior osteophytes result in impingement.
    - Assess for subtalar joint.
  - Anteroposterior, oblique, and lateral weight-bearing views of the foot
    - Assess for concomitant degenerative changes, malalignment.
- Computed tomography
  - Not required to make the diagnosis
  - Study of choice to assess adjacent joint arthritis
- Magnetic resonance imaging
  - Useful to assess for localized osteochondral lesions of the talus or associated tendon disorders, but generally not required in cases of advanced ankle arthritis

Differential Diagnosis

- Charcot (neuropathic) arthropathy: swelling, minimal pain in relation to the destructive bony architectural changes on radiographs

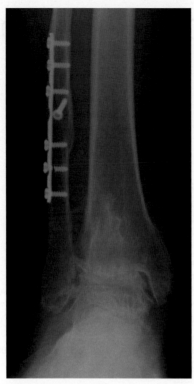

Fig 172.1 Anteroposterior ankle radiograph of a patient demonstrating end-stage ankle arthritis after sustaining an ankle injury 10 years prior. There is loss of tibiotalar joint space, along with medial and lateral osteophyte formation. Plate and screws on the fibula are from original injury 10 years prior.

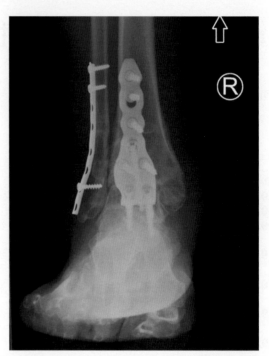

Fig 172.2 Anteroposterior ankle radiograph demonstrating ankle fusion using plate and screws construct. Distal fibula plate and screws are from previous injury which resulted in posttraumatic arthrosis.

- Acute gouty arthritis: acute onset, history of gout, joint effusion
- Subtalar arthritis: pain walking on uneven surfaces, limited and painful hindfoot inversion/eversion, pain localized laterally over sinus tarsi (inferior to the tip of the fibula); diagnostic subtalar injection if source of pain is unclear
- Osteochondral lesion of the talus: paroxysmal pain with locking, catching, or instability; focal defect noted on plain radiographs; magnetic resonance imaging to further evaluate

Treatment

- At diagnosis
  - Initial management is nonoperative.
  - Lifestyle modifications include weight loss in obese patients (joint reactive forces in the ankle are estimated at five times the body weight during normal gait), termination of vigorous activities, and changing to a more sedentary job, if possible.
  - Antiinflammatory medications and intra-articular steroids may be useful for symptomatic management, particularly for acute exacerbations.
  - Injectable viscosupplementation is also an option if steroids are contraindicated or there is a need for to delay surgery. It has not been U.S. Food and Drug Administration (FDA) approved for use in the ankle joint, and reports on efficacy are unclear.

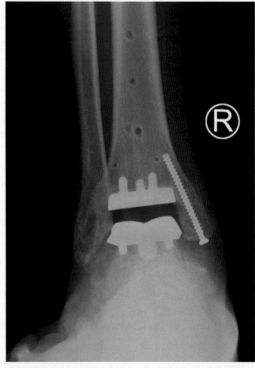

Fig 172.3 Anteroposterior ankle radiograph depicting Infinity total ankle arthroplasty system.

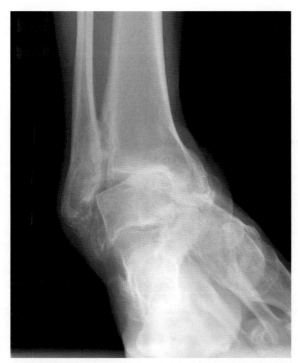

Fig 172.4 Mortise ankle radiograph of a patient with end-stage ankle arthritis. Secondary to chronic instability, the patient developed a severe varus deformity with subchondral sclerosis and obliteration of the medial joint line.

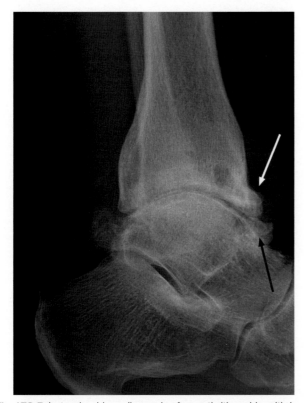

Fig 172.5 Lateral ankle radiograph of an arthritic ankle with large anterior tibial *(white arrow)* and talar *(black arrow)* osteophytes.

- Later
  - Chronic arthritis pain may be managed with mechanical unloading via modified footwear or a brace.
  - Shoe modifications with a rocker-bottom sole and solid ankle cushioned heel may improve gait dynamics and symptoms.
  - A custom polypropylene ankle-foot orthosis or Arizona ankle-foot orthosis brace may provide symptomatic relief, particularly in the setting of deformity or instability.
  - Finally, a trial of immobilization in a short-leg walking cast may provide symptomatic relief and simulate an ankle fusion for patients contemplating surgery.

When to Refer

- Patients with radiographic or clinical evidence of anterior impingement, loose bodies, or osteochondral lesions that may be amenable to open or arthroscopic debridement should be referred.
- Patients with radiographic or clinical malalignment (e.g., previous malunited tibia fracture) may be candidates for surgical realignment procedures.
- Finally, all patients who have end-stage arthritis and debilitating symptoms despite adequate nonoperative management should be referred for consideration for arthrodesis (fusion), joint replacement, or operative joint distraction procedures.

Prognosis

- The use of rigid custom brace (ankle-foot orthosis or Arizona ankle-foot orthosis) can be a very successful treatment choice for patients who are compliant with brace use.
  - Common complaints include difficulty donning the brace, restricted range of motion, shoe-wear difficulty, cosmetic appearance, and pain when out of the brace.
- Ankle arthrodesis is the most reliable surgical intervention with a high rate of fusion and pain relief using current surgical techniques. Ankle arthroplasty has become more popular in recent years as implants and techniques have improved, although long-term outcome studies are lacking.
  - Despite successful fusion, patients can have difficulty with uneven ground, stairs, driving, prone sleeping, and increased risk of arthritis in adjacent joints.
  - Recent gait analysis has shown a more symmetrical gait with reduced limp in patient with ankle replacement compared with fusion.
  - The benefits of an improved gait must be weighed against the less predictable longevity of ankle replacement and the higher complication rate.

Troubleshooting

- Patients should be counseled on risks and benefits of surgery.
  - Fusion results in predictable relief of pain and good preservation of function in many patients. Permanent stiffness results from fusion.
  - Smokers (high risk of fusion failure) and patients with involvement of the adjacent joints are less likely to have a successful outcome with fusion.

- Despite recent advances, ankle replacement remains in the early stages compared with total knee and hip replacement, with far less predictable results and limited long-term outcome studies, and patients should adjust their expectations accordingly.

Patient Instructions

- There are multiple lifestyle modifications that can be made to help alleviate the pain from ankle arthritis.
  - Activities such as swimming, elliptical bike, and seated weight lifting are excellent for physical fitness yet minimize the impact on the ankle.
  - Avoidance of running, uneven ground (sand, grass, and gravel), inclines, and stairs will minimize the discomfort.
  - Walking is encouraged and will not cause the arthritis to worsen.
  - Using shoes with a rocket bottom is very helpful for relieving pain.
  - These can be custom made or purchased over-the-counter at many shoe stores.
  - Use of a boot limits ankle range of motion and will also provide relief during walking.
  - Given the restriction in the range of motion from arthritis, wearing a shoe with a small heel can decrease the pain from the spurs that commonly occur in the front of the ankle.
  - Ice and antiinflammatory medications can help reduce discomfort.

Considerations in Special Populations

- Patients who are obese, diabetic, dysvascular, or smokers are poor candidates for ankle replacement surgery, given the risk of wound complications and risk of amputation. In addition, young patients and those with high-demand occupations may not be appropriate. Ankle fusion is the procedure of choice in this patient population, although each case is evaluated individually. In patients with poor soft-tissue envelope and minimal ankle deformity, arthroscopic ankle fusion is also an option.

Suggested Readings

Coester LM, Saltzman CL, Leupold J, et al. Long-term results following ankle arthrodesis for post-traumatic arthritis. *J Bone Joint Surg Am*. 2001;83:219–228.

Coughlin MJ, Saltzman C, Anderson RB, eds. *Mann's Surgery of the Foot and Ankle*. 9th ed. Philadelphia: Elsevier; 2014.

Knecht SI, Estin M, Callaghan JJ, et al. The agility total ankle arthroplasty. Seven- to sixteen year follow-up. *J Bone Joint Surg Am*. 2004;86: 116–171.

Lawton CD, Butler BA, Dekker RG, et al. Total ankle arthroplasty versus ankle arthrodesis—a comparision of outcomes over the last decade. *J Orthop Surg Res*. 2017;12(1):76.

Myerson MS, ed. *Foot and Ankle Disorders*. Philadelphia: WB Saunders; 2000.

Raikin SM, Rasouli MR, Espandar R, et al. Trends in treatment of advanced ankle arthroplasty by total ankle replacement or ankle fusion. *Foot Ankle Int*. 2013;35:216–224.

Soohoo NF, Zingmond DS, Ko CY. Comparison of reoperation rates following ankle arthrodesis and total ankle arthroplasty. *J Bone Joint Surg Am*. 2007;89A:2143–2149.

Thomas R, Daniels TR, Parker K. Gait analysis and functional outcomes following ankle arthrodesis for isolated ankle arthritis. *J Bone Joint Surg Am*. 2006;88A:526–535.

Thomas RH, Daniels TR. Ankle arthritis. *J Bone Joint Surg Am*. 2003;85A: 923–936.

Chapter 173 Chondral Injuries

Joseph S. Park

ICD-10-CM CODE
M93.279 *Osteochondritis dissecans (unspecified laterality)*

Key Concepts

- Injury to articular cartilage can result in progressive osteoarthritis.
- Articular cartilage damage ranges from softening or fibrillation to separation and detachment from the underlying subchondral bone. In acute trauma, an osteochondral fragment (cartilage plus underlying osseous fragment) can be displaced from the talar dome.
- Chondral lesions of the talus or distal tibia may occur after acute or cumulative trauma to the ankle joint from ligamentous instability.
- High incidence of chondral injuries in ankle fractures (as high as 63%)
- The most common cause of chondral injury is acute trauma, such as an ankle sprain or ankle fracture.
- The talar dome is more often injured than the tibial plafond.

History

- Acute injury
  - Ankle sprain and/or fracture
  - Pain around ankle joint
  - Locking or popping
- Chronic injury
  - Continued or worsening symptoms despite prolonged period of conservative treatment
  - Recurrent swelling and pain with activity
  - Limited ankle range of motion

Physical Examination

- Observation
  - Effusion (intra-articular swelling)
  - Antalgic gait to offload injured ankle
- Palpation
  - Anteromedial and/or anterolateral ankle joint line tenderness
- Range of motion
  - Loss of dorsiflexion/plantarflexion can occur from effusion.
  - Possible locking or popping in conjunction with displaced articular cartilage fragment
- Special tests
  - Assessment of lateral ankle stability with inversion stress and anterior drawer tests

- Varus/valgus stress to the hindfoot may produce medial or lateral talar dome pain.
- Manual testing of peroneal and posterior tibial tendon function to evaluate for concomitant tendon injury

Imaging

- Radiographs: weight-bearing anteroposterior, lateral, and mortise views of the ankle
  - Check for displaced medial or lateral talar dome subchondral bone fragments.
  - Chronic injuries may have medial or lateral cystic lesions in the talus visible on x-ray (XR) (Fig. 173.1).
  - Look for evidence for impingement, including preexisting osteophytes on the anterior distal tibia or talar neck.
- Magnetic resonance imaging
  - Often required to diagnose the chondral lesion
  - Look for the classic bone bruise pattern with possible subchondral cyst formation (Fig. 173.2).
  - Look for additional ligamentous or syndesmotic lesions.
- Computed tomography (CT)
  - Gadolinium arthrography CT arthrogram often reveals the articular cartilage defect (Fig. 173.3).
  - Reveals size and location of osteochondral lesions most accurately
  - Look for underlying cystic lesions to the bone.

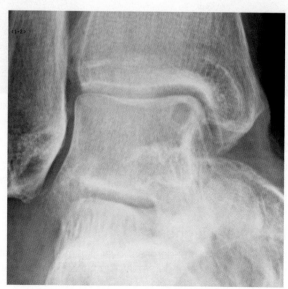

Fig 173.1 Mortise view of the ankle showing a subchondral cystic lesion on the medial talar dome.

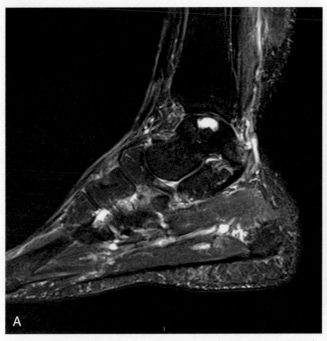

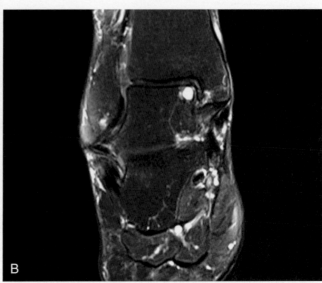

Fig 173.2 (A) T2-weighted sagittal magnetic resonance imaging with chondral irregularity and large subchondral cyst on medial talus. (B) T2-weighted coronal magnetic resonance imaging demonstrating lesion on medial talar shoulder.

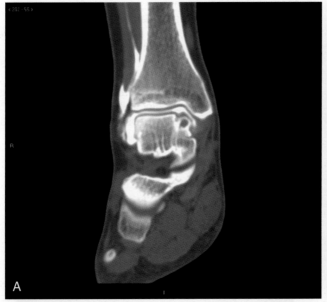

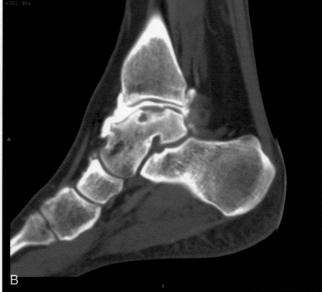

Fig 173.3 (A) Coronal arthrography computed tomography with medial talar dome cartilage lesion (gadolinium entrance) and multicystic subchondral cyst. (B) Sagittal view demonstrating posterocentral location of lesion.

Additional Tests

- Optional infiltration of the ankle joint with local anesthetic and/or cortisone may be used as a diagnostic and therapeutic measure (see Chapter 201).

Differential Diagnosis

- Ankle instability: tenderness over ligaments, possible varus/valgus hindfoot deformity, ligament laxity compared with contralateral side, evidence of global ligamentous laxity
- Avascular necrosis: often pain at rest; differentiate on magnetic resonance imaging

- Osteoarthritis: joint line tenderness, decreased range of motion, XR findings of joint space narrowing, tilt of the talus within mortise
- Ankle impingement: anterolateral tenderness, pain with forced dorsiflexion

Treatment

- At diagnosis
  - Initial treatment of acute chondral injuries includes immobilization of the ankle and non–weight bearing on the involved extremity, combined with analgesia.

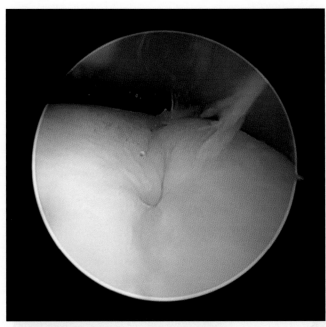

Fig 173.4 Arthroscopic view of medial talar cartilage irregularity.

- Ankle arthroscopy is recommended acutely in the case of restriction of ankle range of motion due to intra-articular step-off or loose body.
- The treatment of choice for an acute osteochondral injury is open reduction and internal fixation if the fragment is displaced and greater than 5 mm in size.
- In the case of smaller unstable subchondral fractures or loose fragments, débridement with microfracture is standard.
- Later
  - Most symptomatic osteochondral lesions are amenable to ankle arthroscopy.
  - The entire articular surface of the talus and tibia should be gently probed to detect changes in surface texture and consistency (Fig. 173.4).
  - If subchondral bone is exposed, débridement, drilling, or microfracture is generally recommended to establish vascular channels with eventual formation of a fibrocartilage surface.
  - For lesions with large subchondral cysts, retrograde drilling and grafting can be considered (Fig. 173.5). Improvement in radiographic appearance of the subchondral cyst can be seen at 6 weeks postoperatively (Fig. 173.6).
  - Patients with persistent symptoms after arthroscopic microfracture may be candidates for restorative techniques, such as autologous chondrocyte implantation or osteochondral grafting. Use of particulated juvenile articular cartilage can also be considered (Fig. 173.7).

When to Refer

- Patients with osteochondral lesions detected on XR or MRI who have failed conservative management in a fixed ankle walker/crutches should be referred for surgical consideration.
- If severe ligamentous instability or tendon injuries are present, earlier referral may be beneficial to prevent further damage to the cartilage surfaces.

Prognosis

- Good, if osteochondral lesions are small (<6 mm)
- Persistent radiologic osteochondral lesions after nonoperative or operative treatment may be asymptomatic.
- Progressive osteoarthritis of the ankle is more likely in larger osteochondral injuries after trauma.
- Treatment of concomitant ankle instability or tendon pathology should be performed with surgical treatment of osteochondral lesions to decrease the chance for recurrence.

Troubleshooting

- The patient should be counseled on the benefits and risks of surgery.
  - Benefits may include restoration of ankle mobility and reconstitution of the cartilage surface with successful return to sports and resolution of pain.
  - Risks include bleeding, infection, nerve injury, loss of motion, persistent pain, recurrence of the osteochondral lesion, and progressive osteoarthritis.

Patient Instructions

- In nonoperative treatment of an acute osteochondral injury, patient education is focused on decreasing the effusion (consider aspiration, start therapy with passive and active ankle motion, use ice and compression).
- Weight bearing is usually started 6 weeks after injury.
- If surgery is planned, follow the instructions of your surgeon.

Considerations in Special Populations

- Inactive, sedentary, or medically compromised patients should be treated nonoperatively. If they have persistent pain, arthroscopic débridement can be considered.
- High-level competitive athletes may benefit from earlier surgical referral for determination of treatment plan/progression for return to play.
- Obese patients should be counseled to consider weight loss before surgery so that biomechanical stress on osteochondral lesion is relieved and the prognosis is improved.
- In the setting of diffuse cartilage loss/advanced arthritis, patients may be considered for arthrodesis or arthroplasty. Arthroscopic treatment may provide relief for limited periods of time.

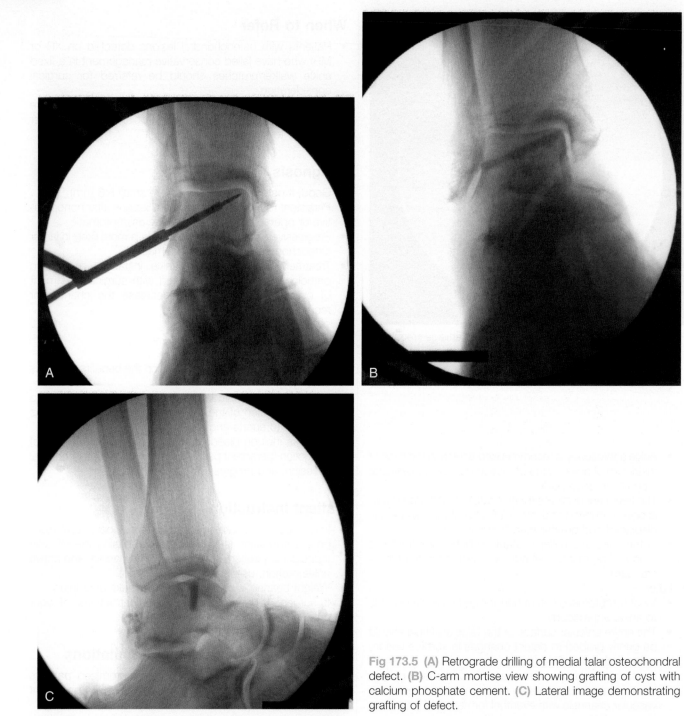

Fig 173.5 (A) Retrograde drilling of medial talar osteochondral defect. (B) C-arm mortise view showing grafting of cyst with calcium phosphate cement. (C) Lateral image demonstrating grafting of defect.

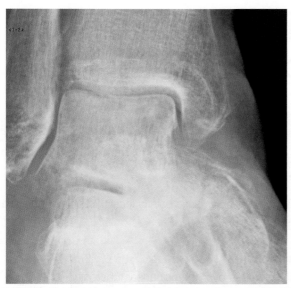

Fig 173.6 Postoperative mortise x-ray showing resolution of medial talar subchondral cyst.

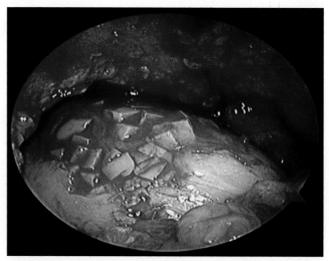

Fig 173.7 Arthroscopic view of particulated juvenile articular cartilage resurfacing of osteochondral defect.

Suggested Readings

Buckwalter JA, Mankin HJ. Articular cartilage: degeneration and osteoarthritis, repair, regeneration and transplantation. *Instr Course Lect*. 1998;47:487–504.

Farmer JM, Martin DF, Boles CA, et al. Chondral and osteochondral injuries. Diagnosis and management. *Clin Sports Med*. 2001;20:299–320.

Gobbi A, Francisco RA, Lubowitz JH, et al. Osteochondral lesions of the talus: randomized controlled trial comparing chondroplasty, microfracture and osteochondral autograft transplantation. *Arthroscopy*. 2002;22:1085–1092.

Hintermann B, Regazzoni P, Lampert C. Arthroscopic findings in acute fractures of the ankle. *J Bone Joint Surg Br*. 2000;82B:345–351.

Japour C, Vohra P, Giorgini R, et al. Ankle arthroscopy: Follow-up study of 33 ankles—effect of physical therapy and obesity. *J Foot Ankle Surg*. 1996;35:199–209.

Lanham NS, Carroll JJ, Cooper MT, et al. A comparison of outcomes of particulated juvenile articular cartilage and bone marrow aspirate concentrate for articular cartilage lesions of the talus. *Foot Ankle Spec*. 2017;10(4):315–321.

Loren GJ, Ferkel RD. Arthroscopic assessment of occult intraarticular injury in acute ankle fractures. *Arthroscopy*. 2002;18:412–421.

Toth AP, Easley ME. Ankle chondral injuries and repair. *Foot Ankle Clin*. 2000;5:799–840.

Ueblacker P, Burkart A, Imhoff AB. Retrograde cartilage transplantation of the proximal and distal tibia. *Arthroscopy*. 2004;20:73–78.

Chapter 174 Posterior Heel Pain/ Chronic Achilles Tendon Disorders

Scott Van Aman, Marissa Jamieson

ICD-10-CM CODES
M76.61 *Right Achilles tendinitis*
M76.62 *Left Achilles tendinitis*
M67.01 *Right Achilles contracture*
M67.02 *Left Achilles contracture*
M77.31 *Right posterior heel exostosis*
M77.32 *Left posterior heel exostosis*

Key Concepts

- Achilles tendinitis can involve peritendinitis (inflammation of the tissue lining the tendon), tendinosis (noninflammatory, atrophic degeneration and thickening of the tendon), or both.
- Tendinitis is classified based on location as insertional (typically older, sedentary patients) or noninsertional (overuse in runners or athletes).
- Conservative treatment of tendinitis has a success rate of approximately 90%.

History

- Insidious onset of pain with activity; may progress to constant pain.
- Pain located in distal posterior/posterolateral heel (insertional) or 2 to 7 cm proximal to the heel (noninsertional) (Fig. 174.1).
- Noninsertional tendinitis occurs primarily in young, active patients.
- Insertional tendinitis is typically seen in middle-aged or elderly patients with a tight heel cord.
- Athletes may report an increase in intensity or volume of training prior to the onset of symptoms.
- History of obesity, spondyloarthropathy, gout, or diffuse idiopathic skeletal hyperostosis (DISH) may predispose to insertional tendinitis.
- Fluoroquinolone use may predispose to Achilles tendinitis/ tendinosis.

Physical Examination
Observation

- Limp

Palpation
Noninsertional

- Tenderness along the Achilles tendon proximal to the heel.
- Peritendinitis is associated with diffuse inflammation, warmth, crepitation, and pain with motion.

- Tendinosis may cause painful focal thickening or nodularity of the tendon.

Insertional

- Tenderness over the calcaneal tuberosity
- Swelling and thickening of the distal Achilles tendon at the insertion on the posterior heel
- Often large bony prominence at the heel insertion that causes irritation with shoe wear

Range of Motion

- Decreased dorsiflexion due to contracture of calf muscles (insertional)
- Painful resisted plantarflexion

Imaging

- Not necessary for most cases of acute tendinitis
- Radiographs
  - Lateral view of the foot may demonstrate a spur on the posterior margin of the calcaneus in insertional tendinitis (Fig. 174.2).
  - Calcification within the tendon may be visible on lateral and oblique views of the foot with chronic tendinitis.
- Magnetic resonance imaging
  - Unnecessary for most nonoperative cases of tendinitis
  - Useful for determining severity of disease and extent of tendon pathology if planning surgical treatment in recalcitrant cases

Differential Diagnosis

- Retro-calcaneal bursitis: inflammation of the bursa between the Achilles and calcaneus
- Haglund disease: enlargement of the posterior-superior tuberosity of the calcaneus, "pump bump"
- Calcaneal stress fracture: exquisite tenderness over the medial and lateral borders of the calcaneus
- Sever disease: calcaneal apophysitis, usually adolescent athletes in running/jumping sports
- Spondyloarthropathy: HLA-B27 positive, diagnosis of psoriatic arthritis, Reiter syndrome, or ankylosing spondylitis
- Posterior tibial, peroneal, or flexor hallucis longus tendinitis: pain along tendon, exacerbated by resisted inversion, eversion, or great toe flexion, respectively

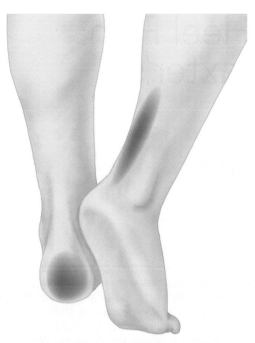

Fig 174.1 Location of insertional versus noninsertional Achilles tendinitis.

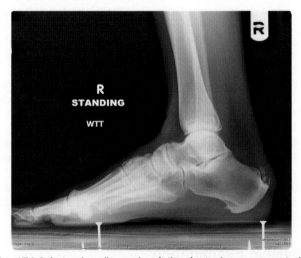

Fig 174.2 Lateral radiograph of the foot shows a posterior calcaneus spur.

Treatment

Acute Tendinitis

- Activity modifications, avoid all offending activities
- Eccentric stretching of the gastrocnemius-soleus complex
- 1-cm heel lift
- Nonsteroidal antiinflammatory drugs

Chronic Tendinitis

- Physical therapy modalities.
- Night splint or full-time use of walking boot with rocker-bottom sole.
- If structural or mechanical abnormalities are present (cavus or pes planus foot, over-pronation), a semirigid orthosis can be used.
- Activity is gradually reinstituted on a pain-free basis.
- Corticosteroid injections are discouraged due to risk of rupture.
- High-energy ultrasound and newer biologic stem cell treatments show promise and continue to gain scientific support as they are more fully studied.

When to Refer

- Patients with recalcitrant tendinitis that has failed several months of conservative treatment should be referred for possible surgical treatment, which may include debridement of diseased tissue, resection of a small portion of the calcaneal tuberosity, and tendon transfer.

Prognosis

- There is a 90% success rate with nonoperative treatment of tendinitis, and most athletes return to their previous level of participation.

Suggested Readings

Kearney R, Costa M. Insertional achilles tendinopathy management: a systematic review. *Foot Ankle Int*. 2010;31:689–694.

Kraeutler M, Purcell JM, Hunt KJ. Chronic achilles tendon ruptures. *Foot Ankle Int*. 2017;38:921–929.

Maffulli N, Via AG, Oliva F. Chronic achilles tendon disorders: tendinopathy and chronic ruptures. *Clin Sports Med*. 2015;34:607–624.

Schon LC, Shores JL, Faro FD, et al. Flexor hallicus longus tendon transfer in treatment of achilles tendinosis. *J Bone Joint Surg*. 2013;95:54–60.

Uquillas CA, Guss MS, Ryan DJ, et al. Everything achilles: knowledge and current concepts in management. *J Bone Joint Surg*. 2015;97: 1187–1195.

Chapter 175 Plantar Heel Pain: Plantar Fasciitis and Baxter's Nerve Entrapment

W. Bret Smith, Corey A. Hamilton, Logan W. Huff

ICD-10-CM CODES
M72.2 *Plantar fascial fibromatosis*
M79.2 *Neuralgia and neuritis, unspecified (Baxter's neuritis)*

Key Concepts

- *Plantar fasciitis* is the term used to describe acute or chronic pain in the anatomic region of the plantar fascia.
- General anatomy: three major bands of the plantar fascia primarily originate from the plantar calcaneus and insert primarily at the plantar plates of the metatarsophalangeal joints (Fig. 175.1).
- The term *fasciitis* refers to an acute inflammatory process, whereas the pathology of true plantar fasciitis is thought to be degeneration as a result of repetitive microtrauma/tears to the plantar aponeurosis. In several cases of tissues collected from surgeries for plantar fasciitis the tissue samples have failed to demonstrate inflammatory cells in histological studies.
- Histological studies have shown that the plantar fascia is well innervated with free and myelinated nerves and plays a role in proprioception and stabilizing movements of the foot.
- Innervation to the foot is via the branches of the posterior tibial nerve. Roughly at the level of the ankle it divides into three branches, the lateral, medial, and calcaneal. The medial and lateral bands continue further in the foot passing deep to the abductor hallucis (Fig. 175.2). Baxter nerve is the first branch of the lateral plantar nerve.
- The combination and coordination of the actions of the Achilles in conjunction with the plantar fascia and first metatarsal-phalangeal (MTP) joint create what is considered a windlass mechanism that assists in stabilizing the arch during the gait cycle (Fig. 175.3).
- The prevalence of this pathology is described to affect between 7% and 10% of the population of the United States, accounting for over 1 million physician outpatient visits.
- Risk factors for plantar fasciitis include but are not limited to: advanced age greater than 50; previously gender was thought to be slanted toward female patients but larger and more recent studies have shown possible male predominance; increased body mass index (BMI) but no specific studies demonstrate a specific number; athletic lifestyles and sedentary lifestyles were studied and demonstrated to be risk factors at the extremes of each lifestyle; pes planus; and several biomechanical studies have shown factors that disturb the energy dissipation in the heel and increase tension in plantar fascia are thought to adversely affect plantar fasciitis.

History

- The diagnosis for plantar fasciitis can be largely concluded with history and physical exam alone. Patients present with typical presentation. Commonly, pain with the first steps of ambulation after a period of rest is present. Usually the patient states that the pain will decrease to an extent after walking, but will begin to insidiously return and progress throughout the day with daily activities and standing.
- Patients may complain of pain in the entirety of the plantar foot, but most commonly the pain is localized to medial tubercle of the calcaneus, or the insertion of the plantar fascia.
- Inflammatory signs and symptoms are usually not present. Patients may present with swelling, edema, and erythema of the plantar aspect, but usually this is minimal.
- Tenderness to compression over the medial or lateral tuberosity should make the clinician wary of other pathology, such as calcaneal stress fracture.

Physical Examination

- Observation
  - In athletic individuals, may present with high arched feet and varus knee alignment
  - In sedentary populations, a higher BMI, pronated feet, and ankle equinus
- Palpation
  - Maximal tenderness at the anteromedial calcaneus; may be exacerbated by passive dorsiflexion or having patient stand on their toes
- Range of motion
  - Midfoot, hindfoot, and ankle range of motion is generally pain free.
  - May have decreased dorsiflexion at the ankle due to Achilles tendon tightness or gastrocnemius contracture.

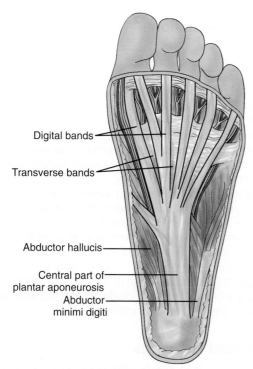

Fig 175.1 Anatomy of the plantar fascia.

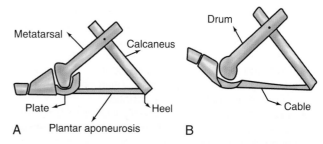

Fig 175.3 (A) The windlass mechanism. (B) The plantar aponeurosis functions like a cable in the windlass mechanism, maintaining the plantar arch.

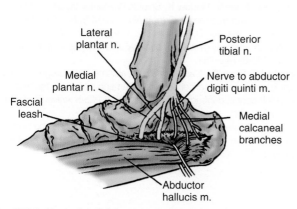

Fig 175.2 Posterior tibial nerve and its branches.

- Special tests
  - Neurologic examination is mandatory, especially if entrapment is suspected of either Baxter's nerve or the tarsal tunnel.
    - Electromyography (EMG) and nerve conduction velocity (NCV) studies may be warranted in cases where nerve entrapment is suspected, or to rule out proximal nerve lesions.
  - Positive Tinel sign can indicate nerve entrapment.

Imaging

- Imaging is not completely indicated, as history and physical exam are highly suggestive of plantar fasciitis, but can assist in ruling out other causes of heel pain.
- X-ray imaging plays a limited role in the acute setting but should be indicated in setting of trauma, pain out of proportion, and recalcitrant pain. Heel spurs on imaging are not necessarily indicative of pathology and are present in many patients without symptoms.
- Magnetic resonance imaging (MRI) is rarely used, with its greatest utility for patients who failed conservative therapy.
- Ultrasound may be diagnostically useful but is very user dependent. It can assist in measuring thickness of fascia for qualitative use and guiding injections.

Differential Diagnosis

- Achilles tendinopathy/enthesopathy: pain with resisted plantar flexion, tenderness over tendon
- Calcaneal stress fracture (patient will likely have a positive compression test of the calcaneus)
- Haglund deformity with or without bursitis: noticeable bump on back of heel; possible insertional Achilles tendinopathy
- Neurologic heel pain: Tarsal tunnel syndrome, heel neuroma, medial plantar nerve compression
- 5-10% have concomitant entrapment of first branch of lateral planter nerve (Baxter's nerve; innervates abductor digiti minimi)
- Other: arthritis, tumor, infection, vascular, calcaneal apophysitis (Sever disease), and fat pad atrophy
- Baxter's neuritis
  - Described as entrapment of the first branch of the lateral plantar nerve
  - Often will have pain similar to plantar fasciitis, but will not respond to standard treatment protocols
  - May have associate paresthesias around the plantar heel region
  - Often will not have an associated Tinel sign
  - Initial treatment is similar to standard plantar fasciitis treatment.

Treatment

- Treatment is broken down into conservative and invasive. Most patients, approximately 80%, receive therapeutic results after conservative measures; however they should be counseled that it may take several months.
- Initial treatment
  - Nonsurgical: Activity modification, antiinflammatories, shoe alterations, dorsiflexion night splints, weight loss, and cast immobilization in severe cases

- Physical therapy: Stretching exercises of plantar fascia and Achilles tendon, plantar fascia massage, intrinsic foot muscle strengthening, ice, and taping
- Shoe modifications: There are a wide variety of customized and prefabricated insole options. Prefabricated full-length arch supports have been shown to be as effective as custom-made orthotics.
- Corticosteroid injection: Usually limited to 2 to 3 per side in a 12-month time frame due to fad pad atrophy and risk of rupture
- Night splints: Splints maintain ankle and foot in a neutral position when patients normally sleep with feet in plantar flexed position.
- Extracorporeal shockwave therapy (ESWT): Not routinely used but has shown to be a valuable option
- Platelet-rich plasma injections have been described; however, results have been inconsistent.
- Surgical intervention
  - Surgical intervention should be reserved for chronic, refractory cases that have failed appropriate conservative treatment for 6 months or longer.
  - Options include plantar fasciotomy (open/endoscopic/percutaneous) or gastrocnemius recession.
  - In certain cases of Baxter's nerve entrapment a full nerve decompression may be required.

When to Refer

- If no improvement is noted within 6 to 12 weeks of appropriate conservative care, the patient should be referred for consideration of more intensive conservative therapies or possibly surgery.
- If neurologic testing suggests entrapment, then early referral is warranted.

Prognosis

- Self-limiting condition, with 90% of patients responding to nonsurgical treatments within 6 to 10 months.

Patient Instructions

- There are certain things a patient can do to try to prevent plantar fasciitis, especially in the case of prior plantar fasciitis:
  - Regularly changing shoes used for running or walking
  - Wearing shoes with good cushioning in the heels and good arch support
  - Weight loss, if overweight
  - Avoiding exercise on hard surfaces and going barefoot
- Medical attention should be sought on an elective basis if any of the classic symptoms of plantar fasciitis are present consistently for 2 to 3 weeks:
  - Gradual onset of mild to moderate heel pain (usually aggravated by the commencement of ambulation and also higher-intensity activities)
- The patient should seek medical help urgently if he/she has the following symptoms:
  - Heel pain that occurs at night or resting
  - Swelling or discoloration of the back of the foot
  - Signs of an infection, including fever, redness, warmth
  - Any other unusual symptoms

Suggested Readings

Caratun R, Rutkowski NA, Finestone HM. Stubborn heel pain: treatment of plantar fasciitis using high-load strength training. *Can Fam Physician*. 2018;64(1):44–46.

Johnson RE, Haas K, Lindow K, Shields R. Plantar fasciitis: what is the diagnosis and treatment? *Orthop Nurs*. 2014;33(4):198–204.

Kirkpatrick J, Yassaie O, Mirjalili SA. The plantar calcaneal spur: a review of anatomy, histology, etiology and key associations. *J Anat*. 2017;230(6):743–751.

Schneider HP, Baca JM, Carpenter BB, et al. American college of foot and ankle surgeons clinical consensus statement: diagnosis and treatment of adult acquired infracalcaneal heel pain. *J Foot Ankle Surg*. 2018;57(2):370–381.

Thomas JL, Christensen JC, Kravitz SR, et al. The diagnosis and treatment of heel pain: a clinical practice guideline-revision 2010. *J Foot Ankle Surg*. 2010;49(3 suppl):S1–S19.

Chapter 176 Compressive Neuropathies: Tarsal Tunnel Syndrome

Jonathan P. Smerek, Minton Truitt Cooper

ICD-10-CM CODES

G57.50	*Tarsal tunnel syndrome*
G57.51	*Tarsal tunnel syndrome, right ankle*
G57.52	*Tarsal tunnel syndrome, left ankle*
G57.53	*Tarsal tunnel syndrome, both ankles*
G57.91	*Neuralgia, right ankle*
G57.92	*Neuralgia, left ankle*

Key Concepts

- Tarsal tunnel syndrome (TTS) results from compression of the posterior tibial nerve and its branches that occurs in the tarsal tunnel, in the posteromedial ankle, and hindfoot.
- TTS is an uncommon disorder, and the diagnosis should not be made without a careful history and examination.
- TTS is more common in females, and there is no age predilection.
- A specific etiology is found in only 60-80% of individuals, and may include a space-occupying lesion, trauma, venous engorgement, or foot deformity (pes planovalgus or severe "flatfoot").
- History is the key to diagnosis.
- Electromyography (EMG) may be unreliable. However, they may be used to supplement history and physical exam, or to rule out more proximal lesions or neuropathy.
- The posterior tibial nerve supplies the majority of the sensation on the plantar foot.
- The tarsal tunnel is a fibro-osseous structure posterior to the medial malleolus and formed by the flexor retinaculum, which originates from the tibia and inserts onto the posterior process of the calcaneus and talus laterally. The retinaculum blends with the sheaths of the posterior tibial tendon, flexor digitorum longus tendon, posterior tibial nerve/artery, and flexor hallucis longus tendon (Fig. 176.1).

History

- Often vague symptoms
- Burning, sharp, electric pain, tingling, or numbness on the plantar foot
- Rest pain common and symptoms often worse at night, with inability to tolerate socks or sheets on the feet
- Radiation of pain proximally to the posteromedial aspect of the distal tibia (Valleix phenomenon)
- Although pain can be worse with activity, symptoms usually do not correlate with the amount or duration of activity.

Physical Examination

- Observation
  - Gait
  - Heel alignment: Observe patient standing from behind with shoes and socks removed; assess heel varus/valgus and note whether arch is high (cavus) or collapsed (planovalgus or "flatfoot").
- Palpation
  - Tenderness along course of the posterior tibial nerve at the level of the ankle coursing distal to the medial malleolus
  - Positive Tinel sign: the patient's symptoms reproduced with gentle percussion along the course of the posterior tibial nerve
  - Palpate for tenderness over the plantar fascia.
- Range of motion
  - Ankle, subtalar, and talonavicular range of motion
- Special tests
  - Tarsal tunnel compression test: Reproducing the patient's symptoms by pressure over the nerve (compress against the posteromedial tibia for 30 seconds) is a highly specific finding (Fig. 176.2).
  - Dorsiflexion eversion test: Ankle is passively maximally dorsiflexed and everted while the metatarsophalangeal joints are dorsiflexed and held for 5 to 10 seconds. This may reproduce or exacerbate symptoms.

Imaging

- Radiographs: weight-bearing anteroposterior, lateral, and oblique/mortise views of the foot/ankle
  - Look for acute and malunited fractures, arthrosis, accessory ossicles, and tarsal coalitions.
- Magnetic resonance imaging (MRI)
  - Useful if radiographs are normal and index of suspicion for a space-occupying lesion of the tarsal tunnel is high (Fig. 176.3)
  - Lesions are more common in pediatric patients.

Additional Tests

- Electrodiagnostic studies: Decreased mixed motor and sensory conduction velocity is the most specific and sensitive for TTS.
  - There is a false-negative rate of at least 10%, so the diagnosis is not eliminated with a normal EMG.

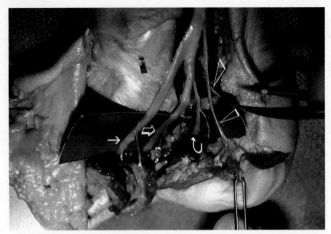

Fig 176.1 Anatomy of the tarsal tunnel demonstrating the boundaries and surrounding structures. *Thin arrow* indicates the medial plantar nerve; *thick arrow* indicates the lateral plantar nerve; *curved arrow* indicates the nerve to the flexor digitorum brevis; *triangles* indicate the medial calcaneal branches.

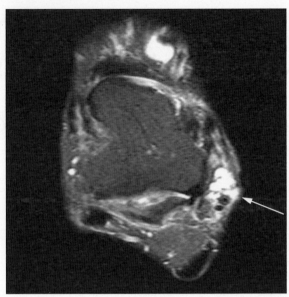

Fig 176.3 Axial T2-weighted magnetic resonance imaging of the ankle demonstrates a multiloculated ganglion cyst *(arrow)* within the tarsal tunnel resulting in compression of the nearby posterior tibial nerve.

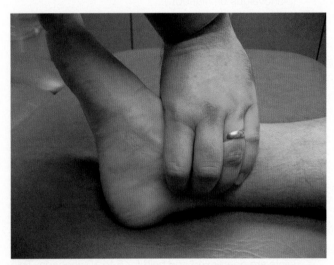

Fig 176.2 Tarsal tunnel compression test demonstrating compression over the posterior tibial nerve in an attempt to recreate the patient's symptoms. The light compression should be held for at least 30 seconds.

- Neurolemma/neuroma/ganglion cyst: fullness in the tarsal tunnel, MRI
- Fracture of the ankle/talus/calcaneus: point tenderness; radiographs and computed tomography
- Rheumatoid arthritis: systemic findings; arthrosis on radiographs
- Tenosynovitis: tenderness over posterior tibial tendon, relieved with rest and immobilization
- Venous varicosities: fullness, varicosities on examination
- Tarsal coalition: limited hindfoot motion; radiographs or MRI
- Crush injury/blunt trauma: history of trauma, highly sensitive overlying skin (allodynia)

Treatment

- At diagnosis
- Unless the patient has a space-occupying lesion compressing the posterior tibial nerve, a prolonged course of conservative management is mandatory.
  - Avoid inciting activities.
  - Some patients may benefit from a course of nonsteroidal antiinflammatory drugs.
  - Physical therapy with adjuvant modalities for desensitization of the posterior tibial nerve may be attempted.
  - In flexible foot deformities, arch supports with a medial heel wedge to take tension off of the nerve may provide significant relief.
  - Neuropathy medications (Neurontin [gabapentin], Lyrica [pregabalin]) may be instituted, but should not be the first line of therapy due to potential side effects.
  - Immobilization with a boot walker or cast is usually not beneficial and may lead to calf atrophy and ankle weakness.

- EMG may also have a high false-positive rate, while nerve conduction studies have a high false-negative rate.
- Studies have demonstrated limited correlation between EMG results and clinical outcomes.
- May rule out peripheral neuropathy, proximal compression, or double crush injury

Differential Diagnosis

- Herniated nucleus pulposus: radiating leg pain, positive straight leg raise, back pain
- Plantar fasciitis: heel pain, worse with first step in morning
- Peripheral vascular disease: claudication, no palpable pulses
- Peripheral neuropathy: stocking-glove pain and numbness, diabetes, EMG

- A trial of a topical neurogenic compounding cream may be beneficial. This is a topical prescription lotion that combines lidocaine, gabapentin, and Voltaren.
- Later
  - Failure of 6 weeks of conservative therapy with no relief of symptoms warrants consideration of a tarsal tunnel injection. This injection can be both therapeutic and diagnostic. For precise placement, this may be done under ultrasound guidance.
  - Failure of at least 3 months of conservative management, including a tarsal tunnel injection, is sufficient to consider surgical intervention for release of the posterior tibial nerve.

When to Refer

- Diagnosis of TTS requires (1) pain and paresthesias in the foot, (2) positive electrodiagnostic studies, and (3) a positive Tinel sign or tarsal tunnel compression test. With two of these findings, the patient may have TTS and should be followed closely.
- Identification of any space occupying lesion with symptoms of TTS

Prognosis

- As many as 75% of patients who undergo release of the posterior tibial nerve can expect nearly complete relief of their symptoms.
- The other 25% do not improve, and in fact can have worsening of their symptoms after attempted surgical release.
- Repeat surgery has extremely poor outcomes due to scarring around the nerve.

- Patients with a space-occupying lesion have a better prognosis and can expect nearly complete resolution of their symptoms with mass excision and release.

Troubleshooting

- Failure to improve with conservative measures warrants a tarsal tunnel injection, which can be both diagnostic and therapeutic.

Patient Instructions

- Patients should be instructed that nerve-related symptoms frequently take many months to resolve and they should expect a slow diminution in symptoms over time.
- Patients should be encouraged to modify their footwear with arch supports and to modify their activity, limiting high-impact exercise, to allow the symptoms to dissipate prior to suggesting any more aggressive treatment.
- Surgery should be only undertaken after at least 3 months of conservative care because surgical outcomes in general are unpredictable. Surgery should not be the first option.

Suggested Readings

DiGiovanni BF, Gould JS. Tarsal tunnel syndrome and related entities. *Foot Ankle Clin*. 1998;3:405–426.

Gould JS. Tarsal tunnel syndrome. *Foot Ankle Clin*. 2011;16(2):275–286.

Pomeroy G, Wilton J, Anthony S. Entrapment neuropathy about the foot and ankle: an update. *J Am Acad Orthop Surg*. 2015;23(1):58–66.

Sammarco GJ, Chang L. Outcome of surgical treatment of tarsal tunnel syndrome. *Foot Ankle Int*. 2003;24:125–131.

Schon LC, Reed MA. Disorders of the nerves. In: Coughlin MJ, eds. *Mann's Surgery of the Foot and Ankle*. 9th ed. Philadelphia: Elsevier; 2014:621–682.

Chapter 177 Adult Flat Foot/ Posterior Tibial Tendon Disorders

Jonathan P. Smerek, Minton Truitt Cooper

ICD-10-CM CODES

M21.40	*Posterior tibialis tendon insufficiency/ dysfunction*
M21.41	*Posterior tibialis tendon insufficiency, right ankle*
M21.42	*Posterior tibialis tendon insufficiency, left ankle*
M76.821	*Posterior tibialis tendon tendonitis, right ankle*
M76.822	*Posterior tibialis tendon tendonitis, left ankle*
M66.871	*Posterior tibialis tendon tear, right ankle*
M66.872	*Posterior tibialis tendon tear, left ankle*
M21.40	*Pes planovalgus, acquired*
M21.41	*Pes planovalgus, acquired right*
M21.42	*Pes planovalgus, acquired left*

Key Concepts

- The posterior tibial tendon (PTT) courses posterior to the medial malleolus and has a broad insertion, with the primary attachment at the plantar medial navicular tuberosity (Fig. 177.1).
- The PTT is the main invertor of the hindfoot, which serves to lock the transverse tarsal joint allowing for a rigid lever arm for push off during gait.
- Chronic insufficiency of the tendon leads to progressive collapse of the longitudinal arch and weakness during heel rise.
- Risk factors for posterior tibial tendon insufficiency (PTTI) include female sex, age over 40, diabetes, hypertension, and obesity.
- Although traumatic injury may occur, it is more commonly a degenerative condition and is often related to long-standing flatfoot deformity.
- Poor vascularity of the PTT as it courses posterior to the medial malleolus leads to poor healing potential and degeneration.
- Complete rupture of the tendon is rare, with failure more commonly due to multiple longitudinal split tears, mucoid degeneration, and loss of normal collagen architecture.

History

- Acute tendinitis
  - Can occur with any mechanism of ankle sprain/lower extremity injury
  - Medial and posteromedial ankle pain and swelling
  - Pain worse with walking, especially on stairs

- Chronic tendinitis
  - Insidious onset with no relation to traumatic event
  - Medial and posteromedial ankle pain with or without swelling
  - The patient may report "collapse" of the arch and progressive flatfoot deformity.
- In cases of pes planovalgus deformity, patients may also experience pain in the lateral hindfoot, around the sinus tarsi, and at the tip of the fibula due to impingement.

Physical Examination

- Observation
  - Gait
  - Heel alignment: Have the patient remove shoes and socks and roll pants to above the knees. Stand behind him/her to observe.
    - Assess varus/valgus of the heel and compare with the contralateral side.
    - Describe the arch as high (cavus) or collapsed (planovalgus or flatfoot).
- Palpation
  - Tenderness along course of the PTT
  - Sinus tarsi tenderness
- Range of motion
  - Ankle, subtalar, and talonavicular range of motion
    - In advanced stages of the disease, the heel valgus may become fixed and not correctable.
  - Assess for gastrocnemius contracture by testing ankle dorsiflexion with the knee extended and flexed. Gastrocnemius contracture, if present, will limit ankle dorsiflexion with the knee extended. Limited dorsiflexion with the knee flexed indicates a contracture of the ankle capsule and Achilles tendon. It is important to hold the heel in a "subtalar neutral" position to truly test dorsiflexion.
- Special tests
  - Single heel rise (Fig. 177.2)
    - Patient stands facing the examiner, holding the examiner's hands for balance.
    - Alternatively, the patient may place his or her hands on the wall for balance.
    - The contralateral leg is elevated, and the patient should be able to elevate on the toes on the affected side. Watch for inversion of the heel during this maneuver as an indication that the PTT is functioning.
    - Inability to do so reflects PTTI.
    - Watch for the patient who cheats and uses his or her arms to push up to initiate the single heel rise.

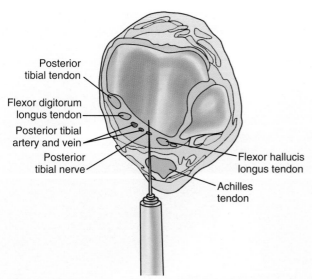

Fig 177.1 Anatomy of the posterior tibial tendon at the medial ankle.

Posterior tibial tendon

Flexor digitorum longus tendon

Posterior tibial artery and vein

Posterior tibial nerve

Flexor hallucis longus tendon

Achilles tendon

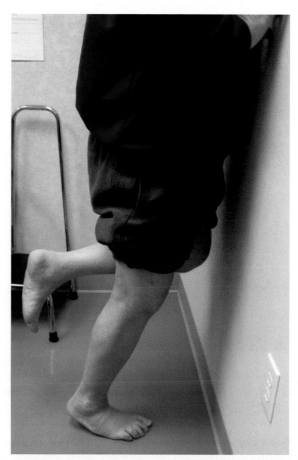

Fig 177.2 Clinical photograph demonstrating a patient with the ability to perform a single heel rise, consistent with an intact and functioning posterior tibial tendon. The contralateral leg should be fully off the ground and the hands lightly on the wall for balance.

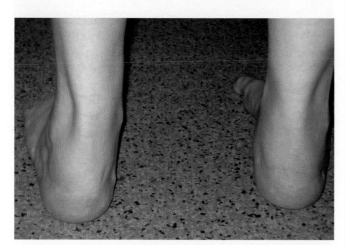

Fig 177.3 Clinical photograph demonstrates increased left heel valgus compared with the normal right side. Also demonstrated is the "too many toes" sign with more of the lesser toes visible in this patient with left posterior tibial tendon insufficiency.

- "Too many toes" sign (Fig. 177.3)
  - With patient standing, observe heel alignment from behind.
  - With PTTI, more of the lesser toes will be visible lateral to the heel due to excessive heel valgus and abduction of the midfoot.

Imaging

- Radiographs
  - Weight-bearing anteroposterior, lateral, and oblique views of the foot
    - Evaluate for arthritis of the talonavicular, subtalar, calcaneocuboid, and midfoot joints.
    - Look for stress fractures.
    - Check for an accessory navicular.
  - Weight-bearing anteroposterior, lateral, and mortise views of the ankle
    - Check for valgus tilting of the talus within the mortise, a sign of long-standing PTTI and deltoid ligament insufficiency.
- Magnetic resonance imaging
  - Not required for diagnosis or planning treatment
  - May assist in narrowing the differential diagnosis if the initial diagnosis of PTTI is not clear
  - Frequently demonstrates multiple longitudinal split tears, thickening, synovitis, and fluid surrounding the diseased tendon (Fig. 177.4)

Differential Diagnosis

- Painful congenital flatfoot deformity: ability to perform repetitive single heel rise, long-standing flatfoot deformity with plantar medial pain
- Painful accessory navicular: tenderness over the navicular tuberosity, ability to perform repetitive single heel rise, evident on radiographs
- Rheumatoid arthritis: systemic findings and arthropathy of multiple joints, decreased joint space with arthrosis on weight-bearing radiographs

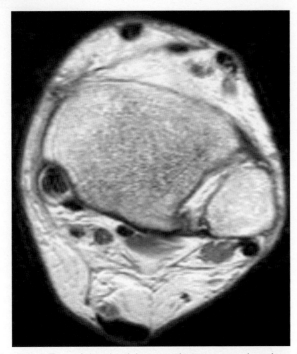

Fig 177.4 T1-weighted axial magnetic resonance imaging at a level just proximal to the ankle joint demonstrates thickening, multiple vertical split tears, and synovitis of a degenerated posterior tibial tendon.

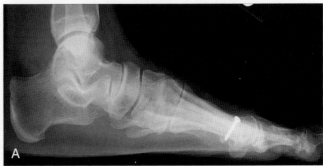
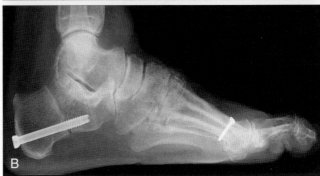

Fig 177.5 Lateral radiographs before (A) and after (B) calcaneal osteotomy and tendon transfer for reconstruction of flatfoot deformity demonstrate re-creation of the longitudinal arch.

- Tarsal coalition: usually long-standing flatfoot deformity, calcaneonavicular or talocalcaneal bony coalition on radiographs
- Osteoarthritis or posttraumatic arthritis of the midfoot/hindfoot: tenderness over the first, second, or third tarsometatarsal or subtalar articulations, flatfoot deformity, joint space narrowing on radiographs

Treatment

- At diagnosis
  - Initial treatment of PTTI focuses on decreasing swelling and synovitis around the PTT.
  - Complete rest of the tendon is accomplished with a tall boot walker or a short leg walking cast to immobilize the ankle and hindfoot. In milder cases, a lace-up ankle brace may provide relief.
  - The patient is encouraged to ice the area of maximum swelling daily and take nonsteroidal antiinflammatory drugs as needed.
  - The patient can be weight bearing as tolerated in the boot or walking cast.
- Later
  - If the patient has significant resolution of symptoms after 4 to 6 weeks of cast or boot immobilization *and* is able to perform a single heel rise repetitively, a less obtrusive support may be used. The patient may try a custom-made or over-the-counter orthosis with a 3-degree medial heel wedge to reduce the work required by the PTT or a PTT dysfunction brace, which incorporates an air bladder into the brace to support the PTT and longitudinal arch.

- Physical therapy may be prescribed once the acute inflammation has subsided.
- Patients who continue to have pain and are unable to perform a single heel rise may be tried on continued boot or cast immobilization. Many will require either a tenosynovectomy or a reconstruction with tendon transfer of the flexor digitorum longus tendon to the navicular to replace the PTT (Fig. 177.5). Most often this will require concomitant osteotomies or fusions to correct alignment.
- Patients with a long-standing flatfoot deformity that is rigid through the subtalar and talonavicular joints may require a hindfoot arthrodesis to correct the deformity and restore the longitudinal arch.

When to Refer

- Patients with persistent pain, tenderness, swelling, and an inability to perform a single heel rise at 6 weeks should be referred to an orthopaedic surgeon. Persistent pain and a nonfunctioning PTT can lead to a long-standing rigid, flatfoot deformity that limits reconstructive options. Magnetic resonance imaging is not required for referral.

Prognosis

- Excellent with aggressive early immobilization, followed by a course of physical therapy
- Patients who develop persistent pain and PTTI do quite well with reconstruction and tendon transfer, although the transferred tendon is never as strong as the healthy, native PTT.

- Patients with rigid flatfoot deformity who require a triple arthrodesis may experience early ankle arthritis.

Troubleshooting

- The benefits of reconstruction usually outweigh the risks because it leads to pain relief, decreased deformity, and return to an active lifestyle.
- The risks of surgical intervention include neuritis, wound complications, infection, and weakness of inversion due to transfer of a weaker tendon to replace the PTT.
- Injection of the tendon and/or tendon sheath with steroids should be avoided because it can lead to tendon rupture.
- Simple suture repair of the tendon has been shown to fail due to the poor vascularity of the tendon.

Patient Instructions

- Patients should be instructed that insufficiency of the tendon holding up the arch has led to the continued pain.
  - Strict rest of the tendon with boot or cast immobilization can lead to marked improvement in symptoms.
  - Surgery may be required if immobilization is unsuccessful.
- Patients should be reassured that magnetic resonance imaging is not required for diagnosis.

Considerations in Special Populations

- Young (younger than 40 years) and very active individuals may benefit from a tenosynovectomy alone.

- In patients with multiple medical comorbidities or who have low demands, long-term bracing with an ankle foot orthosis (Arizona brace) may provide significant relief.
- Elderly and sedentary individuals are likely best treated with a triple arthrodesis due to the rehabilitation required after a reconstruction and tendon transfer.

Suggested Readings

Abousayed MM, Tartaglione JP, Rosenbaum AJ, Dipreta JA. Classifications in brief: Johnson and Strom classification of adult-acquired flatfoot deformity. *Clin Orthop Relat Res*. 2016;474(2):588–593.

Beals TC, Pomeroy GC, Manoli A. Posterior tendon insufficiency: diagnosis and treatment. *J Am Acad Orthop Surg*. 1999;7:112–118.

Deland JT. Adult-acquired flatfoot deformity. *J Am Acad Orthop Surg*. 2008;16(7):399–406.

Haddad SL, Deland JT. Pes planus. In: Coughlin MJ, Saltzman CL, Anderson RB, eds. *Mann's Surgery of the Foot and Ankle*. 9th ed. Philadelphia: Elsevier; 2014:1292–1360.

Kulig K, Reischl SF, Pomrantz AB, et al. Nonsurgical management of posterior tibial tendon dysfunction with orthoses and resistive exercise: a randomized controlled trial. *Phys Ther*. 2009;89(1):26–37.

Thordarson DB. Stage II adult acquired flatfoot deformity: treatment options and indications. In: Nunley JA, et al, eds. *Advanced Reconstruction: Foot and Ankle*. Rosemont, IL: American Academy of Orthopaedic Surgeons; 2004:109–114.

Chapter 178 Hindfoot/Midfoot Arthritis

Tyler W. Fraser, Jesse F. Doty

ICD-10-CM CODES
M19.07+   *Primary OA*
M19.17+   *Post-traumatic OA*

Key Concepts

- Primary osteoarthritis (OA) of the midfoot and hindfoot generally presents in patients more than 50 years old
- Common forms of secondary arthritis of the midfoot and hindfoot include posttraumatic arthritis and inflammatory arthritis (rheumatoid, psoriatic, and gouty)
- Patients present clinically with pain, decreased function, and stiffness
- Primary OA generally follows a progressive chronic course that can sometimes be managed conservatively but may benefit significantly from surgery as pain worsens
- Posttraumatic arthritis and inflammatory arthritis typically have an earlier onset and a higher rate of operative intervention may be necessitated

Anatomy

- Hindfoot: talus and calcaneus bones, and subtalar (ST), talonavicular (TN), and calcaneocuboid (CC) joints
- Midfoot: navicular, cuboid, and cuneiform(s) bones, and tarsometatarsal (Lisfranc) and naviculocuneiform joints

History

- Prior trauma?
  - Approximately 20% of calcaneus and 40% of talus fractures require a second operation for posttraumatic arthritis after initially fixing the fracture
  - Lisfranc injuries
- Pain walking on uneven ground
- Push-off pain, pain exacerbated by activity, achy pain worsening as the day progresses
- Personal or family history of rheumatologic disease?
- Personal history of diabetes and vascular disease?
- Aggravating footwear?
- Subjective change of foot shape? (such as flattening of the arch)

Physical Examination

- Decreased motion of the joints
- Swelling and warmth
- Deformity, loss of longitudinal arch or significantly high arch
- Pain with palpation over joints such as pressure on the tarsometatarsal (TMT) joints
- Often prominent dorsal osteophytes or ganglion cysts may be associated with midfoot arthritis.
- Callous or ulcers
- Sinus tarsi or subfibular pain
- Pain with forefoot abduction, pronation

Imaging

- Weight-bearing radiographs—anteroposterior (AP), 45-degree oblique, and lateral foot, AP or mortise ankle
  - Joint space narrowing, subchondral sclerosis of the joints, osteophytes, loose bodies (Fig. 178.1)
  - Loss of normal alignment such as arch collapse
  - If diabetic, Charcot changes in midfoot may include complete bone resorption and joint destruction
- Advanced imaging: generally reserved for a specialist planning surgery or to identify specific affected joints
  - Computed tomography (CT) scan
    - History of complex fractures, nonunions, and malunions
    - Preoperative planning for significant deformities
  - Bone scan
    - Useful for diagnostic purposes especially in the midfoot, where it can be difficult to determine which joint the pain is emanating from. (Can be coupled with a CT scan—known as a single-photon emission computed tomography [SPECT-CT].)

Differential Diagnosis

- Ankle arthritis
- Osteochondral lesions of the talus
- Charcot arthropathy
- Metatarsalgia
- Posterior tibial tendon or peroneal tendon dysfunction
- Neuropathic pain (most commonly diabetes)
- Vasculopathy

Treatment

- Nonsurgical
  - Weight loss
  - Shoe modifications such as custom insole or graphite plate insoles and avoiding barefoot walking
  - Activity modification to low-impact exercises
  - Antiinflammatories—topical or oral nonsteroidal antiinflammatory drugs (NSAIDs), cryotherapy

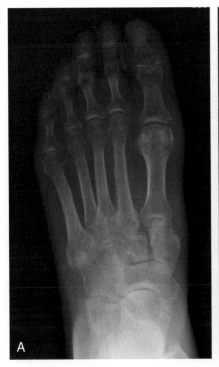
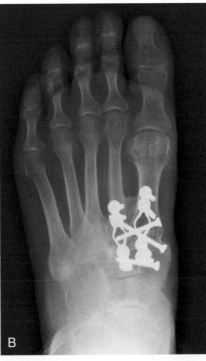

Fig 178.1 (A) Anteroposterior foot radiograph demonstrates a chronic Lisfranc injury that developed posttraumatic midfoot arthritis. (B) Postoperative radiograph demonstrates a successful midfoot fusion.

- Bracing/orthoses, such as Arizona brace or ankle foot orthosis, which further restrict hindfoot/midfoot motion
- Steroid injections—typically fluoroscopic guided—may be used for diagnostic and therapeutic purposes.
- Surgical
  - Arthroscopic debridement for larger joints—questionable efficacy.
  - Osteophyte removal for dorsal midfoot when shoe wear difficulty is primary complaint
  - Fusions (Fig. 178.2)

When to Refer

- Continued pain with conservative treatment
- Unacceptable functional limitations
- Rigid or nonbraceable deformities
- Inflammatory arthropathies
- Neuromuscular disease

Prognosis

- In general, all types of arthritis are progressive, although conservative modalities may be effective for symptomatic relief and delaying the need for operative intervention
- Subtalar (ST) fusion for nontraumatic arthritis has excellent results and at least good results are reported for posttraumatic ST arthritis
- In general, greater than 85% of patients are satisfied after midfoot fusion
- Fusion alters normal biomechanics, and therefore patients may develop arthritis is other areas of the foot
- After surgery, it is common to have some degree of foot pain and fatigue with prolonged activity, although this is usually substantially improved

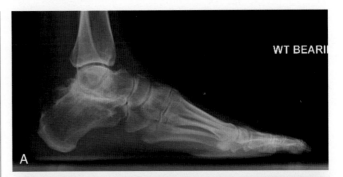
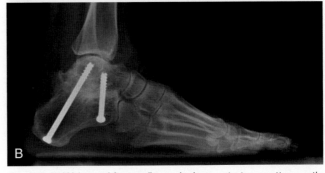

Fig 178.2 (A) Lateral foot radiograph demonstrates posttraumatic arthritis after a calcaneus fracture. (B) Postoperative radiograph demonstrates a successful subtalar fusion.

Patient Instructions

- Patients should be counseled on chronic nature of diagnosis
- Compliance with conservative measures may negate the need for operative intervention

- Smoking cessation is strongly encouraged
  - Smokers have decreased union rates of fusion and higher rates of revision surgery and wound complications
- Comorbidities should be optimized prior to surgery to attempt to minimize complications

Suggested Readings

Davies MB, Rosenfeld PF, Stavrou P. A comprehensive review of subtalar arthrodesis. *Foot Ankle Int*. 2007;28(3):295–297.

Janisse DJ, Janisse E. Shoe modification and the use of orthoses in the treatment of foot and ankle pathology. *J Am Acad Orthop Surg*. 2008;16(3):152–158.

Patel A, Rao S, Nawoczenski D, et al. Midfoot arthritis. *J Am Acad Orthop Surg*. 2010;18(7):417–425.

Sanders DW, Busam M, Hattwick E, et al. Functional outcomes following displaced talar neck fractures. *J Orthop Trauma*. 2004;18:265–270.

Sanders R, Fortin P, DiPasquale T, et al. Operative treatment in 120 displaced intraarticular calcaneal fractures. Results using a prognostic computed tomography scan classi cation. *Clin Orthop*. 1993;290:87–95.

Watson TS, Shurnas PS, Denker J. Treatment of lisfranc joint injury: current concepts. *J Am Acad Orthop Surg*. 2010;18:718–728.

Chapter 179 Peroneal Tendon Disorders

Venkat Perumal, George Lee Wilkinson III

ICD-10-CM CODES
M66.88   *Peroneal tendon tear*
M76.7   *Peroneal tendinitis*
M77.50   *Peroneal tendon subluxation*
M89.8X7   *Os peroneum syndrome*

Key Concepts

- The peroneal tendons serve as the primary evertors/pronators of the foot and play a major role in dynamic ankle stabilization and maintaining proper foot alignment.
- The peroneus brevis and longus run posterior to the lateral malleolus (Fig. 179.1).
  - The longus inserts on the first and second metatarsals as well as the medial cuneiform.
  - The brevis inserts onto the fifth metatarsal base.
- The brevis resides in the fibular groove in between the lateral malleolus and the longus (Fig. 179.2).
- The musculotendinous junction of the longus is located more proximally than that of the brevis.
- The peroneal tendons are held in place by a combination of both the concave shape of the fibula as well as the fibrous peroneal retinaculum.
- An ossicle in the peroneus longus near the base of the fifth metatarsal is known as an os peroneum.
  - This is a normal anatomic variant but can become painful with injury.
- Peroneal tendon injuries can be acute or chronic.
- Peroneal tendon neuromuscular weakness or tears may be associated with a varus hindfoot and cavus forefoot.
- Lateral ankle instability is often seen in conjunction with peroneal pathologies.

History

- Tendon tear
  - Can be acute and mistaken for an ankle sprain, often seen in younger, more active patients
  - Can also be a source of chronic lateral ankle pain, often seen in older, more sedentary patients
  - Swelling and/or ankle instability can be present.
- Tendonitis
  - Occurrence of lateral ankle pain when resuming activity after a period of inaction or when sharply increasing activity level

- Tendon subluxation
  - Reported sensation of "snapping" or "popping"
  - Can be describes as a chronic "giving way" of the ankle
- Os peroneum syndrome
  - May present in the same fashion as an ankle sprain
  - Can be acute or chronic

Physical Examination

- Observation
  - Swelling and ecchymosis following acute injuries
- Palpation
  - Tenderness over course of the tendon either in the fibular groove or distally
  - Tenderness just proximal to the fifth metatarsal base is present in os peroneum syndrome.
- Range of motion and strength
  - Usually normal, but pain or weakness with resisted eversion is common.
  - Pain with toe rise, plantar flexion of first ray, or supination and inversion of the foot is seen in os peroneum syndrome.
- Special tests
  - Assess hindfoot alignment by standing behind the patient to see how the leg is lined up with respect to the heel (Fig. 179.3).
    - A varus heel can lead to peroneal tendonitis or tearing.
  - Assess for peroneal subluxation by moving the ankle from a plantarflexed, inverted position to a dorsiflexed, everted position (Fig. 179.4).
    - Can also sometimes be observed with ankle circumduction

Imaging

- Weight-bearing anterior posterior, mortise, and lateral radiographs of the ankle and foot
  - May have a fleck sign from avulsion of the superior peroneal retinaculum, but often normal from the fibula in peroneal tendon subluxation/dislocation (Fig. 179.5)
  - Recommend comparing with the contralateral foot films if multipartite versus fractured os is present.
- Magnetic resonance imaging (Fig. 179.6)
  - Can help identify tendon tears and any associated ligamentous or bony injuries
  - May help discern whether an os is multipartite or fractured

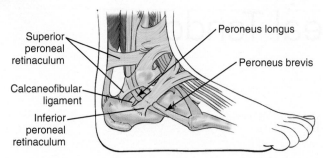

Fig 179.1 Anatomy of the peroneal tendons. Sagittal drawing of the lateral ankle.

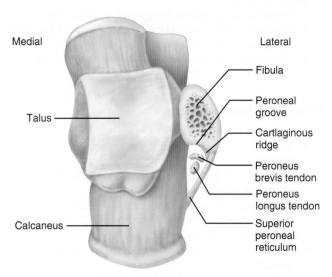

Superior view

Fig 179.2 Relation of the peroneal tendon to the fibula. (Redrawn and modified from Rosenfeld P. Acute and chronic peroneal tendon dislocations. *Foot Ankle Clin*. 2007;12[4]:643–657.)

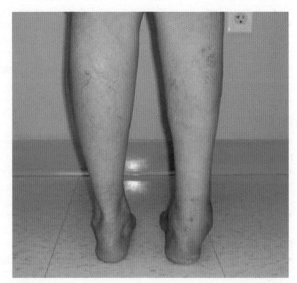

Fig 179.3 Varus alignment of the right heel. Left heel normal alignment.

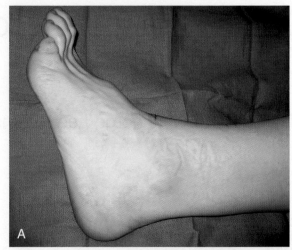

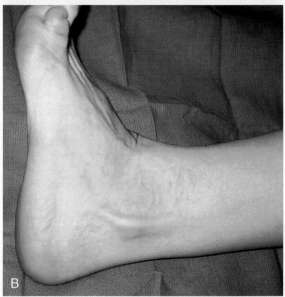

Fig 179.4 Peroneal tendon subluxation. **(A)** With plantar-flexion and inversion, the tendons are reduced in the fibular groove. **(B)** With dorsiflexion and eversion, tendon instability is reproduced. Note the subluxed position of the peroneal tendons.

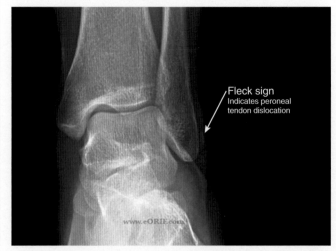

Fleck sign
Indicates peroneal
tendon dislocation

Fig 179.5 Fleck sign on ankle X-ray. (Copyright © 2009–2017 eORIF LLC, www.eORIF.com.)

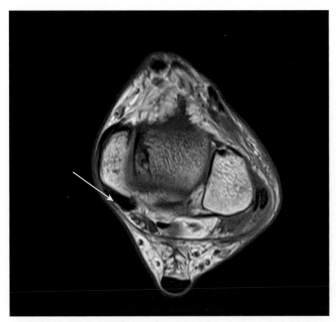

Fig 179.6 MRI showing subluxation/dislocation of both the peroneal tendons *(arrow)*.

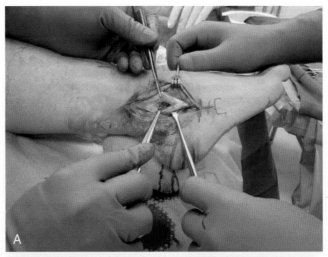

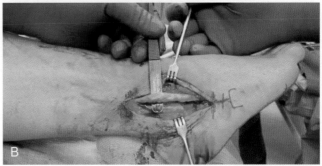

Fig 179.7 **(A)** Peroneal tendon split tear. **(B)** After repair of the peroneal tendon tear.

- Ultrasonography
  - Superior to both MRI and plain films for peroneal tendon subluxation
  - Can also help evaluate for subluxation if done dynamically

Differential Diagnosis

- Ankle sprain
- Ankle fracture
- Arthritis
- Ankle synovitis
- Osteochondral injury of the ankle
- Fracture of the lateral process of the talus
- Fracture of the fifth metatarsal base
- Tarsal coalition
- Neuromuscular disease

Treatment

- Acute peroneal tendon tears and acute, traumatic subluxation of the peroneal tendons benefit from acute surgical intervention.
  - Surgical intervention for peroneal subluxation may involve repair of the peroneal retinaculum with or without fibular groove deepening.
- Chronic peroneal tendon tears are first treated with rest, nonsteroidal antiinflammatory drugs (NSAIDs), and physical therapy.
  - If these do not significantly relieve symptoms, bracing and immobilization can be considered.
  - Surgical intervention may involve repair of the tendons (Fig. 179.7), as well as correction of the cavovarus deformity by a possible lateralizing calcaneal osteotomy

with or without dorsiflexion osteotomy of the first ray to lessen likelihood of recurrence.
- Os peroneum syndrome is treated with immobilization for 1 month.
  - Surgical intervention may involve excision of the os with repair or tenodesis of the peroneus longus.

When to Refer

- Prompt referral to a specialist is appropriate in the case of acute peroneal tear or subluxation.
- Referral is also recommended in the case of chronic tearing or subluxation, but this does not need to occur as quickly as in an acute case.
- Referral for os peroneum syndrome is only recommended after failure of conservative management.

Prognosis

- Surgical repairs of acute injuries generally have an excellent prognosis.
- There is a more guarded prognosis of returning to high-level function for those with chronic tendon injuries.
- Addressing associated pathology such as lateral ankle instability or varus hindfoot concurrently can lead to an improvement in prognosis.

Suggested Readings

Chambers HG. Ankle and foot disorders in skeletally immature athletes. *Orthop Clin North Am*. 2003;34:445–459.

Dombek MF, Lamm BM, Saltrick K, et al. Peroneal tendon tears: a retrospective review. *J Foot Ankle Surg*. 2003;42:250–258.

MacDonald BD, Wertheimer SJ. Bilateral os peroneum fractures: comparison of conservative and surgical treatment and outcomes. *J Foot Ankle Surg*. 1997;36:220–225.

Steel MW, DeOrio JK. Peroneal tendon tears: return to sports after operative treatment. *Foot Ankle Int*. 2007;28:49–54.

Vienne P, Schöniger R, Helmy N, et al. Hindfoot instability in cavovarus deformity: static and dynamic balancing. *Foot Ankle Int*. 2007;28:96–102.

Chapter 180 Morton Neuroma (Plantar Interdigital Neuroma)

Brian D. Powell

ICD-10-CM CODE
G57.6 *Lesion of plantar nerve; Morton metatarsalgia, neuralgia, or neuroma*

Key Concepts (Fig. 180.1)

- Most common in the third web space but infrequently present at the second.
- History and physical examination sufficient for diagnosis.
- Conservative care includes shoe modification, a metatarsal pad, and steroid injections.
- Surgical treatment after failure of conservative care includes excision of the affected nerve.

History

- Pain at the second or third intermetatarsal web space, with the third being more common.
- Neuromas at the first and fourth web space are exceptionally rare, and an alternative diagnosis should be considered.
- Radiating burning and paresthesia into the toes adjacent to the affected toes.
- Occasionally, catching or an uncomfortable mass can be felt in the plantar forefoot.
- Aggravating factors include shoes with elevated heels, a narrow toe box, or repetitive trauma such as long-distance running.
- Pain may be alleviated with removing shoes and massaging feet.

Physical Examination

- Observation
- Weight-bearing evaluation of the foot includes assessment for lesser toe deformities: crossover toe, hammertoe, or claw toe deformity. These contribute to metatarsalgia, which can commonly be mistaken for a plantar interdigital neuroma.
- A normal-appearing foot is common.
- Palpation
- Firm pressure in the affected web space between the metatarsal heads is a hallmark sign (Fig. 180.2). This pain can radiate into the adjacent toes.
- Adjacent metatarsal heads are palpated in isolation to differentiate from metatarsalgia. Pain with direct pressure on the metatarsal head or the metatarsophalangeal joint (MTP) is more indicative of metatarsalgia, synovitis, or a plantar plate rupture.

- Special tests
  - Compression test: Firmly squeeze the metatarsal heads in the medial to lateral direction to compress the neuroma between the metatarsal heads. Applying plantar pressure simultaneously at the affected web space can assist with reproduction of symptoms (Fig. 180.3).
  - Mulder click: A painful "click" with the compression test is indicative of a neuroma and called a Mulder click. Pain and reproduction of symptoms without a click is still indicative of a neuroma but is not considered a positive Mulder sign. This test is not as helpful in recurrent neuromas after surgical intervention.
  - Vertical Lachman test: Grasp the phalanx and firmly place vertical stress on the MTP joint. Reproduction of plantar pain or gross motion/instability is indicative of a plantar plate rupture and not a neuroma.

Imaging

- Radiographs: anteroposterior, lateral, and oblique views of the foot
  - Rule out other causes of forefoot pain: crossover toe, claw toe, MTP dislocation, prior metatarsal trauma, Freiberg infraction (Fig. 180.4), and stress fractures.
- Magnetic resonance imaging
  - Not normally indicated. May be helpful when the diagnosis is ambiguous (Fig. 180.5).
- Ultrasonography
  - More economical alternative to assist in diagnosis
  - Highly operator dependent; leads to potential misdiagnosis

Additional Tests

- Injection (see Chapter 203)
  - A local anesthetic such as 1% lidocaine with 0.5% bupivacaine is typically used.
  - Traditionally a steroid is used with the local anesthetic.
  - Blocking the common digital nerve resulting in reduction of symptoms is diagnostic.
  - Can be performed with ultrasound guidance for improved accuracy

Differential Diagnosis

- Metatarsalgia with contributing lesser toe deformities
- Plantar plate rupture at MTP
- Tarsal tunnel syndrome
- Intractable plantar keratoses (calluses)
- Avascular necrosis of the lesser metatarsal head (Freiberg infraction)

- Soft-tissue mass
- Stress fractures
- Arthritis
- Metatarsal-phalangeal synovitis

Treatment

- First-line conservative treatment includes a soft wide toe box shoe. Addition of a metatarsal pad appropriately

placed proximal to the metatarsal heads may also reduce pressure.
- An injection with 1% lidocaine, 0.25% bupivacaine, and a steroid for persistent symptoms can be used for both treatment and diagnostic purposes.
- Sclerosing alcohol injections with 20% ethanol and 0.25% bupivacaine given every 2 weeks up to five injections with ultrasound guidance have been used. Extreme caution should be observed in the clinical setting without ultrasound

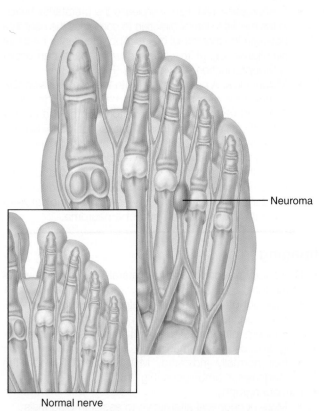

Neuroma

Normal nerve

Fig 180.1 Overview of Morton neuroma.

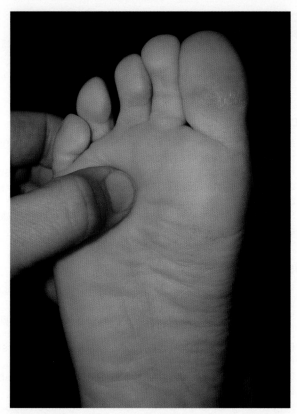

Fig 180.2 Direct palpation of the third web space. It is important not to press on the metatarsal heads or distal to them.

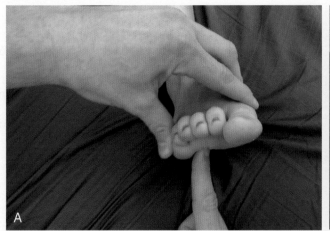

A

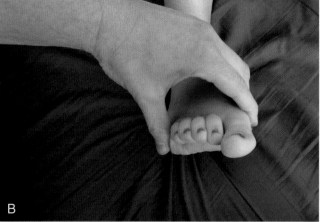

B

Fig 180.3 (A) The compression test is performed by placing the examiner's hands securely on the metatarsal heads and directing pressure centrally from either side. (B) Plantar pressure at the affected web space with a compression test can deliver the dilated nerve between the metatarsal heads and help reproduce symptoms.

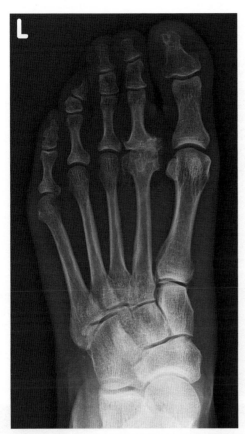

Fig 180.4 Radiograph showing Freiberg infraction. Note the destruction of the second metatarsophalangeal joint and subsequent arthritic wear.

due to high failure rates and morbidity. Although short-term treatment can provide relief, it does not normally provide permanent resolution of symptoms and should not be considered equivocal to surgical intervention.

When to Refer

- Patients with returning or persistent symptoms following conservative treatment can be referred for surgery (Fig. 180.6). Since repeat injections or continuing conservative care does not affect the surgical intervention or outcome, no referral needs to be made until the patient is ready for more aggressive treatment.

Prognosis

- Surgical success rates vary, with the literature suggesting good to excellent results in 50-80% of patients.

Troubleshooting

- If an injection offers no benefit, it is important to seek other diagnoses. Further accuracy can be obtained by having a repeat injection done under ultrasound guidance, which can provide assurance of an incorrect diagnosis.
- Pain relief may not be complete after surgical resection and can result in permanent paresthesia in the toes adjacent to the affected web space.

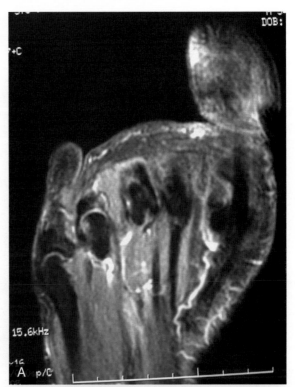

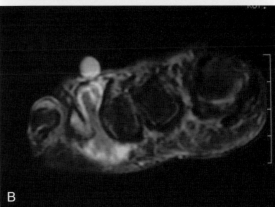

Fig 180.5 Magnetic resonance images of a large Morton neuroma. (A) T1-weighted image demonstrates the enlarged digital nerve between the third and fourth metatarsal heads. (B) T2-weighted image demonstrates the enhanced, inflamed tissue in the same interspace.

- Reasons for failure include incorrect diagnosis, incomplete resection, and scar tissue entrapment.
- Returning symptoms after appropriate surgical care can be indicative of a recurrent neuroma.

Patient Instructions

- Ensure that patients understand the nature of the condition: early surgical intervention does not lead to improved outcomes.
- Conservative care can have improved effectiveness overtime. Thus these measures can be continued until the patient is ready for surgery.

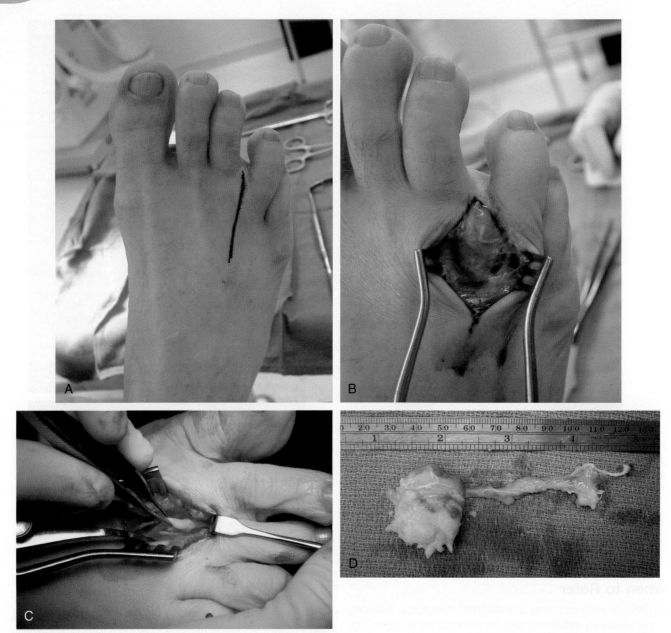

Fig 180.6 Surgical excision of a Morton neuroma. **(A)** Surgical approach. **(B)** Example of massive neuroma in the third web space. **(C)** Example of a smaller Morton neuroma in the second web space, completely freed from surrounding soft tissues, with the dilation visible at the level between the metatarsal heads. **(D)** Resected Morton neuroma, with 3 cm of proximal common digital nerve attached to the resected segment.

Suggested Readings

Betts LO. Morton's metatarsalgia: neuritis of the fourth digital nerve. *Med J Aust*. 1940;1:514.

Bossley CJ, Cairney PC. The intermetatarsophalangeal bursa: its significance in Morton's metatarsalgia. *J Bone Joint Surg Br*. 1980;62B:184–187.

Erickson SJ, Canale PB, Carrera GF, et al. Interdigital (Morton) neuroma: High-resolution MR imaging with a solenoid coil. *Radiology*. 1991;181:833–836.

Greenfield JK, Rea J Jr, Ilfeld FW. Morton's interdigital neuroma: indications for treatment by local injections versus surgery. *Clin Orthop Relat Res*. 1984;185:142–144.

Gurdezi S, White T, Ramesh P. Alcohol injection for Morton's neuroma. *Foot Ankle Int*. 2013;34(8):1064–1067.

Lizano-Díez X, Ginés-Cespedosa A, Alentorn-Geli E, et al. Corticosteroid injection for the treatment of Morton's neuroma: a prospective,

double-blind, randomized, placebo-controlled trial. *Foot Ankle Int*. 2017;38(9):944–951.

Mulder JD. The causative mechanism in Morton's metatarsalgia. *J Bone Joint Surg Br*. 1951;33B:94–95.

Nissen KI. Plantar digital neuritis: Morton's metatarsalgia. *J Bone Joint Surg Br*. 1948;30B:84–94.

Redd RA, Peters VJ, Emery SF, et al. Morton neuroma: sonographic evaluation. *Radiology*. 1989;71:415–417.

Shapiro PP, Shapiro SL. Sonographic evaluation of interdigital neuromas. *Foot Ankle Int*. 1995;16:604–606.

Terk MR, Kwong PK, Suthar M, et al. Morton neuroma: evaluation with MR imaging performed with contrast enhancement and fat suppression. *Radiology*. 1993;189:239–241.

Womack JW, Richardson DR, Murphy AG, et al. Long-term evaluation of interdigital neuroma treated by surgical excision. *Foot Ankle Int*. 2008;29:574–577.

Chapter 181 Hallux Valgus (Bunion)

Alexander D. Conti, Justin J. Ray, Robert D. Santrock

ICD-10-CM CODES
M20.10 *Hallux valgus, acquired, unspecified laterality*
M20.11 *Hallux valgus, acquired, right*
M20.12 *Hallux valgus, acquired, left*
M21.619 *Bunion of unspecified foot*

Key Concepts

- Hallux valgus or "bunion" is a complex positional deformity of the first ray characterized by medial deviation of the first metatarsal and lateral deviation and pronation of the hallux.
- The medial bump or prominence (bunion) may cause considerable pain and altered joint mechanics.
- Predisposing factors include female gender, age, constricting footwear, and family history.
- Concomitant processes associated with hallux valgus include hammertoe deformity, pes planus, Achilles tendon contracture, and metatarsus adductus.
- Nonoperative treatment involves patient education and footwear and activity modifications.
- Operative treatment includes a combination of soft-tissue balancing procedures, proximal or distal metatarsal osteotomies, and fusion of either the first metatarsophalangeal (MTP) or tarsometatarsal (TMT) joint, depending on the severity of the deformity.

History

- Patients commonly present complaining of difficulty with certain types of shoes and pain over the medial eminence (bunion).
- Several intrinsic and extrinsic factors have been identified.
  - Extrinsic factors include constricting footwear.
  - Intrinsic factors include female gender, age, family history, pes planus, metatarsus adductus, Achilles tendon contracture, generalized ligamentous laxity, hypermobility of the first ray, and length of the first metatarsal.
  - Genetics appears to have a major role in hallux valgus. Although the inheritance pattern remains unclear, the suspected pattern is autosomal dominant with incomplete penetrance.
  - Increased prevalence in females (up to 15:1 ratios have been reported)
- Patients may also present with cosmetic concerns, transfer metatarsalgia, or lesser toe deformities.
- Pain in the distribution of the dorsal cutaneous nerve is also common.

Physical Examination

- Patients should be examined in a seated and standing position (standing accentuates deformity).
- Inspection
  - Look for any skin changes, general position of the first ray, and any lesser toe deformities.
  - Assess for any swelling, erythema, or inflamed bursa.
  - Observe for antalgic gait and general lower extremity alignment.
- Palpation
  - Determine the specific location of pain based on history and palpation of the foot.
  - Palpate for areas of focal tenderness, crepitus, arthritic changes, sesamoid tenderness, synovial or bursal thickening, or tenderness related to lesser toe deformities.
- Neurovascular examination
  - Important to rule out neurovascular insufficiency
- Range of motion
  - Of the ankle, subtalar, tarsal, TMT, MTP joints
  - Assess first ray for general range of motion and passive correction of the deformity.
- Special tests
  - Silfverskiöld test: assess for gastrocnemius tightness by examining ankle dorsiflexion with knee flexed versus knee extended.
  - Assess for hypermobility of the first TMT joint (Fig. 181.1).
    - Hold second metatarsal with one hand while other hand holds first metatarsal head and deviates it dorsomedially and then plantar laterally.

Imaging

- Radiographs—weight-bearing anteroposterior (AP), lateral, oblique, and axial sesamoid views
- Hallux valgus angle (HVA)—angle between the long axis of the first metatarsal and first proximal phalanx (Fig. 181.2A)
  - Normal <15 degrees; mild deformity <20 degrees; moderate deformity 20 to 40 degrees; severe deformity >40 degrees
- Intermetatarsal angle (IMA)—angle between the long axis of the first and second metatarsals (see Fig. 181.2A)
  - Normal <9 degrees; mild deformity 9 to 11 degrees; moderate deformity 11 to 16 degrees; severe deformity >16 degrees
- Axial Sesamoid View (see Fig. 181.2B)
  - Evaluate position of sesamoids in relation to cristae of first metatarsal head.
  - Evaluate for subluxation of the sesamoids or rotation of the first metatarsal.

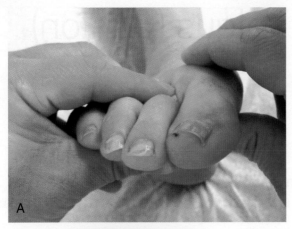

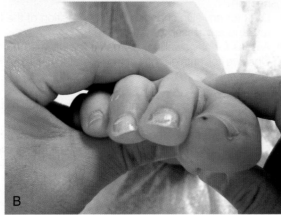

Fig 181.1 Illustration demonstrating how to assess hypermobility of the first tarsometatarsal joint, showing maximal dorsiflexion (A) and plantarflexion (B) in a patient with hypermobility of the first ray.

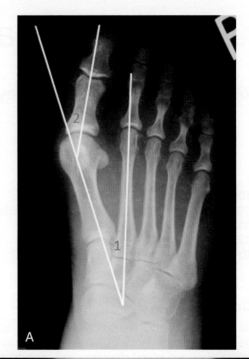

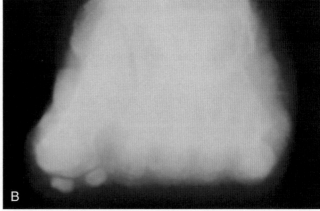

Fig 181.2 (A) Traditional hallux valgus measures on anteroposterior radiographs. The number 1 corresponds to the intermetatarsal angle; the number 2 corresponds to the hallux valgus angle. (B) Shows the axial sesamoid view demonstrating the normal anatomic location of the sesamoids in relation to the crista.

- Distal metatarsal articular angle (DMAA)—angle between the distal articular surface and long axis of the first metatarsal
  - Normal <10 degrees
  - DMAA has proven less reliable than the HVA and IMA in studies.
- Evaluate first MTP joint for evidence of any arthritic changes.

Additional Tests
- Weight-bearing computed tomography (CT) scanning is emerging as a valuable tool to provide a three-dimensional analysis of the deformity.
- Ankle-brachial index and arterial toe pressures if vascular deficit is suspected.

Differential Diagnosis
- Hallux rigidus
- Hallux varus
- Juvenile hallux valgus
- Infection
- Inflammatory arthropathy (gout, psoriasis, rheumatoid arthritis)

Treatment
- Nonoperative treatment
  - May provide pain and symptom relief but cannot correct the deformity.
  - Goals include symptom management, prevention of deformity progression, and decreased pain.
  - Footwear modifications with a wide toe box and activity modifications.
  - Achilles tendon stretching if a contracture is present.
  - Orthotics with medial arch support may provide up to 6 months of symptom relief.
- Surgical treatment
  - Reserved for patients who have failed nonoperative treatment and have persistent problems with shoe wear and pain.

TABLE 181.1 Traditional Radiographic Classification and Treatment of Hallux Valgus Deformity

Severity of Deformity	Hallux Valgus Angle (HVA)	1st to 2nd Intermetatarsal Angle (IMA)	Treatment
Normal	<15°	<9°	None
Mild	<20°	9–11°	Distal osteotomy ± soft-tissue procedure
Moderate	20–40°	11–16°	Proximal osteotomy ± soft-tissue procedure
Severe	>40°	>16°	Proximal osteotomy or 1st tarsometatarsal (TMT) arthrodesis ± soft-tissue procedure

- More than 100 different procedures have been described.
- Cosmetics alone is not an indication for surgical treatment.
- Includes a combination of soft-tissue balancing procedures, distal and proximal metatarsal osteotomies, and fusions of either the first MTP or TMT joints depending on severity and congruity of the deformity.
- Traditionally surgical treatment has been based on the HVA and IMA (Table 181.1):
  - Mild deformity—distal osteotomy ± soft-tissue procedure
  - Moderate deformity—proximal osteotomy ± soft-tissue procedure
  - Severe deformity—proximal osteotomy or first TMT arthrodesis ± soft-tissue procedure
  - In presence of first MTP arthritis, a fusion of the first MTP joint is performed.
- Complications of surgical treatment include infection, recurrence, overcorrection (resulting in hallux varus), avascular necrosis, residual pain, nonunion, or transfer metatarsalgia.

When to Refer

- Patients who have failed nonoperative treatment and have persistent problems with footwear and pain related to hallux valgus should be referred for possible surgical intervention.

Prognosis

- Progression of deformity with age is common in patients with hallux valgus.

- Patients with a congruent deformity (high DMAA) and proper sesamoid location have slower rates of progression.
- Excellent results have been reported with appropriate surgical treatment (80-95% success rate).

Patient Instructions

- Educate patients on realistic expectations and the progressive nature of hallux valgus.
- Patients should be instructed on appropriate footwear (limit constrictive footwear, use shoes with a wide toe box), as well as activity modifications.

Considerations in Special Populations

- Symptomatic hallux valgus is uncommon in the pediatric population.
- Surgical treatment in the pediatric population is associated with high rates of recurrence, possible growth disturbance, and variable clinical outcomes.
- Most surgeons advocate delaying surgery until skeletal maturity is reached.

Suggested Readings

Coughlin MJ, Jones CP. Hallux valgus: demographics, etiology, and radiographic assessment. *Foot Ankle Int*. 2007;28:759–777.

Coughlin MJ, Roger A. Mann Award. Juvenile hallux valgus: etiology and treatment. *Foot Ankle Int*. 1995;16:682–697.

Perera AM, Mason L, Stephens MM. The pathogenesis of hallux valgus. *J Bone Joint Surg*. 2011;93(17):1650–1661.

Robinson AH, Limbers JP. Modern concepts in the treatment of hallux valgus. *J Bone Joint Surg Br*. 2005;87:1038–1045.

Chapter 182 Hallux Rigidus

Carroll P. Jones

ICD-10-CM CODES
M20.22 *Acquired hallux rigidus, left*
M20.21 *Acquired hallux rigidus, right*

Key Concepts

- By definition, degenerative arthritis of the hallux metatarsophalangeal (MTP) joint
- Does **not** include inflammatory arthritis (i.e., gout)
- Second most common pathology affecting the first MTP joint
- Multiple theoretical causes but most often hereditary with an insidious onset
- The progression of arthrosis leads to proliferation of bone (osteophytes) over the dorsal aspect of the metatarsal head and alteration of normal joint kinematics (Fig. 182.1)
- Marginal osteophytes restrict motion and lead to pain (initially) at the extremes of motion
- As the arthritis progresses, the entire articulation may become involved and cause diffuse joint pain
- Generally graded as I (mild), II (moderate), or III (severe)
- Conservative interventions aim to provide space within footwear for the hypertrophied joint, externally restrict painful motion of the first MTP joint, and address the inflammation within the joint
- Surgical interventions include cheilectomy (excision of osteophytes), interposition arthroplasty, prosthetic replacement, and arthrodesis

History

- Localized pain and swelling over dorsum of the first MTP joint, typically atraumatic
- As the arthritis progresses, more diffuse pain and stiffness are characteristic
- Occasionally, lateral (LAT) forefoot pain secondary to offloading the affected first MTP joint may occur
- Pain often presents initially with dorsiflexion (DF) of the great toe, including the toe-off phase of gait
- Aggravating factors (e.g., footwear, repetitive activities) should be identified
- Occurs in two populations: adolescents and adults aged 30 to 70 years of age
- The etiology is unknown, but there are multiple proposed mechanisms
  - Posttraumatic (i.e., severe sprain, fracture)
  - Repetitive microtrauma (i.e., running)
  - Congenital/hereditary: length of first metatarsal, shape of metatarsal head and proximal phalanx, positive family history, osteochondritis dissecans (OCD)

Physical Examination
Critical to Examine Contralateral Foot for Comparison

- Inspection
  - Skin color: localized erythema dorsal aspect of joint may indicate pressure points from footwear irritation over dorsal osteophytes
  - Increased size of joint from dorsal spurring (Fig. 182.2)
  - Ambulation: painful toe-off during gait
  - Swelling localized to hallux MTP
  - Alignment of hallux in axial plane (hallux valgus or varus may also be present)
- Palpation
  - Dorsal bony prominence and tenderness at first MTP
  - Positive Tinel along dorsal medial cutaneous nerve not uncommon
- Range of motion
  - Loss of sagittal range of motion (ROM), typically decreased DF in early phases
  - Pain at the extremes of motion (DF and plantar flexion [PF])
  - Crepitus and pain throughout arc of motion may be present in later stages with more extensive degenerative arthritis

Imaging

- Radiographs
  - Weight-bearing anteroposterior (AP) view: evaluate extent of joint space narrowing, marginal osteophytes, and axial alignment (Fig. 182.3)
  - Weight-bearing LAT view: evaluate for dorsal osteophytes and plantar extent of degeneration (Fig. 182.4)

Additional Tests

- Magnetic resonance imaging (MRI): rarely necessary—helpful for suspected OCD lesion, sesamoiditis, or unusual presentation of hallux MTP pain

Differential Diagnosis

- First MTP joint infection
- Inflammatory arthritis (gout, pseudogout, rheumatoid arthritis)
- Sesamoiditis (pain localized to *plantar* aspect of joint)
- Acute sprain/injury (i.e., turf toe)

Treatment

- Conservative measures recommended as first-line treatment
  - Goals include providing adequate space to accommodate the increased joint size, minimizing painful joint

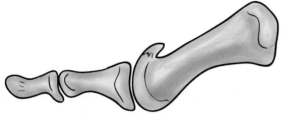

Fig 182.1 Drawing showing lateral view of the first metatarsophalangeal joint with dorsal osteophytes characteristic of hallux rigidus.

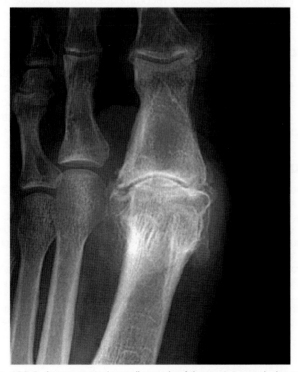

Fig 182.2 Thickening of tissues around the first metatarsophalangeal joint in a patient with severe hallux rigidus.

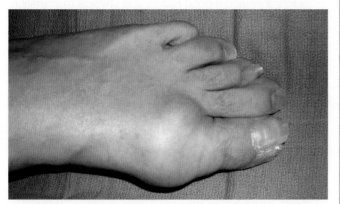

Fig 182.3 Anteroposterior radiograph of the metatarsophalangeal joint with severe hallux rigidus.

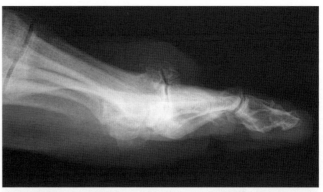

Fig 182.4 Lateral radiograph of the metatarsophalangeal joint demonstrating severe hallux rigidus.

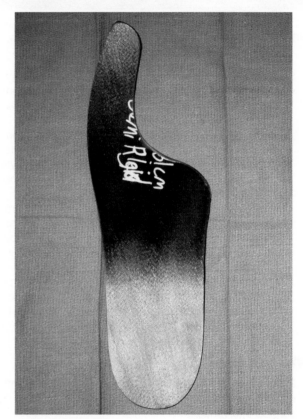

Fig 182.5 Carbon fiber insert with Morton extension limits the amount of flexion at the first metatarsophalangeal joint.

motion, and decreasing inflammation in and around the joint
- Avoid aggravating footwear (tight shoes, high heels) and activities
- Recommend footwear with a wide toe box
- A rocker sole (external shoe modification) or Morton's extension orthotic (insole) to decrease motion (and pain) at the first MTP joint (Fig. 182.5)
- Nonsteroidal antiinflammatory medication and ice
- Corticosteroid injection: diagnostic and therapeutic, and may provide many months of relief; can be repeated every 3 to 4 months if effective

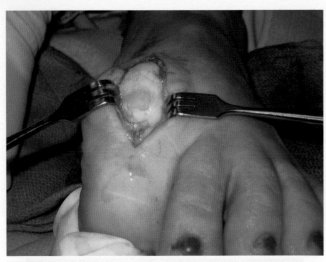

Fig 182.6 Intraoperative image showing loss of metatarsal articular cartilage in advanced hallux rigidus.

- Surgical intervention indicated if conservative measures fail
  - A number of surgical interventions are available depending on the extent of the disease, age, activity level, and expectations of the patient.
    - Cheilectomy: indicated for mild to moderate arthritis and pain primarily overlying the dorsal osteophytes; involves surgical resection of the dorsal osteophytes to improve motion and decompress the dorsal aspect of the joint
    - First MTP joint arthrodesis: indicated for moderate to severe arthritis with (Fig. 182.6) a more diffusely painful and stiff joint; although very effective for pain relief, it will eliminate motion at the joint and limit certain activities and shoe wear
    - Less common surgical interventions include interposition arthroplasty, silicone arthroplasty, nonsilicone prosthetic replacement, and osteotomies of both the metatarsal and proximal phalanges.

When to Refer

- Patients who have persistent symptoms after 6 months of conservative treatment are candidates for referral for surgical intervention.

Prognosis

- Hallux rigidus is a progressive degenerative disease but very treatable.
  - Nonoperative therapies are aimed at slowing progression and providing pain relief.

- Good to excellent results can be expected in patients with dorsal pain and impingement who undergo cheilectomy.
- Patients with advanced degenerative joint disease often require arthrodesis. Despite eliminating the joint, pain relief is very predictable, and most patients remain very functional.
- Complications from surgery are relatively uncommon.

Troubleshooting

- The diagnosis of hallux rigidus is fairly straightforward and in the vast majority of cases is made based on plain radiographs and a good history and physical examination.
- All patients are initially treated conservatively and should be educated regarding the progressive nature of the arthritis and the goal of slowing disease progression. Surgery should only be discussed after an adequate trial of conservative treatment.
- Choosing the ideal surgical procedure (i.e., cheilectomy vs. arthrodesis) is sometimes difficult and is best made by an orthopedic specialist.

Patient Instructions

- Nonoperative treatment of hallux rigidus may include activity modification, ice, shoe modifications, orthotics, medications, and injections in the joint. Multiple treatment methods may need to be combined, and there is no perfect "recipe" for every patient.
- Referral to a specialist is recommended for surgical discussion is conservative treatment is not effective.

Considerations in Special Populations

- Older, lower-demand patients are often ideal candidates for arthrodesis if conservative measures are ineffective.
- Patients with neuromuscular disease and/or spasticity are best treated with arthrodesis if they fail nonoperative modalities.

Suggested Readings

Coughlin M, Shurnas P. Hallux rigidus: demographics, etiology, and radiographic assessment. *Foot Ankle Int*. 2003a;24:731–743.

Coughlin M, Shurnas P. Hallux rigidus: grading and long-term results of operative treatment. *J Bone Joint Surg Am*. 2003b;85A:2072–2088.

Coughlin M, Shurnas P. Hallux rigidus: surgical techniques (cheilectomy and arthrodesis). *J Bone Joint Surg Am*. 2004;86A:119–130.

Hirose CB, Coughlin MJ, Stevens FR. Arthritis of the foot and ankle. In: Coughlin M, Saltzman CL, Anderson RB, eds. *Mann's Surgery of the Foot and Ankle*. 9th ed. Philadelphia: Elsevier; 2014:868–1007.

Mann R, Coughlin M, DuVries H. Hallux rigidus: a review of the literature and a method of treatment. *Clin Orthop Relat Res*. 1979;142:57–63.

Chapter 183 Lesser Toe Deformities

C. Thomas Haytmanek, Jr.

ICD-10-CM CODES
R-M20.41, L-M20.42 *Hammertoe*
R-M20.5X1, L-M20.5X2 *Claw toe and other acquired deformities of toe*

Key Concepts

- Lesser toe deformities include mallet toe, hammertoe, and claw toes; crossover and curly toe deformities; and instability of the metatarsophalangeal (MTP) joints.
- Lesser toe deformities may cause significant pain.
- Conventionally deformities with neurologic etiologies are termed *claw toes*. Those caused by improper footwear are *hammertoes*.
- The etiology may be an anatomic abnormality of the affected toe or an adjacent toe. Neurologic conditions, repetitive injury, inflammatory arthropathies, muscular imbalance between the intrinsic/extrinsic foot musculature, and ill-fitting/high-fashion shoes may also contribute.
- Diagnosis and elimination of causative factors aid in treatment and prognosis.
- Treatment is initially nonoperative with the goal of alleviating symptoms. The aim is to passively stretch or correct supple deformities and cushion or relieve pressure in rigid deformities.

History

- Painful callosities are common in all deformities due to abnormal pressure points.
- Mallet toe, hammertoe, and claw toes: difficulty with shoe wear; pain on tips of toes, dorsal interphalangeal joints (where callosities can form), and plantar callosities.
- MTP joint instability: ill-defined forefoot pain with walking; initially plantar (with plantar plate rupture); generalized synovitis over time; pain precedes deformity.
- Crossover toe deformity: progressive worsening of second toe alignment often seen in conjunction with hallux valgus.
- Curly toe deformity: passively correctable, asymptomatic, overlapping toe in young children; usually bilateral and familial; third and fourth toes most common.

Physical Examination

- Observation
  - Examine patient sitting and standing. When sitting, flexible deformities may be harder to identify.
  - Forefoot/hindfoot malalignment may contribute to toe abnormalities.

- Thick, painful plantar callosities are common (Fig. 183.1).
- Hammertoes (Fig. 183.2): proximal interphalangeal (PIP) joint flexion; frequent MTP joint hyperextension; distal interphalangeal (DIP) joint in a variable position
- Claw toes (Fig. 183.3): The primary deformity is MTP hyperextension and PIP and DIP flexion. Plantar position of the metatarsal head results in painful plantar callosities or ulcers.
- Mallet toes (Fig. 183.4): isolated DIP flexion (attenuation of the terminal extensor tendon leads to unopposed pull of the flexor digitorum longus); callosities at tip of toe or dorsal DIP joint
- Crossover toes (Fig. 183.5): varus, dorsiflexion deformity of the second toe allowing it to lie over the top of the hallux (capsular instability of the second MTP joint); commonly associated with hallux valgus; occasionally lesser toe goes into varus
- MTP joint instability (Fig. 183.6): medial or lateral toe deviation related to tearing of the plantar plate—tested with "drawer maneuver" as noted in figure; compare to unaffected toe to evaluate baseline laxity
- Curly toes (Fig. 183.7): toe flexion, medial deviation (lies under the adjacent toe), and internal rotation (nail faces laterally); caused by tight toe flexor tendon
- Palpation
  - Palpate for tenderness at the metatarsal heads and web spaced to evaluate for interdigital neuroma formation. The plantar fat pad migrates distally as hammer/claw toes develop, contributing to metatarsalgia.
- Range of motion
  - Determine whether deformities are flexible or rigid.
- Special tests
  - Drawer test for MTP joint instability: Grasp the proximal phalanx of the involved toe between the thumb and index finger and pull the toe dorsally; when performed on an unstable MTP joint, this produces dorsal translation and pain (see Fig. 183.6).
  - Assess for associated neurologic or inflammatory conditions (e.g., Charcot-Marie-Tooth disease, rheumatoid arthritis).

Imaging

- Radiographs: weight-bearing anteroposterior, lateral, and oblique views of the foot (Fig. 183.8)
  - Check for concomitant pathology and alternate sources of pain such as arthritis, Freiberg infraction, and fractures.
- Magnetic resonance imaging
  - Not usually required, but can show stress fractures and Freiberg infraction

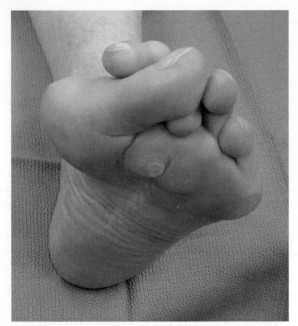

Fig 183.1 Plantar callosities in a patient with multiple severe lesser toe deformities.

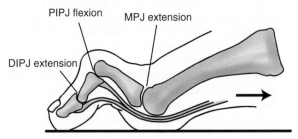

Fig 183.2 Hammertoe deformity. *DIPJ*, Distal interphalangeal joint; *MPJ*, metatarsophalangeal joint; *PIPJ*, proximal interphalangeal joint.

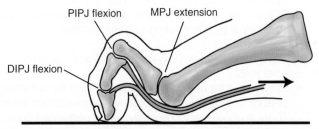

Fig 183.3 Claw toe deformity. *DIPJ*, Distal interphalangeal joint; *MPJ*, metatarsophalangeal joint; *PIPJ*, proximal interphalangeal joint.

Additional Tests

- Diagnostic injection: Local anesthetic and steroid solution can be injected into the MTP joint or around the digital nerve to distinguish between these two common causes of pain.

Differential Diagnosis

- Metatarsal fracture
- Corn

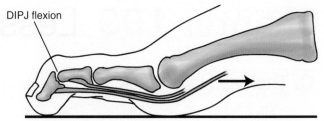

Fig 183.4 Mallet toe deformity. *DIPJ*, Distal interphalangeal joint.

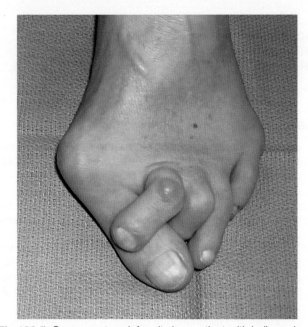

Fig 183.5 Crossover toe deformity in a patient with hallux valgus.

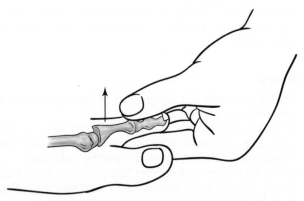

Fig 183.6 Metatarsophalangeal drawer test for the diagnosis of joint instability.

- Interdigital neuroma
- Freiberg infraction
- Stress fracture

Treatment

- At time of diagnosis
  - Conservative management includes activity modification to reduce synovitis, footwear modifications, and accommodative orthotics to relieve pressure and accommodate

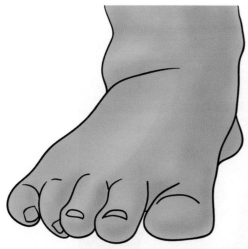

Fig 183.7 Curly toe deformity of the fourth digit.

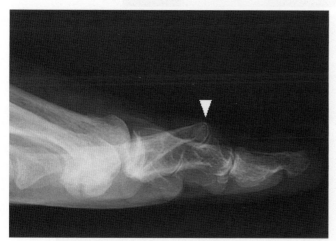

Fig 183.8 Lateral radiograph of patient with second hammertoe deformity *(arrowhead)*.

deformities, passive stretching exercises to keep joints supple, and careful trimming of calluses.

- Nonsteroidal antiinflammatory drugs may decrease pain and inflammation.
- Footwear modifications: Extra-depth shoes with a wide toe box and flat heel prevent crowding of the toes. Patients unwilling to change shoes may have their current leather shoes modified with stretching.
- A firm-soled shoe, with or without a rocker bottom, decreases flexion at the MTP joints.
- Taping of toes to the plantar foot (Fig. 183.9A) or use of a Budin (toe straightening) splint can help alleviate the pain of lesser toes with angular deformity (see Fig. 183.9b).
- Orthotics: A toe crest, pad, or cap may be used to decrease pressure (see Fig. 183.9c).
- Soft insoles with metatarsal pads may decrease the pressure on the affected metatarsal heads.
- Custom accommodative insoles may be beneficial in severe deformity.

- Strengthening of the intrinsic muscles of the foot can help correct muscular imbalances contributing to claw/hammertoe deformity (Figs. 183.10 and 183.11).
- Later
  - If nonsurgical measures fail, surgical realignment may be required.

When to Refer

- Patients with deformities and pain unresponsive to conservative therapy should be referred to an orthopaedic surgeon.

Prognosis

- Conservative management often is all that is required for alleviation of pain and callosities. Curly toe deformities frequently correct spontaneously; stretching and taping have no proven efficacy.

Troubleshooting

- In patients who do not improve, ensure that they have instituted the therapies prescribed. If improper use is noted or decreased compliance is suspected, further education may lead to greater success with nonoperative measures.

Patient Instructions

- Patients should be instructed on the importance of appropriate footwear and the use of recommended orthotics. Position a metatarsal pad just proximal to the metatarsal heads.
- Educate patients on the need for daily foot inspections to check for redness, ulcers, and blisters.

Consideration in Special Populations

- Neuropathic patients may develop unrecognized ulcerations due to insensate feet. These patients need to be further educated about soft-tissue breakdown and the need to inspect their feet daily. Toe strapping and bracing devices may cause pressure sores and should be avoided. Management problems should be referred to an orthopaedic surgeon immediately.
- Vasculopathic patients: Even small amounts of pressure or constriction applied by orthotic devices may lead to digit-threatening ischemia. Use of these devices should be done with extreme care or avoided altogether.
- Rheumatoid arthritics: Because of progressive soft-tissue inflammation and destruction that is a hallmark of the disease, conservative management may not be possible. If optimally managed with pharmacotherapy and footwear/orthotics fail to give relief, referral should be made for surgical options.

Acknowledgment

The author would like to acknowledge Drs. Aaron Hoblet and Eric M. Bluman for their contributions to the previous edition of this chapter.

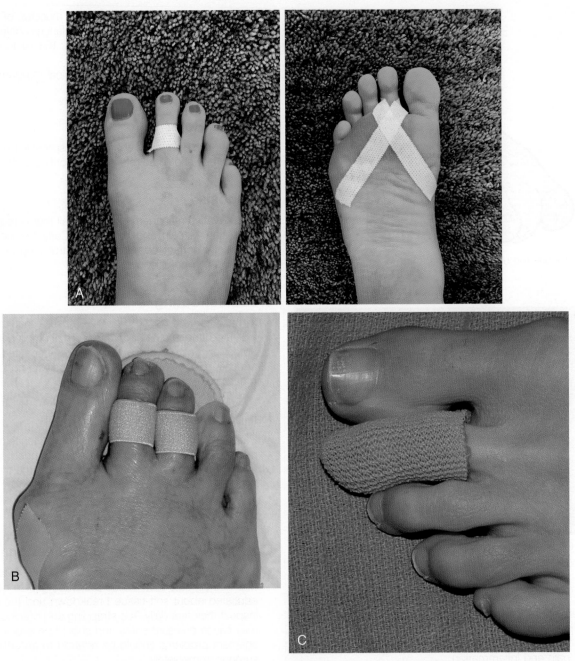

Fig 183.9 Options for hammertoe/crossover toe deformity. **(A)** Example of toe taping with ½" athletic tape. **(B)** Commercial splint for reduction of deformity. **(C)** Silicone toe sleeve for padding of deformity.

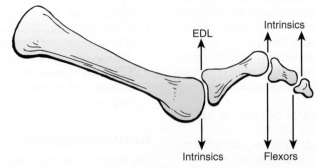

Fig 183.10 Imbalance of the intrinsic and extrinsic foot musculature causes toe deformities. *EDL,* Extensor digitorum longus. (From Coughlin MJ, Mann RA, Saltzman CL. *Surgery of the Foot and Ankle*. 8th ed. Philadelphia: Mosby; 2006.)

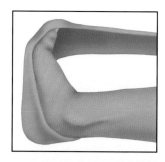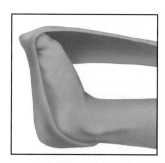

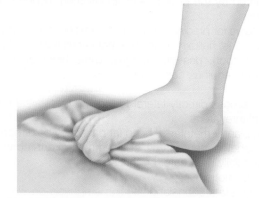

Fig 183.11 Exercised designed to strengthen the foot intrinsic muscles.

Suggested Readings

Coughlin MJ. Lesser-toe abnormalities. *J Bone Joint Surg Am*. 2002;84A: 1446–1469.

Doty JF, Coughlin MJ. Metatarsophalangeal joint instability of the lesser toes and plantar plate deficiency. *J Am Acad Orthop Surg*. 2014;22(4):235–245.

Easley ME, Aydogan U. Lesser toe deformities and bunionettes. In: Thordarson DB, eds. *Foot and Ankle (Orthopedic Surgery Essentials)*. 2nd ed. Philadelphia: Lippincott Williams & Wilkins; 2013:144–174.

Mosca VS. The foot. In: Weinstein SL, Flynn FM, eds. *Lovell and Winter's Pediatric Orthopaedics*. 7th ed. Philadelphia: Wolters Kluwer; 2014:1388–1525.

Myerson MS, Shereff MJ. The pathological anatomy of claw and hammer toes. *J Bone Joint Surg Am*. 1989;71A:45–49.

Thompson GH. Bunions and deformities of the toes in children and adolescents. *J Bone Joint Surg Am*. 1995;77A:1924–1936.

Chapter 184 Bunionette

Minton Truitt Cooper

ICD-10-CM CODE
M21.62X *Bunionette, tailor's bunion*

Key Concepts

- A bunionette is a bony prominence of the fifth metatarsal head, frequently associated with overlying bursitis and a corn.
- Common etiologies include
  - Idiopathic
  - Rheumatoid arthritis
  - Sporting activities (e.g., long-distance running, skiing)
  - Congenitally short, plantarflexed, or dorsiflexed fifth metatarsal
  - Failure or incomplete development of the intermetatarsal ligament
- There are a variety of treatments, including footwear modification, chiropody, and surgery.
- The prognosis is good, with 90% or more success rates.

History

- Bunionettes are a common abnormality, but the majority of cases are asymptomatic.
- Symptoms are most commonly present from adolescence to middle age.
- Pain around the fifth metatarsal head is most commonly lateral but may be dorsolateral or plantar; symptoms are exacerbated by constrictive footwear.
- May have difficulty purchasing footwear, especially if associated with hallux valgus or splaying of the foot
- Patients may report a history of a corn over the affected area.
- There may be history of predisposing features: increased activity, restrictive footwear, other foot deformities, inflammatory or crystalline arthropathy, altered sensation.
- There may be a history of swelling, skin color changes, or even ulceration and infection. If either of the latter two is present, careful attention should be paid to the possibility of diabetes or an inflammatory arthropathy.

Physical Examination

- Observation
  - Gait
  - Obvious bony prominence of the fifth metatarsal head, often with an overlying hyperkeratotic area and possible surrounding erythema due to pressure from constrictive footwear (Fig. 184.1)

- The size of the osseous protuberance may be exacerbated by the presence of an inflamed, hypertrophic bursa.
  - Observe for predisposing foot deformities: hammertoes/claw toes, hallux valgus, intermetatarsal ligament laxity (splay foot), pes planovalgus, varus hindfoot, hallux rigidus, equinus contracture.
- Palpation
  - Tenderness directly lateral to the fifth metatarsal head or plantarlateral
  - The plantar metatarsal head fat pads may be atrophied in diabetes, neuropathy, or inflammatory arthropathies (especially rheumatoid arthritis).
- Range of motion
  - Fifth metatarsophalangeal joint: emphasis on whether the joint is subluxed or dislocated
- Special tests
  - Careful examination for active or healed ulcers and signs of chronic infection
  - Careful neurovascular examination

Imaging

- Radiographs: weight-bearing anteroposterior (with 15-degree cephalic tilt), lateral, and oblique views (Fig. 184.2)
  - The intermetatarsal angle between the fourth and fifth metatarsals (Fig. 184.3) may be increased to more than 10 degrees in symptomatic patients (normal, <8 degrees).
  - The fifth metatarsophalangeal angle averages more than 16 degrees in symptomatic patients (normal, <10 degrees).
  - Lateral bowing of the fifth metatarsal averages 8 degrees in symptomatic patients (normal, <3 degrees). This is also dependent on angulation of the image, as bowing will appear to increase with increasing obliquity of the beam.
  - Bunionettes are classified into four types (Fig. 184.4).
- Magnetic resonance imaging: may be useful with gadolinium enhancement if chronic infection is suspected in the setting of previous ulceration (especially in diabetics)
- CT scan: dual-energy CT scan may be used to evaluate for the presence of a uric acid tophus if gout is suspected.

Differential Diagnosis

- Malunited fracture of the fifth metatarsal shaft: history of trauma, sudden-onset deformity, greater angular deformity
- Bone tumor: extremely rare, rapidly expanding lesion, nocturnal pain, systemic illness, history of other tumors
- Gouty tophus
- Rheumatoid nodule

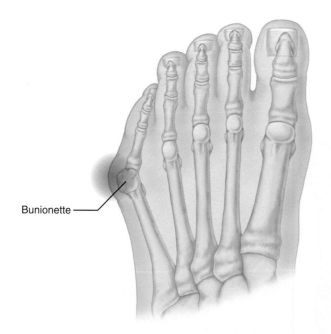

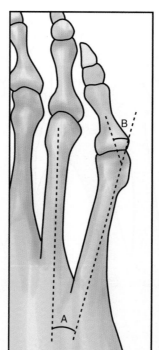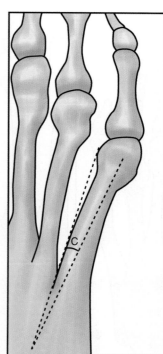

Fig 184.1 A prominent fifth metatarsal head with overlying erythema and bursitis due to bunionette deformity.

Fig 184.3 Schematic diagram depicting radiographic angular measurements in the assessment of a bunionette. A, Fourth-fifth intermetatarsal angle. B, Fifth metatarsophalangeal angle. C, Angle of lateral bowing of the fifth metatarsal.

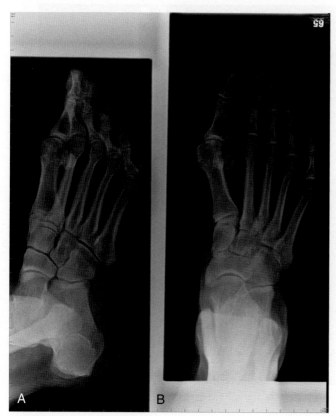

Fig 184.2 Oblique (A) and anteroposterior (B) radiographs of patient with bunionette and hallux valgus deformities with splaying of the foot.

Treatment

- At diagnosis
  - Conservative management consists of footwear modifications and orthoses, callus management, and antiinflammatory medications.
  - Footwear: wide, deep toe box, semirigid shoes without heels and accommodating insole designs (especially in rheumatoid arthritis, diabetes, peripheral neuropathy); padding of the bunionette may also be used as an adjunct.
  - Orthoses: may include hindfoot corrective orthoses if the bunionette is a secondary pathology; midfoot and forefoot orthoses, such as metatarsal pads/bars, have limited success.
  - Chiropody: Paring down of any hyperkeratotic lesions can provide symptomatic relief and should be carried out with caution by experienced practitioners in diabetic patients with neurovascular compromise.
  - Medications: Simple analgesics are first-line treatment in the majority of cases. Nonsteroidal antiinflammatory drugs may lessen the duration of an exacerbation of an inflamed bursa. Disease-modifying agents are of benefit in rheumatoid arthritis and crystalline arthropathy patients.
- Later
  - Patients in whom conservative measures fail may benefit from surgical procedures. Options include exostectomy, head resection, and a variety of metatarsal osteotomies, including chevron osteotomy (Fig. 184.5). Patients may fully weight bear in a stiff-soled postoperative shoe immediately. They continue to wear the shoe for 6 weeks.

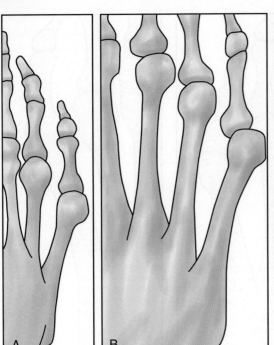

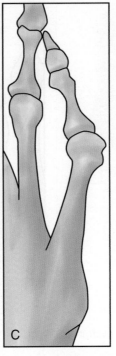

Fig 184.4 Bunionette classification. (A) Type 1: enlargement of the lateral aspect of the fifth metatarsal head. (B) Type 2: lateral bowing of the fifth metatarsal. (C) Type 3: widened fourth-fifth intermetatarsal angle. Type 4 is a combination deformity.

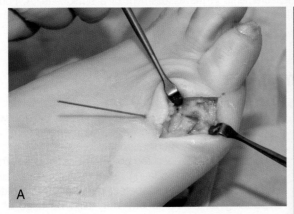

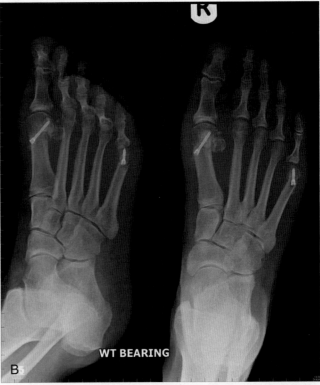

Fig 184.5 Chevron osteotomy. (A) Intraoperative photograph showing displacement of the osteotomy held with guidewire. (B) Radiographs 4 weeks postoperatively of a patient who underwent chevron osteotomies of her bunionette and hallux valgus deformities.

When to Refer

- Athletic patients in whom the deformity and symptoms are unacceptable to their activity level, patients at risk of skin breakdown and possible infection (e.g., those with neuropathic or rheumatoid conditions), and patients in whom conservative measures failed are appropriate for referral.

Prognosis

- Success rates of conservative treatment are difficult to quantify due to the large variety of patients who are affected by this condition. Patient expectations and compliance are critical. However, there is a good chance of success in the nonathletic patient with a bunionette of idiopathic origin.

- Surgical success rates vary from 63% to 90% or more, depending on the technique. Complication rates depend on the patient cohort and vary from 0% to 15%.

Troubleshooting

- Initial treatment should include the wide range of conservative measures.
- Close attention should be paid to the state of the soft tissues in patients with rheumatoid arthritis, diabetes, and neuropathy of any cause.
- Patients should be referred for a surgical consult if conservative measures have failed or are unacceptable to the patient with continued symptoms.

Information for Patients

- A bunionette is a relatively common deformity that is most often idiopathic but may be associated with other foot pathology or generalized systemic disease.
- There are many successful conservative therapies including footwear, in-shoe orthoses, chiropody, and medications.

- Modern surgeries have a high chance of excellent results. The complication rate depends on the general health of the patient.

Suggested Readings

Baumhauer JF, DiGiovanni BF. Osteotomies of the fifth metatarsal. *Foot Ankle Clin*. 2001;6:491–498.

Bertrand T, Parekh SG. Bunionette deformity: etiology, nonsurgical management and lateral exostectomy. *Foot Ankle Clin*. 2011;16(4):679–688.

Cohen BE, Nicholson CW. Bunionette deformity. *J Am Acad Orthop Surg*. 2007;15(5):300–307.

Cooper MT, Coughlin MJ. Subcapital oblique osteotomy for correction of bunionette deformity: medium-term results. *Foot Ankle Int*. 2013;34(10):1376–1380.

Coughlin MJ. Treatment of bunionette deformity with longitudinal diaphyseal osteotomy with distal soft tissue repair. *Foot Ankle*. 1991;11:195–203.

Karasick D. Preoperative assessment of symptomatic bunionette deformity: radiologic findings. *AJR Am J Roentgenol*. 1995;164:147–149.

Kitaoka HB, Holiday AD Jr, Campbell DC II. Distal chevron metatarsal osteotomy for bunionette. *Foot Ankle*. 1991;12:80–85.

Chapter 185 Stress Fractures of the Foot

Scott Van Aman, Marissa Jamieson

ICD-10-CM CODES

M84.374A	*Stress fracture of right metatarsal or foot initial encounter*
M84.374D	*Stress fracture of right metatarsal or foot subsequent encounter*
M84.375A	*Stress fracture of left metatarsal or foot initial encounter*
M84.375D	*Stress fracture of left metatarsal or foot subsequent encounter*
M84.38XA	*Stress fracture of other site initial encounter*
M84.38XD	*Stress fracture of other site subsequent encounter*

Key Concepts

- Stress fractures can affect any bone in the foot but most commonly affect the metatarsals
- Caused by failure of bone to adequately respond and remodel to repetitive stress or abnormal loading patterns
- May also be due to weakened or abnormal bone (related to chronic disease states or osteopenia) that is unable to meet the demands of normal physiologic stresses
- Females are at higher risk, especially those with the female athlete triad of amenorrhea, eating disorders, and low bone mineral density
- Many stress fractures of the foot can be treated conservatively with activity modification and rest
- Underlying causative factors (systemic or mechanical abnormalities) must be addressed
- High-risk stress fractures, including the navicular, talus, and fifth metatarsal, have a propensity to develop into nonunions and require more aggressive treatment

History

- Insidious onset of pain, frequently worsened with activity
- Recent increase or alteration of physical activity, such as beginning a running program or enlisting in boot camp
- A history of prior stress fractures is common
- Important to note predisposing medical conditions
  - Hormonal and/or menstrual abnormalities
  - Osteoporosis/osteopenia

- Low vitamin D
- Anorexia or eating disorders
- Medications (corticosteroids)
- Chronic disease (diabetes or rheumatoid arthritis)
- Certain stress fractures are classically associated with specific activities
  - "March" fractures are second or third metatarsal shaft fracture often seen in military recruits
  - Second metatarsal base fractures are seen in ballerinas who dance *en pointe*

Physical Examination

- Observation
  - Mild swelling or erythema
  - Most will have some pain with weight bearing
  - Check for foot deformity or leg length discrepancy
  - High arch with varus heel may predispose to fifth metatarsal stress fracture (increased lateral column load)
  - Flatfoot deformity with hypermobile first ray may predispose to second metatarsal stress fracture (load transfer)
- Palpation
  - Point tenderness
  - Palpate each metatarsal and tarsal bone individually to localize pain (Fig. 185.1)
  - Squeeze medial/lateral heel to elicit pain related to a calcaneus stress fracture and differentiate from pain over the Achilles insertion (Achilles tendinitis) or plantar heel (plantar fasciitis)
- Range of motion
  - Tight gastrocnemius-soleus complex may predispose to forefoot stress fractures
  - Dorsiflexion of the great toe elicits pain with stress fractures of the sesamoid

Imaging

- Radiographs: standing anteroposterior, lateral, and oblique views of the foot
  - Frequently normal, findings may lag behind clinical symptoms by 2 to 3 weeks
  - If the stress fracture has been present for an extended period of time, may see early callous formation or a distinct fracture line (Fig. 185.2)

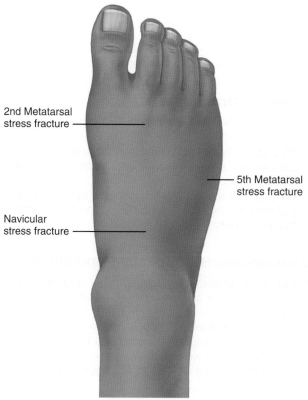

Fig 185.1 Location of pain in common stress fractures of the foot.

2nd Metatarsal stress fracture

5th Metatarsal stress fracture

Navicular stress fracture

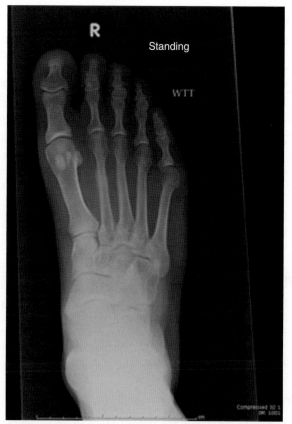

Fig 185.2 Anteroposterior radiograph of the foot showing early callous formation at the second metatarsal shaft.

- If there is a high level of suspicion for stress fracture, particularly in a high-risk area such as the navicular, talus, or proximal fifth metatarsal, proceed with advanced imaging
- Nuclear imaging (bone scan)
  - Increased uptake in region of fracture
  - Highly sensitive but not specific
- Computed tomography
  - Best modality to demonstrate bony anatomy and fracture line orientation
  - Particularly useful for navicular
- Magnetic resonance imaging
  - Most sensitive study
  - Earliest finding is an increase in T2-weighted signal indicating marrow edema (Fig. 185.3)
  - T1-weighted images will demonstrate a linear zone of low signal

Differential Diagnosis

- Synovitis: pain isolated to a specific joint elicited with range of motion, may also have instability at the affected joint
- Arthritis: pain isolated to a specific joint, radiographs reveal loss of joint space, osteophytes, and subchondral sclerosis
- Infection: erythema usually present, common in patients with systemic illness (diabetes)
- Tendinitis: pain located over a major tendon, worsened when the tendon is stressed
- Acute fracture: acute pain with history of traumatic incident

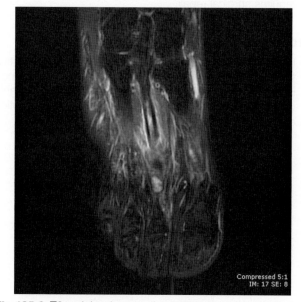

Fig 185.3 T2-weighted magnetic resonance imaging sequence showing edema in a metatarsal shaft indicative of a stress fracture.

Treatment

- Except for high-risk stress fractures, most can be treated initially with conservative management that involves discontinuing any painful activities (such as running)
  - Middle metatarsal shaft stress fractures: hard-soled shoe or fixed ankle walker with gradual return to activity when symptomatically improved (approximately 6 weeks)
  - Calcaneal stress fractures: walking boot or cast, limited activity, heel cups, and stretching of the calf musculature
  - Talus, navicular, and fifth metatarsal base: short leg non–weight-bearing cast for 6 to 8 weeks or primary surgical consideration
- If any deformity (varus or valgus foot) or mechanical abnormality is present, appropriate orthotics should be used to prevent recurrence

When to Refer

- Stress fractures that remain symptomatic despite appropriate nonoperative management
- High-risk fractures (navicular, talus, proximal fifth metatarsal)
- Stress fractures in high-level athletes, as they may benefit from early operative fixation

Prognosis

- Generally good for most healthy patients with healing in 6 to 8 weeks with nonoperative treatment
- High-risk fractures also have a good prognosis when they are diagnosed early and treated appropriately. With delayed treatment, nonunion may develop, which often requires surgical repair.

Troubleshooting

- In patients with stress fractures resistant to conservative treatment, it is imperative to ascertain whether compliance is an issue. Many patients with stress fractures are highly driven athletes who may continue to participate in athletics despite pain.

- In patients with a history of multiple stress fractures, it is prudent to obtain appropriate laboratory workup to rule out metabolic abnormalities.
- Despite appropriate treatment, there is a risk of completion of fracture or refracture if activity is resumed too soon.

Patient Instructions

- Patients should be instructed to discontinue any painful activities.
- Athletes for whom continued conditioning is crucial may participate in alternative low-impact training such as water running or cycling.
- For high-risk stress fractures, patients must be informed that there is a significant risk of delayed healing or nonunion that could possibly require surgery.

Considerations in Special Populations

- High-level athletes may require more aggressive treatment to allow for a faster return to activity and continued conditioning.
- Patients with suspected endocrinopathy should be referred for appropriate diagnostic testing and treatment.
- Diabetic patients will frequently require longer periods of treatment due to a slowed healing response.

Suggested Readings

Greaser MC. Foot and ankle stress fractures in athletes. *Orthop Clin North Am*. 2017;47:809–822.

Mayer SW, Joyner PW, Almekinders LC, Parekh SG. Stress fractures of the foot and ankle in athletes. *Sports Health*. 2014;6:481–491.

McCabe MP, Smyth MP, Richardson DR. Current concepts review: vitamin D and stress fractures. *Foot Ankle Int*. 2012;33:526–533.

Torg JS, Moyer J, Gaughan JP, Boden BP. Management of tarsal navicular stress fractures: conservative versus treatment, a meta-analysis. *Am J Sports Med*. 2010;38:1048–1053.

Welck MJ, Hayes T, Pastides P, et al. Stress fractures of the foot and ankle. *Injury*. 2017;48:1722–1726.

Wright AA, Hegedus EJ, Lenchik L, et al. Diagnostic accuracy of various imaging modalities for suspected lower extremity stress fractures. *Am J Sports Med*. 2016;44:255–263.

Chapter 186 Sesamoid Disorders of the Hallux

Joseph S. Park

ICD-10-CM CODES
M25.80   *Sesamoiditis*
S92.819 *Fracture of sesamoid bone of foot, closed*
M87.876 *Other osteonecrosis, foot*

Key Concepts
- Hallucal sesamoids are an important part of normal static and dynamic foot mechanics.
- The sesamoid complex transmits 50% body weight with stationary weight bearing and as much as 300% during active push-off. These high stresses result in injury and difficulties in healing.
- Stress fractures are the most common injury, occurring frequently in individuals who experience repetitive loading, such as runners and dancers.
- Ten percent of individuals have a bipartite medial sesamoid, which is a normal anatomic variant. In 25% of these individuals, the condition is bilateral. Bipartite lateral sesamoids are rare.
- Treatment involves accurate diagnosis, initial conservative treatment, and surgical intervention in those with refractory symptoms.
- *Sesamoiditis* is a term sometimes used as a diagnosis of exclusion. This condition does not have a clear pathology associated with it and may actually represent chondromalacia or an osteochondral lesion.

History
- Subacute/Chronic: Insidious onset of generalized pain about the metatarsophalangeal (MTP) joint with weight bearing, usually concentrated on the plantar aspect.
- Acute injury can result in fractures with displacement/comminution or significant diastasis within synchondrosis between a bipartite sesamoid.
- Increased pain with passive MTP dorsiflexion or resisted flexion of the MTP joint.
- May walk on lateral border of the foot to offload the medial forefoot. This can lead to secondary metatarsal stress fractures and ankle pain due to this compensatory gait.
- Neuritic symptoms may be described on the plantar aspect of the hallux if swelling results in compression of the plantar nerves.
- Inquire about previous trauma or foot surgery.

Physical Examination
- Observation
  - Erythema and swelling
  - Callus formation
  - Standing foot position: The patient may walk on the lateral column of the foot to avoid pressure on the sesamoids. Cavus foot alignment is associated with first ray plantarflexion and resultant increased pressure on the sesamoids.
  - Hallux alignment: Valgus or varus may gradually develop if the medial or lateral sesamoid is fractured or resected, respectively. Clawing of the hallux can occur with plantar plate injury/sesamoid retraction or significant diastasis of a bipartite sesamoid. This is due to loss of intrinsic function due to disruption of the flexor hallucis brevis complex.
- Palpation
  - Focal tenderness: challenging due to close proximity of the sesamoids to each other and other structures that may generate pain.
  - Tinel sign may be elicited if there is plantar digital nerve compression.
  - Subhallucal sesamoids are located at the plantar interphalangeal joint and may be associated with plantar keratosis.
- Range of motion
  - Increased pain with dorsiflexion, relieved with plantarflexion.
  - Effusion may restrict MTP joint motion.
  - Pain on resisted hallux interphalangeal joint flexion suggests flexor hallucis longus tendinitis or injury.
  - Limitation in ankle range of motion (gastrocnemius or Achilles contracture) can place excessive forces through the sesamoid complex.

Imaging
- Radiographs: anteroposterior, lateral, and oblique views of the foot (centered on the MTP joint) and axial view of the sesamoids
  - Evaluate for bony deformity of the first metatarsal.
  - Evaluate for arthritic changes of the first MTP joint.
  - An axial view aids in evaluation of osteonecrosis, degenerative joint disease of the sesamoids, and plantar exostoses (Fig. 186.1).

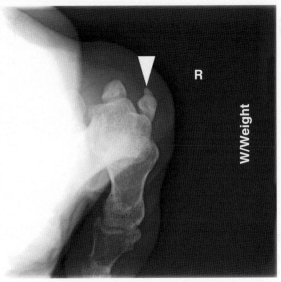

Fig 186.1 Axial sesamoid x-ray demonstrated plantar exostosis of medial sesamoid. *Arrowhead* indicates exostosis of the sesamoid.

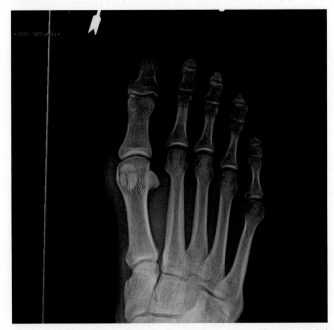

Fig 186.2 AP x-ray of foot demonstrating significant medial sesamoid fracture with significant displacement.

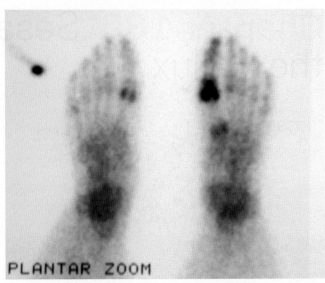

PLANTAR ZOOM

Fig 186.3 Bone scan indicating medial and lateral sesamoid fractures on the *right*. Compare with normal sesamoids on the *left*.

- Magnetic resonance imaging
  - Valuable in evaluation of soft-tissue structures such as plantar plate, cartilage, nerves, and flexor tendons
  - May be a useful adjunct in the workup of osteomyelitis, fracture, osteonecrosis (Fig. 186.4), and tendinitis

Differential Diagnosis

- Acute sesamoid fracture or stress fracture
- Turf toe (plantar plate injury-sesamoid-phalangeal ligament rupture)
- Osteonecrosis
- Digital nerve compression/neuroma
- Degenerative changes of the first MTP joint or sesamoid-metatarsal joint
- Subluxation of hallucal sesamoids
- Plantar keratosis
- Osteomyelitis
- Flexor hallucis longus tendinitis

Treatment

- At diagnosis
  - Conservative treatment should be attempted initially for the majority of sesamoid disorders. Fractures displaced more than 2 mm may eventually heal with fibrous union but could benefit from consideration for surgery. Osteonecrosis of sesamoids with sclerosis and fragmentation seen on plain x-ray may also benefit from early surgical referral. Conservative treatment aims to reduce pressure and stress on the sesamoid complex to allow bony healing and/or resolution of inflammation.
  - Activity modification to avoid high-impact jumping, sprinting, or excessive MTP dorsiflexion
  - Footwear modifications and orthotics: shoe insert with cutout below sesamoids, rocker bottom, metatarsal bar/pad, lateral heel posting; avoid high heels

- Evaluate for fractures and bipartite sesamoids (Fig. 186.2). Diastasis between the poles of a bipartite sesamoid can also signify substantial instability of the plantar complex.
- Proximal retraction of the sesamoids may be seen with a severe turf toe injury.
- Bone scan
  - To distinguish between acute fracture and bipartite sesamoid (Fig. 186.3)
  - May aid in distinguishing between osteonecrosis and sesamoiditis (cold for osteonecrosis)

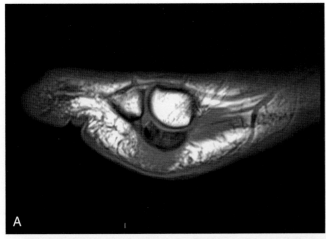

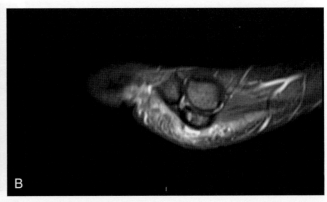

Fig 186.4 (A) T1-weighted sagittal magnetic resonance image showing decreased signal in medial sesamoid, concerning for avascular necrosis. (B) T2-weighted image showing minimal inflammation within medial sesamoid.

- Gastrocnemius/Achilles stretching if equinus deformity (limitation in ankle dorsiflexion) is present. Shaving of plantar keratoses
- Taping to block dorsiflexion of MTP joint to decrease stress on sesamoid complex/plantar plate
- Nonsteroidal antiinflammatory drugs for nonfracture pathology
- Later
  - More intensive conservative treatments can be used if initial attempts are unsuccessful and include casting/non–weight bearing for 6 to 8 weeks. Extend cast out past the great toe to prevent unintended motion at the MTP joint. Use of a heel wedge to offload the forefoot can also be considered in cases of acute fracture/diastasis.

When to Refer

- Immediate consultation for potential surgical treatment is recommended for severely displaced acute fractures or diastasis of bipartite sesamoids. Patients with significant swelling and difficulty or inability to flex the hallux should also be considered for early referral.
- Chronic conditions treated unsuccessfully for more than 3 to 6 months with appropriate conservative measures should also be referred.
  - Surgical options include bone grafting, shaving of prominences, and excision (Fig. 186.5).
  - Patients with associated hallux varus/valgus or arthrosis of the first MTP joint may benefit from realignment or fusion surgery.
  - If significant equinus deformity persists despite therapy/stretching, referral for surgical lengthening (Strayer procedure or Achilles lengthening) can be considered.
- Significant cavus foot alignment may require custom orthotics to help offload the sesamoids.

Prognosis

- Prognosis for most sesamoid disorders is excellent with appropriate conservative measures. Patients with

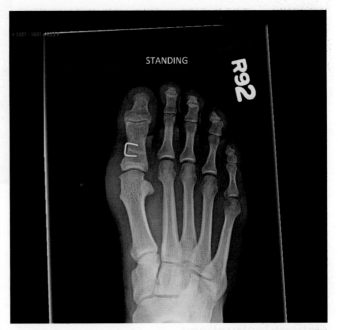

Fig 186.5 Postoperative anteroposterior x-ray after medial sesamoid excision, Akin proximal phalanx osteotomy.

osteonecrosis, disruption of the flexor mechanism, or significant distraction/comminution may require surgical intervention.

Troubleshooting

- Fractures with more than 2 mm displacement are less likely to heal with conservative means.
- Treatment usually consists of excision of the fractured sesamoid, as results are comparable to those of open reduction and internal fixation (Fig. 186.6).
- Osteonecrosis may require prolonged non–weight bearing and may eventually require excision.
- If orthotics do not provide adequate relief, dorsiflexion osteotomy of the first metatarsal may be required to correct

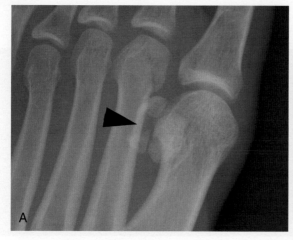

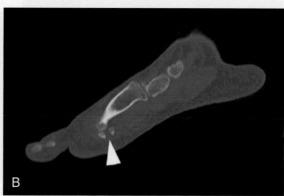

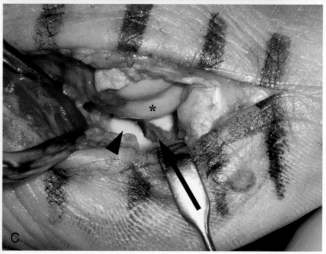

Fig 186.6 (A) Oblique radiograph showing fractured lateral sesamoid with significant displacement. **(B)** Sagittal computed tomography reconstruction. **(C)** Intraoperative photograph of plantar surface of metatarsal head *(asterisk)*, distal fragment of fractured lateral sesamoid *(arrow)*, and articular surface of proximal fragment *(arrowhead)*.

a significant cavus foot deformity. A more comprehensive reconstruction may be required for those patients with severe cavovarus alignment or peroneal tendon dysfunction.

- Equinus deformity may place excessive stress on the sesamoids, and should be considered as a cause of chronic sesamoiditis/overload.

Patient Instructions

- Conservative treatments aim to provide pain relief and immobilization of the hallucal sesamoid complex.
- A decrease or elimination of weight bearing may be needed to allow the injury to heal. This may require orthotics, taping, or cast immobilization with or without crutch weight bearing.
- If the patient has been diagnosed with a sesamoid fracture or osteonecrosis, nonsteroidal antiinflammatory medications should not be taken without first consulting the physician.
- If conservative measures fail, surgery may be required.

Suggested Readings

Axe MJ, Ray RL. Orthotic treatment of sesamoid pain. *Am J Sports Med*. 1998;16:411–416.

Bichara DA, Henn RF, Theodore GH. Sesamoidectomy for hallux sesamoid fracture. *Foot Ankle Int*. 2012;33(9):704–706.

Biedert R, Hintermann B. Stress fractures of the medial great toe sesamoids in athletes. *Foot Ankle Int*. 2003;24:137–141.

Coughlin MJ. Sesamoid pain: causes and surgical treatment. *Instr Course Lect*. 1990;39:23–35.

Dedmond BT, Cory JW, McBryde A. The hallucal sesamoid complex. *J Am Acad Orthop Surg*. 2006;14:745–753.

Richardson EG. Hallucal sesamoid pain: causes and surgical treatment. *J Am Acad Orthop Surg*. 1999;7:270–278.

Richardson EG. Injuries to the hallucal sesamoids in the athlete. *Foot Ankle*. 1987;7:229–244.

Chapter 187 The Diabetic Foot

Justin J. Ray, Alexander D. Conti, Robert D. Santrock

ICD-10-CM CODES
M14.67 *Charcot joint, ankle, and foot*
E11.610 *Type 2 diabetes mellitus with diabetic neuropathic arthropathy*
E11.621 *Type 2 diabetes mellitus with foot ulcer*

Key Concepts

- Diabetes is a metabolic disease characterized by high blood glucose levels.
- More than 30 million Americans have diabetes.
- Diabetic foot problems include foot ulcers, infection, and Charcot arthropathy.
- The etiology is peripheral nerve impairment that leads to loss of protective sensation, autonomic dysfunction, and possible motor deficits.
- Charcot arthropathy is a chronic and progressive process that leads to bone destruction, joint fragmentation, and deformity.
- The loss of protective sensation and excess plantar pressure leads to foot ulcers.

History

- History of peripheral neuropathy
- Pain manifests in approximately 50% of cases; the other 50% are painless due to loss of sensation.
- Charcot arthropathy
  - Early stages include swelling, warmth, and erythema.
  - Later stages involve progressive deformity of the foot with possible ulcer development.
- Diabetic foot ulcer
  - Typically painless ulcer of insidious onset
  - History of bony prominence, skin breakdown, and eventual ulcer development

Physical Examination

- Inspect foot.
  - Look for skin changes, swelling, erythema, ulcers, or structural deformity.
- Evaluate sensation to light touch.
  - Semmes-Weinstein 5.07 monofilament testing to plantar foot
- Evaluate circulation (dorsalis pedis and posterior tibial pulses).
  - Absent pulses require vascular workup; pulses typically strong in Charcot arthropathy.

- Diabetic foot ulcers
  - Evaluate depth of ulcer, presence of infection.
  - Osteomyelitis is likely (67%) if able to probe to bone.
- Special tests:
  - Elevation test: elevate feet above the heart for 1 minute. Erythema will decrease with elevation in Charcot arthropathy, whereas redness persists with infection.
  - Silverskiöld test: assess for gastrocnemius tightness by examining ankle dorsiflexion with knee flexed versus knee extended.

Imaging

- Weight-bearing radiographs of the foot and ankle
  - Charcot arthropathy (Fig. 187.1)
    - Early changes include soft tissue edema and bony fragmentation. Late changes include bony coalescence/remodeling, joint destruction, and decreased edema.
  - Diabetic foot ulcers
    - Assess for fractures, foreign body, subcutaneous emphysema, and arthritis.

Additional Tests

- MRI
  - Usually not necessary but can differentiate abscess from soft tissue swelling
- Bone scan (Tc99m, In 111)
  - Can differentiate osteomyelitis, soft tissue infection, and Charcot arthropathy
- Vascular studies (to evaluate circulation if nonhealing ulcer or weak pulses)
  - Ankle-brachial index (ABI)
    - Normal 1.0; pressures >45 mm Hg necessary for healing potential
  - $TcpO_2$
    - Gold standard to evaluate wound healing potential
    - > 30 mm Hg (or 40 depending on source) indicates good healing potential
- Inflammatory markers
  - White blood cell (WBC) count, erythrocyte sedimentation rate (ESR), and C-reactive protein (CRP) elevated in both infection and acute stage of Charcot arthropathy
- Bone biopsy
  - May be useful in cases of osteomyelitis to guide antibiotic therapy

Differential Diagnosis

- Other neuropathies (Charcot-Marie-Tooth disease, spinal cord neuropathy)

- Soft tissue infection (cellulitis, abscess): drainage; erythema does not improve with elevation
- Gout: painful, increased uric acid, improves with anti-inflammatory medication
- Osteomyelitis: likely if ulcer probes to bone, positive bone scan

Classification

- Diabetic Charcot arthropathy
  - Eichenholtz stages of Charcot arthropathy
    - Stage 0 (pre-fragmentation): swelling, warmth, erythema, no bony changes
    - Stage 1 (fragmentation): swelling, warmth, erythema, bony fragmentation

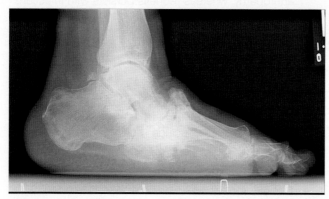

Fig 187.1 Lateral foot radiograph showing collapsed midfoot in Charcot arthropathy.

- Stage 2 (coalescence): decreased edema, bony absorption and coalescence
- Stage 3 (resolution): edema resolved, bony consolidation and remodeling
- Diabetic foot ulcers
  - Depth-ischemia classification modified from Wagner-Meggitt classification (Fig. 187.2)

Treatment

- Medical optimization for wound healing
  - Rigid glycemic control with goal A1c <7.0
  - Optimization of nutrition with goal serum albumin >3.0
- Nonoperative treatment
  - Charcot arthropathy
    - Early stages are best treated with footwear modifications or immobilization in a total contact cast or Charcot restraint orthotic walker (CROW boot; Fig. 187.3).
    - Later stages involve progressive deformity with possible ulceration; these stages may not be amenable to bracing and may require surgery to correct deformity.
  - Diabetic foot ulcers
    - Footwear modifications (offload with custom insoles, rocker bottom soles, etc.)
    - Wound care (offload, create barrier, provide environment for healing)
    - Total contact casting (gold standard to offload plantar surface)
    - Contraindications to casting include infection, poor compliance, poor vascularity

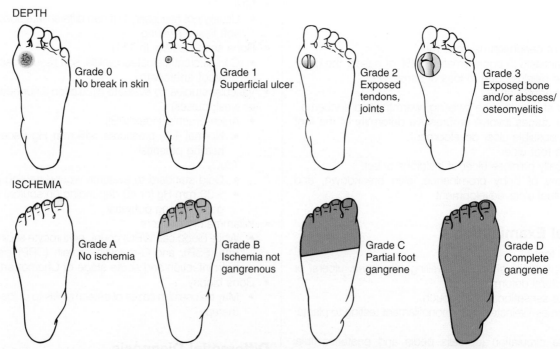

Fig 187.2 Illustration of the depth-ischemia classification of diabetic foot ulcers modified from the Wagner-Meggitt classification. (From Johnson JE, Klein SE, Brodsky JW. Diabetes. In: Coughlin MJ, Saltzman CL, Anderson RB, eds. *Mann's Surgery of the Foot and Ankle*. 9th ed. Philadelphia: Elsevier; 2014. Copyright JW Brodsky, MD, 1998.)

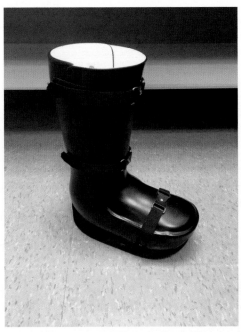

Fig 187.3 The Charcot restraint orthotic walker provides off-loading and stability to a Charcot foot.

- Operative treatment
  - Diabetic Charcot arthropathy
    - Resection of bony prominences and Tendo-Achilles lengthening (TAL)
    - Indicated for early disease with equinus contracture, bony prominences
    - Arthrodesis with or without osteotomies
      - Severe deformity not amenable to bracing
    - Amputation
      - Failed other surgical options, recurrent/uncontrollable infection
  - Diabetic foot ulcer
    - Surgical debridement, antibiotics, topical wound care
      - Indicated for deeper ulcers, associated abscess, or osteomyelitis
    - Resection of bony prominences and TAL
      - Indicated if bony prominence causing pressure ulcer

- Amputation (partial or complete)
  - Indicated for partial or extensive gangrene

When to Refer

- Any diabetic patient who develops foot ulcers, infection, deformity, or unexplained swelling or pain should be referred to a specialist.

Prognosis

- Charcot arthropathy of the foot has a 75% success rate with nonoperative management but eventually results in decreased function and progressive foot deformity.
- If managed with prompt and aggressive treatment, foot ulcers will usually heal. Recurrence may be avoided with proper foot care and footwear.

Troubleshooting

- Education is key to preventing diabetic foot problems and avoiding complications.
- Diabetic patients should be counseled on risks of possible amputation for foot ulcers.

Patient Instructions

- All diabetic patients should receive education on proper foot care and footwear.
- Patients should also be instructed to perform daily foot inspections and wear proper shoes.

Suggested Readings

Anakwenze OA, Milby AH, Gans I, et al. Foot and ankle infections: diagnosis and management. *J Am Acad Orthop Surg*. 2012;20:684–693.

Pinzur MS, Slovenkai MP, Trepman E, et al. Guidelines for diabetic foot care: recommendations endorsed by the diabetes committee of the American Orthopaedic Foot and Ankle Society. *Foot Ankle Int*. 2005;26: 113–119.

Uhl RL, Rosenbaum AJ, DiPreta JA, et al. Diabetes mellitus: musculoskeletal manifestations and perioperative considerations for the orthopaedic surgeon. *J Am Acad Orthop Surg*. 2014;22:183–192.

Van der Ven A, Chapman CB, Bowker JH. Charcot neuroarthropathy of the foot and ankle. *J Am Acad Orthop Surg*. 2009;17:562–571.

Chapter 188 Corns and Calluses

Minton Truitt Cooper, Andrea M. White

ICD-10-CM CODE
L84   *Corns and callosities*

Key Concepts

- Corns and calluses are typically caused by thickening of the keratin layers of the epidermis due to excessive pressure exerted over a bony prominence of the foot.
- Loss of the normal fat pad, improper footwear, toe deformities, increased activity level, and systemic diseases (rheumatoid arthritis) may contribute to the development of corns and calluses.
- Callus refers to a large lesion with undefined boundaries and without a central core.
- Corn refers to a smaller lesion with well-defined boundaries and a central core. Corns are divided into hard and soft corns.
- Nonoperative treatment consists of modifying footwear, paring the excessive keratin layers, and applying padding to alleviate pressure. Patient education is also important.
- Surgery may be indicated to correct bony deformity.
- Corns and calluses have a tendency to recur unless the underlying pathology is properly addressed.

History

- Discomfort in normal footwear or when walking barefoot (advanced corn)
- Inquire about a history of Charcot-Marie-Tooth disease, other neurologic conditions (such as diabetic neuropathy), or systemic disease (rheumatoid arthritis), as these can be causes for the toe deformities associated with corns and calluses.
- May also be associated with older age, female gender, hallux valgus, and prolonged standing.

Physical Examination

- Observation (Fig. 188.1)
  - Calluses are typically located on the plantar aspect of foot, mainly at the metatarsophalangeal joints, but may occur anywhere bony prominence exists.
  - Hard corns are commonly located on the fibular aspect of the fifth toe or dorsal aspect of the proximal interphalangeal (IP) or the distal interphalangeal (DIP) joints.
    - May be associated with hammertoe, mallet toe, or claw toe deformity
    - Hyperkeratotic area with a lighter conical center (without underlying vessels)

- Soft corns present as maceration between the lesser toes, mainly between 4 and 5.
  - A result of the absorption of extreme amounts of moisture from perspiration
  - Sometimes reddish in appearance and may become infected
  - These may be extremely painful.
- Palpation
  - Hard and soft corns eventually become tender.

Imaging

- Usually not necessary for initial treatment; clinical diagnosis
- Radiographs: weight-bearing anteroposterior, lateral, and oblique views of the foot
  - In the case of an ulcerated lesion, may be used to identify osteomyelitis
  - Helpful to view the structural deformities as the cause of the callus or corn

Differential Diagnosis

- Plantar warts: fine capillaries perpendicular to the surface, exhibit punctuate bleeding after trimming
- Skin ulceration: skin layer is destroyed and exposes underlying soft tissues or bone.
- Mycotic infection

Treatment

- At diagnosis
  - Conservative management is appropriate.
    - Reduction of hyperkeratotic area by paring with a scalpel
    - Footwear adaptations (soft-soled shoes with large toe box)
    - Padding of the symptomatic area or to offload excess pressure
    - Toe sleeves or toe crests for dorsal corns on the IP joints of the toes (Fig. 188.2)
    - Instruct patient how to shave the callus/corn with pumice stone after soaking in warm water.
    - Beware of salicylic acid on immunocompromised or neuropathic patients, as this can damage otherwise healthy skin.
- Later
  - If the corn or callus cannot be controlled by conservative measures, surgical intervention may be warranted to correct underlying deformity.

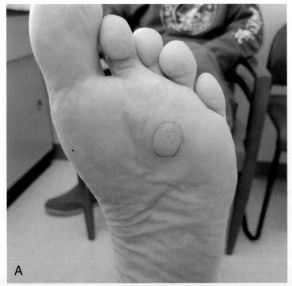

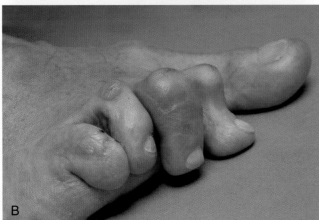

Fig 188.1 **(A)** Clinical photograph of the foot of a patient with callus under the metatarsophalangeal joints. **(B)** Close-up view of the toe deformities that are a cause of corn and callus formation.

When to Refer

- Failure of conservative measures warrants referral to an orthopaedic surgeon. In addition, concern for infection warrants referral.
- Surgical options include correction of the toe deformity and isolated condylectomy.
- Deformity correction varies based on the location of deformity (metatarsal shortening osteotomy for plantar callus vs. hammertoe correction for DIP/IP corns).
- If the examiner is not confident in excluding a true mycotic infection, referral to a dermatologist can be considered.

Prognosis

- Generally good when there is no infection associated with osteomyelitis

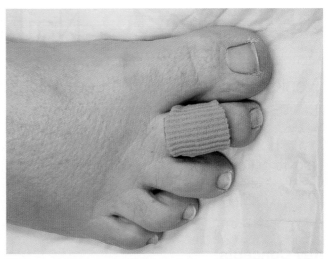

Fig 188.2 Clinical photograph of the foot in a patient with hammertoe wearing a toe sleeve.

Troubleshooting

- Complications include bleeding after trimming the corn or callus, mycotic infection when maceration is not managed adequately, and, in rare cases, deeper infection with osteomyelitis of the phalanx.
- Infection with swelling, redness, and warmth of the toe combined with pain is an absolute indication for immediate referral. Under such circumstances, intravenous antibiotic therapy should be considered.

Patient Instructions

- Patients should be educated about the causes of corns and calluses.
- Shoes should have a wide toe box, be free of any seams over the areas of callus/corn, and be appropriately sized.
- Patients must be instructed in the use of a pumice stone to trim calluses without injuring healthy skin.

Suggested Readings

Freeman DB. Corns and calluses resulting from mechanical hyperkaratosis. *Am Fam Phys*. 2002;65-11:2277–2280.

Jakeman A. The effective management of hyperkeratosis. *Wound Essentials*. 2012;1:65–73.

Spink MJ, Menz HB, Lord SR. Distribution and correlates of plantar hyperkeratotic lesions in older people. *J Foot Ankle Res*. 2009;2:8.

Tlougan BE, Mancini AJ, Mandell JA, et al. Skin conditions in figure skaters, ice-hockey players and speed skaters: part 1—mechanical dermatoses. *Sports Med*. 2011;41(9):709–719.

Chapter 189 Nail Disorders

Venkat Perumal, George Lee Wilkinson III

ICD-10-CM CODES
L60.0 *Ingrowing nail (onychocryptosis)*
B35.1 *Tinea unguium (onychomycosis)*

Key Concepts

- The most common toenail disorder is onychocryptosis.
- Intrinsic factors such as fungal or bacterial infections cause most toenail disorders.
- Other deformities can be caused by mechanical issues.
- Direct trauma can lead to damage to the nail plate and bed.

Onychocryptosis (Ingrowing Nail)

History

- Most likely present on the great toe but can occur in any toes
- Subjective pain along the edge of the nail; worsens in tight-fitting shoes
- Possibility of drainage from beneath the nail
- Admitted improper nail trimming or history of trauma

Physical Examination

- Observation
  - Stage One: erythema, mild edema, irritation of the nail fold, no pus or drainage (Fig. 189.1)
  - Stage Two: increased erythema and edema, hyperplasia of nail fold, active pus or drainage
  - Stage Three: further erythema and edema, granulation tissue, additional hypertrophy of nail fold, increase in signs of active infection
- Palpation
  - Affected nail fold tenderness increases with each stage.
  - In the latter stages, purulence may be expressed from beneath the nail.

Differential Diagnosis

- Onychomycosis: fungal infection of the nail
- Paronychia: superficial infection of the nail fold
- Subungual exostosis: bony growth beneath the nail
- Onychophosis: callus in the nail groove
- Trauma

Treatment

- Stage One: Recommend warm soaks, proper nail trimming, and more accommodative footwear.
- Stage Two: In addition to the above, also consider oral antibiotics and or a partial nail excision under digital block (Fig. 189.2).

- Stage Three: Partial versus complete nail excision and ablation of the nail matrix.

When to Refer

- Recurrent stage three disease or failure of nonoperative treatment

Prognosis

- Recurrence is common.

Patient Instructions

- Explain importance of proper footwear, nail care, and hygiene to patient.

Considerations in Special Populations

- Surgery should be considered sooner in patients at high risk for recurrent infection or sepsis, such as those with total joint replacements or diabetes (Fig. 189.3).

Onychomycosis (Nail Fungal Infection)

History

- Prevalence increases with age and is greatest in those older than 65 years of age.
- Found more often in men than women
- Most common pathogen is Trichophyton rubrum, followed by Trichophyton interdigitale

Physical Examination

- Observation
  - Brittle, deformed, discolored, thickened nail plate (Fig. 189.4)
- Palpation
  - Tenderness may or may not be present.
  - Rough, thickened nail
- Special tests
  - Fungal cultures may be obtained from nail debris.
  - Hyphae may be seen when nail scrapings are examined under light microscopy prepared with potassium hydroxide.

Differential Diagnosis

- Onychocryptosis: ingrown toenail
- Onychogryphosis: significant curling and thickening of the nail plate (Fig. 189.5)
- Psoriasis
- Trauma

Treatment

- Begin with simple debridement and trimming of the nail plate
- Consider topical versus systemic antifungal medications

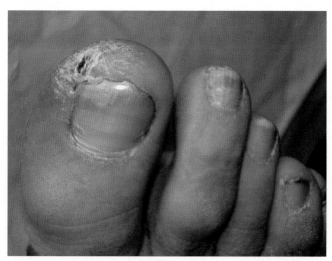

Fig 189.1 Ingrown toenail with medial nail fold penetrated.

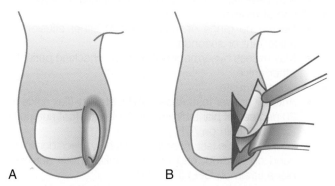

Fig 189.2 (A and B) Partial excision of the nail. (From Nealon TF Jr. Fundamental Skills in Surgery, 4th ed. Philadelphia, WB Saunders, 1994.)

A   B

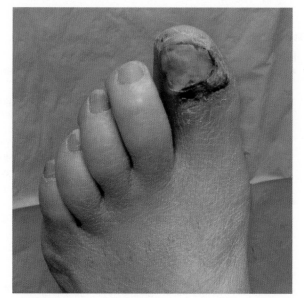

Fig 189.3 Ingrown toenail in a diabetic patient with superinfection.

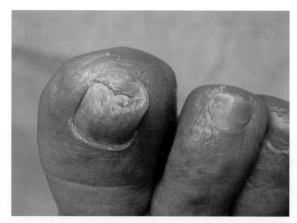

Fig 189.4 Fungal infection of the great toenail. Note the lateral border is also ingrown.

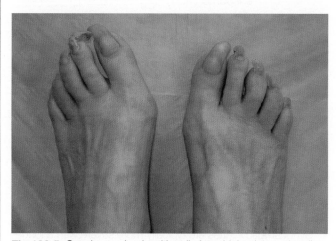

Fig 189.5 Onychogryphosis with nail plate thickening and curling.

When to Refer

- Recalcitrant cases may necessitate nail matrix ablation

Prognosis

- Smaller lesions respond well to conservative treatments.
- Larger lesions do not respond as well to these measures and often require permanent nail removal.

Patient Instructions

- Stress the importance of foot hygiene.

Considerations in Special Populations

- Systemic antifungals are to be avoided in patients with hepatic disease or pregnant women.

Suggested Readings

Alavi A, Woo K, Sibbald RG. Common nail disorders and fungal infections. *Adv Skin Wound Care*. 2007;20:346–357.

Armstrong AD, Hubbard MC, eds. *Essentials of Musculoskeletal Care*. 5th ed. Rosemont, IL: American Academy of Orthopaedic Surgeons; 2016.

Coughlin MJ, Saltzman C, Anderson RB, eds. *Mann's Surgery of the Foot and Ankle*. 9th ed. Philadelphia: Elsevier; 2014.

Mayeaux EJ Jr. Nail disorders. *Prim Care*. 2000;27:333–351.

Chapter 190 Ankle Sprain

W. Bret Smith, Thomas Ergen

ICD-10-CM CODES
S93.401A *Sprain of unspecified ligament of right ankle, initial encounter*
S93.491A *Sprain of other ligament of right ankle, initial encounter*
S93.402A *Sprain of unspecified ligament of left ankle, initial encounter*
S93.492A *Sprain of other ligament of left ankle, initial encounter*

Key Concepts

- Ankle sprains are a very common injury.
- Majority of ankle sprains involve lateral structures.
- Broken down into low ankle sprains and high ankle sprains (syndesmotic injuries)
- Low ankle sprains involve 90% of all ankle sprains.
- Low ankle sprains often involve the anterior talofibular ligament (ATFL) followed by the calcaneofibular ligament (CFL).
- Poor rehabilitation or repeated ankle sprains can lead to ankle instability in 20% of the population.
- Syndesmotic injuries are typically more severe with a longer recovery process.

Anatomy

- Low ankle sprain ligaments
  - ATFL: Prevents anterior translation of the talus relative to the tibia
  - CFL: Prevents inversion of the talus relative to the tibia
  - Posterior talofibular ligament (rarely injured): Prevents posterior translation of the talus relative to the tibia
- High ankle sprain (syndesmosis) ligaments
  - Anterior inferior tibiofibular ligament
  - Posterior inferior tibiofibular ligament
  - Interosseous ligament
  - Inferior transverse ligament
  - Interosseous membrane

History

- Acute
  - Typically occur on an axially loaded foot in plantarflexion and inversion
  - Pain and swelling more commonly located over the lateral ankle
  - Popping or tearing sensation may be present.
- Chronic
  - Recurrent ankle injury with less severe mechanism

Physical Exam

- Observation
  - Look for swelling and ecchymosis along the lateral ankle and distal to lateral malleolus.
  - Effusion of the ankle joint may be present.
  - Cavovarus foot alignment more likely to develop attenuated lateral ligaments that leads to instability
- Palpation
  - Tenderness along the ATFL
  - Tenderness may extend to the CFL.
  - May have tenderness along the peroneal tendons.
  - May have tenderness at distal tip of lateral malleolus.
- Range of motion
  - Decreased range of motion due to either effusion of ankle joint or secondary to pain
  - May assess hypermobility of joint by checking patient's other ankle
- Provocative tests
  - Anterior drawer test: Assess ATFL stability (flex ankle to 20 degrees of plantarflexion and translate foot anteriorly to place strain on ATFL) (Fig. 190.1)
  - Inversion stress test: Assess CFL stability (place dominant hand on hindfoot and dorsiflex ankle; invert ankle to place strain on CFL) (Fig. 190.2)
  - Squeeze test: Assess syndesmosis (squeezing tibia and fibula at midcalf causes pain at ankle)
  - External rotation stress test: Assess syndesmosis (tibia is stabilized proximally and external rotation is applied to foot; pain associated with this maneuver is positive) (Fig. 190.3)

Imaging

- Radiographs:
  - Standard weight-bearing anteroposterior, lateral, and Mortise view
    - Assess for any fractures, avulsion fracture, soft-tissue swelling, osteochondral injuries, syndesmotic widening, tarsal coalition.
    - Ottawa Ankle Rules: X-rays should be ordered on all patients with tenderness along the posterior edge of the tibia/fibula, tip of the medial or lateral malleolus, inability to bear weight, or pain at the base of the fifth metatarsal.
  - Stress views
    - Talar tilt stress: 15 degrees of talar tilt greater than contralateral side is suspicious for injury of CFL.
    - Anterior drawer stress: 5 mm of translation of talus represents an injury to the ATFL.
- Magnetic resonance imaging (MRI):
  - Can show evidence of ligamentous injury (Fig. 190.4A)
  - Reserved for chronic ankle instability with a failed course of conservative treatment

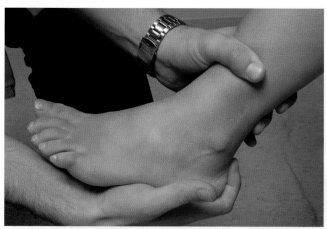

Fig 190.1 Anterior drawer test (anterior talofibular ligament [ATFL]). The hindfoot is grasped with the nondominant hand and the foot is held in plantarflexion. The calcaneus is then pulled anteriorly. Any significant difference when compared with the contralateral side indicates the possibility of ATFL rupture.

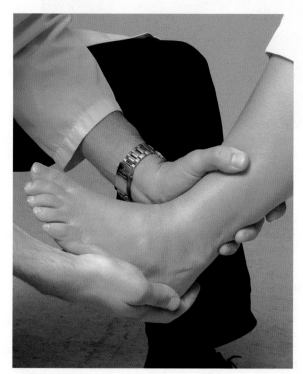

Fig 190.2 Inversion stress test (calcaneofibular ligament). The hindfoot is grasped with the dominant hand and the ankle is held in dorsiflexion. Inversion is performed and talar tilting noted.

- May find associated pathology: Osteochondral lesions (see Fig. 190.4B), syndesmotic injuries, peroneal tendon injuries, loose bodies
- Ultrasound
  - Increasing use in the diagnosis of musculoskeletal injuries
  - May show elongation of the ATFL with anterior drawer stress test applied

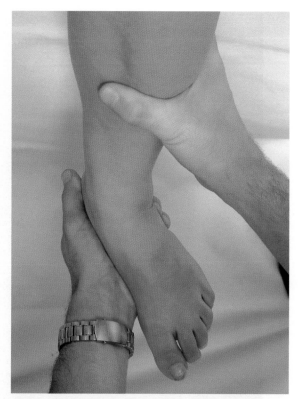

Fig 190.3 External rotation stress test (syndesmosis). The patient is seated with the knee flexed 90 degrees. The tibia is held with the nondominant hand and the foot is externally rotated. Pain provoked in the upper front of the ankle indicates syndesmotic injury.

- May show syndesmotic injury with injury to the interosseous membrane
- Unfortunately, ultrasound continues to be operator dependent with difficulty in interpretation and reproducibility.

Differential Diagnosis

- Fracture of the ankle (medial/lateral/posterior malleolus), talus, or calcaneus: Tenderness, pain with motion, inability to bear weight, swelling, crepitus
- Peroneal tendon subluxation: subluxation of peroneal tendons occurs with resistance to ankle eversion, tenderness, and swelling along peroneal tendons.
- Osteochondral fracture of talar dome
- Osteoarthritis: stiffness and tenderness along the joint line
- Ankle impingement: pain with dorsiflexion of the ankle
- Tarsal coalition: ankle stiffness

Treatment

- Protection (walking boot, weight-bearing soft cast, lace up ankle brace), rest, ice, compression, elevate (3 to 5 days)
- After initial improvement, progress to weight bearing as tolerated
- Improved functional outcomes have been shown with early range of motion with comparable pain scores of continued immobilization.

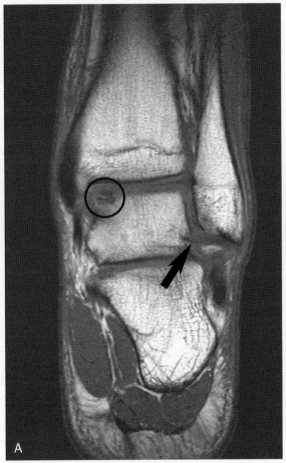
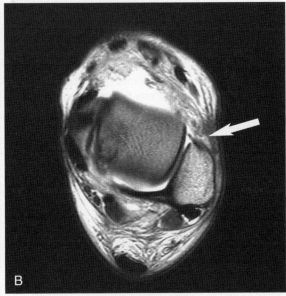

Fig 190.4 **(A)** Coronal magnetic resonance imaging (MRI) reconstruction of the hindfoot in a patient who sustained an ankle sprain. Note the lesion of the lateral ligamentous complex *(arrow)* and the talar dome fracture *(circle)*. **(B)** Axial MRI of the hindfoot of the same patient. The anterior talofibular ligament and calcaneofibular ligament are completely torn *(arrow)*.

- Suspected syndesmotic injuries require longer periods of time for improvement (3 to 4 weeks) compared with simple inversion low ankle sprains.
- Physical therapy and rehabilitation are extremely important in preventing instability and recurrent ankle sprains with recovery of proprioception.
- Nonsteroidal antiinflammatory drugs, either oral or topical, have been shown to be effective in treating pain associated with ankle sprains.

When to Refer

- Patients who failed an appropriate course of conservative management with continued pain or instability, as these patients may be adequate candidates for surgical intervention
  - These patients may need a lateral ligament reconstruction.

Prognosis

- Nonoperative treatment typically results in good to excellent outcomes.
- It is not uncommon for some patients (about 30%) to have pain and swelling that lasts up to 6 months.

- Chronic ankle instability can occur in 20% of patients. These patients may experience improvement after a lateral ligament reconstruction.

Patient Instructions

- Weight bear as tolerated with appropriate protection
- Non–weight bearing for a prolonged period of time is not advised.
- Patient should learn how to do the appropriate proprioceptive exercises from their physical therapist and do them at home.
- MRI should be considered in the patient who continues to be unable to bear weight or has chronic pain.

Suggested Readings

Alonso A, Khoury L, Adams R. Clinical test for ankle syndesmosis injury: reliability and prediction of return to function. *J Orthop Sports Phys Ther*. 1998;27:276–284.

Anderson KJ, LeCocq JF, Clayton ML. Athletic injury to the fibular collateral ligament of the ankle. *Clin Orthop Relat Res*. 1962;23:146–160.

Attarian DE, McCrackin HJ, DeVito DP, et al. Biomechanical characteristics of human ankle ligaments. *Foot Ankle*. 1985;6:54–58.

Bröstrom L. Sprained ankles. I. Anatomic lesions in recent sprains. *Acta Chir Scand*. 1964;128:483–495.

Espinosa N, Smerek JP, Kadakia AR, et al. Operative management of chronic ankle instability: reconstruction with open and percutaneous methods. *Foot Ankle Clin*. 2006;11:547–565.

Henning CE, Egge LN. Cast brace treatment of acute unstable ankle sprain: a preliminary report. *Am J Sports Med*. 1977;5:252–255.

Hertel J. Functional instability following lateral ankle sprain. *Sports Med*. 2000;29:361–371.

Hintermann B. Arthroscopic findings in patients with chronic ankle instability. *Am J Sports Med*. 2002;30:402–409.

Lynch S. Assessment of the injured ankle in the athlete. *J Athl Train*. 2002;37:406–412.

Shawen S, Dworak T, Anderson R. Return to play following ankle sprain and lateral ligament reconstruction. *Clin Sports Med*. 2016;35:697–709.

Yeung MS, Chan KM, So CH, et al. An epidemiological survey on ankle sprain. *Br J Sports Med*. 1994;28:112–116.

Chapter 191 Achilles Tendon Rupture

Scott Van Aman, Marissa Jamieson

ICD-10-CM CODES
S86.011A *Right Achilles tendon rupture initial encounter*
S86.011D *Right Achilles tendon rupture subsequent encounter*
S86.012A *Left Achilles tendon rupture initial encounter*
S86.012D *Left Achilles tendon rupture subsequent encounter*

Key Concepts

- Acute Achilles injuries most commonly occur in middle-aged men participating in episodic athletics ("weekend warriors").
- Acute ruptures are missed initially in up to 25% of patients.
- Active patients typically benefit from operative treatment; however, recent studies have shown that these injuries can be successfully treated nonoperatively.

History

- Rapid eccentric contraction of the gastrocnemius-soleus complex (running, jumping) or strong concentric contraction (explosive plyometrics)
- Sensation of being shot or kicked in the back of the heel often described
- Pain, ecchymosis, cramping, inability to bear weight
- It is important to inquire about prodromal pain prior to injury, which may indicate chronic tendinosis. Sedentary individuals with a history of chronic pain may rupture after minor trauma.
- Fluoroquinolone use or steroid injections may predispose to rupture.
- Patients may also sustain direct laceration of the tendon.

Physical Examination
Observation

- Limp or inability to bear weight
- Ecchymosis and swelling

Palpation

- Palpable defect in the Achilles tendon (usually 2 to 7 cm proximal to insertion); may be subtle with delayed presentation due to hematoma formation (Fig. 191.1)

Range of Motion

- Increased ankle dorsiflexion (may be inhibited by pain)
- Weak plantarflexion; however, patients may have residual ability to plantarflex because the secondary ankle plantarflexors are intact
- Not able to perform a single leg heel raise

Special Tests

- Thompson test (Fig. 191.2)
  - The patient is placed prone with the knee flexed.
  - The calf is squeezed to assess for plantarflexion of the foot.
  - No flexion is considered positive for complete rupture.
  - A false negative may result from squeezing the long toe flexor muscles or posterior tibialis.
- Knee flexion sign
  - The patient is prone and brings the knee from fully extended to 90 degrees of flexion.
  - If the foot falls to neutral dorsiflexion or beyond, considered positive for rupture
  - Must compare to contralateral side

Imaging

- Rarely necessary, diagnosis is primarily clinical
- Radiographs
  - Soft tissue defect can often be appreciated on the lateral view.
- Magnetic resonance imaging
  - Unnecessary for most acute ruptures, unless the diagnosis is unclear
  - May be helpful in differentiating partial and complete tears
  - May be indicated for surgical planning in chronic ruptures or in patients with acute rupture in the setting of chronic tendonitis or tendinopathy
  - Ultrasound may be used to evaluate the Achilles tendon as well

Treatment
Acute Ruptures

- Splint in position of comfort with foot plantarflexed 30 degrees
- Non–weight bearing, ice/elevation to decrease swelling, and oral analgesics

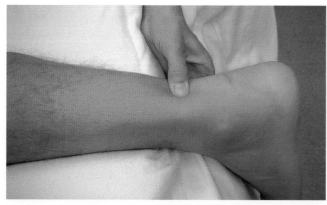

Fig 191.1 Palpation of the Achilles tendon in a patient with an acute injury reveals a defect approximately 2 to 7 cm proximal to the calcaneal tuberosity.

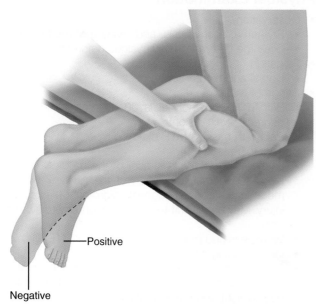

Positive

Negative

Fig 191.2 Thompson test. As the calf muscles are squeezed proximally, the examiner watches for plantarflexion of the foot. In a positive test, as shown here, there is no plantarflexion, indicating an Achilles tendon rupture.

- Active healthy patients may benefit from surgical repair, which may be performed open or percutaneously.
- Nonoperative treatment protocols utilizing functional bracing and early weight bearing have been shown to be effective as well.

Chronic Ruptures

- Immobilization in walking cast or boot
- Healthy, active patients may benefit from surgical intervention involving debridement and secondary repair of the diseased

tendon in combination with lengthening procedures or flexor hallucis longus transfer.
- Sedentary patients may be treated long term with an ankle-foot orthosis.

When to Refer

- Acute ruptures should be referred promptly because repairs are most successful if performed within 2 weeks of injury.
- Patients with chronic ruptures should also be referred for surgical evaluation.

Prognosis

- Good and excellent outcomes have been demonstrated for both operative and nonoperative treatment of acute ruptures.
- The prognosis for chronic rupture is not as good. The primary goal of surgery is a return to normal activities of daily living.

Patient Instructions

- Patients with acute ruptures should be informed early that recovery is lengthy, frequently requiring as long as 6 months to a year to return to normal activity.

Considerations in Special Populations

- Active patients should be counseled that both nonoperative and operative treatment of acute rupture are reasonable treatment options.
- In patients unfit for surgery, nonoperative treatment should be continued indefinitely and may include ankle-foot orthoses to assist with ambulation.
- Diabetes and smoking are significant risk factors for wound complications with surgery; however, this is not a strict contraindication to repair.

Suggested Readings

Chiodo CP, Glazebrook M, Bluman EM, et al. Diagnosis and treatment of acute achilles tendon rupture. *J Am Acad Orthop Surg.* 2010; 18:503–510.

Cooper MT. Acute achilles tendon ruptures. *Clin Sports Med.* 2015;34: 595–606.

Garras DN, Raikin SM, Bhat SB, et al. MRI is unnecessary for diagnosing acute achilles tendon ruptures: clinical diagnostic criteria. *Clin Orthop Relat Res.* 2012;470:2268–2273.

Wilkins R, Bisson LJ. Operative versus nonoperative management of acute achilles tendon ruptures: a quantitative systematic review of randomized controlled trials. *Am J Sports Med.* 2012;40:2154–2160.

Willits K, Amendola A, Bryant D, et al. Operative versus nonoperative treatment of acute achilles tendon ruptures: a multicenter randomized trial using accelerated functional rehabilitation. *J Bone Joint Surg Am.* 2010;92:2767–2775.

Chapter 192 Turf Toe

Joseph S. Park

ICD-10-CM CODES
S93.529A *Sprain, metatarsal phalangeal joint*
S93-123A *Dislocation, metatarsal phalangeal joint*

Key Concepts

- The great toe metatarsophalangeal (MTP) joint is important in gait, push-off, forward drive, running, jumping, and crouching.
- MTP stability is created by the surrounding capsuloligamentous (CL) complex, including the joint capsule, plantar plate, flexor hallucis brevis and sesamoids, and collateral ligaments. The flexor hallucis longus acts as a secondary stabilizer, as it spans both the MTP and interphalangeal (IP) joints (Fig. 192.1). Turf toe, in its strictest definition, is a hyperextension injury to the hallux MTP joint. However, the term has been used for any injury to the hallux MTP joint and represents a spectrum of injuries from mild to severe.
- Turf toe primarily occurs in athletes, particularly football players, and is associated with the increased use of flexible shoe wear and increased traction on artificial turf.
- The injury can be debilitating in athletes who need to perform rapid acceleration and cutting maneuvers.
- Most cases are treated nonoperatively; surgery is rarely required, except for complete tears (Grade 3 injuries) in competitive athletes.

History

- Acute injury
  - Hyperextension injury of the great toe MTP joint with axial loading of the heel and plantarflexed forefoot
  - Limp or inability to bear weight
  - Pain and swelling around the MTP joint, primarily on the plantar surface
  - Collateral ligament injury from valgus/hyperextension force can lead to traumatic hallux valgus.
  - May also result in flexor hallucis longus tendon rupture, tibial or fibular sesamoid fracture, or metatarsal dorsal articular injury
- Chronic injury
  - Difficulty with push-off activities: accelerating, jumping, and running
  - Traumatic hallux valgus deformity if medial collateral ligament complex injured

- Claw toe deformity due to loss of intrinsic flexor hallux brevis function

Physical Examination

- Observation
  - Erythema, ecchymosis, and swelling of the MTP joint
  - Claw toe deformity, hallux valgus deformity
- Palpation
  - Dorsal and plantar tenderness
- Range of motion
  - Stiff MTP joint (normal is 30 degrees of flexion, 80 degrees of extension)
  - Pain with passive MTP extension
- Special tests
  - Lachman test (dorsal stress) of the hallux MTP joint. Increased dorsal translation of the phalanx with the metatarsal stabilized suggests significant plantar plate injury. May be difficult to assess secondary to swelling/pain.
  - Weakness and pain with resisted hallux MTP/IP flexion
  - Injury grading scale
  - Grade 1: stretching or minor tearing of CL complex; minimal pain, swelling, and restricted motion; able to bear weight and return to play
  - Grade 2: partial tear of CL complex; moderate pain, swelling, and restricted motion; can bear weight, but with a limp
  - Grade 3: complete tear of CL complex; severe injuries may show a tibial sesamoid fracture or a dorsal impaction injury of the metatarsal articular surface; severe pain, swelling, and loss of motion; usually unable to bear weight

Imaging

- Radiographs: anteroposterior, lateral, and oblique views of the foot
  - May only demonstrate soft-tissue swelling
  - May see proximal migration or fracture of the sesamoids compared to uninjured side (Fig. 192.2)
  - Bilateral forced (stress) dorsiflexion lateral views may assist in determining migration of the sesamoids, indicating plantar plate rupture or sesamoid diastasis. With complete plantar plate rupture, the sesamoids will not track distally with the proximal phalanx during MTP extension (Fig. 192.3).

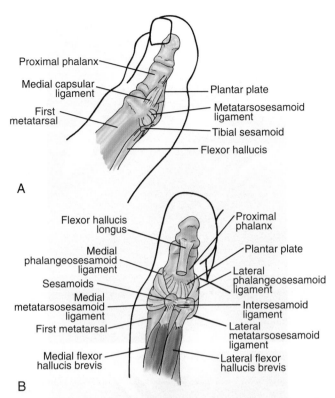

Fig 192.1 Lateral **(A)** and plantar **(B)** views of the hallux metatarsophalangeal joint showing the capsuloligamentous complex.

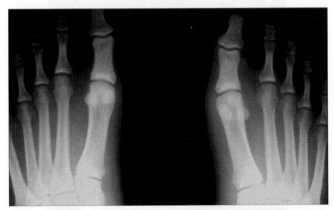

Fig 192.2 Radiograph demonstrating proximal migration of the sesamoids on the right foot. Note the position of the sesamoids on the left foot.

- Magnetic resonance imaging
  - Recommended for grade 2 and 3 injuries, especially in competitive athletes or with higher-energy mechanisms.
  - Evaluates degree of soft-tissue injury and possible articular damage.
  - Sagittal T1- and T2-weighted sequences can demonstrate partial or complete rupture of the plantar plate (sesamoid-phalangeal ligament; Fig. 192.4).

Differential Diagnosis

- Fracture of the great toe metatarsal or phalanges
- Hallux rigidus/valgus
- Sesamoid fracture/avascular necrosis

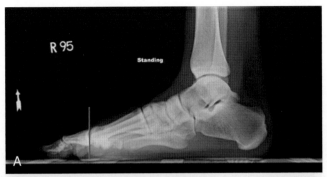

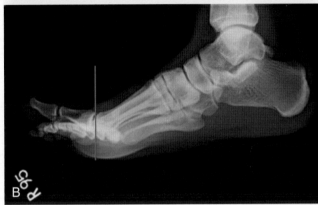

Fig 192.3 (A) Standing lateral XR with red line marking distal aspect of medial sesamoid. **(B)** With dorsiflexion lateral, the medial sesamoid does not track with the proximal phalanx, indicating complete plantar pate rupture.

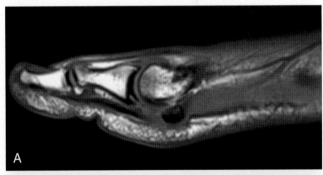

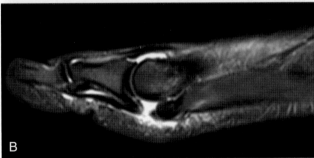

Fig 192.4 (A) T1-weighted sagittal magnetic resonance imaging showing complete rupture of the medial plantar complex and proximal migration of the tibial sesamoid. **(B)** T2-weighted sagittal image demonstrates hallux MTP effusion, complete rupture of plantar plate, and edema within medial FHB muscle belly.

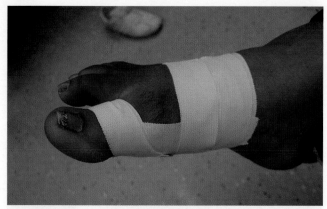

Fig 192.5 Taping procedure for turf toe injury to allow hallux interphalangeal motion but limit metatarsophalangeal dorsiflexion.

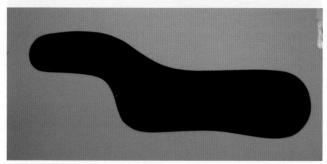

Fig 192.6 Rigid insole (Morton extension) to prevent metatarsophalangeal hyperextension.

Treatment

- At diagnosis
  - Conservative management includes rest, ice, compression, and elevation (RICE); antiinflammatory drugs; and possibly a boot or cast. Turf toe taping provides compression and restricts MTP extension (Fig. 192.5). Taping should not cross the interphalangeal joint. Cortisone and lidocaine injections are contraindicated and may exacerbate chronic turf toe.
  - Grade 1: RICE, taping, stiff-sole shoe, return to play per pain level
  - Grade 2: as for grade 1 plus 2 weeks of rest (weight bearing as tolerated)
  - Grade 3: as for grade 1 plus 6 weeks of rest (non–weight bearing). Surgical treatment should be considered in athletes, especially athletes in cutting/jumping sports.
- Later
  - Return to play is indicated when swelling subsides, flexion strength of the hallux MTP is restored, and painless extension of the MTP joint to 40 degrees (or symmetrical with the opposite side) is achieved. A rigid insole (Morton extension) will allow earlier return by limiting motion (Fig. 192.6). Operative indications include complete medial and lateral plantar plate tears, unstable MTP joint, loose body, medial collateral/capsular rupture (traumatic bunion), and sesamoid fracture or proximal migration.
  - Surgical treatment involves direct repair of the medial and lateral plantar plate (sesamoido-phalangeal ligament)

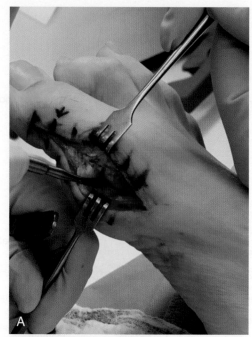

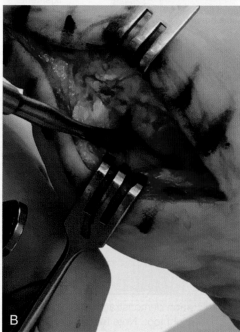

Fig 192.7 (A) Medial approach to plantar plate and medial sesamoid. (B) Freer elevator placed in defect between medial sesamoid and proximal phalanx, indicating complete medial plantar plate rupture. Direct repair can be performed for the majority of acute ruptures.

via a dual approach. Incisions are typically medial (Fig. 192.7) and plantar lateral to approach both sesamoids.

When to Refer

- Referral is indicated if the clinical course does not proceed as expected or there is evidence of significant injury with instability on initial presentation.

- All grade 2 or 3 injuries, especially in elite athletes, should be referred to an orthopaedic foot and ankle surgeon.

Prognosis

- The prognosis is good for incomplete tears. Most turf toe injuries are minor and heal with appropriate care without any functional limitations. Complete ruptures in high-level athletes may benefit from surgical intervention; early MRI and referral is recommended. Return to sport may take 4 to 6 months or more for grade 3 injuries.

Patient Instructions

- Follow-up in a timely manner from the initial injury will allow more rapid diagnosis and initiation of treatment, allowing earlier return to athletic activity.

- Early surgical treatment for grade 3 injuries for elite athletes may allow for more predictable return to sports. Patients with traumatic hallux valgus or claw toe deformity should also be referred for surgical consideration.

Suggested Readings

Anderson RB, Hunt KJ, McCormick JJ. Management of common sports-related injuries about the foot and ankle. *J Am Acad Orthop Surg*. 2010;18:546–556.

Clanton TO, Ford JJ. Turf toe injury. *Clin Sports Med*. 1994;13:731–741.

Mullen JE, O'Malley MJ. Sprains—residual instability of subtalar, Lisfranc, and turf toe. *Clin Sports Med*. 2004;23:97–121.

Sammarco GJ. Turf toe. *Instr Course Lect*. 1993;42:207–212.

Chapter 193 Ankle Fractures

Travis Frantz, Corey Van Hoff

ICD-10-CM CODES
S82.4-8x *Ankle fracture*
S93.0x *Deltoid ligament rupture*
S93.4x *Syndesmotic ligament rupture*

Key Concepts

- Ankle fractures are generally the result of a rotational or angular force on the foot relative to the leg.
- The ankle joint is highly conforming and must transmit large forces over a small surface area. Any abnormal shift of the talus relative to the tibia alters joint pressures and will result in arthrosis.
- It is important to differentiate between stable and unstable ankle fractures. Treatments, surgical or nonsurgical, are based on ankle stability.

History

- Twisting, noncontact injury; less commonly, direct trauma
- Stable fracture: often able to bear weight on the extremity with some discomfort
- Unstable fracture: unable to bear weight on the injured limb; may have an obvious deformity that requires immediate attention, such as reduction

Physical Examination

- Observation
  - Ecchymosis and swelling
  - Fracture blisters may develop later and are a sign of significant soft-tissue trauma. Serum-filled blisters are a sign of superficial skin damage, whereas blood-filled blisters are typically a sign of deeper, more severe soft-tissue injury (Fig. 193.1).
  - Open wounds can be indicative of a possible open fracture (formerly referred to as compound fracture)
  - Deformity or gross malalignment may indicate the presence of fracture-dislocation.
- Palpation
  - Tenderness over the fractured medial and/or lateral malleoli. The medial ankle gutter may be tender if the deltoid ligament has been injured.
- Range of motion
  - Gentle manipulation of the ankle may reveal gross instability and thus an unstable injury.
- Special tests
  - Associated neurovascular injuries are rare but should be ruled out with a careful examination. Pulses can commonly normalize after reduction of a dislocation.

- Compartment syndrome is occasionally associated with high-energy fractures, and if it is suspected on the clinical examination, an orthopaedist should be contacted immediately.

Imaging

- Radiographs: anteroposterior, lateral, and mortise views of the ankle
  - Look for fracture lines and displacement.
  - Mortise view (true anteroposterior view of the ankle) obtained with the foot in 15 to 20 degrees of internal rotation; asymmetry of the clear space, such as medial widening, indicative of injury
- If fracture is identified, obtain anteroposterior and lateral of full-length tibia/fibula.
- If there is an isolated fibula fracture identified, obtain stress radiographs: mortise view with foot externally rotated by manual stress or gravity
  - Helps determine whether the deltoid ligament has been disrupted; medial clear space greater than 3 mm typically an indication of deltoid ligament incompetence
- Computed tomography
  - Quantifies the size of a posterior malleolar fragment in relation to the distal tibial articular surface; helpful for surgical planning in complex fracture patterns (Fig. 193.2)
  - Identifies osteochondral fractures of the talus
- Magnetic resonance imaging
  - Typically not helpful

Differential Diagnosis

- Ankle sprain
- Syndesmotic injury (high ankle sprain)
- Maisonneuve fracture (disruption of distal tibiofibular syndesmosis with concurrent proximal fibular fracture)
- Tibial pilon/plafond fracture
- Osteochondral injury of the talus
- Tarsal bone fracture/dislocation

Treatment

- At diagnosis
  - The ankle is placed in a well-padded, posterior molded splint, and elevated to heart level.
  - Subluxations or frank dislocations are reduced by pulling in-line traction and correcting the deformity.
  - Consider using a hematoma block and/or conscious sedation for severe injuries, if not contraindicated.
  - Mini fluoroscopy unit can be used at the time of reduction to confirm anatomic alignment: the talus should be

centered under the tibia in both the anteroposterior and lateral radiographs.

- The ankle is splinted in situ to hold the reduction: be sure the reduction is near anatomic, as nonanatomic reduction can lead to soft-tissue and skin breakdown.
- If a reduction is performed, a postreduction radiograph is required after splinting to ensure reduction is maintained.
- Open wounds are copiously irrigated with normal saline and dressed with povidone-iodine–soaked gauze. The tetanus immunization is updated, and intravenous antibiotics appropriate for the grade of wound are given (Table 193.1).

- Later
  - Definitive management is by surgical or closed methods (Table 193.2).
  - The primary indications for surgery are unstable bi- or trimalleolar injuries and isolated displaced fractures of the medial malleolus (Fig. 193.3).
  - Surgery is rarely indicated for an isolated fibula fracture without ligamentous injuries (deltoid or syndesmotic) (Fig. 193.4).
  - Nondisplaced/stable fractures can be treated safely with a short leg walking cast or boot for 8 to 12 weeks.
  - Monthly radiographs are used to monitor healing.
- Displaced/unstable fractures should be internally fixed. Even when anatomically reduced, these tend to re-displace and therefore should be treated surgically.
  - Surgical fixation can be performed immediately, as in the case of an open or irreducible fracture.
  - More often, closed fractures can be reduced, splinted, and referred to an orthopaedic surgeon for operative treatment.

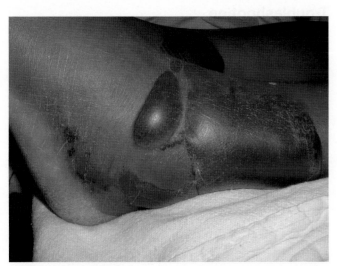

Fig 193.1 Blood-filled fracture blisters are indicative of a deep, dermal soft-tissue injury.

TABLE 193.1 Open Fracture Antibiotic Treatment Algorithm

Gustilo Type	Wound Size	Antibiotic
I	<1 cm	Cephalosporin first-generation
II	1–10 cm	Cephalosporin first-generation
III	>10 cm	Cephalosporin first-generation and gentamicin
Anaerobic contaminant		Add penicillin, clindamycin, or metronidazole (Flagyl)

Some institutions now administering piperacillin/tazobactam alone for Type II and III

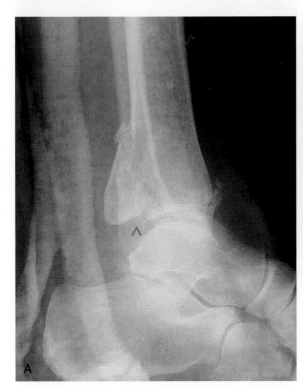

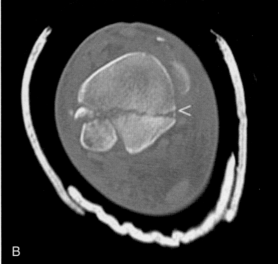

Fig 193.2 (A) Lateral radiograph of a large, displaced posterior malleolar fracture, part of a trimalleolar injury. **(B)** Computed tomography demonstrates the large posterior malleolar fragment *(arrowhead)* involving more than 25% of the articular surface.

- Surgical treatment is often delayed (as long as 1 to 2 weeks) until soft-tissue swelling is reduced (skin wrinkles present) and fracture blisters have healed.

When to Refer

- Unstable ankle fractures (bimalleolar, trimalleolar, deltoid, or syndesmotic disruption) should be referred for surgical treatment (Fig. 193.5). Cases should be referred urgently if there is open fracture, inability to maintain an adequate reduction, or signs of compartment syndrome.
- Isolated displaced fractures of the medial malleolus should also be referred for surgical fixation due to the high incidence of delayed union/nonunion secondary to periosteum interposed in the fracture site with closed treatment.

TABLE 193.2	Examples of Stable and Unstable Ankle Fractures	
Stable	**Unstable**
Isolated lateral malleolus without deltoid or syndesmotic disruption	Lateral malleolus with deltoid and/or syndesmotic disruption
	Isolated displaced (>2 mm) medial or posterior malleolus
	Bi- or trimalleolar fracture
Isolated nondisplaced medial or posterior malleolus	Deltoid and syndesmotic disruption (i.e., Maisonneuve injury with a high fibular fracture)

- Any intra-articular extension of the distal tibia (tibial pilon/plafond fracture) should be referred as well.

Prognosis

- Good to excellent results can be expected for 80-90% of all ankle fractures.
- Stable, nonoperative fractures fair better overall, mainly because the injury sustained was less severe.
- Some unstable fractures, particularly ankle fractures-dislocations, have unrecognized or untreatable injuries to the articular cartilage and may result in early posttraumatic arthritis.

Troubleshooting

- Unstable ankle fractures treated without surgery have a high risk of soft-tissue and skin breakdown, malunion, nonunion, stiffness, chronic pain, and early posttraumatic arthritis.
- The benefits of surgery for an unstable fracture far outweigh the inherent surgical risks, and surgery is highly recommended to restore stability, expedite fracture healing, and improve functional outcome.

Patient Instructions

- Elevation of the injured extremity at heart level is recommended to help control swelling.

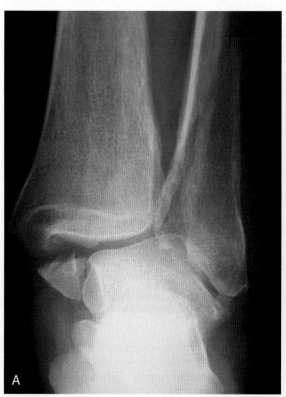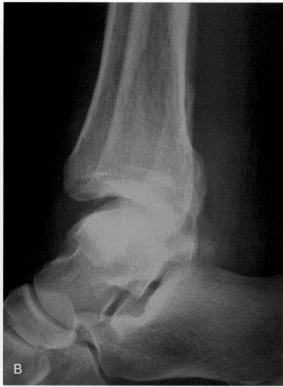

Fig 193.3 Anteroposterior (A) and lateral (B) views of a displaced bimalleolar ankle fracture. This is an unstable injury.

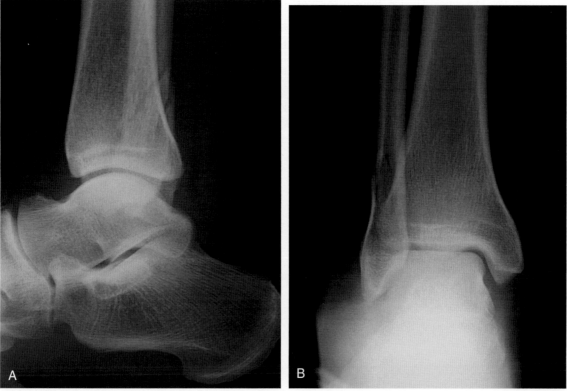

Fig 193.4 Anteroposterior (A) and lateral (B) views of nondisplaced isolated fibula fracture. This is a stable injury and does not require operative intervention.

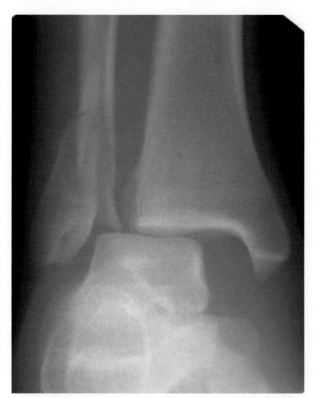

Fig 193.5 Mortise radiograph of a bimalleolar equivalent fracture. The deltoid and syndesmotic ligaments are ruptured. This is an unstable ankle injury and will require operative intervention.

- Weight-bearing restrictions must be strictly obeyed.
  - Unstable injuries require non–weight-bearing limitations, whereas stable fractures are allowed to bear weight as tolerated and not risk further damage once reviewed by the orthopaedist.

Considerations in Special Populations

- Patients with diabetes mellitus, neuropathy, and medical comorbidities such as peripheral vascular disease present a challenge to the treating orthopaedist, with higher rates of wound complications and mechanical failure.
- The elderly and patients with osteoporosis present difficulties with surgical fixation and skin closure secondary to poor bone and soft-tissue quality.
- Care of these special populations is best handled by an orthopaedic surgeon for stable or unstable injuries.

Suggested Readings

Belcher GL, Radomisli TE, Abate JA, et al. Functional outcome analysis of operatively treated malleolar fractures. *J Orthop Trauma.* 1997;11:106–109.

Chaudhary SB, Liporace FA, Gandhi A, et al. Complications of ankle fractures in patients with diabetes. *J Am Acad Orthop Surg.* 2008; 16(3):159–170.

Egol KA, Amirtharajah M, Tejwani NC, et al. Ankle stress test for predicting the need for surgical fixation of isolated fibular fractures. *J Bone Joint Surg Br.* 2004;86:2393–2398.

Gardner MJ, Streubel PN, McCormick JJ, et al. Surgeon practices regarding operative treatment of posterior malleolus fractures. *Foot Ankle Int*. 2011;32(4):120–130.

Irwin TA, Lien J, Kadakia A. Posterior malleolus fracture. *J Am Acad Orthop Surg*. 2013;21(1):32–40.

Jones KB, Maiers-Yelden KA, Marsh JL, et al. Ankle fractures in patients with diabetes mellitus. *J Bone Joint Surg Br*. 2005;87:489–495.

Michelson JD. Ankle fractures resulting from rotational injuries. *J Am Acad Orthop Surg*. 2003;11(6):403–412.

Miller AG, Margules A, Raikin SM. Risk factors for wound complications after ankle fracture surgery. *J Bone Joint Surg Am*. 2012;94(22): 2047–2052.

Tornetta P III, Ostrum RF, Trafton PG. Trimalleolar ankle fracture. *J Orthop Trauma*. 2001;15(8):588–590.

Zalavras C, Thordarson D. Ankle syndesmotic injury. *J Am Acad Orthop Surg*. 2007;15(6):330–339.

Chapter 194 Tarsal Fractures

Travis Frantz, Corey Van Hoff

ICD-10-CM CODES
S92.0x *Calcaneus fracture*
S92.1x *Talus (astragalus) fracture*
S92.2x *Other tarsal fracture*

Key Concepts

- The tarsal bones play a key role in transmitting forces from the ankle to the foot.
- Functionally, the tarsal joints account for the extremes of sagittal motion at the ankle (dorsiflexion/plantarflexion) and are the major location for side-to-side (inversion/eversion) motion.
- The four bones that make up the tarsus (the talus, calcaneus, navicular, and cuboid) are unique in the types of fractures that they sustain and their mechanism of injury.
- Dislocations associated with tarsal fractures must be promptly reduced to prevent pressure necrosis on areas of tented skin.
- Overall, surgical management of displaced tarsal fractures is successful in restoring anatomy and healing the fracture. However, some loss of hindfoot motion should be expected, and heavy labor jobs may not be advised.

History

- Typically fall from height or motor vehicle accident
- Talus fractures: forced dorsiflexion of the foot against the tibia, which can disrupt the posterior ankle joint capsule
- Talar neck fractures most common (50%) (Fig. 194.1)
- High rate of avascular necrosis and nonunion
- Calcaneal fractures: axial loading injury with direct impact to the plantar heel (Fig. 194.2)
- Navicular fractures: twisting injury (Fig. 194.3)
- Cuboid fractures: violent abduction of the forefoot on the hindfoot
  - Often termed nutcracker fractures with compression of the lateral wall of the cuboid (Fig. 194.4)

Physical Examination

- Observation
  - Swelling, fracture blisters, ecchymosis (hindfoot and plantar)
  - Open wounds, indicative of open fracture
  - Deformity or gross malalignment of the hindfoot may indicate a fracture/dislocation.

- Palpation
  - Tenderness in the hindfoot or over the specific tarsal bone fractured
  - Squeeze test identifies occult or stress fracture of the calcaneus; compression of the medial and lateral sides of the calcaneus elicits pain if a fracture is present.
- Special tests
  - Associated neurovascular injuries are rare but should be ruled out with careful examination.
  - Compartment syndrome of the foot is occasionally associated with high-energy crush injuries. If suspected on clinical examination, orthopaedics should be contacted urgently.
  - Occult injuries of the thoracolumbar spine need to be ruled out because they have been associated with tarsal bone fractures.

Imaging

- Radiographs: anteroposterior, lateral, and oblique views of the foot and ankle
- Special radiographic views:
  - Canale/Kelly view (talus): modified anteroposterior view of the foot; allows visualization of the talar neck and evaluates for displacement
  - Harris/axial view (calcaneus): useful in evaluating the calcaneal tuberosity for angulation and shortening
  - Broden view (calcaneus): lateral radiograph with the foot internally rotated and the beam focused on the sinus tarsi; evaluates for displacement of the posterior and middle facet joints
- Computed tomography
  - Necessary for all tarsal fractures; axial, sagittal, and semicoronal images give useful information about fracture pattern, extent of comminution, and preoperative planning (Fig. 194.5)

Differential Diagnosis

- Ankle sprain or fracture
- Osteochondral lesion of the talus
- Subtalar or Chopart joint dislocation
- Lisfranc joint injury

Treatment

- At diagnosis
  - Subluxations or frank dislocations are reduced by flexing the knee (relaxes the Achilles tendon) and pulling in-line traction with the deformity.

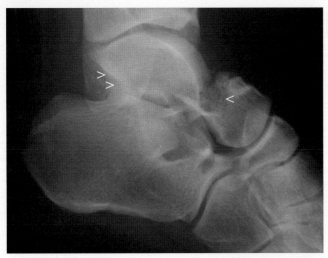

Fig 194.1 Displaced talar neck fracture *(single arrowhead)* with subluxation of the subtalar joint *(double arrowhead)*.

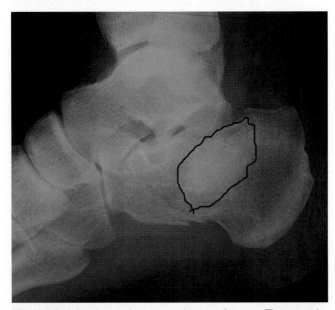

Fig 194.2 Joint depression–type calcaneus fracture. The posterior facet *(outlined in black)* has been depressed and rotated into the calcaneal body.

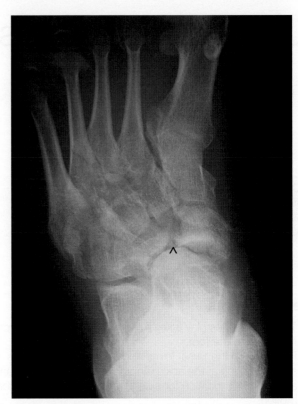

Fig 194.3 Navicular fracture *(arrowhead)* involving the lateral half of the navicular body.

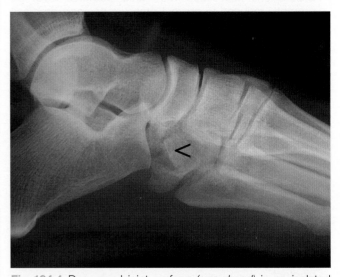

Fig 194.4 Depressed joint surface *(arrowhead)* in an isolated cuboid fracture.

- After closed reduction, the foot is placed in a well-padded posterior molded splint with a stirrup and elevated to heart level. This is sometimes referred to as a "bulky Jones" splint.
- If the fracture is irreducible, immediate open reduction is indicated to prevent pressure necrosis on compromised skin and further damage to the articular cartilage.
- Open wounds are copiously irrigated with normal saline and dressed with povidone-iodine–soaked gauze. The tetanus immunization is updated, and IV antibiotics are given appropriate for the grade of wound.

- Later
  - Definitive management is dependent on the fracture type. In general, nondisplaced fractures are treated with non–weight-bearing immobilization for 6 weeks, followed by a removable walking cast for an additional 4 weeks.
  - Early range of motion may prevent excessive ankle/subtalar stiffness.

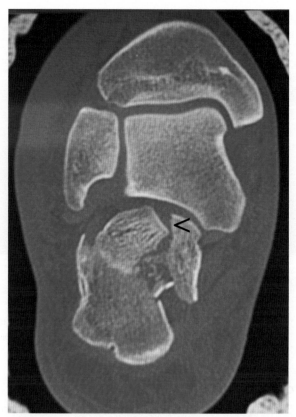

Fig 194.5 Coronal computed tomography image of a joint depression calcaneus fracture. The lateral half of the posterior facet *(arrowhead)* is displaced and rotated.

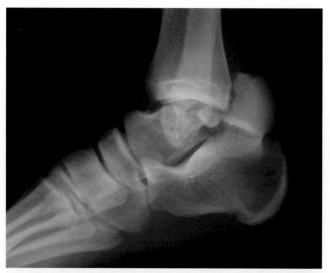

Fig 194.6 Talar neck fracture with a dislocation of the talar body. Emergent surgical reduction is recommended to prevent further soft-tissue compromise.

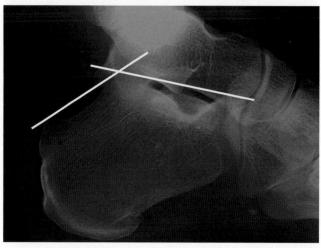

Fig 194.7 Lateral view of a normal calcaneus. A normal Bohler angle (20-40 degrees) is drawn where the white lines intersect.

- Radiographs should be monitored for potential displacement.
- Displaced fractures are typically treated with open reduction and internal fixation.
- Talar neck fracture may require as much as 10 weeks of non–weight bearing.
- Talar neck fractures with dislocation of the talar body are an emergency and require immediate surgical reduction (Fig. 194.6).
- Calcaneus fracture: Fractures with a Bohler angle greater than 20 degrees are treated nonoperatively (Fig. 194.7).
- Surgical treatment of displaced fractures has a high wound complication rate (10-40%).
- Patients with drug/alcohol addiction, mental illness, or neurologic disorders may be unable to cooperate with postoperative protocols and are probably better treated nonoperatively.
- Nicotine use, diabetes, and peripheral vascular disease are also relative contraindications to surgery.
- Severely displaced tongue-type fractures require immediate surgical attention to prevent devastating skin problems (skin necrosis/ulceration) on the posterior heel (Fig. 194.8).
- Navicular fracture: Dorsal chip fractures (capsular avulsion most common) and minimally displaced tuberosity fractures (avulsion of the posterior tibial tendon) are

treated nonoperatively. Body fractures (least common) or displaced tuberosity fractures require open reduction and internal fixation (Fig. 194.9).
- Cuboid fracture: Failure to surgically treat displaced fractures can result in lateral column shortening (pes planus deformity) and painful arthritis (Fig. 194.10).

When to Refer

- All injuries to the tarsal bones can be referred to an orthopaedist. However, those which are open fractures, skin compromising, irreducible, or concerning for compartment syndrome require urgent referral. Others can be seen routinely after using the management guidelines outlined previously.

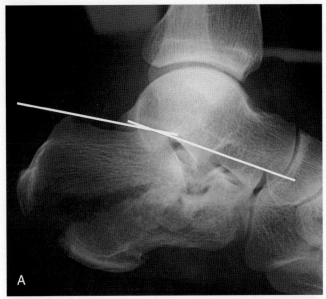

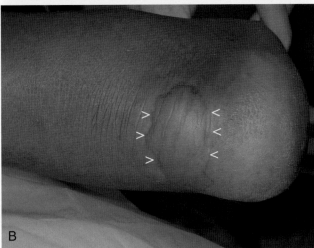

Fig 194.8 (A) Displaced tongue-type calcaneus fracture with flattening of Bohler angle (indicated by crossed *white lines*). **(B)** Posterior heel blister *(arrowheads)* developed immediately after an unreduced tongue-type fracture.

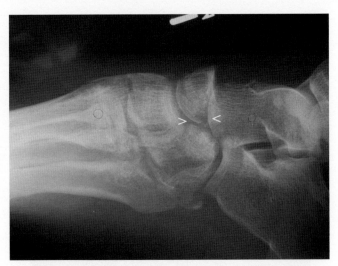

Fig 194.9 Fracture of the navicular body *(arrowheads)* with dorsal subluxation at the talonavicular joint.

of work because they will no longer be able to "trust" their foot and navigate job sites that require climbing ladders or working at heights.

Troubleshooting

- Swelling of the foot/ankle and distortion of the anatomic prominences will make it difficult at times to clinically identify the specific injury. Imaging studies are crucial to the diagnosis.
- Displaced tarsal fractures treated without surgery have a high risk of malunion, nonunion, stiffness, chronic pain, and early posttraumatic arthritis.
- Although the risks of surgery remain high for certain populations, such as open reduction and internal fixation for a calcaneal fracture in high-risk patients, secondary reconstruction at a later date is easier and safer with a well-aligned foot.

Patient Instructions

- Elevation of the injured foot at heart level is recommended to help control swelling.
- Weight-bearing restrictions must be strictly obeyed. Weight bearing on a displaced fracture may risk further damage to an already injured articular surface.

Considerations in Special Populations

- Patients with diabetes mellitus, neuropathy, and medical comorbidities, such as peripheral vascular disease, present a challenge to the treating orthopaedist with higher rates of wound complications and mechanical failure.
- In the diabetic patient, a tarsal bone fracture or dislocation may be the first sign of an evolving neuropathic (Charcot arthropathy) joint. These patients often present with a painless yet severely swollen ankle/foot and deny any trauma. These patients should be referred to an orthopaedist or podiatrist for definitive management.

Prognosis

- The outcomes for nondisplaced tarsal fractures are good. Patients may have occasional stiffness but are able to return to preinjury activities.
- The prognosis for displaced tarsal fractures is guarded, even with anatomic reduction.
  - Many patients develop chronic stiffness with restricted inversion/eversion. Posttraumatic arthritis may develop, resulting in the need for long-term treatment with bracing, nonsteroidal antiinflammatory drugs, cortisone injections, and even surgical arthrodesis.
  - Many tarsal fractures occur in young male laborers, many of whom will never return to their previous line

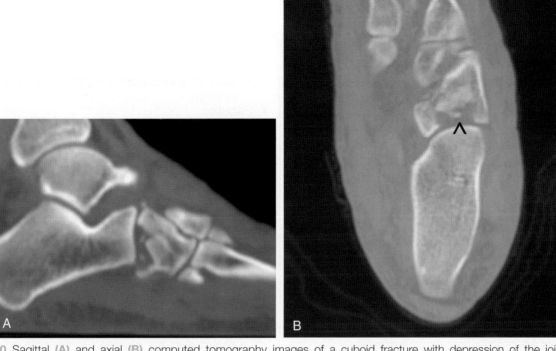

Fig 194.10 Sagittal (A) and axial (B) computed tomography images of a cuboid fracture with depression of the joint surface (arrowhead).

Suggested Readings

Bajammal S, Tornetta P 3rd, Sanders D, et al. Displaced intra-articular calcaneal fractures. *J Orthop Trauma*. 2005;19(5):360–364.

Buckley RE, Tough S. Displaced intra-articular calcaneal fractures. *J Am Acad Orthop Surg*. 2004;12:172–178.

Buckley R, Tough S, McCormack R, et al. Operative compared with nonoperative treatment of displaced intra-articular calcaneus fractures: A prospective, randomized, controlled multicenter trial. *J Bone Joint Surg Am*. 2002;84A:1733–1744.

DiGiovanni CW. Fractures of the navicular. *Foot Ankle Clin*. 2004;9:25–63.

Fortin PT. Balazsy JE: talus fractures: evaluation and treatment. *J Am Acad Orthop Surg*. 2001;9(2):114–127.

Lindvall E, Haidukewych G, DiPasquale T, et al. Open reduction and stable fixation of isolated, displaced talar neck and body fractures. *J Bone Joint Surg Am*. 2004;86(10):2229–2234.

Mihalich RM, Early JS. Management of cuboid crush injuries. *Foot Ankle Clin*. 2006;11:121–126.

Sangeorzan BJ, Benirschke SK, Mosca V, et al. Displaced intra-articular fractures of the tarsal navicular. *J Bone Joint Surg Am*. 1989;71A:1504–1510.

Vallier HA, Nork SE, Barei DP, et al. Talar neck fractures: results and outcomes. *J Bone Joint Surg Am*. 2004;86A:1616–1624.

Vallier HA, Nork SE, Benirschke SK, et al. Surgical treatment of talar body fractures. *J Bone Joint Surg Am*. 2003;85(9):1716–1724.

Chapter 195 Lisfranc Injuries

Minton Truitt Cooper

ICD-10-CM CODE
S93.32X   *Lisfranc (tarsometatarsal) fracture-dislocation*

Key Concepts

- The Lisfranc joint represents the junction between the midfoot and forefoot.
- Three metatarsal-cuneiform articulations (first, second, and third tarsometatarsal joints) and two metatarsal-cuboid articulations (fourth and fifth tarsometatarsal joints) (Fig. 195.1)
- Proper alignment and stability of these joints are essential for normal foot function.
- The Lisfranc joint is very stable because of its bony anatomy and strong ligamentous attachments. The base of the second metatarsal ("keystone") is recessed and locks between the medial and lateral cuneiforms. Plantar ligaments are stronger than dorsal ligaments.
- The Lisfranc ligament is the strongest ligament and runs from the base of the second metatarsal to the medial cuneiform.
- Injuries to this joint range from mild sprains to widely displaced, unstable, debilitating injuries.
  - Injuries can be bony, ligamentous, or a combination of the two.
- As many as 20% of Lisfranc injuries initially go unrecognized. When suspected, weight-bearing and/or stress radiographs are critical.
- Injuries to the tarsometatarsal joints require early accurate diagnosis with prompt anatomic reduction and internal fixation for optimal results. Severe long-term morbidity may occur if injuries are not properly treated at initial presentation.

History

- Mild to severe pain in the midfoot at rest and with weight bearing; may be unable to bear weight
- Acute injury; may be direct or indirect (Fig. 195.2)
  - Direct: crush injury
  - Indirect (more common): axial load in fixed planted foot (football, missed step off curb, landing dance jump) or twisting injury with forceful abduction of forefoot on midfoot (motor-vehicle collision)
- Any traumatic mechanism with significant midfoot pain should raise suspicion of a possible Lisfranc injury.

Physical Examination

- Observation
  - Abrasions, lacerations
  - Bruising (especially medial plantar surface of the foot)
  - Swelling around dorsal midfoot
  - Loss of normal arch or midfoot contour with weight bearing
- Palpation
  - Pain with palpation or manipulation of the tarsometatarsal joints
- Range of motion
  - Passive dorsiflexion and plantarflexion of the metatarsals elicits pain.
  - Stressed pronation/supination or abduction/adduction elicits pain.
- Special tests
  - Careful neurovascular examination emphasizing sensation and perfusion is essential. Lisfranc dislocation can be associated with impingement or laceration of a branch of the dorsalis pedis artery or the deep peroneal nerve, both of which cross dorsally between the base of the first and second metatarsals.
  - Severe swelling, especially in high-energy mechanisms, should alert the physician to possible compartment syndrome of the foot.

Imaging

- Radiographs: anteroposterior, lateral, and oblique views of the foot (Fig. 195.3). Bilateral radiographs are critical in subtle injuries to compare the non-injured anatomic relationships.
  - Should be weight bearing, if possible, to load the ligaments and test their integrity; if not possible, obtain stress views
  - Anteroposterior view: The medial border of the second metatarsal should align with the medial border of the middle cuneiform.
  - Oblique view: The medial border of the fourth metatarsal should align with the medial border of the cuboid.
  - Lateral view: The superior border of the metatarsal base should align with the superior border of the medial cuneiform.
  - Disruption of any these defined relationships is indicative of a Lisfranc injury (Fig. 195.4).
  - Stress views help reveal displacement in subtle cases with spontaneous reduction (Fig. 195.5). Ankle block or sedation may be required.
- Computed tomography
  - Better for discerning minor displacement, associated fractures, comminution, and dislocations. Weight-bearing CT scans are becoming more available and may be helpful.
- Magnetic resonance imaging
  - To assess ligamentous injury.
  - Nuclear medicine bone scans have been used in past; however, these have largely been replaced with CT and MRI.

Fig 195.1 Normal anatomy of tarsometatarsal joints.

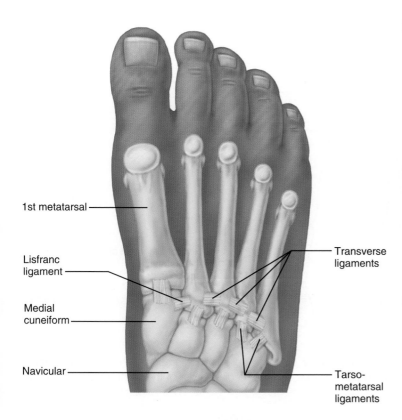

1st metatarsal

Lisfranc ligament

Medial cuneiform

Navicular

Transverse ligaments

Tarso-metatarsal ligaments

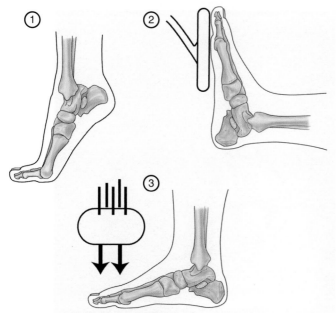

Fig 195.2 Common mechanisms of injury. Axial load in a planted foot (1), motor-vehicle collision trauma (2), direct crush injury (3).

Additional Tests

- Compartment pressure monitoring in selected cases—rare in outpatient setting.

Differential Diagnosis

- Tarsal, metatarsal, or phalangeal fractures of the foot
- Ligamentous injury outside the Lisfranc joint
- Soft-tissue damage around foot without fracture or ligament injury

Treatment

- At diagnosis
  - Initial treatment of a Lisfranc injury focuses on soft-tissue evaluation and diagnosing instability and associated fractures/dislocations.
  - For truly nondisplaced, stable injuries (negative weight-bearing and stress radiographs) with a normal soft-tissue/neurovascular examination, cast immobilization can be used.
  - A non–weight-bearing short leg cast for 6 weeks is followed by a walking cast for an additional 6 weeks until pain and tenderness have resolved.
  - All other injuries should be referred acutely (see the following).
- Later
  - For stable injuries, follow-up weight-bearing radiographs should be repeated at 10 to 14 days. If the injury remains stable (<2 mm displacement) and pain is decreasing, continued cast management with serial repeat radiographs in 2 weeks is recommended.
  - Any evidence of displacement or instability on follow-up examination warrants immediate orthopaedic referral for operative planning.

When to Refer

- When the diagnosis is unclear, it is appropriate to refer to orthopaedic specialist for further evaluation and management.

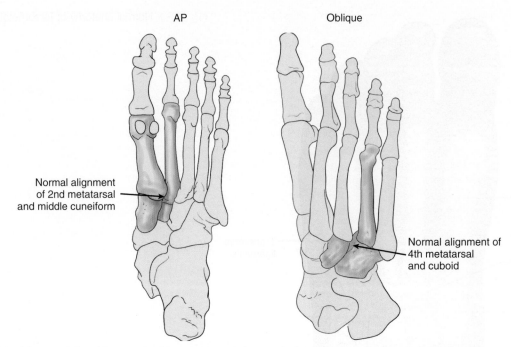

AP

Oblique

Normal alignment
of 2nd metatarsal
and middle cuneiform

Normal alignment of
4th metatarsal
and cuboid

Fig 195.3 Normal bony relationships as would appear on anteroposterior *(AP)* and oblique radiographs. The second metatarsal should align with the medial border of the middle cuneiform on the AP view, and the medial border of the fourth metatarsal should align with the cuboid on the oblique view.

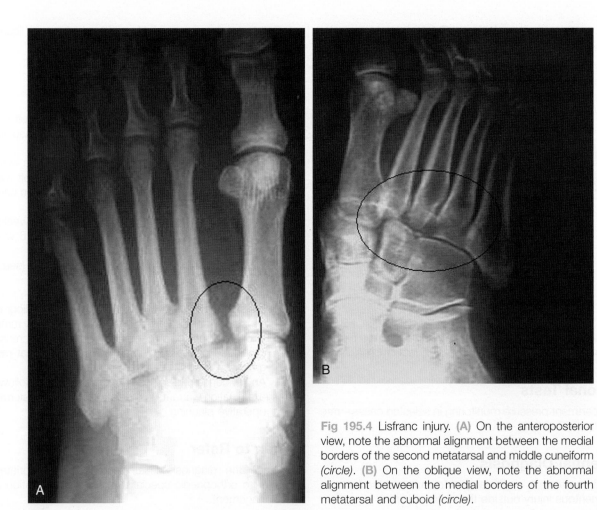

A

B

Fig 195.4 Lisfranc injury. **(A)** On the anteroposterior view, note the abnormal alignment between the medial borders of the second metatarsal and middle cuneiform *(circle)*. **(B)** On the oblique view, note the abnormal alignment between the medial borders of the fourth metatarsal and cuboid *(circle)*.

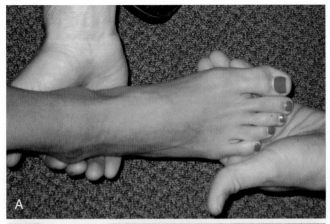

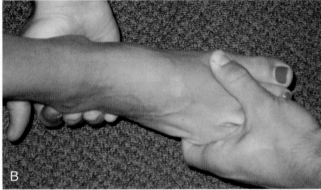

Fig 195.5 **(A)** To obtain a stress view radiograph, stabilize the hindfoot with one hand and grasp the forefoot with the opposite hand. **(B)** With the heel stabilized, place abduction/pronation stress on the forefoot. Widening of more than 2 mm or severe pain indicates a Lisfranc injury.

- Any Lisfranc injury with displacement or instability requires operative intervention and anatomic reduction for optimal results.
- Urgent/emergent referral is essential for any question of compartment syndrome (severe swelling and pain), dislocation, open fracture, or abnormal neurovascular examination.

Prognosis

- As many as 20% of Lisfranc injuries are overlooked, especially in polytrauma patients, with severe long-term morbidity.
- The severity of even subtle Lisfranc injuries is often underestimated, and healing may be prolonged.
- Patients should be provided with an accurate prognosis at the time of diagnosis.
- The best results (95% good to excellent functional recovery) are seen in those patients who undergo open reduction and internal fixation.
- Inadequate reduction or initial damage to the joint surface directly correlates with the development of posttraumatic arthritis.

- Symptoms after Lisfranc injury may persist but continue to subside for several years.

Troubleshooting

- Compartment syndrome usually occurs only with a high-energy Lisfranc fracture-dislocation and should be considered in any injury with severe swelling and a painful, tense foot. Any suspicion warrants immediate orthopaedic evaluation and, if necessary, referral to an emergency department.
- Counsel patients that posttraumatic arthritis is common and related to both the initial injury and the adequacy of reduction. Even in the stable midfoot sprain, recovery often takes several months.
- Be very wary of diagnosing a simple midfoot sprain. If a patient with a foot injury is unable to bear weight or has severe midfoot pain, he or she should be referred for orthopaedic evaluation.
- Standard radiographs may only show slight incongruity of the joint; gross instability may only be seen on stress or weight-bearing views. In any patient with a midfoot sprain, it is essential to obtain such studies to avoid missing an unstable injury.

Patient Instructions

- Instruct patients on the importance of elevation to decrease swelling, weight-bearing restrictions, and orthopaedic follow-up.
- Accurately outlining the prognosis associated with Lisfranc injuries, including a likely prolonged recovery time (immobilization up to 3 to 4 months), is an important component of the treatment plan.

Considerations in Special Populations

- Athletes with traumatic foot injury and resultant midfoot pain should be referred to an orthopaedic specialist for appropriate evaluation.
- Diabetic patients may have an underlying neuropathic (Charcot) arthropathy contributing to the Lisfranc pathology, especially with a history of minimal trauma. These cases require immediate referral to a specialist.

Suggested Readings

Davis E. Lisfranc joint injuries. *Trauma*. 2006;8:225–231.

Desmond EA, Chou LB. Current concepts review: lisfranc injuries. *Foot Ankle Int*. 2006;27:653–660.

Lewis SJ, Anderson RB. Lisfranc injuries in the athlete. *Foot Ankle Int*. 2016;37(12):1374–1380.

Richter M, Wipperman B, Krettek C. Fractures and fracture dislocations of the midfoot: occurrence, causes, and long-term results. *Foot Ankle Int*. 2001;22:392–398.

Seybold JD, Coetzee JC. Lisfranc injuries: when to observe, fix or fuse. *Clin Sports Med*. 2015;34(4):705–723.

Watson TS, Shurnas PS, Denker J. Treatment of lisfranc joint injury: current concepts. *J Am Acad Orthop Surg*. 2010;18(12):718–728.

Chapter 196 Metatarsal Fractures

Jason A. Fogleman, Jesse F. Doty

ICD-10-CM CODE
S92.3*** *Metatarsal fractures*

Key Concepts

- Most isolated metatarsal fractures that are well aligned may be treated nonoperatively with excellent results.
- The fifth metatarsal is most commonly fractured. Usually these are small avulsion fractures off the base of the metatarsal near the Peroneus Brevis insertion, which can be treated symptomatically. Large fractures of the fifth metatarsal base should be evaluated by a specialist.
- Displaced fractures of the first and fifth metatarsals should most likely be referred to a specialist for possible operative intervention.
- The goal of treatment is to maintain alignment and to preserve the arch of the foot with normal weight-bearing distribution under the metatarsal heads.
- An atraumatic history with chronic metatarsal pain likely indicates a stress fracture, which requires special considerations for successful treatment.
- High-risk fractures include the proximal fifth metatarsal, first metatarsal, proximal second metatarsal (Lisfranc joint injury), multiple fractures simultaneously, fractures in diabetics, and any associated joint dislocations.

History

- Injury mechanisms include falls, direct crush, and indirect twisting of the leg with the forefoot in a fixed position. Avulsion fractures of the base of the fifth metatarsal may result from inversion ankle sprains.
- Swelling, pain, and ecchymosis
- Usually able to bear some weight, except in cases of severe trauma
- Stress fractures present with chronic achiness after an antecedent change in exercising regimen or change in footwear.

Physical Examination
Observation

- Antalgic gait
- Swelling, ecchymosis, tenting skin, open wounds?
- Deformity, including rotation, and angulation of toes

Palpation

- Pain is generally elicited directly over the fracture location (Fig. 196.1).

- Careful sensory and vascular examinations to evaluate for neuropathy and vasculopathy that may compromise typical conservative treatment regimens
- Palpate the Lisfranc joint, hindfoot, and ankle to rule out additional injuries.

Imaging

- Radiographs: weight-bearing anteroposterior, lateral, and 45-degree oblique views
  - Check alignment of the metatarsal bases with their respective cuneiforms to rule out Lisfranc joint subluxation.
  - A stress fracture or an acute nondisplaced fracture may not appear for more than 2 weeks on plain radiographs.
- Advanced imaging
  - Computed tomography scan is likely best reserved for a specialist, and may be indicated for complex fractures, nonunions, malunions, multiple fractures, and associated Lisfranc dislocations.
  - Magnetic resonance imaging and bone scan is rarely indicated for acute injuries but may be useful for diagnostic purposes with stress fractures or chronic injuries with multiple normal radiographs.

Differential Diagnosis

- Lisfranc joint injury: pain located at tarsometatarsal joint, exacerbated by pronating/supinating forefoot or midfoot compression
- Midfoot arthritis: pain with palpation pressure over the midfoot joints with an exam similar to Lisfranc injuries but with less acute trauma and a more chronic history of achiness with activity
- Stress reaction: prequel to a stress fracture and treated similarly
- Charcot neuroarthropathy: often diabetic patients with neuropathy and significant swelling and erythema of foot that decreases with elevation

Treatment
At Diagnosis

- Dependent on the metatarsal involved, location (head, neck, shaft, base), and displacement
- Activity restrictions if possible, daily ice therapy, avoid nonsteroidal antiinflammatory drugs (NSAIDs), oral vitamin D supplementation
- Mobilization with a stable weight-bearing platform (i.e., hard-sole shoe, controlled ankle motion [CAM] boot) for walking as tolerated for 6 weeks

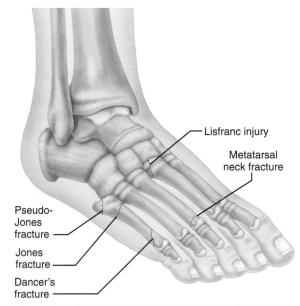

Fig 196.1 Location of common metatarsal fractures.

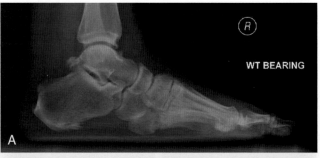

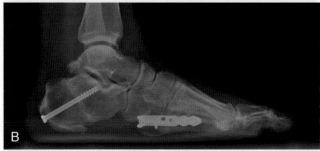

Fig 196.2 (A) Lateral foot radiograph demonstrates a fracture nonunion of the fifth metatarsal at the junction of the diaphysis and metaphysis (Jones fracture). (B) Postoperative radiograph demonstrates a healed fracture treated with a hook plate and screw construct.

- Avulsions of the fifth metatarsal base may be treated with a walking cast or fracture boot until the foot is completely pain free.

Later
- Rarely, metatarsal fractures go on to malunion or nonunion, and surgical osteotomy, bone grafting, and internal fixation may be beneficial (Fig. 196.2).

When to Refer
- Several fracture patterns require referral for surgical consideration.
- Displaced or open fractures
  - Fractures of the first or fifth metatarsals when the proximal fragment is larger than 1 cm (small avulsions are amendable to nonoperative treatment)
  - Multiple metatarsal fractures
  - Questionable Lisfranc joint injury: fixed with screws or fusion of the tarsometatarsal joints depending on the extent of injury
  - Intra-articular fractures, which may lead to posttraumatic arthritis; fixation frequently includes plate and screw constructs
  - Nonunions, malunions, nonhealing stress fractures

Prognosis
- Good, especially for isolated metatarsal shaft fractures.
- Good outcomes can be anticipated for fifth metatarsal base avulsion fractures, although it may be months before preinjury activity level can be anticipated.
- Intra-articular fractures may lead to posttraumatic arthritis.
- Missed Lisfranc joint injuries may lead to devastating arthritic collapse of the arch with chronic pain and deformity.

Troubleshooting
- Optimal glucose control in diabetics, thyroid regulation in hypothyroid patients, and vitamin D supplementation in nearly all patients can prevent nonunions.
- The importance of smoking cessation should be stressed.
- Patients should be counseled on the risks associated with certain fractures, as discussed previously.

Patient Instructions
- Patients should be counseled on appropriate expectations for functional return to exercise, work, and sports.
- Ice and elevation are important acutely to reduce swelling.
- For most fractures, other than isolated metatarsal shaft fractures, patients should be instructed on appropriate crutch, or rolling knee scooter use and the importance of non–weight bearing on the affected limb to allow for proper healing.

Considerations in Special Populations
- Diabetic patients generally require double the length of protected weight-bearing due to delayed healing.
- Diabetic fractures may precipitate Charcot neuroarthropathy. Glucose levels and vitamin D levels may be of particular benefit in diabetic patients.
- Malalignment is poorly tolerated, as altered weight bearing predisposes the patient to the development of skin ulceration or continued pain.
- High-level athletes/dancers and diabetics may benefit from referral to a specialist and possible early surgical fixation.
- Patients with recurrent fractures or chronic injury nonamendable to conservative treatment may benefit from operative intervention (Fig. 196.3).

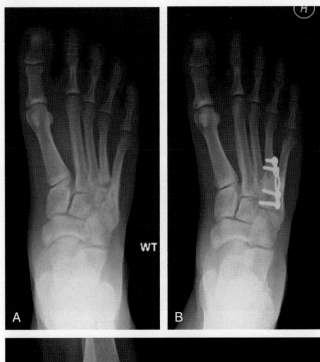

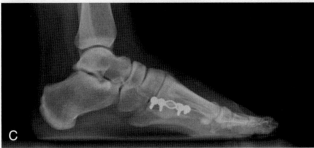

Fig 196.3 (A) Anteroposterior foot radiograph demonstrates a fracture nonunion of the fourth metatarsal diaphysis. **(B)** and **(C)** Postoperative radiographs demonstrate a healed fracture treated with bone grafting and a compression plate construct.

Suggested Readings

Egol K, Walsh M, Rosenblatt K, et al. Avulsion fractures of the fifth metatarsal base: a prospective outcome study. *Foot Ankle Int.* 2007;28:581–583.

Fetzer GB, Wright RW. Metatarsal shaft fractures and fractures of the proximal fifth metatarsal. *Clin Sports Med.* 2006;25:139–150.

Jackson JB, Ellington JK, Anderson RB. Fractures of the midfoot and forefoot. In: Coughlin MJ, Saltzman CL, Anderson RB, eds. *Surgery of the Foot and Ankle.* 9th ed. Philadelphia: Elsevier; 2014:2154.

Jones R. Fracture of the base of the fifth metatarsal bone by indirect violence. *Ann Surg.* 1902;35:697–700.

Kell IP, Glisson RR, Fink C, et al. Intramedullary screw fixation of jones fractures. *Foot Ankle Int.* 2001;22:585–589.

Petrisor BA, Ekrol I, Court-Brown C. The epidemiology of metatarsal fractures. *Foot Ankle Int.* 2006;27:172–174.

Reese K, Litsky A, Kaeding C, et al. Cannulated screw fixation of jones fractures. A clinical and biomechanical study. *Am J Sports Med.* 2004;32:1736–1742.

Schenck RC, Heckman JD. Fractures and dislocations of the forefoot: operative and non-operative treatment. *J Am Acad Orthop Surg.* 1995;3:70–78.

Chapter 197 Phalangeal Fractures of the Foot

Venkat Perumal, George Lee Wilkinson III

ICD-10-CM CODES
S92.4 *Fracture of the great toe*
S92.5 *Fracture of the lesser toe(s)*

Key Concepts

- Phalangeal fractures are caused by direct trauma to a toe.
- Most phalangeal fractures are closed, and are caused by a low-energy injury.
- The most common site of a phalangeal fracture is the fifth digit.
- Nonoperative treatment is sufficient for the majority of phalangeal fractures.
- Surgical intervention may be required for some fractures of the hallux, due to their propensity to cause long-term impairment.

History

- Direct trauma to the toe, followed by pain and swelling in the injured area

Physical Examination

- Observation
  - Look for injury to the nail
  - Assess swelling and/or ecchymosis (Fig. 197.1)
  - Check skin integrity
  - Evaluate angular deformity
- Palpation
  - Feel for tender areas
  - Examine remainder of foot and ankle to exclude additional injury
- Range of motion
  - Mobilize interphalangeal (IP) and metatarsophalangeal (MTP) joints

Imaging

- Anteroposterior, oblique, and lateral radiographs of the toes
  - When the lateral image is being obtained, consider manually elevating the injured toe to image more clearly (Fig. 197.2).
  - Types of toe fractures (Fig. 197.3)

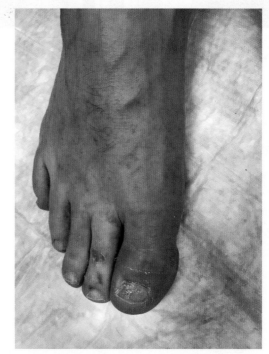

Fig 197.1 Swelling and/or ecchymosis of the toes.

Differential Diagnosis

- Nail bed injury—hematoma beneath the nail; likely normal radiographs (excluding presence of a distal phalanx fracture)
- Paronychia, ingrown toenail—drainage at the nail folds, erythema; normal radiographs
- Freiberg infraction—osteochondrosis of the lesser metatarsal heads (most commonly the second); best visible on anteroposterior radiographs
- MTP joint dislocation—positive drawer sign, tender over the joint; malalignment of joint
- MTP joint synovitis—subacute history; no evidence of fracture, joint deviation on radiographs
- Metatarsalgia—tenderness beneath the MTP joints; no acute abnormalities on radiographs, abnormal MTP joint cascade with relatively long metatarsal(s)

793

8

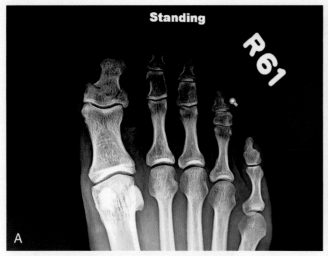

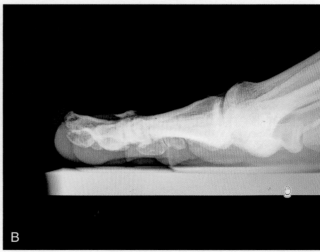

Fig 197.2 (A and B) X-ray great toe fracture.

Fig 197.3 Types of fractures.

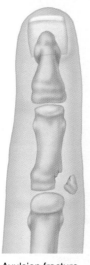

Avulsion fracture

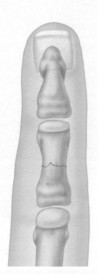

Transverse fracture

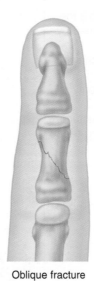

Oblique fracture

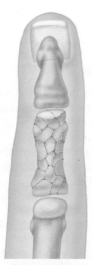

Comminuted/
crush fracture

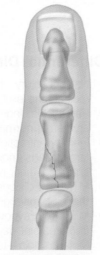

Intraarticular fracture
(in the joint)

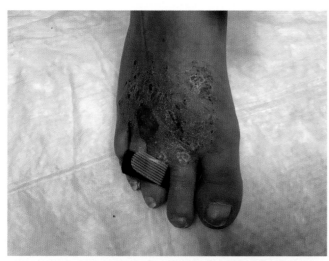

Fig 197.4 Treatment with buddy taping of the injured toe.

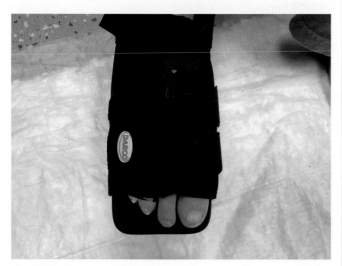

Fig 197.5 Treatment with stiff open-toed shoe. (Courtesy DARCO International, Huntington, West Virginia.)

Treatment

- Reduce fracture with gentle traction under digital block, if necessary
- Buddy tape injured toe to an adjacent toe (Fig. 197.4)
- Immobilize in a stiff, open-toed shoe (Fig. 197.5)
- Return to athletic shoes as pain and swelling allow (2 to 4 weeks)

When to Refer

- Open fractures
- Obvious angular deformity of the toes
- Intra-articular fractures of the MTP joint
- Displaced fractures of the hallux
- Fracture associated with dislocation

Prognosis

- With the majority of these fractures, return to full function is expected, although long-term stiffness and swelling are common.

Patient Instructions

- Recommend that patients reduce their activity level.
- Patients may bear weight as tolerated, but crutches or a cane may be useful immediately following the injury.
- Elevate the foot above the heart to limit swelling.

Considerations in Special Populations

- In diabetics, it is important to monitor for ulcerations when buddy tape is being used.
  - Buddy taping is not recommended in insensate diabetics.
  - The tape should not be overly tight and should be changed regularly.
  - A layer of gauze should be placed between the toes and between the tape and the skin to avoid maceration.

Suggested Readings

Coughlin MJ, Saltzman CL, Anderson RB, eds. *Mann's Surgery of the Foot and Ankle*. 9th ed. Philadelphia: Elsevier; 2014.

Court-Brown CM, Heckman JD, McQueen MM, et al, eds. *Rockwood and Green's Fractures in Adults: Rockwood, Green, and Wilkins' Fractures*. 8th ed. Philadelphia: Wolters Kluwer; 2015.

Chapter 198 Charcot Arthropathy

Carroll P. Jones

ICD-10-CM CODES
M14.671 *Charcot arthropathy, right ankle*
M14.672 *Charcot arthropathy, left ankle*

Key Concepts

- Charcot is a progressive, noninfectious, destructive arthropathy that affects weight-bearing joints in patients with distal peripheral neuropathy (DPN), primarily affecting the foot and ankle.
- Diabetes is the leading cause for DPN in North America and therefore the most common association with Charcot in the United States.
- Charcot affects less than 1% of patients with diabetes.
- Although rare, the most common locations affected, in decreasing order, are (1) midfoot; (2) hindfoot; (3) ankle; (4) forefoot.
- The natural progression of Charcot typically follows three stages, as described by Eichenholtz (1966):
  - Stage I: acute or fragmentation phase
  - Stage II: subacute or coalescence phase
  - Stage III: consolidation and reconstructive phase
- The treatment of Charcot is generally based on the Eichenholtz stage at presentation.
- Etiology of Charcot, despite close correlation with DPN, is unclear but likely a combination of the loss of protective sensation, repetitive trauma, upregulated inflammation, and hypervascularity.
- If untreated, the foot/ankle will develop a deformity, which then causes pressure points that progress to ulceration and ultimately a deep infection (potentially unbeknownst to the insensate patient).

History

- Patients often present with no clear history of significant trauma.
- Because of the neuropathy, pain may be absent or minimal.
- One of the most common complaints is foot swelling, insidious in onset.
- Patients may also note the development of foot/ankle deformity.
- In some cases, the diabetes and/or peripheral neuropathy has not previously been diagnosed—it is critical to pursue these lines of questioning during the history for any patient that presents with unexplained foot/ankle swelling and/or deformity.

Physical Examination

- Inspect both feet and ankles with socks and shoes off, in a standing posture—take note for presence of asymmetric alignment, swelling, and erythema.
- The classic presentation in the acute phase of Charcot is a swollen, warm, erythematous foot (Fig. 198.1)—the edema characteristically IMPROVES with elevation (does NOT improve with cellulitis).
- During inspection, look for calluses, ulcerations, and any bony prominences that may reflect deformity and/or neuropathy.
- Although many patients with Charcot have normal vascularity, always check pedal pulses (dorsalis pedis and posterior tibial).
- Palpate the foot for warmth, a common finding in the early stages of Charcot.
- A 5.07 Semmes Weinstein monofilament is a low-cost, simple, effective way to test for DPN (Fig. 198.2) and an important part of the physical examination.
- Assess all tendon/motor function, especially in the setting of deformity.
- Achilles tightness is common and is important to evaluate.
- Depending on the timing of presentation, the foot/ankle may start to demonstrate lessening of the swelling, warmth, and erythema as the Charcot process goes through healing phases.

Imaging

- Standing radiographs of the foot and ankle are standard.
- Stage I is characterized by fragmentation, fracture, and joint dislocation (Fig. 198.3).
- Stage II demonstrates some degree of bone healing (i.e., callous) and coalescence (Fig. 198.4).
- Stage III shows fully consolidated and healed bone (Fig. 198.5).
- MRI may be helpful if there is a concern for abscess or osteomyelitis.
- CT scan is useful to analyze complex deformity.
- Because Charcot often causes increased bone signal intensity on MRI (false positive for deep infection), a three-phase tagged white blood cell (WBC) scan may be more sensitive to evaluate for osteomyelitis.

Additional Tests

- Complete blood count (CBC), erythrocyte sedimentation rate (ESR), C-reactive protein (CRP) (infection markers)
- For diabetic patients, HgbA1C is helpful to assess compliance and consistency of blood sugar control.

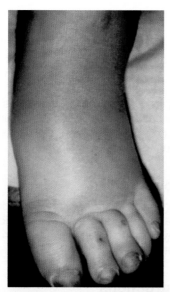

Fig 198.1 Acute presentation of midfoot Charcot arthropathy with a swollen, erythematous foot.

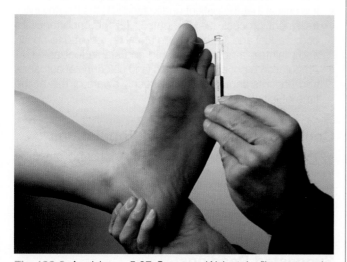

Fig 198.2 Applying a 5.07 Semmes Weinstein filament to the bottom of a foot until it bends—if undetected by the patient, there is a strong likelihood they have distal peripheral neuropathy and lost protective sensation.

- Vitamin D and calcium deficiency are common and should be tested.

Differential Diagnosis

- Cellulitis (elevated glucose and infectious markers)
- Lymphedema

Treatment

- Ideally, during the course of treatment, the foot/ankle is protected until the Charcot process reaches Stage III, and deformity/ulceration is avoided.
- Ultimately, surgically or nonoperatively, the goal is to obtain and maintain a plantigrade (near normally aligned) foot/ankle.

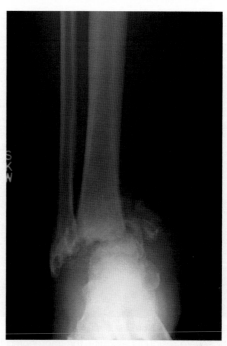

Fig 198.3 Eichenholtz Stage I Charcot of the ankle, anteroposterior view: extensive osteolysis, fracture of the medial malleolus, and subluxation of the tibiotalar articulation.

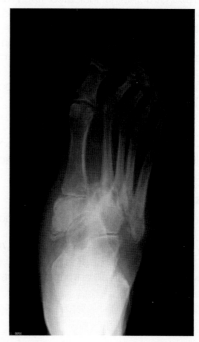

Fig 198.4 Eichenholtz Stage II Charcot of the midfoot, antero-posterior view: note the coalescence of the bone, particularly at the bases of metatarsals 2 to 4 at the tarsometatarsal articulation.

- Early-stage Charcot is treated with cast immobilization and non–weight bearing for up to 3 months.
- Late stage Charcot is addressed with footwear modification and bracing (depending on level and severity of any residual deformity).

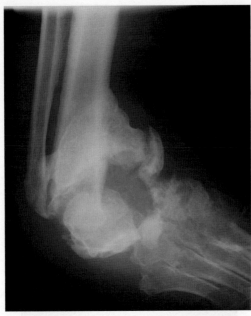

Fig 198.5 Eichenholtz Stage III Charcot of the ankle, AP view: despite the severe residual deformity, the fragmented bone has fully consolidated and matured.

- Surgical reconstruction is indicated if an unbraceable or unshoeable deformity develops during the course of treatment.
- If a callus or ulcers persists or recurs despite immobilization, surgery is often indicated to correct the deformity so that the pressure point will resolve.
- Operative intervention is also necessary if a deep infection develops.

When to Refer

- Almost all cases of Charcot should be referred to a foot/ankle specialist.

Prognosis

- The prognosis of Charcot depends on many factors, many of which the surgeon has no control over.
- Generally speaking, as you move from distal (forefoot) to proximal (ankle), the Charcot process is likely to create a progressively MORE unstable arthropathy, have a HIGHER

likelihood of requiring surgery, and a HIGHER risk of complications, including amputation.
- One of the primary keys to success for Charcot is early recognition and timely treatment, both of which require a heightened sense of awareness from primary care physicians.
- Patient compliance is also critical for a successful outcome—unfortunately patients with diabetic DPN often have difficulty maintaining non–weight bearing restrictions and adhering to strict serum glucose control.

Troubleshooting

- Charcot is an extremely complex, poorly understood condition, and many cases require difficult decision making that should always include thoughtful interaction and feedback from the patient.

Patient Instructions

- One of the most difficult parts about treating Charcot is patient education and managing their expectations.
- It is critical that the patient understands (1) the lengthy initial treatment process (9–12 months); (2) the importance of compliance; and (3) the lifelong attention required to obtain and maintain a normally aligned and stable foot/ankle.
- Amputation is not an uncommon (and unfortunate) outcome, and patients should be made keenly aware of this at the time of initial presentation.

Considerations in Special Populations

- The demographics of patients with Charcot are fairly consistent.
- For patients that have severe deformity and/or active deep infection and poor compliance, amputation (i.e., below-the-knee) is often the wisest plan of action for a reliable outcome.

Suggested Readings

Coughlin MJ, Saltzman CL, Anderson RB, eds. *Mann's Surgery of the Foot and Ankle.* 9th ed. Philadelphia: Elsevier; 2014.

Pinzur MS, Schiff AP. Deformity and clinical outcomes following operative correction of Charcot foot: a new classification with implications for treatment. *Foot Ankle Int.* 2018;39(3):265–270.

Rosenbaum AJ, DiPreta JA. Classifications in brief: Eichenholtz classification of Charcot arthropathy. *Clin Orthop Relat Res.* 2015;473(3):1168–1171.

Chapter 199 Anterior Ankle Impingement

Sonya Ahmed, Alan Shahtaji

ICD-10-CM CODES	
M19.079	*Primary osteoarthritis, unspecified ankle and foot*
M19.179	*Posttraumatic osteoarthritis, unspecified ankle and foot*
M25.70	*Osteophyte, unspecified joint*

Key Concepts

- Ankle pain worse in dorsiflexion
- Also known as "footballer's ankle" or "athlete's ankle" (Fig. 199.1)
- Impingement can be soft-tissue or bone/osteophyte related
- May be a due to repeated, chronic dorsiflexion, or due to a single, acute traumatic event
- Can be anteromedial, which is usually bony mediated, or can be anterolateral, which is usually associated with soft tissue

History

- Determine if acute or chronic, with chronic being those sports with repeated dorsiflexion (such as soccer, gymnastics) and acute with sudden impact injury with loaded or forced dorsiflexion

Physical Examination

Observation

- Localized swelling or bony protrusions, especially anterior ankle joint line
- Scars from previous injuries or tissue hypertrophy
- Surgeries previously
- Pain after activity
- Observe squatting with heels fixed on ground and limited dorsiflexion on affected side

Palpation

- Palpable bony masses or osteophytes
- Tenderness along anterior joint line, especially anterolate or anteromedially
- Pain recreated with forced dorsiflexion
- Bony impingement tends to be more AM (Figs. 199.2 and 199.3)
- Soft-tissue impingement tends to be more AL (Fig. 199.4)
- Possible effusion

Range of Motion

- Loss of maximal dorsiflexion and compared with contralateral side
- Loss of plantarflexions occasionally
- Unable to deep squat single leg equal to contralateral side

Special Tests

- Single squat/impingement sign
- Lunge forward maximally with heel on ground

Imaging

- Radiographs: weight-bearing ankle x-rays, three views, and potentially a plie view or anteromedial impingement view
- Ultrasound: particularly helpful with anterolateral (AL) soft-tissue lesions
  - May add dynamic testing
- Magnetic resonance imaging (MRI): assists in identifying other pathology that can coexist
  - Useful for identifying tissue as source of impingement adhesions
- Computed tomography (CT): best preoperative planning tool for complete localization of osteophytes
  - Identifies talar neck, distal tibia, or both osteophytes

Differential Diagnosis

- Ankle sprain
- Capsular tear
- Ankle loose bodies
- Osteochondral lesion of the talus or tibia
- Distal tibia/talus fracture
- Ankle arthritis
- Ankle arthrofibrosis

Treatment

Nonoperative

- Physical therapy
- Steroid injections potentially for pain relief but not curative
- Activity modification
- Bracing/taping
- Activity modification
- Shoe/orthotic modification if malalignment causing impingement symptoms
- Currently, no evidence for biologics

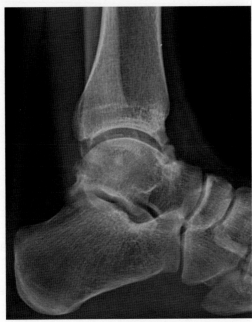

Fig 199.1 Classic lateral radiograph of "footballer's ankle" with bony impingement lesions on the anterior tibia with kissing lesion on the anterior talus.

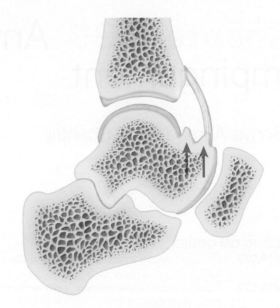

Fig 199.3 Possible talar neck locations for impingement lesions *(arrows)*. (Redrawn from an image provided courtesy of Shi Tang.)

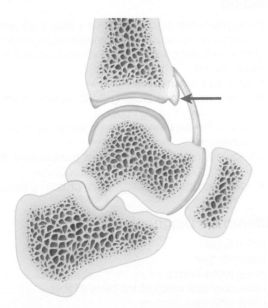

Fig 199.2 Anterior tibial osteophyte *(arrow)*. (Redrawn from an image provided courtesy of Shi Tang.)

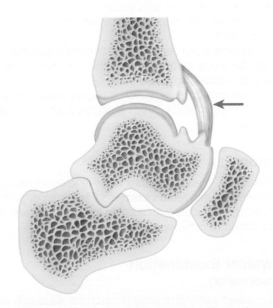

Fig 199.4 Thickened anterior ankle capsule with traction spur *(arrow)*, which can both act as impingement lesions. (Redrawn from an image provided courtesy of Shi Tang.)

Operative

- Ankle arthroscopy
- Open debridement or combination of arthroscopic and open
- Osteoplasty of tibia and talus

When to Refer

- Failed nonoperative management, including attempts at physical therapy (PT) to improve dorsiflexion

- Painful mechanical symptoms
- Unable to return to sport or obtain enough dorsiflexion for activities of daily living (ADLs) (i.e., stairs or job-specific motions; Fig. 199.5)

Prognosis

- Moderate to very successful
- Greater than 70% improvement with lower end of success if concomitant arthritis

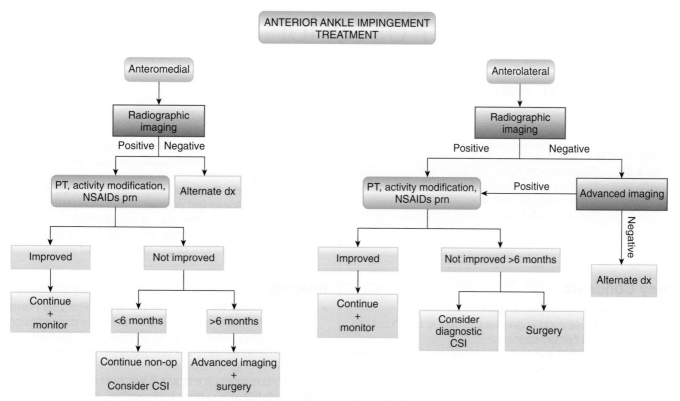

Fig 199.5 Treatment algorithm for anterior ankle impingement. *NSAID*, nonsteroidal antiinflammatory drug. (Courtesy of Turki Tallab.)

Troubleshooting

- Proceed to surgery if failed nonoperative management.
- May use corticosteroid injection (CSI) to assist in diagnosis as well as potential therapeutic benefits.
- Surgery may have modest success due to further fibrosis that may occur and cause recurrent impingement.
- Osteoplasty is not always accessible through the arthroscopic approach.
- Recovery may be slower/delayed with open approach, with inherent risks including nerve injury, stiffness, recurrence.

Patient Information

- Diagnosis is anterior ankle impingement syndrome that can be further divided to anteromedial or anterolateral most commonly.
- Minor injuries over a course of time or an acute injury

- Usually hypertrophy of soft-tissue or bony overgrowth/osteophytes in the front of the ankle causing pain and stiffness
- Initially treat with activity modification, PT, and bracing.
- Imaging can help decipher cause and location, as well as definitively diagnose.
- Can always refer to specialist if nonsurgical management fails

Suggested Readings

van Dijk CN. Anterior and posterior ankle impingement. *Foot Ankle Clin.* 2006;11(3):663–683.

van Dijk CN, Tol JL, Verheven CC. A prospective study of prognostic factors concerning the outcome of arthroscopic surgery for anterior ankle impingement. *Am J Sports Med.* 1997;25(6):737–745.

Vaseenon T, Amendola A. Update on anterior ankle impingement. *Curr Rev Musculoskelet Med.* 2012;5(2):145–150.

Chapter 200 Posterior Impingement

Sonya Ahmed, Alan Shahtaji

ICD-10-CM CODES
M26.82   *Posterior soft-tissue impingement*
S92.13   *Fracture of posterior process of talus*
M65.879 *Other synovitis and tenosynovitis, unspecified ankle and foot*

Key Concepts

- Ankle pain worse in plantar flexion
- Relatively uncommon in general population but increased prevalence in certain sports
- Impingement can be osseous (more common) or soft tissue
- May be a due to repeated plantar flexion or due to a single, acute traumatic event
- Bony contributors include os trigonum or Stieda process (posterolateral process of talus; Figs. 200.1 and 200.2)

History
Chronic

- Those sports featuring repeated plantar flexion, such as dance, ballet (especially en pointe), gymnastics, soccer, and downhill runners
- Also inquire generally:
  - May have history of repeated ankle sprains → anterior laxity → increased impingement posteriorly
  - Previous ankle injuries or surgeries can increase risk for impingement
    - Scar tissue
    - Bony fragments
    - Malalignment

Acute

- Forced plantar flexion injury causing posterior hindfoot or "ankle" pain. May have pain and swelling in hindfoot a few weeks after injury.
- Most commonly a fracture of the posterior process of the talus (Fig. 200.3).

Physical Examination

- Difficult to reproduce symptoms and often hard to diagnose
  - Observation: possibly posterior swelling in retrocalc area or hindfoot. Usually no skin breakdown or dimpling.
  - Palpation: posterior heel or with posterior squeeze behind the ankle. Pain recreated with forced plantarflexion (PF). Pain with en pointe position or heel raise. Palpate flexor hallucis longus (FHL) during great toe motion: if painful, can indicate FHL involvement (Fig. 200.4).

- Range of motion: dorsiflexion normal but may cause a "stretch" feeling. Guarded plantarflexion and potentially less due to pain.
- Special tests: Posterior pinch test with ankle in plantarflexion. Howse test positive when forced plantarflexion and rotation of calcaneus cause pain and symptoms. Guided corticosteriod injection (CSI) or local anesthetic around os trigonum or posterior subtalar joint.

Imaging

- Weight-bearing three views of the ankle. Possible Harris view can be obtained. Possible en pointe or plantarflexion weight-bearing lateral x-ray to evaluate impingement.
  - Can demonstrate prominent Stieda process, os trigonum, osteophytes, or fracture.
- Magnetic resonance imaging (MRI): best exam to evaluate both soft-tissue and bony impingement. Identifies swelling, effusion, bony edema in the os trigonum, as well as soft-tissue impingement and accessory/anomalous structures.
- Ultrasound: can look at tarsal tunnel and identify some soft-tissue pathology as well as bony abnormalities. Dynamic imaging can be utilized. Operator dependent.
- Computed tomography (CT): beneficial in acute vs chronic or os trigonum. Fracture edges versus well-rounded edges.
- Bone scan: can be beneficial if no uptake in os trigonum concluding likely not source of posterior pain.

Differential Diagnosis

- Ankle arthritis
- Subtalar arthritis
- Achilles tendinopathy—insertional, noninsertional, and peritendinitis
- Retrocalcaneal bursitis
- Calcaneal stress fracture
- Avascular necrosis (AVN) talus or calcaneus
- FHL tendinitis
- Posterior tarsal tunnel syndrome

Treatment
Nonoperative

- In general—activity modification to avoid plantar flexion and offload the area of impingement
- Acute injuries may respond to short course of nonsteroidal antiinflammatory drugs (NSAIDs), rest, and immobilization (boot), followed by physiotherapy.
- Chronic injuries have variable success with conservative treatment. Bracing is often not effective.
  - Rest
  - Activity modification

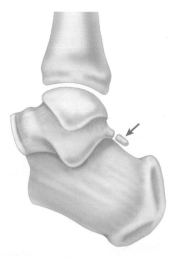

Fig 200.1 Os trigonum. (Redrawn from an image provided courtesy Shi Tang.)

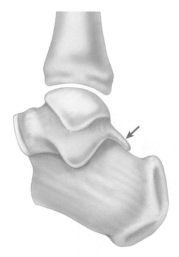

Fig 200.2 Prominent posterior Stieda process. (Redrawn from an image provided courtesy Shi Tang.)

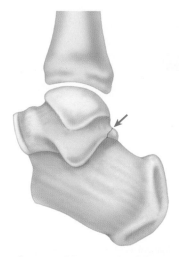

Fig 200.3 Acute fracture of the posterior taller process. (Redrawn from an image provided courtesy Shi Tang.)

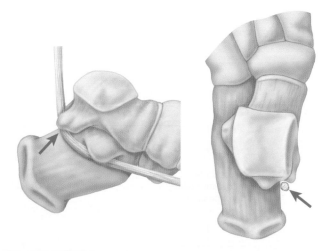

Fig 200.4 FHL tendon (*arrows*) and its proximity to the posterior talar process in the differential diagnosis for posterior ankle impingement. (Redrawn from an image provided courtesy Shi Tang.)

- NSAIDs as needed for pain/inflammation
- Physiotherapy
- Orthotics and footwear modification
- Corticosteroid and/or anesthetic injections may be useful for both diagnostic and therapeutic purposes, and can be done with ultrasound or fluoroscopic guidance. These may also be employed for high-level athletes who need to complete their season before more definitive management (Fig. 200.5).

Operative

- Surgical excision of os trigonum arthroscopically or open
- Concurrent management of FHL tendon and debridement with posteromedial incision or arthroscopically

When to Refer

- When failed nonoperative modalities such as injections or physical therapy after 3 to 6 months of attempts
- When uncertain of diagnosis

Prognosis

- Nonoperative prognosis is 50%. 85% surgical success rates with potentially longer recovery, especially with wound healing with open procedures. Potential sural nerve injuries/neurapraxia possible. Symptoms >2 years have lower likelihood of improvement.

Troubleshooting

- Treat nonoperatively for 3 to 6 months and can use injections for diagnosis and therapeusis.
- Surgery not risk-free, including scarring, nerve injury, and stiffness
- May be done arthroscopically or open, with potentially more complications with open procedure

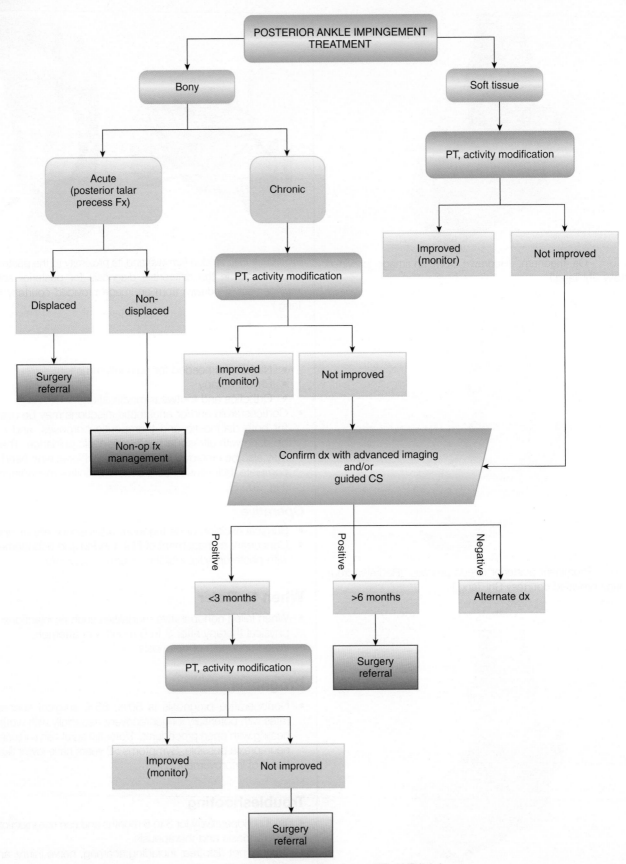

Fig 200.5 Treatment algorithm for posterior ankle impingement. (Courtesy of Turki Tallab.)

Patient Instructions

- Diagnosis is posterior ankle impingement syndrome (PAIS).
- Minor injuries over a course of time or an acute injury
- Usually from a prominent bone or overgrowth of soft tissue in the back of the ankle causing pain when the toe is pointed down
- Initially treat with activity modification, PT, and medications if needed.
- Imaging can help identify the cause of the impingement.
- Sometimes an injection can help confirm the cause of the pain and may treat the problem.
- Can always refer to specialist if nonsurgical management fails

Suggested Readings

Lavery KP, McHale KJ, Rossy WH, Theodore G. Ankle impingement. *J Orthop Surg Res*. 2016;11(1):97.

Maquirriain J. Posterior ankle impingement syndrome. *J Am Acad Orthop Surg*. 2005;13(6):365–371.

Watkins L. *Watkins' Manual of Foot and Ankle Medicine and Surgery*. 4th ed. Philadelphia: Wolters Kluwer; 2017.

Chapter 201 Ankle Aspiration and/or Injection Technique

Venkat Perumal, George Lee Wilkinson III

CPT CODE
20605 *Arthrocentesis, aspiration, and/or injection; intermediate joint or bursa*

Procedure Name

- Ankle aspiration (arthrocentesis) and injection

Equipment

- Sterile tray
- Sterile cup and/or laboratory tubes for aspiration
- Sterile gloves
- Sterile prep solution
- 25-gauge needle and local anesthetic agent if local anesthesia is planned
- Ethyl chloride (optional)
- Injectable agent (steroid or local anesthetic agent)
- 21-gauge injection needle
- 5 to 10 mL injection syringe
- 16 to 18 gauge large-bore aspiration needle
- 10 to 20 mL aspiration syringe
- Stopcock (for combined aspiration and injection)
- Sterile gauze and bandage

Indications

- Injection
  - Osteoarthritis
  - Rheumatoid arthritis
  - Crystalloid deposition disease
- Aspiration
  - Suspected joint infection
  - Gouty arthritis
  - Large painful effusion
  - Loss of motion secondary to effusion

Contraindications

- Injection
  - Impending surgical procedure
  - Overlying skin disease
  - Recent or active joint infection
- Aspiration
  - Generalized sepsis without evidence of infected joint

Technique (Video 201.1)

- The correct limb is identified, and verbal consent is obtained from the patient after discussing risks and benefits (Fig. 201.1).
- Subcutaneous injections of corticosteroids can cause atrophy.
- There is a possibility of injury to the terminal branches of the superficial peroneal or saphenous nerves.
- The medication is prepared on a sterile tray.
- Medication used is left to the discretion of physician; author prefers a cocktail consisting of equal parts of lidocaine with triamcinolone, which is intermediate acting (40 mg/ml).
- A stopcock and extra syringe are added to the tray if aspiration is indicated.
  - While wearing sterile gloves, the sterile prep solution is applied to prepare the skin (Fig. 201.2).
  - Ethyl chloride is administered topically if it is being used (Fig. 201.3).
  - If an aspiration is being performed, a small needle is used to infiltrate the skin with local anesthetic.
  - An aspiration needle is passed into the ankle either medially or laterally.
  - In the **lateral** approach, the needle is inserted between the anterior border of the lateral malleolus and the extensor digitorum longus tendons at the level of the joint line.
  - In the **medial** approach, the needle is directed between the anterior border of the medial malleolus and the medial border of tibialis anterior tendon at the level of the joint line (Fig. 201.4).
- A **posterior** approach is not recommended, as it is difficult and can damage the articular surface.
- Once the needle has passed into the joint capsule, aim across the joint to facilitate the procedure.
- Gentle pressure is then applied to the plunger to aspirate any fluid.
- Synovial fluid obtained here can be sent for cultures, and steroid injections should be avoided.
- A stopcock can be used to allow the same needle to be used for injection once finished with the aspiration.
- Once certain the needle tip is unblocked and in the joint capsule, inject the steroid or local anesthetic preparation.
- Apply dressing (Fig. 201.5).

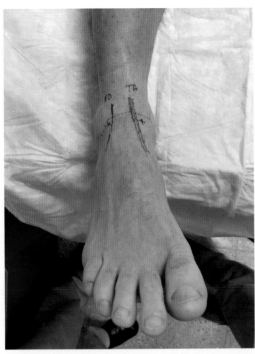

Fig 201.1 Anatomy front of the ankle with time out and marking. Tibialis anterior and extensor digitorum marked.

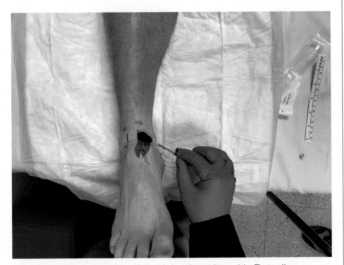

Fig 201.2 Preparation of the injection site with Betadine.

Considerations in Special Populations

- In dark-skinned individuals, skin discoloration can occur.
- A temporary elevation in blood sugar level can occur in diabetic patients.

Troubleshooting

- If you are unable to aspirate any fluid, ensure that you are in the synovial capsule and push the plunger to remove any potential blockages.
- If you feel as if you are bumping the needle into bone, redirect the needle into the joint space.

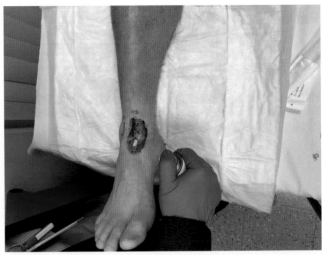

Fig 201.3 Local anesthetic spray application to the injection site.

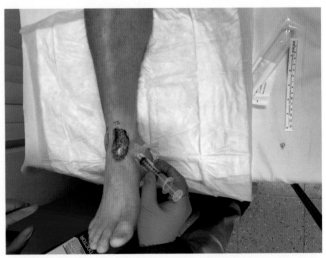

Fig 201.4 Injection of corticosteroid. Anteromedial entry between tibialis anterior tendon and the medial malleolus.

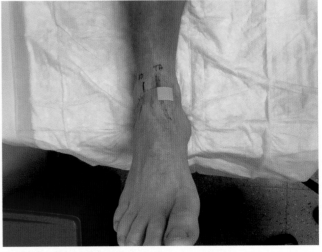

Fig 201.5 Dressing after injection.

Patient Instructions

- Allow the bandage to remain in place for 1 day.
- Use ice to treat and soreness about the site of the injection.
- An increase in pain can occur in the days immediately following the injection, but this usually resolves on its own.
- Patients are to contact the office immediately if an increase in redness, warmth, swelling, or pain occurs, or if they begin to experience fever or chills.

Suggested Readings

Metcalfe S, Reilly I. *Foot and Ankle Injection Techniques. A Practical Guide.* Philadelphia: Elsevier; 2010.

Tallia AF, Cardone DA. Diagnostic and therapeutic injection of the ankle and foot. *Am Fam Physician.* 2003;68(7):1356–1362.

Chapter 202 Plantar Fascia Injection

W. Bret Smith, Matthew J. Pacana

CPT CODES
20550 *Injection(s); single tendon sheath, or ligament, aponeurosis (e.g., plantar "fascia")*
76942 *Ultrasonic guidance for needle placement (e.g., biopsy, aspiration, injection, localization device), imaging supervision and interpretation*

Procedure Name

- Plantar fascia injection

Equipment

- Injection syringe (5–10 mL)
- Needle (22–25 gauge), 1.5 inches
- Local anesthetic agent: Lidocaine (1–2%) or bupivacaine (0.25–0.5%)
- Corticosteroid: triamcinolone acetonide (Kenolog) or methylprednisolone (Depo-Medrol) or Celestone
- Sterile tray
- Sterile gloves
- Sterile prep solution
- Sterile gauze and bandage
- Ultrasound transducer and monitor (6–13 MHz high-frequency linear array US probe)
- Ultrasound jelly and sterile sleeve

Indications

- Symptoms persist after more than 8 weeks of conservative management to decrease inflammation. Conservative measures include stretching, orthotics, nonsteroidal antiinflammatory drugs (NSAIDs, night splinting.

Risks

- Skin atrophy and hypopigmentation, soft-tissue atrophy, infection, bleeding, and failure to provide relief
- Bleeding or bruising can occur in patients with bleeding disorders or those on anticoagulation medicine. Remember to check an International Normalized Ratio (INR) and take appropriate medical history for patients who may have a history of a clotting disorder, have liver failure, or are taking anticoagulation agents.
- Rupture of the plantar fascia may occur in approximately 10% of patients after repeat injection.
- Lateral plantar nerve injury is a possible complication if the local anesthetic is injected either close to or within the nerve itself.
- Minimal risks of ultrasound assistance

Contraindications

- Infection
- Anesthetic allergy
- Steroid allergy

Technique (Video 202.1)

- Obtain verbal/written consent and identify correct foot.
- Prepare the injection supplies: aspirate a mixture of 2 mL of local anesthetic agent and 1 mL of steroid.
- Aseptic technique: The injection site is cleansed with appropriate topical antiseptic such as povidone-iodine or chlorhexidine. The planned site of injection and posterior foot are draped with sterile towels.
- Palpate and locate the most tender spot—usually the anterior aspect of the medial plantar calcaneus (Fig. 202.1). Palpate the most anterior aspect of the medial plantar calcaneal tubercle, and insert the needle at this site.

Ultrasound Guided Injection
Advantages

- Ultrasound allows direct visualization of the plantar structures and may assist in accuracy with proper technique. Some studies demonstrate lower recurrence of similar symptoms.
- Visualization in obese individuals and patients in which there is difficulty palpating point of maximal tenderness.

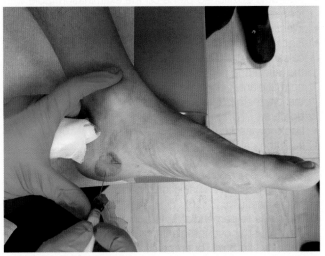

Fig 202.1 Injection of the plantar fascia utilizing a palpation technique. (From Tallia AF, Cardone DA. Diagnostic and therapeutic injection of the ankle and foot. *Am Fam Physician*. 2003;68[7]: 1356–1362.)

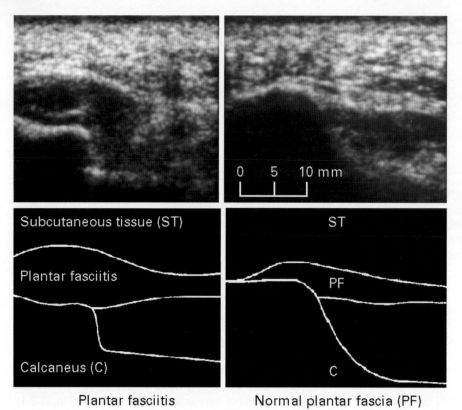

Plantar fasciitis   Normal plantar fascia (PF)

Labels in figure: Subcutaneous tissue (ST), Plantar fasciitis, Calcaneus (C); ST, PF, C; 0 5 10 mm

Fig 202.2 A 7.5 Mhz linear array ultrasound transducer is positioned longitudinally in the midline of the left heel and demonstrates normal plantar fascia with regular fibrillar echotexture. On the right heel, the transducer has been positioned longitudinally over the region of maximal thickness of the plantar fascia, which is grossly thickened with reduced echogenicity. There is loss of definition of fibrillar echotexture and of the fascial borders distal to the anterior border of the calcaneus. (From Kane D, Greaney T, Bresnihan B, Gibney R, FitzGerald O. Ultrasound guided injection of recalcitrant plantar fasciitis. *Ann Rheum Dis*. 1998;57[6]: 383–384.)

Disadvantages

- There is a learning curve to proper ultrasound use. This includes both identifying structures as well as identification of the inserted needle in relation to anatomic structures.

Ultrasound Guided Technique

- Patient is positioned prone on the examination table with foot in dorsiflexion to best define fascial borders.
- Injection site is prepped as described previously.
- Find the longitudinal axis of the heel by looking for the calcaneus, plantar fascia, and changes in echogenicity of the fascia and perifascial edema (Fig. 202.2). On the right, normal plantar fascia demonstrates linear echotexture. On the left, there is thickening, loss of definition, and indistinct borders.
- Look for fascial thickness >4.0 mm about 10 to 15 mm from the calcaneus and mark the thickest portion at skin level.
- Injection is given in an out-of-plane fashion. Injection given in same position as palpation technique on the medial side of the heel (Fig. 202.3).
- Insert needle perpendicular to skin and parallel to the probe aiming just above the plantar fascia (Fig. 202.4).
- Deposit 1 to 3 mL of prepared solution at the level of the plantar fascia, avoiding the fat superficially and the calcaneal insertion to lower the risk of fascial rupture and atrophy.
- Save imaging prior to and after insertion of medicine if able.

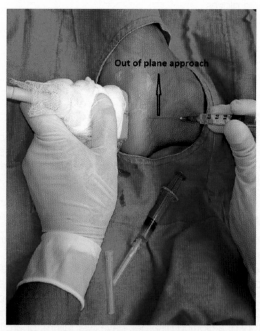

Out of plane approach

Fig 202.3 Out-of-plane injection for plantar fasciitis. The needle is entered in an out-of-plane approach from the medial side. The *arrow* shows the point of needle entry in an out-of-plane approach. (From Nair AS, Sahoo RK. Ultrasound-guided injection for plantar fasciitis: a brief review. *Saudi J Anaesth*. 2016;10[4]:440–443.)

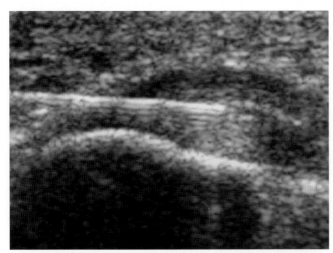

Fig 202.4 Hyperechoic deposit seen in fibers of the plantar fascia. (From Kane D, Greaney T, Bresnihan B, Gibney R, FitzGerald O. Ultrasound guided injection of recalcitrant plantar fasciitis. *Ann Rheum Dis*. 1998;57[6]:383–384.)

Postinjection Care and Instructions

- Remain supine for several minutes and in office for 30 minutes to confirm no adverse reactions to injection.
- Avoid full weight-bearing and strenuous activity for approximately 48 hours postinjection to prevent discomfort.

- Caution patients regarding possible worsening of symptoms 24 to 48 hours after injection, which can be treated with rest, ice, elevation, and antiinflammatory medication like ibuprofen and naproxen.
- Plan for follow-up examination in 3 to 4 weeks.

Suggested Readings

Ball EM, McKeeman HM, Patterson C, et al. Steroid injection for inferior heel pain: a randomised controlled trial. *Ann Rheum Dis*. 2013;72(6):996–1002.

Barkdull TJ, O'Connor FG, McShane JM. Joint and soft tissue aspiration and injection (arthrocentesis). In: Pfenninger JL, Fowler GC, eds. *Pfenninger & Fowler's Procedures for Primary Care*. 3rd ed. Philadelphia: Elsevier; 2011:1303–1321.

Chen CM, Chen JS, Tsai WC, et al. Effectiveness of device-assisted ultrasound-guided steroid injection for treating plantar fasciitis. *Am J Phys Med Rehabil*. 2013;92(7):597–605.

Kane D, Greaney T, Bresnihan B, et al. Ultrasound guided injection of recalcitrant plantar fasciitis. *Ann Rheum Dis*. 1998;57(6):383–384.

McMillan AM, Landorf KB, Gilheany MF, et al. Ultrasound guided corticosteroid injection for plantar fasciitis: randomised controlled trial. *BMJ*. 2012;344:e3260.

Nair A, Sahoo R. Ultrasound-guided injection for plantar fasciitis: a brief review. *Saudi J Anaesth*. 2016;10(4):440–443.

Tsai WC, Wang CL, Tang FT, et al. Treatment of proximal plantar fasciitis with ultrasound-guided steroid injection. *Arch Phys Med Rehabil*. 2000;81(10):1416–1421.

Yucel I, Yazici B, Degirmenci E, et al. Comparison of ultrasound-, palpation-, and scintigraphy-guided steroid injections in the treatment of plantar fasciitis. *Arch Orthop Trauma Surg*. 2009;129(5):695–701.

Chapter 203 Morton Neuroma Injection

Brian D. Powell

CPT CODE
20600 *Arthrocentesis, aspiration and/or injection; small joint or bursa*

Procedure Name

- Morton neuroma injection

Equipment

- 25-gauge injection needle; 1.5-cm length
- Syringe (3–5 mL)
- Local anesthetic (1% lidocaine without epinephrine and 0.25% bupivacaine)
- Steroid solution (methylprednisolone [Depo-Medrol], triamcinolone acetonide [Kenalog], betamethasone [Celestone])
- Sterile tray
- Sterile gloves
- Sterile prep solution
- Ethyl chloride (topical anesthetic)
- Sterile gauze and bandage

Indications

- Painful interdigital neuroma (Morton neuroma) with persistent symptoms
- Commonly used in conjunction with other nonoperative modalities (nonsteroidal antiinflammatory drugs, metatarsal pads, orthoses, wide-toe box shoes)
- Diagnostic tool to confirm interdigital neuroma as the cause of forefoot pain

Contraindications

- Local infection
- Open wound
- Compromised skin

Technique (Video 203.1)

- Verbal consent is obtained, and the correct extremity is identified.
- The patient is positioned supine with the knee supported underneath with a pillow. The ankle is in neutral position.
- The medication mixture of a local anesthetic agent and steroid is prepared on a sterile tray—typically 2 mL of anesthetic agent (1 mL lidocaine and 1 mL bupivacaine) to 1 mL of steroid.
- The area of maximal tenderness is identified dorsal and proximal to the metatarsal heads (Fig. 203.1).
- Ethyl chloride spray (topical anesthetic) can be used for a topical anesthetic as desired.
- The skin is sterilely prepped.
- In a distal to proximal direction, the needle is advanced through the dorsal skin at a 45-degree angle between the metatarsal heads (Fig. 203.2).
- The needle is typically inserted 0.75 to 1 inch, which is slightly plantar to the metatarsal heads.
- Care should be taken to avoid overshooting the neuroma and inadvertently injecting the plantar fat pad, which can result in fat pad atrophy.
- The mixture is injected proximally and distally after the needle tip passes the deep transverse metatarsal ligament (Fig. 203.3).
- Apply a dressing.

Special Considerations

- Complete or partial pain relief is variable, with reported success rates as high as 80%.
- Repeat injections can be successful in alleviating pain, but at the risk of increased complications, including plantar fat pad atrophy, tendon or ligament rupture, dermal thickening, hyperpigmentation of the skin, and infection.
- If the injection fails to alleviate the pain, consider other causes of forefoot pain.

Troubleshooting

- If the metatarsal bone is struck, gently redirect the needle to find the intermetatarsal region.
- Patients with pes planus can be approached with a more perpendicular approach to the axis of the foot, whereas those with high arches will require a more lateral to medial approach to account for the angulation of the metatarsals (Fig. 203.4).

Patient Instructions

- The bandage can be removed later in the day.
- Use ice to treat any local soreness at the site.
- Diabetic patients may notice a slight transient increase in the blood glucose level.
- The physician's office should be called immediately if any purulent drainage, redness, warmth, increased swelling, fevers/chills develops, or if there is a severe increase in pain.

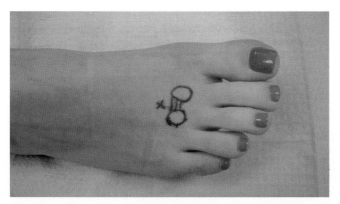

Fig 203.1 The area of maximal tenderness on the dorsum of the forefoot between the metatarsal heads *(marked with an X)*.

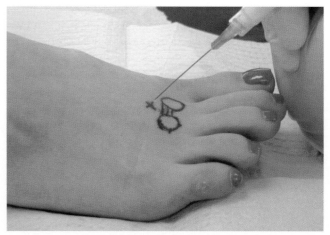

Fig 203.2 Angle of injection on the dorsal surface is shown.

Neuroma Injection

Can be given with local anesthetic without epinephrine and steroid

The nerve runs plantar to metatarsal heads

Avoid injecting the plantar fat pad, it can result in atrophy

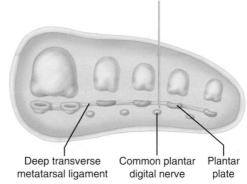

Deep transverse metatarsal ligament   Common plantar digital nerve   Plantar plate

Fig 203.3 Overview of a Morton neuroma injection with a diagram of the relative location of the metatarsal heads, the deep transverse ligament, and the location of the nerve.

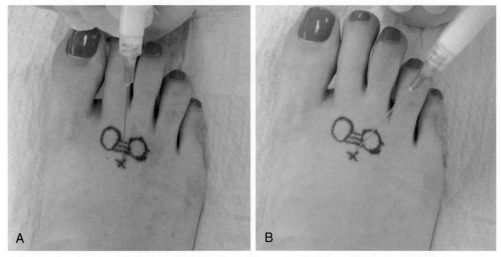

A   B

Fig 203.4 The relative angle of approach for a pes planus foot (A) versus that for a high arch foot (B).

- There may be painful symptoms after the local anesthetic wears off but prior to the steroid taking effect. It can take several days before the desired results are obtained.

Suggested Readings

Miller SD. Technique tip: forefoot pain: diagnosing metatarsophalangeal joint synovitis from interdigital neuroma. *Foot Ankle Int*. 2001;22:914–915.

Rasmussen MR, Kitaoka HB, Patzer GL. Nonoperative treatment of plantar interdigital neuroma with a single corticosteroid injection. *Clin Orthop Relat Res*. 1996;326:188–193.

Weinfeld SB, Myerson MS. Interdigital neuritis: diagnosis and treatment. *J Am Acad Orthop Surg*. 1996;4:328–335.

Chapter 204 Digital Block

Brian D. Powell

CPT CODE
64450 *Injection anesthetic agent; other peripheral nerve or branch*

Procedure Names
- Digital block (foot)
- Toe block

Equipment
- Sterile gloves
- Alcohol swab
- Iodine-based swab
- Ethyl chloride spray
- 10-mL syringe
- 18-gauge needle
- 25-gauge, 1.5-inch needle
- 1% lidocaine *without* epinephrine
- 0.25% bupivacaine *without* epinephrine
- 2 × 2-inch sterile gauze
- Small adhesive bandage

Indications
- Closed reduction of digit
- Nail procedures
- Laceration repair
- Debridement

Contraindications
- Allergy to anesthetic

Technique (Fig. 204.1)
- Mark the digit with your initials, obtain consent, and have an assistant perform a time-out confirming the planned procedure.
- Instruct the patient to lay supine with his or her foot at the edge of the examination table (Fig. 204.2). Place a mark on the dorsal skin on either side of the affected digit at the level of the metatarsal head.
- Using the 18-gauge needle, aspirate 5 mL of each 1% lidocaine without epinephrine and 0.25% bupivacaine without epinephrine into a 10-mL syringe. Aseptically exchange for a 25-gauge needle that is 1.5 inches in length.
- Prepare the dorsal skin over both marks in the usual sterile fashion.
- Use sterile gloves.
- Ethyl chloride spray (freeze spray) can be used as a topical anesthetic if desired.
- Introduce the needle perpendicularly to the skin on one side of the distal metatarsal for the intended toe. Advance the needle just plantar to the level of the metatarsal head (Fig. 204.3). Remember that the digital nerves are located more plantar than dorsal, so be sure that the needle is adequately advanced.
- Aspirate to prevent intravascular injection.
- Inject 3 mL at this location and an additional 2 mL while slowly withdrawing allowing subcutaneous infiltration dorsally proximal to the toe.

Fig 204.1 Overview of a digital block.

Digital Block

Using local anesthetic without epinephrine

Given at the level of the metatarsal heads

Done dorsal to plantar on either side of the metatarsal

The digital nerve is plantar to the metatarsal heads and an adequately sized needle should be used to reach

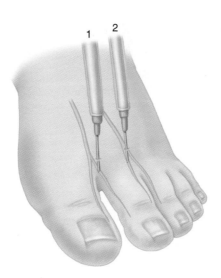

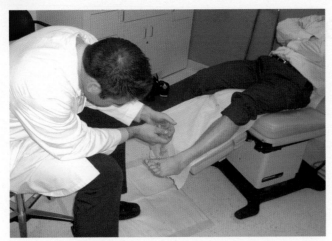

Fig 204.2 Patient and clinician are comfortably positioned for the injections.

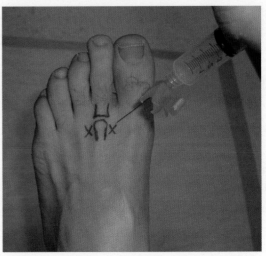

Fig 204.3 The needle should be directed perpendicular to the skin at the level of the metatarsal head.

- Repeat on the other side of the metatarsal head.
- Apply a dressing.

Special Considerations

- Toes adjacent to the injection site can have partial loss of sensation concomitantly. The patient should be reassured that this is normal.
- Use anesthetic agents without epinephrine. Injection of epinephrine near the digits may result in necrosis.

- When applying a dressing to an anesthetized toe, be sure that the dressing is not tight.

Patient Instructions

- Paresthesia can last an hour but may persist into the next day.
- Over-the-counter pain medicine can be used if there is tenderness as the injection site.

Chapter 205 Nail Removal

Joseph S. Park

CPT CODE
11730   *Removal of nail plate, partial or complete*

Procedure Name

- Removal of nail plate

Equipment

- Ethyl chloride (optional)
- 25-gauge needle
- 10-mL injection syringe
- Local anesthetic agent
- Sterile gloves
- Iodine solution
- Sterile fenestrated drape
- Small Penrose drain or wide rubber band
- Two small hemostats
- Periosteal elevator
- Nail splitter
- Iris scissors or equivalent
- Antibiotic ointment
- Sterile dressing
- Matricectomy supplies: electrosurgical unit, sharp instrument or sterile cotton-tip applicators, and phenol solution (88%)

Indications

- Partial removal
  - Onychocryptosis (ingrown toenail)
- Complete removal
  - Onychogryphosis (deformed, curved toenail)
  - Onychomycosis (fungal infection of nail)
  - Chronic or recurrent paronychia
  - Nail bed biopsy

Contraindications

- Nail plate removal:
  - Bleeding disorders: prolonged bleeding time
  - Dysvascular toe: gangrenous toe
  - Concern for malignancy (melanoma)
- Matricectomy: Active infection, cellulitis: All active infections should be eradicated before matricectomy to prevent seeding of deeper tissues or bone.

Technique

- Verbal patient consent is obtained, and the correct toe is identified.
- Chronic lateral onychocryptosis without evidence of deep infection or osteomyelitis will benefit from partial nail excision (Fig. 205.1A).
- Medication and supplies are prepared on a sterile tray or Mayo stand.
- The toe is washed and prepped with povidone-iodine solution, prepping proximal to the level of the metatarsophalangeal joint, and a fenestrated drape is applied.
  - Optional: Have an assistant anesthetize the skin with ethyl chloride at the injection site for a digital block.
- A digital block is performed (see Chapter 204).
  - Optional: Use a sterile rubber band, Penrose drain, or a cut piece of glove clasped tightly with a hemostat to act as a tourniquet at the level of the metatarsophalangeal joint.
- Grasp the toe in your nondominant hand and use a periosteal elevator to separate the eponychial fold (cuticle) from the dorsal aspect of the proximal nail plate.
- Slide the periosteal elevator, iris scissor, or small curved hemostat under the nail plate with gentle dorsal pressure, separating the nail matrix from the nail plate (Fig. 205.1B).
- The nail can now be elevated dorsal to the lateral nail fold (Fig. 205.1C).
- If removing only the lateral or medial fourth of the nail (as for onychocryptosis), incise the nail longitudinally with a nail splitter or strong scissors, taking care to avoid lacerating the underlying nail bed (Fig. 205.1D).
- Grasp the nail with a hemostat; remove the nail plate using gentle traction and elevation.
- If indicated in recurrent cases, perform matricectomy (ablation of germinal matrix) with a curette (Fig. 205.1F), electrocautery, sharp instrument (no. 15 scalpel or Beaver blade), or topical phenol (88% solution applied to germinal matrix with cotton-tipped applicator for 1–2 minutes). Oblique incisions at the medial or lateral edge of the proximal eponychial fold may improve visualization of the germinal matrix.
- Remove the tourniquet. Confirm hemostasis and apply antibiotic ointment or gauze and apply a sterile dressing (Fig. 205.1G and H).

Special Considerations

- Matricectomy decreases the recurrence rate of onychocryptosis but slightly increases the infection rate. Patients should

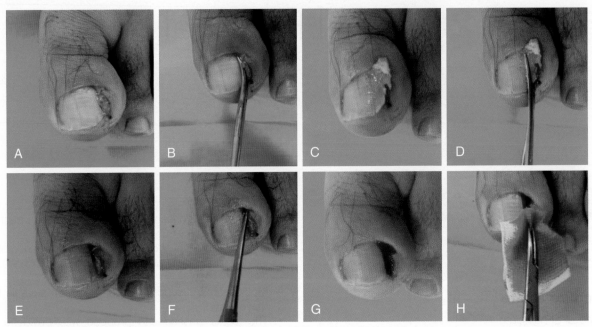

Fig 205.1 (A) Example of an ingrown nail on the lateral margin. (B) Hemostat used to separate the eponychial fold from the nail plate. (C) Hemostat used to bluntly elevate the nail from the nail bed. (D) Nail splitter used to cut nail longitudinally. (E) Nail is removed from underlying nail bed. (F) Curette used to excise nail bed, nail matrix, and granulation tissue. (G) Confirm hemostasis once tourniquet removed. (H) Antibiotic-soaked gauze, followed by compressive sterile dressing. (From Camurcu Y, Sofu H, Issin A, et al. Operative treatment of the ingrown toenail with a less-invasive technique: flashback to the original Winograd technique. *Foot Ankle Spec.* 2017 [Epub ahead of print].)

be counseled that after matricectomy, the nail will not regrow distal to the area of ablation. In the setting of a significant infection or recurrent disease, referral to a foot and ankle specialist should be considered. Formal matricectomy in the operating room may decrease the risk of chronic postoperative infection or osteomyelitis.

- If present, granulation tissue should be debrided back to normal tissue. This will leave a concavity that will gradually fill in over time.
- The development of increasing pain, swelling, or drainage suggests postprocedural infection, which usually responds to oral antibiotics. If there is continued concern for infection, surgical referral should be considered. Plain radiographs may reveal evidence of chronic osteomyelitis (erosions, sclerosis, cortical thickening); MRI may be indicated to evaluate for deep infection/osteomyelitis.
- After performing complete nail plate removal, adhesions may form between the nail fold and matrix, impairing the growth of a new nail plate. Interposing a part of the nail (cleansed with povidone-iodine) or a piece of packaging foil in this space for 3 weeks is recommended to prevent this complication. This material should be placed between the matrix and nail fold and sutured to the proximal nail fold using absorbable suture.

Patient Instructions

- The dressing can be removed in 48 to 72 hours; antibiotic ointment is applied daily for 2 weeks.

- For postprocedural pain, over-the-counter ibuprofen and acetaminophen are generally sufficient. A piece of dental floss under the advancing nail edge should be applied for the next few months to prevent recurrence of ingrown toenail.
- A brief course of oral antibiotics may be utilized after nail removal/ablation if active infection is present.
- If prolonged drainage or infection present, the patient should be seen at regular intervals (<1 week) until the condition improves. Referral to a foot and ankle specialist should be considered if there is no resolution despite local wound care and oral antibiotics.

Suggested Readings

Benjamin RB. Excision of ingrown toenail. In: Benjamin RB, eds. *Atlas of Outpatient and Office Surgery.* 2nd ed. Philadelphia: Lea & Febiger; 1994:357–359.

Kayalar M, Bal E, Toros T, et al. Results of partial matrixectomy for chronic ingrown toenail. *Foot Ankle Int.* 2011;32(9):888–895.

Quill G, Myerson M. A guide to office treatment of ingrown toenails. *Hosp Med.* 1994;30:51–54.

Sanders M. Marginal toenail ablation. In: Kitaoka HB, Ravin D, eds. *Masters Techniques in Orthopaedic Surgery: The Foot and Ankle.* 2nd ed. Philadelphia: Lippincott Williams & Wilkins; 2002:3–10.

Zuber TJ. Ingrown toenail removal. *Am Fam Physician.* 2002;65:2547–2552, 2554.

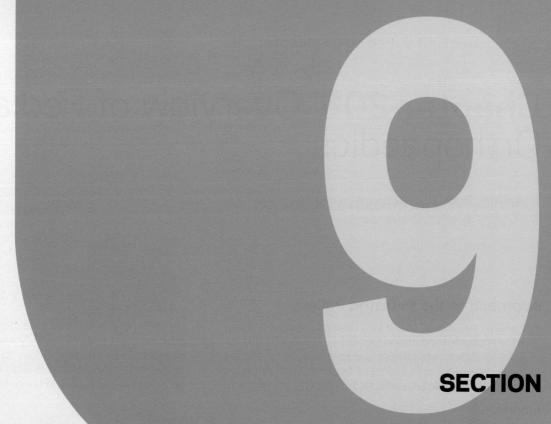

SECTION

9

Pediatric Orthopaedics

Chapter 206 Overview of Pediatric Orthopaedics

Jennifer A. Hart, Keith Bachmann

Approach to the Pediatric Patient

- Pediatric patients provide a very different interaction during an orthopaedic examination than is typical of adult patients. For this reason, we present a unique section to discuss these differences both in general terms and with regard to the conditions that are particular to this patient population.

Infants

- Because infants are unable to communicate their symptoms directly, one is forced to use visual cues and history points provided by the parents to make a diagnosis.
- Crying is nonspecific and may be the result of pain or fear during the examination but can be useful in localizing the problem.
- History and observation of the interaction between the parent(s) and child become even more important in this age group.

Toddlers

- Toddlers can be slightly more descriptive than infants but still do not have the full vocabulary to provide the information needed.
- Toddlers respond well to games (Fig. 206.1), so be firm but creative to make the experience fun and less frightening for them. A simple game of "Simon says" can go a long way to getting a full examination from a cooperative toddler (Fig. 206.2).

Young Children

- Young children can be a difficult group to examine because they have developed the memory necessary to be afraid of health care providers.
- Explain what you are going to do before you do it for every step of the examination. The child will be less frightened if he or she does not feel that he or she is being tricked into something painful. They might also respond to mimicry, allowing them to perform a similar exam or demonstrating on a parent prior to the child.

Adolescents

- For some health care professionals, adolescents prove to be the hardest group to work with because they are often reluctant to communicate personal feelings, including pain and experiences, to someone with whom they are unfamiliar, and the parents are often no longer as deeply informed as they were in the younger children.

- Be open and up front about the examination and the potential diagnoses.
- Be aware of the fact that an adolescent patient is not an adult with the level of maturity necessary to understand everything that you might have to say, but be respectful of the fact that he or she is likely old enough to want to be an active participant in his or her care.

History

- For most young children, the history will come from the parents.
- For cases of trauma, try to find someone who witnessed the injury to collect detailed information regarding when the accident happened, the mechanism of injury, and the forces involved.
- For nontraumatic conditions, ask questions about the timing, apparent location, and frequency of pain. Ask about any patterns the parents have noticed and any history of similar difficulty.
- For many conditions, especially congenital deformities, a detailed pregnancy and birth history will be helpful, as well as information on family members with similar disorders.
- Finally, do not make the mistake of discounting the child's own contributions to the history. Although usually unable to provide the complete history that you need, a child's ability to communicate is often underestimated.

Physical Examination

- Inspection and palpation
  - Inspection should begin the first time that you see the patient, even if that is in the parking lot, waiting room, or the hallway of the office.
  - Useful information regarding gait abnormalities, movement disorders, and parental interaction can be obtained simply by observing the child walking and playing in the examination room (Fig. 206.3).
  - There are a variety of congenital and acquired deformities for which patients seek orthopaedic care. Each deformity should be carefully evaluated and compared with the other side. The use of digital photography or measurement may prove useful for later comparison.
- Range of motion and strength
  - Passive range of motion is much easier to test than active motion in the young child. Be creative and create a game by having the child mimic your own motions to

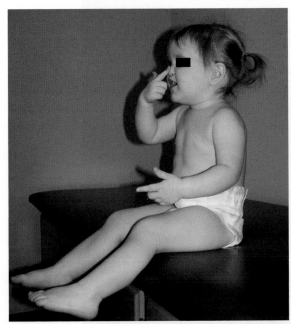

Fig 206.1 Toddlers and young children respond very well to games that can distract them from their natural fear and anxiety.

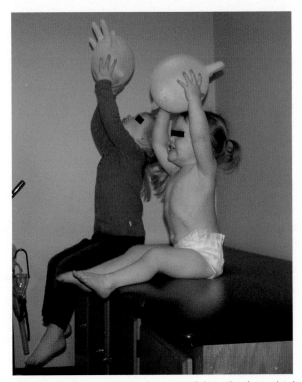

Fig 206.2 "Simon says" can be a useful method to obtain a cooperative toddler examination. Involving a sibling can also ease patient anxiety.

try to get an accurate idea of active joint motion and spasticity with movement.
- Strength can be tested in a similar manner. It may be useful to have one of the parents or caregivers help to demonstrate (Fig. 206.4).

- Special tests
  - Barlow test (Fig. 206.5)
  - Purpose: evaluation for congenital hip instability
  - How to perform: Flex the hips to 90 degrees with the examiner's thumbs along the medial thighs and the index finger along the lateral femur. Apply gentle pressure in the posterior direction at the knee.
  - Positive: indicated by a palpable "clunk" as the hip dislocates
  - Ortolani maneuver (Fig. 206.6)
  - Purpose: evaluation for congenital hip instability
  - How to perform: Gently abduct the hip while pushing anteriorly with the index finger over the greater trochanter.
  - Positive: indicated by a palpable "clunk" as the hip relocates
  - Galeazzi sign (Fig. 206.7)
  - Purpose: evaluation for congenital hip instability resulting in leg length difference after 3 months of age
  - How to perform: Flex the hip to 90 degrees and observe the location of the knees.
  - Positive: indicated by the knee on the affected side being lower
  - Thomas test (Fig. 206.8)
  - Purpose: evaluation for a flexion contracture of the hip
  - How to perform: With the patient lying supine, flex the opposite hip and knee up toward the chest to flatten the lumbar spine and correct anterior pelvic tilt.
  - Positive: indicated by the opposite hip remaining flexed because the patient will be unable to keep it extended on the table
  - Scoliosis (Adams) forward bend test (Fig. 206.9)
  - Purpose: evaluation for scoliosis
  - How to perform: Ask the patient to face away from you and, with his or her arms hanging in front of the body, bend forward as if trying to touch the toes until the spine is parallel with the floor.
  - Positive: indicated by an asymmetry of the rib cage, the degree of which can be measured using a scoliometer

Imaging

- Radiography
  - Evaluating radiographs in pediatric patients involves unique challenges due to the multiple physes in the growing skeleton.
  - Plain radiographs remain the mainstay of initial bony evaluation and, as always, should be ordered in at least two planes.
  - Stress radiographs may be necessary to evaluate for physeal injury as a result of local trauma.
  - Plain radiography is also useful in evaluating bone age when skeletal maturity is in question.
  - Typically a single view of the wrist, hand, and fingers is used and compared with age-related "normals" in an atlas such as that by Greulich and Pyle.
- Magnetic resonance imaging
  - Magnetic resonance imaging has been used with increased frequency to evaluate a variety of pediatric disorders because it can provide information about soft-tissue anatomy that is not as easily assessed with other available studies.

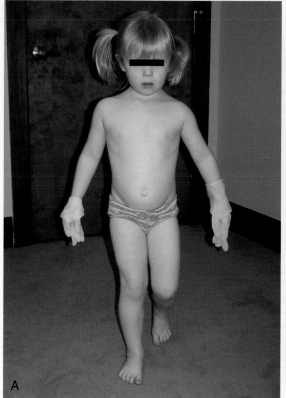

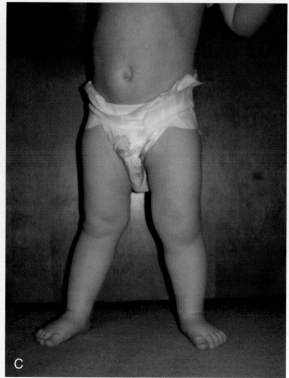

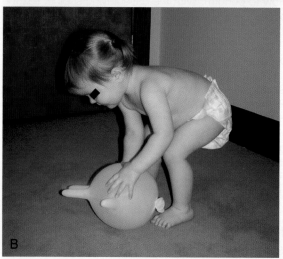

Fig 206.3 Observe the child walking **(A)**, playing **(B)**, and standing normally **(C)** for clues as to pain and movement abnormalities.

Fig 206.4 Having a parent demonstrate the activity can help with evaluation of range of motion and spasticity with movement.

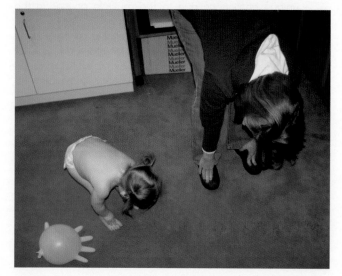

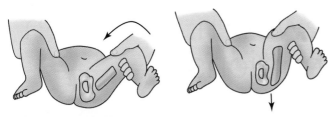

Fig 206.5 Barlow test.

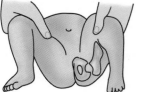

Fig 206.6 Ortolani test.

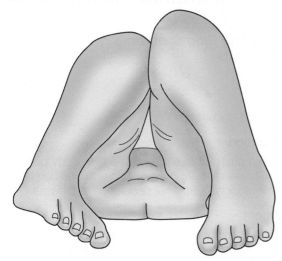

Fig 206.7 Galeazzi sign.

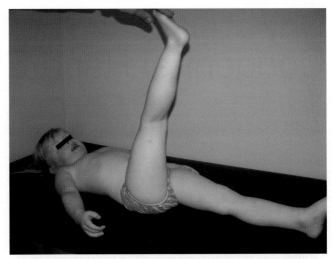

Fig 206.8 Thomas test.

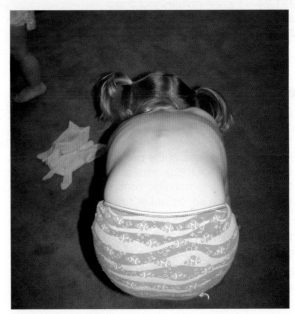

Fig 206.9 Scoliosis (Adams) forward bend test.

- It is especially useful in evaluating joint pathology such as cartilage disorders (osteochondritis dissecans), osteomyelitis, tumors, physeal injury, and soft-tissue spinal abnormalities.
- Computed tomography
  - Computed tomography has a much higher contrast resolution than traditional radiography and is most useful when evaluating traumatic bony lesions (fractures).
  - It also can be useful in evaluating physeal arrest where the three-dimensional anatomy can be better evaluated.
  - Other common uses are to evaluate and measure anatomic bony orientation (i.e., glenoid version, femoral anteversion, or tibial torsion).
- Ultrasonography
  - Ultrasonography is used in pediatric patients because it is safe, easy to perform, and very inexpensive compared with many other available tests.
  - It is primarily useful for evaluating such things as developmental dysplasia of the hip, the presence of joint effusion and hemarthrosis, and evaluating the various "lumps and bumps" that present for evaluation.

- Bone scan
  - Scintigraphy is a useful examination with a high sensitivity for bony abnormalities but a low specificity.
  - It is especially useful for evaluating tumors, bony metastasis, avascular necrosis, and trauma.
  - It can be especially useful in cases of suspected child abuse.

Suggested Readings

Darmonov AV, Zagora S. Clinical screening for congenital dislocation of the hip. *J Bone Joint Surg Am*. 1996;78A:383–388.

Greulich WW, Pyle SI. *Radiographic Atlas of Skeletal Development of the Hand and Wrist*. 2nd ed. Stanford, CA: Stanford University Press; 1959.

Hoppenfeld S. *Physical Examination of the Spine and Extremities*. Norwalk, CT: Appleton & Lange; 1976.

Storer SK, Skaggs DL. Pearls and pitfalls in the evaluation of pediatric congenital and developmental disorders. *Instr Course Lect*. 2006;55:615–623.

Weinstein SL, Flynn JM, eds. *Lovell and Winter's Pediatric Orthopaedics*. 7th ed. Philadelphia: Wolters Kluwer; 2014.

Chapter 207 The Newborn: Common Congenital Hand Conditions

Dan A. Zlotolow

ICD-10-CM CODES
Q70.9   *Syndactyly*
P02.8   *Constriction ring syndrome*
Q69.9   *Polydactyly (duplication)*
M20.00   *Common digital deformities*
M21.24   *Flexion deformity of finger*
M65.31   *Congenital trigger thumb*
Q71.4   *Radial club hand*

Key Concepts

- Congenital hand deformities affect approximately 1 in 500 newborns.
- Parents must grieve for a child with a difference as if they had lost a child (loss of the perfect child).
- Beware of associated anomalies in other organ systems.
- Unless the limb is ischemic or at risk, most children can be referred to a specialist by 3 months of age.

Specific Conditions
Syndactyly (Fig. 207.1)
Key Concepts

- Failure of digital separation
- Frequency is 1 in 2000 births
- More common in males; both hands involved 50% of the time

History

- Apparent at birth
- May have history of other affected family members (autosomal dominant pattern)

Examination

- Fingers may be joined simply by a skin bridge, or conjoined digits may share nail and bone elements.
- The middle/ring web is the most common site.

Studies

- Radiographs may help to define the shared bony elements between the digits.

Associated Conditions

- Sympolydactyly
- Symbrachydactyly
- Chest wall deformities (Poland syndrome)

- Apert syndrome
- Constriction ring syndrome (acrosyndactyly)

Treatment

- Border digits (thumb and small finger) are released sooner to prevent finger deformity (6–9 months of age).
- Central digits can wait until 18 months of age or older if no tethering.

Constriction Ring Syndrome
Key Concepts

- Occurs in 1 in 15,000 births

History

- Sporadic occurrence

Examination

- A deep crease that encircles a digit or body part
- May cause vascular or lymphatic drainage compromise
- Acrosyndactyly (proximal perforation at the web spaces)

Treatment

- If the vascular supply of the body part is compromised, urgent surgical release of the crease is necessary.
- Z-plasties and excision of the bands improve appearance and lymphatic drainage.

Polydactyly (Duplication) (Figs. 207.2 and 207.3)
Key Concepts

- Three types: thumb (preaxial), central, and small finger (postaxial)

History

- Preaxial (thumb) can be associated with other congenital anomalies such as ulnar deficiency.
- Central often has associated syndactyly (sympolydactyly) and has autosomal dominant transmission.
- Postaxial incidence in black population is 1 in 300 births, while incidence in white population is 1 in 3000 births (consider Ellis-van Creveld syndrome).

Treatment

- Thumb duplication requires reconstruction because neither thumb is normal in size and may be sharing or missing elements.
- The central duplication type requires surgical reconstruction.
- Ulnar-side polydactyly may present with a small nubbin or skin tag that can be ligated at the base soon after birth.

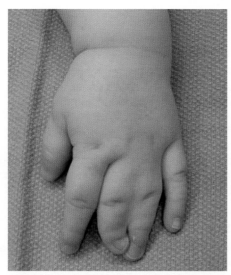

Fig 207.1 Syndactyly. (Courtesy Shriners Hospital of Lexington, Lexington, KY.)

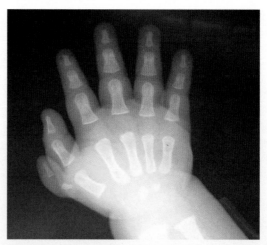

Fig 207.3 Radial polydactyly. (Courtesy Shriners Hospital of Lexington, Lexington, KY.)

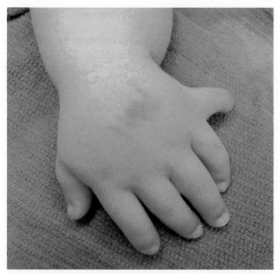

Fig 207.2 Ulnar polydactyly. (Courtesy Shriners Hospital of Lexington, Lexington, KY.)

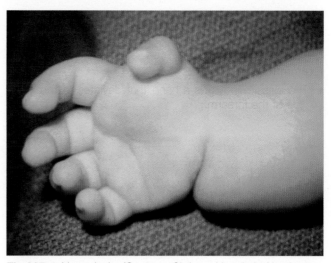

Fig 207.4 Hypoplasia. (Courtesy Shriners Hospital of Lexington, Lexington, KY.)

Common Digital Deformities

- Camptodactyly
  - Flexion deformity of the proximal interphalangeal joint; usually treated by splinting and stretching, unless deformity is severe. Surgical treatment includes volar Z-plasty, flexor digitorum superficialis (FDS) tenotomy, and/or application of a digit widget (Hand Biomechanics Lab, Sacramento, CA)
- Clinodactyly
  - Angular digital deformity thought to be due to an abnormally shaped middle phalanx
  - Treatment is surgical osteotomy if the deformity is severe.
  - Can be seen in as many as 79% of patients with Down syndrome
- Kirner deformity
  - Flexion and angular deformity of the distal phalanx
  - Often bilateral
  - Usually no treatment needed

Common Thumb Conditions

- Hypoplasia
  - "Short thumb," which is staged from type I (small with all anatomic elements present) to type V (total absence)
  - Surgery may be needed for the more severe types (Fig. 207.4).
- Congenital trigger thumb
  - One of the most common pediatric hand conditions seen
  - Presents as a flexion posture of the interphalangeal joint
  - Can be confused with clasped thumb (metacarpophalangeal joint flexion contracture)
  - Many cases resolve by 3 years of age; if not, surgical release gives good functional results.

Radial Clubhand (Fig. 207.5)
Key Concepts

- Four clinical types that vary from a short radial bone to the complete absence of the radius
- Occurs in 1 in 100,000 live births

9

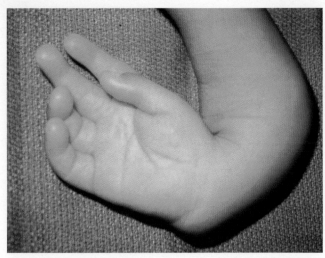

Fig 207.5 Radial clubhand. (Courtesy Shriners Hospital of Lexington, Lexington, KY.)

History
- Fifty percent of cases are bilateral; most cases occur sporadically.

Examination
- The classic finding is a hand that deviates to the radial side of the forearm.

- The remaining ulna is short and bowed; the thumb may be absent.

Associated Conditions
- Aplastic (Fanconi) anemia, thrombocytopenia, and cardiac anomalies, spine anomalies, renal anomalies, tracheo-esophageal fistula, imperforate anus

Treatment
- Depends on the severity of deformity
  - Mild cases respond to stretching and splinting.
  - More severe cases may benefit from surgical repositioning of the hand on the forearm.

Acknowledgment

The author acknowledges Dr. Scott A. Riley who authored this chapter in the previous edition.

Suggested Readings

Flatt AE. *The Care of Congenital Hand Anomalies*. 2nd ed. St. Louis: Quality Medical Publishing; 1994.

Gallant GG, Bora FW Jr. Congenital deformities of the upper extremity. *J Am Acad Orthop Surg*. 1996;4:162–171.

Kozin SH, Zlotolow DA. Common pediatric congenital conditions of the hand. *Plast Reconstr Surg*. 2015;136(2):241e–257e.

Chapter 208 The Newborn: Congenital Lower Extremity Disorders

Mark J. Romness

ICD-10-CM CODES
Q72 *Reduction defects of the lower limb*
Q73 *Reduction defects of unspecified limb*
Q74 *Other congenital malformations of limb(s)*

Key Concepts

- The history and physical examination continue to be the most important tools for assessment.
- Deficiencies of the long bones can range from mild shortening or bowing to complete absence with multiple etiologies (Fig. 208.1).
- Proper diagnosis of the etiology is important for genetic counseling, management, and prediction of progression.
- Isolated hemihyperplasia (previously known as hemihypertrophy) is associated with intra-abdominal tumors in 6% of the cases, including Wilms tumor and hepatoblastoma, so screening exams are required.
- Tibial deficiencies (previously known as tibial hemimelia) are important to distinguish from fibular deficiencies (previously known as fibular hemimelia) in that tibial deficiencies have an autosomal dominant inheritance pattern.

History

- The family often reports some difference noted since birth.
- Major deficiencies are often diagnosed at birth.
- Milder cases may not present until further growth and development uncover the deformity.

Physical Examination

- Accurate assessment of extremity deformity is critical to both diagnosis and treatment.
- All components of the deformity need to be considered, including structural or static deformity and functional or dynamic deformity.
- Structural deformity includes length, rotation, and angular deformity in the frontal, transverse, and sagittal planes.
- Functional impairments include motion, strength, and motor control problems that result in abnormal posturing and an effective deficiency.

Imaging

- Standard radiographs remain the primary method of assessment.

- Full-length standing radiographs (teleroentgenograms) in both the frontal and sagittal planes provide a comprehensive assessment including bone and joint structure, alignment, and length (Fig. 208.2).

Additional Tests

- Genetic evaluation and testing are beneficial for diagnosis and family counseling.
- Isolated hemihyperplasia requires abdominal ultrasound scans every 3 months until 7 years of age and serum alpha-fetoprotein measurement every 3 months until 4 years of age to screen for Wilms tumor and hepatoblastoma.
- Computed tomography and magnetic resonance imaging have specific indications, depending on the condition.
- Computed tomography remains the best instrument to assess bone structure.
- Magnetic resonance imaging provides better definition of cartilage and soft-tissue structures.

Differential Diagnosis

- Hemihyperplasia
  - Be aware of Wilms tumor.
  - Multiple syndromes with hyperplasia:
    - Beckwith-Wiedemann syndrome (BWS)
    - Proteus syndrome
    - Neurofibromatosis Type 1
    - Mosaic trisomy eight
    - Disorders associated with vascular malformations including Klippel-Trenaunay syndrome and megalencephaly-cutis marmorata telangiectatica congenita
- Congenital short femur: proximal femoral focal deficiency
- Tibial deficiencies (hemimelia)
- Fibular deficiencies
- Terminal deficiencies (congenital amputations)
- Posteromedial apex tibial bowing
  - Associated with calcaneovalgus foot deformity
  - Small tibial length discrepancies with growth
- Anterolateral apex tibial bowing
  - Strong association with congenital pseudarthrosis of the tibia and neurofibromatosis (Fig. 208.3)

Treatment
At Diagnosis

- Proper diagnosis
- Family counseling

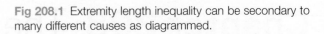

Fig 208.1 Extremity length inequality can be secondary to many different causes as diagrammed.

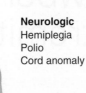

General
Hemihyperplasia
Wilms' and other intra-
   abdominal tumors
Beckwith-Wiedemann
   syndrome (BWS)
Proteus syndrome

Neurologic
Hemiplegia
Polio
Cord anomaly

Joints
Hip dislocation
Contractures

Vascular
Klippel-Trenaunay-Weber
   syndrome (KTWS)
Other vascular anomalies
Cardiac catheterization
Naevi

Physis
Growth arrest secondary
   to trauma, avascular
   necrosis

**Bone deficiencies
and dysplasias**
Ollier's disease
Fibrous dysplasia
Neurofibromatosis

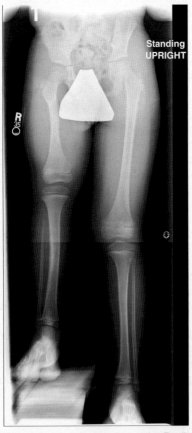

Standing UPRIGHT

Fig 208.2 Full-length standing radiograph. Radiograph taken from hip to ankle gives assessment of bone structure and development, including alignment, length, and formation. This radiograph shows multiple changes associated with a congenital short femur.

- Modifications to accommodate the deformity
  - Shoe lift
  - Bracing to support the extremity

Later
- Monitor change with growth
- Surgery for significant deformity or impairment

When to Refer

- If any significant visual deformity

Prognosis

- Depends on the diagnosis
- Influence on the adjacent joints portends outcome

Troubleshooting

- The small size of infant extremities makes it difficult to determine subtle differences between the limb development and positional influences. If there is sufficient concern, monitor with serial examinations and radiographs.
- Multiple syndromes have associated limb deficiencies, so genetic consult for diagnosis is beneficial to evaluation and treatment.

Patient Instructions

- Tibial deficiencies have an autosomal dominant genetic inheritance pattern.
- Congenital deficiencies are usually not genetic, but genetic counseling may be helpful to confirm this.

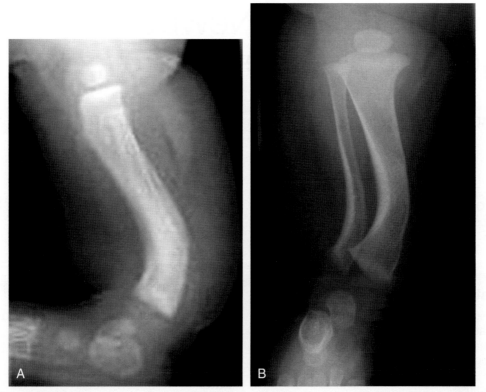

Fig 208.3 Posterior medial tibial bowing. The apex of the deformity is directed in the posterior direction on the lateral view (A) and in the medial direction on the anteroposterior view (B), which is not associated with neurofibromatosis and congenital pseudarthrosis. The amount of deformity in this child will likely be associated with a leg length discrepancy.

Suggested Readings

Edmondson AC, Kalish JM. Overgrowth syndromes. *J Pediatr Genet.* 2015;4(3):136–143.

Finch GD, Dawe CJ. Hemiatrophy. *J Pediatr Orthop.* 2003;23:99–101.

Koman LA, Meyer LC, Warren FH. Proximal femoral focal deficiency: natural history and treatment. *Clin Orthop Relat Res.* 1982;162:135–143.

Schoenecker PL, Capelli AM, Millar EA, et al. Congenital longitudinal deficiency of the tibia. *J Bone Joint Surg Am.* 1989;71A:278–287.

Chapter 209 The Newborn: Congenital Clubfeet

Mark J. Romness

ICD-10-CM CODE
Q66.0 *Congenital talipes equinovarus*

Key Concepts

- Spectrum of equinovarus deformity from mild to severe
- Rarely associated with other anomalies
- Incidence averages 1.24 per 1000 births
- Boys have twice the incidence of girls
- 50% bilateral
- Multifactorial cause
- Less operative treatment than previously when principles developed by Ponseti are followed

History

- Family history of clubfeet
- Clubfeet may be seen in the following neuromuscular conditions:
  - Myelomeningocele (spina bifida)
  - Arthrogryposis
  - Muscular dystrophy
  - Spinal muscular atrophy

Physical Examination (Fig. 209.1)

- Check the spine and hips.
- Rare leg length discrepancy with shortening on the clubfoot side
- Common calf atrophy
- Foot postured in equinus, varus, and adductus
- Limited flexibility to passive range of motion
- Incomplete passive correction to neutral
- Active motor function limited by contractures

Imaging

- Imaging is not required for diagnosis.
- Plain radiographs helpful for atypical foot positions or in complex cases

Differential Diagnosis

- See Tables 209.1 and 209.2.
- Many foot deformities are called clubfeet erroneously.

- The key distinguishing component of the clubfoot is limited dorsiflexion of the hindfoot (Fig. 209.2).

Treatment

At Diagnosis

- Weekly casting for five to six casts (though shorter intervals for casting can be successful)
- Percutaneous tenotomy of Achilles tendon in 80-90%
- Three-week cast after tenotomy
- Brace (foot abduction orthosis) full time for 3 months (Fig. 209.3)

Later

- Foot abduction orthosis at night for up to 4 years of age
- Possible extensive surgical reconstruction if casting not successful
- Transfer of the tibialis anterior for persistent forefoot supination at 3 to 5 years of age in 10% to 20%

When to Refer

- Immediately if rigid for weekly casting
- If not tolerating cast or brace
- Persistent deformity despite casting and bracing

Troubleshooting

- Inability to maintain the cast on the leg, usually due to casting technique
- Inability to keep the foot in the foot abduction orthosis, usually due to a lack of family persistence in maintaining the brace wear schedule or inadequate motion of the foot to tolerate the foot abduction orthosis

Patient Instructions

- Casting is successful in 80% or more of feet if the family adheres to brace wearing.
- Children are expected to walk, run, and play sports at age-appropriate stages.
- Risk for subsequent children
  - Baby boy with clubfoot
    - 1:40 chance for brother
    - Minimal for sister
  - Baby girl with clubfeet
    - 1:16 for brother
    - 1:40 for sister

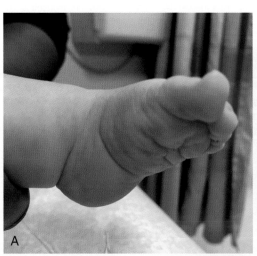
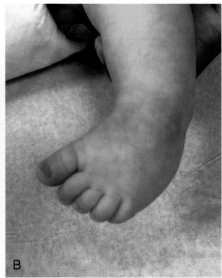

Fig 209.1 (A) and (B), Typical appearance of clubfeet in an infant. Note the high arch for an infant and the varus plus plantarflexed (equinus) position of the heel. The heel pad is less well defined than normal.

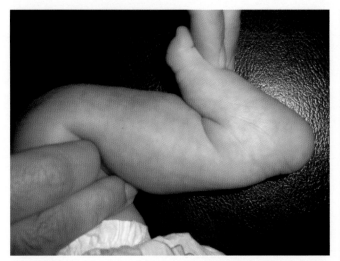

Fig 209.2 A calcaneovalgus foot is hyperdorsiflexed and can often be positioned flush with the anterior shin. A more severe calcaneovalgus deformity may be associated with posterior medial apex bowing of the tibia and limb shortening.

Fig 209.3 The foot abduction orthosis is a variation of the Dennis-Brown bar used frequently in the past and less often now for internal tibial torsion. The clubfoot is externally rotated 70 degrees. The foot abduction orthosis is worn full time for 3 months and then during sleep for as long as 4 years.

TABLE 209.1 Differential Diagnosis

Differential Diagnosis	Differentiating Features
Calcaneovalgus feet	Common at birth with the foot dorsiflexed all the way into the tibia
Metatarsus adductus	Similar forefoot adductus but a mobile hindfoot
Skewfoot	Atypical and more severe form of metatarsus adductus

TABLE 209.2 Foot Positions at Birth

Condition	Forefoot	Midfoot	Hindfoot
Calcaneovalgus	Neutral	Neutral or lateral	Hyperdorsiflexed
Metatarsus adductus	Adduction	Normal	Normal
Skewfoot	Adduction	Lateral	Valgus
Clubfoot	Adduction	Medial	Varus/equinus

- Parent and child with clubfoot
  - 1:4 for siblings

Considerations in Special Populations

- Clubfeet associated with neuromuscular conditions may be more resistant to casting and nonoperative treatment, but casting is still attempted.
- An atypical clubfoot has been described in which the foot is smaller, more deformed, and more rigid than the standard foot and requires special attention for casting and bracing.

Suggested Readings

Morcuende JA, Dolan LA, Dietz FR, Ponseti IV. Radical reduction in the rate of extensive corrective surgery for clubfoot using the Ponseti method. *Pediatrics*. 2004;113:376–380.

Ponseti IV. *Congenital Clubfoot. Fundamentals for Treatment*. Oxford: Oxford University Press; 1996.

Siapkara A, Duncan R. Congenital talipes equinovarus: a review of current management. *J Bone Joint Surg Br*. 2007;89B:995–1000.

Staheli L, Ponseti IV, Morcuende JA, et al: *Clubfoot: Ponseti Management. 3rd ed*. 2009. Available at: https://storage.googleapis.com/global-help-publications/books/help_cfponseti.pdf. Accessed July 13, 2018.

Chapter 210 Toddlers: Nursemaid's Elbow

Justin Kunes, Todd Milbrandt, Scott Riley

ICD-10-CM CODE
S53.006A *Unspecified dislocation of unspecified radial head, initial encounter*

CPT CODE
24640 *Closed reduction of the elbow*

Key Concepts

- The radiocapitellar joint is the key to rotational movement in the forearm and hand.
- It is a secondary restraint to elbow stability.
- Radial head subluxation is a common injury in young children and most common from 2 to 5 years of age.
  - Until this point, the radial head has a spherical shape, and thus the joint is less constrained than the adult's cup-shaped head.

History

- The usual mechanism is a sudden jerking of the upper limb, as when an adult attempts to prevent a child from falling.
  - Elbow extended, forearm pronated position
  - Injury occurs to the annular ligament (restraint for the radial head) and remains interposed in the radiocapitellar joint.
- Most likely to occur in children younger than 4 years of age and rarely in those older than 5 years.
  - May occur in children younger than 6 months of age
- Pain in the elbow; child is hesitant to move elbow

Physical Examination

- Observation
  - Presenting position: forearm pronated, elbow flexed and held at patient's side
  - Skin condition: Look for lacerations, abrasions, and ecchymosis to rule out other conditions (not usually seen in nursemaid's elbow).
- Palpation
  - Tenderness to palpation over the radial head (lateral structure)
  - Feel the medial epicondyle, lateral condyle, and olecranon process for other injuries.

- Range of motion
  - Attempts can be made to passively range the child's elbow if it is tolerated (usually not well tolerated).
- Special tests
  - Neurovascular examination
  - Check the median nerve. The OK sign must show a true O shape, tip to tip, and show an intact anterior interosseous nerve (by demonstrating that the flexor pollicis longus and flexor digitorum profundus tendons are intact) as opposed to the volar pads pinching.
  - Check the ulnar nerve (crossing the patient's fingers and spreading the fingers apart demonstrates intact interosseous innervations).
  - Check the radial nerve (check thumb extension to show that the extensor pollicis longus tendon is intact).
  - Check the radial and ulnar pulses.

Imaging

- Radiographs
  - Obtain two views of the humerus (anteroposterior and lateral), three views of the elbow (anteroposterior, lateral, and oblique), and two views of the forearm (anteroposterior and lateral) (this confirms that there are no other injuries).
  - The center of the radial head and the capitellum should line up normally.
  - Unfortunately, many patients with clinical nursemaid's elbow will have radiographs that are normal in appearance.
- Ultrasound examination
  - Performed prior to manipulation, shows supinator and annular ligament interposed in the radiohumeral joint—"J-sign."
  - After manipulation, J-sign disappears (with normal annular ligament location).

Differential Diagnosis

Please see Table 210.1.
- Congenital radial head dislocation
  - Look for bilateral involvement, no pain, and no trauma.
- Monteggia fracture (fracture of the ulna with associated radial head dislocation)
  - Look for subtle plastic deformation (slight bend without obvious fracture line) of the ulnar shaft or even of the olecranon.
  - Usually associated with severe trauma
- Supracondylar humerus fracture, associated with trauma, ecchymosis, and swelling
  - Anterior and posterior "fat pad" signs on radiographs

TABLE 210.1 Differential Diagnosis

Differential Diagnosis	Differentiating Feature
Congenital radial head dislocation	Look for bilateral involvement; no pain, no trauma
Monteggia fracture (ulna fracture with associated radial head dislocation)	Look for subtle plastic deformation (slight bend without obvious fracture line) of the ulnar shaft or even the olecranon
Supracondylar humerus fracture	Associated with trauma, ecchymosis, and swelling

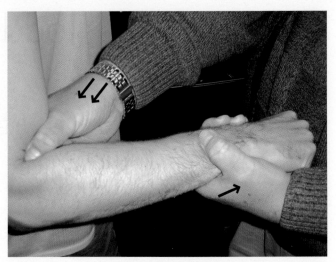

Fig 210.2 Clinical picture showing hand 1 *(single arrow)* and hand 2 *(double arrow)* placement for reduction.

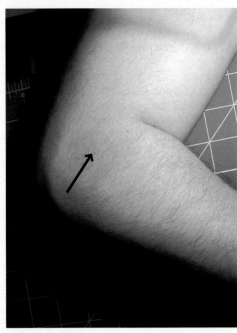

Fig 210.1 Lateral aspect of the elbow with arrow indicating location of the radial head.

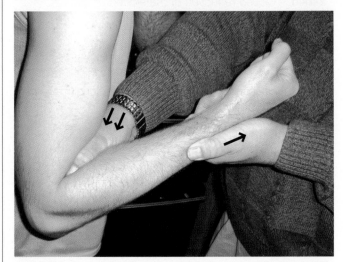

Fig 210.3 Hand 1 *(single arrow)* has now supinated the forearm, whereas hand 2 *(double arrow)* places posterior force on the radial head.

Treatment

- At diagnosis
  - Reduction of nursemaid's elbow (Figs. 210.1 to 210.4)
  - Where to hold the arm and wrist (see Fig. 210.2)
  - One hand at distal forearm (hand 1)
  - Other hand at distal humerus with thumb on radial head (hand 2)
  - *Manipulation I* (see Figs. 210.3 and 210.4) supination-flexion [classic method]
  - Hand 1 flexes and supinates the forearm and gently extends the elbow from 90 to 0 degrees.
  - Hand 2 applies posteriorly directed force on the radial head and feels for reduction of the radial head.
  - Allowing the parent to attempt this reduction while described by the physician over the telephone has been reported; subsequent follow-up is recommended.
  - Immobilization
  - The first episode requires no immobilization unless reduction is delayed more than 12 hours.

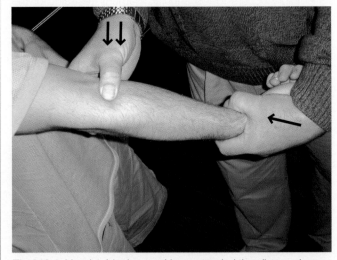

Fig 210.4 Hand 1 *(single arrow)* has extended the elbow, whereas hand 2 *(double arrow)* continues to apply posterior force on the radial head. This completes the reduction maneuver.

- Delayed for more than 12 hours: 10 days in a posterior long arm splint (including hand and wrist), with 90 degrees of elbow flexion and full forearm supination
- Recurrent episodes: After three recurrences, the patient should wear a cast for 3 weeks in the same position as a long arm splint.
- Manipulation II, other technique: Hyperpronation method
- Forearm is hyperpronated while palpating the radial head, no need to flex or extend elbow.
- Postmanipulation care is same as first method.

When to Refer

- Children who develop recurrent subluxation after 3 weeks of cast immobilization should be referred to an orthopaedist comfortable with dealing with pediatric upper extremity injuries.
- Occasionally such children will require surgical intervention to reconstruct the annular ligament to prevent further instability.

Troubleshooting

- Many patients will have reduced on the way to the office.

Patient Instructions

- Have the family watch for the expected recovery after relocation, which is increasing use of the elbow by the child. If this does not occur, then a reevaluation must be performed.
- Most children can return to full activities in approximately 1 week.

Suggested Readings

Choung W, Heinrich SD. Acute annular ligament interposition into the radiocapitellar joint in children (nursemaid's elbow). *J Pediatr Orthop*. 1995;15:454–456.

Dohi D. Confirmed specific ultrasonographic findings of pulled elbow. *J Pediatr Orthop*. 2013;33(8):829–831.

Eismann EA, Cosco ED, Wall EJ. Absence of radiographic abnormalities in nursemaid's elbow. *J Pediatr Orthop*. 2014;34(4):426–431.

García-Mata S, Hidalgo-Ovejero A. Efficacy of reduction maneuvers for "pulled elbow" in children: a prospective study of 115 cases. *J Pediatr Orthop*. 2014;34(4):432–436.

Kaplan RE, Lillis KA. Recurrent nursemaid's elbow (annular ligament displacement) treatment via telephone. *Pediatrics*. 2002;110:171–174.

Newman J. "Nursemaid's elbow" in infants six months and under. *J Emerg Med*. 1985;2:403–404.

Chapter 211 Toddlers: The Limping Child

Janet L. Walker

ICD-10-CM CODE
R26.89 *Other abnormalities of gait and mobility*

Key Concepts

- Seeing your child limp is a scary situation for parents, and the causes of a childhood limp can vary from the very benign to the malignant, from growing pains to septic hip.
- It is crucial that practitioners approach these children in a systematic fashion to not miss or delay the diagnosis to prevent lifelong consequences.
- Examination of the involved limb includes inspection for rashes, redness, warmth, swelling, tenderness, atrophy, and range-of-motion testing of the major joints.
- Observation of the child's gait can give the practitioner insights into the correct diagnosis.
- The tests to order are directed by the findings on physical examination and include blood work for inflammation markers, radiography, ultrasonography for joint effusions, bone scintigraphy, and magnetic resonance imaging.
- Treatment is based on the diagnosis and ranges from simple observation to emergent surgical treatment for infection or slipped capital femoral epiphysis.
- Overall the prognosis is good if the diagnosis is made in a timely manner.

History

- Acute onset
  - May be related to minor trauma
  - May have associated fever and malaise
  - Refusal to bear weight or move extremity (pseudoparalysis)
  - Pain may not be a reported complaint
- Chronic onset
  - Can be associated with premature birth
  - Not usually associated with trauma
  - Pain may be transient throughout the day or night or associated with activities

Physical Examination

- Gait observation
  - Normal gait
  - Normal gait in children can vary by age and neuromuscular development. At the beginnings of a child's gait pattern, typically between 12 and 16 months, the child will have a shorter stride length and a fast cadence.
  - By the age of 7, a child has obtained a mature gait pattern of a smooth and rhythmic cadence with a minimal expenditure of energy.
  - Antalgic gait
  - Antalgic gait is an avoidance pattern with less time in stance phase on the involved extremity. By decreasing the time in single limb stance, the child limits the overall pressure during gait on that limb.
  - Children may simply refuse to walk to prevent pain in the limb, especially if the pain is severe enough and the child's verbal skills are not well developed.
  - Toe walking
  - It can be normal when the child first begins walking but should be bilateral and symmetrical and rapidly extinguished as walking skills are gained.
  - Unilateral tiptoe walking can compensate for leg length.
  - Tiptoe stance can facilitate decreased stance time on a painful extremity during gait and may be used to prevent weight bearing on a painful forefoot.
  - Tiptoe walking can compensate for increased ipsilateral knee or hip flexion.
  - It may indicate a spastic condition involving the gastrocnemius, hamstrings, or hip flexors or weakness in hip and knee extensors in neuromuscular conditions like muscular dystrophy.
  - Trendelenburg gait
  - Children will shift their trunk over the affected hip during stance phase. This lateralizes the center of gravity to reduce forces on the hip that would cause pain. It is also caused by muscle weakness in chronic conditions. This compensatory gait pattern may not hurt the patient.
  - Spastic gait
  - Weakened quadriceps muscles in combination with hamstring tightness can lead to a crouched knee gait in which the knee does not extend, shortening the stride length.
  - If the quadriceps muscles are strong or very spastic, the opposite deformity may be created. This is known as the stiff knee gait pattern in which the child walks with the knees in extension with limited flexion.
  - Other spastic patterns also exist, such as the scissoring gait in which the hip adductors are hypertonic, thus making it difficult during the swing phase of gait. Isolated toe walking may also indicate a spastic process.
- Palpation
  - Warmth or tenderness in the affected extremity may indicate trauma or infection.

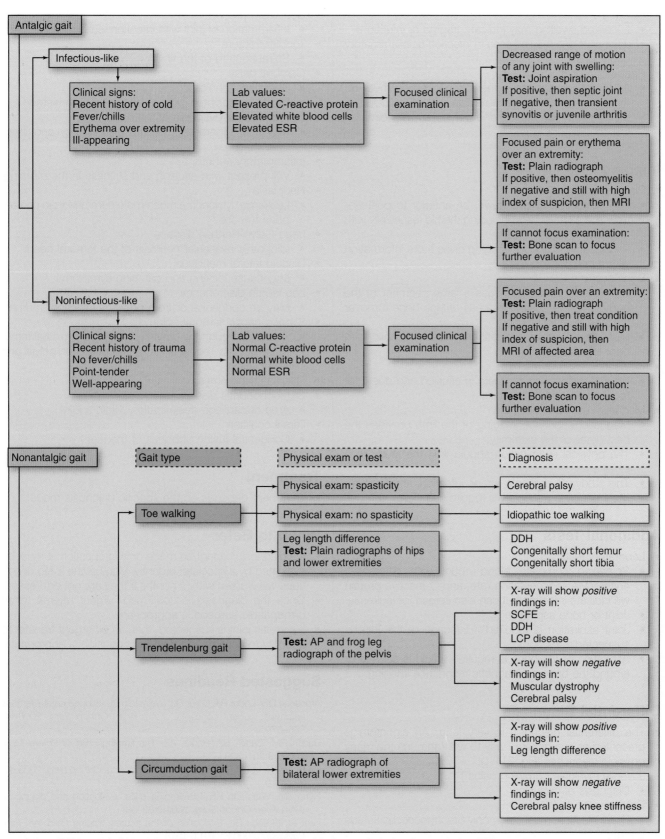

Fig 211.1 Differential diagnosis. *AP,* Anteroposterior; *DDH,* developmental dysplasia of hip; *ESR,* erythrocyte sedimentation rate; *LCP,* Legg-Calvé-Perthes; *SCFE,* slipped capital femoral epiphysis.

- Swelling
  - Localized swelling may indicate trauma or infection.
  - Joint effusions may be seen in infection or inflammatory conditions.
- Range of motion
  - All the affected joints in the leg in question must go through a passive range-of-motion evaluation (including the hip, knee, and ankle) and compared with joints on the contralateral side.

Imaging

- Plain radiographs
  - The entire limb in two views, an anterior to posterior view and a lateral view, including the hip (especially with knee pain)
  - Pelvis, rather than hip, imaging gives more information with a comparison
- Bone scan
  - Can reveal pathology across a large segment of the body; it will be positive in areas of high bone turnover (fracture, tumor, infection)
  - Most helpful when evaluating a nonverbal child with poor localizing signs
- Ultrasound scan of the hip
  - Will determine whether there is effusion and does not require sedation of the patient
- Magnetic resonance imaging
  - Magnetic resonance imaging of the limb provides the best detail of the extremity.
  - The physical examination should limit the study to a small area.
  - This study will delineate tumor, infection, and fracture.
  - Most pediatric patients will require sedation.

Additional Tests

- Laboratory tests
  - Screening complete blood count with differential, erythrocyte sedimentation rate, and C-reactive protein will indicate infection but can also screen for leukemia.
  - Joint or bone aspiration.
  - Joint aspiration is required if infection of the joint is suspected.
  - Aspiration of the bone is required if fluid is seen in or around the bone on magnetic resonance imaging.

Differential Diagnosis

- The differential diagnosis is very long. An algorithm is presented as a suggested way to work through the many possible diagnoses (Fig. 211.1).
- Juvenile myalgias ("growing pains")
  - Diagnosis of exclusion
- Osteomyelitis
  - Bone infection, most commonly *Staphylococcus aureus*
- Discitis
  - Infection of the intervertebral disc, most commonly *Staphylococcus aureus*
- Transient synovitis
  - Inflammation of the joint, usually the hip, without infection

- Septic arthritis
  - Inflammation of joint with infection; surgical emergency
- Toddler fracture
  - Spiral fracture of the tibia
- Cerebral palsy
  - Static encephalopathy
  - Usually associated with an abnormal birth history
- Developmental dysplasia of the hip
  - May see apparent leg length discrepancy and Trendelenburg gait
- Inflammatory arthritis
  - Will present with effusion and stiffness in the morning
- Neoplasia
  - Leukemia, lymphoma much more common than primary bone tumors
- Legg-Calvé-Perthes disease
  - Idiopathic avascular necrosis of the femoral head
- Discoid lateral meniscus
  - May cause locking and catching symptoms
- Leg length discrepancy
  - May be congenital or from previous infection/trauma
- Slipped capital femoral epiphysis
  - Rotation through the growth plate of the proximal femur
  - Must get hip radiographs (anteroposterior pelvis and frog pelvis views)
- Overuse syndromes
- Osteochondritis dissecans
  - Area of cartilage delamination within a joint
- Tarsal coalition
  - Congenital fusion of bones of the feet

Treatment

- Treatment depends on the specific diagnosis made.

When to Refer

- If a diagnosis cannot be made or is in question, it must be evaluated by a specialist urgently. Many of the listed conditions will worsen within months if they are not addressed.
- Once the diagnosis is confirmed, urgent referral to an orthopaedic surgeon is appropriate.
- If a septic joint is suspected, then an emergent transfer to a facility to confirm and treat the condition is appropriate.

Suggested Readings

Aronsson DD, Loder RT, Breur GJ, Weinstein SL. Slipped capital femoral epiphysis: current concepts. *J Am Acad Orthop Surg*. 2006;14: 666–679.

Barkin RM, Barkin SZ, Barkin AZ. The limping child. *J Emerg Med*. 2000;18:331–339.

De Boeck H, Vorlat P. Limping in childhood. *Acta Orthop Belg*. 2003;69: 301–310.

Flynn JM, Widmann RF. The limping child: evaluation and diagnosis. *J Am Acad Orthop Surg*. 2001;9:89–98.

Leet AI, Skaggs DL. Evaluation of the acutely limping child. *Am Fam Physician*. 2000;61:1011–1018.

Leung AK, Lemay JF. The limping child. *J Pediatr Health Care*. 2004;18: 219–223.

Chapter 212 School Age: Legg-Calvé-Perthes Disease

Vishwas R. Talwalkar, Ryan D. Muchow

ICD-10-CM CODES
M91.11 *Juvenile osteochondrosis of head of femur*
M79.609 *Pain in unspecified limb*

Key Concepts

- Idiopathic osteonecrosis of the capital femoral epiphysis causing varying degrees of pain, deformity, gait disturbance, and ultimately risk of premature arthrosis of the hip
- Simultaneously described in 1909 by Legg, Calvé, and Perthes
- Onset of symptoms at ages 2 to 12 years
- Male-to-female ratio of 5:1
- 1 in 4000 incidence
- Ethnic variation exists (rare in African Americans)
- Ten percent to 12% bilateral
- Most patients with skeletal age less than chronologic age
- Proposed etiologies include coagulation disorder, trauma, bone dysplasia, venous hypertension, collagen abnormality, environmental

Disease Course

- Disease progresses through stages described by Waldenström and recently modified by the multicenter International Perthes Study Group.
- The *initial stage* includes the inciting event and inflammation of the hip.
- The *fragmentation stage* starts with subchondral fracture and progresses to loss of structural integrity, significant radiographic irregularity, and shape distortion of the femoral epiphysis. It is usually the most symptomatic phase.
- The *reossification stage* is characterized by increasing new bone formation in the epiphysis, greater structural integrity, and decreasing pain.
- The *remodeling stage* is the final phase that progresses from the completion of reossification to skeletal maturity.

History

- Insidious onset of limp and pain, often a remote traumatic history
- Pain may be localized to the hip, groin, thigh, knee, or entire limb
- Symptoms exacerbated by activity, partially relieved by rest

- Usually several months of symptoms before diagnosis
- Rarely any family history; if present, consider other etiology

Physical Examination

- Examination of the hip usually reveals limited abduction and internal rotation
- Motion is limited by pain early in the disease process and by deformity later
- Trendelenburg gait evident
- Muscle atrophy may also be evident
- Late in the course, fixed adduction deformity and leg length discrepancy may also be seen

Imaging

- Radiographs (AP pelvis and frog-leg lateral pelvis) are most widely used to diagnose, classify, treat, and monitor the disease process.
  - The initial radiographic finding is a relatively smaller femoral epiphysis with an apparently widened joint space.
  - Subsequent findings during the fragmentation phase include increased radiodensity, subchondral fracture (crescent sign), fragmentation of the ossific nucleus, flattening of the ossific nucleus, physeal irregularity, broadening and shortening of the femoral neck, and flattening and widening of the acetabular roof (Figs. 212.1–212.4).
- Magnetic resonance imaging (MRI) is becoming more widely used to establish a diagnosis in the initial stage of disease, to quantify the extent of epiphyseal injury (with perfusion MRI), or to identify intra-articular and cartilage pathology (i.e., labral tears, osteochondritic lesions, articular cartilage injuries) in late deformity
- Technetium-99 bone scan has been described as an additional imaging modality to track reperfusion of the epiphysis.
- Computed tomography, particularly with three-dimensional reconstruction, is useful for assessing shape deformity and for possible osteotomy planning in young adult patients.

Differential Diagnosis (Table 212.1)

- Steroid-induced osteonecrosis
- Postinfectious osteonecrosis
- Multiple epiphyseal dysplasia
- Spondyloepiphyseal dysplasia
- Gaucher disease
- Sickle cell disease

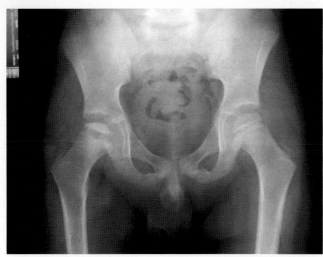

Fig 212.1 Anteroposterior view of the pelvis of a 6-year-old child with lateral pillar C Legg-Calvé-Perthes disease.

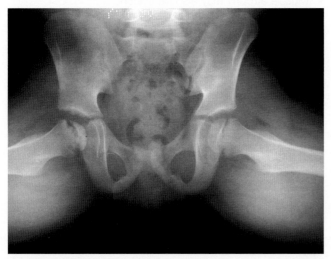

Fig 212.2 Frog leg view of the pelvis of a 6-year-old child with lateral pillar C Legg-Calvé-Perthes disease.

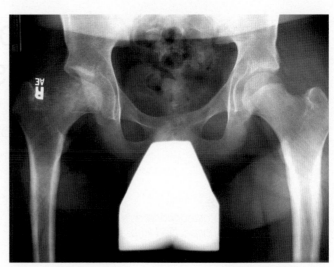

Fig 212.3 Anteroposterior view of the pelvis of the same child shown in Figs. 212.1 and 212.2 at age 15 displaying a Stulberg class IV result.

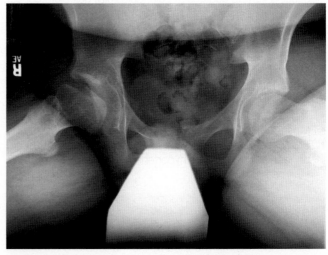

Fig 212.4 Frog leg view of the pelvis of the same child shown in Figs. 212.1 and 212.2 at age 15 displaying a Stulberg class IV result.

TABLE 212.1 Differential Diagnosis

Differential Diagnosis	Differentiating Feature
Steroid-induced osteonecrosis	Bilateral, shoulders and knees involved
Postinfectious osteonecrosis	History of infection
Multiple epiphyseal dysplasia	Bilateral, symmetrical, multiple sites
Spondyloepiphyseal dysplasia	Bilateral symmetrical with spine abnormality
Gaucher disease	Signs of systemic disease
Sickle cell disease	Signs of systemic disease

Classification

- Severity
  - Lateral pillar: currently the most popular and widely applied; measured during the fragmentation phase (Fig. 212.5)
    - A: no loss of height of the lateral one-third of the epiphysis (lateral pillar)
    - B: loss of as much as 50% of the height of the lateral pillar
    - B/C border: preservation of 50% of the lateral pillar height, but abnormal bone quality in the lateral pillar
    - C: more than 50% loss of height of the lateral pillar
  - Catterall: stages I through IV with increasing volume of head deformity

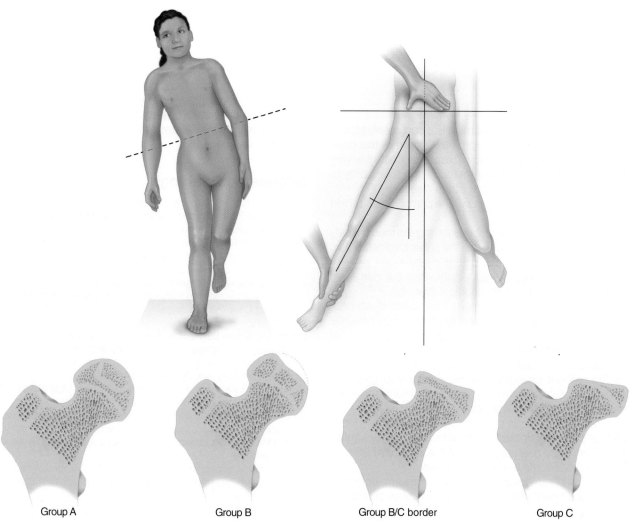

| Group A | Group B | Group B/C border | Group C |

Fig 212.5 Typical physical exam findings and classification systems for Legg-Calvé-Perthes disease. **(A)** Typical Legg-Calvé-Perthes limp, which is a combination of an antalgic gait and a Trendelenburg gait. In the stance phase of gait, the patient leans the body over the involved hip to decrease the force of the abductor muscles and the pressure within the hip joint. **(B)** Hip abduction is best examined in extension with the patient supine. Dropping the uninvolved leg over the side of the examining table helps stabilize the pelvis. **(C)** Lateral pillar classification: *group A,* no loss of height in the lateral pillar; *group B,* partial collapse (<50%) of the lateral pillar; *group B/C border,* intermediate between B and C, approximately 50% collapse, thin pillar, irregular; *group C,* more than 50% collapse of the lateral pillar. ([A and C] From Kim HKW, Herring JA. Legg-Calvé-Perthes disease. In: Herring JA, ed. *Tachdjian's Pediatric Orthopaedics*. 5th ed. Philadelphia: Elsevier; 2014. [B] Redrawn from Herring JA. *Legg-Calvé-Perthes Disease*. Rosemont, IL: American Academy of Orthopaedic Surgeons; 1996. In: Herring JA, ed. *Tachdjian's Pediatric Orthopaedics*. 5th ed. Philadelphia: Elsevier; 2014.)

- Salter-Thompson: A, less than 50% head involvement as determined by the width of the crescent sign; B, more than 50% involvement
- Deformity: measures of sphericity and congruity, measured at skeletal maturity
  - Mose: femoral head sphericity compared with circular overlay
  - Stulberg: measure of femoral head flattening and congruity related to risk of developing arthritis
    - I: spherical
    - II: minimal deformity, spherical head
    - III: ovoid head, congruent hip
    - IV: flat head, congruent hip
    - V: flat head with incongruent hip

Natural History

- In general, outcomes are related to the age at onset and amount of femoral head involvement.
- Many patients do well clinically into the fifth decade of life, but approximately half have hip arthritis at age 50 years.
- More recently, a less favorable natural history has been described for hips classified as lateral pillar B or worse, and those hips graded as Stulberg III or IV.
- Patients with incongruous hips and hinged abduction are at highest risk of premature arthritis developing in the third or fourth decade.
- Patients with age at onset younger than 8 years have the best prognosis, those with age at onset of 8 to 10 years

have an intermediate prognosis, depending on severity of disease, and those older than 10 years have a poor prognosis.

- Patients with lateral pillar C hips have a poor prognosis across all ages.

Treatment

- The goal of all methods of treatment is a congruent, spherical, mobile, pain-free hip. Most hips fall short of this goal.
- Due to the great variability of this disease process, it is very difficult to compare treatment methods and their ability to reliably alter the natural history of the disease.
- The concept of containment is still the primary idea behind treatment.
  - Containment is the idea that maintaining the mechanically softer femoral epiphysis within the spherical acetabulum during the critical phase of the disease can prevent flattening and preserve sphericity while the damaged femoral head regains mechanical integrity.
- Various methods of containment have been described, including abduction casting and bracing, varus proximal femoral osteotomy, redirectional pelvic osteotomy, or combinations of these methods.
- Noncontainment treatment is also performed to reposition the leg without changing the hip relationship (proximal femoral valgus osteotomy) or to accommodate the enlarged femoral head (shelf acetabuloplasty).
- More recently, methods of treatment to address late intra-articular pathology including hip arthroscopy and surgical dislocation have been applied, but the long-term efficacy of these procedures is still under review.
- The use of pharmaceutical agents to prevent deformity and femoral head collapse is a promising area of ongoing research and future intervention, but it is still in the experimental phase.

When to Refer

- Immediate but not emergent referral to an orthopaedic surgeon is indicated for any child with any radiographic abnormality of the hip, persistent complaints of hip pain, abnormal physical examination, or a limp that lasts more than a few days.

Suggested Readings

Herring JA, Kim HT, Browne R. Legg-Calve-Perthes disease. Part I: classification of radiographs with use of the modified lateral Pillar and Stulberg classifications. *J Bone Joint Surg Am*. 2004;86A:2103–2120.

Herring JA, Kim HT, Browne R. Legg-Calve-Perthes disease. Part II: prospective multicenter study of the effect of treatment on outcome. *J Bone Joint Surg Am*. 2004;86A:2121–2134.

Hyman JE, Trupia EP, Wright ML, et al. Interobserver and intraobserver reliability of the modified walsenstrom classification system for staging of Legg-Calvé-Perthes disease. *J Bone Joint Surg Am*. 2015;97(8): 643–650.

Larson AN, Sucato DJ, Herring JA, et al. A prospective multicenter study of Legg-Calvé-Perthes disease: functional and radiographic outcomes of nonoperative treatment at a mean of follow-up of twenty years. *J Bone Joint Surg Am*. 2012;94(7):584–592.

McAndrew MP, Weinstein SL. A long-term follow-up of Legg-Calve-Perthes disease. *J Bone Joint Surg Am*. 1984;66A:860–869.

Salter RB. Experimental and clinical aspects of Perthes' disease. In Proceedings of a Joint Meeting of the American Physicians' Fellowship and the Israeli Orthopaedic Society. *J Bone Joint Surg Br*. 1966;48B: 393–394.

Stulberg SD, Cooperman DR, Wallensten R. The natural history of Legg-Calve-Perthes disease. *J Bone Joint Surg Am*. 1981;63A:1095–1108.

Chapter 213 School Age: Slipped Capital Femoral Epiphysis

Elizabeth W. Hubbard

ICD-10-CM CODES

M93.0	*Slipped upper femoral epiphysis (nontraumatic)*
M93.001	*Slipped upper femoral epiphysis right hip*
M93.002	*Slipped upper femoral epiphysis left hip*
M93.003	*Slipped upper femoral epiphysis unspecified hip*
M93.01	*Acute slipped upper femoral epiphysis (nontraumatic)*
M93.011	*Acute slipped upper femoral epiphysis (nontraumatic) right hip*
M93.012	*Acute slipped upper femoral epiphysis (nontraumatic) left hip*
M93.013	*Acute slipped upper femoral epiphysis (nontraumatic) unspecified hip*
M93.02	*Chronic slipped upper femoral epiphysis (nontraumatic)*
M93.021	*Chronic slipped upper femoral epiphysis (nontraumatic) right hip*
M93.022	*Chronic slipped upper femoral epiphysis (nontraumatic) left hip*
M93.023	*Chronic slipped upper femoral epiphysis (nontraumatic) unspecified hip*
M93.03	*Acute or chronic slipped upper femoral epiphysis (nontraumatic)*
M93.031	*Acute or chronic slipped upper femoral epiphysis (nontraumatic) right hip*
M93.032	*Acute or chronic slipped upper femoral epiphysis (nontraumatic) left hip*
M93.033	*Acute or chronic slipped upper femoral epiphysis (nontraumatic) unspecified hip*

Key Concepts

- Slipped capital femoral epiphysis (SCFE) is a common cause of adolescent hip, groin, thigh, or knee pain.
- This is a disorder of the proximal femoral physis with displacement of the head/neck relationship.
  - Most common: femoral epiphysis is displaced posterior and inferior to the femoral metaphysis.
  - Valgus SCFE: femoral epiphysis is displaced superolaterally relative to the metaphysis.
    - Uncommon
    - More common in females
    - Diagnosis delayed due to symptoms and difficulty making the diagnosis radiographically

- Associated with:
  - Increased body mass index (BMI)
  - Endocrine abnormalities
    - Hypothyroidism
    - Renal osteodystrophy
    - Growth hormone deficiency
    - Hypopituitarism
  - History of radiation treatment to the hip/pelvis
- Diagnosis of a stable slip is frequently delayed due to lack of recognition.
- Treatment is always surgical stabilization, but surgical technique and urgency depend on the slip stability (Fig. 213.1).
- Prophylactic fixation of contralateral hip should be considered in:
  - Atypical SCFE
  - Modified Oxford Bone Age Score of 16, 17, 18 and/or patients with open triradiate cartilage (triradiate score of 1; Fig. 213.2)

History

- Chronic, stable SCFE
  - Obese adolescent with brief history of hip, groin, thigh, or knee pain
  - Patient and/or family notices a progressive limp without toeing of the affected side
- Unstable SCFE
  - Sudden onset of severe hip pain
  - Unable to walk, even on crutches
- Atypical SCFE
  - Symptoms similar to the typical SCFE patient
  - Atypical age range (<10 or >16 years of age)
  - <50% for weight or <10% for height
  - Patients should undergo endocrine and metabolic workup to rule out predisposing condition.

Physical Examination

- Often an overweight or obese adolescent, BMI > 95%
  - Atypical SCFE patient may fall below 50% for weight or 10% for height.
- Patient with an unstable slip is unable to ambulate, even with an assistive device.
- Patient with a stable slip will ambulate with or without an assistive device.
  - Antalgic gait/limp
  - External foot progression angle, asymmetric in unilateral SCFE with the patient out-toeing more on the affected side

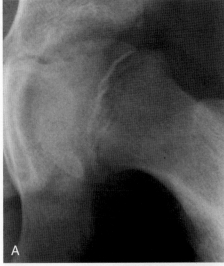

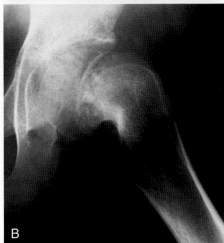

- Cause: Disruption of the proximal femoral physis with displacement of the epiphysis
- Symptoms: Knee, thigh, groin pain; limp versus inability to bear weight
- Classification: Stable vs. unstable
- Treatment: Stable—in situ stabilization with a single screw; Unstable—stabilization with 2 screws vs modified Dunn osteotomy
- Outcomes: avascular necrosis (unstable slips), femoroacetabular impingement, arthritis

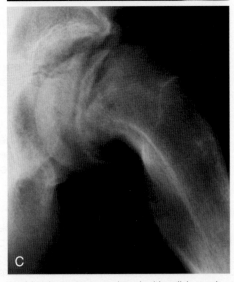

Fig 213.1 (A–C) Radiographic changes associated with mild, moderate, and severe slipped capital femoral epiphysis. (From Herring JA, ed. *Tachdjian's Pediatric Orthopaedics*. 5th ed. Philadelphia, PA: Elsevier; 2014: 632.)

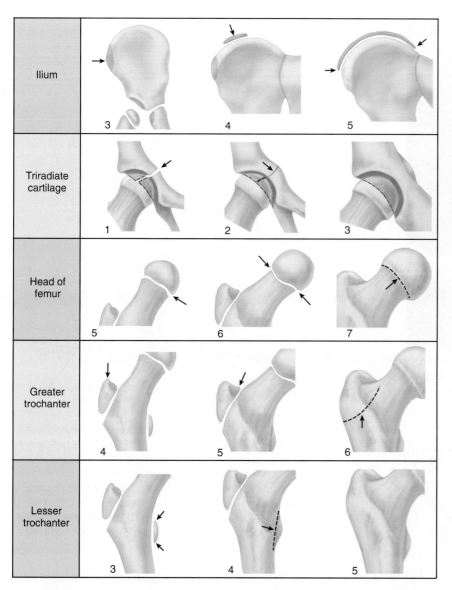

Fig 213.2 Oxford Bone Age Score. To calculate the Oxford Bone Age Score, the radiographic appearance of the physes of the ilium, triradiate cartilage, proximal femur, greater and lesser trochanters are assigned numeric values based on skeletal maturity. A score of 16, 17, or 18 has a PPV for contralateral slip of 92%. A triradiate score of 1 (open) is the signal most predictive radiographic feature for calculating risk of contralateral slip and has a PPV of 89%. *Arrows* indicate the location of the growth apophyses for each section of the pelvis and/ or proximal femur. (Redrawn from Popejoy D, Emara K, Birch J. prediction of contralateral slipped capital femoral epiphysis using the modified Oxford bone age score. *J Pediatr Orthop*. 2012;32[3]:290–294.)

- Will lay with affected leg in an externally rotated position—asymmetric in a unilateral SCFE with more external rotation on the affected side
- Pain with logroll of the affected leg, worse with internal rotation
- Reduced internal hip rotation compared with the contralateral side
- May have obligate abduction and external rotation of hip when flexed

Imaging

- Anteroposterior (AP) and frog lateral of the pelvis
  - Best studies for making the diagnosis
  - Widening of the physis (Fig. 213.3)
  - Osteopenia within the femoral metaphysis
  - Blurring of the proximal femoral metaphysis—due to the overlap of the epiphysis on the metaphysis (Fig. 213.4D and see also Fig. 213.3)

- Displacement of the epiphysis with an interruption in the Klein line (see Fig. 213.4A–C)
- Limited role for magnetic resonance imaging (MRI), computed tomography (CT) or bone scan

Classification

- Functional classification
  - Stable—Patient is able to ambulate, with or without assistive devices
  - Unstable—Patient is unable to ambulate, even with an assistive device
  - Stability correlates with risk of avascular necrosis
    - Stable: avascular necrosis (AVN) risk 0%
    - Unstable: AVN risk 30–47%
- Temporal
  - Acute slip
    - Symptoms present for less than 3 weeks
    - Possible history trauma, may be minor

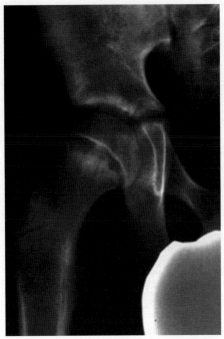

Fig 213.3 Physeal widening in patient with slipped capital femoral epiphysis. Also notice the blurring of the metaphysis and the relative osteopenia of the superior femoral neck.

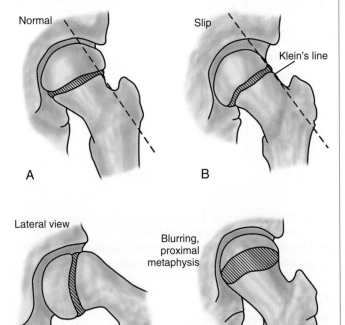

Fig 213.4 Radiographic features of slipped capital femoral epiphysis (SCFE). **(A–C)** Klein line. An interruption in the Klein line on the AP or frog lateral view of the hip is diagnostic of the most common types of SCFE (posterior, inferior displacement of the femoral epiphysis relative to the metaphysis). **(C)** and **(D)** Artistic rendering of physeal widening and blurring of the metaphysis, which are also common radiographic features of SCFE.

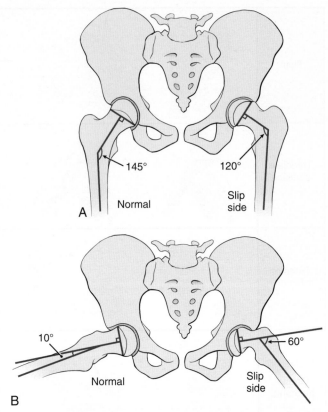

Fig 213.5 (A) and **(B)** Southwick angle. Measure the epiphyseal-diaphyseal angle of bilateral hips on the Frog pelvis radiograph. The slip angle is classified by the difference in this angle between the unaffected and affected sides. A difference of <30 degrees is classified as a mild slip. A difference of 30 to 60 degrees is classified as a moderate slip, and a difference of >60 degrees is classified as a severe slip. (From Herring JA, ed. *Tachdjian's Pediatric Orthopaedics*. 5th ed. Philadelphia, PA: Elsevier; 2014: 632.)

- Chronic slip
  - Symptoms present for greater than 3 weeks
  - Vague history of knee, thigh, buttock, and/or groin pain
- Acute on chronic slip
  - Sudden exacerbation of knee, thigh, buttock, and/or groin pain that has been present for greater than 3 weeks
  - Frequent history of limping followed by sudden increase in symptoms, resulting in an increased difficulty or inability to ambulate
- Slip severity
  - Determined by the Southwick angle–Epiphyseal-metaphyseal angle on frog-leg lateral views compared with opposite side (Fig. 213.5)
  - Mild—less than 30-degree difference
  - Moderate—30–60-degree difference
  - Severe—greater than 60-degree difference

Treatment

- Stable SCFE
  - Prompt in situ fixation with single stainless steel cannulated screw (Fig. 213.6).

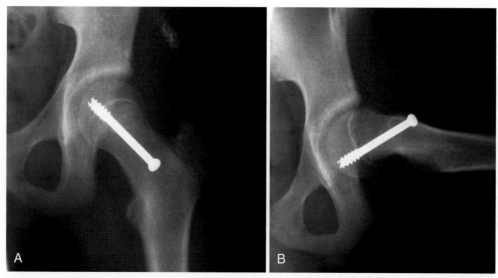

Fig 213.6 (A) and (B) In situ screw fixation of a stable slipped capital femoral epiphysis. The screw should penetrate the physis and epiphysis at a 90-degree angle and should ideally be centered within the epiphysis on both the AP and frog lateral radiographs. At least four screw threads should penetrate the physis to maximize fixation. Immediately after screw placement, multiple fluoroscopic images should be obtained to confirm that the screw does not penetrate the femoral head subchondral bone.

- Place screw perpendicular to orientation of displaced femoral neck in both AP and lateral planes.
- Four screw threads should bridge physis to stabilize the epiphysis.
- Starting point is anterior on femoral neck.
- Need to ensure placement of screw tip in center of femoral head on both views (center-center)
- Before leaving OR, surgeon must assure screw tip does not violate joint.
  - Persistent joint penetration can cause iatrogenic chondrolysis.
- Allowed to weight bear as tolerated or with crutches for 4 to 6 weeks
- Unstable SCFE
  - AVN risk 30–47%
  - Requires urgent surgical stabilization
  - Surgical options:
    - In situ fixation:
      - Two screws provide superior biomechanical stability.
      - Consider gentle reduction maneuver to improve alignment.
      - Arthrotomy for joint decompression, with or without attempted gentle reduction, has been described.
    - Surgical dislocation and modified Dunn osteotomy
      - Performed at select centers by pediatric hip specialists
      - Goal is to improve epiphyseal-metaphyseal alignment and restore near-normal anatomy
      - No long-term clinical outcome studies or randomized clinical trials comparing outcomes of modified Dunn osteotomy with in situ fixation
      - Multicenter study reports 26% rate of postoperative AVN after surgical dislocation and modified Dunn osteotomy.

- Intraoperative monitoring of epiphyseal blood flow
  - Intraoperative monitoring during in situ fixation has been shown to help determine if capsular decompression required during in situ fixation.
    - All stable slips had measurable pulsatile flow to the femoral epiphysis after screw fixation.
    - Unstable slips without detectable flow underwent capsular decompression. Pulsatile flow documented after decompression. No cases of AVN in the postoperative period.
- Atypical SCFE
  - High risk of bilateral slips
  - Consider prophylactic fixation of contralateral hip
- Prophylactic fixation of contralateral hip
  - Modified Oxford Bone Age Score can be utilized to determine risk of contralateral slip in typical and atypical SCFE patients.
  - Score of 16, 17, or 18 has a positive predictive value (PPV) of 96% and negative predictive value (NPV) of 92%.
  - Triradiate score of 1 (open triradiate) has a PPV of 89% and NPV of 96%.

When to Refer

- Immediate referral to orthopaedic surgeon of any patient with SCFE
- Patient with stable SCFE should be made non–weight bearing due to risk of progression to an unstable slip.
- Patients with unstable slip should be admitted to the hospital for urgent/emergent stabilization due to risk of AVN.

Suggested Readings

Escott B, De La Rocha A, Jo CH, et al. Patient-reported health outcomes after in situ percutaneous fixation for slipped capital femoral epiphysis:

an average twenty-year follow-up study. *J Bone Joint Surg Am.* 2015;97:1929–1934.

Katz DA. Slipped capital femoral epiphysis: the importance of early diagnosis. *Pediatr Ann.* 2006;35:102–111.

Lehmann CL, Arons RR, Loder RT, et al. The epidemiology of slipped capital femoral epiphysis: an update. *J Pediatr Orthop.* 2006;26:286–290.

Loder RT. Controversies in slipped capital femoral epiphysis. *Orthop Clin North Am.* 2006;37:211–221, vii.

Loder RT, O'Donnell PW, Didelot WP, et al. Valgus slipped capital femoral epiphysis. *J Pediatr Orthop.* 2006;26L:594–600.

Loder RT, Richards BS, Shapiro PS, et al. Acute slipped capital femoral epiphysis: the importance of physeal stability. *J Bone Joint Surg Am.* 1993;75:1134–1140.

Manoff EM, Banffy MB, Winell JJ. Relationship between body mass index and slipped capital femoral epiphysis. *J Pediatr Orthop.* 2005;25:744–746.

Parsch K, Weller S, Parsch D. Open reduction and smooth Kirschner wire fixation for unstable slipped capital femoral epiphysis. *J Pediatr Orthop.* 2009;29(1):1–8.

Popejoy D, Emara K, Birch J. Prediction of contralateral slipped capital femoral epiphysis using the modified Oxford Bone Age Score. *J Pediatric Orthop.* 2012;32:290–294.

Rahme D, Comley A, Foster B, Cundy P. Consequences of diagnostic delays in slipped capital femoral epiphysis. *J Pediatr Orthop B.* 2006;15:93–97.

Sankar W, Vanderhave K, Matheney T, et al. The modified Dunn procedure for unstable slipped capital femoral epiphysis: a multicenter prospective. *J Bone Joint Surg Am.* 2013;95:585–591.

Schrader T, Jones C, Kaufman A, et al. Intraoperative monitoring of epiphyseal perfusion in slipped capital femoral epiphysis. *J Bone Joint Surg Am.* 2016;98:1030–1040.

Tokmakova K, Stanton RP, Mason DE. Factors influencing the development of osteonecrosis in patients treated for slipped capital femoral epiphysis. *J Bone Joint Surg Am.* 2003;85(5):798–801.

Chapter 214 School Age: Developmental Dysplasia of the Hip

Mark J. Romness

ICD-10-CM CODE
Q65.x *Congenital deformities of the hip*

Key Concepts

- The term *developmental dysplasia of the hip* (DDH) encompasses *all* forms of hip dysplasia, including acetabular dysplasia, instability, subluxation, and dislocation.
- The term *congenital dysplasia of the hip* implies that the deformity was present at birth, which is not always true.
- Teratologic dislocations occur before birth, have more severe deformity, and are often associated with other disorders.
- Instability is present in 0.5% to 1% of babies at birth.
  - Sixty percent recover by 1 week old
  - Eighty-eight percent recover by 2 months old
  - Underdevelopment or dysplasia may persist
- Classic DDH persists in 1 in 1000 births
  - Persistent instability
  - Persistent dislocation
- Diagnosis as early as possible is key to the best outcome.

History

- Perinatal risk factors
  - First-born child
  - Female
    - Eighty percent of DDH patients are female.
    - Female babies twice as likely as males to be breech.
  - Breech position in utero
    - Seventeen percent to 23% of breech babies have DDH.
    - Two percent to 4% of births are breech.
  - Family history
    - Present in 10% to 30% of DDH patients
  - Any condition with intrauterine crowding, including oligohydramnios and twin or multiple birth
- Conditions that may also have DDH associated:
  - Torticollis: 8%
  - Metatarsus adductus: 1.5%
  - Clubfoot or other foot deformities
  - Oligohydramnios
  - Other syndromes or anomalies

Physical Examination

- Asymmetrical inguinal folds
- Klisic line from the greater trochanter to the anterosuperior iliac spine directed below the umbilicus

- The greater trochanter palpable above the Nelaton line connecting the anterosuperior iliac spine and ischial tuberosity
- Decreased hip abduction
- Galeazzi sign of apparent femoral shortening
- Barlow test to subluxate the hip
- Ortolani test to reduce a dislocated hip (Fig. 214.1)
- A simple hip click is not associated with DDH.
- Be aware of bilateral dislocations.
  - Decreased abduction bilaterally
  - Klisic line (trochanter to anterior superior iliac spine—ASIS) points below the umbilicus bilaterally
  - Both greater trochanters above the Nelaton line from ASIS to ischial tuberosity

Imaging

- Ultrasonography: up to 4 months of age
- Anteroposterior radiograph of pelvis if older than 4 months or ossific nucleus present on the ultrasound scan
- Computed tomography or magnetic resonance imaging if additional information is needed, but usually requires sedation
- Additional study: arthrography used to assess reduction intraoperatively

Differential Diagnosis

- See Table 214.1.
- A congenital short femur will have femoral shortening on the Galeazzi test.
- Congenital coxa vara (with a shepherd's crook deformity of the proximal femur) may have decreased abduction.

Treatment

- Close observation of the newborn for spontaneous improvement
- Positioning devices such as a Pavlik harness
- Closed reduction and casting
- Open reduction (Fig. 214.2)

Contraindications to Reduction

- Bilateral dislocation more than 8 years old
- Unilateral with medical contraindications

When to Refer

- Any dislocated hip
- Any unstable hip more than a week old
- Persistent acetabular dysplasia

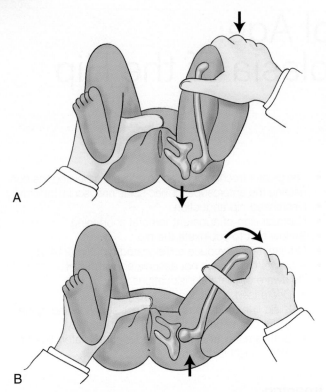

Fig 214.1 (A) Barlow test with posteriorly directed loading of the hip from the flexed and adducted position to try to dislocate or subluxate a reduced hip. **(B)** The Ortolani test with medially directed force at the greater trochanter while the hip is actively abducted to try to reduce a dislocated hip. (Modified from Hüftdysplasie. www.ebenhoeh-dr.com/Schulerseite/Huftdysplasie/huftdysplasie.html. Accessed January 11, 2009.)

TABLE 214.1 Differential Diagnosis

Differential Diagnosis	Differentiating Features	Chapter Reference
Congenital short femur	Femoral shortening on Galeazzi test	208
Congenital coxa vara (with shepherd's crook deformity of the proximal femur)	May have decreased abduction	208

Troubleshooting

- Worse prognosis with delayed diagnosis and treatment
- Hips that are dislocated at rest are more likely to require treatment.

Patient Instructions

- Avoid positioning hips tightly adducted or swaddled.

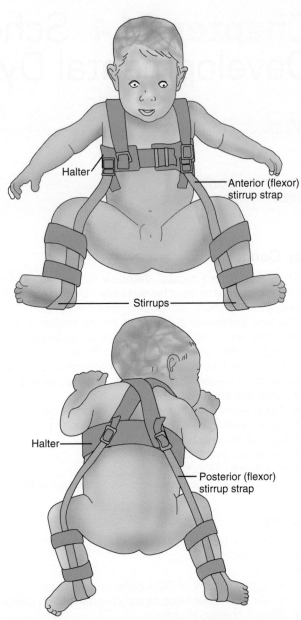

Fig 214.2 Standard strap position of the Pavlik harness to prevent certain hip positions but allow some active motion. The anterior strap prevents hip extension and is set with the hip flexed at 90 to 100 degrees. Overtightening of the anterior strap increases the risk of femoral nerve or artery impingement. The posterior strap prevents adduction and is set to allow hip adduction to 0 degrees or neutral. The posterior strap should not be overtightened in an attempt to pull the hip into a reduced position or the risk of avascular necrosis is increased.

Prognosis

- When detected early, treatment is very successful.

Considerations in Special Populations

- Patients with other conditions of joint laxity such as Down syndrome or Ehlers-Danlos syndrome may require more aggressive treatments.

Suggested Readings

Banta JV, Scrutton D, eds. *Hip Disorders in Childhood*. London: Mac Keith Press; 2004.

Pavlik A. The functional method of treatment using a harness with stirrups as the primary method of conservative therapy for infants with congenital dislocation of the hip. Original 1957. [translated and abridged by Leonard F. Peltier, MD, PhD.]. *Clin Orthop Relat Res*. 1992; 281:4–10.

Weinstein SL, Mubarek SJ, Wenger DR. Developmental hip dysplasia and dislocation: part I. *Instr Course Lect*. 2004;53:523–530.

Weinstein SL, Mubarek SJ, Wenger DR. Developmental hip dysplasia and dislocation: part II. *Instr Course Lect*. 2004;53:531–542.

Chapter 215 School Age: Normal Lower Extremity Anatomic Variants

Michael Hadeed, Keith Bachmann

ICD-10-CM CODES

M21.069	*Valgus deformity, not elsewhere classified, unspecified knee (use for genu valgum)*
M21.169	*Varus deformity, not elsewhere classified, unspecified knee (use for genu varum)*
M21.969	*Unspecified acquired deformity of unspecified lower leg (used for tibial torsion)*
Q65.89	*Other unspecified congenital deformities of hip (used for excess femoral anteversion)*

Key Concepts

- Knowledge of the natural history of lower limb growth is important for any practitioner who evaluates children (Fig. 215.1). It is helpful to evaluate rotation and angulation independently.
- The angular and rotational alignment of the growing child's lower extremity goes through several predictable stages.
- Recognition of normal variations seen in the pediatric lower extremity is key in the accurate assessment of the patient and allows for sound counsel for parents or referring practitioners.
- When the patient's anatomy falls outside of the normal expectations, it may be appropriate to refer them to a specialist.

History

- Any child presenting with a possible lower limb deformity should undergo a complete evaluation.
- This evaluation starts with a thorough history, including:
  - Birth history
  - Dates and age developmental milestone achievement
  - Family history of related illness/congenital abnormalities
  - Any traumas or illness related to that limb

Differential Diagnosis

- In order to differentiate between normal and pathologic anatomy, it is critical to be aware of the typical abnormalities seen.
- This will help guide your exam.

- It is common to group pathologies as they are tested: rotation, angulation, limb length discrepancy.
  - Rotational abnormalities
    - Excessive femoral anteversion
    - Tibial torsion
      - Internal
      - External
  - Angular abnormalities
    - Genu varum
      - Infantile Blount disease (age 2 to 5)
      - Adolescent Blount disease (>10 years old)
    - Genu valgum
    - Tibial bowing
      - Posteromedial (physiologic variant)
      - Anterolateral/anteromedial (pathologic)
    - Metatarsus adductus
  - Limb length discrepancy

Physical Examination

- The physical exam is the key diagnostic tool when evaluating a patient's lower extremity rotation, angulation, and length.
- General physical exam principles:
  - The exam should be performed in a similar routine every time to develop a consistent pattern for easier diagnosis and ensure a comprehensive evaluation.
  - This may be different for each practitioner, and you should develop your own method applicable to your practice.
  - Listed below are the special testing categories for the topics addressed in this chapter; however, be mindful that this is not an exhaustive list of all tests.
- Rotation
  - Hip rotation
    - Hip rotation can be evaluated in the supine position but is best tested in the prone position.
      - The hip should be at neutral, knee flexed to 90 degrees.
      - To assess internal rotation, rotate the legs outward (thigh rotation is internal).
      - To assess external rotation, rotate the legs inward, likely doing one leg at a time or crossing the legs, as they will hit each other.
    - Femoral anteversion can also be appreciated by the classic sitting posture of a "W."

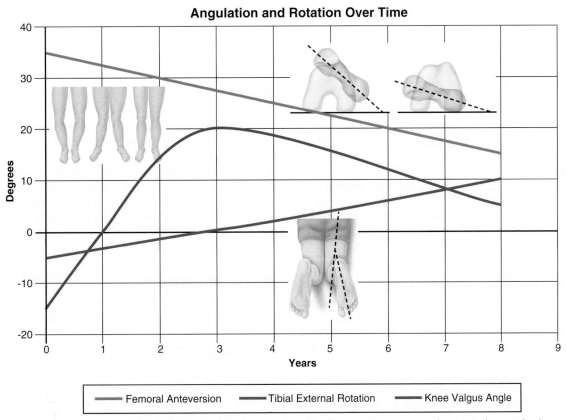

Angulation and Rotation Over Time

y-axis: Degrees (−20 to 40)
x-axis: Years (0 to 9)

— Femoral Anteversion — Tibial External Rotation — Knee Valgus Angle

Fig 215.1 Graph of the normal rotational changes of the lower extremity. The *x*-axis shows age in years; the *y*-axis shows degrees.

- Tibia rotation
  - Tested by assessing the thigh-foot-angle, maintain prone position
  - Knee flexed to 90 degrees; angle is the difference between the thigh and the angle of the axis of the foot.
- Rotation can also be evaluated while standing or during the gait cycle. Global rotation is determined by the foot progression angle or the angle of the axis of the foot relative to the midline.
  - In-toeing causes:
    - Excess femoral anteversion
    - Internal tibial torsion
  - Out-toeing causes:
    - External tibial torsion
    - Relative external tibial torsion due to genu valgum
- Normal values
  - Femoral anteversion
    - At birth, the normal femoral anteversion is typically between 30 and 40 degrees.
    - This will steadily decrease to approximately 15 degrees by skeletal maturity.
    - This transition is often complete by the age of 8.
    - Morphologic variances do not always result in symptoms.
    - When testing the rotation of the hip, the normal values are:
      - Internal rotation—20 to 60 degrees
      - External rotation—30 to 60 degrees

- Tibia rotation (thigh foot angle values)
  - Infants—5 degrees internal rotation (range −30 to 20)
  - 8 years—10 degrees external rotation (range −5 to 30)
- Angulation
  - This is typically measured with the patient supine.
    - Valgus—Determine the distance between the medial ankle malleoli when the legs are in neutral alignment (medial aspect of knee touching, patella facing forward).
      - After age 7, this should be <8 cm—helpful to use same unit of measure for serial evaluation (cm, or marks on a triangle placed between the legs).
    - Varus—Determine the distance between the knees with the legs in neutral alignment (medial malleoli touching, patella pointed forward).
  - Normal values
    - The normal alignment of the knees at birth is approximately 10 to 15 degrees of varus.
    - As the child grows, alignment becomes neutral at approximately 14 months of age.
    - The limb then progresses to maximum physiologic valgus around 3 years old (up to 20 degrees).
    - This gradually decreases to the normal physiologic valgus of ~5 to 7 degrees by age 7.
  - Other considerations
    - Posteromedial tibial bowing can be a normal physiologic variant.

- The apex of the deformity is typically in the distal tibia.
- This often resolves by age 5 to 7.
- Must monitor for leg length discrepancy, may be associated with calcaneovalgus foot.
- Anterolateral or anteromedial bowing indicate a pathologic process.
- Metatarsus adductus is when the forefoot is in an adducted position.
  - The lateral border should be straight, but in this condition it is bent.
- Limb length
  - This can be assessed both supine and standing
  - Supine:
    - It is important to first square the pelvis so as not to throw off your measurement.
    - This can be done by lifting the patient's legs in the air and making sure the pelvis is perpendicular to the exam table.
    - As the legs are brought back down to a standard supine position, the medial malleoli are palpated and the difference between the two is observed.
    - To isolate the femur, you can follow the same procedure, but the knees are flexed and the hips remain flexed.
    - The difference between the femoral condyles is observed (Galeazzi test).
  - Standing
    - Palpate the patient's posterior superior iliac spine while both feet are on the ground.
    - Compare the difference in height between the two points.
    - In addition, blocks of different known sizes may be placed under the shorter limb, stopping when the pelvis is level.
- Normal values
- Leg length discrepancies of 2.5 cm or less are generally well tolerated and do not increase the mechanical work required for ambulation.

Imaging

- Radiographic evaluation may be indicated in children who present with clinical limb asymmetry, short stature, or an abnormality based on the physical exam described previously.
- For rotational deformity: This is difficult to measure with a plain radiograph, and if the in-toeing or out-toeing is causing gait abnormalities, they should be referred for evaluation.
- For angular deformity: Full-length, weight-bearing plain radiographs, centered on the knees, should be the first radiographic imaging obtained.

Acknowledgment

The authors would like to acknowledge Dr. Jasmin McGinty's contributions to this chapter in the previous edition.

Suggested Readings

Engel GM, Staheli LT. The natural history of torsion and other factors influencing gait in childhood. A study of the angle of gait, tibial torsion, knee angle, hip rotation, and development of the arch in normal children. *Clin Orthop Relat Res*. 1974;99:12–17.

Lincoln TL, Suen PW. Common rotational variations in children. *J Am Acad Orthop Surg*. 2003;11(5):312–320.

Sponseller PD. *Handbook of Pediatric Orthopaedics*. 2nd ed. New York: Thieme; 2011.

Weinstein SL, Flynn JM, eds. *Lovell and Winter's Pediatric Orthopaedics*. 7th ed. Philadelphia: Wolters-Kluwer; 2014.

Chapter 216 School Age: Salter-Harris Fractures

Victor Anciano Granadillo, Keith Bachmann

ICD-10-CM CODES
S89.xxx *Salter Harris fracture, lower leg*
S79.xxx *Salter Harris fracture, leg*
S59.xxx *Salter Harris fracture, forearm*
S49.xxx *Salter Harris fracture, arm*

Key Concepts

- Approximately 15% to 30% of childhood fractures involve the physis.
- The risk of growth arrest depends on the site of injury: distal tibia (25%), distal femur (25%), distal ulna (60%), and distal radius (4%).
- Injury classically occurs through the zone of hypertrophy of the physis (zone of provisional calcification), although multiple layers can be involved.
- Salter-Harris classification (Fig. 216.1)
  - Type I: transverse fracture through the physis, more common in younger patients with a thicker physis
  - Type II: fracture line through the physis exiting into the metaphysis. This is the most common type, encompassing approximately 74% of physeal fractures.
  - Type III: transverse fracture line through the physis and exiting into the epiphysis (intra-articular fracture). Should consider posttraumatic arthritis as a sequela, in addition to growth arrest.
  - Type IV: fracture line passes through the metaphysis, physis, and epiphysis
  - Type V: crush injury to the physis, which is usually not apparent initially. This is the rarest of the physeal fractures.
  - Type VI (added by Rang): localized injury to the perichondrium resulting from direct open injury (e.g., lawn mower ankle injuries)
- Fractures create callus quickly, so avoid manipulation and reduction more than 5 days post injury.
- Follow patients for 6 to 12 months after healing to watch for growth arrest (partial or complete). This will be apparent earlier in physes that create more linear growth (distal femur).
- Treatment of physeal growth arrest relies on the location, extent of involvement, and remaining growth.
- Growth arrests are more common in Salter-Harris III, IV, and V fractures because the reserve cell layer is involved.

History
Acute

- Basic trauma history including mechanism of injury, areas of pain or deformity, and other associated injuries or previous injuries to extremity
- It is important to rule out nonaccidental trauma in pediatric fractures. Circumstances surrounding the injury must be obtained especially in younger (<1 year of age) patients.

Chronic or at Follow-Up

- Whether pain exists
- What type of deformity
- Evidence of maturation and amount of growth remaining
  - Age at menarche, adolescent growth spurt, Tanner staging
- Feeling of limb length discrepancy
- Involvement in sports. Some physeal injuries may be due to recurrent microtrauma or overuse.

Physical Examination

- Examination specific to extremity involved
- Acute
  - Observation: deformity and bruising/swelling
  - Palpation: tenderness or crepitus
  - Neurovascular examination
- Chronic or at follow-up
  - Examine for limb length discrepancy
  - Angular deformity

Imaging
Acute

- Radiographs
  - Orthogonal views of the affected joint
- Magnetic resonance imaging
  - Examining for physeal edema and separation in a patient with equivocal initial radiographs
- Computed tomography
  - Aids in assessment of reduction and joint congruence for Salter-Harris III and IV fractures

Follow-Up

- Radiographs
  - Orthogonal views of affected bone and joint
  - Look for Harris growth arrest lines to aid with assessment of growth resumption.

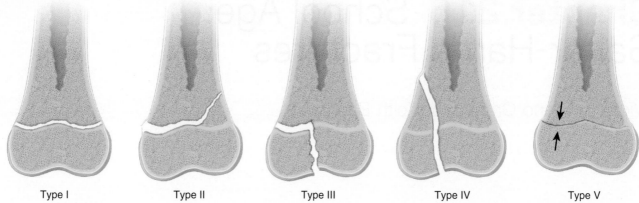

Fig 216.1 Salter-Harris classification of growth plate injuries. (From Herring J. *Tachdjian's Pediatric Orthopaedics.* 4th ed. Philadelphia, PA: Saunders; 2007.)

- Three-foot standing hips to ankles on one cassette with patellas pointing forward to assess mechanical axis alignment and limb length for lower extremity fractures
- Biplanar slot-scanning radiographs may be substituted to limit radiation exposure.
- Left-hand anteroposterior radiograph to assess bone age
- Computed tomography or magnetic resonance imaging to assess physeal closure and determine the percentage of involvement if needed for operative planning or assessment

Differential Diagnosis

- Depends on extremity involved
- All extremities could have fractures of the metaphysis without physeal injury (e.g., distal radius), dislocation of the joint (e.g., shoulder, elbow, hip), ligamentous injury (e.g., knee medial collateral ligament injury), osteochondral injury (e.g., knee), labral or meniscal injury (e.g., hip, shoulder, or knee), infectious process (e.g., osteomyelitis, septic joint), or inflammatory process (e.g., reactive synovitis, juvenile rheumatoid arthritis). With a clear trauma history, infection and inflammatory processes move down the differential list; however, the time frame of the trauma needs to be clarified. Patients who rolled their ankle but were walking and running without issue do not have a fracture when they present with refusal to bear weight 5 days later. They more likely have infection.

Treatment
At Diagnosis

- Depends on fracture and age
- In general, avoid multiple reduction attempts and rigid fixation through the physis. If fixation is necessary, use smooth wires.
- Distal radius and ulna: closed reduction and casting
- Proximal radius (rare, usually fractures thru the metaphysis)
  - Attempt closed reduction; often needs percutaneous or open reduction with or without pinning due to lost motion if fracture left poorly reduced

- Distal humerus
  - Supracondylar humerus fracture: typically metaphyseal
  - Children younger than 18 months may have Salter-Harris I (transphyseal distal humerus fracture), which may look like an elbow dislocation. In this young population, transphyseal injury is much more common. This injury requires closed reduction and percutaneous pinning. Arthrogram is often helpful to aid in diagnosis and to judge joint congruence. Carry a high suspicion of nonaccidental trauma with these injuries.
  - Lateral condyle fracture (see Chapter 228)
- Proximal humerus
  - Observation: This injury rarely needs manipulation despite significant deformity due to the shoulder's great remodeling potential and range of motion.
  - Salter-Harris I more frequent in <5 years, whereas Salter-Harris II are more frequent in >12 years.
  - Operative management tends to be reserved for severely angulated fracture and older children with less remodeling potential or a block to motion.
- Proximal femur
  - Often difficult to distinguish from unstable or acute slipped capital femoral epiphysis (SCFE).
  - Anatomic reduction and fixation; this injury has a very high rate of avascular necrosis (>80% in some series) and should be managed at specialized facilities.
  - Always check contralateral side because SCFE may be bilateral in approximately 25% of cases.
- Distal femur
  - Neurovascular examination important because popliteal vessel injuries can occur (ankle-brachial index)
  - Closed reduction alone usually not sufficient to maintain reduction so fixation usually necessary
  - With Salter-Harris I, crossed pins through physis are necessary if displaced (Fig. 216.2)
  - With Salter-Harris II, reduce and place screws in the metaphyseal fragment (Thurston-Holland fragment) for fixation, avoiding crossing the physis, if possible (Fig. 216.3)
  - Salter-Harris III and IV: screw fixation; articular surface should be congruent

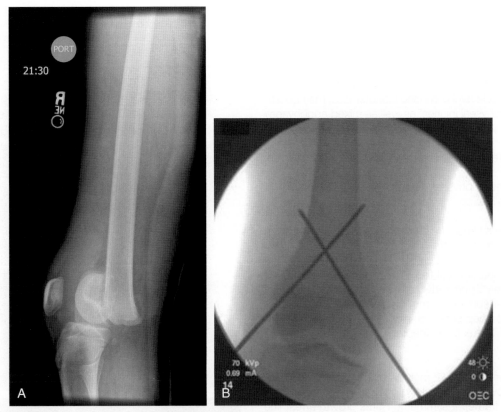

Fig 216.2 **(A)** Salter-Harris I distal femur. **(B)** Salter-Harris I distal femur treated with smooth Kirschner wires.

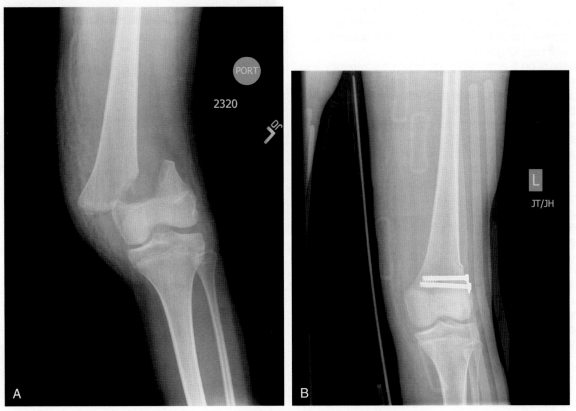

Fig 216.3 **(A)** Salter-Harris II distal femur. **(B)** Salter-Harris II distal femur treated with screws.

- Proximal tibia
  - Injuries through the physis are equivalent to knee dislocations due to tethering of vessels.
    - Careful neurovascular examination is a necessity.
  - Injuries also have a high rate of compartment syndrome.
  - Reduction and pin fixation are usually necessary.
  - Tibial tubercle avulsions (see Chapter 228) may be isolated apophyseal injuries, as well as mixed apophyseal/physeal injuries (Ogden classification).
- Distal fibula
  - Physeal tenderness after "ankle sprain" mechanism common
    - Treat as a physeal fracture with 4 to 6 weeks of immobilization.
- Distal tibia
  - Salter-Harris I and II fractures: typically closed reduction and casting adequate
  - Medial malleolus fracture: usually Salter-Harris IV due to small metaphyseal flag
    - Requires open reduction and screw placement if articular surface >2 mm displacement; usually possible to keep screw epiphyseal
- Triplane and Tillaux (see Chapter 228)

Later

- Must monitor for 6 to 12 months post injury for partial or complete growth arrest (faster growing physes followed for shorter time frame). If symmetric Harris growth arrest line is seen progressing up metaphysis, assume resumption of normal growth.
- Site of injury and mechanism affect likelihood of growth arrest (e.g., growth disturbance rare in the distal radius but common in the distal femur and proximal tibia).
- If complete growth arrest in the lower extremity, must calculate the remaining growth and treat according to anticipated leg length discrepancy.
  - Observation if anticipated leg length discrepancy less than 2 cm
  - Epiphysiodesis of contralateral side at appropriate time if predicted leg length discrepancy 2 to 5 cm
  - Lengthening or shortening procedures if leg length discrepancy more than 5 cm
  - This paradigm may be changing with the relative ease of magnetically actuated lengthening nails.
- If incomplete growth arrest or physeal bar, treatment is based on the remaining growth, percentage of physis involved, and location.
  - Central bars often halt growth, whereas peripheral bars can result in more problematic angular deformity (Fig. 216.4).
  - In general, epiphysiolysis (physeal bar removal) is attempted when less than 50% of the physis is involved (Fig. 216.5).
  - With a potential for angular deformity, the decision must be made whether to complete the partial epiphysiodesis and treat for limb length discrepancy or attempt a bar resection. More central bars are more amenable to attempted resection.

When to Refer

- In the management of acute fractures, referrals are based on the comfort level of the treating physician in

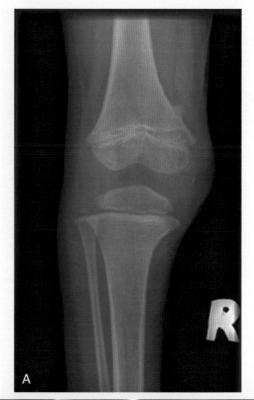

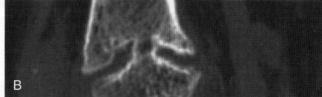

A

B

Fig 216.4 (A) Growth arrest in the distal femur, anteroposterior view: central bar. Note growth lines. (B) Growth arrest in the distal femur: computed tomography scan.

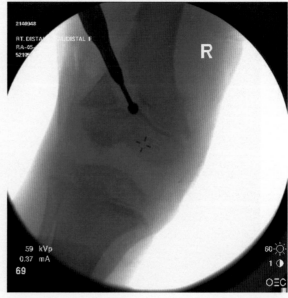

Fig 216.5 Growth arrest treated with physeal bar resection.

managing the fracture. Many fractures in children are nondisplaced.

- In general, distal radius fractures should be able to be treated by most orthopaedic surgeons, whereas fractures of the lower extremities and elbow are usually referred to pediatric trauma centers.
- Monitoring for growth arrest can be completed by community surgeons, whereas addressing leg length discrepancies and angular deformities associated with growth arrest often requires a specialized pediatric orthopaedist.

Prognosis

- Depends on the site of fracture, age of the patient, and energy of the mechanism
- In general, fractures involving the growth plate heal more rapidly (often <4 weeks) and almost never have problems with union.
- Malunion or nonunion is also related to age. Older children closer to end of growth have higher rates of malunion/nonunion.

Troubleshooting

- Attempt only one closed reduction in the emergency department under block or conscious sedation. If this fails, the patient should be paralyzed in the operating room setting.
- Multiple reduction attempts have been associated with growth arrest.

- Use advanced imaging if needed to help with the diagnosis/treatment plan (e.g., distal tibia joint involvement).

Patient Instructions

- Patients and their parents should be aware that any physeal injury has the potential for growth disturbance. The frequency and implications depend on the site of injury, age of the patient (and remaining growth), and the energy of the injury mechanism.
- Fortunately, most physeal injuries do not result in a clinically significant problem.

Suggested Readings

Birch JG. Surgical treatment of physeal bar resection. In: Eilert RE, eds. *Instructional Course Lectures*. Rosemont, IL: American Academy of Orthopaedic Surgeons; 1992:445–450.

Hynes D, O'Brien T. Growth disturbance lines after injury of the distal tibial physis. Their significance in prognosis. *J Bone Joint Surg Br*. 1988;70B:231–233.

Khoshhal KI, Kiefer GN. Physeal bar resection. *J Am Acad Orthop Surg*. 2005;13:47–58.

Peterson HA. Physeal fractures: part 3. Classification. *J Pediatr Orthop*. 1994;14:439–448.

Rathjen KE, Birch JG. Physeal injuries and growth disturbances. In: Beaty JH, Kasser JR, eds. *Rockwood and Wilkins' Fractures in Children*. 7th ed. Philadelphia: Lippincott Williams & Wilkins; 2010.

Salter R, Harris WR. Injuries involving the epiphyseal plate. *J Bone Joint Surg Am*. 1963;45A:587–622.

Chapter 217 School Age: Discoid Meniscus

Catherine A. Logan, Andrea Stracciolini, Mininder S. Kocher

ICD-10-CM CODE
Q68.6 *Congenital discoid meniscus*

Key Concepts

- Discoid meniscus is a congenital variant that characteristically involves abnormal morphology and potential instability of the lateral meniscus.
- The prevalence of bilateral discoid menisci internationally has been estimated to range between 15% and 25%; however, the true prevalence of bilateral discoid menisci is difficult to ascertain due to the large number of asymptomatic cases.
- Discoid menisci are more predisposed to tearing compared to normal menisci, and instability may result secondary to the absence of normal meniscal-capsular attachments.
- Torn or unstable menisci may or may not be symptomatic, including mechanical symptoms, pain, and swelling, which often interfere with function.
- The most commonly utilized classification system was proposed in 1978 by Watanabe et al., which classified discoid menisci based on arthroscopic appearance and stability (Fig. 217.1).
  - Type I (stable, complete discoid meniscus) is stable to arthroscopic probing, block-shaped, and covers the entire tibial plateau.
  - Type II (stable, partial discoid meniscus) is stable to arthroscopic probing and covers up to 80% of the tibial plateau.
  - Type III (unstable discoid meniscus, also called "Wrisburg variant") demonstrates instability on arthroscopic probing due to the complete lack of posterior meniscotibial attachments.

History

- Patients may or may not be symptomatic. Patient presentation is influenced by patient age, discoid meniscus instability type, and the presence or absence of meniscal tearing.
- Children under 10 years of age generally present with intermittent snapping of the knee, often spontaneous in nature, and inability to fully straighten the knee.
- Older children and adolescents may present similarly to an adult with a torn meniscus, including pain and swelling, with or without mechanical symptoms.
- Classic symptoms in the setting of a torn or unstable discoid menisci include mechanical symptoms, pain, and swelling.

- Patients with stable, untorn discoid menisci may have a subtler presentation. These menisci may be asymptomatic or become symptomatic if a tear occurs.

Physical Examination

- A lateral joint line bulge may be apparent, and due to an unstable subluxing lateral meniscus, a clunk may be appreciated during McMurray testing.
- Intra-articular effusion may be present if unstable or torn.
- Lack of knee extension may by be noted on range-of-motion testing

Imaging

- Plain radiographs may be unremarkable; however, radiographic signs may be present in more severe cases, and include:
  - Squaring of the lateral femoral condyle
  - Cupping of the lateral tibial plateau
  - Widening of the lateral joint line up to 11 mm (Fig. 217.2)
  - Hypoplastic lateral tibial spine
- MRI is more helpful in determining if a discoid meniscus is present.
- Of note, Micheli et al. investigated the diagnostic performances of physicians' clinical examination and MRI, and found MRI has a lower sensitivity for diagnosis of lateral discoid meniscus when compared with a physician's physical examination.
- MRI is useful for preoperative planning and may provide valuable information regarding the discoid type, presence or absence of posterior attachments, presence of associated degeneration, and any associated tears (Fig. 217.3).
- Ultrasound (US) may be used to diagnose discoid meniscus. Typical US features include lack of classic triangular shape, abnormally elongated and thick architecture, and heterogeneous central pattern.

Differential Diagnosis

- Meniscal tear, osteochondritis dissecans, chondromalacia patella, tibial or femoral stress injury

Treatment

- Observation is an appropriate treatment choice for asymptomatic or minimally symptomatic discoid menisci. Asymptomatic discoid menisci discovered incidentally on

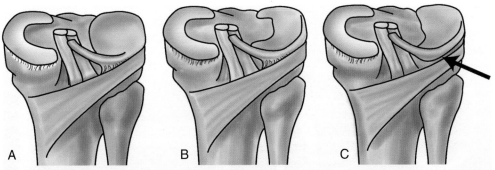

Fig 217.1 Posterior view of the three types of discoid meniscus. Complete **(A)**, incomplete **(B)**, and Wrisberg **(C)** types. Note that the Wrisberg type of discoid meniscus lacks a posterior horn ligamentous attachment to the tibial plateau *(arrow)*, whereas the complete and incomplete types of discoid meniscus have a firm attachment at the posterior horn to the tibial plateau.

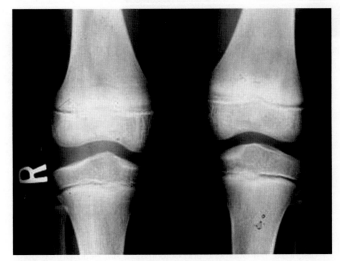

Fig 217.2 Standing anteroposterior view of both knees reveals a widening of the joint space of the right knee compared with the left, which is suggestive of a lateral discoid meniscus. Mild cupping of the lateral aspect of the tibial plateau is also noted.

imaging or during an arthroscopic procedure for a separate pathology are not typically treated unless there is meniscal tearing or instability.

- Surgical intervention is indicated for symptomatic discoid menisci. Historically the treatment of discoid meniscus was complete meniscectomy; however, degenerative changes of the knee joint were noted on follow-up of these postoperative patients.
- Presently surgical treatment emphasizes meniscal rim preservation with arthroscopic saucerization. The purpose of arthroscopic saucerization is to reshape the meniscus and preserve the typical biomechanics of the knee joint.
- Following saucerization, assessment of meniscal stability is performed intraoperatively, with meniscal repair performed as indicated.
- Concomitant central meniscal tears should be treated with partial meniscectomy or repair depending on their size, location, tear pattern, and stability at the time of the saucerization procedure.

When to Refer

- A history of knee locking or the knee joint stuck in flexion on presentation requires immediate referral to an orthopaedic surgeon.
- If the MRI does demonstrate a discoid meniscus, and the patient's symptoms and exam are consistent with discoid meniscus, referral to an orthopaedic surgeon is recommended.

Prognosis

- Favorable outcomes are found in short-term follow-up data for saucerization in the treatment of symptomatic discoid menisci.
- Ogut and colleagues reviewed follow-up results of arthroscopic saucerization performed in 11 knees (average age 11.5 years) with symptomatic discoid lateral meniscus. At the latest follow-up (average duration 4.5 years), nine rated as excellent (no symptoms with full range of motion) and two rated as good (occasional pain).
- Patient age at presentation has proved to be a useful prognostic factor for ultimate clinical outcome. With increasing age, patient-oriented results worsened. Gender, type of discoid lateral meniscus, presence of a meniscal tear, and duration of symptoms did not prove predictive of clinical outcome.
- While the short-term results of saucerization are promising, longer-term studies are necessary to assess for onset of both clinical and radiographic lateral compartment osteoarthritis.

Troubleshooting

- In cases whereby meniscal instability is questionable, dynamic ultrasound may be helpful to evaluate the extrusion of the meniscus into the lateral gutter and to correlate this with knee snapping.

Patient Instructions

- If the discoid meniscus is treated with saucerization without meniscal repair, the patient will be initially partially weight

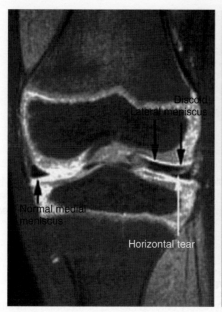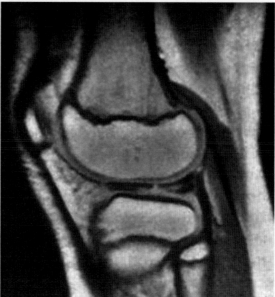

Fig 217.3 Coronal and sagittal views of the knee reveal a lateral discoid meniscus with a horizontal tear.

bearing in a hinged knee brace, followed by a transition to full weight bearing in approximately 1 week.

- Two weeks postoperatively, physical therapy may begin, with progression to return to sport at approximately 8 weeks postoperatively once full knee range of motion and strength is achieved.
- If the patient also undergoes a repair of the discoid meniscus, a longer period of protected weight bearing and a later return to sport should be expected.

Considerations in Special Populations

- In a child less than 10 years of age, symptoms of knee snapping, lateral knee pain, and lack of full extension without knee effusion signify a lateral discoid meniscus until proven otherwise.

Suggested Readings

Ahn JH, Kim KI, Wang JH, et al. Long-term results of arthroscopic reshaping for symptomatic discoid lateral meniscus in children. *Arthroscopy*. 2015;31:867–873.

Good CR, Green DW, Griffith MH, et al. Arthroscopic treatment of symptomatic discoid meniscus in children: classification, technique, and results. *Arthroscopy*. 2007;23:157–163, e1.

Klingele KE, Kocher MS, Hresko MT, et al. Discoid lateral meniscus: prevalence of peripheral rim instability. *J Pediatr Orthop*. 2004;24:79–82.

Kocher MS, DiCanzio J, Zurakowski D, Micheli LJ. Diagnostic performance of clinical examination and selective magnetic resonance imaging in the evaluation of intraarticular knee disorders in children and adolescents. *Am J Sports Med*. 2001;29:292–296.

Kocher MS, Klingele K, Rassman SO. Meniscal disorders: normal, discoid, and cysts. *Orthop Clin North Am*. 2003;34:329–340.

Kocher MS, Logan CA, Kramer DE. Discoid lateral meniscus in children: diagnosis, management, and outcomes. *J Am Acad Orthop Surg*. 2017;25(11):736–743.

Ögüt T, Kesmezacar H, Akgün I, Cansü E. Arthroscopic meniscectomy for discoid lateral meniscus in children and adolescents: 4.5 year follow-up. *J Pediatr Orthop B*. 2003;12(6):390–397.

Yoon KH, Lee SH, Park SY, et al. Meniscus allograft transplantation for discoid lateral meniscus: clinical comparison between discoid lateral meniscus and nondiscoid lateral meniscus. *Arthroscopy*. 2014;30:724–730.

Chapter 218 The Adolescent: Little Leaguer's Shoulder

Mininder S. Kocher, Rebecca Breslow, Michael O'Brien

ICD-10-CM CODES
Proximal humeral epiphysitis/epiphysiolysis, depending on shoulder:
M93.911 *Osteochondropathy, unspecified, right shoulder*
M93.912 *Osteochondropathy, unspecified, left shoulder*

Key Concepts

- Little leaguer's shoulder is a clinical term used to describe proximal humeral pain associated with throwing, typically with radiographic evidence of a widened proximal humeral physis. Chronic changes such as demineralization, sclerosis, or fragmentation of the proximal humeral metaphysis can also be seen.
- Little leaguer's shoulder may be caused by inflammation secondary to overuse or a stress fracture at the proximal humeral physis. The condition is typically self-limited and has been described as proximal humeral epiphysitis, proximal humeral epiphysiolysis, and rotational stress fracture of the proximal humeral epiphyseal plate.
- Little leaguer's shoulder typically occurs in patients between the ages of 11 and 16. Although classically this syndrome occurs in baseball pitchers, it can also arise in a baseball player of any position, racquet sport athletes (i.e., tennis, badminton), swimmers, and even gymnasts.
- With more opportunities for year-round throwing and racquet sports, athletes are frequently on multiple teams or are in tournaments in which multiple games per day or week are expected. Athletes are increasingly more likely to accumulate large numbers of repetitive overhead shoulder motions as they accumulate more sports participation hours per week and per year.

History

- Progressive pain at the proximal humerus with throwing, especially with high-velocity pitches and at higher pitch counts, typically worsening over several months. Furthermore, pitch control and command may be lost as symptoms advance (Fig. 218.1A).
- Pain may occur at any point of the pitching motion, although the highest rotational torque is produced during the late cocking phase of throwing after stride foot contact (SFC). This is the point where there is maximum external rotation (MER) of the shoulder (see Fig. 218.1A).

- Initially, the symptoms of pain resolve over the course of 24 hours. However, increased recovery time is evident as a child continues to throw with this condition.

Physical Examination

- Tenderness to palpation of the proximal humerus, specifically at the lateral aspect
- Discomfort can also be elicited with shoulder abduction at 90 degrees with external or internal rotation against resistance.
- Abduction of the shoulder at 90 degrees against resistance may cause pain.
- There is typically no effusion, muscle atrophy, or loss of active or passive range of motion.

Imaging

- Plain anteroposterior radiographs of both shoulders in internal and external rotation should be taken for comparison (see Fig. 218.1B–E). If initial radiographs are negative and clinical suspicion remains high, MRI may be considered.
- Classically, a widening of the proximal humeral physis will be seen, although symptoms may precede radiographic changes. On occasion, chronic changes such as demineralization, sclerosis, or fragmentation of the proximal humeral metaphysis can also be seen.
- Increasingly, musculoskeletal ultrasound is being used to diagnose this condition. Typical findings are hypoechoic swelling surrounding the shoulder joint suggestive of inflammation surrounding the growth plate.

Differential Diagnosis

- Please see Table 218.1.

Treatment

- Little leaguer's shoulder is typically a benign and self-limited nonoperative condition.
  - Initially, the athlete should be taken out of sports that require any kind of throwing or swinging of the symptomatic shoulder. It is recommended that these activities should be avoided for a total of at least 3 months. In a recent case series, the average time to resolution of symptoms was 2.6 months, with an average time of 4.2 months for return to competition.
  - Immobilization is rarely necessary and may be detrimental. Brief immobilization with a sling may be considered if pain is severe.

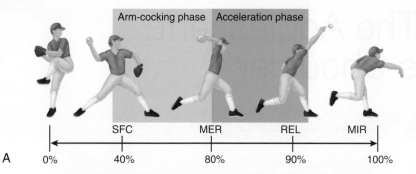

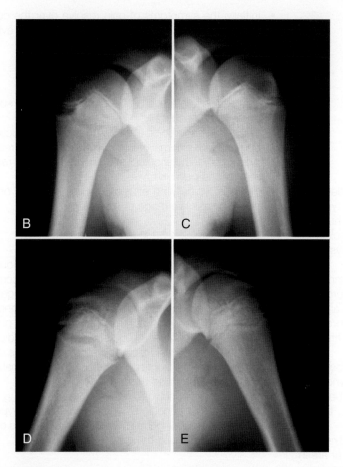

Fig 218.1 (A) The phases of throwing. (B–E) External (B, right shoulder and C, left shoulder) and internal (D, right shoulder and E, left shoulder) rotation anteroposterior comparison radiographs of the proximal humerus show widening of the physis compared with the opposite side. *MER,* Maximum external rotation; *MIR,* maximal internal rotation; *REL,* ball release; *SFC,* stride foot contact. ([A] Redrawn from Osbahr DC, Kim HJ, Dugas JR. Little League shoulder. *Curr Opin Pediatr.* 2010;22:35–40.)

TABLE 218.1 Differential Diagnosis

Differential Diagnosis	Differentiating Feature
Shoulder impingement syndrome	Pain with impingement test
Subacromial bursitis	Pain with impingement test
Rotator cuff tear	Weakness
Labral tear	Positive Speed test, positive O'Brien test
Shoulder instability	Instability on examination
Acromioclavicular joint inflammation	Pain and tenderness over acromioclavicular joint
Biceps tendinitis	Pain and tenderness over biceps tendon

- Later, physical therapy may be started when the patient is asymptomatic, with an emphasis on rotator cuff strength, scapular stability, and improvement in glenohumeral internal rotation deficit (GIRD), if present. When asymptomatic, gradual progressive throwing may be initiated over a 1- to 2-month period. Any return of symptoms during this progression indicates the need to rest and decrease the throwing regimen.
- The decision to allow an athlete to resume throwing should not be based on radiographic evidence of healing, which may take several months. In fact, proximal humeral physeal widening is possibly an adaptive change in throwing athletes and thus may signify a normal finding if not associated with any symptoms.
- Athletes with GIRD are 3.6 times more likely to have symptom recurrence. Correction of GIRD should be part of treatment, to prevent recurrence.

TABLE 218.2 Recommended Maximum Number of Pitches by Age of Athlete

Age (yr)	Maximum Pitches/Game	Pitchers Ages 7–16 Must Adhere to the Following Rest Requirements
<10	75	If a player pitches 61 or more pitches in a day, 3 calendar days of rest must be observed.
11–12	85	If a player pitches 41–60 pitches in a day, 2 calendar days of rest must be observed.
13–16	95	If a player pitches 21–40 pitches in a day, 1 calendar day of rest must be observed.
17–18	105	If a player pitches 1–20 pitches in a day, no calendar day of rest is required before pitching again.

- Optimizing throwing technique and teaching athletes to engage lower body and core strength may be effective in reducing excessive shoulder and elbow stress.

When to Refer

- If the patient continues to have symptoms despite an adequate rest period, then the clinician may need to expand the differential diagnosis and consider referral to a sports medicine specialist. Conditions that are not relieved with rest in the differential diagnosis include shoulder instability, labral tear, and rotator cuff tear.

Prognosis

- If properly diagnosed and treated, little leaguer's shoulder is benign and self-limited.
- More than 90% of athletes who develop this condition are asymptomatic on return to sports.
- Although extremely rare, the most concerning complication is the potential of premature closure of the affected proximal humeral physis.

Troubleshooting

- Physical therapy should be delayed until the patient is completely asymptomatic
- Compliance is essential to a full recovery. Often, adolescents will prematurely become more active and resume throwing or swinging as soon as symptoms of pain have decreased.

Patient Instructions

- Pitch count limitations, rest days between pitching outings, and a gradual increase in the types of pitches thrown are the keys to preventing upper extremity pathology in a young athlete. Listed in Tables 218.2 and 218.3 are the USA Baseball Medical and Safety Advisory Committee's pitching recommendations for injury prevention.

TABLE 218.3 Recommended Minimum Number of Rest Days After Throwing a Certain Number of Pitches

Age (yr)	1 Day of Rest After Throwing (Pitches)	2 Days of Rest After Throwing (Pitches)	3 Days of Rest After Throwing (Pitches)	4 Days of Rest After Throwing (Pitches)
8–10	20	35	45	50
11–12	25	35	55	60
13–14	30	35	55	70
15–16	30	40	60	80
17–18	30	40	60	90

Suggested Readings

Chen FS, Diaz VA, Loebenberg M, Rosen JE. Shoulder and elbow injuries in the skeletally immature athlete. *J Am Acad Orthop Surg*. 2005;13:172–185.

Heyworth BE, Kramer DE, Martin DJ, et al. Trends in the presentation, management and outcomes of little league shoulder. *Am J Sports Med*. 2016;44:1431–1438.

Kocher MS, Waters PM, Micheli LJ. Upper extremity injuries in the paediatric athlete. *Sports Med*. 2000;30:117–135.

Osbahr DC, Kim HJ, Dugas JR. Little league shoulder. *Curr Opin Pediatr*. 2010;22:35–40.

Sabick MB, Kim YK, Torry MR, et al. Biomechanics of the shoulder in youth baseball pitchers: implications for the development of proximal humeral epiphysiolysis and humeral retrotorsion. *Am J Sports Med*. 2005;33:1716–1722.

Chapter 219 The Adolescent: Little Leaguer's Elbow

Michael A. Beasley, Mininder S. Kocher

ICD-10-CM CODES
M24.829 *Little league (leaguer's) elbow*
M77.01 *Medial epicondylitis, right*
M77.02 *Medial epicondylitis, left*

Key Concepts

- Elbow pain is a frequently seen condition with an annual incidence of 20-40% of 9- to 12-year-old baseball players, and 50-70% of adolescent players.
- Little leaguer's elbow is a preventable overuse syndrome stemming from valgus overload seen predominately in skeletally immature throwing athletes.
- Age-dependent range of medial-side injuries from tensile forces with valgus stress
  - Classically refers to medial epicondyle apophysitis in childhood
  - Includes avulsion fractures further into maturity and ligamentous injuries in the skeletally mature athlete
- Throwing motion also creates lateral compressive forces and posterior shear forces.
  - Lateral injuries include osteochondrosis (Panner disease) and osteochondritis dissecans (OCD) of the capitellum or radial head.
  - Posterior injuries include olecranon apophysitis, avulsion fractures, and impingement with osteophyte formation.
- Location of stress and type of injury affected by phase of throwing motion
- Understanding the order of ossification and apophyseal closure is crucial to evaluating radiographs in the developing throwing athlete with elbow pain.
- Prevention and treatment are based on age-appropriate restrictions on throwing, including pitch counts, avoidance of year-round and multiple team training, and possibly focusing on pitch types and proper mechanics.

History

- Chronologic and skeletal age is the initial clue to the differential diagnosis in the throwing athlete with elbow pain.
  - Skeletally immature throwers are more likely to have apophysitis or avulsion fractures, while ligamentous injuries are more common after physeal closure.
- The level of participation in baseball is a crucial history point—positions played, number of months per year in competitive play, number of teams/leagues the player participates in, types of pitches thrown, additional sports played.
- Location(s) of pain is related to forces created by throwing motion (Fig. 219.1).
  - Distracting tension forces created by valgus overload at medial elbow
  - Continued valgus load may create compressive forces at the lateral elbow and shearing forces at the posterior elbow.
- Phases of throwing motion causing pain may help indicate likely diagnoses (Fig. 219.2).
  - Early and late cocking phases create distracting forces at medial elbow.
  - Late cocking and early acceleration create compressive lateral forces.
  - Follow-through may create shear forces into the posterior elbow.
- Onset and duration of pain may suggest nature of injury.
  - Acute onset of symptoms is most consistent with avulsion fracture or ligamentous injury
  - Insidious onset or chronic symptoms more indicative of apophysitis or overuse syndrome
  - Mechanical symptoms of locking, effusions, or decreased range of motion all may indicate loose bodies.
- Family history of osteochondrosis increases likelihood of this diagnosis in other family members.

Physical Examination

- Physical examination of the painful elbow requires assessment for bruising, swelling, range of motion, carrying angle, and muscle bulk, all in comparison to the contralateral nonthrowing elbow.
- Palpation of bony landmarks, including medial epicondyle, lateral epicondyle and radiocapitellar joint, and the olecranon, may best locate pain sites.
  - Palpating from medial epicondyle to sublime tubercle follows the pathway of ulnar collateral ligament (UCL).
- Varus and valgus stress testing throughout a range of flexion/extension helps assess ligamentous stability or "gapping" of joint spaces.
  - Valgus stress testing or "milking maneuver" may best recreate forces of throwing motion.
  - Valgus stress at 30 degrees of flexion is best to assess the stability of the ulnar collateral ligament.
- As the throwing motion involves a complex kinetic chain, the exam must include general evaluation of the neck,

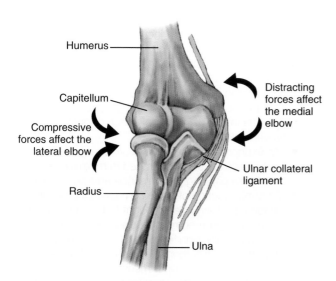

Fig 219.1 Functional anatomy of the elbow.

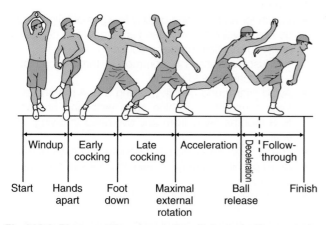

Fig 219.2 Phases of throwing motion. (Adapted with permission from DiGiovine NM, Jobe FW, Pink M, Perry J: An electromyographic analysis of the upper extremity in pitching. *J Shoulder Elbow Surg* 1:15-25, 1992.)

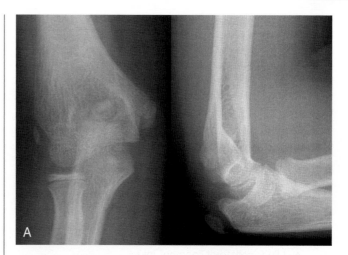

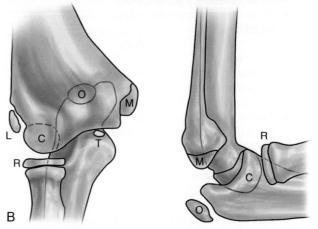

Fig 219.3 Radiographic appearance **(A)** and correlating diagram **(B)** of the six elbow apophyses. The apophyses close by ossification as the elbow matures, with all apophyses completely closed by the mid-teen years in most cases. An understanding of this pattern is crucial in doing a proper reading of plain radiographs. *C,* Capitellum; *L,* lateral epicondyle; *M,* medial epicondyle; *O,* olecranon; *R,* radius; *T,* trochlea. (From (A) and adapted from (B) Benjamin H, Briner W. Little league elbow. *Clin J Sports Med.* 2005;15:37–40.)

shoulder, and wrist, evaluating range of motion, strength, and ligamentous laxity, all compared.
- Medial sided pain, especially if radiating distally into the wrist or if accompanied by numbness, warrants evaluation of the ulnar nerve for subluxation or presence of the Tinel sign in cubital tunnel.

Imaging

- Although little leaguer's elbow is often a clinical diagnosis, imaging is helpful in evaluating the severity of bony or soft-tissue involvement.
- Initial radiographs include anteroposterior, lateral, and oblique views.
  - Stress views may be helpful in evaluating joint line stability.
- Evaluation of radiographs in the skeletally immature athlete requires an understanding of the chronologic order of ossification centers in the elbow (Fig. 219.3).

- The mnemonic CRITOE (*C*apitellum, *R*adius, *I*nternal [medial] epicondyle, *T*rochlea, *O*lecranon, *E*xternal [lateral] epicondyle) is helpful in recalling order of closure.
- Comparison radiographs of the contralateral, nonthrowing arm are helpful in differentiating normal ossification from true injury.
  - Medial pain requires assessment of the medial epicondyle for fragmentation or widening when compared with contralateral side.
  - Lateral pain prompts evaluation for capitellar OCD or Panner disease.
  - Posterior pain may present radiographic evidence of olecranon apophyseal widening or osteophyte formation in the setting of impingement.
- Magnetic resonance imaging (MRI) can be helpful in the setting of both normal and abnormal initial radiographs:
  - Clinical concern for ligamentous injury such as ulnar collateral ligament tear

- Neurologic symptoms and concern for ulnar nerve instability
- Grading severity and assessing stability of OCD lesions
- Evaluating for loose bodies or demonstrating bony stress in impingement syndromes
- Computed tomography (CT) scans may better define fracture displacement and loose body formation.

Differential Diagnosis

- Classically little leaguer's elbow represents medial sided pain, but often is broadly defined to include lateral and posterior sources of elbow pain in throwing athletes
  - Medial pain
    - Medial epicondyle apophysitis
    - Medial epicondyle avulsion fracture
    - Ulnar collateral ligament injury
    - Ulnar nerve entrapment (cubital tunnel syndrome) or instability
    - Common flexor tendon injury
  - Lateral pain
    - Capitellum osteochondritis dissecans (OCD)
    - Capitellum osteochondrosis (Panner disease)
    - Radial head OCD or deformation
    - Lateral extension overload
    - Common extensor tendon injury/lateral epicondylitis (tennis elbow)
  - Posterior pain
    - Olecranon apophysitis
    - Olecranon avulsion fracture
    - Olecranon bursitis
    - Posterior osteophyte formation/impingement
- Differential diagnosis must also include extrinsic causes of elbow pain
  - Stress reactions/fractures in upper extremity
  - Cervical radiculopathy
  - Inflammatory/infectious causes

Treatment

- Little leaguer's elbow in all presentations represents primarily an overuse syndrome; thus prevention efforts and rest from throwing remain the most essential treatment modalities.

- Significant increases in elbow injuries in young throwing athletes have prompted an increased focus on reducing quantity of throwing, especially in pitchers.
  - Pitch count and rest time recommendations vary based on age (Table 219.1).
  - While pitching mechanics, types of pitches thrown, and overall physical fitness and strength are all thought to play a role in risk of injury, only pitch quantity has been a proven risk factor.
    - While unproven, focusing on core strength and proper mechanics are still encouraged to minimize injury and maximize pitching performance and endurance.
    - Early introduction of breaking pitches (curveballs and sliders) has long been thought to be a risk factor for injury, though recurrent studies fail to show this to be statistically significant. It is still strongly recommended by the authors of this chapter that developing pitchers focus on proper mechanics for fastballs and changeups, and delay breaking pitches until 14 years of age or physeal maturation.
- General recommendations for avoiding overuse injuries in throwers
  - Watch for and respond quickly to signs of fatigue, such as loss of velocity, decreased accuracy, and decreased ability to maintain proper mechanics.
    - Muscle soreness is common in throwing athletes; joint pain should not be.
  - Avoid year-round pitching, taking 3 to 4 months away from competitive pitching each year, and at least 2 to 3 months away from any overhead throwing each year.
  - Follow recommended pitch counts and days of rest.
  - Avoid pitching on multiple teams/leagues or overlapping seasons.
  - Avoid use of radar guns, as it may incentivize pitcher simply to throw harder.
  - Pitchers should avoid playing catcher as an alternate position, as it results in higher throw volume.
  - Elbow or shoulder pain in the youth pitcher should prompt removal from the game until evaluated by a sports medicine physician.
  - Encourage multisport involvement rather than baseball sports specialization.

TABLE 219.1 Pitch Count and Rest Time Recommendations by Age

| Age (Years) | Daily Pitch Limit | REQUIRED REST (PITCHES) | | | | | |
		0 Days	1 Days	2 Days	3 Days	4 Days	5 Days
7–8	50	1–20	21–35	36–50	N/A	N/A	N/A
9–10	75	1–20	21–35	36–50	51–65	66+	N/A
11–12	85	1–20	21–35	36–50	51–65	66+	N/A
13–14	95	1–20	21–35	36–50	51–65	66+	N/A
15–16	95	1–30	31–45	46–60	61–75	76+	N/A
17–18	105	1–30	31–45	46–60	61–80	81+	N/A
19–22	120	1–30	31–45	46–60	61–80	81–105	106+

From Pitch Smart MLB and USA Baseball. Guidelines for youth and adolescent pitchers. Available at http://m.mlb.com/pitchsmart/pitching-guidelines.

- Medial injuries
  - Injuries of the medial epicondyle vary widely in presentation and required treatments (Fig. 219.4).
  - Medial epicondylar apophysitis
    - Initiate complete pitching rest for a minimum of 4 to 6 weeks, with consideration of eliminating all throwing if nonpitch throws are painful.
    - Pain relief with ice, massage, and nonsteroidal inflammatory medications.
    - Physical therapy with initial focus on pain relief and maintaining full range of motion to avoid flexion contracture, eventually advancing to strengthening of

entire throwing kinetic chain including core, shoulder, and wrist flexors/extensors.
  - After initial rest period, begin a slow return to throwing program, only progressing if the athlete remains pain-free.
  - Prognosis for classic apophysitis is excellent with an average time to return to pitching of 12 weeks.
- Medial epicondyle avulsion fracture
  - Nondisplaced or minimally displaced fractures are often treated conservatively with brief immobilization and early range of motion beginning at 1 to 2 weeks to avoid flexion contracture.

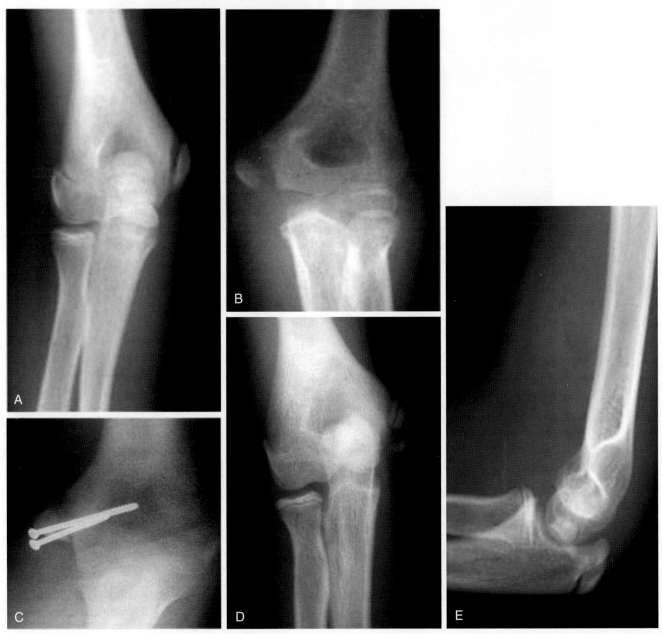

Fig 219.4 Injury patterns of the medial epicondyle. **(A)** Medial epicondyle apophysitis with widening. **(B)** Displaced medial epicondyle fracture requiring open reduction internal fixation I. **(D)** Chronic medial epicondyle apophysitis with fragmentation. **(E)** Entrapment of a displaced medial epicondyle fracture within the elbow joint requiring emergent open reduction internal fixation. (From Klingele K, Kocher M. Little league elbow: valgus overload injury in the paediatric athlete. *Sports Med.* 2002;32:1005–1015.)

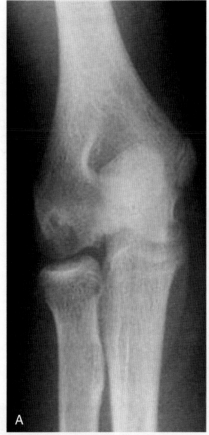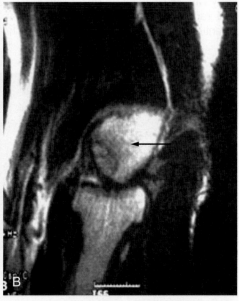

Fig 219.5 Osteochondritis dissecans of the capitellum. **(A)** Anteroposterior radiograph of the elbow reveals a well demarcated subchondral lesion of the capitellum. **(B)** Magnetic resonance imaging demonstrates a stage I lesion *(arrow)* with an intact articular surface. (From Klingele K, Kocher M. Little league elbow: valgus overload injury in the paediatric athlete. *Sports Med.* 2002;32: 1005–1015.)

- Return to throwing program typically begins at 6 weeks or when radiographs demonstrate normal union.
- Displaced fractures typically warrant referral to an orthopaedic surgeon and may require long-arm casting or open reduction and internal fixation.
  - Up to 30-50% are associated with elbow dislocation, and may present with fracture fragment incarceration.
- Lateral injuries
  - Osteochondritis dissecans (OCD) of the capitellum and radial head
    - Treatment guided by initial staging with radiographs and magnetic resonance imaging (MRI) (Fig. 219.5)
    - Stable lesions often treated nonoperatively, often requiring up to 6 months of rest from throwing
      - Six-week interval radiographs and 3-month interval MRIs are used to monitor healing.
    - Unstable lesions, or those failing conservative treatment require surgical management
      - Arthroscopy is associated with decreased operative morbidity and earlier return to play when compared to open arthrotomy.
      - Postoperatively, immediate passive and active range of motion is used to prevent stiffness, with progressive strengthening at 3 months.

- Formal throwing progressing to return to play at 5 to 6 months
- Panner disease (capitellar osteochondrosis)
  - Must be distinguished from capitellar OCD, with Panner disease occurring earlier in childhood than OCD
  - Treatment is conservative, as this is a self-limited condition with excellent prognosis for complete resolution.
  - Rest from throwing and painful activities often quickly resolves symptoms, and return to throwing may be guided by pain, as radiographic findings often lag behind clinical resolution.
- Deformity of the radial head may be seen with repetitive, chronic microtrauma from lateral compressive forces.
  - Treatment is guided by severity and radiographic findings, but typically referral to an orthopaedic surgeon is required for loose body or osteophyte removal, or in severe cases, radial head excision.
- Posterior injuries
  - Olecranon apophyseal injuries
    - Olecranon apophysitis is most common in young throwing athletes and is treated similar to medial epicondyle apophysitis with 3 to 4 weeks initial throwing rest, physical therapy, and progressive return to throwing as tolerated.
      - Most athletes are able to return to play in 6 weeks.

- Olecranon apophysis avulsion fractures seen in adolescent pitchers
  - Nondisplaced or minimally displaced fractures treated with casting
  - Fractures displaced >2 mm require open reduction and internal fixation.
- Extension overload, osteophyte formation, and posterior impingement seen in skeletally mature throwers
  - Failure of initial rest or loose body formation may require open versus arthroscopic surgical debridement

Patient Resources

- The American Academy of Orthopaedic Surgeons has an excellent patient information guide available at http://orthoinfo.aaos.org/topic.cfm?topic=A00328.
- Major League Baseball and USA Baseball provides age appropriate guidelines and recommendations through the Pitch Smart campaign, with resources available at http://pitchsmart.org.

Acknowledgment

The authors would like to acknowledge the contributions from James MacDonald and Olabode Ogunwole in the previous edition of this chapter.

Suggested Readings

Benjamin H, Briner W. Little league elbow. *Clin J Sports Med*. 2005;15: 37–40.

Cain EL Jr, Dugas JR, Wolf RS, Andrews JR. Elbow injuries in throwing athletes: a current concepts review. *Am J Sports Med*. 2003;31:621–635.

Chen F, Diaz VA, Loebenberg M, Rosen JE. Shoulder and elbow injuries in the skeletally immature athlete. *J Am Acad Orthop Surg*. 2005;13:172–185.

Fleisig GS, Andrews JR, Cutter GR, et al. Risk of serious injury for young baseball pitchers: a 10-year prospective study. *Am J Sports Med*. 2011;39:253–257.

Fortenbaugh D, Fleisig GS, Andrews JR. Baseball pitching biomechanics in relation to injury risk and performance. *Sports Health*. 2009;1(4): 314–320.

Grantham WJ, Iyengar JJ, Byram IR, et al. The curveball as a risk factor for injury: a systematic review. *Sports Health*. 2015;7(1):19–26.

Kancherla VK, Caggiano NM, Matullo KS. Elbow injuries in the throwing athlete. *Orthop Clin N Am*. 2014;45:571–585.

Klingele K, Kocher M. Little league elbow: valgus overload injury in the paediatric athlete. *Sports Med*. 2002;32:1005–1015.

Limpisvasti O, ElAttrache NS, Jobe FW. Understanding shoulder and elbow injuries in baseball. *J Am Acad Orthop Surg*. 2007;15: 139–146.

Lyman S, Fleisig GS, Andrews JR, Osinski ED. Effect of pitch type, pitch count, and pitching mechanics on risk of elbow and shoulder pain in youth baseball pitchers. *Am J Sports Med*. 2002;30:463–468.

Olsen S, Fleisig GS, Dun S, et al. Risk factors for shoulder and elbow injuries in adolescent baseball pitchers. *Am J Sports Med*. 2006;34: 905–912.

Chapter 220 The Adolescent: Osteochondritis Dissecans

Mininder S. Kocher, Katherine Victoria Yao, Bridget Quinn

ICD-10-CM CODES

M93.261	*Right knee*
M93.262	*Left knee*
M93.221	*Right elbow*
M93.222	*Left elbow*
93.271	*Right ankle and/or foot*
93.272	*Left ankle and/or foot*
M93.251	*Right hip*
M93.252	*Left hip*

Key Concepts

- The etiology of osteochondritis dissecans (OCD) has been thought of as idiopathic; however, a growing consensus points toward multiple contributors including vascular insufficiency/ischemia, repetitive trauma, abnormal ossification, genetics, or a combination of these factors.
- OCD is a condition affecting the subchondral bone characterized by focal aseptic necrosis and separation of an osteochondral bone fragment with or without articular cartilage involvement.
- The separation of the osteochondral fragment may be present in situ or exhibit an incomplete or complete detachment. Classification of OCD is based on imaging studies (i.e., plain film radiographs, magnetic resonance imaging [MRI], or rarely single-photon emission computed tomography bone scan), surgical findings, and anatomic location of the lesion.
- OCD can also be divided into juvenile and adult forms depending on physeal maturity. The majority of adult OCD cases are secondary to the persistence of an unresolved juvenile OCD lesion, although de novo cases of adult OCD have been described.
- OCD can be present on any joint surface; however, it most commonly involves the knees, elbows, ankles, and hips, in that order. It is extremely rare to have OCD develop in the shoulder or wrist joints.
- Bilateral involvement is reported in as many as 25% of cases.
- If untreated, the long-term sequela is premature degenerative joint disease.

History

- Presentation depends on the stage of the lesion. Early, stable lesions with an intact articular surface may present as vague episodic pain that can be confused with patellofemoral pain in the knee. Later, unstable lesions with disrupted articular surfaces present with more pain, swelling, catching, and locking that can be confused with meniscal tears.
- Clinical presentation of adult OCD is typically insidious, progressive, and unremitting joint discomfort that does not resolve over time and with rest.
- Symptoms of juvenile OCD are classically gradual in onset but fairly nonspecific. Patients may exhibit a joint effusion, locking, or simply poorly localized joint pain that is exacerbated by activity and improves with rest.
- The patient may also report pain with walking and a limp if OCD of the knee, ankle, or hip is present.

Physical Examination
Observation

- Joint effusion may be present.
- An antalgic gait is often seen if OCD involves the lower extremity.

Palpation

- With OCD of the knee, maximal tenderness to palpation is noted over the medial femoral condyle. This can be best felt with the knee in 90 degrees of flexion with pressure directed just medial to the inferior pole of the patella. More than 70% of OCD lesions are found in the posterolateral aspect of the medial femoral condyle.
- With OCD of the elbow, the anterolateral aspect of the capitellum is the most common site of the lesion. This area of the elbow is best palpated with the elbow flexed to 90 degrees.
- With OCD of the ankle, the tibiotalar joint may have diffuse or localized tenderness.
- OCD of the hip may have generalized hip joint pain and tenderness with palpation to surrounding hip flexors and soft tissues.

Range of Motion

- Loss of range of motion may occur secondary to an effusion or a completely detached osteochondral lesion causing locking of the joint.
- Joint movement can be associated with pain and crepitus.

Special Tests

- Wilson sign for OCD of the knee
  - Pain or discomfort with internal rotation of the tibia with the knee in 90 and 30 degrees of flexion

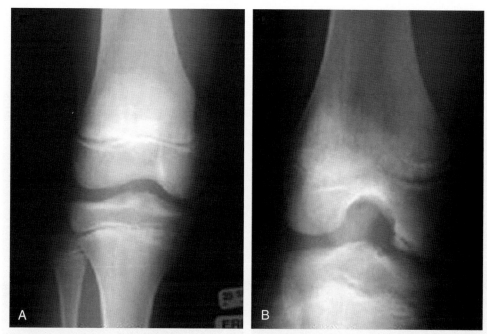

Fig 220.1 (A) Anteroposterior view of the knee does not reveal an osteochondritis dissecans (OCD) lesion in the posterolateral aspect of the medial femoral condyle. However, once a notch view is obtained (B), it is clearly evident that an OCD lesion is present.

- Relief of pain with external rotation of the tibia
- Wilson sign lacks the sensitivity to detect OCD of the knee; however, it is useful as a clinical monitor during treatment.

Imaging
Radiographs
- OCD is indicated by a focal lucency in the articular epiphysis
- For OCD of the knee: anteroposterior, lateral, notch, and sunrise views
  - The notch view will allow for better visualization of the posterior femoral condyle in comparison with the anteroposterior view (Fig. 220.1A and B).
  - More than 70% of OCD lesions are found in the posterolateral aspect of the medial femoral condyle.

Magnetic Resonance Imaging
- If an OCD lesion is found on plain radiographs, an MRI is indicated because it provides vital information regarding prognosis and management.
- MRI will help determine the size of the OCD lesion, the status of the articular cartilage and subchondral bone, the extent of bony edema, the presence of any possible loose bodies, and other knee injuries.

Classification of Osteochondritis Dissecans
- Juvenile OCD is first differentiated from the adult form based on the closure of the physes. In juvenile OCD, the physes remain open, whereas in the adult form, the physes are closed.

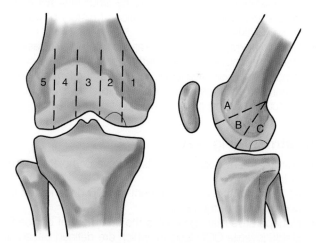

Fig 220.2 Anatomic classification of osteochondritis dissecans of the knee. *1* and *2* are MFC lesions, *3* is a trochlear lesion, and *4* and *5* are lateral femoral condyle lesions. *A* indicates non-weightbearing, and *B* and *C* indicate weight bearing.

- There are different classification schemes based on anatomic location, the stability of the lesion, and imaging modalities (Figs. 220.2 and 220.3).

Differential Diagnosis
- Knee: patellofemoral pain, meniscal tear, normal irregular ossification pattern, avascular necrosis; if trauma: osteochondral impaction fracture.
- Elbow: Panner disease, extensor and/or triceps tendinitis, valgus extension overload syndrome; if trauma: osteochondral impaction fracture, fracture (including avulsion fracture).

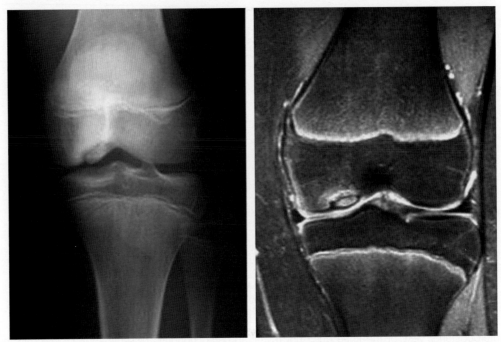

Fig 220.3 Stage 3 juvenile osteochondritis dissecans lesion of the medial femoral condyle. The lesion is clearly demarcated with fluid between the lesion and the subchondral bone.

- Ankle: ankle impingement syndrome, sinus tarsi syndrome, talus stress fracture, tarsal coalition; if history of trauma: chronic ankle sprain.
- Hip: hip flexor tendinitis, dysplasia of the hip with associated instability, Legg-Calve-Perthes disease, slipped capital femoral epiphysis, avascular necrosis of the femoral head, femoral neck stress fracture, hip labral tear; if trauma: fracture (including physeal avulsion fracture).

Treatment (Fig. 220.4)

- The treatment goal of OCD is to have complete healing of the lesion.
- At diagnosis, the initial treatment of OCD depends on the classification of the lesion.
- Nonoperative management is the treatment of choice for stable juvenile OCD lesions, which are defined based on the MRI classification as either stage I or II.
  - The first 6 weeks of treatment involve protected weight-bearing/joint loading, limitation of aggravating activities, and consideration of an immobilization device. This is achieved in the knee via crutches and a knee immobilizer, range-of-motion brace, or unloading brace; in the ankle with crutches and an aircast boot or cast; and in the elbow with temporary early use of a hinged brace (with caution due to risk of elbow stiffness). A plain radiograph should be repeated at the end of this phase to see if there is any healing of the OCD lesion.
  - During the second 6 weeks, the immobilization device is discontinued as the patient is weaned off crutches and advanced to weight bearing as tolerated. Physical therapy is initiated emphasizing range of motion and low-impact muscle strengthening exercises, such as the quadriceps and hamstring in the knee.

- MRI should be repeated to evaluate for healing after a total of 12 weeks of treatment. If there is radiographic and clinical evidence of healing, then the patient is ready to begin the third phase of therapy, which includes sport-specific physical therapy with supervised return to impact activities. The patient is then permitted to gradually return to sports as symptoms allow.
- Evaluation by an orthopaedic surgeon for operative treatment is recommended for the following:
  - Any detached or unstable lesions with MRI classification stage III or higher.
  - Stable lesions that have not healed with 6 to 9 months of nonsurgical treatment.
  - OCD lesions in adolescents approaching physeal closure and adults with OCD lesions
- Surgical treatment options include drilling, fixation, and chondral resurfacing of the OCD lesion

Prognosis

- 66% of stable juvenile OCD lesions will heal within 6 months provided the physes remain open and the patient complies with conservative treatment, including activity modification and immobilization.
- Larger lesions, lesions on the lateral femoral condyle (as opposed to the classical location at the medial femoral condyle), and lesions producing mechanical symptoms are less likely to heal.
- Nonoperatively managed juvenile OCD lesions of MRI classification stage III or higher typically do not heal.
- Patients nearing skeletal maturity are 7.4 times more likely to progress to surgery than those under age 11 years.
- Surgical drilling results in radiographic healing of stable lesions in 86% of adolescents with open physes with

Knee Osteochondral Lesions Treatment

Conservative treatment for stage I and II stable OCD lesions

1. Protect weight bearing x 6 weeks with:
   - Crutches
   - Knee immobilizer brace
2. Wean off crutches and immobilization brace to weight bearing as tolerated for next 6 weeks
3. Initiate physical therapy with focus on range of motion and low-impact muscle strengthening
4. Repeat MRI after 12 weeks

Surgical treatment for stage III and IV unstable OCD lesions

- Microfracture
- Drilling and fixation
- Autograft transfer
- Autologous chondrocyte implant
- Allograft transfer

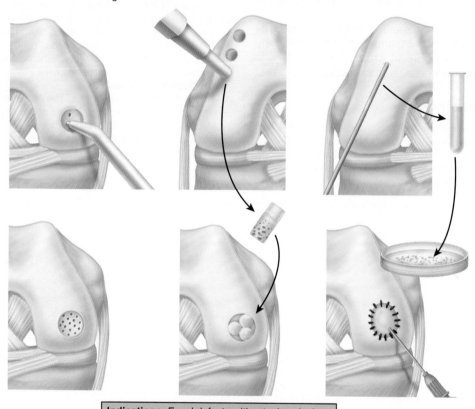

Indications: Focal defects without mirror lesions

Fig 220.4 Treatments for osteochondritis dissecans *(OCD)* of the knee. *MRI,* Magnetic resonance imaging.

significant pain reduction and excellent functional outcomes in 92% to 100% of the cases approximately 8.5 months postoperatively.

- Surgical fixation of unstable juvenile OCD lesions has healing rates of 85% to 100% depending on the type of lesion and fixation techniques used.
- Excision of large fragments should be avoided because this leads to degenerative joint disease. If excision has been performed, chondral resurfacing procedures may be indicated.

Troubleshooting

- Radiographs can be taken at the 6-week mark and MRI performed at the 12-week mark to evaluate the healing of the OCD lesion. A notch view of the knee is helpful in identifying the lesion.

- Persistent pain symptoms and no radiographic improvement often result from poor compliance with treatment in an adolescent patient.
- Protected weight-bearing with slow, gradual advancement is the key to nonoperative therapy.
- If symptoms return after treatment or follow-up radiographs show lesion recurrence, repeated nonoperative treatment can be considered, but counsel with an orthopaedic surgeon is recommended.
- Bilateral involvement is reported in as many as 25% of cases.

Patient Instructions

- Counsel the patient as to the importance of compliance with therapy. Often, adolescents will become more active when symptoms of pain have decreased. However, decreased pain symptoms are not the equivalent of a healed OCD lesion.

- Counsel the patient that complete resolution of the OCD lesion, either nonoperatively or surgically, requires at least 3 to 6 months and can take up to 12 months.
- Unsuccessful treatment of OCD may lead to progressive degenerative joint disease and worsening of pain symptoms.

Considerations in Special Populations

- Adult OCD lesions present typically with insidious, progressive, and unremitting joint discomfort that does not respond to nonsurgical management. Early orthopaedic referral is recommended.
- Nonoperative initial management of stable juvenile OCD lesions is advised. Surgical treatment is indicated for any detached or unstable lesions in which physeal closure is imminent or when nonoperative management has failed.

Suggested Readings

Bauer KL, Polousky JD. Management of osteochondritis dissecans lesions of the knee, elbow and ankle. *Clin Sports Med*. 2017;36:469–487.

Bruns J, Werner M, Habermann C. Osteochondritis dissecans: etiology, pathology, and imaging with a special focus on the knee joint. *Cartilage*. 2017;[Epub ahead of print].

Cahill BR. Osteochondritis dissecans of the knee: treatment of juvenile and adult forms. *J Am Acad Orthop Surg*. 1995;3(4):237–247.

Hefti F, Beguiristain J, Krauspe R, et al. Osteochondritis dissecans: a multicenter study of the European Pediatric Orthopedic Society. *J Pediatr Orthop B*. 1999;8(4):231–245.

Kessler JI, Nikizad H, Shea KG, et al. The demographics and epidemiology of osteochondritis dissecans of the knee in children and adolescents. *Am J Sports Med*. 2014;42(2):320–326.

Kocher MS, Czarnecki JJ, Andersen JS, Micheli LJ. Internal fixation of juvenile osteochondritis dissecans lesions of the knee. *Am J Sports Med*. 2007;35(5):712–718.

Kocher MS, Micheli LJ, Yaniv M, et al. Functional and radiographic outcome of juvenile osteochondritis dissecans of the knee treated with transarticular arthroscopic drilling. *Am J Sports Med*. 2001;29(5):562–566.

Kocher MS, Tucker R, Ganley TJ, Flynn JM. Management of osteochondritis dissecans of the knee. *Am J Sports Med*. 2006;34(7):1181–1191.

McElroy MJ, Riley PM, Tepolt FA, et al. Catcher's knee: posterior femoral condyle juvenile osteochondritis dissecans in children and adolescents. *J Pediatr Orthop*. 2016;[Epub ahead of print].

Wall EJ, Vourazeris J, Myer GD, et al. The healing potential of stable juvenile osteochondritis dissecans knee lesions. *J Bone Joint Surg Am*. 2008;90(12):2655–2664.

Weiss JM, Nikizad H, Shea KG, et al. The incidence of surgery in osteochondritis dissecans in children and adolescents. *Orthop J Sports Med*. 2016;4(3):2325967116635515.

Zanon G, Di Vico G, Marullo M. Osteochondritis dissecans of the knee. *Joints*. 2014;2(1):29–36.

Chapter 221 The Adolescent: Osgood-Schlatter/Sinding-Larsen-Johansson Lesions

Hugo Paquin, Gianmichel Corrado, Mininder S. Kocher

ICD-10-CM CODES
M92.5 *Juvenile osteochondrosis of tibia and fibula (Osgood-Schlatter disorder)*
M92.4 *Juvenile osteochondrosis of patella (Sinding-Larsen-Johansson disorder)*

Key Concepts

- Osgood-Schlatter lesion (OSL) and Sinding-Larsen-Johansson lesion (SLJL) are both disorders of the extensor mechanism of the knee seen typically in active children and adolescents during the time of ossification of characteristic anatomic sites in the knee.
  - Pain results from increased stress at both sites causing inflammation (traction osteochondritis)
- OSL is a disorder of the formation and growth of the proximal tibial apophysis.
  - OSL typically presents with pain and tenderness at the tibial tuberosity with or without a history of local trauma.
  - OSL is a common cause of disability in active adolescents. Some studies have found more than 20% of active 13-year-olds have signs and symptoms of OSL.
- SLJL is a disorder of the normal ossification process involving the inferior pole of the patella.
  - SLJL typically presents with pain and tenderness at the inferior pole of the patella with or without a history of local trauma.
  - SLJL is seen exclusively in children and adolescents with open physes.
  - SLJL is seen less commonly than OSL.
- The diagnosis of both OSL and SLJL is typically made clinically; imaging can occasionally be helpful but often is not necessary initially.
- Treatment of OSL and SLJL is conservative in the majority of cases.
- Symptoms of both disorders are typically self-limited. Late sequelae of OSL and SLJL tend to be mild and insignificant, such as a prominent tibial tuberosity.
- Surgery including excision of painful ossicles is rarely indicated in refractory cases. Surgery is indicated in OSL for complete tibial tubercle avulsion fractures, but this is a rare complication.

History

- OSL and SLJL commonly present as anterior knee pain in children 10 to 15 years of age who participate in running, cutting, and jumping sports such as basketball and soccer.
- OSL and SLJL disorders have been associated with the adolescent growth spurt. Girls typically present at a younger age (mean age of 11.5 years compared with 13 years for boys).
- The onset of pain is typically insidious, but can commonly be associated with trauma. If there has been recent acute trauma, there should be heightened suspicion of a tibial tubercle apophyseal fracture OSL or a sleeve fracture of the patella SLJL.
- Knee pain caused by OSL or SLJL is typically well localized and is not associated with mechanical symptoms such as recurring effusions, locking, and instability.
- Twenty percent to 30% of patients with OSL will report bilateral knee symptoms. If a patient presents with unilateral symptoms, some attention should be paid to the contralateral knee in the history and physical examination.
- A careful review of systems should be done to rule out more insidious etiologies of pain, particularly when the patient presents with unilateral symptoms. A review of systems should include (not exclusively) queries about weight loss, fevers or night sweats, nocturnal pain or pain that awakens a patient, and hip/groin pain.

Physical Examination

- Both knees should be examined, even if the patient is reporting pain exclusively in one knee.
- Inspection
  - Patients may walk with an antalgic gait.
  - There can be swelling over the corresponding anatomic locations (OSL, tibial tubercle; SLJL, and inferior patella).
  - There should be no effusion.
- Palpation
  - There will be tenderness to palpation and palpable swelling over the tibial tubercle in OSL and the inferior pole of the patella in SLJL.
  - There should be no tenderness over the joint line.
- Range of motion
  - There should be full range of motion in the knee.
  - The patient should be able do a straight leg raise and perform active terminal knee extension; if the patient

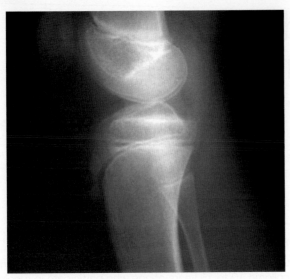

Fig 221.1 Osgood-Schlatter lesion.

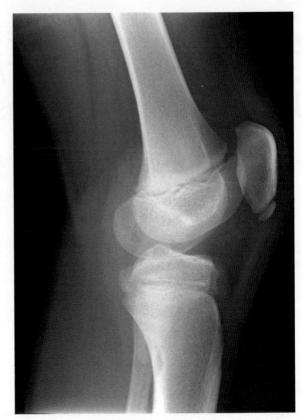

Fig 221.2 Sinding-Larsen-Johansson lesion.

cannot do that, especially if seen in the setting of acute trauma, there may be an associated fracture.
- Flexibility assessment
  - Patients with OSL and SLJL will typically have a marked degree of inflexibility.
  - The popliteal angle (to assess hamstring muscle flexibility) and the Thomas test (to assess hip flexor flexibility) should be done.
- Examination of the hip
  - An examination of the hip should be done to rule out causes of referred pain to the knee.
  - Specifically, the patient should have full and pain-free internal and external range of motion of the hips.

Imaging

- Often imaging is not indicated when OSL or SLJL are the working diagnoses. Clinicians may elect to proceed with treatment and careful follow-up in the majority of cases.
- That being said, plain radiographs can be invaluable in ruling out more insidious etiologies of knee pain (e.g., fractures, osteosarcomas, and osteochondritis dissecans).
- Plain radiographs in OSL may include a four-view series of the affected knee(s), including anteroposterior, lateral, skyline, and notch/tunnel views.
  - The lateral view is especially revealing of the tibial apophysis (Fig. 221.1).
    - May show calcification and thickening of the patellar tendon, irregular ossification of the tibial tubercle, and overlying soft-tissue swelling
  - The notch view can rule out osteochondritis dissecans if that is included in the working differential diagnosis.
  - Comparison views of the contralateral unaffected knee are sometimes helpful, especially if there is significant tibial tubercle fragmentation seen radiographically and the clinician wants to rule out associated fracture.
- Plain radiographs in SLJL likewise may include a four-view series of the affected knee(s).

- Often a radiograph will show a small bone fragment adjacent to the inferior patella; this should be correlated clinically (Fig. 221.2).
- One can see this finding in either SLJL or a patellar sleeve fracture. In the latter, there should be strong clinical evidence such as a significant hemarthrosis and significant disability (e.g., inability to extend the knee).
- Advanced imaging (e.g., magnetic resonance imaging, bone scans, computed tomography) is rarely indicated unless other diagnoses (e.g., stress fractures) are being seriously considered.
  - Ultrasound may be useful as it may show swelling in the soft tissue, cartilage, bursa, and tendon.

Differential Diagnosis

Please see Table 221.1.

Treatment

- Treatment is typically conservative and usually begins with a period of rest or activity modification to decrease a patient's symptoms followed by rehabilitation to address deficits in flexibility and strength (Fig. 221.3).
  - Consideration should be given to provocative activities such as participation in physical education classes or activities requiring kneeling.
- The duration of initial rest is typically 2 to 3 weeks. When the patients are symptom free with activities of daily living, they can return gradually to their sport.

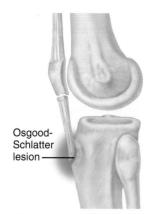

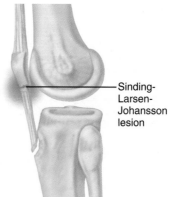

- Growing athletes
- Site of pain
  - OSL: Tibial tuberosity
  - SLJL: Inferior pole of patella
- Xray if trauma or chronic cases
- Treatment conservative
  - Rest/activity modification
  - Strength and flexibility
- Self-limited course

Osgood-Schlatter lesion

Sinding-Larsen-Johansson lesion

Fig 221.3 Osgood-Schlatter and Sinding-Larsen-Johansson.

TABLE 221.1 Differential Diagnosis

Condition	Differentiating Features
Fracture (e.g., tibial tubercle to patella) (see Chapters 163, 164, and 228)	Inability to do terminal extension of leg and significant radiographic abnormalities
Osteogenic sarcoma/osteomyelitis (see Chapters 16 and 20)	Red flags in history, review of systems, and significant radiographic abnormalities
Hoffa disease (see Chapter 153)	Tenderness at different anatomic site
Patellofemoral pain syndrome (see Chapter 153)	More diffuse discomfort
Osteochondritis dissecans (see Chapter 220)	Mechanical symptoms; abnormal notch view typically seen on radiograph
Patellar/quadriceps tendinitis (see Chapter 156)	Skeletally mature individual
Patellar stress fracture (see Chapter 164)	Significant disability; abnormal plain radiographs with or without abnormal bone scan/magnetic resonance imaging
Pre- or infrapatellar bursitis (see Chapter 157)	Significant fluctuance typically seen
Painful multipartite patella (see Chapter 164)	Radiographic abnormality
Referred pain (e.g., slipped capital femoral epiphysis) (see Chapter 213)	Abnormal hip examination; hip radiography abnormal

- Ice therapy should be used liberally. Nonsteroidal antiinflammatory drugs can be considered but should be used sparingly. They should never be taken as premedication so that the patient can engage in activities that have been forbidden or limited.
- Equipment such as protective padding and patellar tendon straps (for SLJL especially) may be useful.
- Quadriceps/hamstring/gastrocnemius muscle strengthening and stretching should be done, in formal physical therapy, with a school athletic trainer, or at home.
- Above all, time is necessary. The natural history of OSL and SLJL is that, in the vast majority of cases, the patient will outgrow the condition without any residual sequelae once skeletal maturity is achieved.
- Avoid cortisone injections.
  - Recent studies suggest potential benefits of prolotherapy with dextrose injections.
- Consider referral when concerned about the following:
  - Possible fracture, especially in the setting of recent acute trauma.
  - Refractory cases; excision of ossicles and tibial tubercle plasty are done in the case of OSL.

Troubleshooting

- Expectations should be managed. Patients and parents can typically expect a waxing and waning course of symptoms corresponding to activity levels during rapid phases of growth in adolescence. Patience is a virtue: The patient will almost inevitably outgrow the disorder.
- Imaging should be performed at times, as in acute trauma, when physical examination findings are atypical, and in prolonged/refractory cases.

Patient Instructions

- Both the American Academy of Orthopaedic Surgeons (https://orthoinfo.aaos.org/en/diseases--conditions/osgood-schlatter-disease-knee-pain/) and the American Academy of Family Practice (https://familydoctor.org/condition/osgood-schlatter-disease/) have excellent Web resources for patients.

Suggested Readings

Circi E, Atalay Y, Beyzadeoglu T. Treatment of Osgood-schlatter disease: review of the literature. *Musculoskelet Surg*. 2017;101(3):195–200.

Patel DR, Villalobos A. Evaluation and management of knee pain in young athletes: overuse injuries of the knee. *Transl Pediatr*. 2017;6(3):190–198.

Smith A. Osgood-schlatter disorder and related extensor mechanism problems. In: Kocher M, Micheli L, eds. *The Pediatric and Adolescent Knee*. Philadelphia: Saunders; 2006.

Topol GA, Podesta LA, Reeves KD, et al. Hyperosmolar dextrose injection for recalcitrant Osgood-schlatter disease. *Pediatrics*. 2011;128(5): e1121–e1128.

Weiss JM, Jordan SS, Andersen JS, et al. Surgical treatment of unresolved Osgood-schlatter disease: ossicle resection with tibial tubercleplasty. *J Pediatr Orthop*. 2007;27:844–847.

Wu M, Fallon R, Heyworth BE. Overuse injuries in the pediatric population. *Sports Med Arthrosc Rev*. 2016;24(4):150–158.

Chapter 222 The Adolescent: Scoliosis

Dennis Q. Chen, Keith Bachmann

ICD-10-CM CODES
M41.12 *Adolescent idiopathic scoliosis*
M41.9 *Scoliosis, unspecified*

Key Concepts

- Scoliosis is a three-dimensional structural spinal deformity involving lateral curvature of the spine in the coronal plane with rotation of the vertebrae in the axial plane.
- Classified broadly as congenital, neuromuscular, syndromic, idiopathic, and spinal curvature due to secondary reasons.
- Adolescent idiopathic scoliosis is the most common and is the focus of this chapter.
- Idiopathic scoliosis is a spinal curve without an identifiable cause.
  - Diagnosis of exclusion
  - Prevalence of curves greater than 10 degrees is 1 to 3 per 100 with an equal proportion of boys to girls.
  - Prevalence of curves greater than 30 degrees is 1 to 3 per 1000 with a 1:8 ratio of boys to girls.
  - Multifactorial etiology: genetic component and also related to multiple syndromes. Presence of a syndrome precludes diagnosis of idiopathic scoliosis.
  - Idiopathic scoliosis classification is based on age at presentation:
    - Infantile, 0 to 3 years (0.5% of idiopathic scoliosis)
    - Juvenile, 4 to 10 years (10.5%)
    - Adolescent, after age 10 (89%)
    - Earlier onset presents more challenges in regard to management that attempts to balance desired growth of the chest with worsening spinal deformity.
- After skeletal maturity, scoliosis curves less than 30 degrees generally do not progress, whereas most curves greater than 50 degrees tend to progress by approximately 1 degree per year.
- Prior to skeletal maturity, the risk of curve progression in idiopathic scoliosis and hence its treatment and prognosis are based on gender, remaining spinal growth, curve type, and magnitude.

History

- Age at onset
- Evidence of maturation
  - Age at menarche, adolescent growth spurt, breast development, signs of puberty
- Presence of back pain
  - Location, intensity, and worsening if any
- Neurologic symptoms
  - Gait abnormalities, weakness, or sensory changes
  - Bowel and bladder difficulties
- Feelings about overall appearance and back shape
  - Posterior chest wall prominence
  - Shoulder asymmetry, postural balance
- Family history: genetic component to this condition, with siblings (seven times more frequently) and children (three times) of patients with scoliosis having a higher incidence

Physical Examination

- Observation
  - Overall body shape (marfanoid, joint hyperlaxity)
  - Note any signs of truncal distortion, including rib or flank prominence, shoulder elevation, flank flattening or indentation, scapular rotation or elevation, and iliac crest prominence or elevation
  - Skin inspection (café au lait spots, hairy patch on back)
  - Pubertal development (Tanner staging)—chaperone if opposite sex patient if this portion of exam is performed.
  - Age and height should be documented on a growth chart to evaluate for peak growth velocity
- Neurologic examination
  - Motor and sensory
  - Reflexes: patellar, Achilles, umbilical, Babinski sign
  - Gait
- Back examination (Fig. 222.1)
  - Palpate spinous processes, paying attention to curve magnitude and rotation, as well as the presence of any step-offs
  - Flexibility with forward, backward, and side bending, noting any asymmetry or limitations in motion
  - Adams forward bend test
  - Scoliometer measurement

Imaging
Radiographs

- Standing posteroanterior 3-foot spine (preferably on one radiograph)
  - Comparison with previous radiographs, if possible
  - Examine vertebral bodies for malformations/symmetry
    - There should be two pedicles at each level.
  - Vertebral rotation: maximum at apex of curve
    - Cobb angles for curve magnitude

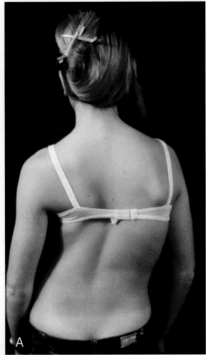

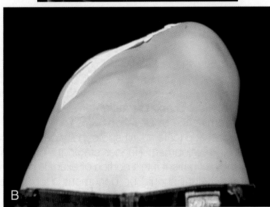

Fig 222.1 Patient with idiopathic scoliosis upright (A) and forward bending (B) test. Note the rotational asymmetry of the back.

- A Cobb angle is measured by selecting the most tilted vertebrae of each curve (end vertebrae).
- Lines are drawn along the superior endplate of the cephalad vertebrae and the inferior endplate of the caudal vertebrae.
- The measurement of these intersecting lines is the Cobb angle (Fig. 222.2).
- Limb length discrepancy (pelvic obliquity while standing)
- Growth remaining
  - Risser sign and triradiate cartilage should be included in scoliosis film, hand film for bone age
- Shape of curvature
  - Sharp versus gradual
  - Apex left versus right
  - Primarily thoracic, lumbar, or both
- Lateral view
  - Useful for assessment of sagittal alignment
  - Examine for vertebral body abnormalities, spondylolysis, and spondylolisthesis.

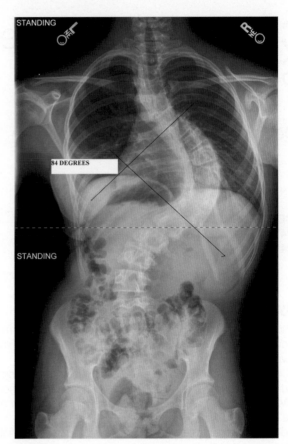

Fig 222.2 Severe adolescent idiopathic scoliosis. Cobb angles of the main curve are drawn. Each curve in the spine would also have a Cobb angle measurement.

- Lack of vertebral rotation or lack of hypokyphosis (look at shape of concave ribs) at the apex may suggest a tumor or intraspinal abnormality as the cause of scoliosis.

Magnetic Resonance Imaging

- Generally not indicated for adolescent idiopathic scoliosis
- Consider magnetic resonance imaging (MRI) in patients with early onset scoliosis (<10 years old), atypical curves (left thoracic, sharp changes), abnormal neurologic exam, rapidly progressing curves, concern for intraspinal pathology (syringomyelia), males, painful scoliosis, or bony tumors (winking owl sign—absent unilateral pedicle).

Computed Tomography Scan

- Useful for complete 3-dimensional evaluation of deformity.
  - Largely being replaced with simultaneous biplanar radiography due to concerns over the large radiation dose from CT.
- If there is concern for bony architecture or evaluation of a congenital deformity, CT still provides the best evaluation of bony architecture. Not routine in idiopathic scoliosis.

Bone Scan

- High-sensitivity scan to find areas of inflammation or stress reaction.
- May show a stress reaction in spondylolisthesis before a defect is seen on the radiograph.

Additional Tests

- Ultrasonography of the kidneys and an echocardiogram should be obtained in cases of congenital scoliosis (VACTERL [vertebral defects, anal atresia, cardiac defects, tracheo-esophageal fistula, renal anomalies, and limb abnormalities]).

Differential Diagnosis

- Leg length discrepancy
  - Unequal pelvic height causes oblique take-off of spine and apparent scoliosis
- Scoliosis due to secondary causes (minimal or no vertebral rotation) (Fig. 222.3)
- Tumor: osteoid osteoma, intradural mass
  - Vertebral destruction, neurologic abnormalities
- Syringomyelia/Chiari malformation
  - Neurologic abnormalities, MRI abnormalities
- Discitis or osteomyelitis
  - Fevers, vertebral changes, significant pain
- Muscle spasm
  - Intermittent back pain; usually a precipitating event
- Scheuermann kyphosis
  - A rigid thoracic hyperkyphosis >45 degrees between three consecutive vertebrae, may be associated with scoliosis
- Spondylolisthesis
  - Anterior slippage of one vertebrae over another, most commonly at L4/L5 and L5/S1

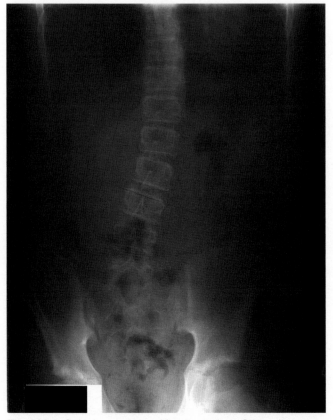

Fig 222.3 Spinal curvature without rotation. Other diagnoses apart from idiopathic scoliosis must be considered.

- Mechanical back pain
  - Long-standing back pain with no other abnormality on radiograph or examination
- Disc herniation
  - Back pain with radicular symptoms
- Congenital scoliosis
  - Abnormalities noted on radiographic examination
- Neuromuscular scoliosis or other syndrome (cerebral palsy)

Treatment

- At diagnosis and later
  - The treatment of scoliosis is based on the type of scoliosis, the magnitude of the curve, the number of years of growth remaining, and the patient's opinion about the shape of his or her back. Although many other factors must be considered, the general goal is to keep curves less than 50 degrees at maturity.
  - Observation is recommended for immature patients with curves less than 25 degrees; no treatment is necessary for mature patients with curves less than 25 degrees.
  - Orthotic management (bracing) is recommended for immature patients with progressing curves between 25 and 45 degrees.
  - Surgical correction of idiopathic scoliosis is considered for curves greater than 45 degrees in immature patients and in curves greater than 50 degrees in mature patients.
  - The treatment of patients with congenital, neuromuscular, and syndrome-associated scoliosis and those with idiopathic curves who are younger than 10 years of age presents a number of controversies. These patients should be treated at specialized facilities.
  - The goals of surgical treatment are to prevent progression and to improve spinal alignment and balance. The hips and shoulders should be level and the head over the sacrum while maintaining sagittal alignment. The spine is corrected and maintained in position with bony anchors (screws, hooks, and sublaminar bands/wires) attached to rods while the biologic process of fusion occurs. Strategies include fusion with and without instrumentation anteriorly, posteriorly, or both depending on the curve type, patient's age, and surgeon preference (Fig. 222.4).

When to Refer

- Any child under 10 years of age with a curve greater than 10 degrees, left thoracic curves, neurologic abnormalities, or significant pain should be referred within 1 month.
- A child older than the age of 10 can be referred at any time for evaluation, but more expedited referral is appropriate once the curve reaches 20 to 25 degrees.

Prognosis

- In untreated scoliosis, curves less than 30 degrees do not progress after skeletal maturity, whereas most curves greater than 50 degrees continue to progress. The progression is approximately 1 degree per year, although this number is variable based on curve location and patient.

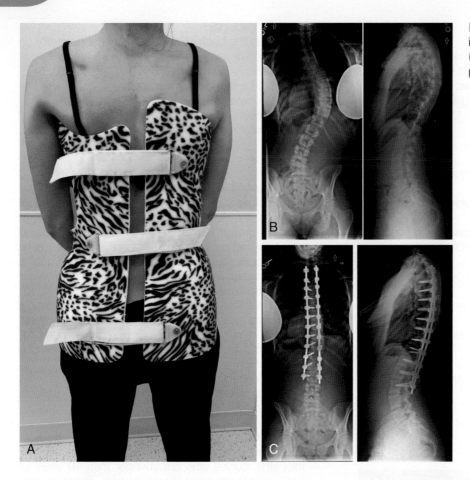

Fig 222.4 Management of adolescent idiopathic scoliosis with brace treatment (A) and pre- and postoperative images of posterior spinal fusion (B) and (C).

- In patients with severe thoracic curves (90 to 100 degrees), there is an increased risk of cardiac and pulmonary complications.
  - However, an increased mortality rate has not been found in long-term studies of patients with adolescent idiopathic scoliosis.
  - Some studies show a slightly higher rate of back pain in patients with adolescent idiopathic scoliosis.
- Scoliosis has also been found to be a risk factor for psychosocial issues and health-compromising behavior. However, there have been no studies comparing treated and untreated patients with scoliosis and their rates of back pain and self-image.
- The techniques for correction and fusion change quickly, and long-term results have not been obtained for the newest techniques. However, with older technology, good results have been found at 20-year follow-up.

Troubleshooting

- The patient should be counseled on the benefits and risks of treatment and nontreatment.
- Bracing is the current standard of care to limit curve progression during growth and compliant use of the brace is the only proven nonoperative treatment to prevent curve progression.
  - However, it can be difficult to convince image-conscious teenagers that bracing can be beneficial.

- Surgical correction with fusion is the only proven method of improving the shape of the back and halting curve progression.
- Risks of surgery include bleeding, nonunion, infection, and nerve injury. Significant nerve complications occur in less than 1% of cases.
- Scoliosis is associated with multiple other conditions including Marfan syndrome, neurofibromatosis, muscular dystrophy, and various tumors. The practitioner must be watchful for these other diagnoses, which often require further workup and treatment.

Information for Patients

- Scoliosis is a curvature of the spine with rotation of the vertebrae.
- Scoliotic curves of more than 50 degrees after maturity tend to continue to progress, so the goal is to prevent curves from reaching 50 degrees.
- Bracing is the only proven nonoperative treatment that may prevent curve progression. Bracing will not correct the scoliosis: the goal is to halt the curve in its current position and size.
- Surgical correction and fusion with instrumentation is the only proven treatment that corrects scoliosis and prevents progression.
- Even when a curve is less than 50 degrees, a patient may still be unhappy with his or her appearance and request surgical correction.

- Patients with scoliosis should be aware that their siblings and eventual children have an increased risk of scoliosis and should be examined in early adolescence.

Considerations in Special Populations

- Scoliosis can be related to neurologic conditions, muscular abnormalities, and global syndromes. This long list of diagnoses would typically have other signs, symptoms, and physical manifestations in addition to scoliosis. Usually these varying diagnoses are treated at tertiary care facilities with special expertise in the management of patients with complex multisystem problems. The caregiver who treats these patients should be familiar with the nonspinal manifestations of these conditions.
- Congenital scoliosis is due to skeletal abnormalities of the spine that are present at birth. These anomalies are broadly classified as a failure of formation or of segmentation (or both) during vertebral development.
  - It is important to identify associated anomalies with a thorough evaluation of the neurologic, cardiovascular, and genitourinary system including a good neurologic and cardiac physical examination and a renal ultrasound scan and echocardiogram.
  - Treatment is based on the age of the patient, progression of the curve, location, and type of anomaly.
  - The options for surgical treatment include in situ fusion and resection with correction of the deformity.
- Infantile idiopathic scoliosis may be associated with neural axis abnormalities, plagiocephaly, hip dysplasia, congenital heart disease, and mental retardation. It usually (90% of cases) resolves spontaneously. Cases that do not resolve may be treated with corrective casting and/or bracing.
- Juvenile scoliosis is often progressive and has the potential for severe trunk deformity and eventual cardiac or pulmonary compromise.
  - Curves that reach 30 degrees are usually progressive if left untreated.

Suggested Readings

Basu PS, Elsebaie H, Noordeen MH. Congenital spinal deformity: a comprehensive assessment at presentation. *Spine*. 2002;27:2255–2259.

Dickson JH, Mirkovic S, Noble PC, et al. Results of operative treatment of idiopathic scoliosis in adults. *J Bone Joint Surg Am*. 1995;77A: 513–523.

El-Hawary R, Chukwunyerenwa C. Update on evaluation and treatment of scoliosis. *Pediatr Clin North Am*. 2014;61:1223–1241.

Lenke LG, Betz RR, Harms J, et al. Adolescent idiopathic scoliosis: A new classification to determine extent of spinal arthrodesis. *J Bone Joint Surg Am*. 2001;83A:1169–1181.

Little DG, Song KM, Katz D, et al. Relationship of peak height velocity to other maturity indicators in idiopathic scoliosis in girls. *J Bone Joint Surg Am*. 2000;82A:685–693.

Montgomery F, Willner S. The natural history of idiopathic scoliosis: incidence of treatment in 15 cohorts of children born between 1963 and 1977. *Spine*. 1997;22:772–774.

Negrini S, Minozzi S, Bettany-Saltikov J, et al. Braces for idiopathic scoliosis in adolescents. *Spine*. 2016;41:1813–1825.

Thompson RM, Hubbard EW, Jo CH, et al. Brace success is related to curve type in patients with adolescent idiopathic scoliosis. *J Bone Joint Surg Am*. 2017;99(11):923–928.

Chapter 223 The Adolescent: Spondylolysis and Spondylolisthesis

Elizabeth W. Hubbard

ICD-10-CM CODES

M43.0	*Spondylolysis*
M43.00	*Site unspecified*
M43.01	*Occipito-atlanto-axial region*
M43.02	*Cervical region*
M43.03	*Cervicothoracic region*
M43.04	*Thoracic region*
M43.05	*Thoracolumbar region*
M43.06	*Lumbar region*
M43.07	*Lumbosacral region*
M43.08	*Spondylolysis, sacral and sacrococcygeal region*
M43.09	*Multiple sites in spine*
M43.1	*Spondylolisthesis*
M43.10	*Site unspecified*
M43.11	*Occipito-atlanto-axial region*
M43.12	*Cervical region*
M43.13	*Cervicothoracic region*
M43.14	*Thoracic region*
M43.15	*Thoracolumbar region*
M43.16	*Lumbar region*
M43.17	*Lumbosacral region*
M43.18	*Spondylolysis, sacral and sacrococcygeal region*
M43.19	*Multiple sites in spine*

Key Concepts

- Spondylolysis and spondylolisthesis are two of the most common causes of low back pain in children older than 10 years of age.
  - Rarely seen before the age of 5 years
  - Prevalence is 6% overall but is reportedly as high as 15% to 47% in the adolescent athlete with low back pain.
  - More common in:
    - Males (6:1 male-to-female ratio)
    - Athletes participating in sports that require hyperextension and loading of the spine (gymnastics, football, weight lifting, soccer, wrestling, and diving)
- Spondylolysis is an acquired condition caused by repetitive hyperextension of the lumbar spine resulting in a stress reaction or fracture of the pars interarticularis, most commonly at L5.

- Spondylolisthesis is the forward translation of one vertebra on the adjacent caudal vertebra, most frequently seen between L5 and S1.
- Classified by type (Wiltse-Newman) and amount of displacement (Myerding)
- Treatment depends on slip severity as determined by the Myerding classification (Fig. 223.1)

History

- Activity-related low back pain
  - Insidious in nature
  - Occasional radiation to buttock or posterior thigh
  - Night pain unusual
- Radicular symptoms or sacral anesthesia with bowel and bladder dysfunction seen in high-grade slips.
- Inquire about type of sporting activity
  - Gymnastics, football, wrestling, weight lifting, diving, soccer

Physical Examination

- Paraspinal tenderness and spasm
- Limited lumbar mobility and pain with hyperextension
- Loss of normal lumbar lordosis
- Tight hamstrings
- Late findings
  - Waddling gait
  - Increased hip and knee flexion
  - Reduced stride length
- High-grade slip
  - Lumbosacral kyphosis
  - Palpable step-off between L4 and L5 spinous process
- Scoliosis can be seen secondary to muscle spasm or in a patient with spondyloptosis.
- Rare neurologic findings
  - Positive straight leg raise
  - Weakness, particularly of the extensor hallucis longus muscle (L5)
  - Cauda equina with bladder dysfunction and sacral anesthesia in cases of severe or dysplastic slip

Imaging
Radiographs

- Anteroposterior and lateral standing views of the spine on a scoliosis cassette

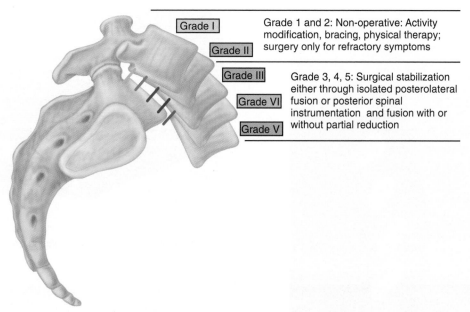

Grade I

Grade II

Grade 1 and 2: Non-operative: Activity modification, bracing, physical therapy; surgery only for refractory symptoms

Grade III

Grade VI

Grade V

Grade 3, 4, 5: Surgical stabilization either through isolated posterolateral fusion or posterior spinal instrumentation and fusion with or without partial reduction

Fig 223.1 Treatment of spondylolysis/spondylolisthesis based on the Meyerding classification. Meyerding classification of spondylolisthesis: Grade I, 0% to 25%; grade II, 26% to 50%; grade III, 51% to 75%; grade IV, 76% to 100%. Spondylolysis and grade 1 and 2 spondylolisthesis can be treated nonoperatively. Grades 3, 4, and 5 spondylolisthesis require surgical management due to the risk of slip progression.

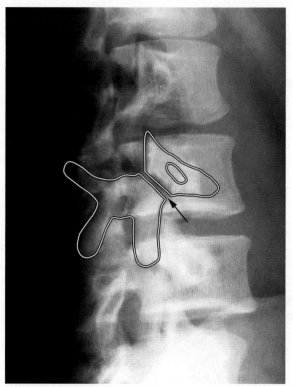

Fig 223.2 "Scottie dog" sign showing fracture *(arrow)* through the pars interarticularis at L4-L5 seen on an oblique radiograph.

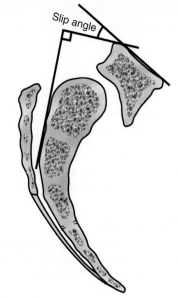

Fig 223.3 Slip angle.

- Lateral view of lumbosacral junction
  - Most sensitive view
  - Quantify the amount of forward displacement (Myerding classification) (see Fig. 223.1)
  - Quantify the amount of lumbosacral kyphosis as measured by the slip angle (Fig. 223.3)

Bone Scan

- Helpful early in the disease course
  - Increased activity at the pars interarticularis
  - Single-photon emission computed tomography (SPECT) has historically been deemed the best means for

- Oblique x-rays have been shown to be helpful in diagnosing unilateral pars defects, but utility overall has been questioned in light of the additional cost and radiation exposure
  - Look for Scottie dog sign (fracture of the pars interarticularis) (Fig. 223.2)

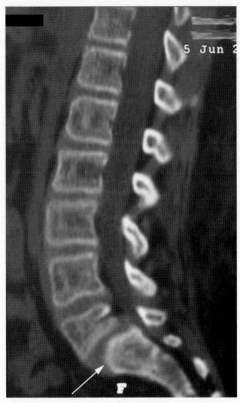

Fig 223.4 Sagittal reconstruction computed tomography of dysplastic spondylolisthesis (note rounded sacrum, *arrow*) and stenosis.

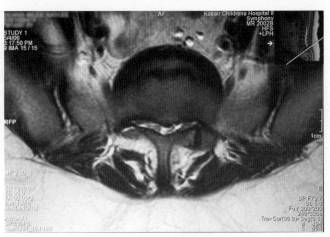

Fig 223.5 Magnetic resonance imaging revealing severe stenosis at S1 in a dysplastic slip.

identifying spondylolysis when radiographs are normal. However, recent literature suggests that SPECT scans provide significantly more radiation without significant diagnostic benefit when compared to two-view x-rays and either magnetic resonance imaging (MRI) or computed tomography (CT) as advanced imaging.

• Contraindicated in an asymptomatic patient with a long-standing defect

Computed Tomography

• Thin-cut CT is more sensitive than plane radiographs
  • Helpful in delineating anatomy (Fig. 223.4)
• Serial CTs are not warranted in patients who are improving clinically

Magnetic Resonance Imaging

• Useful in the acute setting; CT may be more beneficial for patients with chronic symptoms. Best study to evaluate nerve root compression, disc abnormalities, or stenosis or to rule out other sources of back pain such as tumor and infection (Fig. 223.5)

Classification
Wiltse-Newman Classification

• Grade I: dysplastic (congenital), 14% to 21% of the cases, abnormality of the lumbosacral articulation, poorly formed pars interarticularis, abnormal facets, and dome-shaped sacral promontory

• Grade II: isthmic, results from defect in the par interarticularis
  • Grade IIA: disruption of the pars as a result of stress fracture, most common subtype
  • Grade IIB: elongation of the pars without disruption (repeated healed microfractures)
• Grade IIC: acute fracture through the pars (rare)
• Grade III: degenerative
• Grade IV: traumatic
• Grade V: pathologic

Meyerding Classification (see Fig. 223.1)

• Radiographic system for measuring the amount of translation of the cranial vertebra on the caudal vertebra
• The superior endplate of the caudal vertebra is divided into quadrants, and the amount of translation is noted based on the quadrant where the posterior aspect of the cranial body is located.
  • Grade I translation, as much as 25%; grade II, 26% to 50%; grade III, 51% to 75%; and grade IV, 76% to 100%
  • Spondyloptosis describes the complete anterior displacement of the vertebral body on the adjacent caudal segment.

Treatment
Conservative Treatment

• Observation
  • Asymptomatic patients with spondylolysis or spondylolisthesis grade I or II
  • Majority of children
  • Goal of treatment should be alleviation of symptoms rather than bony union. Therefore, serial CT or MRIs are not warranted when patients are improving clinically.
• Physical therapy
  • For symptomatic patients with spondylolysis or grade I or II spondylolisthesis
  • Focus on pain reduction and return to function.
  • Abdominal and core back strengthening, stretching of lumbodorsal and hamstring muscles

- Bracing
  - No large, high-level studies evaluate the effectiveness of bracing in spondylolysis and low-grade spondylolisthesis.
  - Small studies suggest that a hard thoracolumbosacral orthosis (TLSO)-type brace is more effective in relieving symptoms than a soft corset
  - Full-time bracing with a TLSO with physiologic lordosis for 6 to 12 weeks until resolution of symptoms
  - Follow with 4 to 6 weeks of rest and bracing followed by a reconditioning program with gradual resumption of sporting activities.
- Monitoring of patient
  - The rate of slip progression is low for patients with symptomatic spondylolysis.
  - Dysplastic slips need to be monitored with serial radiographs due to a greater risk of slip progression.

Surgical Treatment

- Indications
  - A patient with mild slips (grade I or II) and uncontrolled pain after at least 6 months of conservative measures
  - Slippage of greater than 50% on initial evaluation
  - Young patient with progressive dysplastic spondylolisthesis, slip angle greater than 30 degrees, or significant nerve root irritation or cauda equina
- Direct repair of the pars defect
  - Symptomatic spondylolysis without listhesis
  - Preserve motion segment
- Noninstrumented posterolateral fusion
  - Gold standard
  - L5-S1 for low-grade slip, L4-S1 for higher-grade slip (>50% translation)
  - Excision of posterior elements of L5 (Gill procedure) not recommended and can lead to slip progression
  - Postoperative casting or bracing to reduce slip angle and until fusion is solid
- Instrumented spinal fusion
  - With wide decompression
  - *In situ* arthrodesis versus partial or complete reduction:
    - Reduction increases the risk of neurologic injury
    - The need for reduction is controversial
  - Better environment for fusion by limiting motion and restoring spinal balance
- Anterior spinal fusion
  - May be indicated in high-grade slips to improve fusion rate

When to Refer

- Symptomatic patients with failure of conservative measures
- Young patients with dysplastic slips
- Any patient with neurologic findings

Patient Instructions

- Most cases respond to physical therapy.
- Young patients with dysplastic spondylolysis or spondylolisthesis need to be monitored for progression of the slip with radiographs every 6 months.
- Surgery is recommended for severe slips, unrelenting pain, or neurologic symptoms.

Acknowledgment

The author would like to acknowledge Dr. Henry J. Iwinski, Jr., Dr. Vishwas Talwalkar, and Dr. Todd Milbrandt for their contributions to the previous edition of this chapter.

Suggested Readings

Beck NA, Miller R, Baldwin K, et al. Do oblique views add value in the diagnosis of spondylolysis in adolescents? *J Bone Joint Surg.* 2013;95:e65 (1-7).

Blanda J, Bethem D, Moats W, Lew M. Defects of pars interarticularis in athletes: A protocol for nonoperative treatment. *J Spinal Disord.* 1993;6:406–411.

Crawford CH, Ledonio CGT, Shay Bess R, et al. Current evidence regarding the surgical and nonsurgical treatment of pediatric lumbar spondylolysis: a report from the scoliosis research society evidence-based medicine committee. *Spine Deform.* 2015;3:30–44.

Fredrickson BE, Baker D, McHolick WJ, et al. The natural history of spondylolysis and spondylolisthesis. *J Bone Joint Surg Am.* 1984;66A:699–707.

Harris IE, Weinstein SL. Long-term follow-up of patients with grade III and IV spondylolisthesis. Treatment with and without posterior fusion. *J Bone Joint Surg Am.* 1987;69A:960–969.

Lamberg T, Remes V, Helenius I, et al. Uninstrumented in situ fusion for high-grade childhood and adolescent isthmic spondylolisthesis: Long-term outcome. *J Bone Joint Surg Am.* 2007;89A:512–518.

Meyerding HW. Spondylolisthesis. *Surg Gynecol Obstet.* 1932;54:371–377.

Poussa M, Schlenzka D, Seitsalo S, et al. Surgical treatment of severe isthmic spondylolisthesis in adolescents. Reduction or fusion in situ. *Spine.* 1993;18:894–901.

Sairyo K, Sakai T, Yasui N, et al. Conservative treatment for pediatric lumbar spondylolysis to achieve bone healing using a hard brace: what type and how long? *J Neurosurg Spine.* 2012;16:610–614.

Tofte JN, CarlLee TL, Holte AJ, et al. Imaging in pediatric spondylolysis. *Spine.* 2017;42(10):777–782.

Wiltse LL, Newman PH, Macnab I. Classification of spondylolysis and spondylolisthesis. *Clin Orthop Relat Res.* 1976;117:23–29.

Chapter 224 The Adolescent: Pediatric Discitis

Elizabeth W. Hubbard

ICD-10-CM CODES

M46.3	*Infection of the intervertebral disc*
M46.30	*Site unspecified*
M46.31	*Occipito-atlanto-axial region*
M46.32	*Cervical region*
M46.33	*Cervicothoracic region*
M46.34	*Thoracic region*
M46.35	*Thoracolumbar region*
M46.36	*Lumbar region*
M46.37	*Lumbosacral region*
M46.38	*Sacral and sacrococcygeal region*
M46.4	*Discitis, unspecified*
M46.40	*Site unspecified*
M46.41	*Occipito-atlanto-axial region*
M46.42	*Cervical region*
M46.43	*Cervicothoracic region*
M46.44	*Thoracic region*
M46.45	*Thoracolumbar region*
M46.46	*Lumbar region*
M46.47	*Lumbosacral region*
M46.48	*Sacral and sacrococcygeal region*

Key Concepts

- Discitis is an inflammatory condition of the intervertebral disc. It is also referred to as spondylodiscitis when adjacent vertebral bodies are involved.
- Once felt to be separate entities, discitis and vertebral osteomyelitis are thought to represent a spectrum of the same disease pathology with most infections starting at the endplate and spreading into the disc and/or the vertebral body.
- Approximately 2% of pediatric bone infections annually are due to nontuberculous spondylodiscitis.
- The cause is usually infection, but no organism is identified in more than 25% of cases.
- Trimodal distribution of patients: neonates/infants, toddlers, and young teenagers
- The most common organism in developed countries is *Staphylococcus aureus,* followed by *Kingella kingae* and *Streptococcus*. There are isolated reports of other rare bacteria.
  - *Escherichia coli*, *Proteus*, and *Pseudomonas* are more common after invasive procedures.

- *Salmonella* may be present in the setting of a sickle cell patient.
  - A fungus or tuberculosis cause may be present in immunocompromised patients.
  - No viral isolates have been reported in the literature.
- The classic cause is tuberculosis, especially in underdeveloped countries.
- Commonly affects lumbar and thoracic spine but can occur at any spine level.
- Disease process more destructive in infants.
  - Most often treated with antibiotics. Surgery is indicated when an abscess is seen on advanced imaging or if symptoms do not improve after several days of rest and antibiotic therapy (Fig. 224.1).

History

- The most common presentation is back pain (50%) or a change in gait (limp).
- Symptoms may have a gradual onset and last for weeks.
- May or may not present with a history of fever (<30% with a fever of >100.3°F reported)
- Presentation is related to age and verbal skills
  - Patients younger than 2 to 6 years of age may demonstrate an inability to stay in a seated position, refusal to bear weight (refusal to sit, crawl, or walk depending on ambulatory status), or a gait disturbance.
  - Older children/adolescents will commonly report back, pelvis, or abdominal pain; some may report extremity pain arising from irritated nerve roots. Patients may report abdominal pain due to referred pain from a retroperitoneal abscess.
  - Rare presentation of neurologic changes such as muscle weakness, sensory changes, and incontinence
  - Rare presentation of a septic patient
- Discitis should be considered in the differential diagnosis in pediatric patients with a gait abnormality with no apparent lower extremity clinical findings.
- Delays in diagnosis for as long as 4 to 6 months have been reported because of the benign appearance of the patient.
- Neonates (<6 months of age) are most likely to have a severe presentation with sepsis and multiple foci of infection are common. Significant vertebral destruction with subsequent spinal deformity, including severe kyphosis, is possible.

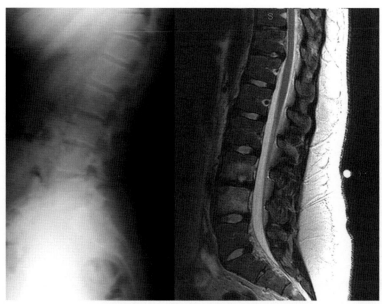

- **Most common cause:** Staphylococcus aureus
- **Symptoms:** Limp or refusal to weight bear, limited active spine flexion, back and/or abdominal pain
- **Diagnosis:** MRI; laboratory studies including CBC, ESR, and CRP
- **Treatment:** Empiric IV followed by oral therapy for S. aureus; needle biopsy or aspiration for failure to respond to empiric treatment; surgical debridement for failure to respond to antibiotic therapy

Fig 224.1 Sagittal cut of magnetic resonance imaging (MRI) of the spine in a pediatric patient with discitis and vertebral osteomyelitis (spondylodiscitis). The diagnostic and treatment algorithm to pediatric spondylodiscitis is dictated above. *CBC*, Complete blood count; *CRP*, C-reactive protein; *ESR*, erythrocyte sedimentation rate.

Physical Examination

- Variable presentation of fever
- Children younger than 3 years may refuse to bear weight on either leg, refuse to walk, or refuse to crawl, depending on their ambulatory status.
- Patients may find relief of symptoms when they are lying supine.
- Patients will usually avoid flexing/extending the spine to perform simple activities such as picking up an object and bending the neck to look down at the ground or extending to look up at the ceiling.
- It is important to test the range of motion of the hip, knee, and spine.
- Pain to palpation may be appreciated along symptomatic regions of the axial spine.
- Rarely, neurologic changes, such as lower extremity weakness, may be seen.
- Must assess for intraabdominal or retroperitoneal process.

Imaging
Plain Radiographs

- Initial films at onset of symptoms are often benign.
- Posteroanterior and lateral x-rays of the entire spine should be obtained.
  - Standing preferred
  - Seated or supine adequate if standing x-rays cannot be obtained
- Subtle loss of disc height is the earliest radiographic finding (Fig. 224.2).
- Certain infections and osteomyelitis may show destructive lesions on plain films (cavitary tuberculosis).

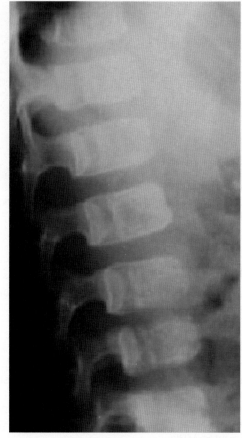

Fig 224.2 Plain radiograph showing narrowed disc space.

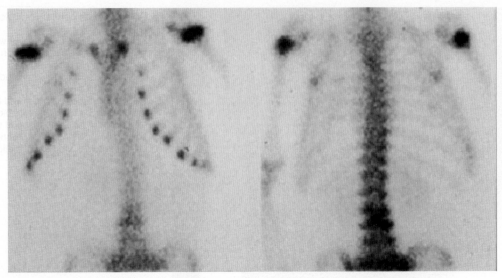

Fig 224.3 Increased lumbar tracer uptake on bone scan.

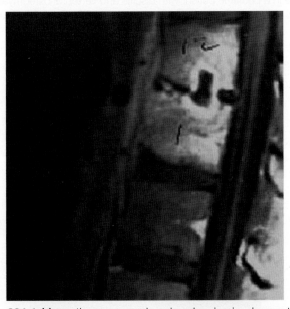

Fig 224.4 Magnetic resonance imaging showing involvement of vertebral bodies.

Bone Scan

- Can localize lesions to the spine; advanced studies are needed to differentiate infection versus other processes (Fig. 224.3)

Magnetic Resonance Imaging

- Early MRI reduces a delay in diagnosis.
- More than 95% of patients with discitis show abnormal findings.
- Edema and suppuration are illustrated by a high-intensity signal on T2-weighted MRIs and a low-intensity signal on T1-weighted MRIs.
- Young patients often need to be sedated for MRI (Fig. 224.4).

Computed Tomography Scan

- Useful for bony analysis and can show fluid collection, but limited soft-tissue examination

Additional Tests

- Laboratory tests are mandatory, but often normal or only slightly elevated.
    - Complete blood count, erythrocyte sedimentation rate (ESR), C-reactive protein (CRP)
    - White blood cell count (WBC) can be normal in as many as 40% of patients with discitis; ESR and CRP are elevated in as many as 80% of patients.
    - CRP is the most sensitive and is often elevated in acute infections; CRP should normalize in 10 to 14 days in patients who are responding to treatment.
    - ESR may be normal in an acute infection and often takes longer to normalize after treatment than CRP.
    - When elevated at the initial diagnosis, serial ESR and CRP values are helpful in monitoring patient response to infection.
    - Blood cultures should be sent, but are often negative.
    - Urinalysis may also help distinguish between gastro-intestinal and genitourinary processes.
- Aspiration: only in cases of an unusual clinical course or failure to respond to initial empiric therapy
    - As many as 60% of aspirations isolate no bacteria.
    - Performed under fluoroscopic or computed tomography guidance
    - If fluid collection is identified, fine-needle aspiration can be performed with guidance.

Differential Diagnosis

- Septic arthritis (hip, knee, and ankle) or toxic synovitis
- Osteomyelitis of the lower extremity
- Sacroiliitis
- Fracture (lower extremity, pelvis, and vertebrae)
- Spondyloarthropathy, including ankylosing spondylitis

TABLE 224.1 Differential Diagnosis

Condition	Feature
Discitis	Back pain, refusal to walk, gait disturbance
Tumor	Neurologic involvement, localized unrelenting night pain
Hip pathology: septic arthritis/ toxic synovitis	Vague hip or knee pain; refusal to walk or gait disturbance; unable to bear weight; fever; elevated C-reactive protein, erythrocyte sedimentation rate, complete blood count
Stress fracture, spondylolysis	Classic: teenager with repetitive activities, pain relieved with rest

- Spondylolysis and/or spondylolisthesis
- Tumor
- See Table 224.1

Treatment
At Diagnosis

- Initial treatment includes bed rest, empiric antistaphylococcal IV antibiotics for 5 to 14 days plus oral antibiotics for 2 to 6 weeks and nonsteroidal antiinflammatory drugs
  - Duration of treatment can be guided by clinical and laboratory response and by initial duration of symptoms and initial MRI findings regarding inflammation and scope of infection
- Bracing or casting can help with pain relief and may help prevent spinal deformity in younger patients with more extensive vertebral involvement.
- Expect clinical response within 2 to 3 days; otherwise consider aspiration or further imaging.
- Surgery is indicated when an abscess is seen on advanced imaging or if symptoms do not improve after several days of rest and antibiotic therapy.

Later

- Continued clinical surveillance until CRP and ESR normalize
- Disc height may remain diminished or even proceed to fusion, but patients are often asymptomatic.

Prognosis

- Generally good unless there is significant bony destruction

When to Refer

- Referral to a pediatric orthopaedist should be made as soon as the diagnosis is made or suspected. A physician with access to an infectious disease specialist would be preferred.

Troubleshooting

- Beware the child with new-onset neurologic symptoms or lack of response to therapy. Both could signal that the organism is not being adequately treated or the process is something other than discitis.
- Bracing is sometimes necessary for 3 to 6 weeks for comfort.

Acknowledgment

The author would like to acknowledge Dr. Michael P. Horan, Dr. Todd Milbrandt, Dr. Henry J. Iwinski, Jr., and Dr. Vishwas Talwalkar for their contributions to the previous edition of this chapter.

Suggested Readings

Brown R, Hussain M, McHugh K, et al. Discitis in young children. *J Bone Joint Surg Br*. 2001;83-B:106–111.

Chandrasenan J, Klezl Z, Bommireddy R, et al. Spondylodiscitis in children: a retrospective series. *J Bone Joint Surg Br*. 2011;93-B:1122–1125.

Dormans JP, Moroz L. Infection and tumors of the spine in children. *J Bone Joint Surg Am*. 2007;89A(suppl 1):79–97.

Early SD, Kay RM, Tolo VT. Childhood discitis. *J Am Acad Orthop Surg*. 2003;11:413–420.

Eismont FJ, Bohlman HH, Soni PL, et al. Vertebral osteomyelitis in infants. *J Bone Joint Surg Br*. 1982;64B:32–35.

Fernandez M, Carrol CL, Baker CJ. Discitis and vertebral osteomyelitis in children: an 18-year review. *Pediatrics*. 2000;105:1299–1304.

Karabouta Z, Bisbinas I, Davidson A, Goldsworthy L. Discitis in toddlers: a case series and review. *Acta Paediatr*. 2005;94:1516–1518.

Ring D, Johnston CE, Wenger D. Pyogenic infectious spondylitis in children: the convergence of discitis and vertebral osteomyelitis. *J Pediatr Orthop*. 1995;15:652–660.

Tay BK, Deckey J, Hu SS. Spinal infections. *J Am Acad Orthop Surg*. 2002;10:188–197.

Waizy H, Heckel M, Seller K, et al. Remodeling of the spine in spondylodiscitis of children at age 3 years or younger. *Arch Orthop Trauma Surg*. 2007;127:403–407.

Chapter 225 The Adolescent: Pelvic Avulsion Fractures

Michael Hadeed, Keith Bachmann

ICD-10-CM CODES
S.32.309A *Unspecified fracture of unspecified ilium, initial encounter for closed fracture*
S.32.609A *Unspecified fracture of unspecified ischium, initial encounter for closed fracture*

Key Concepts

- Pelvic avulsion fractures are uncommon injuries that typically occur in adolescents and young adults participating in athletics.
- Injury occurs during a violent muscle contracture or eccentric contracture as in floor exercises in gymnastics or kicking in soccer.
- Fractures occur at secondary ossification centers because these points are weaker than the musculotendinous attachments.
- The most common sites of injury are the adductor muscle attachments to the ischial tuberosity (IT), the sartorius muscle attachment to the anterior superior iliac spine (ASIS), and the attachment of the direct head of the rectus femoris muscle to the anterior inferior iliac spine (AIIS) (Fig. 225.1).
- Other less common sites include the lesser trochanter (LT) and iliac crest (IC).
- Treatment generally entails rest with a gradual return to activities and rarely requires surgical intervention.

History

- Acute injury
  - Athletic activities with a severe muscle strain (e.g., groin pull); the patient may report hearing a "pop."
  - IT injuries associated with a hamstring stretch as in gymnastic floor exercises, ASIS and AIIS associated with swinging a baseball bat and high kicking as in soccer, IC associated with abrupt changes in direction or in power serves such as in tennis; LT associated with hip flexors
  - Immediate shooting pain, focal tenderness, swelling around the site of injury
  - Inability or difficulty bearing weight
- Chronic injury
  - Repetitive activities without a clear history of a traumatic event
  - Pain with limited joint motion that progresses over time

Physical Examination

- Observation
  - Focal swelling and ecchymosis
  - Inability to bear weight
- Palpation
  - Focal tenderness at fracture site
- Range of motion and motor strength
  - May be limited secondary to pain
  - More likely to be painful with active motion as the muscle contraction puts increased stress on the avulsion site
- Special examinations: based on the anatomy involved, maximal stretch or active contraction of the muscle involved will reproduce symptoms.
  - Ischial avulsion (hamstrings or the adductors)
    - Hamstrings contribute to hip extension and knee flexion
    - Adductors contribute to adduction of the hip/leg
  - ASIS avulsion (testing the sartorius)
    - Origin, ASIS; insertion, pes anserinus (proximal medial tibia)
    - Contributes to flexion, abduction, and external rotation of the hip
  - AIIS avulsion (testing the direct head of the rectus femoris)
    - Origin, AIIS; insertion, proximal pole of the patella (part of the quad tendon)
    - Contributes to hip flexion and knee extension
  - IC (testing the external oblique musculature)
  - LT (testing the iliopsoas)
    - Contributes to hip flexion

Imaging
Radiographs

- Anteroposterior (AP) view of the pelvis
  - Check for symmetry on the contralateral hemipelvis.
  - Look for subtle signs of soft-tissue swelling and evidence of nondisplaced or minimally displaced fractures.
  - Careful attention must be paid at the sites of the various apophyses.
  - Common sites of injury are the IT, ASIS, and AIIS. Less common sites are the IC and LT.
- AP/frog leg lateral view of the hip
  - Rule out other possible diagnoses (e.g., slipped capital femoral epiphysis)
  - May give better dedicated resolution of the hip

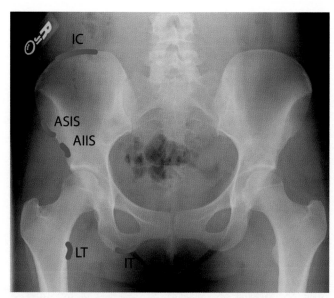

Fig 225.1 Plain radiograph of an adolescent patient demonstrating the common sites associated with pelvic avulsion fractures. *AIIS*, Anterior inferior iliac spine; *ASIS*, anterior superior iliac spine; *IC*, iliac crest; *IT*, ischial tuberosity; *LT*, lesser trochanter.

- False profile view can help assess AIIS
- Iliac oblique (part of the Judet series) may help assess ASIS

Magnetic Resonance Imaging

- In the case of a nondisplaced fracture, bone marrow edema may be evident as well as a fracture line not seen on plain radiographs, but magnetic resonance imaging is rarely indicated to make this diagnosis.

Additional Tests

- In a chronic and sometimes an acute setting in which an athletic injury may be in doubt, other tests to rule out infection, rheumatologic conditions, and neoplasm may be indicated.
  - The evaluation of these etiologies is beyond the scope of this chapter, but you could consider lab testing to include complete blood count with differential, erythrocyte sedimentation rate, C-reactive protein, rheumatoid factor, antinuclear antibody, and Lyme titers.

Differential Diagnosis

- Muscle strain (see Chapters 130 and 132)
  - Similar history and presentation without evidence of fracture
- Slipped capital femoral epiphysis (see Chapter 213)
  - More prevalent in younger teens and preteens
  - May or may not be able to bear weight
  - Can also be activity related
  - May present as knee pain
- Septic arthritis/osteomyelitis (see Chapter 16)
  - Fever, elevated white blood cell count, erythrocyte sedimentation rate, C-reactive protein, inability to bear weight
  - Recent history of upper respiratory infection

- Lyme disease
  - History of tick exposure and bull's-eye rash
  - Insidious onset
  - Knee involvement more common
- Rheumatologic disease
  - Hip pain may be the initial presenting symptom
  - History of other joint pain and other systemic symptoms
  - No trauma or activity-related pain
- Neoplastic disease (see Chapter 20)
  - Radiographs may reveal significant findings
  - Evaluate complete blood count and differential
  - Other constitutional signs

Treatment

- Initial treatment protocol
  - Initial treatment focuses on rest with the hip in a relaxed position of least tension on the muscle groups involved.
  - Crutches are recommended for at least 2 weeks with a gradual return to weight bearing and sports-related activity.
  - Rehabilitation should be guided by clinical and radiographic recovery.
  - A premature return to activity may cause reinjury and prolong the overall recovery time of 6 weeks to several months.
- Operative management
  - Rarely indicated
  - Occasionally considered if fracture displacement is >2 to 3 cm

When to Refer

- Pelvic avulsion fractures typically can be managed with conservative measures. If displacement is greater than 2 cm on radiographs, consider early referral for possible surgical intervention.
- If follow-up shows evidence of a fracture nonunion (e.g., persistent pain and serial radiographs demonstrating a lack of fracture healing), refer the patient for specialist evaluation.
- If long-term follow-up shows radiographs with exuberant callus and the patient has symptoms of painful myositis ossificans, consider referral for specialist evaluation.

Prognosis

- Good with conservative measures
- Surgery is rarely indicated
- Most athletes are able to return to full activities, with disability mostly occurring in patients with ischial avulsions.

Troubleshooting

- Patients and families should be counseled on the time to recovery with conservative measures. Full recovery and return to full activity may take several months.
- It should be stressed that surgery is rarely indicated, even in displaced fractures. It may only be advocated in cases of fracture nonunion, which would be defined as a failure to heal by conservative measures.

Patient Instructions

- The patient should rest the hip in a position of comfort to decrease strain on the muscle groups involved in the avulsion fracture.
- Non-weight bearing for 2 weeks with crutches
- Weight bearing can begin after 2 weeks.
- Guidance of a physical therapist may be helpful.
- Sports-directed therapy should be gradually introduced.
- Any significant pain during rehabilitation should delay the advancement of therapy to prevent reaggravation of the injury.
- Repeat clinical examinations and radiographs are necessary to monitor the progress of healing.
- Once healed, ensure that an appropriate stretching regimen is instituted for the muscle groups involved on both sides.

Considerations in Special Populations

- High-level athletes need to understand that although a quick return to play may be desired, careful and cautious rehabilitation is necessary to obtain full healing.

Acknowledgment

The authors would like to acknowledge Dr. Michael Kwon for his contributions to the previous edition of this chapter.

Suggested Readings

Ferbach SK, Wilkinson RH. Avulsion injuries to the pelvis and proximal femur. *AJR Am J Roentgenol*. 1981;137:581–584.

Kaneyama S, Yoshida K, Matsushima S, et al. A surgical approach for an avulsion fracture of the ischial tuberosity: a case report. *J Orthop Trauma*. 2006;20:363–365.

McCarthy J, Herman MJ, Sankar WN. Pelvic and acetabular fractures. In: Flynn JM, Skaggs DL, Waters PM, eds. *Rockwood and Wilkins' Fractures in Children*. 8th ed. Philadelphia: Wolters Kluwer; 2015:921–952.

Metzmaker JN, Pappas AM. Avulsion fracture of the pelvis. *Am J Sports Med*. 1985;13:349–358.

Rosenberg N, Noiman M, Edelson G. Avulsion fractures of the anterior superior iliac spine in adolescents. *J Orthop Trauma*. 1996;10:440–443.

Rossi F, Dragoni S. Acute avulsion fractures of the pelvis in adolescent competitive athletes: prevalence, location and sports distribution of 203 cases collected. *Skeletal Radiol*. 2001;30:127–131.

Sawyer JR, Spence DD. Fractures and dislocations in children. In: Azar FM, Beaty JH, Canale ST, eds. *Campbell's Operative Orthopaedics*. 13th ed. Philadelphia: Elsevier; 2017:1423–1569.

Sundar M, Carty H. Avulsion fractures of the pelvis in children: a report of 32 fractures and their outcome. *Skeletal Radiol*. 1994;23:85–90.

Vandervliet EJ, Vanhoenacker FM, Snoeckx A, et al. Sports-related acute and chronic avulsion injuries in children and adolescents with special emphasis on tennis. *Br J Sports Med*. 2007;41:827–831.

White KK, Williams SK, Mubarak SJ. Definition of two types of anterior superior iliac spine avulsion fractures. *J Pediatr Orthop*. 2002;22:578–582.

Willis RB, Kocher MS, Ganley TJ. Sports medicine in the growing child. In: Weinstein SL, Flynn JM, eds. *Lovell and Winter's Pediatric Orthopaedics*. 7th ed. Philadelphia: Lippincott Williams & Wilkins; 2014:1596–1660.

Chapter 226 The Adolescent: Cavus Foot

Mark J. Romness

ICD-10-CM CODES
M21.6X *Other acquired deformities of foot*
M21.96 *Unspecified acquired deformity of lower leg*

Key Concepts

- Progressive cavus foot deformity may be the first sign of other pathologic conditions that must be identified with hereditary sensorimotor neuropathy type I (Charcot-Marie-Tooth), the most prevalent neuromuscular cause.
- Treatment for the foot is generally symptomatic.

History

- A family history of any neurologic condition should be defined.
- Clinical signs rarely manifest before age 3 years.
- A visual deformity or a limp is the common symptom in the young child.
- Pain or shoe wear problems occur later.
- Neurologic problems such as bowel or bladder incontinence and subtle weakness signs such as problems with stairs must be asked about specifically.

Physical Examination

- The foot shows a progression of deformity.
  - Toe dorsiflexion and clawing
  - Plantar fascia contraction and increased arch height
  - First metatarsal plantarflexion
  - Asymmetric muscle weakening, especially of the peroneals
  - Hindfoot varus as the first metatarsal plantarflexion increases
  - Rigidity of the foot with maturity (Fig. 226.1)
- Comprehensive neurologic examination, including tone assessment, reflexes, strength, and motor control
- Spine examination for scoliosis or other deformity
- Lower extremity examination to assess length, alignment, and development

Imaging

- Plain radiographs define the degree and location of the deformity.
  - Standing radiographs are recommended.

- The position of the calcaneus is usually dorsiflexed relative to the tibia, indicating that the Achilles tendon is not shortened.
- Magnetic resonance imaging of the spinal axis, including the entire spinal cord if upper motor neuron findings are present
  - Magnetic resonance imaging of the brain if indicated by symptoms and findings

Additional Tests

- Nerve conduction studies may help to classify the condition.
- Serology studies
  - Hereditary sensorimotor neuropathy type IA is inherited in an autosomal dominant manner and is caused by duplication of the gene for peripheral myelin protein 22 *(PMP-22)* in chromosome region 17p11.2.
  - More than 18 genes and 11 additional loci harboring candidate genes have been associated with hereditary sensorimotor neuropathy and related peripheral neuropathies.

Differential Diagnosis

- Many conditions have been associated with cavus foot deformity and are grouped by cause in Box 226.1.
- Hereditary sensorimotor neuropathy type I is the most prevalent neuromuscular cause and is commonly known as Charcot-Marie-Tooth disease type I.

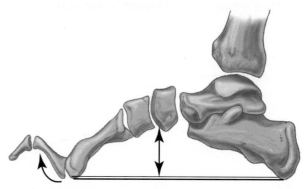

Fig 226.1 Cavus foot. Lateral view of the foot demonstrating the clawing of the toes, plantar fascia contraction, and increased arch height leading to first metatarsal plantarflexion. (From Sabir M, Lyttle D: Pathogenesis of pes cavus in Charcot-Marie-Tooth disease, *Clin Orthop Relat Res* 175:173-178, 1983.)

BOX 226.1 Conditions Associated with Cavus Foot Deformity Grouped by Cause

Central Nervous System

Spastic hemiplegia
Friedreich ataxia
Brain tumors

Spinal Abnormalities

Diastematomyelia
Myelodysplasia
Syringomyelia
Poliomyelitis
Spinal cord tumors
Intrathecal lipoma
Tethered cord syndrome
Guillain-Barré syndrome

Peripheral Nerves

Hereditary sensorimotor neuropathy
Polyneuritis
Small muscular atrophy
Atypical polyneuritis
Neuromuscular choristoma

Other Causes

Isolated injuries to selected nerves, muscles, and
    tendons
Clubfoot or residual clubfoot deformity
Idiopathic

Modified from Schwend RM, Drennan JC. Cavus foot deformity in children. *J Am Acad Orthop Surg.* 2003;11(3):201–211.

Treatment

At Diagnosis

- Determination of the cause if there is one
- Maintain flexibility with stretching as possible
- Shoe modifications or foot orthosis if symptomatic

Later

- Flexibility of the deformity determines treatment options
- Surgical reconstruction if severely symptomatic

When to Refer

- If unable to determine the etiology
- If foot is rigid or symptomatic

Prognosis

- Depends on the etiology but usually progressive deformity and stiffness
- Most forms are treatable and do not prevent light-duty daily activities.

Troubleshooting

- Many of the conditions that cause cavus foot deformity also cause scoliosis and hip dysplasia.

Patient Instructions

- There is no effective medical treatment to prevent progression of hereditary sensorimotor neuropathy (Charcot-Marie-Tooth disease).
- Hereditary sensorimotor neuropathy types Ia and II are autosomal dominant and type Ix is X-linked dominant.

Considerations in Special Populations

- Before skeletal maturity of the foot there is usually more flexibility.
- A rigid foot with skeletal maturity is less likely to respond to nonoperative treatment for severe symptoms.

Suggested Readings

Aktas S, Sussman MD. The radiological analysis of pes cavus deformity in Charcot Marie Tooth disease. *J Pediatr Orthop B.* 2000;9:137–140.

Mosca VS. The cavus foot. *J Pediatr Orthop.* 2001;21:423–424.

Olney B. Treatment of the cavus foot. Deformity in the pediatric patient with Charcot-Marie-Tooth. *Foot Ankle Clin.* 2000;5:305–315.

Saifi GM, Szigeti K, Snipes GJ, et al. Molecular mechanisms, diagnosis, and rational approaches to management of and therapy for Charcot-Marie-Tooth disease and related peripheral neuropathies. *J Investig Med.* 2003;51:261–283.

Schwend RH, Drennan JC. Cavus foot deformity in children. *J Am Acad Orthop Surg.* 2003;11:201–211.

Chapter 227 The Adolescent: Tarsal Coalition

Mark J. Romness

ICD-10-CM CODE
Q66.89 *Other specified congenital deformities of feet*

Key Concepts

- Tarsal coalition is due to the failure of the bones in the foot to separate completely during formation.
- Depending on the position of the coalition, there may be stiffness, deformity, or pain.
- Asymptomatic coalitions may not need treatment.
- Symptomatic coalitions often need surgery.
- The most common types are calcaneonavicular and talocalcaneal coalitions (Fig. 227.1).
- Coalitions should be considered with any ankle sprains.

History

- Clinical signs rarely manifest before preadolescent age.
- The initial symptom is a limp or pain.
- Pain is usually dorsolateral or medial.

Physical Examination

- Asymmetric position of the foot in standing position
- Usually more valgus or pronation of the foot with a coalition
- Decreased motion actively and passively
- Lack of arch accentuation and heel varus on tip-toe position (Fig. 227.2)
- A bony prominence below the medial malleolus for a talocalcaneal coalition
- Tenderness at the area of the coalition
  - Lateral at the sinus tarsi for a calcaneonavicular coalition
  - Medial just below the malleolus for a talocalcaneal coalition

Imaging

- Plain radiographs may be diagnostic, but special views must be ordered.
  - An oblique radiograph of the foot shows most calcaneonavicular coalitions (Fig. 227.3).
  - The axial view of the calcaneus may show a talocalcaneal coalition, but usually computed tomography or magnetic resonance imaging is necessary.
- Computed tomography is more accurate than magnetic resonance imaging for the diagnosis.
- A bone scan is rarely necessary but may be helpful in equivocal cases.

Additional Tests

- Serology studies and nerve conduction studies should be considered if there is no definitive coalition radiographically and there is a suggestion of muscle disease or a neuropathy.

Differential Diagnosis

- The historical term of peroneal spastic flatfoot for coalition is thought to describe the secondary contracture of the peroneal tendons, but primary contracture of the peroneals may occur and mimic a coalition.
- Conditions such as juvenile idiopathic arthritis that can affect the subtalar joint may have similar complaints and presentation.
- Muscle disease or a neuropathy should be considered but is usually associated with an opposite position (cavovarus) of the foot.

Treatment
At Diagnosis

- Proper diagnosis
- Symptomatic treatment with limited activity, inserts or orthoses, antiinflammatory medication, and immobilization in a boot or cast

Later

- Monitor the foot position with growth.
- Consider surgery for significant deformity or pain.

When to Refer

- Persistent pain despite symptomatic treatment
- Significant deformity or stiffness/rigidity

Prognosis

- Depends on the location and extent of the coalition
- Calcaneonavicular coalitions have better prognosis than talocalcaneal coalitions
- More initial deformity and rigidity have worse prognosis

Troubleshooting

- Magnetic resonance imaging may not detect the coalition.
- Secondary changes in the adjacent joints, such as beaking of the talar head, may be misinterpreted as the primary condition if appropriate radiographic views are not obtained.

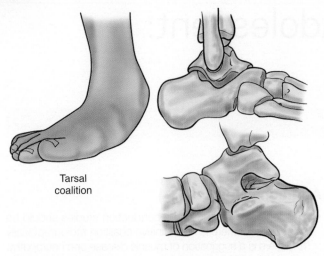

Fig 227.1 Coalitions. A more severe foot position is shown on the *left.* Calcaneonavicular coalition is demonstrated at *top right.* Talocalcaneal coalition is demonstrated at *bottom right.*

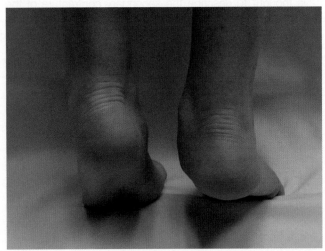

Fig 227.2 Feet in tip-toe position. The right foot with a coalition does not correct out of pronation, but the left does with restoration of the arch and hindfoot varus in tip-toe position.

Patient Instructions

- Bilateral involvement is present in 50% to 60% of cases, and studies of the opposite foot are indicated if clinical evidence is present.
- Asymptomatic feet with only mild deformity do not require treatment.

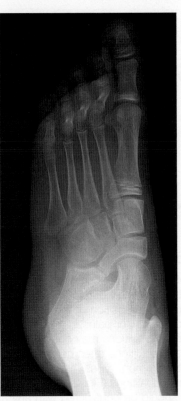

Fig 227.3 Oblique radiograph of the foot with a well-defined calcaneonavicular coalition.

Considerations in Special Populations

- Tarsal coalitions are present in some genetic conditions, such as fibular deficiencies (hemimelia; see Chapter 208), clubfoot, Apert syndrome, and Nievergelt-Pearlman syndrome.

Suggested Readings

Drennan JC. Tarsal coalitions. *Instr Course Lect.* 1996;45:323–329.
Gonzalez P, Kumar SJ. Calcaneonavicular coalition treated by resection and interposition of the extensor digitorum brevis muscle. *J Bone Joint Surg Am.* 1990;72A:71–77.
McCormack TJ, Olney B, Asher M. Talocalcaneal coalition resection: a 10-year follow-up. *J Pediatr Orthop.* 1997;17:13–15.
Mosier KM, Asher M. Tarsal coalitions and peroneal spastic flat foot: A review. *J Bone Joint Surg Am.* 1984;66A:976–984.
Takakura Y, Sugimoto K, Tanaka Y, Tamai S. Symptomatic talocalcaneal coalition: its clinical significance and treatment. *Clin Orthop Relat Res.* 1991;269:249–256.

Chapter 228 The Adolescent: Special Fractures in Pediatrics

Victor Anciano Granadillo, Keith Bachmann

ICD-10-CM CODES

S42.41	*Supracondylar fracture*
S42.43	*Lateral condyle fracture*
S82.15	*Tibial tubercle fracture*
S82.11	*Tibial spine fracture*
S82.89	*Distal tibial intra-articular fracture (triplane and Tillaux)*

Common Fractures: Elbow (Supracondylar and Lateral Condyle Fractures)

Key Concepts

- Elbow fractures common in pediatrics
- Supracondylar humerus fractures
  - Neurovascular injury common in type 3 supracondylar humerus fractures (most displaced), with 15% of cases involving nerve injury and as many as 20% without pulse (although often the hand remains perfused)
  - Avoid cubitus varus deformity with supracondylar fractures.
  - Compartment syndrome higher when treated with closed reduction, hyperflexion, and without pinning
  - Temporary splinting should avoid hyperflexion due to risk of compartment syndrome.
  - Two divergent pins are usually sufficient for fixation (especially with type 2 fracture). Iatrogenic ulnar nerve injury is associated with medial pins.
- Lateral condyle fractures
  - Intra-articular fractures need anatomic reduction of the articular surface.
  - Risk of nonunion that is decreased by fixation
  - Prolonged casting may be necessary, often for 6 weeks.

History

- Acute: basic trauma history including mechanism of injury, areas of pain or deformity, and other associated injuries or previous injuries to extremity
- Always consider nonaccidental trauma in children with stories that are not consistent with injury pattern or in children whose injuries occurred while unattended.

Physical Examination

- Observation: deformity, bruising/swelling, skin condition
- Brachialis/puckered sign: antecubital fossa ecchymosis with skin dimpling: associated with bone spike in brachialis muscle.
- Palpation: tenderness or crepitus at fracture site, as well as in the forearm and shoulder
- Neurovascular examination critical: anterior interosseous nerve (AIN) palsy is the most commonly encountered nerve injury in supracondylar fractures but all upper extremity nerves at risk.

Imaging

- Radiographs
  - Anteroposterior and lateral views of elbow
    - The anterior humeral line should intersect the capitellum on a true lateral view.
    - The radial shaft should point to the capitellum on all views; if not, the radiocapitellar joint is dislocated.
    - Baumann angle (humeral capitellar angle) should be in valgus and typically greater than 9 degrees.
    - A posterior fat pad seen on a lateral view may denote an occult fracture.
  - Oblique elbow radiographs (internal oblique) helpful if high index of suspicion of lateral condyle fracture
- Arthrography helpful if suspect transphyseal fractures or with fractures involving the articular surface in the operating room

Differential Diagnosis

- Please see Table 228.1.

Treatment

Supracondylar Humerus Fracture

- At diagnosis
  - If hand not perfused, traction/flexion often adequate to restore capillary refill
    - If remains poorly perfused, emergent operative treatment necessary
  - Splint in 30 to 50 degrees of flexion to avoid compartment syndrome when hyperflexed.

TABLE 228.1 Differential Diagnosis: Common Injuries of the Elbow

Differential Diagnosis	Differentiation Features
Other fractures Supracondylar Lateral condyle Radial neck Medial condyle Olecranon	Location of pain and tenderness, radiographic differences
Elbow dislocation	Radiographic differences: radial head not aligned with the capitellum
Osteochondral injury	Persistent discomfort (often after elbow dislocation), radiographic diagnosis difficult; joint incongruity noted on magnetic resonance imaging

- Later
  - Closed treatment and casting in 90 degrees of flexion in nondisplaced fractures and those in which the anterior humeral line touches the capitellum with a normal valgus Baumann angle
  - Closed reduction and percutaneous pinning for displaced fractures and fractures in extension (anterior humeral line does not touch the capitellum) and in varus
    - Crossed pins (increased risk of iatrogenic ulnar nerve injury) versus lateral-only pins.
    - Two lateral pins are usually sufficient.
    - No difference in stability between three lateral pins and crossed pins (Fig. 228.1).
  - Open reduction reserved for open fractures, fractures unable to be reduced due to interposed tissue, and those without a pulse
    - Management of pulseless hand:
      - Pulseless, pink, warm well-perfused hands require emergent closed reduction and percutaneous pinning (CRPP) with possible vascular consultation/reconstruction

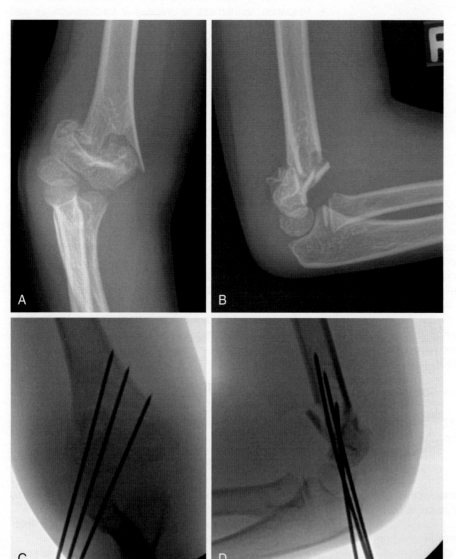

Fig 228.1 (A) Anteroposterior (AP) radiograph of type 3 supracondylar humerus fracture. **(B)** Lateral radiograph of type 3 supracondylar humerus fracture. **(C)** AP fluoroscopic view of closed reduction and percutaneous pinning of supracondylar fracture with three lateral pins. **(D)** Lateral fluoroscopic view of closed reduction and percutaneous pinning of supracondylar fracture with three lateral pins.

When to Refer

- Emergent transfer for cold, nonperfused extremity, or neurologic deficit
- Transfer to treating facility with displaced fractures
- Refer within 24 hours for nondisplaced or minimally displaced fractures.

Prognosis

- Generally excellent
- Healing problems are very rare.
- Stiffness after immobilization can improve for as long as 2 years after casting or pinning.
- Most cases of neuropraxia resolve spontaneously.

Lateral Condyle Fracture
At Diagnosis

- Splint
- Nondisplaced (≤2 mm) fractures with an intact articular surface can be treated nonoperatively with casting. Weekly evaluation with x-ray may be needed to evaluate for displacement. Internal oblique views better characterize lateral column.
- Cast nondisplaced fractures with elbow at 90 degrees.
- Classifications according to involvement of trochlea (Milch) or displacement (Weiss).

Later

- Greater than 2 mm of displacement, operative treatment is indicated.
- If the articular surface is intact (ultrasound, arthrogram), percutaneous pinning is adequate.
- With significant displacement, open reduction, anatomic reduction of the articular surface, and pinning are needed (Fig. 228.2).
  - Do not dissect posteriorly; lateral trochlea blood supply comes from the posterior nonarticular portion.
- May take 4 to 6 weeks to heal

When to Refer

- At diagnosis: Late presenting lateral condyle fractures are often difficult to treat and have a high risk of nonunion and cubitus valgus.

Prognosis

- Usually heal well but increased risk of complications including nonunion, late fracture displacement, and cubitus valgus due to intra-articular nature of fracture
- Patients may experience a prominence laterally after an open reduction.
- Stiffness can be a problem after open reduction and prolonged casting.

Troubleshooting

- Vascular compromise relatively uncommon.
  - With perfused hand, acceptable to watch even without a pulse
  - With cold, pulseless hand, emergent reduction needed (and sometimes vascular surgery)
- Nerve injuries relatively uncommon with lateral condyle fractures (either caused by the injury or iatrogenic).

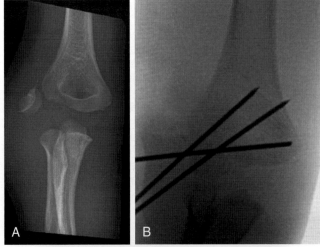

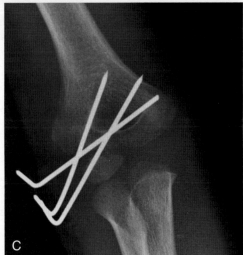

Fig 228.2 Displaced lateral condyle fracture requiring open reduction and percutaneous pinning. **(A)** Displaced fracture. **(B)** Intraoperative fluoroscopy demonstrating reduction and pin fixation. **(C)** Healing demonstrated at 4 weeks just prior to pin removal.

- Like supracondylar neuropraxias, these tend to resolve spontaneously.

Patient Instructions

- Warn patients about the risks of nonunion and stiffness with lateral condyle fractures, as well as a likely prominence laterally on the elbow.

Special Fractures: Knee (Tibial Spine and Tibial Tubercle Fractures)

Key Concepts

- The tibial spine fracture has a mechanism of injury similar to the anterior cruciate ligament in skeletally mature patients earning the moniker of the "pediatric anterior cruciate ligament (ACL) equivalent"

- Despite this, ACL tears are actually more common even among pediatric patients
- If more than 2 mm of displacement, the anterior horn of medial or lateral meniscus may be interposed, and surgical reduction and fixation may be necessary.
- Tibial tubercle fractures are injuries of the anterior proximal tibial apophysis.
- Typically occurs in teenage boys (near skeletal maturity), usually during a jumping sport
- Fixation is typically necessary due to the pull of the extensor mechanism.
- Associated with compartment syndrome despite being a low-energy injury due to the anterior recurrent tibial artery.

History

- See anterior/posterior cruciate ligament injury and extensor mechanism injuries.
- Acute: age of patient, basic trauma history including the mechanism of injury, areas of pain or deformity, and other associated injuries or previous injuries to extremity

Physical Examination

- See anterior/posterior cruciate ligament injury and extensor mechanism injuries.
- Observation: deformity, bruising/swelling, effusion
- Palpation: tenderness, crepitus, effusion
- Range of motion, if able
- Full knee extension is the reduction maneuver for tibial spine fractures. Operative management is usually based on reducible versus nonreducible fracture patterns.
- Assess whether extensor mechanism is intact.

Imaging

- Radiographs: anteroposterior and lateral views of the knee
- Computed tomography or magnetic resonance imaging confirms the diagnosis or the amount of displacement of the tibial spine fracture.
- Meyers and Mckeever classification of tibial spine fractures is based on displacement of the fracture.
- Ogden classification of tibial tubercle fractures is based on involvement of the proximal tibia physis.

Differential Diagnosis

- Please see Table 228.2.

Treatment
Tibial Spine Fracture (Fig. 228.3)
At Diagnosis

- Extension with knee immobilization or cast often reduces fracture
  - If any question, obtain advanced imaging

Later

- If minimal displacement: 3 to 4 weeks in extension followed by range of motion

TABLE 228.2 Differential Diagnosis: Special Injuries of the Knee

Differential Diagnosis	Differentiating Features
Anterior/posterior cruciate ligament tear	Positive Lachman test, knee instability, radiographs negative for fracture, magnetic resonance imaging diagnostic
Patellar sleeve fracture	Extensor mechanism disrupted, patellar tenderness, patellar fracture noted on radiograph
Meniscal tear	Joint line tenderness, mechanical symptoms, magnetic resonance imaging diagnostic
Patellar dislocation	History of kneecap "popping out," medial patellar tenderness, apprehension with lateral patellar translation
Proximal tibial fracture	Proximal tibial pain and tenderness, swelling, radiographs diagnostic
Osgood-Schlatter disease	Chronic knee pain localized over tibial tubercle, intact extensor mechanism

- If displaced (>2 mm with knee extended), the tibial spine should be repaired to its origin
  - Can be performed arthroscopically or open depending on surgeon's preference
  - Fixation options include suture, cannulated screws, and pins.
  - Blocks to reductions include anterior horn of medial meniscus (most common), anterior horn of lateral meniscus, intermeniscal ligament, or fracture fragments (comminuted fractures)

When to Refer

- If the examiner has any concern about management, the patient should be placed in a knee immobilizer and evaluated within 3 to 5 days.

Prognosis

- Generally good
- The tibial spine typically heals well.
- Due to stretching of the anterior cruciate ligament, there may be some laxity to the knee after treatment. This does not appear to be clinically significant and may even improve with growth.
- Arthrofibrosis most common complication after any surgical approach, arthroscopic or open.

Tibial Tubercle Fracture (Fig. 228.4)
At Diagnosis

- Knee immobilizer
- Watch for compartment syndrome due to injury to the recurrent anterior tibial artery.
- Extensor mechanism deficiency is common in more severe fractures.

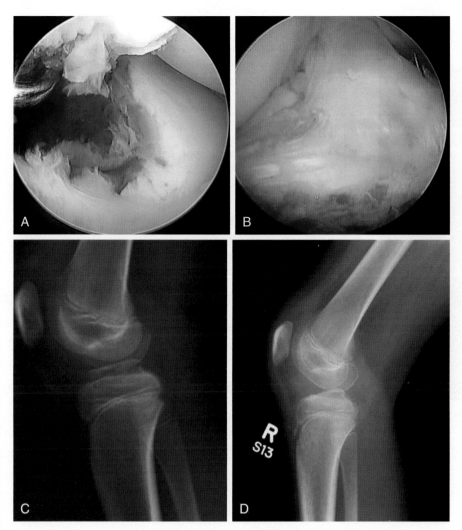

Fig 228.3 (A) Arthroscopic image of prereduced tibial spine fracture fragment. (B) Arthroscopic image of reduced fracture fragment. (C) Preoperative x-ray of displaced tibial spine fracture. (D) Postoperative x-ray of fixed tibial spine fracture.

Later

- Typically, operative fixation needed; screws usually adequate. Smooth K-wires may be used in younger children (usually those with more than 3 to 4 years remaining to skeletal maturity) (Fig. 228.5).
- If extends to the joint, may have associated meniscal or ligamentous injury and needs anatomic reduction of the articular surface either arthroscopic assisted or open

When to Refer

- If the examiner has any concern about management, the patient should be placed in a knee immobilizer and evaluated within 3 to 5 days.

Prognosis

- Bone healing is typically good.
- Despite the fact that this is a physeal injury, clinically significant growth arrest is unusual due to the lack of remaining growth.
- However, in children with 1 year or more of growth remaining, watch for partial physeal arrest.
- Most common deformity associated with tibial tubercle fractures is recurvatum deformity.

Troubleshooting

- In a younger child with tibial tubercle fractures, clinically relevant growth disturbance is possible and results in difficult-to-treat recurvatum deformity.
- Complete physeal closure or consider growth modulation electively if any growth deformity is noted. Consider physeal closure of the contralateral side if clinically relevant limb length difference will result.

Special Fractures: Ankle (Triplane and Tillaux Fractures)

Key Concepts

- Transitional fractures (Tillaux and triplane) occur due to the asymmetric closure of the distal tibial physis during early adolescence.
- Distal tibia physis ossifies asymmetrically in the following order: (1) central, (2) medial, (3) lateral
- A triplane fracture typically has a sagittal fracture line through the epiphysis, a transverse fracture line through the physis, and a coronal fracture line through the metaphysis (Fig. 228.6).

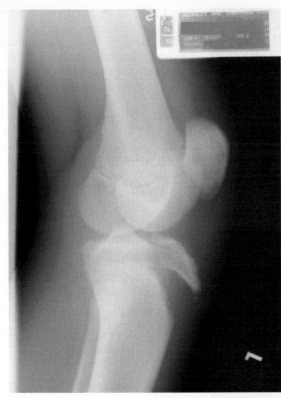

Fig 228.4 Displaced tibial tubercle fracture.

- A Tillaux fracture occurs when the anterolateral portion of the distal tibial epiphysis (the last portion of the physis to close) is avulsed anteriorly by a pull from the anterior inferior tibiofibular ligament.
- Both fractures require anatomic reduction of the articular surface.

History

- Acute: age of the patient, basic trauma history including mechanism of injury, areas of pain or deformity, and other associated injuries or previous injuries to extremity

Physical Examination

- Observation: deformity, bruising/swelling, skin condition
- Palpation: tenderness or crepitus at the fracture
- Neurovascular examination

Imaging

- Radiographs: anteroposterior, lateral, and mortise views of the ankle. Anteroposterior (AP)/lateral views of entire tibia/fibula.
- Triplane fractures are Salter-Harris IV fractures in essence. However, in different views, they will appear as either Salter-Harris II (lateral view) or Salter-Harris III (AP view)
- Fibula often fractured with triplane fractures
- Computed tomography helpful in determining joint congruence and need for open reduction

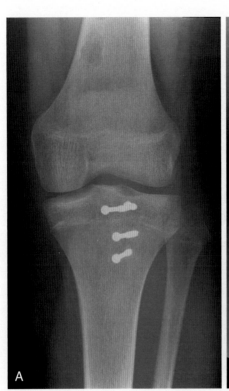

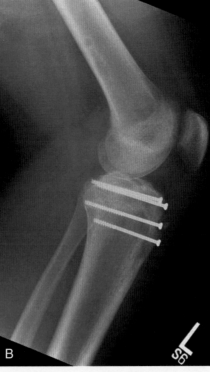

Fig 228.5 (A) Anteroposterior radiographic view of a fixed tibial tubercle fracture with screws. (B) Lateral radiographic view of a fixed tibial tubercle fracture with screws.

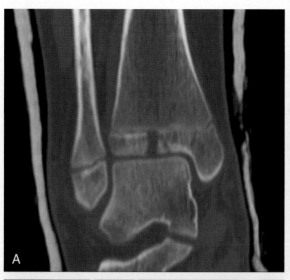

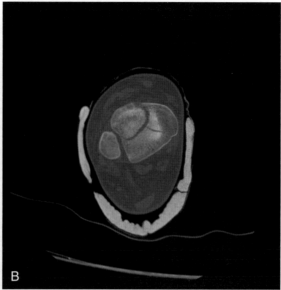

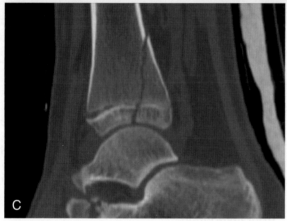

Fig 228.6 (A) Triplane fracture preoperative computed tomography: coronal image showing sagittal plane fracture through the epiphysis. (B) Triplane fracture preoperative computed tomography: axial image showing transverse plane fracture through the physis. (C) Triplane fracture preoperative computed tomography: sagittal image showing coronal plane fracture through the metaphysis.

Differential Diagnosis

- Please see Table 228.3.

Treatment
Triplane and Tillaux Fractures
At Diagnosis

- Can attempt closed reduction and casting; usual maneuver is anterior translation of the ankle with internal rotation; long leg cast is necessary to control rotation
- Perform computed tomography to determine joint congruity.
- Triplane fractures can be lateral triplane, medial triplane, or intramalleolar triplane. Lateral triplane fractures are the most common. Intramalleolar triplane fractures are the most uncommon; they involve an epiphyseal fracture line that exits through the medial malleolus.

Later

- With more than 2 mm of displacement and any articular step-off, open reduction is necessary; some displacement of the metaphysis is acceptable.

TABLE 228.3	Differential Diagnosis: Special Injuries of the Ankle
Differential Diagnosis	**Differentiating Features**
Ankle sprain	Tenderness isolated on soft tissue, no fracture on radiographs
Medial or lateral malleolar fracture	Tenderness at bone, fracture noted on radiographs
Osteochondritis dissecans lesion of the ankle	Often more chronic history of pain, radiographic abnormality, magnetic resonance imaging diagnostic
Nonarticular fractures of the distal tibia	Deformity and radiographic findings

- Intraepiphyseal screw fixation to close down the articular surface in a triplane fracture ± fixation of the Thurston-Holland fragment of the metaphysis (Fig. 228.7).
- Screw fixation for Tillaux fractures also recommended after open reduction (Fig. 228.8)—if medial physis is closing, can direct screw more obliquely

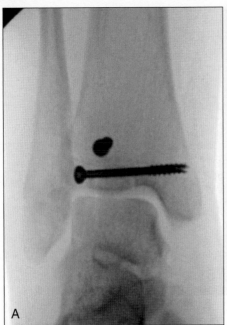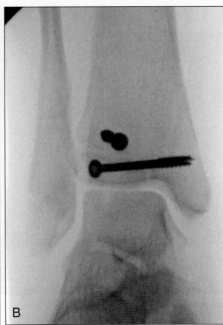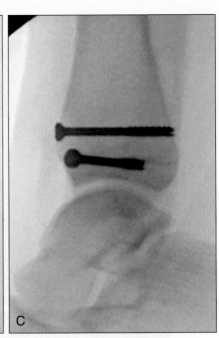

Fig 228.7 **(A)** Anteroposterior radiograph of a triplane fracture treated with open reduction and internal fixation. **(B)** Mortise view radiograph of a triplane fracture treated with open reduction and internal fixation. **(C)** Lateral radiograph of a triplane fracture treated with open reduction and internal fixation. (From Keeler KA, Luhmann SJ. Triplane fractures. In: Kocher MS, Millis MB, eds. *Operative Techniques: Pediatric Orthopaedic Surgery*. Philadelphia, PA: Elsevier; 2011:553–564.)

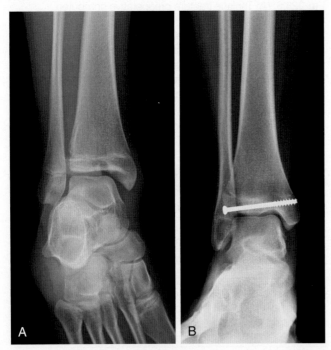

Fig 228.8 **(A)** Preoperative radiograph of a displaced Tillaux fracture. **(B)** Radiograph after open reduction and screw fixation for Tillaux fracture.

When to Refer

- If any question of reduction or decision making

Prognosis

- Heals well generally—follow epiphyseal fracture line given joint involvement

- Increased risk of arthritis, but this risk can be decreased with good anatomic joint reduction
- Growth arrest or deformity not usually a problem because of the fact that fractures occur during growth plate closure. Still monitor if growth remaining or based on patient age.

Troubleshooting

- Articular congruence key to a good long-term result
- Screws in the epiphysis may change the articular cartilage joint mechanics, so consider screw removal after healing.

Suggested Readings

Abzug JM, Herman MJ. Management of supracondylar humerus fractures in children: current concepts. *J Am Acad Orthop Surg*. 2012; 20(2):69–77.

Finnbogason T, Karlsson G, Lindberg L, Mortensson W. Nondisplaced and minimally displaced fractures of the lateral humeral condyle in children: a prospective radiographic investigation of fracture stability. *J Pediatr Orthop*. 1995;15:422–425.

LaFrance RM, Giordano B, Goldblatt J, et al. Pediatric tibial eminence fractures: evaluation and management. *J Am Acad Orthop Surg*. 2010; 18(7):395–405.

Little RM, Milewski MD. Physeal fractures about the knee. *Curr Rev Musculoskelet Med*. 2016;9(4):478–486.

Mosier SM, Stanitski CL. Acute tibial tubercle avulsion fractures. *J Pediatr Orthop*. 2004;24:181–184.

Skaggs DL. Elbow fractures in children: diagnosis and management. *J Am Acad Orthop Surg*. 1997;5:303–312.

Skaggs DL, Hale JM, Bassett J, et al. Operative treatment of supracondylar fractures of the humerus in children: the consequences of pin placement. *J Bone Joint Surg Am*. 2001;83A:735–740.

Wuerz TH, Gurd DP. Pediatric ankle fracture. *J Am Acad Orthop Surg*. 2013;21(4):234–244.

Chapter 229 The Adolescent: Metabolic Bone Diseases: Osteogenesis Imperfecta/Rickets

Leigh-Ann Lather, Keith Bachmann

ICD-10-CM CODES
Q78.0 *Osteogenesis imperfecta*
E55.0 *Rickets*
E55.9 *Vitamin D deficiency*

Key Concepts
Osteoporosis

- Bone fragility with increased risk of fracture.
- Etiology: see Table 229.1
- May result from loss of bone, but more commonly is due to failure to accrue enough bone mineral content for size. Low bone mass in childhood has serious implications for lifelong health.

Osteogenesis Imperfecta

- Rare disorder, 1:20,000 live births (Fig. 229.1)
- The vast majority are disorders of type 1 collagen. *All* collagen-containing tissues are affected.

Metabolic bone disease/secondary osteoporosis (Fig. 229.2)
- Several etiologic factors may act alone or in combination. All causes ultimately lead to calcium or phosphate levels that are lower than those required to create the crystalline component of bone. Anything that causes decreased intake of calcium, phosphorus, or vitamin D, or the malabsorption or increased excretion of those nutrients can cause low bone density. See Tables 229.1 and 229.2.
- *Rickets* refers to deficient mineralization of the growth plate and *osteomalacia* is impaired mineralization of the bone matrix. Only osteomalacia can exist after skeletal maturity.

History
Osteoporosis

- Presence of a vertebral compression fracture in the absence of local disease or high-energy trauma.
- Two long-bone fractures by age 10 years, OR three long-bone fractures by age 19 years and a bone mineral density (BMD) Z-score ≤ −2.0.

TABLE 229.1 Causes of Osteoporosis in Children

Primary Causes	Secondary Causes
Osteogenesis imperfecta	Metabolic bone disease: rickets and osteomalacia
Connective tissue disorders: Marfan, Ehlers Danlos syndromes	Undernourished, low body weight, malabsorption: eating disorders, celiac disease, CF
Osteoporosis pseudoglioma (blindness)	Inflammatory state: JIA, IBD, SLE
Fibrous dysplasia	Meds: Glucocorticoids, anticonvulsants
Juvenile idiopathic osteoporosis	Endocrine: GH deficiency, disordered puberty, thyroid disorders
Bruck syndrome (OI + joint contractures)	Reduced mobility: CP, MMC, Duchenne MD

CF, cystic fibrosis; *CP,* cerebral palsy; *GH,* growth hormone deficiency; *IBD,* inflammatory bowel disease; *JIA,* juvenile idiopathic arthritis; *MD,* muscular dystrophy; *MMC,* myelomeningocele; *SLE,* systemic lupus erythematosis.

TABLE 229.2 Classification of Rickets Based on Resulting Deficiency[a]

Calcium	Phosphorus	Alkaline Phosphatase
Vitamin D deficiency	*X-linked hypophosphatemia*	Hypophosphatasia
Calcium + vitamin D deficiency	Renal tubular abnormalities	
Gastrointestinal rickets (malabsorption)	e.g., Fanconi syndrome	
End-stage renal disease		
1αhydroxylase deficiency (vitamin D resistant)		
Isolated calcium deficiency		

[a]Only the italicized deficiencies are common.

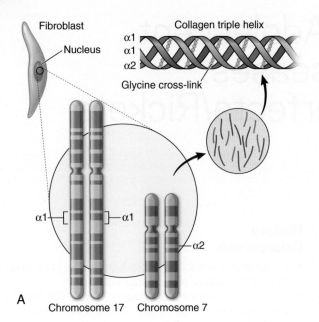

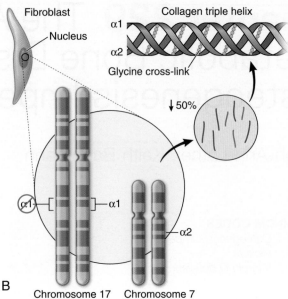

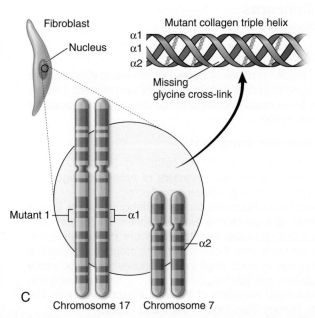

Fig 229.1 Schematic representing normal and abnormal collagen formation. (A) Normal triple-helix collagen formation. (B) A stop codon in one of the *COL1A1* genes results in production of less collagen, characteristic of osteogenesis imperfecta (OI) type I. (C) Mutation in *COL1A1* or *COL1A2* results in poor cross linking and production of reduced amounts of collagen that is qualitatively abnormal: typical of OI types II–IV. (From Kim HKW. Metabolic and endocrine bone diseases. In: Herring J, ed. *Tachdjian's Pediatric Orthopaedics: From the Texas Scottish Rite Hospital for Children*, 5th ed. Philadelphia: Elsevier; 2014:582–642, Fig. 42.26.)

- A BMD *Z*-score > −2.0 does not preclude the diagnosis of osteoporosis if there is clinical bone fragility.

Osteogenesis Imperfecta

- Patient presents with a family history of osteogenesis imperfecta (OI), or with a history of multiple fractures without appropriate trauma
- Depends on type of OI: type 1 presents at toddler/preschool age with spiral and transverse fractures, type II is lethal typically at birth, type III is severe and presents with multiple fractures at birth, and type IV overlaps with type III but has a variable phenotype. More types are classified.

Metabolic Bone Disease

- Extraskeletal symptoms of rickets (Table 229.3)
- Dietary history is essential. Estimate intake of calcium and vitamin D–rich foods.
- X-linked hypophosphatemia: X-linked dominant, but one-third are sporadic mutations
  - Most common inherited cause of rickets. Incidence 1:20,000.
- Vitamin D deficiency (nutritional rickets) (Table 229.4)
  - Vitamin D is essential for calcium absorption, homeostasis, and bone health. Sunlight (UVB) is necessary for

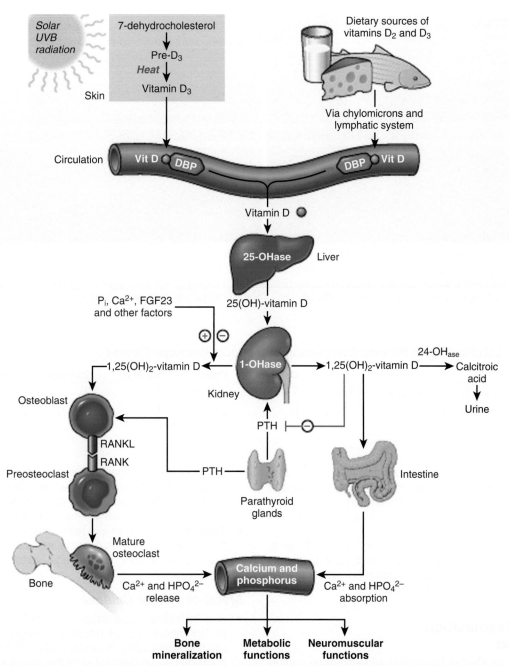

Fig 229.2 Schematic overview of vitamin D and calcium metabolism. *DBP,* vitamin D binding protein; *FGF,* fibroblast growth factor; *PTH,* parathyroid hormone; *RANKL,* receptor activator of nuclear factor kappa-B ligand. (From Kumar V, Fausto N, Aster J, Abbas A, eds. *Robbins and Cotran Pathologic Basis of Disease,* 8th ed. Philadelphia: Elsevier; 2010.)

TABLE 229.3 Extraskeletal Symptoms of Rickets

Hypocalcemia "CATs Go numb"	Hypophosphatemia
Convulsions	Muscle weakness
Arrhythmias	Mental status (or mood) change
Tetany	Low cardiac output
Paresthesias	Unstable cell membranes → hemolysis, rhabdomyolysis
Hypotonia, infections, sweating, bone pain	Decreased WBC function → infections

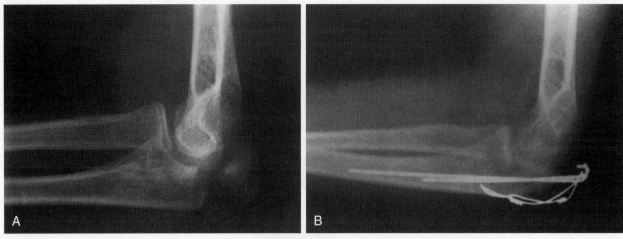

Fig 229.3 (A) and **(B)** Olecranon avulsion fracture in a patient with osteogenesis imperfecta (OI). An otherwise uncommon injury in children, especially as an avulsion fracture (from pull of triceps alone) that should prompt evaluation for OI or other bone metabolism defects. (From Kim HKW. Metabolic and endocrine bone diseases. In: Herring J, ed. *Tachdjian's Pediatric Orthopaedics: From the Texas Scottish Rite Hospital for Children*, 5th ed. Philadelphia: Elsevier; 2014:582–642, Fig. 42.35.)

TABLE 229.4 Lab Findings in Rickets: Comparison of the Most Common Causes

Type	Calcium	Phos	Alk Phos	25-OH D	PTH	Urine Ca
Vitamin D deficiency (leads to calcipenic rickets)	↑ or N	↓ or N	↑	↓	↑	↓ or N
X-linked hypophosphatemia	N	↓↓	↑	N	N	↓

synthesis of the prohormone, which is then converted to the active form by normally functioning liver and kidneys. Only 10% of vitamin D comes from the diet unless it is a fortified food or a supplement. Vitamin D deficiency is on the rise.

- Risk factors: premature or exclusively breast-fed infants, dark skin, northern latitudes, house-bound, obesity, conditions of malabsorption, and medications (certain anticonvulsants and glucocorticoids).

Physical Examination
Osteoporosis

- Dependent on whether presenting with long-bone fracture or may present with back pain due to vertebral compression fractures

Osteogenesis Imperfecta

- **Type I:** Usually presents in toddler/preschool age with spiral and transverse fractures (legs > arms) but can present at any age, blue sclera persist > age 1 year, nondeforming, average adult height, ± dentinogenesis, 50% are deaf by the third decade of life.
  - Olecranon avulsion fractures and patella fractures should prompt evaluation for OI (Fig. 229.3).
- **Type II:** Lethal. Crumpled femurs, ribs, and intracranial hemorrhages at birth.
- **Type III:** Severe, rare, autosomal recessive. Various gene defects lead to qualitatively *abnormal* collagen. Multiple fractures occur during delivery and in infancy. Dysmorphic

triangular facies, +dentinogenesis, short stature, severe bowing deformities of legs, must be handled with extreme care. Most need a wheelchair for mobility. Vertebral compression fractures lead to severe scoliosis and kyphosis.
- **Type IV:** Moderate/severe with variable phenotype. Much overlap with type III. Autosomal recessive, abnormal collagen, short stature, bowed legs, vertebral compression fractures.

Metabolic Bone Disease

- Skeletal findings of *advanced* rickets include delayed closure of fontanelles, frontal bossing, enlarged costochondral junctions particularly at wrists, ankles, and ribs, flared ribs, bowing or varus deformities of the legs in walking children (Fig. 229.4). Seen earliest/most easily at the distal ulna and above or below the knee joint on x-ray.

Imaging/Laboratory

- Initial lab screening: Comprehensive metabolic panel, magnesium, phosphorus, 25(OH) Vit D. Add parathyroid hormone (PTH) if there is osteopenia *without* rickets.
- *Caution*: Calcipenic rickets and pseudoglioma rickets are not always associated with low serum levels of calcium or phosphorus.
- Serum 25(OH) Vit D is the best indicator of vitamin D status and stores in the body.
- Dual-energy X-ray absorptiometry (DXA) for age >8 years should only be performed at a pediatric referral center with experience in bone densitometry.

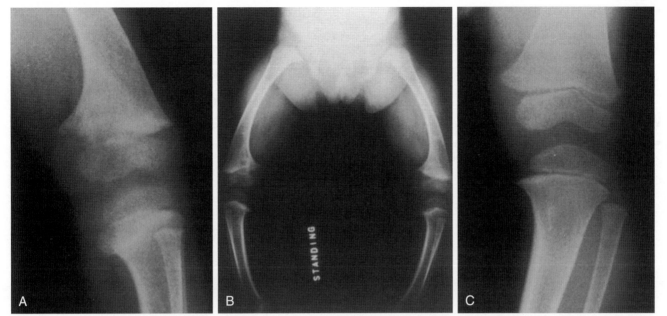

Fig 229.4 Radiographic display of rickets. **(A)** Genu varum with widened physes of the distal femur and proximal tibia. **(B)** Standing alignment with severe genu varum and widened physes. **(C)** Resolution of the physeal changes after treatment, may still require surgical correction of the deformity but now the risk of recurrence due to persistent metabolic deficiency is eliminated. (From Kim HKW. Metabolic and endocrine bone diseases. In: Herring J, ed. *Tachdjian's Pediatric Orthopaedics: From the Texas Scottish Rite Hospital for Children*, 5th ed. Philadelphia: Elsevier; 2014:582–642, Fig. 42.4.)

TABLE 229.5 Vitamin D Status and Treatment

Status	25(OH)D serum	Treatment with Vitamin D (oral)	
Sufficient (treat with a supplement if risk factors for low vitamin D level are present)	>20 ng/mL	400 IU/day 600 IU/day 1–2000 IU/day	Birth–1 yr 1 yr–adult if obese
Insufficient	15–20 ng/mL	5000 IU/day for 6 weeks, then 1000 IU/day ongoing.	
Deficient	≤15 ng/mL	5000 IU/day for 6 weeks, OR 50,000 IU/day once a week for 6 weeks + 1000 IU/day ongoing	

Differential Diagnosis

- Nonaccidental trauma (NAT) and OI: OI is rare and NAT is sadly common. Regardless of genetic testing results, NAT is likely if history, exam, and imaging support that diagnosis. Diagnosing OI does not exclude the possibility of NAT.
- Juvenile idiopathic osteoporosis is a diagnosis of exclusion.
  - Onset 2 to 3 years prior to puberty. The patient presents with metaphyseal fractures or back pain and vertebral compression fracture. Often resolves after puberty.

Treatment

- Osteogenesis imperfecta
  - Treatment for all types requires optimal nutrition and low-impact safe exercise to prevent secondary osteoporosis, shorter casting periods for fractures (just long enough for fracture stability), and physical therapy (PT) in a pool. Refer to a pediatric orthopaedist for comanagement. Bisphosphonates are indicated only for severe types (intravenous or oral); decreases pain and fractures, improves BMD).

Metabolic Bone Disease

- Rickets must be treated according to the underlying cause before any surgical correction of leg deformities can be successful.
- Combined vitamin D and calcium dietary deficiency is also common. Only 10% of girls and 25% of boys age 9 to 17 get the recommended daily allowance (RDA) of 1300 mg of calcium.
  - Vitamin D supplementation (Table 229.5)
  - Referral to an endocrinologist or rheumatology bone specialist for initiation of bisphosphonates/more aggressive supplementation

- X-linked hypophosphatemia
  - Leads to isolated renal phosphate wasting and an inappropriately low or normal kidney production of 1.25-dihydroxy vitamin D3.
    - Treatment is oral phosphate and calcitriol (active vitamin D3).

When to Refer

- Multiple fractures, low-energy fractures, vertebral compression fracture, osteopenia on x-ray, family history of metabolic bone disease.

Suggested Readings

Burnei G, Vlad C, Georgescu I, et al. Osteogenesis imperfecta: diagnosis and treatment. *J Am Acad Orthop Surg*. 2008;16:356–366.

Howard AW, Alman BA. Metabolic and endocrine abnormalities. In: Weinstein SL, Flynn JM, eds. *Lovell and Winter's Pediatric Orthopaedics*. 7th ed. Philadelphia: Lippincott, Williams & Wilkins; 2014:140–176.

Shaw NJ. Management of osteoporosis in children. *Eur J Endocrinol*. 2008;159:S33–S39.

Tortolani PJ, McCarthy EF, Sponseller PD. Bone mineral density deficiency in children. *J Am Acad Orthop Surg*. 2002;10:57–66.

Index

Page numbers followed by "*f*" indicate figures, "*t*" indicate tables, and "*b*" indicate boxes.

Index

Index

Index

Index

Index

Index

Index

Index